PRINCIPLES & PRACTICE
OF POINT-OF-CARE TESTING

PRINCIPLES & PRACTICE OF POINT-OF-CARE TESTING

Edited by

GERALD J. KOST, M.D., Ph.D.

Director, POCT·CTR^SM (Point-of-Care Testing Center for Teaching and Research)
Professor, Medical Pathology
Faculty, Biomedical Engineering
University of California-Davis School of Medicine
Director, Clinical Chemistry
University of California-Davis Health System
Davis, California

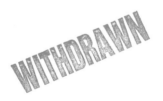
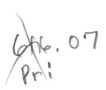
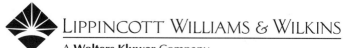
LIPPINCOTT WILLIAMS & WILKINS
A **Wolters Kluwer** Company
Philadelphia · Baltimore · New York · London
Buenos Aires · Hong Kong · Sydney · Tokyo

Acquisitions Editor: Ruth W. Weinberg
Developmental Editor: Stacey L Baze
Production Editor: Janice G. Stangel
Manufacturing Manager: Benjamin Rivera
Cover Designer: Angela L. Kost
Compositor: Lippincott Williams & Wilkins Desktop Division
Printer: Maple Press

Library of Congress Cataloging-in-Publication Data

Principles & practice of point-of-care testing / edited by Gerald J. Kost.
    p. ;cm.
  Includes bibliographical references and index.
  ISBN 0-7817-3156-9
    1. Function tests (Medicine) 2. Diagnosis, Laboratory. I. Title: Principles and practice of point-of-care testing. II. Kost, Gerald J.
  [DNLM: 1 Point-of-Care Systems. 2. Delivery of Health Care—organization & administration. 3. Diagnostic Techniques and Procedures. 4. Patient Care Planning. W84.7 P957 2002]
  RC71.8 .P747 2002
  6616.07′54—dc21

                                              2001050741

Care has been taken to confirm the accuracy of the information presented and to describe generally accepted practices. However, the authors, editor, and publisher are not responsible for errors or omissions or for any consequences from application of the information in this book and make no warranty, expressed or implied, with respect to the currency, completeness, or accuracy of the contents of the publication. Application of this information in a particular situation remains the professional responsibility of the practitioner.

The authors, editor, and publisher have exerted every effort to ensure that drug selection and dosage set forth in this text are in accordance with current recommendations and practice at the time of publication. However, in view of ongoing research, changes in government regulations, and the constant flow of information relating to drug therapy and drug reactions, the reader is urged to check the package insert for each drug for any change in indications and dosage and for added warnings and precautions. This is particularly important when the recommended agent is a new or infrequently employed drug.

Some drugs and medical devices presented in this publication have Food and Drug Administration (FDA) clearance for limited use in restricted research settings. It is the responsibility of the health care provider to ascertain the FDA status of each drug or device planned for use in their clinical practice.

10 9 8 7 6 5 4 3 2 1

To my wife, Angela, for her enduring love and my children,
Christopher and Laurie, for their enthusiasm and inspiration.

To my father, Edward, and mother, Ora, for encouraging me to think and be creative.
To my aunt, Margaret, and uncle, John, for their support of my education.

To my mentors and colleagues for teaching me to strive for excellence.

CONTENTS

CONTRIBUTING AUTHORS

Rosanna Abbate, M.D. Full Professor of Internal Medicine, Department of Medicine, Surgery, and Critical Care, University of Florence; and Chief, Thrombosis Centre, Careggi Hospital, Florence, Italy

Raymond D. Aller, M.D. Clinical Professor, Department of Pathology, Emory University, Atlanta, Georgia; and Vice-President, Medical Affairs Information, MDS Laboratory Services, Nashville, Tennessee

Erika B. Ammirati, R.A.C., M.T. (A.S.C.P.) President, Ammirati Regulatory Consulting, Los Altos, California

Bob Anders, M.D. Healthwyse, Palo Alto, California

Marcy Anderson, M.S., M.T. (A.S.C.P.) Senior Clinical Specialist, Medical Automation Systems, Charlottesville, Virginia

Jack E. Ansell, M.D. Professor, Department of Medicine, Boston University Medical School; and Vice-Chair for Clinical Affairs, Department of Medicine, Boston Medical Center, Boston, Massachusetts

Fred S. Apple, Ph.D. Professor, Department of Laboratory Medicine and Pathology, University of Minnesota School of Medicine; and Medical Director, Clinical Laboratories, Department of Laboratory Medicine and Pathology, Hennepin County Medical Center, Minneapolis, Minnesota

Phillip R. Bach, Ph.D. Clinical Assistant Professor, Department of Pathology, University of Utah School of Medicine; and Director of Chemistry, Department of Pathology, Primary Children's Medical Center, Salt Lake City, Utah

Daniel M. Baer, M.D. Professor Emeritus, Department of Pathology, Oregon Health and Sciences University; and Consultant, Department of Pathology and Laboratory Medicine, VA Medical Center, Portland, Oregon

C. Robert Baisden, M.D. Professor and Chief of Clinical Pathology and Emeritus, Department of Pathology, Medical College of Georgia; and Pathologist, Medical College of Georgia, Inc., Augusta, Georgia

Jan Bakker, M.D., Ph.D. Consultant, Julius Center for Patient Oriented Research, University Medical Center Utrecht; and Chief, Department of Intensive Care, Isala Clinics, The Netherlands

John T. Benjamin, M.D. Charbonnier Professor of Pediatrics, Department of Pediatrics, Medical College of Georgia, Children's Medical Center; and Chief, Section of General Pediatrics, Medical College of Georgia Children's Medical Center, Augusta, Georgia

John W. Berkenbosch, M.D. Assistant Professor, Department of Child Health, University of Missouri-Columbia, Children's Hospital, University of Missouri Health Care, Columbia, Missouri

Kenneth E. Blick, Ph.D. Professor, Department of Pathology, University of Oklahoma Health Sciences Center; Director, Laboratory Information Systems; and Director, Endocrine Laboratories, University Health Partners, Oklahoma City, Oklahoma

Dirk Boecker, M.D., Ph.D. President, Pelikan Technologies, Inc., Palo Alto, California

Joanne M. Born, B.S., M.T. (A.S.C.P.) The Joint Commission on Accreditation of Healthcare Organization, Lombard, Illinois

Sean E. Bourke, M.D. Attending Physician, Department of Emergency Medicine, Wilford Hall Medical Center, Lackland Air Force Base, Texas

Willem Brinkert, M.D. Fellow, Department of Anesthesiology, University Medical Center Nijmegen, Nijmegen, The Netherlands; and Research Fellow, Department of Intensive Care, Gelre Hospital Lukas, The Netherlands

Joan Bullock, M.D. Supervisor, Operating Room Laboratory, Department of Anesthesiology, University of California-Davis Medical Center, Davis, California

Debra L. Case-Cromer, R.N., M.S. Coordinator of Education, Department of Nursing Administration, The Johns Hopkins Hospital, Baltimore, Maryland

David Chou, M.D. Associate Professor, Department of Laboratory Medicine, University of Washington; and Director of Informatics, University of Washington and Harborview Medical Centers, Seattle, Washington

Andrea A. Conti, M.D., M.P.H. Research Assistant, Department of Internal Medicine and Cardiology, University of Florence; and Internal Medicine Consultant, Cardiology Unit, Don Gnocchi Foundation, Florence, Italy

George J. Despotis, M.D. Associate Professor, Departments of Anesthesiology, Pathology, and Immunology, Washington University School of Medicine, St. Louis, Missouri

Patricia I. Donovan, R.N., B.S.N. Manager of Patient Care and Quality Assurance, Department of Surgery, Yale University School of Medicine, New Haven, Connecticut

Sheila G. Dunn, D.A., M.T. (A.S.C.P.) President /CEO, Quality America, Inc., Asheville, North Carolina

Sharon S. Ehrmeyer, Ph.D., M.T. (A.S.C.P.) Professor, Department of Pathology and Laboratory Medicine, University of Wisconsin Medical School, Madison, Wisconsin

Daniel L. Feeback, Ph.D. Head, Muscle Research Laboratory, Human Adaptation and Countermeasures Office, NASA-Johnson Space Center, Houston, Texas

Eva Fremner, M.D. Coordinator, Laboratorie Medicine, Östergotland, Sweden

Isabel Gauss, M.T. (A.S.C.P.) Department of Clinical Pathology, William Beaumont Hospital, Royal Oak, Michigan

Ryan E. Grueber, B.S., R.R.T. Supervisor of Education and Research, Respiratory Care Services, University of Missouri, Columbia, Missouri

Steven Gutman, M.D., M.B.A. Director, Division of Clinical Laboratory Devices, Food and Drug Administration, Rockville, Maryland

Neil A. Halpern, M.D., F.A.C.P., F.C.C.P., F.C.C.M. Professor of Medicine in Clinical Anesthesiology, Department of Anesthesiology, Professor of Clinical Medicine, Department of Medicine, Weill Medical College of Cornell University; and Chief, Critical Care Medicine Service, Department of Anesthesiology and Critical Care Medicine, Memorial Sloan-Kettering Cancer Center, New York, New York

A. Douglas Hirst, F.R.C.Path. Department Head, Department of Biochemistry & Immunology, Bradford Royal Infirmary, Bradford, England

Paul A. H. Holloway, Ph.D., B.M., B.Ch. Honorary Reader in Medicine and Consultant Chemical Pathologist in Intensive Care, Nuffield Department of Medicine, University of Oxford; and Consultant Chemical Pathologist, Ealing Hospital NHS Trust, Middlesex, England

Alexander J. Indrikovs, M.D., M.B.A. Associate Professor, Department of Pathology and Clinical Laboratory Sciences, University of Texas Medical Branch; and Director, Blood Bank Division, University of Texas Medical Branch at Galveston, Galveston, Texas

Holly B. Jimison, Ph.D. Medical Informatics Investigator, Kaiser Permanente Center for Health Research, Portland, Oregon

Jay B. Jones, Ph.D., D.A.B.C.C. Director of Chemistry and Regional Laboratories, Department of Laboratory Medicine, Geisinger Health System, Danville, Pennsylvania

Shaun B. Jones, M.D. Program Manager, Pathogen Countermeasures, Defense Advanced Research Projects Agency, Arlington, Virginia

Tadashi Kawai, M.D., Ph.D. Professor Emeritus, Department of Laboratory Medicine, Jichi Medical School; and Medical Director, International Clinical Pathology Center, Tokyo, Japan

Frederick L. Kiechle, M.D., Ph.D. Associate Professor, Department of Pathology, Wayne State University School of Medicine, Detroit, Michigan; and Medical Director, Beaumont Reference Lab, and Chairman, Department of Clinical Pathology, William Beaumont Hospital, Royal Oak, Michigan

James A. King, M.D., F.A.C.E.P., Ltc, U.S.A.F., M.C. Chairman, Department of Emergency Medicine, Wilford Hall Medical Center, Lackland Air Force Base, Texas

Judy Kirby, R.N., M.S. Nurse Informaticist, Department of Pediatric Pulmonary Medicine, Stanford Cystic Fibrosis Center, Palo Alto, California

J. Douglas Kirk, M.D., F.A.C.E.P. Associate Professor, Department of Internal Medicine - Division of Emergency Medicine, University of California; and Assistant Chief, Department of Emergency Medicine, University of California Davis Medical Center, Sacramento, California

Gerald J. Kost, M.D., Ph.D., F.A.C.B. Director, POCT•CTR^{SM} (Point-of-Care Testing Center for Teaching and Research); Professor, Medical Pathology; and Faculty, Biomedical Engineering, University of California-Davis School of Medicine; and Director, Clinical Chemistry, University of California-Davis Health System, Davis, California

Ronald H. Laessig, Ph.D. Professor, Department of Population Health Sciences, University of Wisconsin; and Director, State Laboratory of Hygiene, University of Wisconsin, Madison, Wisconsin

Lasse Larsson, M.D., Ph.D. Associate Professor, Department of Biomedicine and Surgery, University of Linkoping; and Director, Point-of-Care Testing Division, Laboratoriemedicin Ostergotland, Linkoping, Sweden

Joan Logue, B.S., M.T. (A.S.C.P.) Principal, Health Systems Concepts, Inc., Longwood, Florida

Alessandra Lombardi, M.D. Researcher, Department of Internal Medicine and Cardiology, University of Florence; and Clinical Assistant, Thrombosis Centre, Careggi Hospital, Florence, Italy

Richard F. Louie, B.S. Post-Graduate Researcher, Point-of-Care Testing Center for Teaching and Research, Department of Medical Pathology, University of California-Davis School of Medicine, Davis, California

Alan S. Maisel, M.D. Professor of Medicine, Department of Medicine, University of California at San Diego; and Director, Coronary Care Unit, Veterans Affairs Medical Center, San Diego, California

Robyn Medeiros, B.S., M.T. (A.S.C.P.), C.L.S. QA/ POCT Education Manager, Clinical Laboratory, El Camino Hospital, Mountain View, California

Ronald C. McGlennen, M.D. Associate Professor, Department of Laboratory Medicine and Pathology, University of Minnesota; and Medical Director, Molecular Diagnostics Laboratory, Fairview University Medical Center, Minneapolis, Minnesota

James H. Nichols, Ph.D., D.A.B.C.C., F.A.C.B. Medical Director of Clinical Chemistry, Department of Pathology, Baystate Health System, Springfield, Massachusetts

Ching-Nan Ou, Ph.D. Professor of Clinical Pathology, Department of Pathology, Baylor College of Medicine; and Director of Clinical Chemistry, Department of Pathology, Texas Children's Hospital, Houston, Texas

David H. Pedersen, M.T. (A.S.C.P.) Point-of-Care Supervisor, Clinical Laboratory, Primary Children's Medical Center, Salt Lake City, Utah

Jeffrey Perry Commercial Project Scientist, Medical Department, Agilent Technologies Laboratories, Palo Alto, California

Rhonda M. Pikelny, B.S., C.L.S. (NCA), M.T. (A.S.C.P.) Quality Assurance Coordinator, Laboratory Services, Group Health Cooperative, Seattle, Washington

Stephanie Storto Poe, R.N., M.S.cN. Coordinator, Nursing Clinical Quality, Department of Nursing, The Johns Hopkins Hospital, Baltimore, Maryland

Daniela Poli, M.D. Clinical Researcher, Thrombosis Centre, Careggi Hospital, Florence, Italy

Domenico Prisco, M.D. Associate Professor of Internal Medicine, Department of Medical and Surgical Critical Area, University of Florence; and Consultant, Thrombosis Centre, Careggi Hospital, Florence, Italy

Theodore J. Pysher, M.D. Professor, Department of Pathology, University of Utah School of Medicine; and Director of Laboratories, Department of Pathology, Primary Children's Medical Center, Salt Lake City, Utah

Kimber Creager Richter, M.D. Deputy Director for Clinical and Review Policy, Center for Devices and Radiological Health, Food and Drug Administration, Rockville, Maryland

Thomas F. Ruhlen, M.D. Associate Pathologist, Physicians Reference Laboratory, Overland Park, Kansas; and Medical Director, Laboratory Services, Olathe Medical Center, Olathe, Kansas

Paula J. Santrach, M.D. Assistant Professor, Department of Laboratory Medicine, Mayo Medical School; and Co-Director, Hospital Clinical Laboratories, Department of Laboratory Medicine and Pathology, Mayo Clinic, Rochester, Minnesota

Richard M. Satava, M.D. Professor, Department of Surgery, Yale University School of Medicine; and Faculty Surgeon, Department of Surgery, Yale-New Haven Hospital, New Haven, Connecticut

Selma S.J. Schieveld, M.D. Research Fellow, Department of Intensive Care, Gelre Hospital Lukas, The Netherlands

Waldemar A. Schmidt, M.D., Ph.D. Professor, Department of Pathology, Oregon Health and Sciences University, Portland, Oregon

Michael B. Smith, M.D. Assistant Professor, Department of Pathology, University of Texas Medical Branch; and Director, Division of Clinical Microbiology, Department of Pathology, University of Texas Medical Branch, Galveston, Texas

Scott M. Smith, Ph.D. Nutritionist, Human Adaptation and Countermeasures Office, NASA-Johnson Space Center, Houston, Texas

Lori J. Sokoll, Ph.D. Assistant Professor, Department of Pathology, The Johns Hopkins University; and Associate Director, Division of Clinical Chemistry, Department of Pathology, The Johns Hopkins Hospital, Baltimore, Maryland

Stephanie Spingarn, M.D. Director of Clinical Pathology, Department of Pathology, Sentara Norfolk General Hospital, Norfolk, Virginia

Zuping Tang, M.D.   Research Associate, Point-of-Care Testing Center for Teaching and Research, Department of Medical Pathology, University of California-Davis School of Medicine, Davis, California

Noriyuki Tatsumi, M.D.   Professor, Department of Clinical and Laboratory Medicine, Osaka City University Medical School, Osaka, Japan

Joseph D. Tobias, M.D.   Professor, Department of Anesthesiology and Pediatrics, Vice-Chairman, Department of Anesthesiology, and Director, Division of Pediatric Anesthesia/Pediatric Critical Care, University of Missouri, Columbia, Missouri

John G. Toffaletti, Ph.D.   Associate Professor, Department of Pathology; and Director of Blood Gas Services, Department of Clinical Laboratories, Duke University Medical Center, Durham, North Carolina

Laura A. Townsend-Collymore, M.S., M.T. (A.S.C.P.)   Assistant Director of Pathology Administration, Texas Children's Hospital, Houston, Texas

Nam K. Tran   Research Assistant, Point-of-Care Testing Center for Teaching and Research, University of California-Davis School of Medicine, Davis, California

Robert Udelsman, M.D., M.B.A., F.A.C.S.   Professor and Chairman, Department of Surgery, Yale University School of Medicine; and Chief, Department of Surgery, Yale-New Haven Hospital, New Haven, Connecticut

Michael R. Visnich   Chief Executive Officer, Hometestmed.com, Quality Assured Services, Inc., Orlando, Florida

Gail L. Woods, M.D.   Associate Director, Department of Medical Communications, Merck and Company, Inc., Blue Bell, Pennsylvania

Alan H. B. Wu, Ph.D.   Professor, Department of Laboratory Medicine, University of Connecticut, Farmington, Connecticut; and Director, Clinical Chemistry, Department of Pathology and Laboratory Medicine, Hartford Hospital, Hartford, Connecticut

Lou Ann Wyer, M.T. (A.S.C.P.)   Clinical Specialist, POCT/QM, Department of Laboratory Services, Sentara Healthcare, Norfolk, Virginia

Stephen E. Zweig, Ph.D.   CEO and President, CliniSense Corporation, Los Gatos, California

PREFACE

A treatise for a new field must accomplish three distinct goals: explication of fundamental principles, explanation of clinical practice, and exposition of exciting advances. In achieving these goals, the contributors to *Principles & Practice of Point-of-Care Testing* produced a comprehensive and authoritative compendium of current knowledge of point-of-care testing (POCT), defined as testing at or near the site of patient care. The authors shared a vision of improved patient care and attained a high level of scholarship, while producing an easily-read and useful book.

The shift in the focus of diagnostic testing to the site of patient care is only part of the story. This book documents a larger evolution, transformation, and translocation of the ownership of medical care to the physician, bedside, and patient. Medicine must become less remote and managed care, if it lasts, less dehumanizing. Advisors nominated authors who foster a spirit of change and exemplify leadership. We encouraged the authors, selected from several laboratory and clinical specialties, to carefully and succinctly state, with experimental proof and clinical evidence where possible, their approach to the use of POCT in patient management and therapy. The variety inherent in POCT is a challenge that requires a broad perspective. We did not discourage the inevitable diversity of viewpoints.

Forty focused chapters and fifteen innovative cases mutually compliment each other to teach by means of guiding theory and practical examples applied to the complex systems of modern healthcare. The review process was extensive and not unlike that found in peer-reviewed literature. We took the reviews seriously. Readers will benefit from the patience of the contributors, all of whom revised and perfected their chapters. Barbara Meierhenry, Senior Editor at UCD, deserves special thanks for editing and polishing each of the fifteen case studies, which appear in tandem with related chapters, a format chosen to underscore the basic tenants of diagnosis, management, and therapy from the viewpoint of actual POCT users.

The structure of the book provides the reader with a solid footing in basic methods (Part I. Introduction), interpretative practice (Part II. Point-of-Care Testing in the Hospital and Clinical Practice), and practical management (Part III. Point-of-Care Testing in the Health System, Community, and Field). Parts IV (Management, Performance, Accreditation, and Education) and V (Information, Connectivity, and Knowledge Systems) offer depth that helps health system leaders to direct, coordinate, and integrate state-of-the-art POCT programs. Part VI (Economics, Outcomes, and Optimization) elevates the conceptual level of POCT so that readers will have the knowledge tools they need to cost-effectively improve patient outcomes while preventing potential medical errors. Useful resources in the book include 188 clear illustrations, 161 detailed tables, and more than 3,000 references. The appendices summarize investigative work (Appendix I. Effects of POCT on Time, Process, Decision Making, Treatment, and Outcome) and collate economic analyses (Appendix II. The Economics of Point-of-Care Testing) in settings as varied as academic medical centers, home care clinics, and remote field rescue.

Gerald J. Kost, M.D., Ph.D.

ACKNOWLEDGMENTS

Ultimately, a good book is the product of extensive collaboration of authors, reviewers, editors, artists, librarians, the publisher, and even patients. We thank the University of California for its support of faculty scholarship. Our students perpetually pose stimulating questions and generate creative ideas. The Carlson Health Sciences Library, Interlibrary Loan Department, and the University of California Digital Library provided invaluable bibliographic research for the book. We thank Angela Kost for helping to design the book cover. We thank Claudia Graham, Senior Artist at UCD, for her clever graphics. Ruth Weinberg, Executive Editor at Lippincott Williams & Wilkins, kept the project on track. Researchers at the POCT·CTR[SM] both reviewed and contributed original materials. We thank the individual authors of chapters and cases for their creativity and pride in the completion and production of this book. Above all, we thank our patients, to whom we owe compassion and faith that their participation in POCT will lead to better lives for us all.

PART

I

INTRODUCTION

GOALS, GUIDELINES, AND PRINCIPLES FOR POINT-OF-CARE TESTING

GERALD J. KOST

GOALS

Point-of-care testing (POCT) must be both medically efficacious and economically sound. Hence, *an important fundamental goal of point-of-care testing is to improve medical and economic outcomes.* Another goal is *rapid response.* Therapeutic turnaround time (TTAT), the time from test ordering to patient treatment, assesses the clinical significance of rapid response. TTAT is discussed in Chapter 2. The objective of this chapter is to introduce a cohesive set of principles for the professional practice of POCT testing as a starting point for the detailed discussions in the chapters that follow.

GUIDELINES

Table 1.1 lists guidelines, principles, and standards (GPS) documents for POCT and whole-blood analysis (1–71). These documents appeal to the reader's judgment, resourcefulness, and common sense. They are not instruction manuals but, instead, can be adapted to the unique needs and different environments of healthcare systems (Fig. 1.1). Table 1.2 groups the principles shared by the GPS documents in Table 1.1 into sets with common themes. This chapter summarizes those POCT principles and explains how the themes relate broadly to patient care. GPS documents outdate quickly. As a general rule, they should be reassessed for validity every 3 years (72).

DEFINITION

Point-of-care testing is testing at or near the site of patient care. After more than 10 years of descriptive use, this definition was codified when a group of multidisciplinary physicians, professionals, and leaders met at the national meeting of the Society of Critical Care Medicine in 1994 and selected this phrase and definition from several competing alternatives. Later, representatives from this group and co-authors published a clarifying position paper (41). POCT has become part of common usage in the public domain because of its immediate ability to convey the exact meaning of what those in the medical field are doing—testing at the point of care.

OPTIMIZATION

The first set of principles (Table 1.2A) helps to optimize patient outcomes. POCT generates evidence-based medical decisions that enhance medical efficacy. For example, whole-blood analysis facilitates medical decisions that reduce patient acuity, criticality, morbidity, and mortality during life-threatening crises and emergency resuscitations for which the standard of care demands test results within 5 minutes. There is no time for specimen centrifugation. In these situations, fast test results speed medical decisions essential for immediate treatment.

Decision criteria and thresholds can be used to launch rules for the optimization of treatment and monitoring. The rules can be bounding and, ideally, also quantitative within specified medical settings, such as the transplant center, operating room, emergency department, and intensive care unit. Several of the chapters in this book discuss how to incorporate POCT into *rule-based* performance maps, treatment algorithms, integrative strategies, care paths, and protocols. These rule-based approaches can improve even well-established POCT programs.

The collaborative care team (41) manages outcomes by using both qualitative and quantitative surrogates that help to optimize POCT (see Chapter 40). The following are the clinical objectives of outcomes surrogates: (a) to improve or change clinical strategies, identify important or provide earlier diagnoses, accelerate diagnostic/therapeutic processes, and enhance diagnostic insight or resolve diagnostic uncertainty; (b) to decrease the length of stay, time in critical care, duration of surgery, or physician, nursing, and patient time spent on medical tasks; (c) to launch a new therapy; modify the speed, timing, or costs of treatment; or alter the intensity of therapy; (d) to eliminate, stop, start, or speed interventions; and (e) to prevent patient crises.

Practical objectives are as follows: (a) to reduce or eliminate transfusions, iatrogenic anemia, or drug use; (b) to increase efficiency in anesthesia, surgery, or transplantation; (c) to streamline critical care paths, critical procedures, emergency care, or patient throughput and improve patient access to medical services; (d) to diminish the need for ancillary services, replace obsolete technologies or approaches, or avoid patient hazards; (e) to reduce follow-up testing; (f) to accelerate hospital admission or discharge and reduce the number or

TABLE 1.1. GUIDELINES, PRINCIPLES, AND STANDARDS FOR POCT AND WHOLE-BLOOD ANALYSIS

Ref(s)	Year	Author	Organization(s)	Purpose
1	1977	Kost	NA	Relation of surface pH monitored *in vivo* to whole-blood pH measured *in vitro*
2	1981	Fraser and Geary	AACB	Guidelines for tests outside laboratories
3,4	1981	McMillan and Cook	ACB, ACP, RCP	Performance of chemical pathology assays outside the laboratory
5	1987	Vanderlinde et al.	AACC	Quality stat laboratory services
6	1988	Marks	ACB	Provision of near-patient testing facilities
7	1988	Price et al.	ACB	Extralaboratory blood glucose measurement policy
8	1990	Kost and Shirey	KO	Whole-blood testing at cardiac transplant centers and U.S. hospitals
9	1990	Wimberley et al.	IFCC	Guidelines for transcutaneous P_{O_2} and P_{CO_2} measurement
10–13	1991/2	Boink et al.	IFCC	Sampling, transport, and storage for the determination of the concentration of ionized calcium in whole blood, plasma, and serum
14	1992	Dybkaer et al.	ECCLS	Good practice in decentralized analytical clinical measurement
15	1992	NA	JWGEQA	Guidelines for near-patient testing and procedures by nonpathology staff
16	1993	Kost	KO	Impact of whole-blood analyzers on cardiac and critical care, and axioms of POCT
17	1993	Kost and Lathrop	KO	Guidelines for designing hybrid labs and POCT for patient-focused care
18	1993	Moran et al.	NCCLS (C32)	Blood gases, electrolytes, and related analytes in whole blood
19	1993	NA	ACB	Guidelines for implementation of near-patient testing
20	1994 2002[a]	Barr et al. Sachs	NCCLS (C30)	Ancillary (bedside) blood glucose testing in acute and chronic care facilities
21	1994	Burnett et al.	IFCC	Whole blood sampling, transport, and storage for simultaneous determination of pH, blood gases, and electrolytes
22	1995	NA	ECRI	Guidance regarding POCT and decentralized testing alternatives
23	1995	England et al.	NPTWP	Guidelines for near-patient hematology testing
24	1995	Goodnough and Despotis	NA	Practice guidelines for surgical blood management
25	1995 2001[a]	Graham et al. D'Orazio	NCCLS (C31)	Ionized calcium determinations: precollection variables, specimen choice, collection, and handling
26	1995	Kost	POCT•CTR	Guidelines for improving medical and economic outcomes with POCT
27	1995	NA	NZIMLS/CSLT	Guidelines for hospitals for near-patient testing
28	1996	Crook	NA	Minimum standards for near-patient testing
29	1997	Pilon et al.	NA	Practice guideline for arterial blood gas measurement in the ICU
30–32	1998	Jansen et al.	WGHQSA	Essential criteria for POCT quality systems
33	1998	Kost et al.	Multicenter	Error tolerances for clinical performance of point-of-care glucose monitoring
34	1998	Kost	POCT•CTR	Principles of optimizing POCT in clinical systems management
35	1999	Barr et al.	NCCLS (AST4)	Blood glucose testing in settings without laboratory support
36	1999	Briedigkeit et al.	DGKC, DGLM	Principles that should be observed when introducing POCT
37	1999	Freedman	NA	General recommendations for laboratory practitioners of POCT
38	1999	Goldsmith et al.	NCCLS (AST2)	Point-of-care *in vitro* diagnostic (IVD) testing for primarily nonlaboratory users
39	1999	Hudson et al.	DCRI	Cardiac markers and POCT
40	1999	Janssen et al.	DACC	Views on professional standards and the role of the clinical chemist in POCT
41	1999	Kost et al.	CCLCIG	Guidelines and recommendations for POCT and the clinical–laboratory interface
42	1999	NA	WGEM	Recommendations for decentralized testing
43	1999	Panteghini et al.	IFCC/CSMCD	Use of biochemical markers in acute coronary syndromes, including POCT
44	1999	Phillips et al.	NCCLS (EP18)	Quality management for unit-use testing
45	1999	Wu et al.	NACB	Recommendations for cardiac markers in coronary diseases, including POCT
46,47	2000	Braunwald et al.	ACC/AHA	Guidelines for management of unstable angina and NSTEMI and for the use of POCT
48	2000	Burnett et al.	NCCLS (C46)	Blood gas and pH analysis and related measurements
49,50	2000 2001[b]	CIC	CIC NCCLS[b] (POCT1)	Standards for connectivity of POCT systems and interfaces
51	2000	Cummings	UHC	Clinical practice guidelines for use of cardiac injury markers at the point of care
52	2000	Delaney et al.	NA	Standards for evaluation of near-patient tests in primary care
53	2000	NA	JWGQA	Guidelines to assist managers and staff on components of POCT programs
54	2000	Kirby	PPHB	Guidance for HIV POCT using simple and rapid HIV test kits
55	2000	Kost et al.	POCT•CTR	Practice guidelines for processing specimens for whole-blood analysis
56	2000	Kost	POCT•CTR	Operator lockout features to improve the performance of blood glucose POCT
57	2000	McCabe and Tonniges	NSTF	Newborn screening and decisions regarding tests and testing technology
58	2001	Burnett et al.	WGSE, IFCC	Recommendation on reporting results for blood glucose
59	2001	Haeney	NA	Setting standards for pathology service support to emergency services
60	2001	Hicks et al.	NA	Recommendations and opinions for the use of POCT from a 1999 symposium

TABLE 1.1. *(continued)*

Ref(s)	Year	Author	Organization(s)	Purpose
61	2001	Kost	POCT•CTR	Optimized systems for preventing medical errors in POCT
62	2001	Whitley et al.	SUUT (EP18)	Establishing a quality management system for unit-use testing
63	2001	Wu et al.	NACB	Recommendations for emergency toxicology, including breath alcohol POCT
64	UD	NA	FDA	CLIA 1988 criteria for waiver
65	UD	Hackett	FDA	Review criteria for assessment of invasive blood glucose monitoring
66,69	UD	TC 212	ISO (15197)	Performance criteria for *in vitro* blood glucose monitoring systems
67,69	UD	TC 212	ISO (15196)	Determination of analytical performance goals based on medical needs
68,69	UD	TC 212	ISO (17593)	Measurement performance criteria for self testing of oral anticoagulation therapy
70	UD	Joist et al.	NCCLS (H49)	Point-of-care hemostasis/coagulation testing
71	UD	TBN	NCCLS	Quality model system for offering diagnostic tests in nonlaboratory settings

AACB, Australian Association of Clinical Biochemists; AACC, American Association for Clinical Chemistry; ACB, Association of Clinical Biochemists (England); ACP, Association of Clinical Pathologists (England); CAD, coronary artery disease; CIC, Connectivity Industry Consortium (U.S.); CCLCIG, Cape Cod Laboratory-Clinical Interface Group (U.S.); CSLT, Canadian Society of Laboratory Technologists; CSMCD, Committee on Standardization of Markers of Cardiac Damage; DACC, Dutch Association of Clinical Chemistry (Netherlands); DCRI, Duke Clinical Research Institute (U.S.); DGKC, Deutsche Gesellschaft fur Klinische Chemie; DGLM, Deutsche Gesellschaft fur Laboratoriumsmedizin; ECCLS, European Committee for Clinical Laboratory Standards; ECRI, Emergency Care Research Institute; FDA, U.S. Food and Drug Administration; IFCC, International Federation of Clinical Chemistry; ISO, International Organization for Standardization (Switzerland); JWGEQA, Joint Working Group on External Quality Assessment (England); JWGQA, Joint Working Group on Quality Assurance (England); KO, Knowledge Optimization (Davis, CA); NA, no author or not applicable; NACB, National Academy of Clinical Biochemistry (U.S.); NCCLS, National Committee for Clinical Laboratory Standards (U.S.); NPTWP, Near Patient Testing Working Party (England); NSTEMI, non-ST-segment elevation myocardial infarction; NSTF, Newborn Screening Task Force; NZIMLS, New Zealand Institute of Medical Laboratory Science; POCT, point-of-care testing; POCT•CTR, Point-of-Care Testing Center for Teaching and Research (University of California, Davis); PPHB, Population and Public Health Branch, Health Canada; RCP, Royal College of Pathologists (England); SUUT, Subcommittee on Unit-Use Testing (NCCLS); TBN, to be named; UD, under development; UHC, University Health System Consortium (U.S.); WGEM, Working Group of the Education and Management Division of the IFCC (Europe); WGHQSA, Working Group on Harmonisation of Quality Systems and Accreditation, European Community Confederation of Clinical Chemistry. For government documents, please see the agency web page, such as www.fda.gov, for the FDA.
*a*See reference for NCCLS update information.
*b*Developed and written by the CIC; published by NCCLS as POCT1-A.

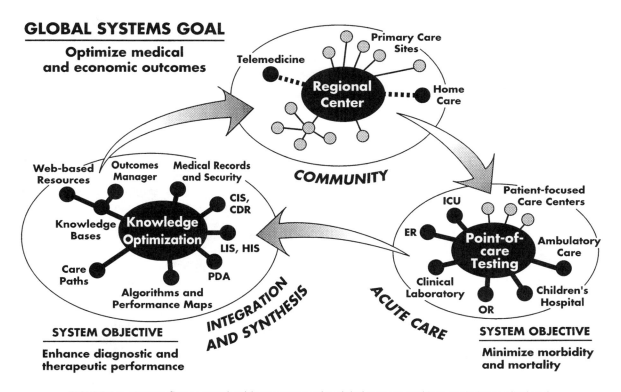

FIGURE 1.1. Twenty-first century healthcare system. The global systems goal is to optimize medical and economic outcomes. The objective of acute care is to minimize morbidity and mortality. Integration and synthesis lead to knowledge optimization. Information flows perpetually. Point-of-care testing enhances diagnostic and therapeutic performance. CDR, clinical data repository; CIS, clinical information system; ER, emergency room; HIS, hospital information system; LIS, laboratory information system; OR, operating room; and PDA, personal digital assistant.

TABLE 1.2. SHARED PRINCIPLES FOR POCT

A. Optimize patient outcomes
Generate data for evidence-based decisions that enhance medical efficiency and efficacy
Provide rapid response, especially in life-threatening crises and emergency resuscitations
Embed POCT in integrative strategies, treatment algorithms, performance maps, and care paths
Employ clinical surrogates to facilitate outcomes tracking, management, and optimization

B. Actuate critical linkages
Blend bedside, near-patient, and satellite laboratory approaches and staff
Use whole-blood methods and reconcile test results with main laboratory results
Conserve blood volume, minimize transfused blood products, and reduce infections
Implement connectivity standards and fully computerize point-of-care informatics

C. Integrate diagnostic testing
Customize test clusters for patient-focused services at the point of care
Deliver effective therapeutic turnaround time (time from test order to patient treatment)
Eliminate delays, lag time, and obsolescence of test results
Compare test results from point-of-care sites and participate in proficiency surveys
Establish consensus critical limits and report critical test results immediately

D. Hybridize strategies and staff
Adopt collaborative leadership for joint laboratorian-clinician leadership and management
Tailor *in vitro, ex vivo,* and *in vivo* modalities to the speed of changes of variables
Synthesize *in vitro* biochemical data with monitoring and physiological observations
Assess the cost-effectiveness of alternate testing sites and modalities
Manage scarce medical and economic resources to maximally benefit the health system

E. Guarantee excellent performance
Appoint a director and a coordinator of POCT and define lines of authority
Select and standardize testing methods for uniformity and technical integrity
Improve the performance and consistency of all testing modalities
Monitor the quality control and proficiency testing programs
Achieve on-site performance comparable to or better than laboratory performance

F. Reduce risk and medical errors
Minimize medicolegal risk proactively through strong leadership
Identify sentinel events, investigate root causes, and improve prevention systems
Validate operators (and lock out non-validated operators)
Require operators to perform quality control (and lock out operators who omit QC)
Assure security, safety, and safeguards for staff, data, and patients

G. Educate point-of-care leaders, staff, operators, students, and patients
Appoint faculty academicians who teach and perform POCT research
Sustain a professional continuing education program in the field of POCT
Train patients how to self-monitor (e.g., glucose) and manage illness
Accredit professional services, credential trainees, and assess skills at least annually

POCT, point-of-care testing; QC, quality control.

frequency of critical care and other admissions; and (g) to advance the quality of care. In addition, each health system will have site-specific objectives for optimization custom-tailored to patient care.

LINKAGE

The objective of linkages is to optimize overall operations of the health system (Fig. 1.1). Linkage principles (Table 1.2B) focus on diagnostic testing services and the acute care hospital, where POCT, including near-patient testing and satellite laboratories, are intensely integrated. For example, biosensor-based whole-blood analysis and other whole-blood methods link medical accuracy, clinical efficiency, blood conservation, and outcomes. In premature infants and newborns, blood conservation is crucial to avoid unnecessary transfusions and the attendant risks, "hidden" costs, and "downstream" poor outcomes.

Direct (undiluted) whole-blood analyses with ion-selective electrodes (ISEs) and substrate-specific electrodes (SSEs) reflect analyte activities and eliminate measurement artifacts caused by volume displacement in hyperlipidemic, hyperproteinemic, or hyperviscous samples. For example, the use of direct whole-blood measurements is indicated for critically ill children and young diabetics and adults, who may manifest these conditions. Whole-blood analysis also conserves blood volume (73). Thus, testing method, blood conservation, patient outcomes, and financial costs are inexorably linked and should be jointly optimized.

Simultaneous measurements using one whole-blood microsample decrease the frequency of venous and arterial punctures for individual tests, eliminate errors from nonequivalent sample matrices (e.g., whole blood, plasma, and serum) derived from multiple arterial and venous sites, and eliminate time-consuming processing steps (e.g., centrifuging, splitting, transporting, and distributing). For broad consistency, POC test results can be reconciled with main (or regional) laboratory test results and vice versa. Because physiologic changes occur continuously in blood specimens *in vitro,* within-hospital standardization of POC test results must be performed with minimum time delays, preferably at the bedside.

Point-of-care testing produces immediate knowledge, but that knowledge must be readily available throughout the health system. Informatics interfacing should accommodate *in vitro* POC instruments for diagnostic testing as well as *ex vivo* and *in vivo* systems for patient monitoring in critical care areas. *Connectivity* (bidirectional communication between computerized information systems and remote devices) of POC instruments, computerized resources, and clinical information systems within and between health system sites is pivotal to global optimization.

INTEGRATION

Table 1-2C lists principles that integrate diagnostic services and medical information. POCT and patient focusing (17) promote an integrated clinical approach and whole-systems thinking in a learning organization. Well-targeted clusters of essential tests for critical indications boost efficiency. Expanding test menus and device modularity will mean that several test clusters are available to integrate vital functions and their diagnostic pivots or physiologic indicators. A key principle is to choose test clusters cleverly to streamline the efficiency of diagnostic and therapeutic processes, to conserve critical resources, and generally to enhance performance.

One should tailor POCT to fulfill physician and patient-focusing objectives and priorities for TTAT (see Chapter 2). Lag time renders data obsolete before the results can be used in clinical diagnosis, interpretation, or treatment. Testing methods at different POC sites need to be consistent to eliminate sudden ("delta") shifts, which may appear real to the clinician, in analyte levels and artifacts. Agreement can be validated by means of frequent intramural comparisons and proficiency testing.

The standard of care and accreditation agencies require critical results to be reported immediately according to established consensus protocols that apply uniformly to the main laboratory and to the point of care. Lack of effective communication of critical results obtained at distributed testing sites (including reference laboratories) can lead to significant financial loss from medical malpractice. See Chapter 2 for a discussion of how POCT can help improve the availability of critical test results.

HYBRIDIZATION

The hybrid laboratory is distributed but integrated testing (see Chapter 2). Collaborative integration of whole-blood analyzers at the point of care created the hybrid laboratory. Hybridization principles (Table 1.2D) encourage timeliness and efficacious use of alternative modalities available for rapid-response testing. For example, specimens obtained at appropriate time intervals for *in vitro* testing will capture pathophysiologic instabilities and detect abnormalities that are potentially harmful to the patient, diagnostically revealing, and treatable.

When patient conditions and variables change quickly, combining *in vitro* testing with *ex vivo* or *in vivo* patient monitoring will result in optimal detection and tracking of pathophysiologic events and mechanisms. Noninvasive monitoring should be used whenever possible, particularly in premature infants and newborns, who have extremely small blood volume. Protocols should be established that blend *in vitro*, *ex vivo*, and *in vivo* systems in different critical care settings. By combining these systems, measurements can span medical decision levels and critical time periods.

Synthesis of POC test results and patient monitoring data with other biochemical data and physiologic observations will improve the continuity and efficacy of therapeutic decisions. Synthesis is most likely to occur when testing strategies are designed to detect unexpected or sudden changes in analytes, indicate life-threatening abnormalities, identify analyte linkages and new patterns, and monitor therapeutic variables and outcomes.

Handheld, portable, transportable, mobile, robotic, and backup POCT systems should be used when and where medically necessary, including airborne and rescue missions. POCT should be integrated in disaster-preparedness plans and include two to four levels of redundancy for untimely failures in critical care. Important clinical observations (e.g., intravenous therapy, ventilation, anticoagulation, sampling site) can be noted when the specimen is obtained to enhance the value of interpretation of test results for diagnosis and treatment.

Synthesis also enhances medical and economic efficiency through comparison of alternative modalities of testing. The focus should be on *relative*, that is, *marginal* cost-effectiveness and efficiencies for coordination of multisite patient-centered testing and patient monitoring. The effect of POCT can be analyzed by weighing the costs of POCT against the benefits of physician efficiency and improved patient outcomes.

It is important to identify the strategic alternatives that best integrate POCT with assessed needs and shared functions of highest priority to the critical care area, patient-focused care center, medical center, and health system. In addition, well-defined alternatives must be selected from the viewpoint of needs fulfillment and maximum value for the entire institution and must optimize whole-systems outcomes.

PERFORMANCE

The rapid evolution of POC technologies calls for flexible, adaptable, and strong leadership by the POCT director and coordinator, who ideally are outcomes managers. A multidisciplinary team led by these persons will design quality paths, define and review quality performance indicators (monitors), and coordinate POCT in the health system and regional network. Performance principles (Table 1.2E) configure change processes through a cooperative multidisciplinary partnership that will plan, authorize, implement, take responsibility, and be accountable for continuously improving performance.

The staff of the hybrid laboratory will provide leadership for continuous performance improvement. The quality improvement program encompasses (a) *in vitro, ex vivo,* and *in vivo* systems; (b) patient results recording, validating, reporting, and tracking; (c) patient testing programs (e.g., glucose meters); (d) policies relevant to federal regulations, state requirements, and professional standards; and (e) other relevant performance factors, including updating.

It is essential to use actual patient outcomes and proven economic effectiveness as performance criteria to ensure that POCT supports a uniformly high level of care throughout the health system. POC systems must provide quality at least commensurate with or exceeding expectations for the intended clinical use. Therefore, satisfaction surveys are also valid tools with which to assess the success of POCT programs. Ultimately, the performance of POCT systems should match or beat that of laboratory systems when assessed relative to real-time analyte levels *in vivo*.

Team leadership draws on physicians, nurses, clinical partners, clinical pathologists, laboratory specialists, clinical engineers, research bioengineers, and system administrators to (a) formulate instrument evaluation criteria; (b) select or approve POC devices and avoid unnecessary duplication; (c) define the POC test menus, clinical sites, and test uses, such as screening, diagnosis, treatment, monitoring, or confirmation and ruling disease in or out; and (d) adopt a reasonable span of control for POC sites.

The team also (a) reviews needs, costs, and reimbursement; (b) administrates written quality assurance policies, detailed procedure manuals, protocols, and communications; (c) supervises quality performance for POCT; (d) revokes testing privileges if performance is not satisfactory; and (e) designates persons, including qualified POC operators with assigned authority, jurisdiction, responsibility, and accountability.

The POCT coordinator and nursing staff are crucial to ensuring that performance principles are included in clinical policies and that POCT operators follow the policies. Performance functions supervised by the POCT coordinator include proficiency testing (extramural surveys, internal blind sample comparisons, and their review), remedial actions, problem solving (complaint investigation), instrument evaluation, scheduled instrument maintenance, reagents and standards management, universal precautions, and biohazard and safety precautions (including Occupational Safety and Health Administration requirements).

A POCT coordinator's technical staff (a) validates the clinical performance of methods, instruments, or systems; (b) verifies calibration routines or automated algorithms initially when received, at least twice per year thereafter, and when major changes occur (e.g., new biosensor, software, calibrator lot, or quality perturbation); (c) designs flexible approaches for different degrees of user adjustment, new device types, and progressive designs (e.g., self-contained multiple-use systems and single-use disposable cartridges); and (d) verifies the equivalency of results obtained with identical or different instrument systems, biosensors, or methods at different sites of POCT.

The POCT coordinator and supervised clinical associates oversee patient preparation, specimen processing (e.g., collection, handling, and, if necessary, preservation), prompt results reporting, results signatures, confidentiality, documentation, audits of patient results, operator performance verification, certification, and other appropriate quality performance tasks, including the use of newer quality tools, such as electronic, internal parallel, and intelligent quality control (QC).

In addition, the POCT coordinator's team must (a) include valid statistical comparisons; (b) determine analytic accuracy, precision, sensitivity, specificity (interferences), linearity, analytic and clinical measurement ranges, and acceptable reportable range, including the low-to-high critical spans; and (c) for biosensor-based measurements, be aware of drift, response time, selectivity, reproducibility, and artifacts. For some devices, such as handheld glucose meters, technical rules-based operation is safest. Clear policies, hands-on training, and periodic review assure excellent quality.

Quality control, performed each day of testing, each 24 hours, or more frequently (e.g., each shift for blood gases and pH) as required by regulations or changes in conditions, provides immediate feedback as to whether the analytic process (operator, technology, and test) is performing satisfactorily. A written plan is needed for reviewing and assessing QC results (preferably weekly), archiving QC records (typically two or more years), and correlating patient results for each testing event.

Clinicians have high expectations for on-site accuracy and precision comparable to that achieved in the main laboratory. POCT instruments should be highly accurate and precise. Therefore, it is important to define and document the reportable limits of analytes and parameters determined with POCT instruments or systems; to develop an efficient protocol for follow-up or referral of samples with analytic errors, unusual results, or results in critical spans outside the reportable limits; and to evaluate false-positive and false-negative results by reviewing clinical diagnoses and outcomes.

For some devices, professional judgment and experience will be necessary to decide what, if any, degree of inaccuracy or imprecision is acceptable in tradeoff for speed, accessibility, or other features. For consistency, it also is important to establish clinical criteria, performance protocols, and operator routines for *ex vivo* and *in vivo* monitoring systems and to determine analyte relationships to *in vitro* measurements to improve the consistency of clinical interpretation.

RISK

Risk assessment is part of any POCT program or new initiative. Risk reduction is proactive, draws on common sense, closes loops, and encourages rethinking and redesigning of systems to prevent future errors. Principles that reduce risk and medical errors (Table 1.2F) target instrument formats (e.g., transportable, portable, and handheld) for *in vitro* testing as well as monitoring systems. For details regarding performance expectations for monitoring systems, please see references 74 and 75 and Chapters 6 and 17.

The POCT committee establishes a risk practice plan that focuses on liability issues, defines strategic policies, and reduces the vulnerability to external interventions (legal actions). The committee proactively reduces liability by identifying, assessing, analyzing, monitoring, tracking, and treating risks at the point of service. Error reduction demands identification of sentinel events and root cause analysis to improve systems fundamentally. Errors can be reduced by identifying trained supervisors and users of POCT; reviewing the access requirements periodically; and allowing only personnel authorized for POCT to perform tests, operate instruments, use robotic laboratories, and perform remote review.

General principles of error reduction include (a) avoiding postanalytic error by fully integrating POC observations (including test results, patient identity, date and time, medical status, clinical site, conditions of specimen collection, when the test was performed, reference interval, and other important information) with the patient's (electronic) medical record; (b) linking POCT with communications, computerized information systems, and new informatics (e.g., wireless alerting and reporting); and (c) implementing connectivity standards.

A systems approach (61) can be used to lock out nonvalidated operators or those not performing quality procedures. Institute of Medicine guidelines (76,77) for error reduction highlight the importance of assuring security, safety, and safeguards for operators, data, and patients involved in POCT. Chapter 40 describes a unified systems approach to error prevention, which was based on a United States national survey and a consensus process involving expert opinion and POC professionals (61).

EDUCATION

Education principles (Table 1.2G) apply broadly to directors, coordinators, staff, operators, patients, and students. For centers with academic programs, these principles recommend recognizing POCT as the new discipline, that it is, integrating POCT into curricula, and developing didactic programs for directors, POCT coordinators, physicians, nurses, and patients who perform self-monitoring.

It is essential to include important learning objectives such as patient outcomes, medical indications for testing, anticipated results, clinical interpretation and significance, critical limits, principles of instrument operation, patient conditions, specimen requirements, biohazard precautions, test performance, methods limitations, interfering substances, quality assurance (QA), QC, and results documentation. An aggressive education and competency program will help streamline all aspects of the POCT program.

To achieve educational objectives, design a competency plan to certify hospital personnel (laboratorians, nurses, and physicians) to perform POCT and its preanalytic, analytic, and postanalytic tasks. Train in the preparation of procedure manuals that include these and other important entries (e.g., formulae, reference intervals, and annual review). Periodically update knowledge and skills, observe the competency of instrument operators where they perform the testing, and document proficiency with written, oral, or practical examinations. Provide librarianship to assure that the process steps of the POCT program are well documented; these include, for example, calibration procedures and joint review of QC, results, and proficiency testing.

Licensing and accreditation requirements, such as those of the College of American Pathologists and the Joint Commission for Accreditation of Healthcare Organizations (described in detail elsewhere in this book), must be followed and records maintained that include the correct lengths of times. Fulfillment of these basic objectives facilitates accreditation processes.

The POCT program must adhere to state and federal statutes, as well as specific accreditation requirements for POCT and for blood gas and critical care testing. When appropriate,

request revisions or exceptions to be made as warranted because good regulations evolve and improve in quality over time if feedback is offered.

GPS NAVIGATION—THE JOURNEY AND CHALLENGE

Improved medical and economic outcomes represent necessary and sufficient driving forces for the future practice of POCT. As the growth rate of new instruments, test clusters, and medical applications increases, POCT will become ubiquitous in hospitals and society. Rapid growth warrants careful consideration of why, how, when, where, and what POCT will be used.

The standard of care places POCT at the center of integrated diagnosis, monitoring, and therapy for critically ill patients. Emergencies, such as cardiopulmonary resuscitation, demand immediate access to diagnostic information. POCT may be lifesaving. Hence, TTAT should be just a few minutes. TTAT standards require continual input from nurses and physicians.

The GPS documents will help to establish sound principles for the practice of POCT. Careful and systematic guidance will benefit practitioners and patients alike. Table 1.3 recommends several points to consider when navigating GPS documents. Fortunately, the GPS documents summarized in Table 1.1 provide helpful assistance in a variety of medical settings.

As consensus guidelines and adaptive POCT systems appear, the standard of care will evolve to encompass several more POCT applications locally and globally. POCT has the prospect of promoting equitable health care throughout the world (Fig. 1.2). Well-informed practitioners will have the challenge and responsibility of interpreting and implementing these standards in their individual settings.

TABLE 1.3. HOW TO NAVIGATE GPS DOCUMENTS

Assess	Was there a current (within 3 years), thorough, and critical literature review?
Determine	Are the recommendations substantiated by evidence and referenced to sources?
Gauge	Are instructions detailed, explicit, extensive, and specific enough to follow?
Measure	Are barriers to implementation too many, high, costly, or risky to overcome?
Seek	Are there better alternatives and decision strategies for their selection?
Discern	Can the recommendations be adapted (not merely adopted) to local practice patterns?
Justify	Is there sufficient need locally and clinically for the new policies?
Balance	Does the cost appear reasonable to the community and hospital?
Anticipate	Based on their beliefs, will physicians, patients, and staff accept the changes?
Project	Is there a high probability of improving medical, economic, and social outcomes?
Judge	Does the standard of care medically or legally obligate the change?
Reward	Are the net benefits to physicians and the health system substantial?

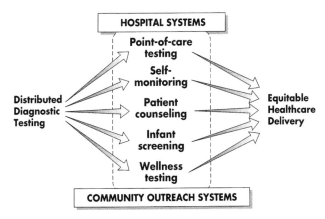

FIGURE 1.2. The point-of-care testing (POCT) systems filter. The future prospect of distributed diagnostic testing is equitable healthcare delivery as medical knowledge shifts to patients who are empowered for prevention, monitoring, and self-care.

Our current knowledge of shared principles for POCT draws on more than two decades of pioneering contributions by creative investigations to a bright new field. They help to ensure that POCT embraces superior professional ethics on its journey through twenty-first century medicine.

ACKNOWLEDGMENTS

I am indebted to the creative students and colleagues who contributed to this work and sincerely thank Claudia Graham for her artistry. Figure and table concepts used courtesy of Knowledge Optimization, Davis, CA, U.S.A.

REFERENCES

1. Kost GJ. Utilization of surface pH electrodes to establish a new relationship for muscle surface pH, venous pH, and arterial pH. *Proceedings of the San Diego Biomedical Symposium* 1977;16:25–33.
2. Fraser CG, Geary TD. Guidelines for the performance of clinical biochemistry tests outside laboratories. *Clin Biochem Res* 1981;2:24–25.
3. McMillan M, Cook J. Chemical pathology on the ward. *Lancet* 1987; 1:487.
4. Anderson JR, Linsell WD, Mitchell FM. Guidelines on the performance of chemical pathology assays outside the laboratory. *BMJ* 1981; 282:743.
5. Vanderlinde RE, Goodwin J, Koch D, et al. *Guidelines for providing quality stat laboratory services.* Washington, DC: AACC Press, 1987:26 pp.
6. Marks V. Essential considerations in the provision of near-patient testing facilities. *Ann Clin Biochem* 1988;25:220–225.
7. Price CP, Burrin JM, Nattrass M. Extra-laboratory blood glucose measurement: a policy statement. *Diabet Med* 1988;5:705–709.
8. Kost GJ, Shirey TL. New whole-blood testing for laboratory support of critical care at cardiac transplant centers and US hospitals. *Arch Pathol Lab Med* 1990;114:865–868.
9. Wimberley PD, Burnett RW, Covington AK, et al. Guidelines for transcutaneous PO_2 and PCO_2 measurement. *J Int Fed Clin Chem* 1990;2:128–135.
10. Boink ABTJ, Buckley BM, Christiansen TF, et al. IFCC recommendation on sampling, transport, and storage for the determination of the concentration of ionized calcium in whole blood, plasma, and serum. *Ann Biol Clin* 1991;49:434–438.
11. Boink ABTJ, Buckley BM, Christiansen TF, et al. IFCC recommendation on sampling, transport, and storage for the determination of the concentration of ionized calcium in whole blood, plasma, and serum. *Clin Chim Acta* 1991;202:S13–S22.
12. Boink ABTJ, Buckley BM, Christiansen TF, et al. IFCC recommendation on sampling, transport, and storage for the determination of the concentration of ionized calcium in whole blood, plasma, and serum. *Eur J Clin Chem Clin Biochem* 1991;29:767–772.
13. Boink ABTJ, Buckley BM, Christiansen TF, et al. IFCC recommendation on sampling, transport, and storage for the determination of the concentration of ionized calcium in whole blood, plasma, and serum. *J International Federation Clin Chem* 1992;4:147–152.
14. Dybkaer R, Martin DV, Rowan RM. Good practice in decentralized analytical clinical measurement. *Scand J Clin Lab Invest* 1992; 209(Suppl):1–116.
15. Joint Working Group (JWG) on External Quality Assessment (EQA) in Pathology. *Guidelines on the control of near-patient tests (NPT) and procedures performed on patients by non-pathology staff.* Liverpool, England: JWGEQA, Mast House, 1992.
16. Kost GJ. New whole blood analyzers and their impact on cardiac and critical care. *Crit Rev Clin Lab Sci* 1993;30:153–202.
17. Kost GJ, Lathrop JP. Designing diagnostic testing for patient-focused care. *Med Laboratory Observer* 1993;25(9S):16–26.
18. Moran RF, Bergkuist C, Graham GA, et al. *Considerations in the simultaneous measurement of blood gases, electrolytes, and related analytes in whole blood.* Wayne, PA: National Committee for Clinical Laboratory Standards. Document C32-P, 1993.
19. Association of Clinical Biochemists. *Guidelines for implementation of near-patient testing.* London, England: Royal Society of Chemistry, 1993.
20. Barr JT, Betschart J, Bracey A, et al. *Ancillary (bedside) blood glucose testing in acute and chronic care facilities.* Wayne, PA: National Committee for Clinical Laboratory Standards. Document C30-A, 1994. [Sachs D, chair, update C30-A2, 2002.]
21. Burnett RW, Covington AK, Fogh-Andersen N, et al. Recommendations on whole blood sampling, transport, and storage for simultaneous determination of pH, blood gases, and electrolytes. International Federation of Clinical Chemistry Scientific Division. *J Intl Fed Clin Chem* 1994;6:115–120.
22. Emergency Care Research Institute. Guidance article. "Point-of-care" laboratory testing: is decentralized testing the best alternative for your hospital? *Health Devices* 1995;24:173–207.
23. England JM, Hyde K, Lewis M, et al. Guide-lines for near patient testing: haematology. *Clin Lab Haematol* 1995;17:301–310.
24. Goodnough LT, Despotis GJ. Establishing practice guidelines for surgical blood management. *Am J Surg* 1995;170(Suppl 6A):16S–20S.
25. Graham GA, D'Orazio P, Bergkuist C, et al. *Ionized calcium determinations: precollection variables, specimen choice, collection, and handling.* Wayne, PA: National Committee for Clinical Laboratory Standards. Document C31-A, 1995. [D'Orazio P, chair, update C31-A2, 2001.]
26. Kost GJ. Guidelines for point-of-care testing: improving patient outcomes. Pathology Patterns. *Am J Clin Pathol* 1995;104(Suppl 1): S111–S127.
27. Near patient testing. Recommended guidelines for hospitals—August, 1992. *Can J Med Tech* 1995;57:74–75, and Canadian Society of Laboratory Technologists Position Statement. Point-of-care laboratory testing. *Can J Med Tech* 1995;57:75.
28. Crook M. Minimum standards should be set for near patient testing. *BMJ* 1996;312:1157.
29. Pilon CS, Leathley M, London R, et al. Practice guideline for arterial blood gas measurement in the intensive care unit decreases numbers and increases appropriateness of tests. *Crit Care Med* 1997;25: 1308–1313.
30. Jansen RTP, Blaton V, Burnett D, et al. Additional essential criteria for quality systems of medical laboratories. *Clin Chem Lab Med* 1998;36: 249–252.

31. Jansen RT. Point-of-care testing. *Clin Chem Lab Med* 1999;37:991.

32. Jansen RT. Point-of-care testing. *Clin Chem Lab Med* 2000;38:261.

33. Kost GJ, Vu HT, Lee JH, et al. Multicenter study of oxygen-insensitive handheld glucose point-of-care testing in critical care/hospital/ambulatory patients in the United States and Canada. *Crit Care Med* 1998;26:581–590.

34. Kost GJ. Optimizing point-of-care testing in clinical systems management. *Clin Manage Lab Rev* 1998;12:353–363.

35. Barr JT, Betschart J, Kiechle FL, et al. *Blood glucose testing in settings without laboratory support.* Wayne, PA: National Committee for Clinical Laboratory Standards, Document AST4-A, 1999.

36. Briedigkeit L, Muller-Plathe O, Schlebusch H, et al. Recommendations of the German working group on medical laboratory testing (AML) on the introduction and quality assurance procedures for point-of-care testing (POCT) in hospitals. *Clin Chem Lab Med* 1999;37:919–925.

37. Freedman DB. Guidelines on point-of-care testing. In: Price CP, Hicks JM, eds. *Point-of-Care Testing.* Washington, DC: AACC Press, 1999:197–212.

38. Goldsmith BM, Travers EM, Lamb LS, et al. *Point-of-care in vitro diagnostic (IVD) testing.* Wayne, PA: National Committee for Clinical Laboratory Standards. Document AST2-A, 1999.

39. Hudson MP, Christenson RH, Newby LK, et al. Cardiac markers: point of care testing. *Clin Chim Acta* 1999;284:223–237.

40. Janssen HW, Bookelman H, Dols JL, et al. Point-of-care testing: the views of the working group of the Dutch Association of Clinical Chemistry. *Clin Chem Lab Med* 1999;37:675–680.

41. Kost GJ, Ehrmeyer SS, Chernow B, et al. The laboratory-clinical interface: point-of-care testing. *Chest* 1999;115:1140–1154.

42. Group de travail "Point of care testing" de la division "Education and Management" de l'IFCC. Recommandations pour la mise en place d'analyses declocalisees. *Ann Biol Clin* 1999;57:232–236.

43. Panteghini M, Apple FS, Christenson RH, et al. Use of biochemical markers in acute coronary syndromes. *Clin Chem Lab Med* 1999;37:687–693.

44. Phillips DL, Santrach PJ, Anderson R, et al. *Quality management for unit-use testing.* Wayne, PA: National Committee for Clinical Laboratory Standards. Document EP-18-P, 1999.

45. Wu AHB, Apple FS, Gibler WB, et al. National Academy of Clinical Biochemistry standards for laboratory practice: recommendations for the use of cardiac markers in coronary diseases. *Clin Chem* 1999;45:1104–1121.

46. Braunwald E, Antman EM, Beasley JW, et al. ACC/AHA guidelines for the management of patients with unstable angina and non-ST-segment elevation myocardial infarction: executive summary and recommendations. *Circulation* 2000;102:1193–1209.

47. Braunwald E, Antman EM, Beasley JW, et al. ACC/AHA guidelines for the management of patients with unstable angina and non-ST-segment elevation myocardial infarction: a report of the American College of Cardiology/American Heart Association task force on practice guidelines (Committee on the Management of Patients with Unstable Angina). *J Am Coll Cardiol* 2000;36:970–1056.

48. Burnett RW, Ehrmeyer SS, Moran RF, et al. *Blood gas and pH analysis and related measurements.* Wayne, PA: National Committee for Clinical Laboratory Standards. Document C46-P, 2000.

49. Connectivity Industry Consortium. *AACC milestone status.* Connectivity Industry Consortium, 2000:50 pp. Available at: www.pocic.org. Accessed November 14, 2001.

50. Connectivity Industry Consortium. *Standards documents (Access Point, Device Messaging Layer, Observation Reporting Interface, et al.).* Connectivity Industry Consortium, 2001. Wayne, PA: National Committee for Clinical Laboratory Standards. Document POCT1-A, 2001. Available at: www.poccic.org. Accessed November 14, 2001.

51. Cummings JP. *POC tests for cardiac injury markers.* Oak Brook, IL: University Health System Consortium, 2000:38 pp.

52. Delaney B, Wilson S, Fitzmaurice D, et al. Near-patient tests in primary care: setting the standards for evaluation. *J Health Serv Res Policy* 2000;5:37–41.

53. Guidelines. Near to patient or point of care testing. *Clin Lab Haematol* 2000;22:185–188.

54. Kirby DL, Major CJ, Steben MH, et al. Point-of-care HIV testing using simple/rapid HIV test kits: guidance for health-care professionals. *Canada Commun Dis Rep* 2000;26:49–59.

55. Kost GJ, Nguyen TH, Tang Z. Whole-blood glucose and lactate: tri-layer biosensors, drug interference, metabolism, and practice guidelines. *Arch Pathol Lab Med* 2000;124:1128–1134.

56. Kost GJ. *Using operator lockout to improve the performance of point-of-care blood glucose monitoring.* Milpitas, CA: LifeScan, 2000:8 pp.

57. McCabe E, Tonniges T. Newborn screening: a blueprint for the future. *Pediatrics* 2000;106(2 Suppl):382–427.

58. Burnett RW, D'Orazio P, Fogh-Anderson N, et al. IFCC recommendation on reporting results for blood glucose. International Federation of Clinical Chemistry, Scientific Division, Working Group on Selective Electrodes. *Clin Chim Acta* 2001;307:205–209.

59. Haeney M. Setting standards for pathology service support to emergency services. *J R Soc Med* 2001;94(Suppl 39):26–30.

60. Hicks JM, Haeckel R, Price CP, et al. Recommendations and opinions for the use of point-of-care testing for hospitals and primary care: summary of a 1999 symposium. *Clin Chim Acta* 2001;303:1–17.

61. Kost GJ. Preventing errors in point-of-care testing: security, validation, performance, safeguards, and connectivity. *Arch Pathol Lab Med* 2001;125:1307–1315.

62. Whitley RJ, Santrach PJ, Phillips DL. Establishing a quality management system for unit-use testing based on NCCLS proposed guideline (EP18-P). *Clin Chim Acta* 2001;307:145–149.

63. Wu AH, Broussard LA, Hoffman RS, et al. Recommendations for the use of laboratory tests to support the impaired and overdosed patient from the emergency department. National Academy of Clinical Biochemistry, 2001. Available at: http://www.nacb.org/emergency/Toxicology_LMPG.htm. Accessed November 14, 2001.

64. Food and Drug Administration. Guidance for clinical laboratory improvement amendments of 1988 (CLIA) criteria for waiver for industry and FDA. Available at: http://www.fda.gov/cdrh/ode/guidance/1147.pdf. (Under development).

65. Hackett J. Review criteria for assessment of invasive blood glucose monitoring *in vitro* diagnostic devices which use glucose oxidase, dehydrogenase, or hexokinase methodology. Division of Clinical Laboratory Devices, Food and Drug Administration. Available at: http://www.fda.gov. (Under development).

66. International Standards Organization (ISO) TC 212, WG 3. American National Standards Institute (ANSI) Secretariat. *Determination of performance criteria for in vitro blood glucose monitoring systems for management of human diabetes mellitus.* Geneva, Switzerland: International Organization for Standardization. Document ISO/DIS 15197, 2001:26 pp. Draft international standard (DIS). Under development.

67. International Standards Organization (ISO) TC 212, WG 3. *Determination of analytical performance goals based on medical needs.* Geneva, Switzerland: International Organization for Standardization; Document ISO/CD 15196. Under development.

68. International Standards Organization (ISO) TC 212, WG 3. *Performance criteria for measurement systems for self testing of oral anticoagulation therapy.* Geneva, Switzerland: International Organization for Standardization; Document ISO/NW 17593. Under development.

69. Kallner A. International standards in laboratory medicine. *Clin Chim Acta* 2001;307:181–186.

70. Joist JH, Ansell J, Despotis G, et al. *Point-of-care hemostasis/coagulation testing.* Wayne, PA: National Committee for Clinical Laboratory Standards. Document H49-UD, 2001. Under development.

71. National Committee for Clinical Laboratory Standards (NCCLS). *Application of a quality model system for offering diagnostic tests in non-laboratory settings.* Wayne, PA: NCCLS. Under development.

72. Shekelle PG, Ortiz E, Rhodes S, et al. Validity of the Agency for Healthcare research and quality clinical practice guidelines: how quickly do they become outdated? *JAMA* 2001;286:1461–1467.

73. Salem M, Chernow B, Burke R, et al. Bedside diagnostic testing: its accuracy, rapidity, and utility in blood conservation. *JAMA* 1991;226:382–389.

74. Kost GJ, Hague C. Current status of critical care testing and patient monitoring: pathology patterns. *Am J Clin Pathol* 1995;104(Suppl1):S2–S17.

75. Kost GJ, Hague C. *In vitro, ex vivo*, and *in vivo* biosensor systems. In: Kost GJ, ed. *Clinical laboratory automation, robotics and optimization.* New York: John Wiley and Sons, 1996:648–753.

76. Kohn LT, Corrigan JM, Donaldson MS, eds. Committee on Quality of Health Care in America, Institute of Medicine. *To err is human: building a safer health system.* Washington, DC: National Academy Press, 2000:287 pp.

77. Richardson WL, Berwick DM, Bisgard JC, et al. *Crossing the quality chasm: a new health system for the 21st century.* Washington, DC: National Academy Press, 2001:pp. 337.

THE HYBRID LABORATORY, THERAPEUTIC TURNAROUND TIME, CRITICAL LIMITS, PERFORMANCE MAPS, AND KNOWLEDGE OPTIMIZATION®

GERALD J. KOST

INTRODUCTION AND GOAL

The goal of this chapter is to present the principles and practice of the hybrid laboratory. This chapter (a) introduces the "test cluster symphony," (b) summarizes evidence showing that point-of-care testing (POCT) improves rapid response, (c) illustrates the importance of therapeutic turnaround time (TTAT) and timeliness, (d) presents the rationale for temporal and diagnostic–therapeutic (Dx-Rx) process optimization, (e) discusses the value of physician capture, (f) explains how POCT performance maps alleviate problems associated with emergency notification of critical results, and (g) outlines the total quality principle for POCT. These concepts form the foundation for improving the efficiency and efficacy of POCT. The unique requirements of POCT sites (Table 2.1) require collaborative interfacing of medical specialists (1). Therefore, we conclude with a multidisciplinary model of integration and synthesis called Knowledge Optimization®.

THE HYBRID LABORATORY

The hybrid laboratory is *distributed but clinically integrated testing*. Bedside and near-patient testing, customized test clusters, minimized TTAT, optimized temporal and Dx-Rx processes, the total quality principle, collaborative teamwork, increased productivity, and especially evidence-based decision making and improved outcomes constitute the hallmarks of the hybrid laboratory (Table 2.2) (2–4). Conversely, these factors represent important driving forces behind POCT.

Doing more with less while doing it faster ("managed" care!) produces an "infinite loop"—a cycle of ever increasing demand for scarce medical resources (Fig. 2.1). Eventually, performance is pushed to the limit. Hospitals caught in the cycle saturate with critically ill patients. Shifts in patient populations force

health systems to grow maximally efficient and, simultaneously, care paths to become maximally efficacious. Whether or not managed care survives, the new health care economy calls for clinically integrated testing guided by hybrid laboratory principles.

Three fundamental "roots" of modern POCT, first invented, then innovated and pioneered clinically, were miniaturized biosensor-based, whole-blood analysis, on-site hemostasis testing, and glucose monitoring (5). Historically, accurate activity-based biosensors enabled medically essential whole-blood test clusters to be performed quickly in the operating room, intensive care unit, and emergency department (Fig. 2.2). Success in critical care, timeliness, and physician satisfaction were strong motivators propelling testing to the bedside.

Invention and innovation created compact transportable, portable, and handheld point-of-care (POC) instruments that simultaneously measure electrolytes, such as Ca^{2+}, K^+, Na^+, Cl^-, and Mg^{2+}, blood gases (PO_2 and PCO_2), pH, and hematocrit or hemoglobin, followed by the addition of metabolites, such as glucose, lactate, urea nitrogen, creatinine, and then, other important analytes (e.g., O_2 saturation and co-oximetry). In parallel, hematology, hemostasis, and focused test clusters, such as cardiac injury [e.g., cardiac troponin I and T, myocardial muscle creatine kinase isoenzyme (CK-MB) mass, and myoglobin] and function (e.g., brain natriuretic peptide) markers also migrated to the POC.

Rapid response and flexibility engendered clinician efficiency and enthusiasm, two powerful factors perpetuating the POCT paradigm shift (Fig. 2.3). Universal access to fast testing empowers physicians, nurses, and patients. Compact POC devices are appearing in the doctor's "black bag" along with the stethoscope and ophthalmoscope. POCT data are part of bedside evaluation of the patient. Immediate access to information increases awareness of the patient's metabolic status and improves opportunities for discovery and self-education.

TABLE 2.1. HYBRID LABORATORY SETTINGS AND SITES OF POINT-OF-CARE TESTING

Hospital (acute care center)
  Bedside (alternate/alternative, ancillary, decentralized, distributed, waived)
  Critical care workstation in the OR, CCU, ER, NICU, PICU, and ICU
  Ex vivo and *in vivo* systems
  Modular plug-in for intensive care systems
  Near-patient (permanent, temporary, mobile)
  Patient-focused care center
  Patient monitoring station and personal monitor
  Procedure suite (e.g., cardiac catheterization suite)
  Satellite laboratory
  Side laboratory and ward
  Trauma center
  Triage and holding area
Outpatient
  Clinic and specialty care center (e.g., dialysis center, intravenous drug unit)
  Community outreach (e.g., cholesterol)
  Home (e.g., self-monitoring of blood glucose)
  Industrial (e.g., chemical exposure, drug check, hazard)
  Patient-focused care facility (e.g., ambulatory surgery, chronic care, heart center)
  Pharmacy, drugstore, and megamarket
  Physician office
  Primary care and regional network
  Urgent care center
  Wellness testing area (e.g., screening)
Rescue and unique locations
  Automatic testing machine and robotic module
  Backpacking, camping, and mountain climbing
  Emergency ground vehicle (e.g., ambulance)
  Helicopter and fixed-wing aircraft for patient transport (adult, pediatric)
  Military field operation, command station, battlefield, and transport
  Patient travel including remote and inaccessible locations
  Points of disaster and emergency rescue
  Remote health outposts and outreach centers
  Roadside check for driving while under the influence of alcohol
  Ship, submarine, submersible, and other nauticals
  Space shuttle, space station, and planetary exploration

OR, operating room; CCU, critical care unit; ER, emergency room; NICU, neonatal intensive care unit; PICU, pediatric intensive care unit; ICU, intensive care unit.

TABLE 2.2. THE HYBRID LABORATORY: EMERGENCE, CHARACTERISTICS, AND FUTURE

Conventional Laboratory	Hybrid laboratory	
	Millennium	Future
Centralized	Patient focused	Hybridized
Separate samples	Critical care profile	Test cluster symphony
Multiple material transfers	Process simplicity	Information connectivity
Confusion from disjoint and dispersed results	Whole-blood priority and volume conservation	Blended *in vitro*, *ex vivo*, and *in vivo* modalities
Slow, high-volume panels	Fewer, more important tests faster	Selective, treatment-targeted adaptive systems
Discrete QC and manual verification	Semiautomated and electronic QC	Parallel process QC and standardization
Data overload	Diagnostic synthesis	Knowledge kernels
Laboratory turnaround time	Therapeutic turnaround time	Real-time biochemical and physiologic observations
Cost analysis by function	Cost effectiveness from patient outcomes	Maximum medical and economic benefits
Discretely organized	Carefully integrated	Fully optimized

QC, quality control.

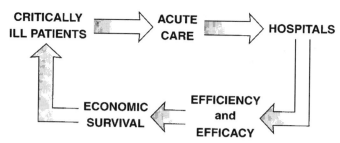

FIGURE 2.1. The "infinite loop" of healthcare systems. Critically ill patients in acute care force hospitals to improve efficiency and efficacy to survive economically. Improved performance attracts even more acutely ill patients. The cycle is perpetual. Fast diagnostic testing and optimized collaborative strategies decrease length of stay and conserve scarce resources.

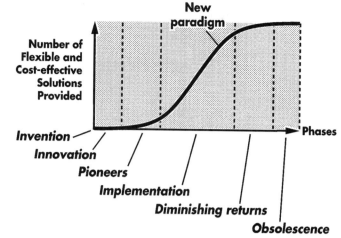

FIGURE 2.3. The point-of-care testing paradigm shift. (Used with the permisssion of Knowledge Optimization and the Archives of Pathology and Laboratory Medicine.)

Home POCT satisfies the consumer's need to know and manage personal medical care.

In the past two decades, microprocessors and microcomputers facilitated POCT growth. Analogous to the rapid and widespread proliferation of personal computers, the use of POCT has become nearly ubiquitous. A variety of instrument formats satisfy special needs. Progressive shifts in tests from conventional instrument platforms to whole-blood, biosensor-based, and micromechanism-nanoscale devices can be expected, especially in acute and urgent care settings where prompt treatment of the patient has great value.

Technologic advances will bring increasing numbers of quantitative tests to the bedside in the next five to ten years. There also are new qualitative tests and novel applications from disciplines such as molecular diagnostics. Continued rapid growth depends on problem-solving advances, however, such as nanofabrication, expanded test menus, connectivity, parallel-process quality control (QC), information synthesis, and improved cost effectiveness. Without these advances, the POCT paradigm shift will yield diminishing returns and become obsolete.

An essential principle of the hybrid laboratory is minimization of the area under the "criticality function" (Fig. 2.4) so that patients spend little time at high risk. Speed of action requires integration, synthesis, and optimization. Expensive resources

deplete rapidly during rescue and critical care. Saving time saves money. POCT promotes cost effectiveness in these settings because efficient diagnosis and efficacious treatment improve outcomes and spare resources.

Another important hybrid laboratory principle is temporal and Dx-Rx process optimization. *Well-directed* POCT targets rapidly changing analytes and allows immediate therapeutic intervention. Pressured physicians do not want to wait for test results. Delays can cause harm to patients. A fully hybridized approach is temporally optimized by integrating *in vitro*, *ex vivo*, and *in vivo* testing modalities (6,7) and by integrating a well-trained *hybrid staff*, who will engage in collaborative teamwork and creative enterprise to apply POCT for Dx-Rx process optimization at the bedside. Therefore, the hybrid laboratory perpetually *shifts the focus to the point of care* (2–4).

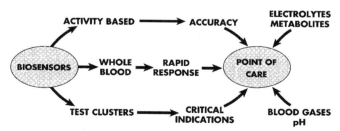

FIGURE 2.2. Biosensors ⇒ point-of-care testing.

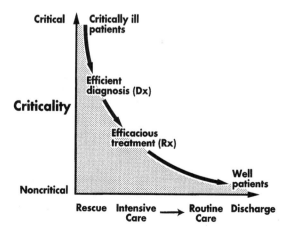

FIGURE 2.4. The criticality function.

TABLE 2.3. THE TEST CLUSTER SYMPHONY: VITAL FUNCTIONS AND DIAGNOSTIC PIVOTS

Vital Function	Diagnostic Pivots–Physiologic Indicators
Energy	Glucose
	Hemoglobin
	P_{O_2}
	O_2 saturation
Conduction	Potassium
	Sodium
	Ionized magnesium
	Ionized calcium
Contraction	Ionized calcium
	Ionized magnesium
Perfusion	Lactate
Acid–base	pH
	P_{CO_2}
	CO_2 content
	End-tidal CO_2 tension
	Bicarbonate
Osmolality	Measured osmolality
	Calculated osmolality
Hemostasis	Hematocrit
	Prothrombin time (PT), international normalized ratio (INR)
	Activated partial thromboplastin time (aPTT)
	Activated clotting time (ACT)
	Platelet count and function
	D-dimer
Homeostasis	Creatinine, urea nitrogen
	White blood cell count
	Chloride
	Inorganic phosphate
	B-type natriuretic peptide (BNP and pro-BNP)
	CO-oximetry variables
	Glycosylated hemoglobin, fructosamine, microalbumin
Biomarker	Cardiac injury and risk (myoglobin, CK-MB mass/isoforms, troponin I/T)
	Lipids (cholesterol, HDL, LDL, triglycerides)
	Cancer (prostate-specific antigen)
Stroke	Trauma (S100 [brain injury marker])
	Bone formation and resorption
Detection	Infection, sepsis, inflammation, and drugs (blood, CSF, body fluids, urine)
Birthing	Antenatal screening (genetic disorders)
	Prenatal testing (urine protein, plasma glucose)
	Delivery monitoring (fetal heart rate, newborn bilirubin)

CK-MB, myocardial muscle creatine kinase isoenzyme; HDL, high-density lipoprotein; LDL, low-density lipoprotein; CSF, cerebrospinal fluid.

THE TEST CLUSTER SYMPHONY™

Let us use the analogy of the symphony. Test clusters will serve as the instruments played by hybrid staff (the performers). Physicians select test clusters for their value as diagnostic pivots of vital functions in Dx-Rx processes (Table 2.3). Test cluster results reveal the status of vital functions through fundamental pathophysiologic mechanisms.

What if there is an accelerando? The quicker the decision is made, the more important POCT is in diagnosis, monitoring, and therapy. Fewer, more important tests that match clinical objectives improve efficiency. Faster, smaller, and smarter POCT devices allow physicians to integrate knowledge of the patient's condition in the shortest possible time and take action. Actions are synchronized, like musicians in a symphony.

Featured ensembles, that is, tightly focused test clusters, fulfill medical needs by shifting the basis for medical decision-making from empirical judgment to evidence-based medicine (Fig. 2.5). A POC orchestra . . . *a poco, a poco.* . . performs well in this metaphor, shifting attention to test cluster analysis and focusing on the most important medical themes.

The melodic texture of the composition unfolds, and awareness heightens. Knowledge of pathophysiology from test cluster results is timely, interactive, and dynamic—in tempo with critical problem solving.

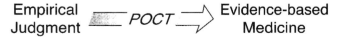

FIGURE 2.5. Transforming empiricism into evidence.

DYNAMIC RESPONSE, IMMEDIATE KNOWLEDGE, AND THE FIFTH DIMENSION

Working harder and faster in the conventional laboratory might improve response time somewhat, but it does not solve the major problems, which are products of an old paradigm that is not wrong but instead is incomplete, with dilemmas symptomatic of obsolescence. Disjoint laboratory divisions, dispersed test results, and discontinuous time domains confuse physicians and cause delays (Fig. 2.6). POCT solves these problems.

Specimens deteriorate because of sample splitting and lag time before analysis in physically separated laboratory sections. Data, once obtained, may be out of date or irrelevant. Physicians may not realize that the data are obsolete, not synchronized with current treatment, and therefore potentially hazardous if the patient is unstable. Outliers are difficult to predict. They distract both clinicians and laboratorians and may impede life-saving treatment.

Clinicians who experience POCT expect superior performance. Appendix I of this book summarizes studies showing that POCT minimizes response time, eliminates process steps, enhances decision-making, and improves treatment options. Efficiency streamlines triage, conserves blood, decreases length of stay, and improves outcomes. The appendix to this chapter presents the concept of dynamic response. Briefly, once turnaround time is minimized, subsequent increases appear huge to the clinician. The directional dynamic explains why the immediacy of POCT irreversibly changes the clinician's mindset.

Timely data are needed for accurate calculation of derived parameters, such as anion gap, strong ion difference, and base excess, and for the determination of prognosis, severity, and cost effectiveness. POCT information density (data produced per unit of time) is high and peaks early (Fig. 2.6). The availability of fewer, more important tests done faster potentially reduces the total testing burden (the integrated time-adjusted area under the curves in Fig. 2.6). POCT consistently accelerates the information cycle and creates immediate knowledge. This immediacy of knowledge, the "fifth dimension" of the hybrid laboratory, helps practitioners to optimize patient care efficiently.

THERAPEUTIC TURNAROUND TIME

A fundamental principle of the hybrid laboratory is the continuity of preanalytic, analytic, and postanalytic events as measured by TTAT (1,4,8–11). TTAT is defined as the time from test ordering to receipt of results by the clinical team, plus the time needed to start, stop, or modify treatment (Fig. 2.7). Clinicians prefer to obtain test results, explain therapeutic rationale, and treat patients in the same episode. Timely information increases physician efficiency and may shorten the patient's stay. The patient's perception of responsive care encourages wellness.

Whole-blood analysis and POCT decrease TTAT. The logic of shorter TTAT is that early treatment, especially of critically ill patients, helps to decrease the time from treatment to outcome

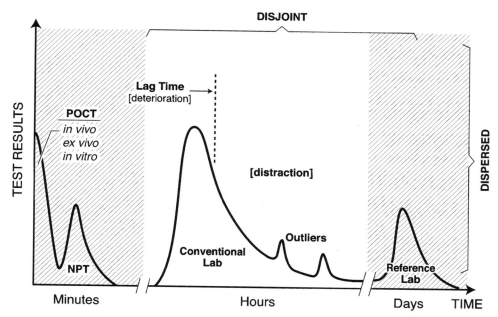

FIGURE 2.6. Space–time continuity and the diagnostic testing process. Point-of-care testing synchronizes test results and physiologic observations at the bedside, where immediate knowledge of sudden or unexpected changes in the patient's status is most valuable. When testing is performed far from the patient, the fidelity, reliability, and continuity of information degrade because test results are disjointed, dispersed, and delayed. Lag time can deteriorate specimen integrity. Splitting disaggregates test results and may diminish awareness. Outliers can interfere with critical clinical decisions.

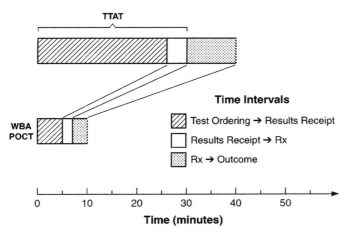

FIGURE 2.7. Therapeutic turnaround time (TTAT). The TTAT is the time from test ordering to appropriate treatment (Rx). Point-of-care testing (POCT) and whole-blood analysis (WBA) shorten TTAT. The interval from Rx to outcome typically also decreases, thereby improving care.

POCT. Evaluation correlates (right frame) showed that timeliness, convenience, labor conservation, and, most importantly, improved patient care were the principal components correlated with the higher satisfaction rating.

Fast TTAT accelerates clinical decision-making and Dx-Rx processes. Quick evidence-based Dx-Rx processes improve intermediate outcomes. Therefore, temporal optimization links rapid response and clinical outcomes. In settings where speed is not critical, the POC coordinator can negotiate response times specific to each clinical unit but also should decrease the volume and the TTAT of conventional testing. Mohammad and colleagues (13) showed that fast TTAT works well as an enterprise strategy, metric surrogate, and performance goal for near-patient testing.

TEMPORAL AND DIAGNOSTIC—THERAPEUTIC PROCESS OPTIMIZATION

The axioms (2,4,5) of the hybrid laboratory state that diagnostic efficiency increases as response time decreases and the cluster effectiveness of tests increases. For a critical test cluster, optimum response time is achieved when the combination of analysis time and transit time, a function of the distance of the measurement from the patient, is minimized. Fast test results avoid empiric treatment, inefficient delays, physiologic obsolescence, and unnecessary cycles of unproductive testing.

Whole-blood analysis decreases response time by eliminating specimen centrifugation and other preanalytic steps. Process simplicity reduces waste and errors. Current guidelines (see Chapter 1) recommend the availability of rapid response testing with a TTAT of a few minutes during emergencies, such as cardiopulmonary resuscitation. The temporal sequence of test results

and generally, improves the patient's condition or at least helps diminish complications and unforeseen problems that delay favorable outcomes, prolong care, and waste valuable medical and financial resources. Therefore, TTAT is an essential metric surrogate for tracking the efficiency and efficacy of POCT.

Figure 2.8 illustrates the results of clinical research by Kilgore and colleagues (12), who demonstrated the validity of TTAT and the benefits of shortening it. POCT significantly decreased median TTAT in the cardiac intensive care unit and at the bedside (left frame in the figure) compared with the central laboratory. Overall satisfaction ratings (middle frame) were higher for

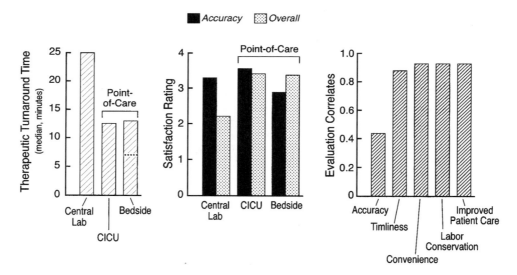

FIGURE 2.8. Fast therapeutic turnaround time (TTAT) improves patient care. In intensive care, point-of-care testing (POCT) significantly decreased TTAT ($p < 0.0001$) and prompted treatment changes more often. The dashed line (bedside) is the time required for physician decision-making and the interval above it for diagnostic testing. Overall satisfaction was higher with POCT. Principal components analysis showed that timeliness correlated most closely with improved patient care, labor conservation, and convenience. (Drawn from research results published in 12. Kilgore ML, Steindel SJ, Smith JA. Evaluating stat testing options in an academic health center: therapeutic turnaround time and staff satisfaction. *Clin Chem* 1998;44:1597–1603.)

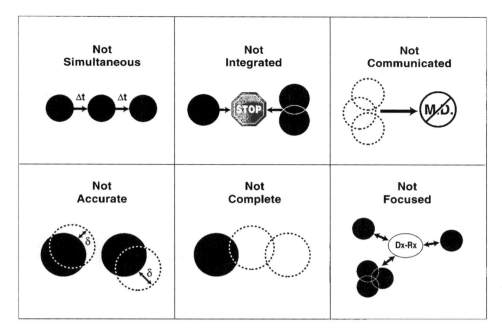

FIGURE 2.9. Knowledge mosaics. In the top row, lack of temporal optimization cause external defects. Test results are not simultaneous, integrated, or communicated. In the bottom row, diagnostic–therapeutic (Dx-Rx) processes are not optimized. Test results are inaccurate, incomplete, or poorly focused. Point-of-care testing repositions the tiles to create holistic knowledge mosaics.

defines primary and secondary medical events and their causality. Fast POCT allows simultaneous temporal and Dx-Rx process optimization. The POCT paradigm breaks with the conventional laboratory approach by solving major process problems.

Remapping of medical knowledge improves patient care and outcomes. Figure 2.9 shows, by the scattering of the tiles in the top row, that if testing is not temporally optimized, it will not be simultaneous, integrated, and communicated. Patient care becomes slow, discontinuous, inefficient, and expensive. Dx-Rx processes will not be optimized (bottom row) if test results are not accurate, complete, and focused. POCT synchronizes and realigns knowledge mosaics to reduce fractionation, prevent discontinuities, and reduce errors.

Therefore, two additional fundamental principles of the hybrid laboratory are that (a) testing must be simultaneous, integrated, and communicated promptly and continuously, that is, temporally optimized; and (b) test results must be accurate, complete, and focused to optimize Dx-Rx processes.

PHYSICIAN CAPTURE™

The objective of physician capture (Fig. 2.10) is to allow physicians to make decisions to start, stop, or modify therapy as soon as possible before adverse outcomes occur (2–5). POCT produces evidence fast enough to capture physicians' thoughts (at

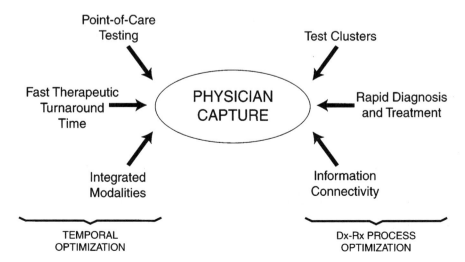

FIGURE 2.10. Physician capture—physical or mental. Key elements of physician capture are fast therapeutic turnaround time (left) and rapid diagnosis and treatment (right). The elements on the left generate temporal optimization; on the right, diagnostic–therapeutic process optimization. Whether the physician is at the bedside or telecommunicating orders, physician capture is a practical optimizer that helps improve medical and economic outcomes.

the bedside or elsewhere) during critical moments, to enable simultaneous biochemical and physiologic observations, and to supply answers to questions while they are still in mind. In Figure 2.10, elements on the left save time (temporal optimization), whereas those on the right eliminate guesswork during the testing of hypotheses (Dx-Rx process optimization). Quick resolution of hypotheses is crucial.

The rate of change of the patient's status and analyte levels often determines the level of interest of nurses and physicians. Fast TTAT (left, Fig. 2.10) enables rapid diagnosis and treatment (right). Integrated *in vitro, ex vivo,* and *in vivo* modalities and information connectivity facilitate evidence-based medical practice at the bedside. POCT engenders awareness, investigation, consultation, and feedback to close knowledge loops (14). Therefore, physician capture is a practical performance and outcomes optimizer.

CRITICAL LIMITS AND PERFORMANCE MAPS™

Failure to notify physicians of critical test results in a timely fashion represents a serious problem in complex and busy healthcare systems. Emergency notification systems for critical test results are required in all hospitals. Critical limits define the boundaries of the low and high life-threatening values of laboratory test results (15–19). Critical results are those that fall outside these two levels. POCT avoids problems associated with emergency notification of critical results.

Hyponatremia is the single most common electrolyte disturbance in hospitalized patients (20). The objectives of treatment are to restore the sodium level at a safe rate and to treat the underlying disease (21). Consider, for example, the flow of information during an episode of acute hyponatremia (Fig. 2.11). Indecision as to what discrete low critical limit to select yields a potentially dysfunctional sequence of events that can produce high risk and poor outcomes. Hospitals select different critical limit thresholds (dashed lines) for emergency notification. Even within the same health system, thresholds may not be consistent.

The sequence to the right in Figure 2.11 may be complicated by misleading pseudohyponatremia (22–36) or by external defects, such as no action for undetected decreases in sodium levels, unsuccessful emergency notification of clinicians, or inability to rule out pseudohyponatremia. Rate-limiting steps in this awkward sequence increase the chances of encephalopathy, seizures, and respiratory failure, especially in vulnerable patients, such as children or women during or following surgery, who may experience prolonged hospitalization and poor outcomes (37–47). Empiric treatment is dangerous and should not be undertaken (21).

Compare the performance map (Fig. 2.12) design for the operating room and critical care settings where whole-blood analysis is available on site. POCT obviates the analytic problem of pseudohyponatremia and also provides the speed necessary to optimize the feedback loop of critical knowledge required for sodium repletion at a safe rate until a normal or near-normal sodium level can be restored. See Enquist (20), Zaloga and colleagues (21), and Fraser and Arieff (44) for discussion of appropriate repletion rates. A similar integrated strategy can be used for hypernatremia (48).

The Dx-Rx process optimization (left bracket) and temporal optimization (bottom bracket) help to prevent costly poor outcomes associated with acute hyponatremia. Ultimately, feedback loops will automate integrated therapeutic protocols (Fig. 2.13) for detection, monitoring, and treatment of patients with critical problems such as acute hyponatremia.

Sodium is a medical surrogate of sublethal and lethal events (see Chapter 40). Immediate knowledge of sodium levels through the use of POCT links temporal optimization and Dx-Rx process optimization. This linkage enhances medical synthesis and speeds decision-making. Cost effectiveness derives from the prevention of serious sequelae or from their early detection and resolution through evidence-based treatment conducted in a timely manner.

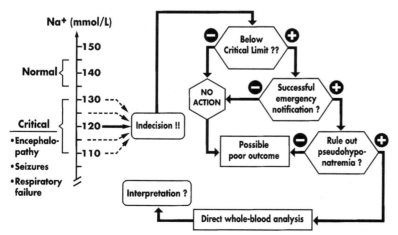

FIGURE 2.11. Emergency notification of critical test results for sodium. External defects in critical result notification occur frequently and are dangerous. This flowchart illustrates the potential mechanisms of errors. The vertical scale shows normal (135–145 mmol/L) and critical (mean 120 mmol/L) sodium levels (15,18). Please see Figure 2.12 and the text explanation of how point-of-care testing can help improve performance.

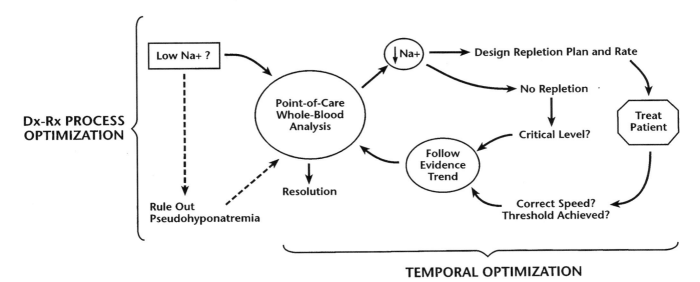

FIGURE 2.12. Performance map for acute hyponatremia.

THE TOTAL QUALITY PRINCIPLE FOR POINT-OF-CARE TESTING

In an industrial model, quality may be what consumers desire, endorse, or buy; in health care, quality is what is good for patients and must be based on the standard of care, societal guidelines, access, and equity. The use of POCT in diverse and complex settings (Table 2.1) warrants careful consideration of the basis and strategy for enhancing performance.

Good quality practices transcend federal, state, and local statutory requirements. The Clinical Laboratory Improvement Amendments of 1988 (CLIA, 1988) imposed graded regulatory requirements based on the level of test complexity (the "complexity model") rather than on the location of diagnostic testing, so-called site neutrality. Revisions of statutes are inevitable, but the concept of site neutrality is likely to remain a permanent feature for the foreseeable future.

Therefore, based on the concept of site neutrality, the *total quality principle* for POCT (10,11,49) means empowering professionals (50) who proactively integrate QC, quality monitors,

proficiency testing, and performance improvement into one patient-focused package that meets customer needs *irrespective of where the diagnostic testing is performed.*

The goal of the total quality principle for POCT is to improve the integrated outcomes of the diagnostic testing process. This principle can be implemented by using total quality management to produce organizational alignment. Each institution designs its own performance-improvement program, monitors, and oversight. Surveying quality monitors, perpetually assessing trends, and continuously devising new ways to improve quality will enhance POCT performance.

PRACTICAL AND PROGRESSIVE STRATEGIES TO OPTIMIZE POINT-OF-CARE TESTING

Medicine now faces increasingly tough competition in the marketplace. Fiscal constraints challenge our ability to provide the highest quality patient care. Present problems associated with the conventional laboratory are a product of that paradigm. We cannot solve significant problems at the same level of thinking used when older paradigms were created. Clinical teams must conserve resources and simultaneously improve outcomes. Shorter hospital stays, particularly shorter critical care episodes, are essential.

This urgency calls for collaborative hybrid teams (Table 2.4) for POCT. Nurses often perform substantial POCT and can contribute significantly to the teams. The POC coordinator, who supervises operations, quality, and staff on a daily basis, and other team members serve as vigilant outcomes managers. Practical and progressive strategies (Table 2.5) guide the drastic changes engulfing healthcare systems. Outcomes management at all levels fulfills one of the important visions of the hybrid laboratory for the future.

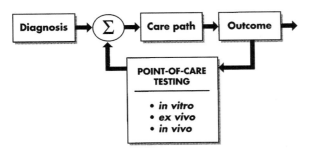

FIGURE 2.13. Feedback system for continuous monitoring and therapy.

TABLE 2.4. HYBRID LABORATORY TEAM AND LEADERSHIP

Title	Functions
Director of point-of-care testing	Sets goals, has authority, and is accountable
Point-of-care coordinator	Supervises operations, quality, and staff
Connectivity consultant	Supports computerized and wireless communications
Bioengineering research group	Develops novel new measurements and instruments
Multidisciplinary strategies committee	Assures clinical interfaces and minimizes risk
Certified and validated hybrid staff	Performs point-of-care testing
Outcomes (performance) manager	Optimizes medical and economic outcomes

TABLE 2.5. PRACTICAL AND PROGRESSIVE STRATEGIES TO OPTIMIZE POINT-OF-CARE TESTING (POCT)

Establish critical care and patient-focused test clusters
    Fulfill clinical objectives by selecting key tests
    Combine tests in clusters to improve efficiency
    Monitor vital functions using diagnostic pivots
Select instruments designed for POCT
    Use direct whole-blood methods
    Eliminate centrifugation
    Conserve blood
Maximize connectivity and minimize response time
    Adopt connectivity standards
    Create patient proximity to reduce specimen transit time
    Report results immediately
Prevent medical errors
    Train and certify POCT instrument operators and renew annually
    Implement security, validation, performance, and emergency systems
    Assure safeguards and privacy
Optimize systems to improve performance
    Follow the total quality principle for POCT
    Employ temporal and Dx-Rx process optimization
    Integrate and synthesize to optimize knowledge
Target critical opportunities
    Identify surrogates of sublethal and lethal events
    Track quantitative metrics for efficiency and efficacy
    Improve medical and economic outcomes

MAPPING THE FUTURE

Discovery Challenge

The future of POCT presents exciting challenges (Table 2.6). Some milestones, such as wireless connectivity, are on the horizon, whereas others, such as noninvasive monitoring, will take decades to perfect. Still others are yet to be discovered. Nonetheless, POCT has established a new standard for rapid-response diagnostic testing, which is expected in the practice of critical

TABLE 2.6. THE FUTURE OF POINT-OF-CARE TESTING

No reagents (continuous)
No samples (noninvasive)
No delays (real-time monitoring)
No discontinuities (wireless connectivity)
Efficient (integrated)
Cost-effective (benefits > costs)
Efficacious (improves outcome)

care medicine and, increasingly, in other specialties and medical settings. The immediacy of test results is especially valuable in guiding emergency interventions when there is little or no knowledge of the patient's medical condition.

Therapeutic Turnaround Time Standard

During resuscitations and critical emergencies, a TTAT of 5 minutes represents the standard of care (1,9). Besides speed, well-directed POCT targets medical surrogates of sublethal and lethal events to reduce morbidity and mortality. POCT conserves patient blood volume, thereby decreasing the need for transfusions, diminishing the risks of reactions and infections, and eliminating unanticipated "downstream" and "hidden" costs. Prevention of adverse outcomes benefits the entire health system. Therefore, POCT has much to offer right now.

Holistic Monitoring

Ex vivo and *in vivo* monitoring augment *in vitro* testing by producing a continuous, or nearly continuous, stream of information. Monitoring finds use in settings where urgency limits quick gathering together of discrete, disjoint data. Much research is needed to automate closed-loop feedback systems using *in vitro*, *ex vivo*, and *in vivo* monitoring to guide therapy. Ultimately, judicious and cost-effective combinations of these modalities will lead, despite technologic hurdles, to improved quality of patient care through simultaneous biochemical and physiologic observations.

Human Performance

For the clinician, enhanced personal performance depends on accelerated cognitive function and decision-making and on elimination of poorly focused, unnecessary, and obsolete data. Knowledge mosaics (Fig. 2.9) illustrate how testing should be simultaneous, integrated, communicated, accurate, complete, and focused. Pressed to become more efficient, physicians desperately need integrated and synthesized information for optimal diagnosis and therapy.

Global Effort

The most useful POCT clusters carefully target critical indications, based on medical necessity. As relevancy of testing increases, the total volume of testing should decrease. Necessity inspires the discovery of appropriate new POCT diagnostic pivots (e.g., platelet function tests, coronary ischemia prognosticators, and stroke survival indicators), critical decision thresholds, and care strategies that improve outcomes and avoid excessive costs. Cost-effective solutions are needed in both developed and emerging countries.

Hybrid Laboratory

Optimally directed POCT is not only distributed but is clinically integrated. It is easy to justify the use of POCT in critical care settings where cost effectiveness derives mainly from competition for scarce resources. POCT facilitates immediate evidence-based medical decisions in the operating room, intensive care unit, and other critical care settings. Outcomes managers can map POCT into these areas first while assessing the efficacy of the resulting changes in practice patterns.

Adaptive POCT Systems

Clinical optimization derives from the knowledge of critical perturbations, vital functions, and shifting surrogates, such as dangerous elevations (e.g., K^+ in arrhythmias), unanticipated changes (Na^+ in encephalopathy), temporal trends (lactate in shock), specific biomarkers (cTnI in coronary occlusion), Dx-Rx patterns (Ca^{2+} in cardiac decomposition), surgical endpoints (parathyroid hormone in parathyroidectomy), and treatment monitors (prothrombin time and activated partial thromboplastin time in anticoagulation). POCT treatment algorithms, performance maps, integrative strategies, care paths, and new knowledge structures (14) facilitate rapid synthesis of information in adaptive POCT systems.

Knowledge Transfer

Outcomes optimization forms a solid basis for establishing POCT priorities for the support of critical care. The clini-cian–laboratorian of the future provides health care directly as an outcomes manager in the hybrid laboratory. The challenge is how to synthesize immediate diagnostic information most efficiently and effectively. The focus shifts to immediate knowledge and patterns of change. POCT is a *knowledge technology*. POCT creates immediate new knowledge that is medically valuable in critical care and other medical settings.

KNOWLEDGE OPTIMIZATION

Let us apply a simple principle: Outcomes integrate preceding effects. Therefore, *integrate to improve outcomes*. Patient-focused POCT is efficient and efficacious when integrated into performance maps, treatment algorithms, care paths, and other clever strategies using appropriately targeted test clusters tuned to critical limit priorities (Fig. 2.14A). Systems (51) also should be tuned for time- and process-optimized, evidence-based patient care (Fig. 2.14B). Optimization prospectively synthesizes knowledge components. Therefore, integration and synthesis optimize knowledge (Fig. 2.14C).

Temporal optimization tracks disease evolution and compresses its resolution, based on the fact that biochemical variables are coupled, fundamentally, to pathophysiologic changes at the cellular level and, ultimately, to patient survival and outcomes. Optimized Dx-Rx processes prevent critical problems through early and accurate detection. Together, integration and synthesis are synergistic for diagnosis, management, and treatment. POCT points beyond simple efficiency to knowledge optimization in medical practice.

ACKNOWLEDGMENTS

I am indebted to the creative students and colleagues who contributed to this work and sincerely thank Claudia Graham for her artistry. Figure and table concepts used courtesy of Knowledge Optimization, Davis, CA, U.S.A.

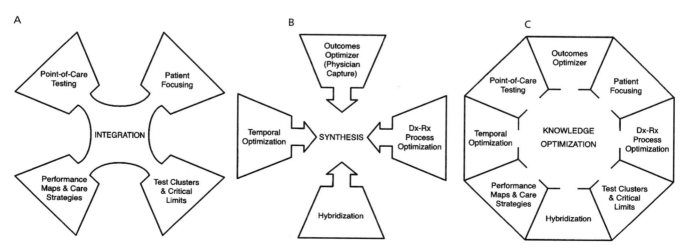

FIGURE 2.14. Integration ∪ synthesis ⇒ knowledge optimization. The union (∪) of integration (**A**) and synthesis (**B**) yields knowledge optimization (**C**).

CHAPTER 2 APPENDIX: DYNAMIC RESPONSE

Dynamic response is the change in process response time. This appendix illustrates how point-of-care testing (POCT) affects dynamic response and its perception.

Definitions

TAT_1 is turnaround time before change, TAT_2, after change. Dynamic response, ΔTAT, is $|TAT_2 - TAT_1|$. The vertical bars mean absolute value, that is, ΔTAT is positive. $TAT_M = (TAT_1 + TAT_2)/2$. δ_{CL} is the percent change in TAT from the viewpoint of the clinical laboratory, and δ_{POC}, from the viewpoint of the point of care. The perception index (pi), Π, is $[TAT_{NEW}/TAT_{OLD}]$. Turnaround times are in minutes. Two methods for determining the effects of changes in ΔTAT are described next.

Method 1

TAT_1 appears in the denominator for δ_{CL}, and TAT_2, for δ_{POC}, when calculating the percent change in TAT:

$$\delta_{CL} = (\Delta TAT/TAT_1)(100\%)$$

$$\delta_{POC} = (\Delta TAT/TAT_2)(100\%)$$

Method 2

TAT_M is used in the denominator:

$$\delta = [(\Delta TAT/TAT_M)(100\%)]$$

and in this case,

$$\delta = \delta_{CL} = \delta_{POC}$$

When $\Delta TAT < TAT_M$, $\delta < 100\%$, and when $\Delta TAT > TAT_M$, $\delta > 100\%$. ΔTAT is equal to TAT_M when $TAT_1 - TAT_2 = (TAT_1 + TAT_2)/2$, or $TAT_2 = TAT_1/3$, that is, when performance improvements decrease TAT by two-thirds. For continuous monitoring, let $\delta = \partial(TAT)/\partial t$.

Forward Dynamic Sequence

If the clinical laboratory TAT_1 of 30 is improved by 10 to 20, TAT_2 is 20, and ΔTAT is 10. The percent improvement, $\delta_{CL} = [(30-20)/30](100\%) = 33\%$ and $\Pi = 0.67$. If testing subsequently shifts to the point of care where TAT_2 is 5, then (with TAT_1 of 20), $\delta_{CL} = 75\%$ and $\Pi = 0.25$. From the clinical laboratory viewpoint, there are incremental improvements of 33% and 75%. Overall, $\delta_{CL} = 83\%$ and $\Pi = (5/30) = 0.17$. Perception indices are less than one; however, clinicians are pleased with the improvements. Incremental and overall values of δ are 40, 120, and 143% (Method 2).

Reverse Dynamic Sequence

From the physician's perspective at the point of care, if POCT were taken away and TAT increased from 5 to 20, $\delta_{POC} = [(20-5)/5](100\%) = 300\%$, and $\Pi = 4$! TAT without POCT would be four times worse! Further degradation from 20 to 30 yields $\delta_{POC} = 50\%$ and $\Pi = 1.5$. Overall, $\delta_{POC} = 500\%$ and $\Pi = 6$, a

TABLE A2.1. CHANGES IN PARAMETERS FOLLOWING SEQUENTIAL BINARY CHANGES IN ΔTAT TO 2 MINUTES, THE ANALYSIS TIME COMMONLY ACHIEVED BY POINT-OF-CARE INSTRUMENTS

Site	TAT_1	TAT_2	ΔTAT	Forward ↓ δ_{CL}	Forward ↓ Π	Reverse ↑ δ_{POC}	Reverse ↑ Π	δ
Clinical lab	64	32	32	50%	0.50	100%	2.0	67%
↓↑	32	16	16	"	"	"	"	"
↓↑	16	8	8	"	"	"	"	"
↓↑	8	4	4	"	"	"	"	"
POCT	4	2	2	"	"	"	"	"
Overall	64	2	62	97%	0.03125	31x	32x	188%

sixfold deterioration in TAT. Clinicians perceive a huge setback and are not happy! Satisfaction plummets when TAT exceeds one hour, an outdated standard, which some laboratorians still accept. Corresponding forward and reverse values of Π are reciprocals, that is, $1/0.25 = 4$, $1/0.67 = 1.5$, and $1/0.17 = 6$, after allowing for rounding error. Values of δ are unchanged.

Table A2-1 illustrates changes in parameters following sequential binary changes in ΔTAT to 2 minutes, the analysis time commonly achieved by POC instruments.

Appendix Conclusions

Comparisons of relative changes in TAT appear psychologically dynamic with hysteresis because of viewpoint. POCT improves TAT "irreversibly." Clinicians do not want to give up fast access to diagnostic data once they experience the immediacy of POCT. POCT also eliminates extremely delayed test results ("outliers"), which are the nemesis of batch testing and the bane of critical care. Like a chain reaction, the elimination of outliers improves performance in complementary activities. Improvements in dynamic TAT are enduring. Clinical value is magnified by perception.

REFERENCES

1. Kost GJ, Ehrmeyer SS, Chernow B, et al. The laboratory-clinical interface: point-of-care testing. *Chest* 1999;115:1140–1154.
2. Kost GJ. The hybrid laboratory: shifting the focus to the point of care. *Medical Laboratory Observer* 1992;24(9 Suppl):17–28.
3. Kost GJ. The hybrid laboratory: the clinical laboratory of the 1990's is a synthesis of the old and the new. *Arch Pathol Lab Med* 1992;116:1002–1003.
4. Kost GJ. Point-of-care testing ⇒ The hybrid laboratory ⇒ Knowledge optimization. In: Kost GJ, ed. *Handbook of clinical automation, robotics, and optimization.* New York: John Wiley and Sons, 1996:757–838.
5. Kost GJ. New whole blood analyzers and their impact on cardiac and critical care. *Crit Rev Clin Lab Sci* 1993;30:153–202.
6. Kost GJ, Hague C. The current and future status of critical care testing and patient monitoring. Pathology Patterns. *Am J Clin Pathol* 1995;104(Suppl 1):S2–S17.
7. Kost GJ, Hague C. *In vitro, ex vivo,* and *in vivo* biosensor systems. In: Kost GJ, ed. *Handbook of clinical automation, robotics, and optimization.* New York: John Wiley and Sons, 1996:648–753.
8. Kost GJ. The role of new whole-blood analytic techniques in critical care. *Clin Chem* 1989;35:1232–1233.

9. Kost GJ. Guidelines for point-of-care testing: Improving patient outcomes: Pathology Patterns. *Am J Clin Pathol* 1995;104(Suppl 1): S111–S127.

10. Kost GJ. Point-of-care testing in intensive care. In: Tobin MJ, ed. *Principles and practice of intensive care monitoring.* New York: McGraw-Hill, 1998:1267–1296.

11. Kost GJ. Point-of-care testing. In: Meyers RA, ed. *Encyclopedia of analytical chemistry: instrumentation and applications.* New York: John Wiley & Sons, 2000:1603–1625.

12. Kilgore ML, Steindel SJ, Smith JA. Evaluating stat testing options in an academic health center: therapeutic turnaround time and staff satisfaction. *Clin Chem* 1998;44:1597–1603.

13. Mohammad AA, Summers H, Burchfield JE, et al. STAT turnaround time: satellite and point-to-point testing. *Lab Med* 1996;27:684–688.

14. Kost GJ. Artificial intelligence and new knowledge structures. In: Kost GJ, ed. *Handbook of clinical automation, robotics, and optimization.* New York: John Wiley and Sons, 1996:149–193.

15. Kost GJ. Critical limits for urgent clinician notification at US medical centers. *JAMA* 1990;263:704–707.

16. Kost GJ. Critical limits for emergency clinician notification at United States children's hospitals. *Pediatrics* 1991;88:597–603.

17. Kost GJ. The significance of ionized calcium in cardiac and critical care: availability and critical limits at US medical centers and children's hospitals. *Arch Pathol Lab Med* 1993;117:890–896.

18. Kost GJ. Using critical limits to improve patient outcome. *Medical Laboratory Observer* 1993;25:22–27.

19. Kost GJ. Designing critical limit systems for knowledge optimization. *Arch Pathol Lab Med* 1996;120:616–618.

20. Engquist A. From plasma [Na⁺] to diagnosis and treatment. *Acta Anesthesiol Scand* 1995;39(Suppl 107):273–279.

21. Zaloga GP, Kirby RR, Bernards WC, et al. Fluid and Electrolytes. In: Civetta JM, Taylor RW, Kirby RR, eds. *Critical care.* Philadelphia: Lippincott–Raven, 1997:413–442.

22. Forrest ARW, Shenkin A. Dangerous pseudohyponatremia. *Lancet* 1980; 2:1256.

23. Frier BM, Steer CR, Baird JD, et al. Misleading plasma electrolytes in diabetic children with severe hyperlipidemia. *Arch Dis Child* 1980;55: 771–775.

24. Nanji AA, Blank DW. Pseudohyponatremia and hyperviscosity. *J Clin Pathol* 1983;36:834–835.

25. Pain RW. Test and teach (41). Diagnosis: hypertriglyceridemia with pseudohyponatremia in acute and chronic alcoholism. *Pathology* 1983; 15:233,331–334.

26. Aw TC, Keichle FL. Pseudohyponatremia. *Am J Emerg Med* 1985;3: 236–239.

27. Howard JM, Reed J. Pseudohyponatremia in acute hyperlipemic pancreatitis: a potential pitfall in therapy. *Arch Surg* 1985;120: 1053–1055.

28. Weisberg LS. Pseudohyponatremia: a reappraisal. *Am J Med* 1989;86: 315–318.

29. Kost GJ. Accurate and efficient diagnosis of hyperosmolar coma. *Audio-Digest Internal Medicine* 1991;38(10).

30. Grateau G, Bachmeyer C, Taulera O, et al. Pseudohyponatremia and pseudohyperphosphatemia in a patient with human immunodeficiency virus infection. *Nephron* 1993;46:640.

31. Vaswani SK, Sprague R. Pseudohyponatremia in multiple myeloma. *South Med J* 1993;86:251–252.

32. Olivero JJ. Case in point: pseudohyponatremia due to hyperproteinemia in multiple myeloma. *Hosp Pract* 1994;29:61.

33. Sachs C, Levillain P. The real cause of discrepancy between plasma sodium results obtained by ISE and "dilution" techniques: an error in the dilution factor. *AACC Electrolyte/Blood Gas Division Newsletter* 1994;9:2–4.

34. Lawn N, Wijdicks EF, Burritt MF. Intravenous immune globulin and pseudohyponatremia. *N Engl J Med* 1998;339:632.

35. Ng SK. Intravenous immunoglobulin infusion causing pseudohyponatremia. *Lupus* 1999;8:488–490.

36. Rosenthal R, Koelz A, Vogelbach P. Pseudohyponatremia. Schweizerische Medizinische Wochenschrift, *J Suisse Med* 2000;130:161.

37. Ayus JC, Wheeler JM, Arieff AI. Postoperative hyponatremic encephalopathy in menstruant women. *Ann Intern Med* 1992;117:891–897.

38. Singhi S, Dhawan A. Frequency and significance of electrolyte abnormalities in pneumonia. *Indian Pediatr* 1992;29:734–740.

39. Singhi S, Prasad SV, Chugh KS. Hyponatremia in sick children: a marker of serious illness. *Indian Pediatr* 1994;31:19–25.

40. Ayus JC, Arieff AI. Pulmonary complications of hyponatremic encephalopathy: noncardiac pulmonary edema and hypercapnic respiratory failure. *Chest* 1995;107:517–521.

41. Ayus CJ, Arieff AI. Brain damage and postoperative hyponatremia: the role of gender. *Neurology* 1996;46:323–328.

42. Ayus JC, Arieff AI. Hyponatremia and myelinolysis. *Ann Intern Med* 1997;127:163.

43. Ayus JC, Arieff AI. Postoperative hyponatremia. *Ann Intern Med* 1997; 126:1005–1006.

44. Fraser CL, Arieff AI. Epidemiology, pathophysiology, and management of hyponatremic encephalopathy. *Am J Med* 1997;102:67–77.

45. Laureno R, Karp B. Myelinolysis after correction of hyponatremia. *Ann Intern Med* 1997;126:57–62.

46. Arieff AI. Postoperative hyponatremic encephalopathy following elective surgery in children. *Paediatr Anesth* 1998;81:1–4.

47. Arieff AI, Ayus JC. Hyponatremia. *N Engl J Med* 2000;343:886.

48. Palevsky PM, Bhagrath R, Greenberg A. Hypernatremia in hospitalized patients. *Ann Intern Med* 1996;124:197–203.

49. Kost GJ. Planning and implementing point-of-care systems. In: Tobin MJ, ed. *Principles and practice of intensive care monitoring.* New York: McGraw-Hill, 1998:1297–1328.

50. Kost GJ, Lathrop JP. Designing diagnostic testing for patient-focused care. *Medical Laboratory Observer* 1993;25(9 Suppl):16–26.

51. Kost GJ. The clinical systems manager: optimizing point-of-care testing. *Clinical Laboratory Management Rev* 1998;12:353–363.

3

PRINCIPLES OF ANTICOAGULATION AND SAMPLE TRANSPORT FOR POINT-OF-CARE ANALYTES

JOHN G. TOFFALETTI

As the need for statistical analysis and reporting of these test results has increased, old problems remain and new challenges emerge in proper sample collection and transport. Some of these pitfalls are illustrated in Figure 3.1 and are discussed in this chapter.

ELECTROLYTES

Sodium and Potassium

Although serum, heparinized plasma, and whole blood are used for sodium and potassium analysis, heparinized whole blood is the preferred sample for point-of-care analysis. Because the concentration of sodium in erythrocytes is only 10% that in plasma, hemolysis does not cause significant changes in the plasma sodium result unless hemolysis is severe, in which case the sodium result may be decreased.

It is well known that potassium is in much higher concentration in cells than in plasma. Thus, hemolysis will increase the potassium result by 0.6% for every 10 mg per deciliter increase in hemoglobin. Less obvious is that coagulation, temperature, and glycolysis also can affect the potassium result. The rupturing of platelets during coagulation will increase the potassium result by 0.1 to 0.7 mmol per liter, depending on the platelet count (1). If the whole-blood sample cannot be analyzed immediately, leakage of potassium eventually can alter the result, increasing by 0.1 to 0.2 mmol per liter each hour. Icing the sample, which inhibits glycolysis and promotes leakage of potassium from the cells, enhances this effect to 0.4 mmol per liter each hour at 4°C (2). In near-patient analyses, where heparinized blood at room temperature is analyzed within 15 min after collection, these effects should be minimal.

Another consideration is that skeletal muscle activity causes potassium efflux from cells. Therefore, excessive clenching of the fist prior to venipuncture should be minimal, and the tourniquet should be released as blood is drawn. In extreme cases, potassium can increase by up to 2 mmol per liter (1).

Ionized Calcium and Magnesium

Whereas both serum and whole blood have been used for ionized calcium analysis, the need to measure ionized calcium rapidly during surgery and other critical care settings effectively limits the sample to anticoagulated whole blood. Citrate, oxalate, and ethylenediametetraacetic acid (EDTA) lower the ionized calcium or magnesium result by binding to calcium and magnesium. Although heparin is a polyanion that also binds calcium ions, the effect of heparin is much less than for the other anions listed previously, and heparin is currently the only acceptable anticoagulant for ionized calcium and magnesium testing. As an example, 15 U per milliliter of heparin (typical for evacuated collection tubes) lowers ionized calcium by 0.03 mmol per liter or less (3). Because blood-gas syringes may contain 25 U heparin per milliliter or more, special modified heparins are now widely used. These include (a) very low heparin (about 2.8 U/mL) dispersed in a special "puff" of inert material designed to dissolve rapidly and prevent coagulation; (b) electrolyte-balanced heparin that contains calcium and other ions that effectively occupy the cation-binding sites on heparin to minimize changes in ionized calcium in the blood. This material can cause a bias at either very low or very high ionized calcium concentrations, however; (c) a blend of lithium heparin and zinc heparin offsets the interference to ionized calcium results. Because zinc ions have been reported to interfere with magnesium measurements (4), this product has been reformulated to minimize this effect (5). Although self-prepared syringes containing sodium heparin solution have been reported to affect ionized magnesium measurements minimally compared with dry balanced heparin (6), the variability among users to expel completely excess liquid heparin could cause significant bias.

A recent report studied the effects of several heparin anticoagulants and fill volumes on both ionized calcium and ionized magnesium measurements. In full syringes, mean changes in ionized calcium or magnesium were less than 0.01 mmol per liter over the range of typically encountered concentrations. In half-full syringes, ionized calcium and ionized magnesium were affected no more than about 0.01 mmol per liter by most syringes, although ionized calcium was lowered about 0.03 mmol/L in one brand of syringe (5). At very high concentrations of ionized calcium (>1.95 mmol per liter) and ionized magnesium (>0.95 mmol/L), a few effects in the range of 0.02 to 0.06 mmol per liter were noted. The clinical impact of these changes should be minimal at these very high concentrations, however.

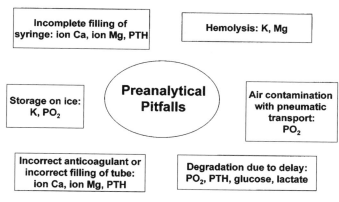

FIGURE 3.1. Preanalytic pitfalls.

It is interesting to note that results on serum indicate that the clotting process affected the ionized calcium and magnesium results more than any of the heparinized syringe products tested (5).

It is desirable for the sample to be collected and analyzed anaerobically. By preventing loss of carbon dioxide, changes in sample pH are minimized, which otherwise could alter protein binding of calcium ions and change the ionized calcium concentration. For example, if pH decreases by 0.1 U, ionized calcium increases by about 0.05 mmol per liter and vice versa (7). Ionized magnesium also increases with pH, but to a lesser extent (0.02 mmol/L per 0.1 U decrease of pH) than does ionized calcium (8). In addition, hemolysis should be avoided during sample collection.

Currently, ionized magnesium testing is usually not available, especially in near-patient applications. Whereas the clinical and biochemical importance of magnesium is well established, the intracellular/extracellular distribution of magnesium complicates interpretation of blood measurements of magnesium, both total and ionized (9). As they point out, it is the clinical consequences of hypomagnesemia that require treatment, not the concentration.

CARBOHYDRATES

Glucose

For a variety of reasons, both physiologic and methodologic, whole-blood glucose results are about 12% lower than plasma glucose results. Whereas most near-patient meters are calibrated to whole blood, both our data and the data of others show that meters actually correlate more closely to plasma than to whole blood (10). Because point-of-care test results are supposed to agree with laboratory tests results, this is a desirable goal.

Glycolysis continues in whole blood after it is collected, decreasing glucose by 5% to 7% (5–10 mg/dL) in 1 hour. The rate of decrease is related to the number of leukocytes and bacteria in the sample. Once separated from cells, glucose in sterile serum is stable for 8 hours at 25°C and for 72 hours at 4°C (11). Plasma contains some leukocytes and is therefore slightly less stable than serum. The addition of glycolytic inhibitors, such as

fluoride, can stabilize a sample for up to 3 days at room temperature. Fluoride inhibits the glycolytic enzyme enolase by forming a complex with a magnesium ion, phosphate ion, and the enzyme. Because fluoride often is combined with the anticoagulant oxalate in sample collection tubes, samples containing this mixture are not suitable for several other chemistry tests, such as enzymes and electrolytes. Unless the patient has a very high leukocyte count, it is probably not necessary to use a collection tube containing fluoride if the sample is analyzed within 60 minutes after blood collection. In patients with high leukocyte counts, however, blood glucose can decrease by up to 65 mg per deciliter each per hour (11).

Especially with point-of-care glucose measurements on whole blood, hematocrit appears to affect the results. In a study of five glucose meters using both low and high glucose concentrations, the measured glucose declined as hematocrit increased (10). Although biases are small and clinically insignificant for the usually encountered hematocrits (0.25–0.45), as hematocrit exceeds 0.50, the underestimation of glucose concentrations can become unacceptable. Although this underestimation may be enhanced by glycolysis because of the higher proportion of red cells and leukocytes in these samples, a higher hematocrit appears to affect directly the readings of these glucose meters (10).

Lactate

Lactate is produced from pyruvate as a by-product of glucose metabolism when anaerobic conditions lead to insufficient nicotinamide-adenine dinucleotide (NAD) for pyruvate to enter into the tricarboxylic acid (TCA) cycle and oxidative phosphorylation (12). Because erythrocytes have no mitochondria, lactate is a normal product of glycolysis. Consequently, lactate increases rapidly in whole-blood samples at room temperature, with no glycolytic inhibitors present. In whole blood at room temperature, lactate increases by 0.5 mmol per liter (a 30%–50% increase) in only 30 minutes. Ice storage slows this increase to about 0.05 mmol per liter in 30 minutes (13), whereas fluoride/oxalate slows the increase to about 0.1 mmol per liter in 30 minutes at room temperature (14). Clearly, in near-patient applications where ordinary heparin is used, lactate must be measured within 5 minutes.

BLOOD GASES

pH, P_{CO_2}, and P_{O_2}

Blood-gas measurements (pH, P_{CO_2}, and P_{O_2}) are done exclusively on heparinized whole-blood samples, usually of arterial origin. These tests, especially P_{O_2}, are among the most sensitive to preanalytic effects, including collection technique, volume of (liquid) anticoagulant used, exposure to air and air bubbles, time of sample handling, and temperature and agitation of the sample.

Anaerobic collection technique is essential to successful blood gas measurements. Because air has a much lower P_{CO_2} and (typically) higher P_{O_2} than blood, exposure of the blood at any time can alter these results.

Blood-gas samples are best collected with dry heparin anticoagulants in syringes of 1 mL or greater. Liquid heparin in sufficient volume can alter the P_{CO_2} result (1). This becomes a problem either when syringes are incompletely filled or when too much liquid heparin is left in the syringe. Although many samples are collected in small (pediatric) tubes, even greater care must be taken because the effects of dilution and exposure are greater for a small sample volume.

Air bubbles are easily entrapped when blood is collected in a syringe. Whereas this may have minimal effect if the air bubble is not disturbed, it can have a significant effect on P_{O_2} if the sample is agitated either by mixing or especially by transport in a pneumatic tube (15). This is especially significant when P_{O_2} is 70 to 100 mm Hg, where a 0.2-mL air bubble can increase P_{O_2} by 30 mm Hg. At a high P_{O_2}, the combination of an air bubble and pneumatic transport can lower P_{O_2} by 100 mm Hg. Clearly, it is extremely important to remove all air bubbles when transporting blood-gas samples by pneumatic tube.

An additional problem when a blood-gas sample remains at room temperature is that the blood-gas values can change markedly when analysis is delayed over 15 minutes. In 1 hour at room temperature, the pH decreases by 0.02 to 0.03, P_{CO_2} increases by 1 mm Hg, and P_{O_2} decreases by 2 mm Hg (1). These changes are caused by cellular metabolism and can be enhanced at higher temperatures or if the sample has a high white cell count.

Ice storage of blood samples can minimize these changes. For blood samples collected in plastic syringes, however, P_{O_2} actually can increase significantly for the following reasons: Plastic is permeable to oxygen, hemoglobin greatly increases its affinity for oxygen at cold temperatures, and blood ultimately is analyzed at 37°C, which releases the oxygen from hemoglobin (16). In the report cited, P_{O_2} increased from 101 to 110 mm Hg after 30 minutes of ice storage. This effect varies depending on the initial P_{O_2}.

A recent report found that changes in P_{O_2}, P_{CO_2}, and pH were about three times lower in samples stored on ice than in those at 22°C. Rapid increases in P_{O_2} were observed for samples stored on ice with an initial P_{O_2} between 50 and 250 mm Hg, and decreases were noted for samples with an initial P_{O_2} over 250 mm Hg. This report concluded that samples with an initial P_{O_2} between 50 and 250 mm Hg stored on ice should be analyzed within 30 minutes. The magnitude of change in P_{O_2} for samples kept on ice depended on their hemoglobin capacity for buffering oxygen, which is inversely related to the oxygen saturation level of hemoglobin (17).

An additional factor to be considered is the effect of artificial oxygen carriers or hemoglobin substitutes on laboratory tests. A perflubron emulsion was reported to have large effects on co-oximetry results (18). This effect, apparently caused by turbidity, was later minimized by a suitable algorithm (19). A bovine hemoglobin-based oxygen carrier was reported to affect several chemistry tests, although it did not affect hematology tests, coagulation tests, or blood-bank tests (20). If the use of these additives becomes widespread, until the interferences can be eliminated, it may be necessary for the laboratory to be notified of such samples from patients receiving blood substitutes.

HORMONES

Intraoperative Parathyroid Hormone

Over the last few years, parathyroid hormone (PTH) has emerged as a somewhat unusual test in the point-of-care category. Rapid (<15 min) measurements of PTH now are used as a guide for surgically removing an appropriate amount of parathyroid tissue to correct primary hyperparathyroidism (21,22). The issue of anticoagulants is important because the stability of PTH in blood at room temperature is enhanced markedly by the use of ethylenediametetraacetic acid (EDTA) (23). If the blood collection tubes containing EDTA are not completely filled (half-filled or less), the higher concentration of EDTA can falsely lower the PTH concentration (24).

CONCLUSIONS

A significant advantage for near-patient testing is that the effects of agitation during sample transport, time delays before cell separation or analysis, and temperature effects may be eliminated when the sample is analyzed within minutes (or seconds) after being collected.

- Novel preparations of heparin have minimized or eliminated the effects of standard heparin on some laboratory tests, especially ionized calcium and ionized magnesium.
- Incomplete filling of syringes containing novel preparations of heparin or tubes containing EDTA can cause clinically significant interferences with tests such as ionized calcium and magnesium and PTH.
- Whereas hematocrits between 0.25 and 0.50 have little effect, hematocrits above 0.50 lower the apparent glucose result of handheld glucose meters.
- P_{O_2} remains an analyte that is influenced by air contamination, cellular metabolism, and cold absorption through plastic syringes.
- Intraoperative measurements of PTH have become a routine practice at many hospitals and may represent a prototype for stat use of other tests in surgical procedures.
- The clinical laboratory must work cooperatively with nurses, perfusionists, anesthetists, respiratory therapists, physicians, and other personnel who collect and analyze samples at off-site locations to ensure that optimal sample collection and handling procedures are followed.

REFERENCES

1. Scott MG, Heusel JW, LeGrys VA, et al. Electrolytes and blood gases. In: Burtis CA, Ashwood ER, eds. *Tietz textbook of clinical chemistry*, 3rd ed. Philadelphia: WB Saunders, 1999:1056–1092.
2. Fleisher M, Gladstone M, Crystal D, et al. Two whole-blood multi-analyte analyzers evaluated. *Clin Chem* 1989;35:1532–1535.
3. Toffaletti JG. Ionized calcium. In: Pesce AJ, Kaplan LA, eds. *Methods in clinical chemistry*. St Louis, MO: CV Mosby, 1987:1010–1020.
4. Toffaletti JG. Use of novel preparations of heparin to eliminate interference in ionized calcium measurements: have all the problems been solved? *Clin Chem* 1994;40:508–509.

5. Toffaletti JG, Wildermann RF. The effects of heparin anticoagulants and fill volume in blood gas syringes on ionized calcium and magnesium measurements. *Clin Chim Acta* 2001;304:147–151.

6. Chantler J, Cox DJA. Self-prepared heparinized syringes for measuring ionized magnesium in critical care patients. *Br J Anaesth* 1999;83:810–812.

7. Endres DB, Rude RK. Mineral and bone metabolism. In: Burtis CA, Ashwood ER, eds. *Tietz textbook of clinical chemistry*, 3rd ed. Philadelphia: WB Saunders, 1999:1395–1457.

8. Wang S, Sedor FA, Toffaletti JG. Effects of pH changes in serum or heparinized blood or measurements of ionized Ca and ionized Mg. *Clin Chem* 2001;47(abst):A83.

9. Foley C, Zaritsky A. Should we measure ionized magnesium? *Crit Care Med* 1998;26:1949–1950.

10. Chance JJ, Li DJ, Jones KA, et al. Technical evaluation of five glucose meters with data management capabilities. *Am J Clin Pathol* 1999;111:547–556.

11. Sacks DB. Carbohydrates. In: Burtis CA, Ashwood ER, eds. *Tietz textbook of clinical chemistry*, 3rd ed. Philadelphia: WB Saunders, 1999:750–808.

12. Toffaletti JG. Blood lactate: biochemistry, laboratory methods, and clinical interpretation. *CRC Crit Rev Clin Lab Sci* 1991;28: 253–268.

13. Toffaletti JG, Hammes ME, Gray R, et al. Lactate measured in diluted and undiluted whole blood and plasma: comparison of methods and effect of hematocrit. *Clin Chem* 1992;38: 2430–2434.

14. Astles R, Williams CP, Sedor F. Stability of plasma lactate *in vitro* in the presence of antiglycolytic agents. *Clin Chem* 1994;40:1327–1330.

15. Astles JR, Lubarsky D, Loun B, et al. Pneumatic transport exacerbates interference of room air contamination in blood gas samples. *Arch Pathol Lab Med* 1996;120:642–647.

16. Mahoney JJ, Harvey JA, Wong RJ, et al. Changes in oxygen measurements when whole blood is stored in iced plastic or glass syringes. *Clin Chem* 1991;37:1244–1248.

17. Beaulieu M, Lapointe Y, Vinet B. Stability of PO_2, PCO_2, and pH in fresh blood samples stored in a plastic syringe with low heparin in relation to various blood-gas and hematological parameters. *Clin Biochem* 1999;32:101–107.

18. Shephard AP, Steinke JM. CO-oximetry interference by perflubron emulsion: comparison of hemolyzing and nonhemolyzing instruments. *Clin Chem* 1998;44:2183–2190.

19. Toffaletti JG, Wildermann RF. Use of turbidity-correction algorithm eliminates the effect of perflubron emulsion on CO-oximeter results. *Clin Chem* 2000;46:136–137.

20. Wolthius A, Peek D, Scholten R, et al. Effect of the hemoglobin-based oxygen carrier HBOC-201 on laboratory instrumentation: Cobas Integra, Chiron Blood Gas Analyzer 840, Sysmex SE-9000 and BCT. *Clin Chem Lab Med* 1999;37:71–76.

21. Garner SC, Leight GS. Initial experience with intraoperative PTH determinations in the surgical management of 130 consecutive cases of primary hyperparathyroidism. *Surgery* 1999;126:1132–1138.

22. Wiens FH, Balko JA, Hsu RM, Byrd W, Snyder WH. Intraoperative vs central laboratory PTH testing during parathyroidectomy surgery. *Lab Management* 2000;31:616–621.

23. Immulite Intact PTH package insert. Diagnostic Products Corporation, April 1999, Los Angeles, CA.

24. Immulite technical bulletin 1152. Diagnostic Products Corporation, November 2000, Los Angeles, CA.

4

MOLECULAR DIAGNOSTICS AT THE POINT OF CARE

RONALD C. MCGLENNEN

DEFINITION OF MOLECULAR DIAGNOSTICS

The past two decades have revealed a revolution in cellular and molecular biology and with it a vastly greater understanding of the nature of human physiology and disease. The advent of technical breakthroughs in molecular biology led to the emergence of simple protocols for testing genetic material as well as for a host of cellular and extracellular proteins. To a large extent, these innovations in molecular biology have been made possible by the characterization and optimization of specialized molecular tools, which are themselves the products of recombinant DNA technology. One invention of the technique is called the polymerase chain reaction, or PCR. The key ingredient in this biochemical reaction is *Taq* polymerase, discovered by accident as a consequence to asking the question of how microbial organisms can survive in extreme environments, such as the very high temperatures found in hot springs, like those in Yellowstone National Park (1). The observation that bacteria can proliferate in thermal conditions that would denature the enzymes and ultimately kill eukaryotic cells demonstrates that nature has created natural reagents that can accommodate highly precise biochemical processes for extreme environments. *Taq* polymerase is an enzyme that mediates the polymerization of nucleotide triphosphates into the elongating chain of DNA and, to a lesser extent, RNA. Through a process of repeated heating and cooling, double-stranded DNA undergoes strand denaturation and reannealing accompanied by activation and relative inactivation of *Taq* polymerase (2). The result is the replication of a segment of the original DNA template to an exponential copy number. In practice, the utility of PCR is that it results in the manufacture of a quantity of a precise sequence of DNA, sufficient that it can be analyzed by any of a number of simple laboratory techniques.

Through the use of recombinant DNA technologies, cloned versions of the gene for *Taq* polymerase can be manipulated in such a way as to improve on useful qualities, such as its thermal stability, nucleotide processivity and long-term stability (2–4). The strategy for the molecular improvement of these reagents, which will be discussed in detail later, subsequently were assembled into a variety of simple-to-use kits. The mode of operation for most molecular diagnostics laboratories today is a reliance on these commercial kits.

Such is the definition of modern molecular diagnostics, in which the routine use of techniques involving recombinant enzymes (e.g., *Taq* polymerase and a variety of other bacterial-derived enzymes) that precisely cut DNA at a known nucleotide sequence are used for the purpose of routine patient-care diagnostics. In a practical sense, Table 4.1 illustrates a working definition of molecular diagnostics as involving the characterization of human disease by examination of nucleic acid, both DNA as well as RNA, for the purpose of patient care. In a functional sense, molecular diagnostics can be broken down into testing for disorders, either inherited or constitutional. These diseases include those for which the gene mutations are well characterized, such as cystic fibrosis, phenylketonuria, Huntington disease, and muscular dystrophy (5). Testing for acquired diseases such as cancer is another area in the realm of molecular diagnostics. At many institutions, routine testing for novel genetic markers, such as bcr-*abl*, associated with chronic myelogenous leukemia, point mutations in the *ras* oncogene, associated with a large number of solid tumors, and the analysis of point mutations in the *p53* gene have become routine (6). A third is in the detection of infectious disease, including bacteria, fungi, as well as many viruses (7). A clear advantage of using molecular genetic techniques to characterize infectious disease is that it does not rely on more costly, time-consuming, less specific culture-based methods (8). A fourth category is unique to the field of molecular diagnostics and is termed *genetic predisposition testing*. The analysis of genes such as breast cancer 1 gene (*BRCA-1*) exemplifies this emerging area of medicine wherein patients will be able to seek testing, and hence information, about the probability of developing such devastating diseases as breast cancer. In addition, patients will have available the necessary resources to prevent its development (9).

The introduction of molecular diagnostics into the clinical laboratory has been to improve diagnostic sensitivity and specificity. Based on the use of current methods and instrumentation, these assays are considerably more costly, require more time, and lack standardized quality measures and controls. In a practical sense, for only a handful of tests is molecular genetics the front-line choice for making a diagnosis. Correspondingly, gene-based diagnostics often serves as an adjunct strategy to more conventional means of testing, such as biochemical testing and histopathology. In this era of cost containment, with particular

TABLE 4.1. DEFINITION OF MOLECULAR DIAGNOSTICS

Molecular diagnostics, broadly defined, is the characterization of human disease by analyzing nucleic
acids, both DNA and RNA, which are the template for all proteins, for sequence variations that
cause disease.
The types of testing performed in molecular diagnostics include the following:
  Constitutional or inherited disorders
  Acquired disease, such as cancer
  Infectious disease
  Genetic predisposition syndromes
Molecular diagnostics offers improved sensitivity and specificity, but these assays have special
requirements to ensure quality performance.
Molecular diagnostics complements other types of clinical testing: morphologic diagnosis, flow
cytometry, biochemical analysis, and other functional types of clinical testing.

emphasis on minimizing the cost of laboratory testing, molecular diagnostics remains an esoteric discipline. The promise of molecular diagnostics testing is intimately tied to our ability to develop instrumentation that will significantly reduce the cost of this type of testing as well as to make it more commonly available. One goal would be to realize a point-of-care (POC) technology that could serve any physician's office and potentially consumer-based, at-home venues. The purpose of this chapter is to outline some of the current technologies destined to improve the performance of molecular diagnostics testing and to examine the challenges for future technical innovation; special emphasis is given to microchip-based devices and their complementary testing procedures.

OVERVIEW OF THE OPERATIONAL BREAKDOWN OF MOLECULAR DIAGNOSTICS

Before discussing how to adapt current molecular diagnostics to the POC paradigm, we first must review the basic operational steps involved in the execution of any molecular genetic test. In the case of any nucleic acid–based test, there are four distinct operational steps: (a) specimen procurement, (b) nucleic acid extraction and characterization, (c) nucleic acid amplification and manipulation and (d) product detection and analysis (Fig. 4.1). For each of these operations, both conventional and emerging or "cutting edge" technologies exist, typically in a stand-alone format. In contrast to other, more mature areas of the clinical lab-

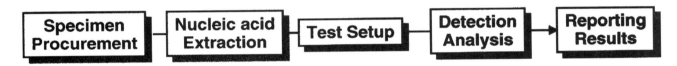

Specimen Procurement	Nucleic acid Extraction	Test Setup	Detection Analysis	Reporting Results

•Sample of blood, tissue or other cellular material
  •Accession sample
  •Specify test to be performed
  •Manual cell separation
•Point of Care Solution
  •Minaturize sample:20µL of blood, cell scrape or body fluid

•DNA or RNA extraction by manual or automated methods
  •Salt precipitation
  •Proteinase K digestion
  •Alcohol precipitation
  •Rehydration and dilution
•Point of Care Solution
  •Continuous flow fluidics
  •Miniaturized cell separator
  •Sample collection on solid support system

•Set up specific test assay: Southern transfer for genomic DNA, amplification based reaction (PCR, LCR) for most others
•Point of Care Solution
  •Chip based thermocycler

•Detection of DNA product by gel or capillary electrophoresis. Variation on above detection systems include:
  •Automated fluorescence detection, e.g. ABI DNA analyzers, LiCor and Visible Genetics
  •Real-time detection by fluorescence or electrochemical reactions, e.g. Taqman, Light cycler
•Point of Care Solution
  •Microaddressable arrays
  •Electromechanical biosensors
  •Electrochemical biosensors

•Integration of analytic results with interpretation report generation.
•Point of Care Solution
  •Miniaturized or hand held analytic instrumentation with integration of assay control and information processing on a portable computer

FIGURE 4.1. Operational schema of a molecular diagnostics laboratory.

oratory, such as clinical chemistry, molecular diagnostics lacks significant automation of these operational steps. In the meantime, most clinical molecular genetics laboratories strive to perform each of these operational steps in the most efficient and cost-conserving manner while using a combination of technologies, some of which are commercial and some are "home brew." At best, molecular genetic testing in its state can import "piece-meal" automation and integration strategies.

Specimen Procurement

The wide variety of molecular genetic tests also necessitates the use of numerous sample types. In the case of most forms of genetic testing for constitutional diseases, blood is the most commonly sought tissue type. There is no particular reason not to use other forms of tissue; simple cellular scrapes, a sample of hair follicle, and a wide host of other body fluids will also work. Additionally, most molecular genetic tests involve the use of enzymatic amplification techniques, such as PCR, that also permit the use of samples that have been previously fixed by conventional means such as formalin, alcohol, or paraffin embedding. In addition to the variation in sample types, specimen procurement is also the single most important step in the assurance of a high-quality result. Subscribing to the age-old adage "garbage in equals garbage out," careful attention to quality (preservation of high molecular DNA or RNA), purity, and concentration are paramount to improving the efficiency and reliability of the analytic steps of the complete testing schema. For a particular molecular genetic test, determination as to whether DNA, RNA, or both types of nucleic acid are required should be considered. Although most preservatives used in blood collection are satisfactory for the differential extraction of both RNA or DNA, most other types of tissue preservation, including flash freezing, formalin fixation, and other techniques commonly used in anatomic pathology, are usually unsatisfactory for routine retrieval of RNA.

In addition to the technical aspects of specimen procurement is the consideration that not all tissue samples are representative of the disease process. One example is in the testing of genes involved in cancer, such as the mutational analysis of the tumor suppressor gene *p53*. In the process of malignant transformation, the *p53* gene commonly accumulates point mutations in a series of exons that encode for important protein function. Malignant tissues, however, are typically comprised of a mixture of stromal and inflammatory cells, which typically do not harbor mutations in *p53*. The net effect is a relative dilution of the mutant *p53* signal. Strategies for evaluating cancer genes either must include methods for improving the sensitivity of current detection methods or ways to enrich for the target genes in samples that are genetically heterogeneous. These practical aspects of specimen collection, in consideration of new technologies described later to make specimen procurement simpler and cheaper, need to be engineered and optimized.

Cost containment is the most important aspect of specimen procurement. Techniques such as PCR, and to a lesser degree Southern transfer, are inherently sensitive and generally not reliant on the amount of collected sample. Despite this, the laboratory typically is presented with anywhere between 8 to 10 mL of whole blood. The cost to process this or smaller volumes constitutes the single largest expense in gene-based testing (5). Inclusive of materials such as syringes, needles, the glass vacuum tube with preservative, and the expense of packing material for transport, sample collection may cost as much as $10 to $12 (Fig. 4.2). Commensurate with the quantity of specimen is the issue of patient satisfaction and safety. As an example, too often large volumes of blood are collected from newborns when no more than the equivalent of one droplet (20 µL) of whole blood is necessary to perform a high-quality analysis. Important to the future of molecular genetic testing is to identify materials or techniques that can greatly reduce the amount of specimen required so that there is also a reduction in the waste and asso-

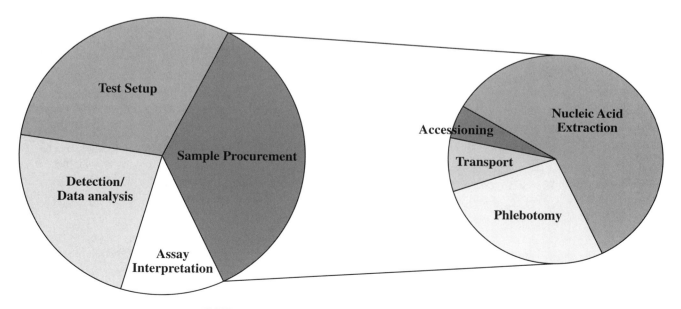

FIGURE 4.2. Distribution of costs in molecular genetic testing.

ciated cost with each of the subsequent operational steps involved in the testing.

Alternative sample collection strategies, such as specially treated filter paper, use of body fluids such as urine, or even swabs taken from specific body sites, are not only adequate but, as will be shown later, preferred. In the future, specimen procurement will be designed as a part of an integrated genetic testing format, which may include a simple collection device or possibly a microchip-based technology that can be installed secondarily into the instrument.

One advantage of sampling for gene-based testing is that DNA and RNA are very durable and can be retrieved from most environments. This fact relates favorably to the ideal of POC testing for molecular genetics in that even with current technology, sample procurement can be optimized for nearly any context. Thus, the potential of using a fingerprick sampling of blood, urine, stool, or a buccal scrape as an over-the-counter collection device for testing on site in a physician's office, a pharmacy, or other retail outlet already is being realized. The prospect of consumers purchasing a kit as an at-home test is an example of how a simple collection system can result in a high-quality analytic result.

Nucleic Acid Extraction

The new tools for molecular biology provide a myriad of ways to manipulate DNA and RNA and increasingly are being used for routine medical diagnostics. Correspondingly, knowledge about the *in vivo* processes by which DNA and RNA are replicated, processed, and repaired continue to provide insights as to how we can more efficiently use these materials in routine assays. In the clinical laboratory, considerations of cost, uniformity, and reproducibility in the performance of nucleic acid extraction are paramount. Therefore, a complete understanding of the principal steps by which genomic DNA and total cellular RNA are extracted is essential to appreciate what material is best for specific genetic assays. The intent of this chapter is to provide an overview of the basic biochemical procedures involved in processing nucleic acid for clinical genetic testing and, correspondingly, to use these considerations as to how they might then first be automated and potentially used in a POC setting.

Extraction of genomic DNA from eukaryotic cells is the most laborious and costly operation in molecular diagnostics (Fig. 4.2). Usually, whole blood collected by means of venipuncture is the source of the sample. For several reasons, using whole blood for genetic testing is more complicated than would be the ideal material. First, blood involves proportionally a great deal of waste material (i.e., red blood cells, plasma, and water). Of the total volume processed, only 1 in 10,000 cells in whole blood are nucleated, which is the source of genomic DNA. Table 4.2 outlines the basic steps involved in the extraction of high-molecular-weight genomic DNA from whole-blood sources. The first step involves removal of the red cell fraction as well as the large majority of the volume of plasma and water. In its simplest form, removal of the red blood cells can be achieved by differentially lysing the red blood cells into a homogeneous solution. This leaves the nucleated white blood cells intact, which can be pelleted by centrifugation. Several types of commercial kits use

TABLE 4.2. OUTLINE OF NUCLEIC ACID EXTRACTION

Conventional nucleic acid isolation
  Collect specimen by venipuncture (blood) or tissue (fresh or frozen)
  DNA and RNA
    Lyse the cell and nucleus
    Remove DNA from histone packaging
    Proteinase K digestion of protein
    Precipitate protein with high concentration of salt
  RNA only
    Treatment with RNAse free DNAase
  Common means to concentrate nucleic acid
    Alcohol precipitate
    Phenol–chloroform extraction
    Rehydration in a neutral pH buffer
    Quantitation by spectrophotometry
Extraction from solid support (paper)
  Collect specimen (droplet of blood, touch prep or mucosal scrape)
  DNA
    Dry specimen on paper
    Rinse paper sample in wash buffer (removal of globin proteins)
    Dry paper

a hypotonic solution for red blood cell lysis. Complete removal of the hemoglobin from the sedimented white cells is essential because this protein is a pronounced inhibitor of PCR, specifically interfering with the binding of *Taq* polymerase to the template (10,11). Hence, any technique involving the use of whole blood as a source of tissue necessitates a robust way to remove hemoglobin and other globin-type proteins.

The next step in nucleic acid extraction is the lysis of the white blood cell membranes and solubilization of the cytoplasmic proteins and the contents of nucleus. A mild, nonionic detergent serves to dissolve the cell membranes and denatures most cellular proteins. Addition of chelating agents, such as EDTA, are important for the removal of divalent ions, which are required for the action of endogenous nucleases, enzymes that otherwise will degrade DNA and RNA and therefore destroy the specimen. The next step typically involves the addition of a nonspecific proteinase, such as proteinase K, which further digests cytoplasmic proteins and nucleoproteins. The latter include histones that are tightly associated with chromosomal DNA. Adequate removal of protein, with or without the addition of proteolytic digestion, requires heat and time (45°C for one to several hours). Additionally, to achieve highly purified samples of nucleic acid, organic solvents, such as combinations of phenol chloroform and isoamyl alcohol, can be added; these work by deprotonation of proteins and act to tear these tightly associated nucleosome proteins from chromosomal DNA. The first generation of automated nucleic acid extractors were based on a standard protocol of cell lysis, protein removal, and precipitation using salt-based buffers but include using phenol and chloroform for the final cleanup step. This is accomplished in an instrument configured with a complex system of fluid conduits and valves and a mechanism to agitate the samples as they are passed through a series of reactor vessels (Fig. 4.3A).

Obviously, the requirements of these extraction steps—adding enzymes, heating, and using organic solvents—all preclude the possibility of making this procedure simple and portable. Finally, at the conclusion of these steps, the result is a

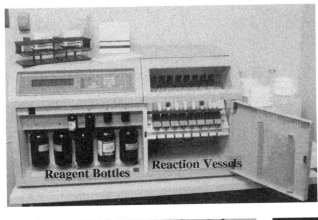

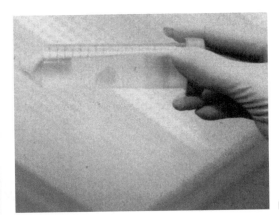

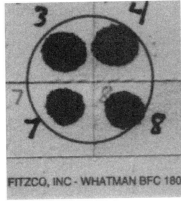

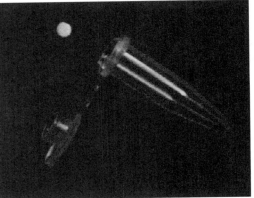

FIGURE 4.3. Methodologies in nucleic acid extraction. **A**: An early generation automated nucleic acid instrument (Perkin-Elmer Applied Biosystems Inc., Foster City, CA, U.S.A.). **B**: Precipitated high-molecular-weight DNA in ethanol. **C**: Sample procurement on chemically treated analytic-grade paper product called FTA. **D**: Small punches of samples processed on FTA paper are read for enzymatic amplification.

turbid mixture of denatured proteins and other cellular materials in a solution of nucleic acid and salts. Adding salt, followed by centrifugation to pellet this material, easily precipitates the protein fraction. What remains is a clear aqueous phase that contains both DNA and RNA in solution. The final step is nucleic acid precipitation, which occurs with the addition of isopropanol or ethanol. The tell-tale formation of stringy, white–yellow material is evidence of DNA precipitation, which in turn can be collected by spooling (around a glass rod) or centrifugation at high speed, which causes the stringy DNA material to pellet at the bottom of the tube (Fig. 4.3B). Before the sample can be used for subsequent testing, high-molecular-weight DNA must be hydrated in an aqueous buffer, which can take up to several hours.

In general, working with RNA extraction from whole blood or any other tissue source is more difficult than with DNA. The most significant challenge is to avoid degradation of RNA by endogenous cellular enzymes, which are very robust and ubiquitous throughout the laboratory. Second, most protocols seek to remove RNA from a solution of DNA and RNA by differential precipitation or sequestration. Adjusting the pH of the extraction solution after removal of the protein and salt does this. Alternatively, the cell lysis solution can be suspended in a gradient of cesium chloride followed by ultracentrifugation. Under

these conditions, genomic DNA is buoyant and will float, whereas the RNA will pellet to the bottom of the tube. Ultracentrifugation is much more costly and labor intensive, but the result is a highly purified form of RNA, which greatly improves the reliability of these assays. With the advent of amplification technologies, specifically reverse transcriptase PCR (RT-PCR), the need for such highly purified template has been diminished.

In the clinical laboratory, the drive to reduce the cost of nucleic acid extraction has created the need for a variety of new products that also greatly simplify the process of genomic DNA as well as RNA isolation. Typically, these products involve the use of specialized reagents that are proprietary and additional paraphernalia, such as spin columns, specially prepared filter papers, Sepharose, or other polymeric beads, some combined with specific "capture" molecules (12–17). One product called FTA shows promise for routine applications in the molecular diagnostic laboratory (Fig. 4-3C, D) (16,17). The process involves a specially prepared analytic-grade paper impregnated with a solution that preserves the integrity of the genomic DNA from most mechanical and environmental insults. Wet samples applied to the paper hydrate the materials in the paper, which cause the cells to lyse on contact. Various chemicals on the paper also work to inhibit both endogenous and contaminating microbial sources of degradation. After the paper with the sample is dried, the high-molecular-weight genomic DNA is entrapped and tightly bound to the paper fibers. In the laboratory, the paper samples are readied for testing following a series of simple rinsing steps. In the case of PCR-based testing, a small punch of the paper then serves as the source of template DNA for the subsequent amplification reaction.

Another application of this product is to use an additional reagent to remove high-molecular-weight DNA, which can secondarily be digested with restriction endonucleases and used in subsequent restriction fragment-linked polymorphism (RFLP) testing. Variations on this theme involve inserting the paper on a plateau in a small polypropylene centrifuge tube. When the sample of blood or tissue is applied, it can be spun against the paper, and the subsequent lysis and wash steps can occur in one or two additional steps. Drying the paper within the context of the centrifuge tube, followed by the addition of the PCR cocktail mixture, enzyme, and primer allows for the sample collection, nucleic acid extraction, and PCR production in a single device. Alternatively, spin column devices for nucleic acid extraction use various types of matrix polymers to capture nucleic acid liberated from lysed cells. Genomic DNA is released from the matrix material following incubation with a specific elution buffer, much the way chemical analytes are liberated from the column using liquid chromatography. The solvated DNA then can be taken directly to gene amplification or some other means of characterizing specific DNA sequences.

A new product called Xtra Bind™ uses a solid-phase nucleic acid binding material into a one-step extraction process. The binding material has unique properties that capture both RNA and DNA in a single-stranded conformation. Depending on the selected buffer, DNA can be preferentially captured, and as little as 10 µL of blood can be used for assays that look for even low-copy-number genes. A noted advantage of this system is that the captured DNA is stabilized and covalently linked to the surface. This feature eliminates the need to transfer the sample to a new container for the next step of gene amplification.

Novel methods for RNA extraction include combining cell lysis, nuclease inhibition, and protein denaturation in a single reagent buffer (18). RNA can be captured out of the aqueous phase and subsequently removed by the addition of magnetic beads coated with thymidine oligonucleotides (oligo dT) that bind to the polyadenylated tails of messenger RNA (19). This technique is a way to obtain highly purified messenger RNA in a two-step extraction procedure.

To execute any of the preceding techniques for use in the clinical laboratory requires the skill of a trained medical technologist. In consideration of sample procurement for POC testing, nucleic acid extraction will need to be made much easier, perhaps simplifying it to only a single-step process. Until then, however, several points can be made about nucleic acid purification that may serve as a starting point for those with ideas about how to package new technologies: (a) nucleic acid extraction typically is simple and involves no more than two or three steps, most of which can be multiplexed into a single liquid phase; (b) purified nucleic acids are extremely durable and tolerant to harsh environmental conditions such as desiccation, exposure to light, heat, and even chemical degradation; and (c) for most examples of molecular genetic testing, only very little DNA or

RNA is required for successful amplification. Hence, in the overall scheme of genetic testing for POC, the step of nucleic acid extraction is well suited for miniaturization.

DNA Amplification and Manipulation

This section refers to the use of a variety of novel techniques for manipulating nucleic acid for the purpose of analyzing specific regions within those samples, whether they are a gene or a noncoding sequence, that specifically relates to the diagnosis of genetic disease or human identity. What are now considered conventional methods, including Southern transfer, northern blotting, as well as other simple hybridization techniques like slot blot, dot blot, and reverse dot blots, are still very much in use in clinical molecular genetics laboratories. Particularly in testing for diseases with complex genetics, these techniques will continue to be used because they have the advantage of being robust and unambiguous. By contrast, concerns about amplification-based techniques, including the risk of cross-contamination with amplified DNA, the dependence on instruments such as a thermocycler, and the general problem of optimizing the conditions for each reaction, remain as challenges to the laboratory first endeavoring into molecular diagnostics.

The practicality of being able to use only minute amounts of sample, however, and the versatility of techniques such as PCR point to the fact that these are the methods of choice as POC technologies emerge. Moreover, there are now many choices of method, including the ligase chain reaction (LCR or LDR), Q-beta replicase, rolling circle replication, Invader, and self-sustained sequence replication (20–22). Hence, the advent of PCR and related technologies has revolutionized the field of clinical molecular genetics (Fig. 4.4). The premise of this technique is that a DNA polymerase obtained from a bacterium called *Thermophilus aquaticus* can be used to produce exponential quantities of a specific DNA sequence by subjecting template DNA to repeated heating and cooling in a device called a *thermocycler*. Figure 4.4A and B outlines the essential ingredients and the biochemical mechanism by which PCR is achieved. Today, the experience with PCR is great, with the vast majority of laboratories using this technique routinely in the performance of a wide variety of diagnostically useful tests, including detection of infectious organisms, markers for oncology, and constitutional genetic disorders. Specialized laboratories also use PCR for paternity and forensic testing. Because PCR is robust and tolerant of harsh environmental situations, it is also innately adaptable to a variety of ways of performing the technique, including conducting the reaction in miniature on a microchip. Referring to Table 4.3, a list of conditions that need to be optimized for routine clinical molecular genetic testing is the same as that for other platforms, including microchips. It is important to remember, however, that PCR, and similarly other enzymatic amplification methods, are used only to generate sufficient amounts of a specific sequence so that they can be secondarily analyzed for the presence or absence of disease-specific changes or mutations.

In addition to PCR several other methods of amplifying specific DNA sequences bear discussion. On completing the sequencing of the human genome, attention now is focused on

- **Template-Genomic DNA**
- **Oligonucleotide Primers; 20-30 nucleotides long complementary to the DNA to be amplified**

  5' GAACTAGGTACTGAATGCAACCGTATCT 3'
  CTTGATCCAT

                            AACCGTATCT
  3' CTTGATCCATGACTTACGTTGGCATAGA 5'

- **Buffer containing dNTP's**
- **Taq I DNA polymerase; thermostable to 95°C**
- **Temperature cycler**

A

FIGURE 4.4. The polymerase chain reaction. **A**: Essential ingredients in the polymerase chain reaction. **B**: Illustration of the process of polymerase chain reaction based amplification of genomic or template DNA.

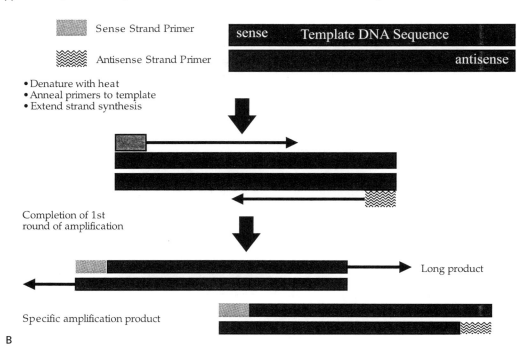

B

the cataloging of differences in the nucleotide sequence that exist between individuals as well as to understanding their relationship to disease predisposition. Many of the variations in the human genome are single-nucleotide polymorphisms, or SNPs. Several new gene amplification technologies show particular promise for SNP analysis. One system, known as Invader™, is based on the action of the enzyme cleavase and has been commercialized into a series of kits for some of the most common genetic tests. The simplicity of this "cookbook" procedure has the potential of making gene-based testing available to a larger number of laboratories not presently versed in molecular diagnostics.

TABLE 4.3. PCR OPTIMIZATION

Reaction Variable	Test Range	Step Size	Change Noted
Annealing temperature	45–62°C	2–3°C	No primer multimers
DNA polymerase buffer (pH, KCl)	8.3–9.2 pH 1.0–2.5 mM	0.5 U	Decrease nonspecific amplification
Units of DNA polymerase/rxn	0.5–3.0 U/rxn	0.5 U/100 μL rxn	Higher yield of product Less nonspecific product
MgCl$_2$ concentration	1.25–3.0 mM		
Additives (glycerol, DMSO, gelatin)	Variable	0.25 mM	Enhance avidity of enzyme for template
Each primer concentration	0.2–2.0 μM	0.5 μM	Higher product yield, less primer reduces multimers

PCR, polymerase chain reaction; DMSO, dimethyl sulfoxide; KCl, potassium chloride; MgCl$_2$, magnesium chloride.

In the process of PCR and other *in vitro* polymerase reactions, there is often damage to the 5′-end of single DNA strands, which is not observed with *in vivo* DNA replication. Cleavases, another class of bacterially derived nucleases, function to remove nucleotides from the 5′ and 3′ ends of DNA chains (23). The products of this enzymatic digestion are typically single nucleotides, but short oligonucleotides are also generated. Thus, in addition to the exonuclease activity (cutting enzymes that work on the end of nucleotide strands), these enzymes function as endonucleases. Importantly, the finding of a 5′-endonuclease activity inherent to *Taq* polymerase complexes was shown to be dependent on recognition of molecular structures rather than on the recognition of a certain nucleotide sequence. The same is true of the various cleavases that have been identified.

Hairpin structures are one type of DNA conformation recognized by cleavase. The method called cleavage fragment-length polymorphism analysis (CFLPA) was introduced several years ago as a strategy to take advantage of the pattern of DNA fragments resulting from cleavage of hairpin structures surrounding a known DNA sequence (24). The assay consisted of digestion of single-stranded DNA by endonuclease Cleavase I, a thermostable, sequence-specific member of this family of endonucleases. When the DNA digested by cleavase is electrophoresed in a denaturing gel, the pattern of fragments is diagnostic of the sequence of the sample DNA.

The Invader™ assay takes advantage of a three-dimensional structure that results when single-stranded sample DNA is hybridized to a mutation-specific primer and a so-called Invader oligonucleotide probe (25). The combination of these three components creates a structure of two overlapping duplexes and a single-stranded flap sequence, which is a structure recognized by cleavase. Endonucleolytic digestion of the probe liberates the flap at or near the site of overlap liberating this flap into the reaction solution (26). In the specific case of the Invader assay, the technology involves use of a fluorochrome-labeled oligonucleotide probe that lies near a fluorescent quencher molecule. This double-fluorochrome label strategy is called *F*luorescent *R*esonant *E*nergy *T*ransfer, or FRET. The use of FRET reagents is an increasingly common theme in bioanalytic assays. On cleavage of the flap, the fluorescent label is liberated from the quencher molecule, resulting in increasing fluorescence of the reaction solution. A single denaturation step and repeated annealing of new oligonucleotide probe results in a linear accumulation fluorescence, which is measured spectrophotometrically as an endpoint reaction. Hence, the Invader technology involves identification of a specific DNA sequence by the liberation of a fluorescent reporter molecule without amplifying the template or target DNA. The relationship between the oligonucleotide probe, the Invader primer, and the sample template is very specific, and thus this strategy has proven to be of high diagnostic precision. The simplicity of the Invader assay setup and the fact that no specialized equipment is required support the notion that technologies of this type may well become the method of choice when molecular genetics from the large central laboratory are applied to the POC.

Detection and Analysis

The most commonly used analytic technique in the genetics laboratory is gel electrophoresis. For more than two decades, various preparations of polymer-based gel systems, such as agarose and polyacrylamide, have been used to isolate and separate restriction-cut and PCR-amplified DNA. Several variables can be controlled in routine gel electrophoresis to meet the requirements of the test, including the running temperature, the ionic strength of the buffer, and other chemical compounds that either denature or leave double-stranded the DNA as it migrates through the gel. Table 4.4 outlines some of the specific types of analytic techniques that use gel electrophoresis as the underlying principle for detecting DNA products. More recently, the use of capillary electrophoresis has been examined as a means to achieve high-throughput analysis for PCR-derived DNA. Capillary electrophoresis is similar to gel electrophoresis, except the separation medium is confined to a small glass capillary.

Recent innovations in automation technology to detect amplified DNA are most often variations on the theme of gel electrophoresis or capillary electrophoresis (Table 4.5). Once

TABLE 4.4. COMMON ANALYTIC TECHNIQUES IN MOLECULAR DIAGNOSTICS

Genomic DNA as template
    Southern transfer—evaluation of digested genomic DNA
    Northern blot—evaluation of cellular RNA
    Western blot—evaluation of cellular and extracellular protein
Amplification-based methods
    Polymerase chain reaction (PCR)-amplification of small regions of nucleic acids by a thermostable DNA polymerase
    Reverse-transcriptase polymerase chain reaction: (RT-PCR)-Two step amplification process beginning with cellular RNA. Reverse transcriptase first convert RNA to cDNA, followed by exponential amplification of cDNA to DNA by taq polymerase
    Ligase chain reaction/detection reaction (LCR/LDR)-Exponential or arithmetic amplification of two sequence specific primers 'fused' together by a thermostable DNA ligase
    Q beta replicase
    Isothermic amplification enzymes such as are used in the Invader™ assay
    DNA sequencing: addition of dideoxynucleotides to each of 4 PCR reactions to create termination reaction products. When these DNA products are separated, the size differentials between them can be inferred as the DNA nucleotide sequence

TABLE 4.5. ANALYTIC METHODS BASED ON FRAGMENT SIZE SEPARATION

Gel electrophoresis
  Standard gel electrophoresis in agarose or polyacrylamide—Separation of DNA fragment generated by PCR or other amplification methods in a uniform electric field through a sieving medium
  Automated gel electrophoresis with real time fluorescence detection—Use of fluorochrome labeled DNA fragments separated in a denaturing polyacrylamide gel. Detection is based on continuous scanning of the gel by a low intensity laser and measurement of the resulting emitted fluorescence.
  Single stranded conformational polymorphisms—Denaturation of the double stranded DNA fragments.
  Denaturing gradient gel electrophoresis—Denaturation of the double stranded DNA fragments in the gel medium. Mutations inherent to the samples are detected by alterations in the pattern of fragment migration.
  Heteroduplex analysis—Heat denaturation, followed by controlled renaturation of double stranded DNA fragments before separation on a nondenaturing gel. Detection of mutations is based on alteration in the pattern of fragment migration.
Capillary electrophoresis
  Separation of fluorescently labeled DNA fragments though a single or multiplexed capillary. Detection is based on laser induced fluorescence emission at a point distal on the capillary.
Methods based on fragment detection *in situ*
  TaqMan™ detection system
  LightCycle® realtime fluorescence detection

PCR, polymerase chain reaction.

fragments are separated, they can be visualized. Conventional protocols employ chemicals like ethidium bromide to stain DNA, but these compounds are gradually being replaced by fluorescent dyes. Fluorescence detection involves scanning the gel or the capillary continuously with a low-intensity laser as the DNA products migrate through the gel matrix. The detection is achieved by capturing the emitted fluorescence on a photodiode or a charge-coupled device (CCD). Incorporating several fluorescent dyes that emit at various wavelengths makes it possible to analyze multiple DNA products simultaneously. Hence, the schematic of electrophoretic separation and visualization, whether manually or in an automated format, is the way most genetic testing is performed. Automation of this system introduces a means of interpreting the fluorescent data through a software algorithm that can catalog the signal strength and position to derive the fragment size and quantity. The addition of an autosampler, which draws a small volume of the PCR product and loads it onto the medium, is most useful in the analysis of low-complexity genetic tests, such as SNPs, in which the result is a uniform sized DNA fragment.

Most automated DNA analyzers in use in the clinical laboratory are based on endpoint determination (Table 4.5). A new advance in the molecular genetics laboratory involves real-time detection of a DNA fragment, and is based on the repeated measurement of fluorescence or an electrochemical signal during the PCR reaction. Real-time detection systems make quantitative analysis possible. One such technique, referred to as *Taqman* technology, takes advantage of properties of the exonuclease activity inherent to *Taq* polymerase (27). In this method, *Taq* polymerase binds to the DNA primer and begins to replicate the template DNA in a 5′ to 3′ direction. A third FRET oligonucleotide primer/probe is positioned to overlay the point mutation. Similar to the Invader assay, as long as the FRET primer/probe remains intact, the emission spectra of one fluorochrome will

quench the spectra of the other. As *Taq* creates the elongating DNA strand, it will encounter the opposing probe, wherein the 5′-exonuclease activity of *Taq* will act to cleave the terminal nucleotides from one end of the FRET. This cleavage liberates each of the fluorochromes into solution, along with the disinhibition of their respective fluorescent emissions. Fluorescence detectors in contact with the reaction tube or optical fibers placed into the reaction fluid monitor the fluorescence of the sample in real time.

Capture of fluorochrome-labeled PCR product onto internally color-coded microbeads is the basis of Luminex technology (28). A variety of beads, each of a different color, are assigned to a specific oligonucleotide probe, and hence the system is amenable to multiplexing reactions for multiple gene or mutations within a single gene. Quantitation is also possible because the magnitude of the surface reaction is a function of the amount of bound PCR product. To perform a test, the color-coded microspheres, reporter molecules, and sample are combined. This mixture then is injected into an instrument that uses microfluidics to align the microspheres in single file where lasers illuminate the colors inside and on the surface of each microsphere. Next, advanced optics capture the color signals. Finally, digital-signal processing translates the signals into real-time, quantitative data for each reaction. In one application, six different viral or control PCR products were coupled to six microsphere sets. The surface oligonucleotide probes were biotinylated, and the viral amplicons were detected with fluorescent streptavidin. The method is very sensitive and has a lower limit of detection of 50 virions per milliliter and 3 logs of dynamic range.

Variations on the theme of combining the amplification and detection phases into a single operational step are at the heart of innovation in new technology for genetic testing. Drawing from the advantages of other recombinant enzymes, such as thermal stable ligase and isothermic polymerases, may permit the testing of several gene markers simultaneously and may eliminate the need for a thermocycling device. Strand displacement amplification, developed by BD Biosciences, is one such system that combines the action of a unique isothermal polymerase and a restriction enzyme to create single-stranded DNA products. The fact that once genetic testing was imagined to be *at least* a four-step operational schema in which assay setup and subsequent analysis were separate steps soon may give way to protocols that combine operations into a one- or two-step system. When such systems are available, the prospect of simple and efficient POC testing (POCT) for genetics can be realized.

INTERPRETATION AND REPORTING

The use of genetic information for patient care is still sufficiently novel that having expert interpretation of the data and construction of a thoughtful report is essential. In most cases, molecular diagnostics laboratories are dedicated to the performance of complex genetic tests that involve interpretation of a variety of genetic abnormalities, including point mutations, deletions, rearrangements, and gene loss by scientists or physicians specifically trained in molecular genetics. Whereas the interpretation of a well-done genetic test is easy, the complexity of each of the analytic operations and the chance of error in any of the manual steps make the practicality of an automated interpretation high risk. A variety of simple genetic analyses with high clinical utility, however, do serve as models of where automated interpretation and reporting can be explored. Factor V *Leiden* is the specific name of a mutation with a high incidence in the white population. When this mutation is present, patients are at an increased risk for deep vein thrombosis and other vascular complications (Fig. 4.5A). Factor V *Leiden* results from a single point mutation in the gene for the factor V protein, a pivotal component in the cascade of biochemical events that determine intravascular clot formation and clot dissolution (Fig. 4.5B) (29). Several investigators have attempted to automate molecular genetic testing for factor V *Leiden* in the hope that this simple model system will lead to strategies for other POCT applications (30–33).

In its simplest form, factor V *Leiden* testing involves interpretation of a PCR-based assay that falls into one of three categories: (a) homozygote normal (i.e., no mutation), (b) heterozygote mutant, and (c) homozygote mutant. Figure 4.5C illustrates how, using a conventional gel electrophoresis methodology, the factor V *Leiden* test can be performed such that the presence or absence of a band of a prescribed molecular weight is diagnostic of each and every one of the three potential genetic outcomes. Figure 4.5D–F also shows the proposed manner in which these same genetic outcomes could be adapted to an automated interpretation system that requires nothing more than the generation of a simple yes or no readout and hence the elimination of a need for specialized physician interpretation. Third-Wave Technologies (Madison, WI, U.S.A.) has commercialized a simple and high-throughput kit for factor V *Leiden* based on the Invader assay. In this case, the result is presented in the form of a spreadsheet, whereas a series of software-encoded scripts

determine the genotype automatically. In turn, these data can be exported directly into a report form, with only a minimal need to review the raw data. Although this means of data handling is a marked simplification of the days of manually interpreting gels, the overall requirement for specialized laboratory personnel and equipment prevents classifying this technology as ready for POC. As discussed in the subsequent section, the promise of several new and promising technologies centered on miniaturization may lead to the eventual test bed of a fully automated genetic analysis system.

Opportunities for Molecular Diagnostics Instrumentation at the Point of Care

Despite the requirements of time and manual operations of extraction, amplification, and analysis, nucleic acid-based testing is really quite simple and typically robust. Correspondingly, this simplicity translates into the wide versatility of applications for molecular genetic testing. As a material, DNA is very durable and tolerant to mechanical stress as well as to heat, cold, and desiccation. For many applications, DNA can be retrieved from harsh environments and still can be amplified with efficiency and high fidelity. In terms of durability and robustness, the potential for DNA-based POCT is great; however, in terms of the requirements of time, operator skill, and lack of automation, the story is quite different.

The amount of time involved in molecular diagnostic testing is considerable. In routine practice, most molecular tests require several days to complete, and results are reported in 5 to 7 days. Fortunately, in the marketing of most genetic disease, the turnaround time of molecular testing is rarely an issue. By contrast, for areas of clinical medicine with a routine need for bedside diagnostics, molecular-based testing does not yet compete with other methods common to the clinical chemistry laboratory. In the interim, however, we are left to use the basic operational format of specimen collection, nucleic acid extraction, analytic test performance, and interpretation, usually in a turnaround time measuring in hours and, one would hope, no more than 1 or 2 days. Table 4.6 lists a series of specific examples of genetic tests that require rapid turnaround time and consequently may have a significant impact on therapeutic decision-making. This list is by no means complete, but it attempts to catalog the types of clinical situations for which the investment in a genetic diagnosis overshadows the disadvantages of cost and turnaround time when these tests are compared with more conventional biochemical measures.

In addition to applications for constitutional genetic disorders, oncology, and infectious diseases, molecular diagnostics plays an important role in settings outside the health care system. One area is in forensic testing, where retrieval of DNA from the crime scene is used to identify persons involved in a crime. Forensic laboratories routinely use special techniques and simple tools to retrieve samples such as blood or tissue from locations where they are likely to have been dried, heated, diluted with water and other chemicals, or mechanically disrupted. In this setting, case specimen procurement typically involves the rehydration of blood spots from materials, which then are secondarily collected onto a swab and transported in

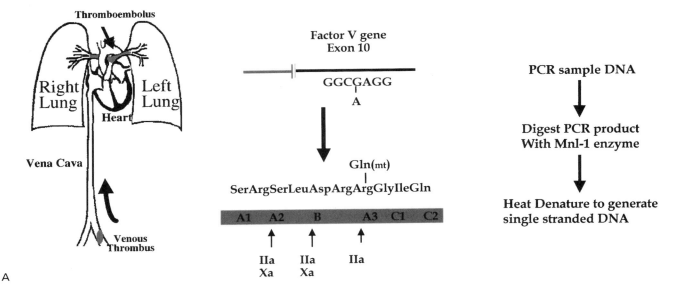

A

B,C

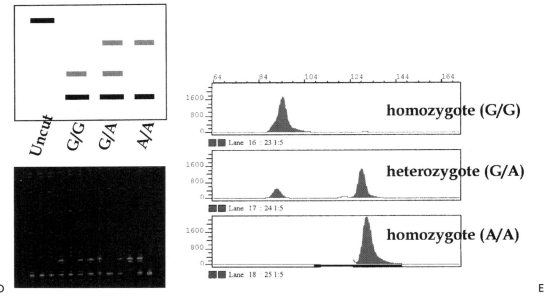

D

E

F

FIGURE 4.5. A: Thrombophilia is a common medical condition relating to the predisposition to form intravascular thrombi. **B**: The factor V *Leiden* mutation is a single nucleotide substitution (G → A) that encodes the amino acid substitution Asn → Gln in the factor V protein. **C**: The algorithm for polymerase chain reaction (PCR) detection of factor V *Leiden.* In the PCR reaction, fluorochrome end-labeled oligonucleotide primers are used to amplify sample template DNA. A fraction of the end product then is digested with the restriction endonuclease MnI-1, a cleavage site that is destroyed in the presence of the point mutation. This product then is electrophoresed on a denaturing polyacrylamide gel. **D**: Schematic of the detection of the fluorescent product of digestion of the PCR reaction derived DNA. **E**: The output of the automated fluorescent detection system. **F**: The histogram presents the signal data as numeric ratios. The numeric ratios are linked to interpretative macros, which interpret the diagnosis and monitor quality control.

TABLE 4.6. GENETIC TESTS WITH HIGH CLINICAL IMPACT, RAPID TURNAROUND

Test	Clinical Need	Conventional Analytic Approach	Advantage/Opportunity of POC Test
Constitutional genetic disorder			
Factor V Leiden	Major factor is venous clotting predisposition	PCR amplification followed by detection restriction digestion and electrophoresis	Rapid turnaround (1–5 hs) would impact on postsurgical care. May be a required test before prescription of birth control or hormone supplements
Factor II polymorphism	Second major cause of clotting predisposition	PCR amplification followed by detection restriction digestion and electrophoresis	Same as for factor V Leiden
Mutational analysis of rantidine receptor gene	Diagnosis of malignant hyperthermia	PCR amplification followed by sequence analysis of high probability exons and introns	Ability to identify heterozygotes would mandate the selection of anethestic agents
Molecular detection of pathogens			
Tuberculosis	Diagnosis from body fluids	PCR of extracted sample DNA, or Q-beta replicase or RT-PCR of extracted bacterial ribosomal RNA	Rapid or immediate diagnostic test would permit prescription of necessary treatment in the context of clinic or for population screening
Bacterial infections	Diagnosis from various body sites and fluids, e.g., Neisseria meningitis	PCR of extracted sample DNA, or Q-beta replicase or RT-PCR of extracted bacterial ribosomal RNA	Early diagnosis may be lifesaving. Determination of a positive test mandates treatment of infected person and close contacts
Viral infection associated with acute clinical syndromes	e.g., rhinovirus, other GI or respiratory viruses; detection and diagnosis confirmation	PCR or RT-PCR amplification of conserved gene sequence, followed by detection by automated cap. or gel electrophoresis	Point of care testing for septicemia could be lifesaving. Detection of precise species could direct choice of therapy
Viral infection associated with chronic clinical course	e.g., Hepatitis C virus; monitoring of viral levels in blood	PCR or RT-PCR amplification of conserved gene sequence, followed by detection by automated capsule or gel	Detection of common viral agents could direct physician to guide dosing of antiviral therapies. Measurement of viral titers may be prognostic
Molecular testing of cancer			
Leukemia chromosomal translocation	Diagnosis or monitoring of minimal residual disease with chimeric gene transcripts, e.g., PML-RARα associated with promyelocytic leukemia	RT-PCR of extracted total cellular or messenger RNA from a representation sample. Detection is typically by gel electrophoresis identifying a specific size amplification product	From example, rapid diagnosis of this type of leukemia (1–3 hs) may be lifesaving in the initiation of treatment of choice

POC, point of care; PCR, polymerase chain reaction; RT-PCR, reverse transcriptase-polymerase chain reaction; GI, gastrointestinal; PML, RARα, promyelocytic leukemia-retinoic acid receptor alpha.

either a liquid media or on a solid support system such as FTA paper. Once in the laboratory, high-quality DNA can be retrieved, but typically at very low concentrations. Amplification of so-called satellite genetic markers consisting of varying lengths of tandem repeating DNA sequences by PCR then are secondarily size-separated by gel electrophoresis or capillary electrophoresis. In an effort to achieve the highest sensitivity and specificity in testing, forensic investigators often have been the leaders in innovations of molecular genetic technology. Their methods are proven to be exquisitely sensitive even when working with a minute amount of sample. Specificity relates to confidence in the data to identify two individuals based on the combination of genetic alleles. In the prosecution of most violent crimes, the submission of PCR-amplified DNA evidence has become a routine practice. In the United States, nearly all 50 states now accept the results of DNA-based identification data.

Another area where molecular genetic testing has found great utility is in environmental testing. The most common application of environmental testing involves using samples obtained from sites contaminated by hazardous materials, whether that is in the hospital or in the outdoor environment. PCR or other gene-amplification technologies then are used to amplify gene segments from microbial organisms, considered valid indicators of a source of contamination. In the area of public health, using filter paper-based swabs collected from patients or locations throughout a health care facility facilitates investigation of the source of drug-resistant bacteria, such as methicillin-resistant streptococci. Samples then are tested for the plasmid-based genes these bacteria carry, which impart their resistance to the most commonly used antibiotic medications.

Based on a similar concept, home-based diagnostic kits designed to detect certain infectious agents are becoming available for use by consumers in the comfort and confidentiality of their own home. One such product, called Home Access, involves a self-administered collection of a small quantity of blood spotted onto filter paper. The filter paper is subsequently addressed into a postmarked envelope and is sent to a central laboratory, where testing for the human immunodeficiency virus (HIV) is performed. The validation of this assay has been demonstrated many times and is included in several references (34,35). In this example, the POCT of testing is only in the specimen collection. The analytic components of this test are performed through a registered and U.S. Food and Drug Administration (FDA)-approved central laboratory. Trained health care professionals provide interpretation of the data and presentation to the consumer in a confidential and supportive manner by telephone. The invention of an at-home test for HIV, based on molecular genetic methods, is certain to lead to many other test platforms. It is noteworthy that the motivation for these products is born out of the consumer's need to know and desire to have diagnostic testing made simple and convenient.

A related application for molecular diagnostics testing has been embraced by several governments as a means to monitor for the production of weapons of mass destruction. Around the world, several national governments are involved in developing technologies for the rapid and on-site identification of microorganisms that are the causes of the human forms of the disease anthrax, vibrio cholera, tularemia, bubonic plague, and a host of lethal and chronic viral illnesses (36–38). In this situation, the intended goal is rapid retrieval of trace evidence of these pathogens from potential weapons manufacturing facilities as well as contaminated munitions sites. The ability to process specimens as well as to execute the test at the inspection site is for the protection of personnel near that site but also for purposes of supporting foreign policy by being able to verify the presence and deny the proliferation of these illegal weapons.

Not all gene-based testing for microorganisms is focused on detecting or preventing disease; it also focuses on industrial applications where microbes are used to improve society or make medicine. From the vantage of the size of investments, the largest driver for POC gene-based technology is in the discovery and development of new pharmaceutical products. In 1997, 5.4 billion dollars was invested in biotechnology research and development, with more than 35% of those companies focused on gene discovery or refinement of molecular biological techniques. It is hoped that these, along with other enabling technologies such as combinatorial chemistry, will serve to lower the costs of finding new drugs and bringing them to market (39–42).

Collectively, this diverse group of applications for molecular diagnostics will be major drivers for technologies leading to POC instrumentation. Although these opportunities appear great and the economic gains a justification for their pursuit, the technical hurdles that lie in the path of achieving total system integration are great. As discussed in the subsequent sections, a major hope of POC instrumentation for molecular diagnostics is directed at the use of silicon-based microchips. Appreciation of this technology involves an overview of what is involved in the production of these devices and where the future lies in the integration of these "DNA chips with microelectronics, microfluidics, and packaging constraints."

Emergence of Technologies for Miniaturization of Molecular Diagnostics

Cost reduction is a major driving force to improve the performance of molecular diagnostics. As discussed earlier, to appreciate where costs accumulate in the operational schema of genetic testing requires a whole system analysis inclusive of sample collection. Based on current technology, molecular diagnostic laboratories have worked to optimize each of the operational steps (Fig. 4.1), and through a combination of efforts involving computerization or piecemeal integration, the overall testing schema can be "semiautomated" (43). Commensurate with the current practice of molecular diagnostics, however, is the emergence of engineering research directed at creating a fully integrated testing system (44). This research has led principally to the conclusion that miniaturization comparable to the size of today's computer chips will afford the greatest likelihood of achieving this integration and at the same time significantly decrease costs (45).

In the past 10 years, there has been a major effort to develop microminiaturized devices to support biochemical testing, including PCR (46). In the effort to create a highly portable and inexpensive gene amplification and detection system, there has been a need to converge expertise from at least two scientific areas for which there previously has been no practical connection. The first is in the area of biotechnology, with its focus on refinement of the molecular biology and the *in vitro* application of key biochemical processes. The second area is electrical engineering, both material science and computers, with a specific focus on the design of microelectronic components and microelectromechanical systems, or MEMS. Collectively, these two groups are working in the relatively new discipline of biomedical engineering. The interface between these two disciplines has led to some exciting new ideas that only in the last few years are being realized as devices with potential commercial viability.

Bioengineering is the broad-based term used to describe the application of research tools found in the recombinant DNA laboratory toward the purpose of developing more refined biologic materials and reagents. An earlier section discussed the use of *Taq* polymerase, which is a bioengineered product derived from bacteria found in nature in places like a hot spring. Using *Taq* polymerase as an example, a number of valuable properties have been engineered into this commercially available enzyme.

Taq polymerase is derived from thermophilous *aquaticus*, a species of bacteria found to live in waters at 70 to 75°C. Compared with DNA polymerases from eukaryotic cells, *Taq* polymerase has optimal activity at these high temperatures. For years, *Taq* polymerase has been used in the research laboratory as a means to amplify a segment of a template DNA with high fidelity. The process involves repeated heating to denature the double-stranded conformation of native DNA and is followed by a moderate cooling phase during which short stretches of DNA, called *primers*, can bind and initiate the replication of the template. This is followed by an intermediate heating step to a temperature at which the enzyme is optimally active. This repeated heating and cooling process, called *thermocycling*, is the basis of PCR. Experience with PCR has shown that a number of chemical additives can be added to the reaction mixture, which greatly improves the performance of this enzyme. Characteristics such as processivity, or the ability to process large strands or strips of unique as well as repetitive DNA sequence, can be improved by adding such agents as nonionic detergents and mild denaturants, which increase the binding avidity of the enzyme for the DNA strand. Commercial buffer solutions have optimized the performance of *Taq* and other similar enzymes by adding dimethyl sulfoxide (DMSO), formamide, and sodium dodecyl sulfate (SDS). Other observations point to the fact that *Taq* polymerase also possesses certain "exonuclease activity." Typically, exonuclease activity would be an unfavorable characteristic of this enzyme because it usually destroys or removes basis from the elongating DNA strand in a five-prime to three-prime orientation. Genetic manipulation of the portion of the *Taq* polymerase gene that encodes for exonuclease activity resulted in a recombinant enzyme with improved processivity and diminished exonuclease activity (47). Taking advantage of the inherent exonuclease activity of *Taq* is the basis for the design of the Taqman™ technology. Other genetic modifications of *Taq* polymerases have improved the native enzyme's precision in reading the DNA template. This so-called proofreading and repair capability permits the generation of very long fragments of amplified DNA, or amplicons (48). This version of thermostabile polymerase is one with significant utility in the diagnostic arena. Lastly, efforts are afoot to improve the long-term storage and tolerance of *Taq* polymerase to varied reaction conditions. The importance of this modification is that the enzyme could be more useful in the preparation of prepackaged reaction solutions, which require only sample template DNA to be activated. These reagents will be critical to the assembly of one-step PCR kits that can be thermocycled in a simple benchtop or POC genetic testing instrument.

A second area of discovery is focused on the exploitation of silicon-based microchips as a platform for building an integrated genetic testing system. Amalgamation with a personal computer controller, this work is leading to POCT for molecular diagnostics. Much of the development has evolved from the field of MEMS (49), which is a means to make microminiaturized actuators and sensors by processes identical to those used to fabricate microelectronic chips. Physical sensors are the primary commercial application of MEMS, although new approaches toward combining the mechanical features of MEMS with biologic materials are laying the foundation for a whole new class of biosensors. MEMS married to microelectronic circuitry is referred to as *smart sensor systems* because they can be controlled according to which are robust and can be fitted easily into highly portable and inexpensive handheld and benchtop instrumentation.

Much of the progress in MEMS technology is borrowed from the optimization of techniques used in the integrated circuit technology arena, with the promise of miniaturization and batch fabrication. Fabrication of MEMS sensors is based on the processes of photolithography, surface micromachining, and deposition of novel materials on silicon. An analogy to the creation of a MEMS device can be found in the construction of a house. Before a house can be constructed, blueprints of the structure need to be drawn by a draftsperson, who will outline a template designating the position of the walls and other key elements in that structure. Similarly, the process of photolithography leads to a series of masks, each outlining one layer within the MEMS structure. Each photo mask is projected onto the surface of a silicon wafer, resulting in a pattern of shadows and lighted areas. Photoresists are epoxy-type materials used in photolithography to protect and deprotect differentially areas of the silicon wafer. Exposure of specific wavelengths of light causes these epoxys to "cure" by cross-linking or, in the shadowed areas, to be vulnerable to dissolution by organic solvents. The result of photolithography is to leave a footprint for each sequential step and the precise location for the placement of materials on the wafer, much like a bricklayer might first place the foundation with bricks and cement in preparation for the footings of the vertical walls.

Another process in MEMS fabrication is deposition of thin films. Typically, this involves the use of high temperatures and mixtures of gases bathing the surface of the silicon wafer for precisely defined times and pressures. The result is a deposition of materials, which have either electrical or structural properties useful to the finished device. *Micromachining* refers to the use of a variety of techniques, including dry or wet etching procedures, to remove differentially materials from the silicon wafer or previously laid-down thin films. Micromachining is performed in concert with serial photolithography steps to create the structures with intricate details, including vertical wall and freestanding beams or diaphragms, as well as to prepare planer surfaces for subsequent deposition of metals or biochemical layers

The utility of MEMS in creating an integrated genetic device is highly focused on two broad areas. The first is in the creation of miniaturized chambers in which to carry out biochemical reactions such as PCR. The next section presents a review of the various technologies involving MEMS or MEMS-like devices for gene amplification. The second area in which MEMS is employed includes the creation of unique sensors. Collectively referred to as *biosensors*, the advent of microaddressable arrays or DNA chips has been among the most remarkable and exciting areas of opportunity in the whole of the biotechnology industry. In addition to these DNA chips, numerous more classic sensor technologies are being evaluated as potential biosensors. One particularly exciting opportunity in the use of these other MEMS sensors is their compatibility with integrated microelectronic circuitry. With the goal of creating an integrated genetic testing system, which can be scaled to a device no larger than a postage stamp, the need to provide control of these sensing or actuating elements mandates comparably sized electronic controller units. These high-bred sensor systems, or "smart sensors," are also compatible with commonly available controlling software elements such as might be found in any personal computer. The following section presents an overview of the industry's current sensor technologies.

DNA Chip Technologies

As is often the case with breakthrough technologies, there is a great deal of hyperbole surrounding the development of micrometer- and even nanometer-scaled chip technologies, popularly known as *DNA* or *genetic chips*. In this case, however, much of this optimism is certainly justified, considering that in just a few short years basic research has led to a number of products that are at or near the commercial phase of their development. In this chapter, the focus is on the delivery of DNA or other forms of gene-based testing for POC medicine. Developers of DNA chips believe that in the near future these technologies will enable clinicians—and in some cases patients themselves—to detect quickly and inexpensively the presence of a wide variety of genetic-based diseases and conditions, including acquired immunodeficiency syndrome (AIDS), Alzheimer's disease, cystic fibrosis, and several forms of cancer. In other arenas, this technology also will make it possible to develop inexpensive strategies for screening new pharmaceutical agents and new gene discoveries associated with hitherto uncharacterized diseases. In the meantime, however, considerable work needs to be done to make these technologies useful and robust as well as inexpensive to the end user. To date, a few companies have commercialized DNA chip products, but many more underlying scientific principles remain to be discovered before these devices are ready for routine clinical use. The following section outlines some of the underlying technologic principles involved in these microfabricated biochips and presents a critical review of their respective capabilities today and in the near future.

As discussed in the earlier section, much of the DNA chip technology is based on advances in MEMS and microelectronics. A third component to this mix of technologies includes insights as to how biochemical reagents and fluids interact in these microenvironments, with particular emphasis on biocompatibility and changes in simple physical properties of fluids when confined to very small spaces.

Microcapillary Electrophoresis

One of the first applications of microfabrication technology for bioanalysis were attempts to demonstrate the flow of fluid containing certain key analytes through microcapillary channels cre-

ated from glass or plastic. The microfabricated devices are used in a manner identical to the mesoscale version of multichannel capillary electrophoresis, in which capillaries measure between 1 and 3 mm in diameter. These chips are constructed from glass, plastic, and silicon and have microchannels that are typically 50 to 100 μ in diameter. Using conventional photolithography and surface micromachining, several investigators have shown how they can confine up to 2 m of micromachined capillary into a space no larger than that of a postage stamp. At the proximal end of these microcapillaries is a fluid reservoir in continuity with microelectrodes that provide the electromotive force (50). Through the application of a voltage across these two electrodes, fluid will flow across the length of the microchannel, and dissolved analytes will separate according to their electrophoretic mobility and the counterbalanced electro-osmotic flow (Fig. 4.6) (51). A technology developed by Caliper Technologies (Mountain View, CA) incorporates the use of what is called *electrokinetic flow*. Electrokinetic flow involves the coordinated movement of fluid columns electrophoretically across intersecting microcapillaries by way of differential application of voltage across electrodes specific for each (52–54). In this way, several fluid reservoirs can be combined, each containing separate buffer solutions and sample reservoirs. By coordinated application of current to each of these electrodes, there can be the appropriate mixing of several buffers and the sample in a coordinated flow that results in electrophoretic separation across the longest length of capillary (54). This approach is the so-called "lab on a chip," and it has the potential to involve several analytic assays to be combined in a very small and low-cost platform. Figure 4.7 is an illustration of the Caliper labchip, which is now available commercially.

A simpler version of a microcapillary electrophoresis device has been tested in several important clinical assays, including detection of the bcr-*abl* gene transcripts associated with chronic myelogenous leukemia, the factor V *Leiden* mutation assay, as well as a multiplexed reaction to detect mutations in the cystic

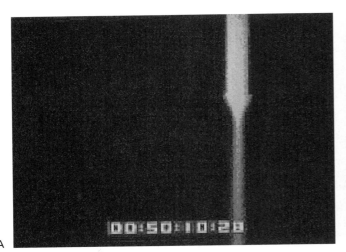

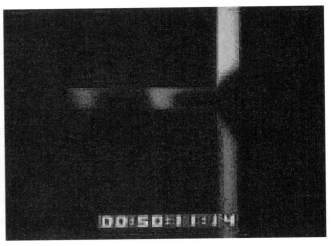

A

B

FIGURE 4.6. Microcapillary electrophoresis and electrokinetic flow. **A:** Fluid carrying a fluorescent material is being electro-osmotically pumped from top to bottom through an intersection of channels measuring 80 × 10 at the rate of approximately 1 nanoliter (a nanoliter is one billionth of a liter) per second. **B:** Electrokinetic flow occurs when the direction of electric fields is changed to produce a significant voltage drop right to left and a smaller one in the upward and downward directions.

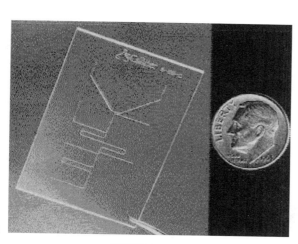
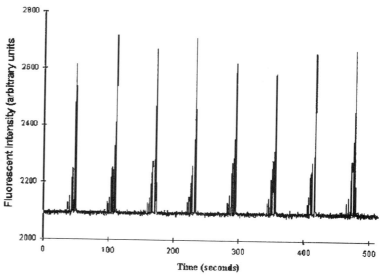

A   B

FIGURE 4.7. A: Labchip, from Caliper Technologies (Palo Alto, CA, U.S.A.). Caliper has employed manufacturing methods from the electronics industry to produce miniature, integrated biochemical processing systems. The design features interconnected channels etched into glass, silicon, quartz, or plastic. **B**: The graph illustrates separation of fragments produced by Hae III digestion of bacteriophage ØX174 DNA.

fibrosis gene (51,55,56). In each case, the clear advantage of microcapillary electrophoresis is its high throughput capability. Table 4.7 summarizes the various DNA fragment detection modalities, some of which have been adapted to a silicon chip platform. Of note, only the microcapillary-chip and the microaddressable-array–based devices are available for clinical practice.

Microaddressable Arrays

When the popular press refers to DNA chips, in most cases they are referring to variations on the theme of microaddressable arrays (Fig. 4.8). Microaddressable arrays or DNA arrays represent a unique combination of technologies wherein microfabrication of silicon is combined with unique ways of affixing gene

TABLE 4.7. SUMMARY OF MICROCHIP DETECTION MODALITIES

Type of Biochip	Technical Principle	Stage of Development
Microcapillary electrophoresis	Separation of DNA fragments created by PCR or other means of amplification by electrophoresis in a microfabricated capillary 1–30 µM in diameter	Commercialized by Cepheid and Caliper Technologies
DNA hybridization chip	Synthesis or site directed affixation of oligonucleotide probes onto chip surface. Detection is achieved by laser-induced fluorescence or hybridized PCR product	Commercialized by Affymetrix for several diagnostic tests including HIV, *p53* and *BRCA-1* Other manufacturers either involved in the research market or are awaiting FDA approval
Surface acoustic wave sensor (SAW)	Detection of change in the propagation of a surface wave from transmitter to receiver through a molecular binding domain	Research device developed at the University of California, Berkeley
Surface plasmon resonance (SPR)	Detection of the evanescent wave propagated from the interface of a reflecting metal to which is bound a hybridized DNA duplex	Commercialized as a benchtop instrument by BIAcore, a division of Pharacia-Upjohn. Microchip based version under development
Electromechanical MEMS sensor	Detection of mass loading, either by shift in resonant frequency or static flex of a piezoelectric transducer	Under development in research laboratories, including Naval Research Laboratories
Mass spectrometer on-a-chip	Reduction of the components of an electrospray or time-of-flight mass spectrometer to a silicon chip format	University of Minnesota Research device based in part on retrofitting miniaturized components into a conventional instrument

PCR, polymerase chain reaction; HIV, human immunodeficiency; FDA, U.S. Food and Drug Administration.

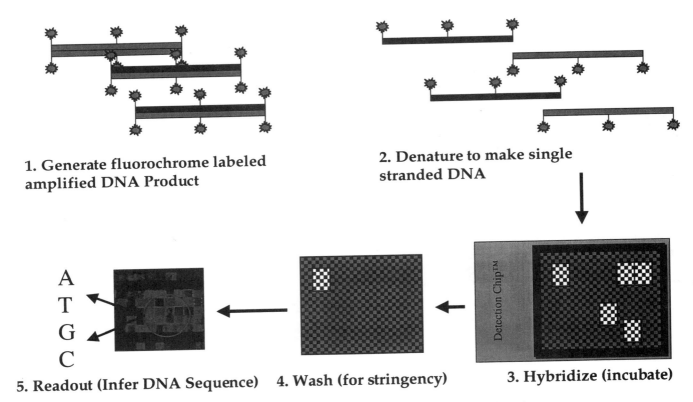

1. Generate fluorochrome labeled amplified DNA Product

2. Denature to make single stranded DNA

5. Readout (Infer DNA Sequence)   **4. Wash (for stringency)**   **3. Hybridize (incubate)**

FIGURE 4.8. Schematic of the use of microaddressable arrays for genetic testing.

probes to a solid support system. The vanguard of this technology is based on research performed by Fodor and colleagues, dating to the middle 1980s, wherein conventional photolithography was used to construct oligonucleotide DNA probes directly from a silicon microchip surface (57,58). This so-called light-directed chemical synthesis encompasses two mature technologies: semiconductor-based photolithography and solid-phase chemical synthesis. Synthesis linkers modified with photochemically removable protection groups are attached to the silicon substrate (Fig. 4.9). Light is directed through a photolithographic mask to specific areas of the synthetic surface to affect localized photo-deprotection. The first of a series of chemical building blocks, for example, a photo-protected amino acid or hydroxyl, incubated with the surface and chemical coupling occurs at those sites, which have been illuminated in the preceding step. Next, light is directed to a different region of the substrate through a new photo mask, and the chemical cycle is repeated. Complicated strategies can be employed that will generate a large number of oligonucleotide probes in a minimum number of chemical steps. For example, only $4 \times N$ chemical steps can produce a complete set of $4N$ oligonucleotides of length N or any subset of the array. The pattern of illumination and the order of chemical reactants prescribe the synthesis of these products and their precise location on the chip. An alternative to photolithography is laser directed from the surface of a digitally directed micromirror array to photoactivate the surface of the DNA chip with pinpoint accuracy. This method is referred to as *maskless microarray fabrication*. The promise of this

technique is rapidly changeable chip configurations and a marked reduction in the cost of chip manufacture (59).

Affymetrix Corporation (Santa Clara, CA) uses light-directed chemical synthesis to create its series of microaddressable arrays called Genechip™. The chip platform in the Affymetrix system serves as a convenient sample module that is "interpreted" in the benchtop fluidics and optical station. Affymetrix's HIV Genechip is designed to detect mutations in the HIV protease as well as in the virus' reverse transcriptase gene (60). Additional

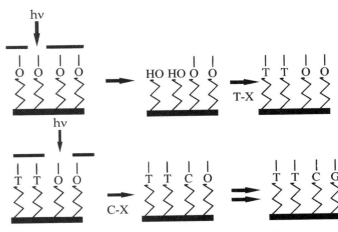

FIGURE 4.9. Method of DNA chip fabrication using light-directed chemical synthesis.

products, including gene chip arrays for p53 and SNPs for genes encoding proteins involved in drugs are now available (61). Recently, Affymetrix focused on the development of very high-density DNA arrays, which contain probes for up to 64,000 genes. Less dense and more clinically useful chips for the genetic analysis of large genes with a multiplicity of known point mutations, such as *BRCA-1*, as well as in characterization of bacterial pathogens are under investigation (62,63).

Alternative strategies for affixing oligonucleotide gene probes to a silicon surface have been accomplished by companies such as Nanogen Corporation (La Jolla, CA, U.S.A.) and Genometrix (Woodlands, TX). Nanogen involves the off-chip synthesis of oligonucleotide probes that are secondarily directed to microelectrodes through electrostatic attraction (64,65). By differentially turning on each of these electrodes, different oligonucleotide probes can be directed to a precise location on the chip. Genometrix's approach involves the deposition of off-chip synthesized oligonucleotide probes through a microjet dispensing system to predetermined locations on the chip (66,67). Deposition of 5'-thiolated oligonucleotides onto glass slides using a bubble jet printer has been shown to be a very low cost yet robust technique amenable for use with home-brew assays (68).

One problem with these DNA chips is the fact that only a single nucleotide difference determines whether normal and mutant PCR products will hybridize to their cognate probes on the chip. The result is an inherently low signal-to-noise relationship and, correspondingly, a genotyping assay that is difficult to interpret. An alternative method developed by Barany and colleagues exploits the ability of the ligase detection reaction (LDR) system to discriminate differences in the nucleotide sequence of the sample DNA prior to its hybridization on the chip (69). In this case, a series of two primers align on one DNA strand overlying a point mutation. The LDR chemistry, through a thermostabile ligase, fuses the two primers together only if there is perfect nucleotide complementarity. Attached to the end of one of the ligase primers is a generic oligonucleotide called a *zip code*. Each zip code is designed so as not to interact with the sample DNA; at the same time, the library of zip codes all share very similar melting point characteristics. This approach greatly simplifies the process of optimizing the condition by which the products of the LDR reaction are hybridized to the chip because each zip code is hybridized with identical avidity. A positive test is detected when the product of the ligation reaction binds to the chip via the hybridization of the zip code and its immobilized complement (Fig. 4.10). In this case, the geographic localization of the product to the chip serves only to indicate that the very specific mutation detection reaction took place. Based on this universal platform, several diagnostic chips have been devel-

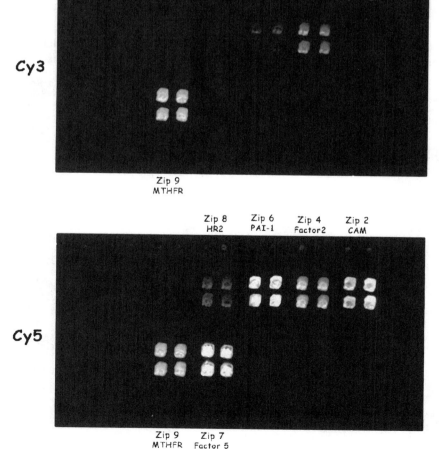

FIGURE 4.10. Zip code DNA microarray. Photograph of the captured fluorescent image of the zip code array for a series of genetic markers in the evaluation of inherited thrombophilia. The top panel is the image of the fluorochrome Cy-3 detecting the normal gene sequence. The bottom panel is the image of Cy-5 detecting the mutant gene signal.

oped that demonstrate the feasibility of this system to multiplex the analysis of several genes into a single test (70–73).

Despite the fact that there are now numerous studies describing applications of DNA microarrays for research, most methods are neither simple nor cost-effective enough to be used in routine clinical testing. In most cases, the principal problems relate to using single nucleotide difference to hybridize DNA to a probe and then to render an unambiguous genotype. Concerns over the manufacture of the chips themselves, however, remain and include the best ways to optimize the probe density, the durability of the attachment chemistry, and the effect of the probe sequence on its accessibility to hybridization (74,75). When these assay conditions are well controlled, it is possible to use microarray data to deduce the DNA sequence of the amplification product in a high throughput format (76,77).

Motorola Life Sciences (Pasadena, CA, U.S.A.) is developing a system that aims to provide direct electronic detection of DNA hybridization on a chip. The essence of this company's approach is that the DNA probe is attached to electrode pads on the chip through molecular wires (made of a phenylacetylene polymer) (78). After hybridization, DNA linked to a ferrocene redox label is added. When the voltage is raised, a detectable current flows through the system. The aim of this approach is to be able to undergo direct DNA detection in an amplification-free system (79). For a typical clinical sample, that would mean detecting around 10,000 copies of a particular target DNA sequence. Current prototypes of this device are not that sensitive, with detection limits of around 10^7 copies.

CHIP-BASED BIOSENSORS FOR NUCLEIC ACID DETECTION

The evolution of MEMS technology led to the development of a number of biosensors based on physical characteristics of biologic phenomena. Surface plasmon resonance is a technique in which nonamplified DNA sample can be detected directly. Surface plasmon resonance (SPR) is based on intermolecular changes in the refractive index over time taken at the surface of the sensor (80,81). In this technique, a DNA template, amplified or not amplified, is hybridized in a small reservoir containing an optical interface bound with specific oligonucleotide DNA probes. Through the process of complementary-based hybridization, light illuminated through the sensor base will be refracted at an angle greater than in those sensors not demonstrating specific hybridization (82). This process can be calibrated by varying the temperature and is dependent somewhat on time. The specific conditions and kinetics of this interaction, in turn, are characteristic of the degree of sequence complementarity between the DNA template and the cognate probe. Work by Nilsson and colleagues demonstrated the utility of SPR in the detection of clinical samples amplified by PCR for a series of clinically relevant gene markers, including *p53* (83).

Change in the optical path length also has been demonstrated to be an effective means of showing DNA hybridization on a silicon microchip interferometer (84). An *interferometer* is a device consisting of an array of microsized pillars or finger-like projections that are created by etching deep into a silicon wafer.

1. Etch silicon wafer by RIE and fill it with PSG by LPCVD.

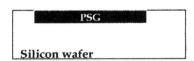

2. Deposit Low stress Si₃N₄ and polysilicon by LPCVD.

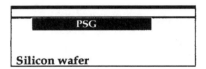

3. Deposit PZT thin film by MOD and top electrode by sputtering.

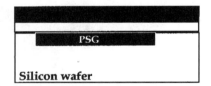

4. Patterning top electrode & PZT and bottom electrode by ion milling and deposit encapsulation layer.

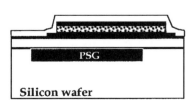

5. Etching holes through PSG by RIE to etch PSG and patterning the beam structure.

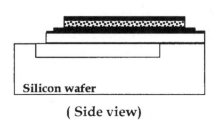 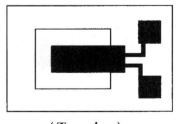

(Side view)   (Top view)

FIGURE 4.11. Process for microfabrication of a microelectromechanical system (MEMS) microcantilever. The process involves the deposition of materials, such as polysilicon, that will be removed at a later point. The design outlined employs the piezoelectric material, lead zirconate titanate, or PZT, which acts as a transducer of force created by the binding of biomolecules to the surface of the device.

Incident light shown onto this area of micropillars will be reflected backward at a predictable angle of efferent light. When the effective thickness of these individual pillars is increased because of a coating of first DNA probes and secondarily hybridized product to the DNA probes, there is a change in the effective path length of this light, creating what are called Perot-Fabry fringes (85). The shift in the angle of the efferent light is proportional to the quantity of DNA hybridized to the affixed probes and thus is an effective way to quantitate DNA. This is achieved because of the specificity of DNA to hybridize only when complete complementarity is maintained.

Exploitation of true MEMS devices only recently have been demonstrated to function as a biosensor (Fig. 4.11). In its truer sense, MEMS devices take advantage of certain mechanical properties of structures that have homologs in the macroscale world. One such device is a so-called *quartz microbalance*, in which bulk monocrystalline quartz or a microfabricated cantilever-like structure is combined biochemically with certain probes of a known mass (86,87). Quartz, having piezoelectric properties, can be put into a high-frequency oscillatory mode in which the frequency of this oscillation is dependent on the mass of the structure. In this case, DNA probes serve as a receptor, which then hybridizes its cognate DNA template, resulting in a structure of increased mass

over that of devices not containing bound DNA (88). The resulting device has a resonant frequency that is shifted downward or lower than those not displaying specific strand hybridization. A quartz microbalance array has been constructed and has been demonstrated to show the high sensitivity of DNA hybridization to as little as 10^{-18} M or approximately 10^{-12} g of target DNA (89). Other researchers have constructed a surface acoustic wave (SAW) sensor employing thin-film piezoelectric materials (90–92). In this case, DNA probes or other biomolecules are immobilized onto a planar surface and set into oscillatory mode by virtue of a microfabricated transmitter on the opposite side is a microfabricated receiver. Broadcast of an oscillatory signal across the piezoelectric field is met at the receiver in a known time, which is dependent on any impedance of that transmitted signal, such as that created by bound DNA. Wang and colleagues demonstrated the utility of the so-called flexural plate wave sensor for the detection of serum-based proteins through their affinity to bind to a monoclonal antibody affixed to the piezoelectric sensor surface (93). McGlennen and colleagues demonstrated how other types of piezoelectric thin films can be applied to structures such as microfabricated diaphragms or microcantilevers that detect mass changes with DNA hybridization (Fig. 4.12). In this case, the microcantilever is set into a fixed oscilla-

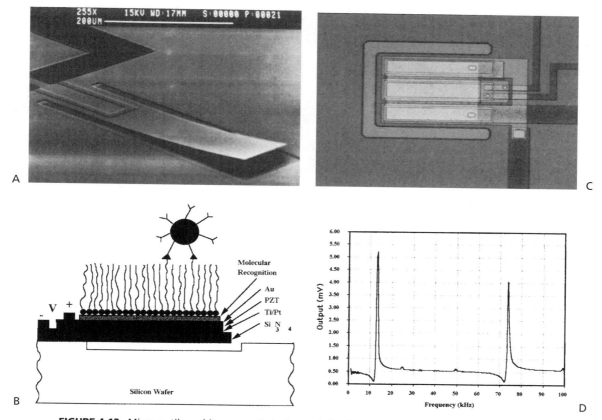

FIGURE 4.12. Microcantilever biosensors. **A**: A piezoresistive device that measures bound material as a function of the change in electrical resistance of a piezoresistive element. **B**: Schematic of a micro-electromechanical system (MEMS) microcantilever biosensor. The surface, prepared with a molecular recognition material, can be adapted for detection of nucleic acid, peptides, proteins, or microparticulate. **C**: Top view of a piezoelectric microcantilever. **D**: One mode of operation is to apply a voltage to the cantilever that sets up an oscillation that is adjusted to its fundamental resonant frequency. Material bound to the surface increases the mass of the oscillating body and produces a shift of the resonant frequency downward in a predictable way.

tory mode that is altered when hybridization between PCR-derived DNA and its cognate oligonucleotide probe takes place. These devices are sensitive to picograms of mass loading but demonstrate the added advantage of their compatibility with on-chip microelectronic circuitry. Taken in total, these sensor systems can achieve high sensitivities not previously observed with addressable array-based approaches, which in turn can be directly linked to microelectronic circuitry resulting in a device that is highly compact and very inexpensive to manufacture.

Each of the preceding approaches involves in some way exploitation of either physical properties inherent to the DNA or the capability of light-based detection systems to resolve isolated areas of DNA hybridization. The last sensor system to be discussed involves the combination of complex nonliving biological systems with a silicon microchip interface, creating what is touted to be a truly universal platform for biosensors of the future.

Cornell and colleagues reported a biosensor that uses an artificial ion channel. This device takes advantage of the sensitive discrimination of naturally occurring receptor systems and the resolution of natural and artificial biomembranes to transduce and amplify signals in highly compact and reproducible systems (94). Briefly, a lipid bilayer is constructed and mixed with a known quantity of the artificial antibiotic gramicidin. Gramicidin exists in a homodimeric form wherein both monomers of the protein reside in a linear conformation. Intact homodimeric gramicidin permits the flow of cations across the lipid membrane through a central pore. To function as a biosensor, one subunit of gramicidin is covalently linked to a specific cellular receptor, such as thyroid-releasing hormone receptor or a hapten directed against some analyte. Another hapten is tethered directed to the lipid membrane. When a ligand, such as thyroid-releasing hormone, binds to its cognate receptor, there is competition between the tethered hapten and the one linked to gramicidin. The result is a disruption in the formation and continuity of the gramicidin transmembrane pores with a net loss of positively charged ions flowing across the membrane through the central pore. Detection of this change in current can occur through a simple connection of a galvanometer, which measures the absolute loss or decrease in current flow and additionally can record the phenomenon as a function of time.

The opportunity to use any of the above listed biosensors is indeed great. By design, many of these approaches can be adapted to a variety of test types, and each has the promise of high sensitivity and specificity. The possibility for miniaturization is also apparent, but the commercial application of these technologies in this case for POC testing in gene-based diagnostics remains to be realized. The greatest challenges lie, however, in the integration of sensing technologies with those "front-end events," such as sample preparation and, in the case of PCR, thermocycler-based assays. The following section discusses what efforts are presently under way in an attempt to integrate chip-based detection systems into a format that involves these other key components.

BRINGING NUCLEIC ACID AND GENE TESTING TO POINT-OF CARE TESTING

The earlier sections of this chapter focused on research and development of novel biosensor platforms. These concepts detail the many ways that nucleic acid-based testing can be done on a microminiaturized format. This section focuses on those efforts, both in the research phase as well as commercialized devices, to assemble an integrated gene testing instrument inclusive of operations for specimen processing, enzymatic amplification, and product detection. To date, the number of research groups and companies dedicated to this process is small but growing rapidly (Table 4.8) (95,96). Moreover, many of these devices are

TABLE 4.8. COMPARISON OF BIOCHIP COMPANIES

Company	Technical Program/Approach
Affymetrix	Genechip arrays, high-density probes per chip
Amersham Pharmacia Biotech	CY3 and CY5 fluorescent dyes for detection by molecular array scanners
Caliper Technologies	Lab-on-a-chip microfluidic technology
Cepheid	Microfluidics for clinical diagnostic applications
Gene Logic	READS microarray technology for expression profiles
Hewlett-Packard	Array scanners
Hyseq	Sequencing by hybridization chips for expression analysis and diagnostics
Micronics	Microfluidics technology development
Millennium Pharmaceuticals	Expression analysis molecular arrays
Molecular Dynamic	Medium density DNA chip (1.5 K spots/chip)
Mosiac Technologies	Acryite polyacrylamide gel arrays
Oncormed	Tumor diagnostics for *p53* using Affymetrix Genechip
Orchid Biocomputer	3-D microfluidic chip for parallel synthesis and screening
PE Applied Biosystems	Integrated genetic testing system focused on single nucleotide polymorphism mapping
Sarnoff Corporation	Microfluidics technology development
Sequana Therapeutics	Variable density DNA chips
Sequanom	Spectrochips for DNA diagnostics by mass spectroscopy
Soane Biosciences	Multiplexed chip for DNA sequencing and fragment analysis
Synteni	Gene expression microarrays (small or medium density platforms)
Xenometrix	Gene expression profiling by microarrays

3-D, three-dimensional.

still very much in their developmental phase, with the key components in beta testing or on the near-term horizon. Thus, the opportunity to evaluate a miniaturized integrated genetic testing system for POC delivery is either just beginning or is still in blueprint phase.

Currently, several compelling integrated technology platforms have been assembled that clearly demonstrate that each of the operational steps of genetic testing done on conventional instrumentation also can be done on a chip or combination of chips. Most advanced among these efforts is a product under development by Cepheid Corporation (Sunnyvale, CA, U.S.A.). Cepheid's MicroBE analyzer is the product of nearly 15 years of development. Derived from research at national laboratories as well as academic institutions, it focuses on two key steps in the genetic testing format, namely, a miniaturized thermal cycling device and an integrated detection system (97,98).

Based on support from the U.S. Department of Defense, Cepheid has demonstrated and optimized the performance of a microchip-based thermal cycling device. This component has its origins from Lawrence Livermore Laboratories (Livermore, CA), where Dr. Allen Northrup was a principal engineer in this project. In brief, the thermal cycling element in the MicroBE analyzer involves the fabrication of a silicon-based heating element and enclosed reservoir. Early work by Dr. Northrup and others demonstrated the importance of pacification of the surface of the silicon microchip to ensure compatibility with reactants in the PCR mixture (99,100). Subsequent prototype development focused on the creation of a plastic insert or sleeve surrounded by a silicon microchip-heating element. The clear advantage of this approach is that silicon, having a high heat capacity, can quickly respond to the input of electric power to heat the microreactor to the appropriate temperatures in the minimal amount of time (101). Similarly, because the entire device is very small and hence its thermal mass slight, the necessary cooling element occurs with near-equal speed. Early data with side-by-side comparisons of the microchip-based thermocycler versus conventional PCR thermocyclers demonstrated that the quality, quantity, and reliability of these miniaturized systems often exceeded that of conventional bench-top instrumentation (102). Importantly, however, the conventional PCR results, consisting of approximately 20 to 35 repetitive cycles of heating and cooling, could be achieved in as little as 30 minutes or less. A focus on the microprocessing control elements demonstrated that this time could be shortened to even less than 20 minutes for certain types of high-efficiency PCR.

Variations on the theme of a silicon chip heater have been described by a number of groups, including researchers at Perkin-Elmer Applied Biosystems (Foster City, CA, U.S.A.). This group's approach was to combine the flexibility of silicon microdevices to be fabricated in large quantities in a multiple-reaction chamber format. Consequently, they produced several devices containing various numbers of reaction wells, ranging from 6 to 48. This group also compared the performance of various reaction volumes, that is, 9 μL to as little as 0.5 μL for the total PCR reaction. Devices have been constructed not only from silicone but also from glass; more recently, attempts have been made in certain types of plastic, such as polycarbonate. In each case, these materials proved to support efficient PCR

amplification of template DNA, typically in much reduced times from that of conventional instrumentation (103).

Efforts by Polla and colleagues demonstrated another version of a silicon chip-based thermocycler wherein secondary treatment of the surface with compounds, such as bovine serum albumin as well as a variety of polymeric materials that increase surface hydrophobicity, work very well with PCR chemistry (104). Their work also focused on the integration of various thermal sensing elements, including microfabricated thermodiodes, thermal couples, and placement of Peltier-type coolers. Recently, exploitation of other silicon processing materials, such as various types of photoresistant materials used to protect and deprotect silicon structures during various chemical etching and metallization steps, also can be used to construct precisely defined reservoirs, channels, valves, and seals (Fig. 4.13A) (105). Use of the materials offers a convenient and cost-effective means to link structurally multiple chip components with interconnecting microfluidic elements on a single piece of silicon (Fig. 4.13B) (106).

Regardless of the performance of individual components in the integrated genetic testing system, the key to success in the commercialization, and hence the success in their application to POC gene-based testing, is the issue related to sample processing and microfluidics (107–109). Modern DNA diagnostic assays face mounting demands to detect organisms or DNA mutations at very low concentrations, often less than 100 copies per milliliter of raw biologic sample, such as blood or urine. Such sensitivities set fundamental physical limitations on the minimum quantities of starting material that will prove to be clinically useful. For example, with PCR, a 50- to 100-μL reaction containing 20 to 100 ng of sample DNA typically can detect as few as 20 copies of a target sequence. In cases where the requirement is to achieve much higher levels of sensitivity, such as often is the case in assays for infectious agents, either new detection modalities are required or a greater amount of sample needs to be processed. In the latter case, the advantages of using microchip-based instrumentation, with its inherent limitations to handle minute quantities of sample, are at odds with these clinical demands of high sensitivity in PCR-based assays. Hence, the consideration of sample processing, and microfluidic control in microchip-based integrated systems requires further discussion.

Under ideal conditions, microchip-based thermocyclers and detection systems are capable of processing sample sizes as small as 0.5 μL. In the clinical laboratory, and more importantly in other environments such as POCT at the bedside or possibly even in at-home applications, the interface between the human hand and the struggle to work with such minute volumes will result in avoidance of these new chip-based technologies. Again, Cepheid Corporation is committed to developing and implementing fluidic systems that attempt to bridge the gap between the easy-to-use large-sample volumes to the world of microstructures and microarrays. Their work is focused on attacking this problem in two fronts. First, their chip-based thermal cycling technology is based on performing high-throughput PCR on relatively large samples. Their beta-tested prototype system can work with volumes as large as 100 μL, which are comparable to those used in conventional molecular

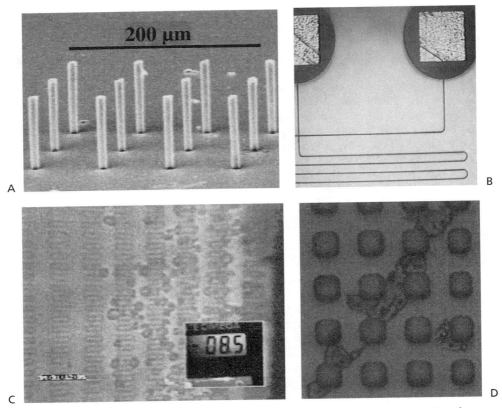

FIGURE 4.13. Various microelectromechanical system (MEMS) Microfluidic Devices. **A**: Use of epoxy resin to create intricate structures, such as the micropillars. **B**: A microcapillary electrophoresis chip created from silicon. **C**: Microfabricated cell separator demonstrates nonturbulent fluid through which cells of different density are sequestered. **D**: The same chip can be used to capture nucleated cells, which stick to the surface material, typically silicon or silicon nitride.

diagnostic laboratories (Fig. 4.13C). This is accomplished first by developing sample-processing modules, which can handle large volumes of liquid sample in a flow through format. Specifically, they have developed a DNA capture chip consisting of a dense array of microfabricated silicone pillars. Early work by Carlson and colleagues demonstrated that anticoagulated whole blood flowing across such a structure would tend to passively permit the flow of red blood cells through the microstructure, where they could be captured and removed as waste (110). White blood cells being inherently sticky finding the silicone surface to be abnormal would tend to be retained and actually stick to the surface (Fig. 4.13D). This process involves a simple flow-through step, the marked enrichment of whole blood such that only the nucleated cellular components are retained. Secondary steps, including flushing the chip with lysis buffers, electrical biasing to retain negatively charged DNA, and rinsing steps, all can be introduced to the device via prepackaged or stored extraction reagents. The net result is retention of high-molecular-weight and high-integrity genomic DNA from samples ranging in volume from 1 to 10 mL.

Transport of the enriched DNA fraction and other fluid elements following extraction has been the focus of several groups, including Caliper Technologies and Aclara Biosciences. As previously discussed, Caliper's trademarked "lab on a chip" approach is based on conventional microfabrication techniques of etching in both glass as well as in silicon to create a network of well-defined microcapillary conduits. Caliper has focused on the use of electrophoresis in electrokinetic control of fluid flow across the chip to deliver samples to distinct biochemical stations where individual assays are taken place in a microreservoir format. Devices developed by Aclara Biosciences focused on single-use flexible 96-well microplates, where each reservoir is connected to a series of microcapillaries. The company's proprietary microfluidics technology enables the accurate measurement, dispensing, and mixing of minute quantities of liquid with volumes as small as 10 to 0.1 μL. Plastic microchips are used that also involve controlling elements and are trademarked under the name Lab Card™.

The challenge to understand the dynamic properties of fluids at this microscale is one that also points to some clear advantages. In general, the creation of microcapillary channels with a cross-sectional dimension as small as 100 μ defines an environment in which fluid typically flows in a laminar (nonturbulent) manner. Hence, fluid can be made to flow at higher velocities (108,111). This phenomenon has a profound impact on the performance of these integrated devices, not only because of the speed by which the assay is completed, but also that certain benefits of the pattern by which certain molecules are diffused in a laminar flow environment can be exploited. In particular, certain molecules are differentially removed laminar fluid streams, resulting in the enrichment of certain molecular species. On the negative side, laminar flow diminishes the opportunity for sample and reagent mixing, which happens readily when turbulent flow occurs in larger-volume streams. One solution to this problem is a so-called lamination of fluids, or the formation of multiple plumes of fluid, which increase the interaction of solutions of different ionic concentrations and viscosity.

Lastly, microfluidic channels and reservoirs are inherently fraught with problems related to the formation of bubbles (50). Whether in the case of PCR reactants within a thermal cycling chamber or the conduction of fluids between chip components in the integrated device, bubbles can prevent as well as occlude the system to completeness. Hence, the central challenge in the development of these systems is to create the optimized interface between the operator and fluid components of the device in the effort to prevent or remove any types of bubbles consequent to pipetting or the motion of the fluid.

In contemplation of POC instruments for genetic testing, the design of the user interface is as important as the functioning of the internal components. In this regard, several investigative groups focused on ways to present minute quantities of fluid to a miniaturized genetic testing system. The approach by Cepheid and others is to accept that the handling of small amounts of fluid by the human hand is in fact a very difficult task. Rather, their system emphasizes the presentation of sample volumes scaled for the subsequent analytic steps; their approach is to embrace the concept of continuous-flow sampling. By this it is meant that only the useful material is collected from a larger volume of sample that is processed. This is achieved by segregating from the main flow of sample only the useful cellular components; the remainder is filtered through as waste. This concept is similar to the process of continuous flow used in other manufacturing industries. In this setting, the system splits sample fluid into smaller streams or regions, such as in heat exchangers, nozzles, arrays, or perforated plates (because fluid-processing strategy must be based on the principle of assuring that every fluid molecule is subjected to the same microenvironment). This same approach can be applied to biochemical analysis in a microchip format. In the case of genetic testing, small portions of the fluid flowing sample can be reacted or otherwise processed at each site as the sample stream passes through the reactor environment. In such a case, this might represent a miniaturized thermocycler device. Reagents can be added to the sample stream at appropriate points along the flow path. Several investigators demonstrated this to work using MEMS-based or microfabricated micropumps (109,112). On completion of the thermal cycling process, the PCR reaction fluid is allowed to flow further along the flow path, perhaps then passing in front of a fluorescence detector or in other cases allowed to react and hybridize on a DNA array-based detection chip. By combining these modalities, a continuous microfluidic flow process is created, and each of the operational steps involved in genetic testing can be accomplished in a fully automated, hands-off platform.

Beyond the concerns of microfluidics, the clear advantage of the microchip-based gene testing system is its adaptability to simple operational control elements. In most cases, a desktop personal computer is sufficient. MEMS and other microelectronic chip devices can be controlled by common software packages, such as LabView™, sold through National Instruments, or those written by a programmer familiar with computer codes such as C++ language. In this way, many versions and embodiments of controlling software can be developed cheaply and can be readily adapted to specific applications. Through a series of simple driven button controls, the sensing elements of the chip can be controlled and programmed to meet the optimal conditions of the biochemical reaction. Other prototype devices for performing complete genetic testing, inclusive of the power supply, the sample presentation port, and each of the microchip components, can be conveniently packaged into a credit card–sized device that might be packaged into a Personal Computer Memory Card International Association (PCMCIA) card format like that typically used for lap-top computer fax-modem devices. This has been demonstrated and can be produced cheaply (about $100), which in many applications might be less than the cost of gene testing through conventional hospital-based molecular diagnostic laboratories.

CONCLUSIONS

Although the prospects for an integrated gene testing device appear to be close at hand, a great deal of testing needs to be done before these systems are ready for use in the patient care environment. The first steps toward molecular diagnostics at the POC have been in the refinement and reduction to simpler formats of the basic methods of nucleic acid extraction and DNA amplification. DNA extraction has been simplified to work on paper and in one-step processes in microtiter plates. To a large extent, improvements in methods to amplify DNA correspond to the bioengineering of these enzymes to work better *in vitro* and to exploit particular functional characteristics. This is true of the newer chemistry platforms, including cleavase, strand displacement, and more robust versions of PCR. The second steps leading to genetics for POC lay in the evolution of new instrumentations that are simpler to use and integrate what has been a series of distinct and separate processes involved in gene testing. Here the emphasis has been on the miniaturization of detection systems, most notably in the form of microaddressable arrays. Although DNA chips are very small, each system typically requires large and expensive instrumentation to use. Several commercial versions of these chips have been approved for clinical assays, but none show any distinct advantages over in-house versions of microarrays, which are clearly lower cost. The prospect of using industrial processes akin to the manufacture of electronic chips is being studied in the form of MEMS-based biosensors. These devices are early in their development cycle but have the potential to be configured into miniature total-analysis systems that combine all the operational steps in gene testing, and hence could be used at the POC. Like microarrays, these devices presently lack the reliability for clinical use and remain largely a research tool.

The pathway to molecular diagnostics at the POC is only at the planning stage; but experience in using molecular genetics in a large reference laboratory suggests that the first steps on that path lead to the introduction of these techniques and the routine use of these tests into the much larger number of moderate-to low-complexity clinical laboratories. In parallel with the maturing of the genetic assays to easy-to-use kits and continued improvements in miniaturized instrumentation, application of molecular genetics testing for physician offices and even consumer outlets may be only a few years away.

REFERENCES

1. Brock TD, Freeze H. Thermus aquaticus gen. n. and sp. n., a non-sporulating extreme thermophile. *J Bacteriol* 1969;98:289–297.
2. Mullis KB, Faloona FA. Specific synthesis of DNA *in vitro* via a polymerase-catalyzed chain reaction. *Methods Enzymol* 1987;155: 335–350.
3. Tindall KR, Kunkel TA. Fidelity of DNA synthesis by the Thermus aquaticus DNA polymerase. *Biochemistry* 1988;27:6008–6013.
4. Jandreski MA. Novel methods of DNA analysis. *Clin Lab Med* 1995; 15:817–837.
5. Eng C, Vijg J. Genetic testing: the problems and the promise. *Nat Biotechnol* 1997;15:422–426.
6. Morgan GJ, Pratt G. Modern molecular diagnostics and the management of haematological malignancies. *Clin Lab Haematol* 1998;20: 135–141.
7. Tang YW, Procop GW, Persing DH. Molecular diagnostics of infectious diseases. *Clin Chem* 1997;43:2021–2038.
8. Baselski VS. The role of molecular diagnostics in the clinical microbiology laboratory. *Clin Lab Med* 1996;16:49–60.
9. Mackay J. The role of genetic testing in breast cancer by the year 2000. *Cancer Treat Rev* 1997;23:S13–S22.
10. Wiedbrauk DL, Werner JC, Drevon AM. Inhibition of PCR by aqueous and vitreous fluids. *J Clin Microbiol* 1995;33:2643–2646.
11. Belec L, Authier J, Eliezer-Vanerot MC, et al. Myoglobin as a polymerase chain reaction (PCR) inhibitor: a limitation for PCR from skeletal muscle tissue avoided by the use of Thermus thermophilus polymerase. *Muscle Nerve* 1998;21:1064–1067.
12. Greenspoon SA, Scarpetta MA, Drayton ML, et al. QIAamp spin columns as a method of DNA isolation for forensic casework. *J Forensic Sci* 1998;43:1024–1030.
13. Harding JD, Gebeyehu G, Bebee R, et al. Rapid isolation of DNA from complex biological samples using a novel capture reagent—methidium-spermine-sepharose. *Nucleic Acids Res* 1989;17: 6947–6958.
14. Lin HJ, Tanwandee T, Hollinger FB. Improved methods for quantification of human immunodeficiency virus type 1 RNA and hepatitis C virus RNA in blood using spin column technology and chemiluminescent assays of PCR products. *J Med Virol* 1997;51:56–63.
15. Pederson NE. Spin-column chromatography for DNA purification. *Anal Biochem* 1996;239:117–118.
16. Raskin S, Phillips JA, Kaplan G, et al. Cystic fibrosis genotyping by direct PCR analysis of Guthrie blood spots. *PCR Methods & Applications* 1992;2:154–156.
17. Rogers C, Burgoyne L. Bacterial typing: storing and processing of stabilized reference bacteria for polymerase chain reaction without preparing DNA—an example of an automatable procedure. *Anal Biochem* 1997;247:223–227.
18. Nickoloff JA. Sepharose spin column chromatography: a fast, nontoxic replacement for phenol:chloroform extraction/ethanol precipitation. *Mol Biotechnol* 1994;1:105–108.
19. Beaulieux F, See DM, Leparc-Goffart I, et al. Use of magnetic beads versus guanidium thiocyanate-phenol-chloroform RNA extraction followed by polymerase chain reaction for the rapid, sensitive detection of enterovirus RNA. *Res Virol* 1997;148:11–15.
20. Brown D, Gold L. RNA replication by Q beta replicase: a working model. *Proc Natl Acad Sci USA* 1996;93:11558–11562.
21. Burg JL, Cahill PB, Kutter M, et al. Real-time fluorescence detection of RNA amplified by Q beta replicase. *Anal Biochem* 1995;230: 263–272.
22. Barany F, Gelfand DH. Cloning, overexpression and nucleotide sequence of a thermostable DNA ligase-encoding gene. *Gene* 1991; 109:1–11.
23. Lyamichev V, Brow MA, Varvel VE, et al. Comparison of the 5′ nuclease activities of taq DNA polymerase and its isolated nuclease domain. *Proc Natl Acad Sci USA* 1999;96:6143–6148.
24. Rossetti S, Englisch S, Bresin E, et al. Detection of mutations in human genes by a new rapid method: cleavage fragment length polymorphism analysis (CFLPA). *Mol Cell Probes* 1997;11:155–160.
25. Kwiatkowski RW, Lyamichev V, de Arruda M, et al. Clinical, genetic, and pharmacogenetic applications of the Invader assay. *Molecular Diagnosis* 1999;4:353–364.
26. Lyamichev V, Mast AL, Hall JG, et al. Polymorphism identification and quantitative detection of genomic DNA by invasive cleavage of oligonucleotide probes. *Nat Biotechnol* 1999;17:292–296.
27. Desjardin LE, Chen Y, Perkins MD, et al. Comparison of the ABI 7700 system (TaqMan) and competitive PCR for quantification of IS6110 DNA in sputum during treatment of tuberculosis. *J Clin Microbiol* 1998;36:1964–1968.
28. Colinas RJ, Bellisario R, Pass KA. Multiplexed genotyping of beta-globin variants from PCR-amplified newborn blood spot DNA by hybridization with allele-specific oligodeoxynucleotides coupled to an array of fluorescent microspheres. *Clin Chem* 2000;46:996–998.
29. Dahlback B. Molecular genetics of venous thromboembolism [Review]. *Ann Med* 1995;27:187–192.
30. Enayat MS, Williams MD, Hill FG. Further simplifications of the factor V: Q506 mutation detection test [Letter, Comment]. *Blood Coagul Fibrinolysis* 1997;8:205.
31. Zehnder JL, Benson RC, Cheng S. A microplate allele-specific oligonucleotide hybridization assay for detection of factor V Leiden. *Diagn Mol Pathol* 1997;6:347–352.
32. Lay MJ, Wittwer CT. Real-time fluorescence genotyping of factor V Leiden during rapid-cycle PCR. *Clin Chem* 1997;43:2262–2267.
33. Gomez E, van der Poel SC, Jansen JH, et al. Rapid simultaneous screening of factor V leiden and G20210A prothrombin variant by multiplex polymerase chain reaction on whole blood [Letter]. *Blood* 1998;91:2208–2209.
34. Stryker J, Coates TJ. Home access HIV testing: what took so long? [Editorial; Comment]. *Arch Intern Med* 1997;157:261–262.
35. Frank AP, Wandell MG, Headings MD, et al. Anonymous HIV testing using home collection and telemedicine counseling: a multicenter evaluation. *Arch Intern Med* 1997;157:309–314.
36. Ramisse V, Patra G, Garrigue H, et al. Identification and characterization of Bacillus anthracis by multiplex PCR analysis of sequences on plasmids pXO1 and pXO2 and chromosomal DNA. *FEMS Microbiol Lett* 1996;145:9–16.
37. Shlyakhov E, Rubinstein E: Anthraxin skin testing: an alternative method for anthrax vaccine and post-vaccinal immunity assessment. *Zentralbl Veterinarmed [B]* 1996;43:483–488.
38. Wiener SL. Strategies for the prevention of a successful biological warfare aerosol attack. *Mil Med* 1996;161:251–256.
39. Persidis A. Pharmacogenomics and diagnostics. *Nat Biotechnol* 1998; 16:791–792.
40. Drews J, Ryser S. The role of innovation in drug development. *Nat Biotechnol* 1997;15:1318–1319.
41. Drews J. Genomic sciences and the medicine of tomorrow. *Nat Biotechnol* 1996;14:1516–1518.
42. Agris CH. Patenting DNA sequences. *Nat Biotechnol* 1998;16:877.
43. Chehab FF. Molecular diagnostics: past, present, and future. *Hum Mutat* 1993;2:331–337.
44. Beugelsdijk TJ. The future of laboratory automation. *Genet Anal* 1991;8:217–220.
45. Marshall A, Hodgson J. DNA chips: an array of possibilities. *Nat Biotechnol* 1998;16:27–31.
46. McGlennen RC. Miniaturization technologies for molecular diagnostics [Review]. *Clin Chem* 2001;47:393–402.
47. Merkens LS, Bryan SK, Moses RE. Inactivation of the 5′-3′ exonu-

cleace of Thermus aquaticus DNA polymerase. *Biochim Biophys Acta* 1995;1264:243–248.

48. Hanaki K, Odawara T, Nakajima N, et al. Two different reactions involved in the primer/template-independent polymerization of dATP and dTTP by Taq DNA polymerase. *Biochem Biophys Res Commun* 1998;244:210–219.

49. Joseph H, Swafford B, Terry S. Medical applications for MEMS devices. *Proceedings of the International Symposium on Test and Measurement,* 1997:399–404.

50. Wilding P, Pfahler J, Bau HH, et al. Manipulation and flow of biological fluids in straight channels micromachined in silicon. *Clin Chem* 1994;40:43–47.

51. Righetti PG, Gelfi C. Capillary electrophoresis of DNA for molecular diagnostics. *Electrophoresis* 1997;18:1709–1714.

52. Kutter JP, Jacobson SC, Ramsey JM. Integrated microchip device with electrokinetically controlled solvent mixing for isocratic and gradient elution in micellar electrokinetic chromatography. *Anal Chem* 1997;69:5165–5171.

53. Jacobson SC, Ramsey JM. Electrokinetic focusing in microfabricated channel structures. *Anal Chem* 1997;69:3212–3217.

54. Jacobson SC, Ramsey JM. Integrated microdevice for DNA restriction fragment analysis. *Anal Chem* 1996;68:720–723.

55. Kearney PP, Aumatell A. Rapid diagnosis of chronic myeloid leukaemia by linking PCR to capillary gel electrophoresis. *Clin Lab Haematol* 1997;19:261–266.

56. Audrezet MP, Costes B, Ghanem N, et al. Screening for cystic fibrosis in dried blood spots of newborns. *Mol Cell Probes* 1993;7:497–502.

57. Pease AC, Solas D, Sullivan EJ, et al. Light-generated oligonucleotide arrays for rapid DNA sequence analysis. *Proc Natl Acad Sci USA* 1994;91:5022–5026.

58. Fodor SP, Read JL, Pirrung MC, et al. Light-directed, spatially addressable parallel chemical synthesis. *Science* 1991;251:767–773.

59. Singh-Gasson S, Green RD, Yue Y, et al. Maskless fabrication of light-directed oligonucleotide microarrays using a digital micromirror array. *Nat Biotechnol* 1999;17:974–978.

60. Lipshutz RJ, Morris D, Chee M, et al. Using oligonucleotide probe arrays to access genetic diversity. *Biotechniques* 1995;19:442–447.

61. Anonymous. To affinity . . . and beyond [Editorial; Comment]. *Nat Genet* 1996;14:367–370.

62. Lipshutz RJ, Fodor SP, Gingeras TR, et al. High density synthetic oligonucleotide arrays. *Nat Genet* 1999;21:20–24.

63. Hacia JG, Brody LC, Chee MS, et al. Detection of heterozygous mutations in BRCA1 using high density oligonucleotide arrays and two-colour fluorescence analysis. *Nat Genet* 1996;14:441–447.

64. Sosnowski RG, Tu E, Butler WF, et al. Rapid determination of single base mismatch mutations in DNA hybrids by direct electric field control. *Proc Natl Acad Sci USA* 1997;94:1119–1123.

65. Edman CF, Raymond DE, Wu DJ, et al. Electric field directed nucleic acid hybridization on microchips. *Nucleic Acids Res* 1997;25:4907–4914.

66. Eggers M, Hogan M, Reich RK, et al. A microchip for quantitative detection of molecules utilizing luminescent and radioisotope reporter groups. *Biotechniques* 1994;17:516–525.

67. Lamture JB, Beattie KL, Burke BE, et al. Direct detection of nucleic acid hybridization on the surface of a charge coupled device. *Nucleic Acids Res* 1994;22:2121–2125.

68. Okamoto T, Suzuki T, Yamamoto N. Microarray fabrication with covalent attachment of DNA using bubble jet technology. *Nat Biotechnol* 2000;18:438–441.

69. Barany F. Genetic disease detection and DNA amplification using cloned thermostable ligase. *Proc Natl Acad Sci USA* 1991;88:189–193.

70. Gerry NP, Witowski NE, Day J, et al. Universal DNA array with polymerase chain reaction/ligase detection reaction (PCR/LDR) for multiplex detection of low abundance mutations. *J Mol Biol* 1999;292:251-262.

71. Witowski NE, Leiendecker-Foster C, Gerry NP, et al. Microarray-based detection of select cardiovascular disease markers. *Biotechniques* 2000;29:936-938, 940, 942.

72. Favis R, Barany F. Mutation detection in K-ras, BRCA1, BRCA2, and p53 using PCR/LDR and a universal DNA microarray. *Ann NY Acad Sci* 2000;906:39–43.

73. Favis R, Day JP, Gerry NP, et al. Universal DNA array detection of small insertions and deletions in BRCA1 and BRCA2. *Nat Biotechnol* 2000;18:561–564.

74. Southern EM, Maskos U, Elder JK. Analyzing and comparing nucleic acid sequences by hybridization to arrays of oligonucleotides: evaluation using experimental models. *Genomics* 1992;13:1008–1017.

75. Southern E, Mir K, Shchepinov M. Molecular interactions on microarrays. *Nat Genet* 1999;21:5–9.

76. Drmanac R, Labat I, Brukner I, et al. Sequencing of megabase plus DNA by hybridization: theory of the method. *Genomics* 1989;4:114–128.

77. Drmanac S, Kita D, Labat I, et al. Accurate sequencing by hybridization for DNA diagnostics and individual genomics. *Nat Biotechnol* 1998;16:54–58.

78. Hodgson J. Shrinking DNA diagnostics to fill the markets of the future. *Nat Biotechnol* 1998;16:725–727.

79. Henke C. DNA-chip technologies. Part 3: what does the future hold? *IVD Technology* 1999;7:37–42.

80. Lawrence CR, Geddes NJ, Furlong DN, et al. Surface plasmon resonance studies of immunoreactions utilizing disposable diffraction gratings. *Biosens Bioelectron* 1996;11:389–400.

81. Millot M-C, Vals T, Martin F, et al. Surface plasmon resonance response of a polymer-coated biochemical sensor. *Proceedings of SPIE, the International Society for Optical Engineering,* 1995:2331.

82. Kai E, Sawata S, Ikebukuro K, et al. Detection of PCR products in solution using surface plasmon resonance. *Anal Chem* 1999;71:796–800.

83. Nilsson P, Persson B, Larsson A, et al. Detection of mutations in PCR products from clinical samples by surface plasmon resonance. *J Mol Recognit* 1997;10:7–17.

84. Thust M, Schoening MJ, Frohnhoff S, et al. Porous silicon as a substrate material for potentiometric biosensors. *Measurement Science & Technology* 1996;7:26–29.

85. Lin VSY, Motesharei K, Dancil KP, et al. A porous silicon-based optical interferometric biosensor. *Science* 1997;278:840–843.

86. Thundat T, Oden PI, Warmack RJ. Microcantilever sensors [Review]. *Microscale Thermophysical Engineering* 1997;1:185–199.

87. Tuller HL, Mlcak R. Inorganic sensors utilizing MEMS and microelectronic technologies [Review]. *Current Opinion in Solid State & Materials Science* 1998;3:501–504.

88. Fauver ME, Dunaway DL, Lilienfeld DH, et al. Microfabricated cantilevers for measurement of subcellular and molecular forces. *IEEE Trans Biomed Eng* 1998;45:891–898.

89. Caruso F, Rodda E. Quartz crystal microbalance study of DNA immobilization and hybridization for nucleic acid sensor development. *Anal Chem* 1997;69:2043–2049.

90. Hussain I, Kumar A, Mangiaracina A, et al. Fabrication of piezoelectric sensors for biomedical applications: materials for Smart Systems II. *Proceedings of the Materials Research Society Symposium,* 1997:459.

91. Zhai J, Cui H, Yang R. DNA based biosensors. *Biotechnol Adv* 1997;15:43–58.

92. Kondoh J, Matsui Y, Shiokawa S, et al. Enzyme-immobilized SH-SAW biosensor. *Sensors & Actuators B Chemical* 1994;199–203.

93. Wang AW, Radwan K, White RM, et al. A silicon-based ultrasonic immunoassay for detection of breast cancer antigens. Transducers 97. *Proceedings of the 1997 International Conference on Solid-State Sensors and Actuators,* 1997:191–194.

94. Cornell BA, Braach-Maksvytis VL, King LG, et al. A biosensor that uses ion-channel switches. *Nature* 1997;387:580–583.

95. Persidis A. Biochips. *Nat Biotechnol* 1998;16:981–983.

96. Persidis A. Biotechnologies to watch. *Nat Biotechnol* 1997;15:1409–1411.

97. Henke C. DNA-chip technologies: state of the art and competing technologies. *IVD Technology* 1998;4:35–44.

98. Petersen K, McMillan W, Kovacs G, et al. The promise of miniaturized clinical diagnostic systems. *IVD Technology* 1998;6:43–49.

99. Northrup MA, Gonzalez C, Hadley D, et al. A MEMS-based miniature DNA analysis system. *Transducer 95'* 1995:764–767.

100. Shoffner MA, Cheng J, Hvichia GE, et al. Chip PCR I. Surface passivation of Microfabricated silicon-glass chips for PCR. *Nucleic Acids Res* 1996;24:375–379.

101. Eggers M, Ehrlich D. A review of microfabricated devices for gene-based diagnostics. *Hematol Pathol* 1995;9:1–15.

102. Cheng J, Shoffner MA, Hvichia GE, et al. Chip PCR. II. Investigation of different PCR amplification systems in microfabricated silicon-glass chips. *Nucleic Acids Res* 1996;24:380–385.

103. Taylor TB, St. John PM, Albin M. DNA analysis on microchips. In: *Micro Total Analysis Systems '98*, Kluwer Academic Publishers, The Netherlands. 1998:261–266.

104. Hsich S, Smith A, Markus, et al. Fabrication and structural characterization of a resonant frequency. *Smart Materials and Structures.* 2001;10:252–263.

105. Despont M, Lorenz H, Fahrni N, et al. High-aspect-ratio, ultrathick, negative-tone near-UV photoresist for MEMS applications. *Proceedings of the IEEE Micro Electro Mechanical Systems*, 1997: 518–522.

106. Burns MA, Mastrangelo CH, Sammarco TS, et al. Microfabricated structures for integrated DNA analysis. *Proc Natl Acad Sci USA* 1996; 93:5556–5561.

107. Zengerle R, Sandmaier H. Microfluidics. *Proceedings of the International Symposium on Micro Machine and Human Science,* 1996:13–20.

108. Mastrangelo CH, Burns MA, Burke DT. Microfabricated devices for genetic diagnostics. *Proc IEEE* 1998;86:1769–1787.

109. Schomburg WK, Fahrenberg J, Maas D, et al. Active valves and pumps for microfluidics. *Journal of Micromechanics & Microengineering* 1993;3:216–218.

110. Carlson RH, Gabel CV, Chan S, et al. Self-sorting of white blood cells in a lattice. *Physical Review Letters* 1997;15:2149–2152.

111. Gravesen P, Branebjerg J, Jensen OS. Microfluidics—a review. *Journal of Micromechanics & Microengineering* 1993;3:168–182.

112. Freiherr G. Micromachines making headway in medical applications. *Medical Device & Diagnostic Industry* 1997;19:50–52.

5

DRY REAGENT PROTHROMBIN TIME AND OTHER HEMOSTASIS METHODS

STEPHEN E. ZWEIG

Point-of-care (POC) tests for hemostasis (blood coagulation) have become increasingly important in recent years. This chapter presents an overview of the wide variety of different diagnostic tests for coagulation that are presently in clinical use. We then focus on an overview of some of the technical, quality control, clinical, and regulatory considerations behind the most commonly used coagulation test, the prothrombin time (PT) test.

REVIEW OF HEMOSTASIS BIOCHEMISTRY

Hemostasis is a complex biological process that can be perturbed by many different disease states and drug therapies. Rapid assessment of a patient's hemostatic state is imperative in many different clinical situations. As a result, POC tests for hemostasis are becoming a routine part of modern health care.

Hemostasis is controlled by a number of biochemical pathways, primarily involving proteolytic enzymes. These are the *intrinsic* coagulation pathway (heparin sensitive, surface triggered, composed of factors XII, XI, IX, and VII), the *extrinsic* coagulation pathway (heparin insensitive, thromboplastin triggered, composed of factor VII), and the *common* pathway (composed of factors X, V, prothrombin, and fibrinogen). These pathways, and their associated clot formation and degradation, are in turn regulated by a number of other coagulation-related enzymes (1).

Because hemostasis is complex, it can be monitored by a variety of tests. Each test monitors the performance of a different part of the coagulation pathway. A graph showing an overview of the biochemistry of hemostasis and some of the tests used to monitor hemostasis is shown in Figure 5.1.

COMMONLY USED HEMOSTASIS TESTS

Depending on the clinical indication, different types of diagnostic tests are used. An overview (2) of the various types of hemostasis diagnostic tests, their indications, applications, and limitations is shown in Table 5.1.

Point-of-Care Hemostasis Tests

Although hemostasis tests originated as central laboratory tests, clinical technology now has enabled a number of them to be implemented as POC tests. Some of these POC tests are shown (3) in Table 5.2.

Prothrombin Time Testing

To focus more specifically on some of the technical, quality assurance, and regulatory considerations involved in POC hemostasis tests, we have chosen prothrombin time (PT) as an example. PT is the most frequently performed hemostasis test because, unlike the other hemostasis tests, which are used primarily for hospitalized patients, PT testing is used for the routine monitoring of patients on oral anticoagulants, such as warfarin or coumadin.

Warfarin is indicated for many disease conditions, including atrial fibrillation (AF), mechanical heart valves, and deep vein thrombosis (4). Currently, about 2.5 million patients in the United States are receiving warfarin treatment, and this number is expanding at an annual rate of about 15%.

Warfarin is a vitamin K antagonist, which inhibits the activity of vitamin K–dependent coagulation factors in the extrinsic coagulation pathway (e.g., factors II, VII, and X). Although warfarin is highly effective, it is notoriously challenging to use. It has a narrow therapeutic range and requires frequent monitoring and dosage adjustment. Its pharmacokinetic half-life is variable but averages about 2 days (5).

Prothrombin time testing is an important POC test because the cost and poor access of central-site testing discourage the frequency of PT testing required for optimal anticoagulation management and thus can compromise patient outcomes. For example, a 1995 government patient outcomes research team (PORT) study estimated that, for AF alone, 40,000 strokes per year could be prevented if AF patients were properly treated with warfarin (6). As a result, there is significant medical interest in portable, low-cost, easy-to-use, PT devices suitable for the POC environment and also for patient performed self-tests in the home environment.

It should be noted that numerous parallels exist between POC testing of PT in the early 2000s and POC (home) blood glucose testing in the early 1980s. Home blood glucose tests are in many ways the prototypical POC test. Twenty years ago, when they were first introduced, they were somewhat controversial in the clinical community and had to overcome skepticism about their safety and efficacy. The Diabetes Control and Complication Trials (DCCT) (7), however, as well as other

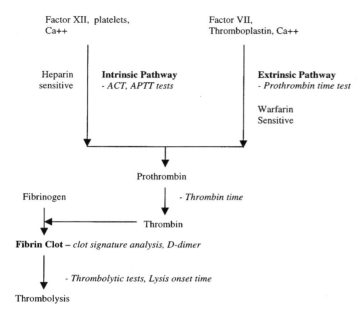

FIGURE 5.1. Simplified model of the intrinsic and extrinsic coagulation pathways involved in common hemostasis clinical tests. Schematic showing the major intrinsic and extrinsic coagulation pathways involved in hemostasis and some of the associated clinical tests.

large-scale clinical trials, clearly demonstrated that the devices significantly improved patient outcomes. Thus, over a 20-year period, home blood glucose testing became the standard of care for diabetic patients. Although DCCT-like trials are extremely complex and expensive and likely to be beyond the means of private industry to finance, DCCT-like trials have been proposed for home PT testing as well (8).

Point-of-Care Prothrombin Time Tests

The development of POC tests of PT has lagged behind the development of blood glucose tests by almost a generation; this is due to a number of factors. Blood glucose tests measure the level of a single, well-defined, nontemperature-sensitive analyte (glucose) that is present in high concentration. By contrast, PT measures the function of a more complex enzymatic pathway, where each enzyme is present in a variable amount, has a temperature-sensitive reaction profile, and is present at levels far below the levels of glucose in whole blood. Not surprisingly, POC tests of PT have been technically challenging for manufacturers to develop.

An additional factor has been the more difficult regulatory environment. After blood glucose tests were first developed, government requirements for safety, accuracy, and ease of use

TABLE 5.1. COMMONLY USED HEMOSTASIS, THROMBOLYSIS, AND THROMBOSIS TESTS

Diagnostic Pivots	Indications, Applications, and Limitations
Activated clotting time (ACT, ACT-Plus)	Surgery, invasive procedures, hemodialysis, arteriovenous and venovenous dialysis
ACT>= target threshold (e.g., 400 s)	CPB, PCTA (high heparin levels strong contact activator in reagents)
ACT<= target threshold	ECMO, stents, catheter sheath removal, pharmacologic agents (low heparin levels, moderate activator)
Activated partial thromboplastin time	Heparin anticoagulation monitoring—indications listed above (low heparin levels), intrinsic coagulation screening, and monitoring treatment (e.g., hemophilia A)
Clot signature analysis (CSA), TEG, others	Transplantation, CPB, protracted surgery
D-dimer (XL-FDP)	Qualitative only, quantitative under development; DIC, PE, deep venous thrombisis, preeclampsia, reactive fibrinolysis
Fibrinogen	Preanalytic processing required; under development for whole blood at point of care; thrombolytic therapy; 1° (congenital) and 2° (acquired consumptive coagulopathy—DIC, liver disease), hypofibrinogenemia; after surgery, ECMO
Heparin dose-response	Improved precision in monitoring anticoagulation and relative insensitivity to hemodilution and hypothermia; various heparin management systems/panels
Platelet count and function	Transfusion therapy, drug effects, screening for acquired and congenital platelet problems
Prothrombin time (PT), INR	Warfarin anticoagulation monitoring, extrinsic coagulation screening—bedside, clinics, physician office laboratory, home monitoring, other settings
Thrombin time (TT, HNTT, HiTT)	Determining or predicting response to thrombolytics, tracking lytic state; tests for thrombolytics (e.g. streptokinase, TPA, urokinase) and LOT are under development or in clinical trials
Thrombolysis	Determining or predicting response to thrombolytics, tracking lytic state; tests for thrombolytics (e.g. streptokinase, TPA, urokinase) and LOT are under development and clinical trials
Thrombosis	Suggested in acute myocardial infarction, PE, stroke; clinical validation and point-of-care test pending

CPB, cardiopulmonary bypass; PCTA, percutaneous coronary transluminal angioplasty; ECMO, extracorporeal membrane oxygenation; TEG, thromboelastography; XL-FDP, crosslinked fibrin degradation product; DIC, disseminated intravascular coagulation; PE, pulmonary embolism; INR, international normalized ratio; TPA, tissue plasminogen activator; LOT, lysis onset time.

TABLE 5.2. HEMOSTASIS TECHNOLOGIES FOR POINT-OF-CARE TESTING

Manufacturer	Tests	Device	Principle	Detected Clotting Parameter
American Diagnostica (Greenwich, CT, U.S.A.)	D-dimer (qualitative)	SimpliRed	Hemagglutination	Agglutination of antibody coated red cells
American Labor (Raleigh, NC, U.S.A.)	PT, aPTT, platelet function	CoaCARD APACT	Turbidity	Detection of change in optical density during mechanical mixing
Avocet Medical (San Jose, CA, U.S.A.)	PT	AvoSure PT	Optical observation of rhodamine-110 fluorescence	Thrombin generation with fluorescent substrate
Roche/Boehringer Mannheim (Indianapolis, IN, U.S.A.)	PT, aPTT	CoaguChek Plus and Pro	Optical pattern recognition	Change in laser interference pattern from slowing of red cell motion;
	PT	Coaguchek	Optical observations of paramagnetic iron oxide particle motion	Slowing of motion of paramagnetic iron oxide particles in pulsating magnetic field
Cardiovascular Diagnostics (Raleigh, NC, U.S.A.)	PT, PT-ONE, aPTT, HMT, LOT Platelet function	TAS	Optical observations of paramagnetic iron oxide particle motion	Same as above; thrombolysis releases particles and restores motion for LOT
Dade International (Miami, FL, U.S.A.)	Platelet function	PFA-100	Pressure	Change in pressure across porous aperture when platelet aggregates occlude openings
HemoSense (Milpitas, CA, U.S.A.)	PT	INR (in development)	Electrochemical	Detection of electrochemical changes as sample coagulates
LifeScan (Milpitas, CA, U.S.A.)	PT	Rubicon (in development)	Optical	Optical changes as sample coagulates
International Technidyne (Edison, NJ, U.S.A.)	ACT, FIB, AMS, PT, aPTT, TT, HNTT, HiTT, ACT-Plus, and LR PT, aPTT	Hemochron series Hemochron Jr. Pro Time	Magnet position Fluid oscillation	Detection of change in magnet position in a slowly rotating reagent-filled tube; Optical detection of slowing of oscillatory motion in a test channel
Medtronic HemoTec (Parker, CO, U.S.A.)	PT, aPTT, HMS, LRACT, HRACT, HemoSTATUS	ACT II HepconHMS	Plunger motion	Optical detection of change in the fall rate of a plunger assembly that is raised and lowered

PT, prothrombin time; aPTT, activated partial thromboplastin time; HMT, hematocrit; LOT, lysis onset time; PFA-100, phosphonoformatic acid 100; INR, international normalized ratio; ACT, activated coagulation time; FIB, fibrinogen; AMS, altered mental status; TT, thromboplastin time; HNTT, *heparin neutralized thrombin time*; HiTT, high-dose thrombin time; LR, *activated clotting time low range*; LRACT, *low range activated clotting time*; HRACT, *high range activated clotting time.*

became more stringent on an almost yearly basis, at times outpacing available technology in the field. Although somewhat more stringent requirements now apply to blood glucose monitors as well, these monitors were able to develop to a relatively mature state first. By contrast, POC tests of PT tests must enter the market at a much higher degree of maturity.

Technical Principles

Several principles are common for all POC tests of PT. The tests work with fingerstick samples, possibly obtained by unskilled users. Thus, the ease of sample application and the ability to function with minimal sample sizes are important considerations.

The PT test itself typically takes place in a plastic cartridge or test strip reaction element. The reaction element must not distort the coagulation reaction and typically will be made of a coagulation neutral material (9). Because the PT test is temperature sensitive, keeping the reaction element at a temperature at which the reaction kinetics are highest, typically around 37 - 40°C, enhances test precision. At this reaction-speed maximum,

small perturbations in temperature have only a small effect on the PT reaction (10), and thus temperature effects are minimized.

The reaction element typically contains thromboplastin (which is necessary to initiate coagulation), additional agents to modulate the PT reaction, a detection system, and appropriate instrumentation to read the reaction.

The various instruments used for POC testing of PT have a number of elements in common (11,12). These devices typically use a stage with a heated optics block, a microprocessor, and display means to output the results of the test. Optionally, the devices may also contain a time and date clock, an onboard database storing past patient results, a printer interface, and a modem or computer interface (13). Usually the display prompts and user interface are simplified to promote ease of use. To promote portability, the devices typically use both AC adapter power and battery power.

By contrast, larger differences exist between the reagents used for the various POC tests of PT. Each test has a slightly different biochemistry, which can act to influence the accuracy and clinical utility of the assay. Some of these biochemical issues are discussed in the following sections.

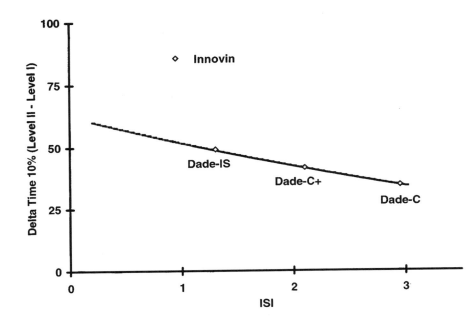

FIGURE 5.2. Effect of r-DNA thromboplastin on the sensitivity of point-of-care prothrombin time (PT) assays. Effect of different thromboplastins on a point-of-care PT assay. Membrane-based reaction test strips were made with thromboplastins with International Sensitivity Index (ISI) values ranging from 0.92 (Dade Innovin recombinant DNA thromboplastin) to 2.8 (Dade C rabbit brain thromboplastin). These were treated with Sigma level I (international normalized ratio, or INR of 1.0) and level II (INR 3.0) controls. As the sensitivity of the thromboplastin decreased (higher ISI), the sensitivity, or Δ, of the point-of-care PT assay also decreased. Note the high sensitivity achieved using the r-DNA thromboplastin.

Thromboplastin

Thromboplastin is a naturally occurring lipoprotein released by the endothelium when cellular damage occurs. It interacts with coagulation factor VII to stimulate the extrinsic coagulation pathway (14). All PT tests rely on this interaction between thromboplastin and factor VII. Point-of-care PT tests use thromboplastin stored in a reaction element in a dry form and are thus often referred to as *dry-reagent tests*.

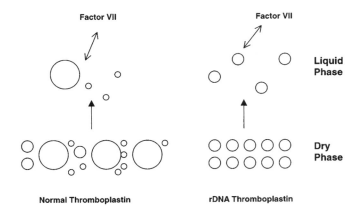

FIGURE 5.3. Effect of r-DNA thromboplastin on a dry-reagent prothrombin time (PT) test. Schematic showing the difference between normal thromboplastin and r-DNA thromboplastin in a point-of-care PT test. Normal thromboplastin consists of a heterogeneous mixture of thromboplastin micelles, with a poorly defined phase transition between the dry state and the fully hydrated liquid state. By contrast, r-DNA thromboplastin has a more uniform micelle population and has a sharper phase transition between the dry state and the fully hydrated liquid state. As a result, the factor VII component of the sample sees a more uniformly reacting thromboplastin population, and acts in a more well-defined manner.

Although in theory there is concern that natural thromboplastin released as a result of tissue damage from a fingerstick might interfere with a dry reagent PT test, in practice no such effect is observed (15).

These dry-reagent PT tests differ from liquid-phase PT tests in one important manner. In a liquid-phase PT test, the thromboplastin is predissolved in the liquid phase, and the factor VII component of the sample comes into contact with fully hydrated and stable thromboplastin. By contrast, in a dry-reagent PT test, the thromboplastin is stored in a dry state and is hydrated while in full contact with the factor VII component of the sample. As a result, the factor VII component of a sample in a dry-reagent PT test is exposed to a wide variety of intermediate thromboplastin conformational states while the thromboplastin rehydrates. These "intermediate transition states" can act to distort the PT reaction unless the system and thromboplastin are selected to minimize this effect. This is shown in Figures 5.2 and 5.3.

Using a thromboplastin that has a sharp phase transition between the dry state and the liquid state can minimize this effect (16). Synthetically relipidated recombinant DNA (r-DNA) thromboplastin typically consists of a very uniform population of micelles, each of which can transition from the dry state to a liquid state in a consistent way. For this reason, r-DNA thromboplastins help improve the accuracy of point-of-care PT tests.

At present, some point-of-care PT devices use r-DNA thromboplastin, and some use natural thromboplastin.

Calcium

Fresh fingerstick samples typically contain enough calcium to initiate coagulation without the need for additional calcium in the reaction cartridge. If use with citrate anticoagulated proficiency samples, plasma, or venous blood is desired, extra calcium may be added to the reaction cartridge to overcome the effect of the citrate anticoagulant. Some POC testing of PT devices contain added calcium, and some do not.

Heparin Antagonists

Many patients receiving oral anticoagulants may be in transition from heparin treatment. Heparin can interfere with the PT reaction. To reduce the effect of this heparin interference, the reaction cartridge may contain a heparin antagonist such as Polybrene (Sigma-Aldrich, Saint Louis, MO) (17). Different POC PT tests may contain different levels and types of heparin antagonists and thus may differ in their relative susceptibility to heparin interference.

Coagulation Detection Means

Coagulation detection means can include red cells endogenous to the fingerstick sample (18), magnetic microparticles (19), fibrin-mediated viscosity change (20), fluorescent thrombin substrates (21), and electrochemical agents (22). All have the common purpose of enabling the system to detect when the onset of coagulation has occurred. Detection methods range from laser light scattering, optical observation of magnetically oscillating microparticles, pressure-induced movement, onset of fluorescence, and onset of electrochemical change.

Algorithms

The algorithm necessary to transform the data from a dry-reagent PT test into an international normalized ratio (INR) value may or may not resemble the classic liquid-phase PT reaction equations. This is because the data collected may be quite different. The classic PT reaction measures the time elapsed between the onset of coagulation and the first unambiguous detection of clot activity. By contrast, because of the effects of thromboplastin rehydration, dry-reagent PT tests may take longer for coagulation to initiate. Additionally, it is common for dry-reagent PT tests to take data beyond the initial onset of coagulation and then to determine the initial onset of coagulation by extrapolation or interpolation techniques.

Although all POC dry-reagent PT tests should output results that agree with liquid-based laboratory reference PT tests, the internal calculations that each assay uses are typically individualized to that specific system.

Calibration

Point-of-care PT tests are typically factory calibrated. To do this, the manufacturer will calibrate relative to a standard laboratory reference system that is itself calibrated by the best available methods. Ideally, the system should be traceable to World Health Organization (WHO) International Reference Preparation (IRP) thromboplastin, which is the only recognized world standard (23). The present official IRP, rTF/95, is a pure synthetic recombinant human thromboplastin.

Each batch of reagents is subjected to a series of clinical tests with the laboratory reference standard. In these tests, the results from a patient's fingerstick sample on the POC instrument are compared with the fresh citrate anticoagulated plasma results (obtained from a venous draw from the same patient) on the laboratory reference standard. The instrument calibration setting is chosen to match best the results from the POC PT device with the reference standard.

Under proper storage conditions, this factory calibration is expected to remain constant until the test reagent cartridge exceeds its expiration date. Indeed, the expiration date is normally defined as the time in which a reagent cartridge, when stored according to the product instructions for use, continues to perform within the tolerances specified during factory calibration.

The factory-determined calibration setting for the reagent cartridge is communicated to a PT device by manual setting of calibration codes, photo-optical reading of optical patterns encoded on a reagent cartridge, an electronic calibration chip, or a combination of these.

It should be noted that, despite efforts to standardize PT tests by use of the INR system, significant calibration and performance differences still exist between central laboratory PT tests (24–27). Although these differences in central laboratory calibration and performance exist even if no POC devices are used, POC tests of PT tend to bring these issues to the forefront. The normal tendency is to believe that whenever a discrepancy between a POC PT device and a central laboratory PT test exists, the POC device must be in error. Because POC tests of PT use fresh samples, thus avoiding most preanalytical errors, this is often not the case. Whenever possible, when comparative studies are done, it is recommended that the reference samples be handled carefully and that preferably more than one reference instrument be used.

Quality Control

Scientific Considerations

Although daily testing with two levels of liquid quality control (QC) reagents (daily liquid QC) is normal for laboratory-based PT tests, such tests can more than triple the costs and time required to do a PT test and can thus impose a considerable burden on POC PT users. As a result, there is considerable interest in finding alternate QC methods that can ensure test quality while lessening the burden on the user (28).

At an abstract level, QC is done on a reagent-instrument system to detect failures in the reagent, instrument, or user mode of operation. If the function of each individual system component can be adequately verified without the time and expense of daily liquid QC testing, daily liquid QC testing is redundant. Such a process of elucidating all system failure modes, examining their root cause, and methods of detection is called a *failure modes and effects analysis* (FMEA). The U.S. Food and Drug Administration (FDA) now requires FMEA analysis as an essential part of design control for all modern medical devices. To show that daily liquid QC is redundant and that alternate QC methods are sufficient, a complete FMEA analysis should be conducted on the reagent, instrument, and various modes of user interaction. Typically, such FMEA analysis will show that a comprehensive alternate QC program must provide separate tests for all these components.

Alternate QC methodologies presently used include unitized "high-low" controls built into the reagent cartridge (29), use of electronic controls (30), and use of a combination of electronic controls with ancillary alternate QC controls that assess reagent status, such as integrating time and temperature indicators and humidity indicators (31).

Reagent Quality Control

Dry reagents, such as the typically used POC tests of PT, differ from liquid reagents in a number of ways. Liquid reagents typically are stored in a lyophilized form in small vials, each vial usually containing enough reagent for 20 to 100 tests. Every few days, a new vial is opened, a clinician adds a measured amount of water or buffer, and the reagent is allowed to rehydrate. As a result, liquid reagents can vary on a day-to-day basis, depending on the pipetting skill of the particular user and on that day's reagent storage conditions. Here it is standard laboratory practice to do at least two QC tests on each day's batch of reagents. Typically, this will be one test with a "low" QC liquid control, followed by one test with a "high" QC liquid control. This helps to spot reconstitution errors and improperly adjusted equipment.

By contrast, POC PT dry reagents are manufactured in very large batches (usually 50,000 or more tests per lot) and are subjected to a very high degree of manufacturer internal QC and process control (usually involving about 1,000 QC tests per lot). The manufacturer tests for consistency within the lot and assigns an expiration date to the lot, such that to a high degree of statistical certainty, all reagent tests within the lot will perform to the manufacturer's label claims for accuracy until the lot reaches its expiration date. Typically, the manufacturer then individually packs in foil each reagent test to guard against environmental factors such as light and humidity.

Under such conditions, dry-reagent tests do not need to be reconstituted by users on a day-to-day basis and thus can avoid the issues of day-to-day reconstitution variability that plague liquid-reagent tests. In practice, only two factors—excessive storage temperature or breach of foil integrity resulting from improper handling, both of which are beyond the control of the manufacturer—typically degrade unit-packed dry-reagent tests.

In the past, issues of excessive storage temperature were handled by printing a maximum storage temperature warning and an expiration date on the test strip box. A simple printed warning can fail, however, if, unknown to the user, the recommended storage temperature is exceeded during transportation or storage. This can happen if test reagents are inadvertently left on a loading dock, stored in a car trunk, or such. More recently, some manufacturers have included integrating time and temperature indicators on their reagents. Such integrating time and temperature indicators give the user a visual indication whenever recommended storage conditions have been exceeded. To do this, the temperature-stability properties of the reagent are first extensively characterized, and a suitable time-temperature indicator is designed that closely matches the thermal stability of the reagent. A properly designed indi-cator will give a visual warning before the reagent becomes significantly impaired.

In a similar manner, some manufacturers also now pack indicating desiccant with each individual reagent foil pack. This can warn the user if improper handling has damaged the foil pack.

Instrument Quality Control

Early electronic controls did not fully mimic the response of a test strip reacting with a sample and thus did not fully test all aspects of a meter's function. By contrast, more modern electronic controls attempt to mimic fully all aspects of a test-strip reaction, including the subtle changes that occur when the reactions are run at improper temperatures. Although simple to use, the technology behind these controls is fairly complex. A schematic showing the principles of operation for a modern POC PT electronic control (EC) (32) is shown in Figure 5.4. To illustrate more clearly the complexity behind modern electronic controls, the technical aspects of this particular control are discussed in some detail.

Figure 5.4 shows a schematic diagram of a modern EC interacting with an AvoSure PT meter optics block. The AvoSure PT meter's optics block consists of an electrically heated support stage 27, containing an optical window 30 through which light 22 emitted from the meter's light source 21 can pass. The meter additionally contains an optional fluorescence filter 24 and a photodetector 26. In normal use, meter light 22 travels through the optics window 30 and illuminates the EC's fluorescent reagent target. Fluorescent light 23 travels through filter 24 and after filtration illuminates photodetector 26. The meter is controlled by a microprocessor 29, which initiates test timing in response to inputs from strip detect and sample detection electrodes 28.

The EC has an optical shutter 12, placed on a circuit board 10, which interfaces with the AvoSure PT meter's optics block. The EC additionally contains electrodes 14 that interact with the strip detect and blood detect electrodes 28 on the AvoSure PT meter's optics block 20. The EC also contains a thermocouple 11 that performs an independent measurement of the temperature of the meter's heated optics block 27.

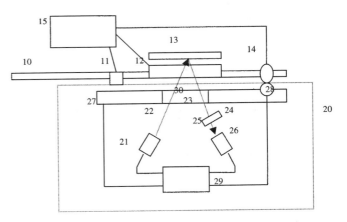

FIGURE 5.4. Modern point-of-care electronic control.

The optical shutter has a backing **13** consisting of Rhodamine 110 mixed with epoxy. The Rhodamine 110 retains its normal fluorescence activity when mixed with the epoxy, and the epoxy provides a way to affix the Rhodamine 110 to the back of the optical shutter **12** in a durable and permanent manner.

The active elements on the circuit board are controlled by a Texas Instruments TSS400-S3 sensor signal processor **15**, which is a combination microcontroller, liquid crystal display driver, and A/D converter. The TSS400 additionally contains 2K bytes of programmable EEPROM, which contains the algorithm needed to drive the system.

When turned on (switches not shown), the EC initially turns the optical shutter to a fully opaque mode. Electrodes **14** connecting to the strip present sensors **28** on the meter's optics block **20** are switched to conducting mode (resistance was lowered) to allow the Avocet Meter to detect that a test strip was inserted into the optics block. The meter then initiates a warmup sequence.

On reaching proper temperature, the meter then sends a signal via its sensor electrodes **28** to the EC electrodes **14** to inform the EC that the meter is now warmed up. After the EC is informed that the meter is now ready to proceed, the EC then reduces the resistance across a second set of electrodes **14a** (not shown), which interact with the blood present sensors **28a** (not shown) on the meter's optics block. This resistance drop normally is used to signal the application of blood to the reagent strip. Here it is used to signal the meter to proceed even though no blood has actually been applied.

The microcontroller **15** on the EC consults an algorithm and selectively switches the liquid crystal optical shutter **12** to an increasingly transparent mode as a function of a number of variables, including time, the setting of the EC (e.g., Level I or II control, etc.), and the temperature of the meter's optics stage **27** as measured by temperature sensor **11**. The meter optical system **20** observes the fluorescent backing **13** through the optical shutter **12** and observes a progressive increase in overall fluorescence as a function of time and temperature.

Quality Control for U.S. Professional Tests and Ex-U.S. Home Tests

The FMEA-based alternate QC approach is generally understood by most regulatory agencies and is accepted for home PT tests outside the United States (Canada, Europe, and elsewhere) and for POC PT tests in the United States that are conducted by health care professionals. Typically, such a FMEA-based alternate QC approach will call for daily use of electronic controls and daily observations of the reagent time-temperature indicators and humidity indicators (if any). On a less frequent basis, typically for each new lot of reagents, two levels of liquid controls also are used as an overall system check.

Quality Control for Home Prothrombin Time Tests in the United States

The drawback of the FMEA approach is that this analysis requires a deep understanding of each system's specific technology. Although the system's manufacturer may possess such understanding and may be able to document it in detail, such documents are, by necessity, complex to review. Additionally, acceptance of the FMEA approach requires "trust," for example, an assumption that the system's manufacturer will, in fact, follow its legally mandated internal manufacturing process controls. As a result, irrespective of any type of scientific FMEA analysis, high-frequency liquid control use for most home PT devices is presently mandated by U.S. regulatory agencies (33). This has the net effect of requiring home users to expend more than 66% of their test reagents in QC testing for each day of use. Counting the cost of liquid controls, these regulations raise the cost per day of testing from $6.00 to $26.00.

Although these regulations are well meaning, it is not clear whether the present U.S. QC regulations on home PT systems are in the best interests of overall public health. To illustrate this point, a smoke detector analogy may be appropriate. When they work, smoke detectors save lives, but smoke detectors sometimes fail. A hypothetical smoke detector QC regulation requiring everyone to test their smoke detectors each day by first building a small fire and then building a large fire would find these failed units. The burden of such QC testing, however, would discourage nearly everyone from installing smoke detectors in the first place. Thus, in this example, such a QC regulation would have the unwanted effect of decreasing overall public safety.

Clearly, a sound QC regulatory approach must consider both the burden (costs, frequency of injury resulting from QC barriers to testing) and the benefits (frequency of injury that could be prevented by QC) of mandated QC protocols. Attempts should be made to quantify both factors, with the goal of finding a balance that best promotes overall public health.

Clinical Aspects

At present, there are three primary ways to manage prothrombin time testing: (a) *routine care*—infrequent care done by clinicians who do not specialize in PT testing and warfarin management; (b) *anticoagulation clinics*—high-volume PT testing done by clinicians who specialize in PT testing and warfarin management; and (c) *patient self-testing* using POC PT tests. The results from each testing modality, in terms of the frequency that a typical patient tests in a clinically tolerable (34) range, taken from the work of Chiquette and colleagues (35) and Bernardo (36), is shown in Table 5.3. A number of other studies (37,38) also showed that patient self-testing improves the percentage of time that a patient is in the correct therapeutic range from about 50% (routine care) to about 80%. Samsa and Matchar (8) reviewed the work in this area.

The data suggest that patient self-testing is superior to other testing modalities. A major reason for this is that self-testing enables PT tests to be performed at a higher frequency. This higher frequency more closely matches the pharmacokinetics of warfarin, enabling deviations to be spotted and corrected quickly.

TABLE 5.3. PERCENTAGE OF PATIENT TESTS BETWEEN INR 2–5 FOR ROUTINE CARE, ANTICOAGULATION CLINIC, AND PATIENT-SELF-TESTING[a]

	Routine Care (Chiquette)	Anticoagulation Clinic (Chiquette)	Patient self-testing (Bernardo)
Average test frequency	10.7 tests/yr	12.6 tests/yr	52 tests/yr
% tests below INR 2.0: at risk of stroke	23.8%	13%	12.3%
% tests between INR 2.0–5.0	57.2%	72%	86.6%
% tests above INR 5.0: at risk of hemorrhage	19%	15%	4.6%

INR, international normalized ratio.
[a]In this study, the percentage of tests falling within three clinically relevant INR regions, INR <2.0, INR 2–5, and INR >5.0 was compared using the results from two different clinical studies. The routine care Vs anticoagulation clinic care data were taken from the high-INR-target (heart-valve) population of Table 2 in Chiquette E, Amato MG, Bussey HI. Comparison of an anticoagulation clinic with usual health care. *Arch Intern Med* 1998; 158: 1641–1647, with permission, where the percentage of tests between INR 2–5 = 100 – (% tests <INR 2.0 + %tests > INR 5.0). The patient self-testing data were taken from the high-INR-target heart-valve patient population of Table 3 in Bernardo A. Post-conference session: experience with patient self-management of oral anticoagulation. *Journal of Thrombosis and Thrombolysis* 1996; 2: 321–325, with permission.

Regulatory Aspects

In the United States, the regulatory aspects of POC PT tests are quite complex. In contrast to the first blood glucose monitoring devices, which were developed prior to 1976 and the implementation of the FDA medical device amendments, and thus received a regulatory "grandfather" status, POC PT tests are regulated much more stringently.

Historically, POC PT devices in the United States have been required to go through two to three cycles of FDA 510(k) review. The first 510(k) cycle, for professional use clearance, is typically designed to demonstrate that the device can give adequate performance, relative to a predicate device and reference system, in the hands of skilled, trained, medical professionals. On clearance, such devices may be sold to larger clinics and laboratories that comply with the Clinical Laboratory Improvement Act (CLIA) regulations for moderately complex devices.

To be marketed for physician's office use, or prescription home use, POC PT devices historically have been required to go through a second 510(k) cycle of clinical testing. This second 510(k) is designed to demonstrate that a large population of average lay users can maintain proficiency with the device over a significant period. The trials also are used to prove that the device is robust enough to operate under home conditions for extended periods and return clinically acceptable results. On this second 510(k) premarket clearance, the device is cleared for home use. To obtain a waiver for professional use under the CLIA 1988 regulations, a third 510(k) has been required. This third 510(k) combines the two previous 510(k) submissions into one file. At this point, the product is CLIA waived, and it then may be used by the average health care professional. Historically, the road to full approval has been a long, difficult, and uncertain process, which few companies have successfully completed. Fortunately, the FDA has recently started attempts to bring more order and coherence to this area (39).

Reimbursement for POC PT devices is presently in a state of flux. Although other countries, such as Germany, reimburse for patient use of POC PT devices (40), U.S. government reimbursement has been more problematic. Historically, the U.S.

Health Care Finance Administration (HCFA) reimbursement policies have been oriented toward hospital and clinic PT tests. Reimbursement has been constrained by stipulations that the PT testing be done in either a laboratory that is physically connected to a hospital (either on hospital grounds or through a connecting passage), or they may be done in a laboratory under supervision of the treating physician. Numerous other constraints have further hindered flexibility (41). Historically, home PT testing has not been reimbursed by HCFA, and this lack of reimbursement was cited by Roche Diagnostics as the primary reason behind its decision in late 2000 to withdraw its home-use CoaguChek PT device from the U.S. market (42). HCFA is presently reviewing its policies in this area. In the near future, it is hoped that this *de facto* national noncoverage policy, which has been in effect from the approval of the first home PT devices in 1997 to the date of this writing (2001), will be corrected.

CONCLUSIONS

Because hemostasis is of profound medical importance, and because hemostasis can be modulated very quickly by many therapeutic regimens and disease states, POC tests for hemostasis will become increasingly important to medicine in future years. Such tests, however, are technically demanding and are subjected to a high degree of regulatory scrutiny. Thus, progress cannot be taken for granted. To promote work in this area, it will be important that the needs of clinicians and patients be translated into both appropriate technology and appropriate regulatory requirements. In the United States, the field has clearly suffered from overregulation, which has imposed significant barriers to innovation and has restricted access to lifesaving technology.

Although POC PT testing has encountered many regulatory barriers in the United States, it is beginning to make headway in Europe, particularly in Germany. In 1997, there were about 14,000 German patients doing PT self-testing. By 1999, after only 2 years, this grew to about 53,000 patients (43), and growth has continued since then.

Early German adoption of this practice has been facilitated by a number of factors, including government reimbursement, quicker regulatory approval, and regulations permitting patient self-management without the requirement of daily liquid QC testing.

Typical studies have shown that for low-dose anticoagulation, patient self-testing helps to move a large percentage of anticoagulated patients from the subtherapeutic range to the therapeutic range. For high-dose anticoagulation, patient self-testing can help prevent patients from drifting into the overly anticoagulated range.

Other new technologies have encountered initial regulatory obstacles and have overcome them (44). The clinical advantages of POC hemostasis tests, in particular, home PT tests, are compelling. Over the next generation, it is likely that POC PT testing will follow the same trends that blood glucose testing did in the past generation. Because POC PT testing enables superior control of anticoagulation, it is likely to become the future standard of care for oral anticoagulants.

It is hoped that other POC hemostasis tests will benefit from the pioneering efforts of POC PT testing. As technology improves, regulations become more streamlined and reimbursement issues are resolved, the next generation of hemostasis diagnostics should be increasingly able to make important contributions to medical care.

REFERENCES

1. Colman RW, Marder VJ, Salzman EW, et al. Overview of hemostasis. In: Colman MJ, Hirsh J, Marder VJ, et al., eds. *Hemostasis and thrombosis*. Philadelphia: JB Lippincott, 1987:3–17.
2. Kost GJ. Point-of-care testing in intensive care. In: Tobin MJ, ed. *Principles and practice of intensive care monitoring*. New York: McGraw-Hill, 1998, 1267–1296.
3. Kost GJ. Planning and implementing of point-of-care testing systems. In: Tobin MJ, ed. *Principles and practice of intensive care monitoring*. New York: McGraw-Hill, 1997, 1297–1328.
4. Hirsh J. Oral anticoagulant drugs. *N Engl J Med* 1991;324:1865–1875.
5. White RH, McKittrick T, Hutchinson R, et al. Temporary discontinuation of warfarin therapy: changes in the international normalized ratio. *Ann Intern Med* 1995;122:40–42.
6. Matchar DB, et al. Stroke PORT released early, touting warfarin. U.S. government AHCPR patient outcomes research team (PORT) press release. *Medical Outcomes & Guidelines Alert* Sept. 28, 1995.
7. Anonymous. The absence of a glycemic threshold for the development of long-term complications: the perspective of the Diabetes Control and Complications Trial. *Diabetes* 1996;10:1289–1298.
8. Samsa GP, Matchar DB. Relationship between test frequency and outcomes of anticoagulation: a literature review and commentary with implications for the design of randomized trials of patient self-management. *Journal of Thrombosis and Thrombolysis* 2000;9:283–292.
9. Zweig SE. Test article and method for performing blood coagulation assays. U.S. Patent 5,418,143. 1995.
10. Daka JN, Poon R, Hinberg I. Effects of temperature and viscosity on prothrombin times of blood. *J Invest Surgery* 1991;4:279–290.
11. Lucas F, Duncan A, Jay R, et al. A novel whole blood capillary technic for measuring the prothrombin time. *Am J Clin Pathol* 1987;88:442–446.
12. Rose VL, Dermott SC, Murray BF, et al.. Decentralized testing for prothrombin time and activated partial thromboplastin time using a dry chemistry portable analyzer. *Arch Pathol Lab Med* 1993;117:611–618.
13. Aller RD. Coagulation analysis at the point of care. *CAP Today* 1999;13:65–70
14. Nemerson Y. Tissue factor and hemostasis. *Blood* 1988;1:1–8.
15. Quien ET, Morales E, Cisar LA, et al. Plasma tissue factor antigen levels in capillary whole blood and venous blood: effect of tissue factor on prothrombin time. *Am J Hematol* 1997;55:193–198.
16. Zweig SE, Sharma S, Meyer BG. Test articles for performing dry reagent prothrombin time assays. U.S. Patent 5,418,141. 1995.
17. Cumming AM, Jones GR, Wensley RT, et al. *In vitro* neutralization of heparin in plasma prior to the activated partial thromboplastin time test: an assessment of four heparin antagonists and two anion exchange resins. *Thromb Res* 1986;41:43–56.
18. Hillman RS, Cobb ME, Allen JD, et al. Capillary flow device. U.S. Patent 5300779. 1994.
19. Oberardt B. Reaction system element and method for performing prothrombin time assay. US Patent 4,849,340. 1989.
20. Chusack R, Laduca FM, Samo RJ. Blood coagulation time test apparatus and method. U.S. Patent 5,302,348. 1994.
21. Zweig SE, Meyer BG, Sharma S, et al. Membrane-based, dry-reagent, prothrombin time tests. *Biomedical Instrum Technol* 1996;30:245–256.
22. Jina AN. Method and device for measuring blood coagulation or lysis by viscosity changes. U.S. Patent 6,046,051. 2000.
23. Tripodi A, Chantarangkul V, Negri B, et al. International Collaborative Study of the Calibration of a Proposed Reference Preparation for Thromboplastin, Human Recombinant, Plain. *Thromb Haemost* 1998;79:439–443.
24. Critchfield GC, Bennett ST. The international normalized ratio and uncertainty – validation of a probabilistic model. *Am J Clin Pathol* 1994;102:115–122.
25. Ng VL, et al. Highly sensitive thromboplastins do not improve INR precision. *Am J Clin Pathol* 1998;109:338–346.
26. Cunningham MT, Johnson GF, Pennell BJ, et al. The reliability of manufacturer-determined, instrument-specific international sensitivity index values for calculating the international normalized ratio. *Am J Clin Pathol* 1994;102:128–133.
27. Kitchen S, Jennings I, Woods TA, et al. Two recombinant tissue factor reagents compared to conventional thromboplastins for determination of international normalized ratio: a thirty-three laboratory collaborative study. *Thromb Hemostasis* 1996;76:372–376.
28. Fairweather RB, et al. College of American Pathologists Conference XXXI on Laboratory Monitoring of Anticoagulant Therapy. *Arch Pathol Lab Med* 1998;122:768–781.
29. Gavin M, et al. Portable prothrombin time test apparatus and associated method of performing a prothrombin time test 1997. U.S. patent 5,591,403. 1997.
30. Coaguchek system, Roche/Boehringer Mannheim. U.S. Food and Drug Administration 510K, no. K930454, 1993.
31. Avocet PT system, Avocet Medical, Inc. Food and Drug Administration, 510K no. K980839, 1998.
32. Zweig SE, Meyer BG, Downey TD. Verification device for optical clinical assay systems. World Health Organization. PCT international publication number WO 99/12008, 1999.
33. O'Leary TM, Calvin MA, Gutman S, et al. Hematology and Pathology Devices Panel of the Medical Devices Advisory Committee. Miller Reporting Company, Inc., Washington D.C., September 5, 1997.
34. Rosendall FR, van der Meer FJM, Cannegieter SC. Management of anticoagulant therapy: the dutch experience. *Journal of Thrombosis and Thrombolysis* 1996;2:265–269.
35. Chiquette E, Amato MG, Bussey HI. Comparison of an anticoagulation clinic with usual health care. *Arch Intern Med* 1998;158:1641–1647.
36. Bernardo A. Post-conference session: experience with patient self-management of oral anticoagulation. *Journal of Thrombosis and Thrombolysis* 1996;2:321–325.
37. Zerback R, Horstkotte D. Patient self-monitoring in follow-up of long term anticoagulant therapy. *Z Kardiol* 1998;87(Suppl 4):68–74.
38. Hasenkam JM, Kimose HH, Knudsen L, et al. Self management of oral anticoagulation therapy after heart valve replacement. *Eur J Cardiothorac Surg* 1997;11:935–942.
39. U.S. Food and Drug Administration (FDA). FDA guidance docu-

ment. Guidance for Clinical Laboratory Improvement Amendments of 1988 (CLIA). Criteria for waiver. Draft guidance for industry and FDA. Not for implementation, 2001.

40. Taborski U, Muller-Berghaus G. State-of-the-art patient self-management for control of oral anticoagulation. *Semin Thromb Hemost* 1999; 25:43–47.

41. Hughes RA. Workshop: reimbursement for anticoagulation services. *Journal of Thrombosis and Thrombolysis* 1996;2:301–304.

42. Health Care Finance Administration. Raising curtain on PT self-testing. Roche Bows out prior to showtime. The Gray Sheet, August 28, 2000:3–4.

43. Wenzel E. Self-control and self-management of oral anticoagulant therapy: state of the art in Germany. First ENAT (European Network on Anticoagulant Treatment) conference. 1999, Bologna, Italy.

44. British Parliament. Locomotive on Highways Act ("Red Flag Law"). Self-propelled vehicles on public highways must be preceded by a man on foot carrying a red flag to warn oncoming horse drawn vehicles. 1865.

6

PRINCIPLES AND PERFORMANCE OF POINT-OF-CARE TESTING INSTRUMENTS

ZUPING TANG
RICHARD F. LOUIE
GERALD J. KOST

Point-of-care testing (POCT) instruments are defined as diagnostic medical devices used at or near the site of patient care. The sites include the bedside, operating room (OR), emergency department (ED), intensive care unit (ICU), and satellite laboratories or nonhospital settings such as the field and home. POCT instruments provide near real-time analysis and rapid test results. Immediate results reduce therapeutic turnaround time, shorten length of hospital stay, and potentially improve patient outcomes (1–10). POCT instruments are designed to be user friendly and generally to be operated by nonlaboratory personnel. The instruments are generally equipped with a test menu that can provide vital physiologic indications of the patient's health (11,12). Test menus and clusters vary among POCT instruments and may include testing of electrolytes, hematocrit, blood gases [partial pressure of oxygen (PO_2) and partial pressure of carbon dioxide (PCO_2)], pH, metabolites (creatinine, glucose, lactate, urea nitrogen), cardiac injury markers, hemostasis indicators, drugs of abuse, infectious disease markers, and molecular diagnostics. These instruments often are used to diagnose disease and to monitor the efficacy of treatment. The objectives of this chapter are (a) to describe the characteristics and formats of POCT instruments, (b) to discuss their analytical principles, (c) to provide an overview of performance criteria, (d) to present a selection and evaluation process for POCT instruments, and (e) to outline emerging technologies.

INSTRUMENT FORMATS

Point-of-care testing instruments can be grouped into different categories based on their format and detection principle. Table 6.1 compares the common characteristics of POCT instrument formats. Tables 6.2 through 6.5 list examples of instruments in each of the categories; however, the instruments listed are approximately categorized. Some could be grouped into more than one format. Table 6.6 summarizes *ex vivo*, *in vivo*, and noninvasive instruments. The tables list only examples and are not meant to be all inclusive.

Transportable

Table 6.2 lists transportable instruments. These instruments are generally heavy and large. They can be placed on bench tops or on carts for mobile use (13,14). Transportable instruments require a conventional (AC) power source but may be equipped with a battery backup for short-term use, such as a few minutes of operation when an AC source is not readily accessible. The size of transportable instruments allows for multiple sensors and detectors to be incorporated and for a broad test menu. Several analytic measurements can be made on a single sample. Most transportable instrument platforms allow the operator to customize the tests, selecting individual tests from the batch. This customization of tests can minimize and conserve the volume of blood needed per analysis cycle. Transportable instruments operate with liquid reagents, calibrators, and buffers. Some transportable instruments involving blood gas analysis may or may not have external gas tanks for blood gas calibration.

Transportable instruments may utilize various specimens, including whole blood, plasma, serum, urine, cerebrospinal fluid (CSF) samples, and others. The samples typically are aspirated into the testing chamber automatically by the instrument, thereby reducing dependence on operator technique and manual sample processing steps. Some transportable instruments require manual sample introduction. For example, the Ciba-Corning 278 (Bayer Diagnostics, Tarrytown, NY, U.S.A.) blood-gas analyzer requires the operator to inject the sample into a reservoir, from which the analyzer automatically draws a suitable volume for testing.

Different analytic principles are used for analysis of analytes. These include potentiometry (ion-selective electrodes), amperometry (substrate-specific electrodes), conductometry (electric conductance electrodes), optical method (optical sensors/optodes), and immunochemistry (Table 6.2). The testing methodologies and principles are discussed in further detail in Section 3 of this book. The electrodes and sensors, such as sodium and PO_2, are compartmentalized and removable, allowing operators or manufacturers to replace, customize, or expand the instrument test cluster.

Transportable instruments have automatic internal one- and two-point calibration that is performed periodically. Some

TABLE 6.1. CHARACTERISTICS OF POINT-OF-CARE TESTING INSTRUMENTS

Characteristic	Transportable	Portable	Handheld	Immunodetection Device
Size	Large	Medium	Small or miniature	Medium to miniature
Power source	Conventional	Conventional or batteries	Batteries	Variable to none
Mobility	Low	Medium	High	High
Test option/menu	Operator-defined/multitest	Fixed/single- to multitest	Fixed/limited	Fixed/single- to multitest
Sample type	WB, P, S, U, CSF	WB, P, S, U	WB	WB, U, saliva
Sample volume	Adjustable	Not adjustable	Not adjustable	Not adjustable
Sampling method	Automatic	Automatic/manual	Manual	Manual
Calibration	Algorithmic	Periodic or prior to testing	Built-in	Not applicable
Connectivity	Available	Possibly available	Limited	None
Password security	Available	Possibly available	Limited	None
Waste storage	Self-contained biohazard storage	Self-contained biohazard storage	Biohazard storage instrument dependent	Biohazard storage instrument dependent

WB, whole blood; P, plasma; S, serum; U, urine; CSF, cerebrospinal fluid.

TABLE 6.2. TRANSPORTABLE INSTRUMENTS[a]

Instrument	Analytes	Analytical Principle	Manufacturer
Piccolo[b]	Na, K, CK, Tco$_2$, UA, glucose, cholesterol, ALP, ALT, AST, GGT, AMY, ALB, TP, Tbil, urea nitrogen, CRE	Spectrophotometry	Abaxis (Union City, CA, U.S.A.)
Micros CRP[c]	C-reactive protein, Hb, WBC, RBC, Hct, platelet	Immunoturbidometry, spectrophotometry	Abx Diagnostics (Irvine, CA, U.S.A.)
AVL OMNI[d,e]	Po$_2$, Pco$_2$, pH, Na$^+$, K$^+$, Ca^{2+}, Cl$^-$, Hct, Hb, urea nitrogen, glucose, lactate, creatinine, Co-oximetry	Potentiometry, amperometry, conductometry, spectrophotometry	AVL Scientific/Roche (Roswell, GA, U.S.A.)
Rapid Lab 800 series[d]	Po$_2$ Pco$_2$, pH, Na$^+$, K$^+$, Ca^{2+}, Cl$^-$, glucose, lactate, Co-oximetry	Potentiometry, amperometry, optical reflectance	Bayer Diagnostics (Norwood, MA, U.S.A.)
RapidPoint 400	Po$_2$, Pco$_2$, pH, Na$^+$, K$^+$, Ca^{2+}, Cl$^-$, Hct, glucose	Potentiometry, amperometry, conductometry	Bayer Diagnostics (Tarrytown, NY, U.S.A.)
Synthesis 35	Po$_2$, Pco$_2$, pH, Na$^+$, K$^+$, Ca^{2+}/Cl$^-$/glucose Hct, glucose, Co-oximetry	Potentiometry, amperometry, conductometry	Instrumentation Laboratory (Lexington, MA, U.S.A.)
EasyBloodGas	pH, Po$_2$, Pco$_2$	Potentiometry, amperometry	Medica (Bedford, MA, U.S.A.)
pHOX Plus C	pH, Pco$_2$, Po$_2$, SO$_2$, Hct, Hb, Na$^+$, K$^+$, glucose, Ca^{2+}, Cl$^-$	Potentiometry, amperometry, conductometry, optical reflectance	Nova Biomedical (Waltham, MA, U.S.A.)
pHOX Plus L	pH, Pco$_2$, Po$_2$, SO$_2$, Hct, Hb, Na$^+$, K$^+$, glucose, lactate, Ca^{2+} / Cl$^-$	Potentiometry, amperometry, conductometry, optical reflectance	Nova Biomedical
Stat Profile M/M7[d]	Po$_2$, Pco$_2$, pH, SO$_2$, Na$^+$, K$^+$, Ca^{2+}, Cl$^-$, Hct, urea nitrogen, glucose, lactate, Mg^{2+} / creatinine, Co-oximetry	Potentiometry, amperometry, conductometry, optical reflectance	Nova Biomedical
Nova series (16)	Na$^+$, K$^+$, Cl$^-$, Hct, Tco$_2$, Hct, urea nitrogen, glucose, creatinine	Potentiometry, amperometry, conductometry, optical reflectance	Nova Biomedical
ABL 700	Po$_2$, Pco$_2$, pH, Na$^+$, K$^+$, Ca^{2+}, Cl$^-$, Hct, Hb, glucose, lactate, Co-oximetry	Potentiometry, amperometry, optical reflectance	Radiometer America (Westlake, OH, U.S.A.)
NPT™7	Po$_2$, Pco$_2$, pH, SO$_2$, Hb, Co-oximetry	Infrared spectroscopy, phosphorescence decay, optical absorbance	Radiometer America
YSI 2300 Stat Plus	Glucose, lactate	Amperometry	Yellow Springs Instrument (Yellow Springs, OH, U.S.A.)

Po$_2$, partial pressure oxygen; Pco$_2$, partial pressure carbon dioxide; WBC, white blood cell; RBC, red blood cell; Hct, hematocrit; Hb, hemoglobin; SO$_2$, oxygen saturation; Tco$_2$, total carbon dioxide; UA, uric acid; ALP, alkaline phosphatase; ALT, alanine aminotransferase; AST, asparate transaminase; GGT, gamma-glutamyl transferase; AMY, amylase; ALB, albumin; TP, total protein; Tbil, total bilirubin; CRE, creatinine.
[a]Data in table were compiled in September 2001. Please refer to vendor for latest information. Co-oximetry is available as a modular add-on on some whole-blood analyzers.
[b]Test menu is test disc dependent.
[c]Under development, is tenfold increase in sensitivity of the C-reactive protein test.
[d]Co-oximetry available as a modular add-on.
[e]AVL OMNI test cluster is instrument model dependent.

TABLE 6.3. PORTABLE INSTRUMENTS[a]

Instrument	Analytes	Analytical Principle	Manufacturer
Ultegra RPFA	Rapid platelet function assay	Microparticle aggregation	Accumetrics (San Diego, CA, U.S.A.)
IRMA SL (series 2000)[b]	Po_2, Pco_2, pH, Na^+, K^+, Ca^{2+}, Hct, Cl^-, urea nitrogen, [glucose]	Potentiometry, amperometry, conductometry	Agilent Technologies (St. Paul, MN, U.S.A.)
CoaCard APACT	PT, aPTT, platelet function	Turbidity	American Labor (Raleigh, NC, U.S.A.)
TAS	PT, PT-ONE/NC, aPTT, HMT, LOT	Particle motion	Cardiovascular Diagnostics (Raleigh, NC, U.S.A.)
AVL OPTI/OPTI-R	Po_2, Pco_2, pH, Na^+, K^+, Ca^{2+}, Cl^-	Optical fluorescence	AVL Scientific/Roche (Roswell, GA, U.S.A.)
Rapidpoint Coag	PT, aPTT, HMT	Impedance of particle motion	Bayer Diagnostics (Tarrytown, NY, U.S.A.)
DCA 2000	HbA1c	Latex agglutination inhibition	Bayer Diagnostics
Clinitek 50[c]	Leukocytes, glucose, bilirubin, ketone, nitrate, pH, protein, urobilinogen, blood, albumin, creatinine	Optical method	Bayer Diagnostics
CareSide Analyzer[e]	Na^+, K^+, Cl^-, Mg^{2+}, urea nitrogen, alkaline phosphatase, Tco_2, cholesterol, CK-MB, creatinine, glucose, LDH, total bilirubin, triglycerides, uric acid, lactate[d], PT[d], iCa[2+], aPTT[d], Hb[d], Hct[d]	Spectral transmittance, reflectance, electrochemical	CareSide (Culver City, CA, U.S.A.)
LDX system[e]	Total cholesterol, HDL, triglycerides, glucose, lipid profile, ALT	Optical reflectance	Cholestech (Hayward, CA, U.S.A.)
Whole blood aggregometer	Platelet function	Impedance	Chronolog (Havertown, PA, U.S.A.)
PFA-100	Platelet function	Pressure	Dade International (Miami, FL, U.S.A.)
Stat-Site	Acetaminophens, blood ketones, glucose, total cholesterol, hemoglobin	Enzymatic, colorimetry, reflectance photometry	GDS Technologies (Elkhart, IN, U.S.A.)
HemoSite	Hemoglobin	Colorimetry, reflectance photometry	GDS
HemoCue B-Hemoglobin	Hb	Absorbance photometry	HemoCue (Mission Viejo, CA, U.S.A.)
HemoCue B-Glucose	Glucose	Absorbance photometry	HemoCue
Gem Premier 3000	Po_2, Pco_2, pH, Na^+, K^+, Ca^{2+}, Hct, glucose[d], lactate[d]	Potentiometry, amperometry, conductometry	Instrumentation Laboratory (Lexington, MA, U.S.A.)
Gem PCL	PT, ACT, aPTT, ACT-LR	Mechanical endpoint clotting detection	Instrumentation Laboratory
Hemochron response	PT, aPTT, ACT, HiTT, TT, HNTT, FIB, HRT, PRT	Mechanical clot detection	International Technidyne (Edison, NJ, U.S.A.)
Hemochron series	FIB, AMS, PT, aPTT, TT, HNTT, HiTT	Magnet position	International
Hemochron Jr. Signature	ACT-LR, ACT[+], aPTT, PT, citrate PT	Fluid oscillation/optical clot detection	International
Pro Time microcoagulation system	PT, INR	Fluid oscillation/optical clot detection	International
ACT II Plunger HepconHMS	PT, aPTT, HMS, ACT-LR, ACT-HR, HR-HTC, Hemo-STATUS	Motion	Medtronic HemoTec (Parker, CO, U.S.A.)
A1cNow	HbA[1c]	Optical reflectance	Metrika (Sunnyvale, CA, U.S.A.)
NycoCard	HbA[1c]	Optical reflectance	Primus (Kansas City, MO, U.S.A.)
ABL 70 Series	Po_2, Pco_2, pH, Na^+, K^+, Ca^{2+}, Hct	Potentiometry, conductometry	Radiometer America (Westlake, OH, U.S.A.)
Chemstrip 101	Leukocytes, glucose, bilirubin, ketone, nitrate, pH, protein, urobilinogen, blood	Reflectance photometry	Roche Diagnostics (Indianapolis, IN, U.S.A.)
CoaguChek Plus	PT, aPTT	Pattern recognition	Roche Diagnostics
CoaguChek Pro DM	PT, aPTT, ACT	Laser photometry to detect change in blood flow	Roche Diagnostics
CoaguChek	PT, INR	Particle motion/reflectance photometry	Roche Diagnostics

Hct, hematocrit; IRMA, immediate response mobile analysis; TAS, thrombolytic assessment system; PFA, platelet function assay; PT, prothrombin time; aPTT, activated partial thromboplastin time; HMT, heparin management test; LOT, lysis onset time; HbA1c, hemoglobin A1c; Tco_2, total carbon dioxide; CK-MB, myocardial muscle creatine kinase isoenzyme; LDH, lactate dehydrogenase; iCa[2+], ionized calcium; Hb, hemoglobin; HDL, high-density lipoprotein; ALT, alanine aminotransferase; ACT, activated clotting time; ACT-LR, low-range ACT; HiTT, high-dose thrombin time; TT, thrombin time; HNTT, heparin-neutralized thrombin time; FIB, fibrinogen; HRT, heparin response time; PRT, protamine response time; AMS, anticoagulation management system; INR, international normalized ratio; ACT-HR, high-range ACT.
[a]Data in table were compiled in September 2001. Please refer to vendor for latest information.
[b]IRMA test cluster capability is cartridge dependent. Module SureStepPro required for glucose testing.
[c]Measured analytes are test strip–type dependent.
[d]The tests are under development.
[e]The available tests are cartridge dependent.

TABLE 6.4. HANDHELD INSTRUMENTS[a]

Instrument	Analytes	Analytical Principle	Manufacturer
i-STAT[b]	Po_2, Pco_2, pH, Na^+, K^+, Ca^{2+}, Cl^-, Hct, urea nitrogen, glucose, lactate, creatinine	Potentiometry, amperometry	Abbott Diagnostics (Abbott Park, IL, U.S.A.)
Precision PCx	Glucose	Amperometry	Abbott
Precision Xtra[c]	Glucose, ketones	Amperometry	Abbott
At Last	Glucose	Photometry	Amira Medical (Scotts Valley, CA, U.S.A.)
Glucometer Elite XL	Glucose	Amperometry	Bayer Diagnostics (Elkhart, IN, U.S.A.)
POC PT	PT	Electrochemical	Hemosense (Milpitas, CA, U.S.A.)
INRatio	PT, INR	Impedance / electrochemical	Hemosense
SureStepFlexx	Glucose	Reflectance photometry	LifeScan (Milpitas, CA, U.S.A.)
SureStepPro	Glucose	Reflectance photometry	LifeScan
One Touch Hospital	Glucose	Reflectance photometry	LifeScan
FastTake	Glucose	Amperometry	LifeScan
In Charge	Glucose	Reflectance photometry	LXN Corporation (San Diego, CA, U.S.A.)
ExpressView	Glucose	Reflectance photometry	LXN Corporation
BioScanner 2000	Glucose	Reflectance photometry	Polymer Technology Systems (Indianapolis, IN, U.S.A.)
Accu-Chek Advantage H	Glucose	Amperometry	Roche Diagnostics (Indianapolis, IN, U.S.A.)
Accu-Chek Comfort Curve	Glucose	Amperometry	Roche Diagnostics
FreeStyle	Glucose	Amperometry	TheraSense (Alameda, CA, U.S.A.)
Prestige Smart System	Glucose	Reflectance photometry	Walgreens (Deerfield, IL, U.S.A.)

Hct, hematocrit; PT, prothrombin time; INR, international normalized ratio.
[a]Data in table were compiled in September 2001. Please refer to vendor for latest information.
[b]i-STAT test cluster capability is cartridge dependent.
[c]A separate test strip is used for testing ketones.

instruments, such as the ABL 700 blood-gas/chemistry analyzer (Table 6.2) use low-pressure internal gas tanks for calibration. Others, such as the pHOx Plus, have eliminated gas tanks altogether in place of liquid calibration. A few instruments use pretonometered liquid calibration materials, whereas others calibrate blood-gas measurements using electronic zeroing and room air. Instruments with external gas tanks have added size and bulk, which decrease the instrument's mobility. Low-pressure internal gas tanks not only reduce peripheral components but also decrease hazards. Some instruments provide 1- or 2-point calibration options based on the operator's requirement. They also have an interrupt option during the calibration cycle to allow operators immediate access to the instrument for sample measurements. Transportable instruments generally are maintenance free, with the occasional replenishing of reagents, such as buffer and calibration solutions.

Built-in biohazard containers allow easy disposal of waste and minimize operator exposure to bio-contaminants. Transportable instruments are equipped with advanced data management software that enables test results to be connected directly to the hospital-computerized databases [i.e., hospital/laboratory information system (HIS/LIS)]. Transportable instruments typically are stationed in the OR, ED, ICU, and satellite laboratories.

Automatic and Intelligent Quality Control

The purpose of quality control (QC) testing is to monitor and evaluate the overall quality of the analytical testing process to ensure the reliability and accuracy of patient test results. QC materials contain the analyte to be tested. The concentrations can be low, normal, and high. The different concentrations

assess the instrument performance over the ranges that may be observed in patient samples. Ampules of aqueous QC solutions are commonly used. The conventional method for QC testing is manual external introduction of aqueous QC solutions. Some of the latest transportable instruments come equipped with automatic QC testing features. These instruments automatically draw sample from the ampules or bottles onboard the instrument at an operator-defined schedule. Automatic QC testing makes maintenance of the instrument more user friendly. Automatic QC ensures QC testing is performed routinely and helps reduce the workload of the operator.

Intelligent quality control (iQC) is an example of a new QC check feature. This technology is used on the Piccolo system (Table 6.2). iQC verifies the chemistry, optics, and electronics functions of the analyzer during each run. Because no operator interaction is required, QC standards are met independently of the operator's skill level. Whole-blood, plasma, or serum sample is introduced directly into the single-use, self-contained reagent test disc, where sample preparation, including separation of whole blood, is handled automatically. All reactions, including analyte, reagent, and instrument QC testing, occur in solution in cuvettes on the periphery of the disc. The Piccolo generates flashes of full-spectrum white light and measures absorption for each reaction at multiple wavelengths, from ultraviolet to near infrared. iQC verifies the composition and delivery within the disc of all substances participating in the reactions (chemistry), validates the performance of the light-generating and detection components (optics), and audits the conversion of the light absorbance into digital values for use in mathematical algorithms (electronics). The iQC feature on the Piccolo system monitors the levels of hemolysis, lipemia, and icterus (jaundice)

TABLE 6.5. IMMUNODETECTION DEVICES AND TESTS[a]

Instrument	Analytes	Analytical Principle	Manufacturer
Murex SUDS HIV-1	HIV-antibody	Enzyme-linked immunosorbent assay	Abbott Diagnostics (Abbott Park, IL, U.S.A.)
ACON® DOA	Morphine, heroin, marijuana, cocaine, amphetamine, methamphetamine, phencyclidine	Chromatographic immunoassay	ACON Laboratories (San Diego, CA, U.S.A.)
ACON® HBsAg	HBsAg	Chromatographic	ACON Laboratories
ACON® HIV ½	HIV antibody	Chromatographic	ACON Laboratories
ACON® Syphilis	TP antibody	Chromatographic	ACON Laboratories
Microtiter (poc test pending)	Thrombus precursor protein (TpP)	Enzyme-linked immunosorbent assay	American Biogenetic Sciences (Copiague, NY, U.S.A.)
SimpliRed	D-dimer	Hemagglutination	American Diagnostica (Greenwich, CT, U.S.A.)
MiniQuant	D-dimer	Immunoturbidometry	Biopool International (Ventura, CA, U.S.A.)
Triage®			
Drugs of abuse panel	Amphetamines/methamphetamines, barbituates, benzodiazepines, cocaine, methadone, opiates, THC, tricyclic antidepressants	Competitive immunoassay	Biosite Diagnostics (San Diego, CA, U.S.A.)
Cardiac panel	Troponin I, CK-MB mass, and myoglobin	Fluorescence immunoassay	Biosite Diagnostics
BNP test	B-type natriuretic peptide	Fluorescence immunoassay	Biosite Diagnostics
Stratus™ CS	Troponin I, CK-MB mass, and myoglobin	Dendrimer enhanced radial particle immunoassay	Dade-Behring (Newark, DE, U.S.A.)
EZ-Screen	Amphetamines, cocaine, opiates, THC, PCP, barbituates	Solid phase enzyme immunoassay	Editek (Burlington, NJ, U.S.A.)
Alpha-Dx	Troponin I, CK, CK-MB, and myoglobin	Fluorescent immunoassay	First Medical (Mountain View, CA, U.S.A.)
I.D.Block	Amphetamines, cocaine, opiates, barbituates	Solid-phase enzyme immunoassay	International Diagnostic Systems, (St. Joseph, MI, U.S.A.)
BioSign PSA II-WB[c]	Prostate specific antigen	Solid-phase immunochromatography	Princeton BioMeditech (Princeton, NJ, U.S.A.)
Osteomark NTx	Bone resorption marker (NTx)[b]	Competitive immunoassay spectrophotometry	Ostex International (Seattle, WA, U.S.A.)
Poly stat			Polymedco (Cortlandt Manor, NY, U.S.A.)
Strep A	Group A streptococcal antigen	Two-site sandwich immunoassay	
Mono	Mononucleosis heterophile antibodies	Sandwich solid phase gold conjugate immunoassay	Polymedco
H. pylori	IgG specific for *Helicobacter pylori*	Chromatographic immunoassay	Polymedco
hCG	hCG	Chromatographic immunoassay	Polymedco
BTA Stat	Bladder tumor associated antigen, hCFHrp	Chromatographic immunoassay	Polymedco
QuickVue	Influenza, Strep A, *H. pylori, Chlamydia*	Lateral-flow immunoassay, antibody-labled immunoassay	Quidel, (San Diego, CA, U.S.A.)
CARDS	Mononucleosis	Color immunochromatographic assay	Quidel
Metra BAP	Bone-specific alkaline phosphatase	Enzyme-linked immunosorbent assay	Quidel
CardiacT Rapid Assay	Cardiac troponin T	Monoclonal antibody, double sandwich immunoassay with a poly (streptavidin)-biotin capture system and gold sol as a particle label	Roche Diagnostics (Indianapolis, IN, U.S.A.)
Testcup-er	Amphetamines, cocaine, morphine, barbituates, benzodiazepines	Microparticle capture inhibition	Roche
Chemstrip Micral	Microalbumin	Chromatographic Immunoassay	Roche
Abuscreen Ontrak	Amphetamines, cocaine, opiates, THC, PCP, barbituates, benzodiazepine	Latex agglutination inhibition	Roche Diagnostics Systems (Branchburg, NJ, U.S.A.)
Cardiac STATus	Troponin I, CK-MB, Myoglobin	Solid-phase chromatographic immunoassay	Spectral (White Stone, VA, U.S.A.)
First Check	Amphetamines, cocaine, opiates, THC, PCP, barbituates, benzodiazepines	Microparticle capture immunoassay	Worldwide Medical (Irvine, CA, U.S.A.)

BNP, brain natriuretic peptide; HBsAg, hepatitis B surface antigen; HIV, human immunodeficiency; DOA, drugs of abuse; THC, tetrahydracannabinol; PCP, phencyclidine; TP, IgG, immunoglobulin G.
[a]Data in table were compiled in September 2001. Please refer to vendor for latest information.
[b]Cross-linked N-telopeptides of type I collagen (NTx).
[c]Device not for sale in U.S. market.

TABLE 6.6. *EX VIVO, IN VIVO*, AND NONINVASIVE POCT INSTRUMENTS*a*

A. *Ex Vivo* and *In Vivo* POCT Instruments

Manufacturer	Instrument	Monitor Type	Measurements	Analytical Principle
Agilent Technologies (St. Paul, MN, U.S.A.) www.agilent.com	Trendcare Paratrend Neotrend	*In vivo* Vascular Vascular	pH, PO_2, PCO_2, temperature	Fiberoptic chemical
VIA Medical (San Diego, CA, U.S.A.) www.viamedical.com	VIA ABG VIA LVM	*Ex vivo* Withdraw/reinfuse	pH, PO_2, PCO_2, Na+, K+, hematocrit	Electrochemical
	VIA GLU	*Ex vivo* Withdraw/reinfuse	Glucose	Electrochemical
MiniMed (Northridge, CA, U.S.A.) www.minimed.com	Continuous glucose monitoring system	*In vivo* Subcutaneous	Glucose	Electrochemical
Optical Sensors (Minneapolis, MN, U.S.A.) www.opsi.com	SensiCath*b*	*Ex vivo* Withdraw/reinfuse	pH, PO_2, PCO_2	Fiberoptic chemical

B. Novel Noninvasive POCT Instruments

Manufacturer	Instrument	Test Location	Measurement	Analytical Principle
Optical Sensors (Minneapolis, MN, U.S.A.) www.opsi.com	Capno Probe SL	Sublingual	Sublingual PCO_2 (perfusion test)	Fiberoptic
Cygnus (Redwood City, CA, U.S.A.) www.cygn.com	GlucoWatch Biographer	Transcutaneous (wristwatch)	Glucose	Reverse Iontophoresis, Electrochemical
Aspect Medical (Natick, MA, U.S.A.) www.aspectms.com	Bispectral Index	Transcutaneous (forehead sensor pad)	Brain waves (EEG)	Power distribution spectral and phase analysis
Nonin (Plymouth, MN, U.S.A.) www.nonin.com	Pulse oximeter carbon dioxide detector (9840 series)	Transcutaneous (finger adapter) Airway adapter	Oxygen saturation, carbon dioxide level	Optical absorption
SpectRx (Norcross, GA, U.S.A.) www.spectrx.com	BiliChek	Transcutaneous (forehead)	Bilirubin	Multiwavelength spectral analysis

POCT, point-of-care testing; EEG, electroencephalogram; ABG, arterial blood gas; GLU, glucose; LVM, low-volume mode; Temp, temperature.
*a*Data in table were compiled in September 2001. Please refer to vendor for latest information.
*b*The SensiCath system is no longer marketed or manufacturered.

in the sample. If these levels exceed the instrument operating limits, the accuracy of measurements will be compromised. The instrument will suppress the result and print an asterisk followed by one or more letters indicating the sources of the interferences. In addition, the printed result card shows the levels of the hemolysis, lipemia, and icterus in the sample. A single chemistry or the entire panel is suppressed if uncharacteristic performance is detected, and an error message is displayed on the analyzer's four-line light emitting diode (LED) display. The system QC data are compiled for each run and stored in the analyzer memory with the run results. These data can be recalled and printed.

The QualityGuard is a built-in QC and quality assurance system that automatically monitors parameters associated with the quality of the test results on the NPT7 analyzer (Table 6.2). QualityGuard is composed of three components, a system check, measuring check, and two-level check. The system check evaluates the power supply, voltage, the onboard computer system, temperatures of the spectrophotometer and measuring chambers, and the mechanical cuvettes delivery system in the analyzer on a continuous basis. The measuring check evaluates the quality of the cuvettes, the measuring process, and checks the sample for clots and air bubbles. The two-level check is a feature that simulates quantitative values at two levels. The simulated values are determined by optical detection before each measurement. Based on the three checks, the QualityGuard determines whether the NPT7 analyzer is operating properly (15).

Portable

Table 6.3 lists portable instruments. Portable instruments range in size from that of a personal computer to nearly a handheld device. The modest size increases the mobility and allows easier access to patients. The instruments operate with power adapters or battery sources. Most portable whole-blood chemistry analyzers use disposable cartridge/cuvette technology. The electrodes/sensors and reagents are built and packaged within the cartridges/cuvettes. Unlike the transportable instruments, the cartridge/cuvette, electrodes/sensors, and reagents are disposable after use. The number and types of tests available on a cartridge/cuvette depend on the electrodes/sensors and reagents/chemicals/enzymes available on the cartridges and on the device. Expansion of the test menu requires the purchase of a cartridge with those sensors available. The test menu can include electrolytes, metabolites, blood gases, and hemostasis indicators. Cartridges are packaged as either single- or multiple-use units. A multiuse cartridge may provide a few hundred measurements.

Testing is performed with whole-blood samples. Samples are introduced either automatically or manually. With manual sample introduction, the quality and performance of testing are dependent on the operator technique and procedure. Selection of the testing modes, either adult or neonate mode, can influence the required test sample volume. The principles of measurement of portable instruments include potentiometry, amperometry, conductometry, optical method, and immunoassay systems.

The calibration of whole-blood chemistry systems differs between single-use and multiple-use cartridges. For the single-use cartridge systems, such as in the immediate response mobile analysis (IRMA) blood gas analyzer (Table 6.3), calibration is performed on each cartridge just prior to its use, as opposed to the frequent calibrations on transportable systems. On the other hand, calibration on multiple-use cartridge systems, such as the GEM Premier blood gas analyzer, closely parallels that of the transportable systems. Calibration on the multiple-use cartridges is performed periodically at predefined intervals and between patient sample measurements until all available tests on the cartridge have been used. Once depleted of all tests, the cartridge is removed and disposed. Multiple-use cartridges typically are prepackaged with an ample supply of calibration agents and reagents for the number of available patient tests (about 150–300 tests) or the operating life (about 2–4 weeks) of the cartridges. Portable instruments that perform blood gas measurements generally lack internal or external gas tanks for calibration. Instead, the cartridges may be packaged with pretonometered calibration solutions that are stored in impervious bags. In a few systems, such as the GEM Premier, gas calibration is performed using room air.

Portable instruments generally are equipped with data-management software that allows test results to be downloaded into hospital databases. Portable instruments are used in the OR, ED, and ICU but also can be used in physician offices, ambulances, and rescue helicopters, where space limitations and power constraints demand a smaller, battery-operated device.

Electronic Quality Control

Electronic quality control (EQC) testing is a unique state-of-the-art feature that is available on many portable and handheld instrument formats. EQC is a quality management tool that supplements the traditional liquid QC procedures in the evaluation of the optics, electronic, and computational components of the system. EQC uses a surrogate or reference cartridge that simulates the analytic process to assess the response of the sensors, such as with color filters or solutions for optical sensors. EQC, however, does not validate the performance and functionality of the cartridge lot used for testing (16–18). EQC is not designed to replace liquid QC testing, but it functions to detect internal system fail-

ures, such as the electronics and sensor response, which potentially could invalidate the entire testing process.

Handheld

Table 6.4 lists handheld instruments. These instruments are highly mobile for bedside use in patient care. Whole-blood samples are used for testing. The test menu on these instruments varies with test strip design, reagents, and sensor availability. The instruments have limited tests, generally to a specific analyte (e.g., glucose or prothrombin time). The electrodes and biosensors are constructed into the test strips. Dry-reagent chemistry technology often is used for glucose meter testing, in which the catalytic enzymes are immobilized in a dry form on the test strips. Usually stabilizers are added to maintain favorable pH and enzyme activity. The dry reagents in the test strips are activated on reconstitution with the test sample.

Handheld instruments do not have internal calibration but have several electronic verification steps. EQC check is used on several handheld instruments. Liquid controls are used to assess instrument, operator, and test-strip lot performance. Some handheld instruments lack the capability and or the data management software compatible for interfacing and downloading of test results to hospital databases. Operators of handheld devices may be exposed to biohazards because of the lack of a waste storage or containment unit. Handheld instruments are used in hospital settings and, because of their unique size, can be used conveniently at home and in virtually all settings, limited only by manufacturers' constraints on ambient physical extremes.

Immunodetection Units

Table 6.5 lists cassette- and test strip–based immunoassay point-of-care devices. The format of these testing units can be characterized as miniature or equivalent in size to a handheld instrument. These devices, however, can be as large as a portable instrument when the external detector system used for quantitating results is included. Immunodetection devices come as stand-alone or detector-dependent formats. Stand-alone formats are applied to qualitative tests, where a positive or negative indicator is visually read. For detector-dependent systems, the test cassettes or test strips are inserted into a detector system after sample application for quantitation. The indicators, such as the color labels or fluorescent labels on the antibody or antigen, are optically assayed. A variety of immunoassay methods are used in point-of-care devices, such as fluorescence immunoassay, chromatographic immunoassay, and enzyme-linked immunosorbent assay. The intensity of the indicator achieved is proportional to the concentration of the analyte. The assays can be performed with whole blood, plasma, urine, or saliva samples.

Immunodetection devices are used for testing and screening of antigens or antibodies for infectious diseases (e.g., human immunodeficiency virus, or HIV), endogenous substances [e.g., human chorionic gonadotropin (hCG) and microalbumin], cardiac injury markers (e.g., cardiac troponin I and T, myoglobin, and creatine kinase-MB), bone-resorption markers (e.g., crosslinked N-telopeptides of type 1 collagen, or NTx), tumor markers [e.g., prostate-specific antigen (PSA) and bladder tumor–associated antigen (hCFHrp)], and drugs of abuse (e.g., amphetamines). Because the immunoassay devices are used for screening and testing, it is often recommended that positive results be confirmed with an established laboratory technique before implementing treatment.

The detachability of the immunoassay units (e.g., cassettes, dipstick, and test strip) from the detector system allows the operator to take the units to the patients. Samples are collected and applied and then returned to the detector system for quantitation. For example, in the Cardiac T Rapid Assay/reader system (Table 6.5), the operator applies the blood sample onto the cassette and then places the cassette on the reader for quantitation. The detachability of the test cassettes increases the flexibility and application of the testing. The detector system could be left on a cart in front of the patient's room while the nurse or medical technologist brings the test strip or cassette into the patient room. No calibration is needed for stand-alone systems. Immunoassay test units are used in clinics, EDs, law-enforcement facilities, and in patients' homes.

Ex Vivo, In Vivo, and Noninvasive Point-of-Care Testing Instruments

Table 6.6 lists *ex vivo*, *in vivo*, and noninvasive POCT instruments. Unlike *in vitro* diagnostic instruments, *ex vivo* and *in vivo* (in-line) monitors fall into a separate category of instrumentation. *Ex vivo* and *in vivo* monitors have the potential for continuous and frequent patient monitoring. The sensors and electrodes for *ex vivo* or *in vivo* monitors are housed either external to the patient in a "device-control center" or in a microporous tubing that is fed through an indwelling line into the radial artery for monitoring. Calibration on these *ex vivo* and *in vivo* monitors initially is performed *in vitro* and subsequently *ex vivo* or *in vivo* at intermittent cycles. For some devices, no additional calibration is performed after the first *in vitro* calibration. Whole-blood or interstitial-fluid samples are tested on *ex vivo* and *in vivo* monitors.

Noninvasive devices offer a method for monitoring the blood chemistry without the need for blood collection by venipuncture or fingerstick. Table 6.6 lists examples of novel noninvasive devices. One device is the GlucoWatch Biographer, which transcutaneously monitors the glucose level in the interstitial fluid. Another device is the BiliChek system. It is a noninvasive monitor for bilirubin that has been applied to monitoring neonates at risk for development of hyperbilirubinemia. There is also a device used to measure sweat for ruling out cystic fibrosis. The testing principles applied to *ex vivo*, *in vivo*, and noninvasive devices include new methods, such as reverse iontophoresis, coupled to potentiometry, amperometry, and optical methods. Some of the analytes tested with these systems include blood gases, pH, sodium, potassium, glucose, bilirubin, and O_2 saturation. *Ex vivo* and *in vivo* monitors can be used in the ICUs and surgery departments for trend monitoring in place of serial *in vitro* blood testing. Besides the hospital, noninvasive devices also can be found in the home setting.

ANALYTICAL PRINCIPLES OF POINT-OF-CARE TESTING INSTRUMENTS

The intent of this section is to discuss common analytic principles, including potentiometry, amperometry, conductometry, optical method, and immunoassay.

Potentiometry

Potentiometry is the measurement of the electric potential difference between two electrodes in an electrochemical cell. The potential difference is logarithmically proportional to the electrolyte activity (concentration). One of the electrodes serves as the reference, and the other (e.g., ion-selective electrode, or ISE) is specific and selective for the ion measured. Ion-selective electrodes typically have a membrane at one end of the electrode. The membrane contains ionophores that are specific for the ion of interest. The ionophore selectively extracts the analyte (ion) when the membrane surface is in contact with the sample. Ideally, the electrode membrane should have a high-selectivity coefficient for one specific type of cation or anion. A low selectivity indicates the membrane is not specific for the ion measured and that other ions potentially could interfere. The displacement of the ion creates an electric potential difference across the membrane, between the sample and the internal standard solution. The membrane potential can be measured through the circuit of the reference and ion-selective electrode.

An ISE is used for electrolyte and pH measurements. The pH is measured using a hydrogen ion(H^+)-selective glass electrode. H^+ in the blood sample diffuses into the H^+-selective glass membrane, creating change in the potential between the buffer and the test sample. The change in electric potential is measured with respect to a reference electrode of constant potential. The Nernst equation [$\Delta E = (RT)/(ZF) \ln (H^+)/(H^+)_{ref}$], where R is the gas constant; T, temperature; Z, ion coefficient; and F, Faraday's constant, is used to correlate the change in electric potential with change in the ratio of the H^+ ions in the internal standard solution. The pH is calculated by the Henderson–Hasselbalch equation: pH = pKa + log $[H^+]/[H^+]_{ref}$. The pH electrodes can be constructed with different membranes, such as a polymer-based membrane. The polymeric membrane contains a lipophilic tertiary amine compound (e.g., tridodecylamine). The tridodecylamine serves as a selective proton ionophore within the membrane (19). The test principles are similar with the pH glass electrode.

Blood P_{CO_2} also is determined by using the H^+-selective principle in the Stowe–Severinghaus electrode. The CO_2 dissolved in the blood diffuses across a semipermeable membrane covering the glass electrode. The change in the pH of the buffer under the membrane is measured. The pH change is calibrated to the P_{CO_2} level in the blood. P_{CO_2} also can be tested with polymer-based membrane H+-selective electrode (19).

Total carbon dioxide content (T_{CO_2}) is measured similarly. Testing of T_{CO_2}, however, involves an acidification step that causes the release of the different forms of CO_2 in the blood sample. The released CO_2 (gas phase) diffuses across the electrode semipermeable membrane into the buffer, where the CO_2 reacts to form H_2CO_3. The carbonic acid (H_2CO_3) dissociates into H^+ and bicarbonate (HCO_3^-). The pH change in the buffer is measured using the preceding method. The change in the pH is calibrated to the total CO_2 level in the blood. Clinically, potentiometry can be used for the measurement of several other electrolytes, such as Na^+, Ca^{2+}, Cl^-, K^+, and Mg^{2+}.

Error Sources in Potentiometry

In potentiometry, the electric potential is logarithmically proportional to the activity of the electrolyte measured. Therefore, small errors in the measured potential can produce large errors in the results. These errors will affect both accuracy and precision. For example, if there is a change in the ion concentration (activity), there will be a corresponding change in the electric potential. If $\Delta E = E_2 - E_1$, it follows from the Nernst equation that $\Delta E = [(RT \ln 10)/(ZF)] \log[$ratio of the activities$]$, where R is the gas constant ($8.31431 JK^{-1} mol^{-1}$), T is the absolute temperature (K, Kelvin), $\ln 10$ is the natural log of 10 (2.303), F is the Faraday constant ($96487 C mol^{-1}$), and Z is the valence (charge) of the ion. When ΔE is 1 mV, T is 310.15K (37°C), and Z is 1, the ratio of the activities will be equal to $\log^{-1}[1 mV/61.54 mV] = 1.038$. Hence, a ±1-mV change in the measured potential is equivalent to approximately a ±4% change in the reported value. The reference electrode alone can introduce uncertainty of up to ±0.5 mV from junction potential, sample matrix, and boundary layer phenomena where the electrolyte enters the sample flow path. This is equivalent to a change in accuracy of approximately ±2% for monovalent ions (i.e., $Z = 1$ and $\log^{-1}[0.5 mV/61.54] \sim 1.019$) or approximately ±4% for divalent ions (i.e., $Z = 2$ and $\log^{-1}[0.5 mV/30.77 mV] \sim 1.038$). Instabilities during the electronic measurement of the potential of the electrochemical cell (ISE:reference electrode) and electric noise coming from electrode modules or *in vivo* probes detract from the precision of the analyte readings.

An ISE responds to the free anions and cations. The activity of the free ions is influenced by the pH, and the pH affects the equilibrium of free and protein-bound ions through competition between H^+ and the free ions for the protein-binding sites. For example, changes in pH affect the equilibrium of Ca^{2+} and equilibrium of Mg^{2+}. Increase in pH can lower the concentrations of free Ca^{2+} or Mg^{2+}, which result in decreased measured levels of free calcium and free magnesium (20–22). The dependency of the level of ionized Mg^{2+} on pH was described by Ising and colleagues (21) and was expressed with the *Siggaard-Andersen equation* (23): $iMg^{2+} (pH) = iMg^{2+} (7.4) \cdot 10^{x(7.4 - pH)}$, where x is the correction factor for the pH change. The equation provides a correction for the bias in iMg^{2+} attributed to the pH change in the sample. Equation-based corrections, however, are not necessarily valid in critically ill patients. Another factor that could affect the measurement of Mg^{2+} is the lack of selectivity of the ionophore in the membrane. Other bivalent ions, such as Ca^{2+} and Zn^{2+}, may also bind to the ionophore (24,25). Additionally, direct whole-blood analysis obviates the need to rule out pseudohyponatremia, an error that can arise with indirect measurement due to hyperlipidemia or hyperproteinemia (26–40).

Amperometry

Amperometry is measurement of the electric current flowing through an electrochemical sensor circuit when a constant poten-

tial is applied to the electrodes. The electrochemical sensor consists of two electrodes, an anode where oxidation occurs and a cathode where reduction occurs. A selectively permeable membrane surrounds the end of the sensor. The membrane has two functions: (a) to prevent proteins or other oxidants from accessing the cathode surface and (b) to limit the diffusion zone (41). The membrane can be constructed with different materials, such as cellulose acetate (42) or nafion (43,44) for selectivity of the membrane. The substrates and analytes of interest diffuse through the membrane to the electrodes. The oxidation–reduction reaction releases electrons. The electrons form a current under the electric potential applied. The amplitude of the current is linearly proportional to the substrate level in the cell. Clinically, the amperometric method has been used in the measurement of PO_2, urea nitrogen, glucose, lactate, creatinine, ketones, and other substances.

An example of amperometry is measurement of the partial pressure of oxygen (PO_2) using the Clark electrode. The Clark electrode consists of a silver–silver chloride anode and a platinum cathode. One end of the electrode is covered with a membrane that is permeable to oxygen but impermeable to reducible ions. O_2 in blood sample can diffuse across the membrane onto the cathode surface. At the anode, the chloride ion from the buffer solution reacts with the silver anode to form silver chloride. The reaction releases electrons under the potential of approximately 0.6 V provided by the analyzer. The electrons are transferred to the cathode, where the electrons reduce the oxygen. The current generated in the process is proportional to the PO_2 in the sample.

Enzymes can be embedded on a membrane to catalyze substrates for amperometric testing. When the membrane surface is exposed to a blood sample, the enzyme catalyzes the oxidation–reduction reaction of the substrate in the sample. During the chemical reaction, electrons are released. The current formed is measured and is proportional to the level of the substrate in the sample. Below is an illustration of the reaction mechanism for amperometric measurement of creatinine:

$$\text{Creatinine} + H_2O \rightarrow \text{creatine} \qquad [1]$$

$$\text{Creatine} + H_2O \rightarrow \text{sarcosine} + \text{urea} \qquad [2]$$

$$\text{Sarcosine} + O_2 + H_2O \rightarrow \text{formaldehyde} + \text{glycine} + H_2O_2 \, [3]$$

$$H_2O_2 \rightarrow O_2 + 2H^+ + 2e^- \qquad [4]$$

The creatinine substrate-specific electrode (SSE) uses three enzymes: creatinine amidohydrolase [Eq. 1], creatine amidohydrolase [Eq. 2], and sarcosine oxidase [Eq. 3]. These enzymes are immobilized in the SSE membrane. When creatinine diffuses across the membrane, the enzymes catalyze the conversion of creatinine into the end product of formaldehyde, glycine, and peroxide [Eq. 1–3]. The hydrogen peroxide (H_2O_2) is then oxidized on the platinum electrode, which is maintained at a constant voltage [Eq. 4]. The current produced is linearly related to the creatinine concentration.

Error Sources in Amperometry

Amperometric measurements are related to the transfer of electrons. Substances that interfere with the production or the transfer of the electrons from the oxidation–reduction reaction can affect measurements. For example, acetaminophen, analgesic–antipyretics, and anti-inflammatory agents can diffuse across the porous membrane to the electrode surface, where it could be directly oxidized, producing an interfering current that increases glucose reading (45–47). Ascorbic acid, a strong reducing substance, is oxidized at the electrode surface, resulting in the production of more electrons and the generation of more current (48,49).

Conductometry

Conductometry is the measurement of the impedance of the current flow in a fluid. The current is carried by the electrolytes in the solution under an applied potential. The current flow is determined by the viscosity of blood, the concentration and size of the charge-carrying substances (electrolytes) in the solution, and the strength of the electric potential. Impedance in the current flow is generally related to either a decreased concentration of electrolytes or an increased level of nonconductive or less conductive substances in the fluid. To measure the conductivity, two electric conductance sensors (ECS) are placed in contact with the fluid and on opposite ends or sides. An alternating voltage then is applied to the electrodes or sensors, and the conductivity (impedance) of the current through the fluid is recorded and calculated.

Clinically, conductometry is used for hematocrit measurements on whole-blood analyzers. Red blood cells (RBCs) are nonconductive, and electrolytes in blood are conductive. With the same test sample size, an increase in the proportion of RBCs in the test samples will decrease the proportion of plasma electrolytes in the test samples. Therefore, the conductivity of current through the blood is lowered. The impedance of the conductivity of current is measured, and the hematocrit levels can be calculated. Important to note is that normally electrolytes, especially sodium levels, are measured simultaneously. This is to take into account the potential effect of elevated electrolytes (such as sodium and potassium) on the conductivity in the blood.

Error Sources in Conductometry

Changes in the osmolality can affect conductometry measurements. Osmolality is largely determined by sodium concentrations (50). Clinically, sodium concentrations vary in critically ill patients. A study (51) showed that hematocrit measurements with conductometry reported lower results than with the microcentrifuge packed-cell volume (PCV) technique. This study was performed using blood samples from patients who received large transfusions of processed autologous blood. The study determined that the difference in the hematocrit measurement was because of high levels of sodium and chloride ions in the autologous infusates. The increase in electrolyte concentration increases conductivity and lowers the impedance in the sample, thus resulting in a lowered hematocrit level.

Changes in the protein concentration in whole-blood samples also could affect hematocrit measurements using the conductometry method (52). Increases in blood total-protein concentration could increase hematocrit readings because protein molecules in plasma are poorly conducting particles. The poor conductivity increases the impedance, therefore increasing the hematocrit reading. Mannitol pulls the water from blood cells and thus can increase the plasma volume. The increase in the plasma volume increases the conductivity; that is, a decrease in the impedance resulted in lowered hematocrit readings (53). Hematocrit determined by conductometry method must be interpreted with caution in critically ill patients, particularly those who receive intravenous therapy and blood products.

An alternative method for hematocrit determination in these patients is to use an electronic-particle counting (EPC) approach of the blood cells. The Coulter Z1 (Beckman Coulter, Fullerton, CA, U.S.A.) system is an example of an electronic particle counter. The EPC principle is based on measurement of the changes in the electric resistance produced by nonconductive or less conductive particles suspended in an electrolyte solution (salt solution). Applied to RBC counting, the cells suspended in the salt solution are forced through a tiny orifice. The conductivity across the orifice is lowered as the cells pass through. Each time a cell passes through the orifice, the resistance increases, which can be measured with two electrodes placed on either side of the orifice. This causes a spike in the electric potential difference between the electrodes. This method requires test sample to be diluted (dilution 1:6,250) with isotonic saline. The purpose of the sample dilution is to minimize the effects of protein or electrolyte components in plasma (52). The conventional microcapillary hematocrit test is another alterative to hematocrit measurements.

Optical Methods

Optical testing technologies are available for POCT and include optical reflectance, absorbance, fluorescence, and multi-wavelength spectrophotometry. Optical reflectance and absorbance measure the change in the color between the incident light and the reflected or absorbed light. This testing process involves a chemical oxidation–reduction reaction. As an analyte is oxidized, electrons are generated. The electrons oxidize the chromogen (colorless dye) to develop a color. The color intensity is proportional to the concentration of the analyte. The color intensity is measured by determining the reflectance and absorbance of a specific incident wavelength of light. The light intensity can be altered by light absorption or reflectance. Optical reflectance and absorbance technology have been widely used for glucose measurements.

Optical fluorescence and luminescence measure photons emitted from molecules making the transition from an excited to a ground state. For example, Na^+ and K^+ ions can be measured using fiberoptic chemical sensors (optodes). The optodes consist of fluorescent dyes and optical fibers. Optodes are encased by a semipermeable membrane, which contains recognition elements (*ionophores*). The ionophores are linked to fluorescence dyes and are selected for the analyte tested. As the ions pass through the membrane, they are bound to the ionophores. When exposed to light of a particular wavelength, the dye molecules are excited and emit photons. For example, as Na^+ concentration increases, the ionophores bind larger amounts of ions. The intensity of the emitted fluorescence varies proportionately with the concentration of the ions (Na^+, K^+). Optical reflectance technology also has been used in the measurement of P_{O_2}, P_{CO_2}, and pH (54–56).

Multi-wavelength spectrophotometry has been used for co-oximetry testing. For example, the NOVA pHOX Co-oximeter uses seven wavelengths to detect the oxyhemoglobin (O_2Hb), deoxy or reduced hemoglobin (HHb), carboxyhemoglobin (COHb), methemoglobin (MetHb), and sulfhemoglobin (SulfHb). The analyzer aspirates a whole-blood sample (approximately 100 μL) and lyses the RBCs. The fluid containing hemoglobin released from the lysed RBCs is drawn into an optical cuvette. Sensors are placed on opposite sides of the cuvette. Seven predefined wavelengths are transmitted through the sample. The absorbance of the lights at each wavelength is calculated. The sample absorbance is correlated to hemoglobin concentrations using an equation based on Beer's Law (57).

Dry-Reagent Biosensors

Dry-reagent based biosensors share principles of amperometric and optical testing methods. Both test methods incorporate membrane technology and enzyme-catalyzed reactions. Dry-reagent biosensors incorporate chemical reagents, such as enzymes, reagents, and buffers, onto test strips in an inactive (dry) form. The inactive reagents become activated on reconstitution with the blood sample. This technology has been used for measuring hemostasis indicators, such as prothrombin time. *In vitro* blood glucose monitoring systems are another example where dry-reagent biosensor technology are used. The monitor consists of a meter and a test-strip component. The meter can measure the current generated or the color developed during the chemical reactions that occur in the test strips. The typical construction of glucose meter test strips is a multilayer structure with two electrodes (test and reference) and a membrane coated with catalytic enzyme (Fig. 6.1).

Amperometric Glucose Test Strip

Figure 6.1 illustrates the architecture and the reaction principle of a glucose dehydrogenase-based electrochemical assay. The test strip (Accu-Chek Comfort Curve, lower left) comprises multiple components: a sample observation window, hydrophilic layer, and reagent layer. Between the top and bottom plastic layers are two palladium electrodes, one that serves as a working electrode and the other as an auxiliary electrode. The hydrophilic layer functions to direct the flow of sample (blood or aqueous controls) over the reagent layer. Glucose dehydrogenase, the primary component in the reagent layer, catalyzes the oxidation of glucose, which is present in the sample. During the reaction, ferricyanide is reduced to ferrocyanide. After a specific delay, the meter applies 300 mV across the test strip, and in the process ferrocyanide is reoxidized to ferricyanide (58). The meter converts the current generated from the sample to a corresponding glucose value (usually expressed in mg/dL).

Optical-based Glucose Test Strip

Optical-based glucose test strips are constructed without electrodes. Figure 6-2 shows the principle of the photometric method for glucose testing on SureStepPro system (Table 6.4).

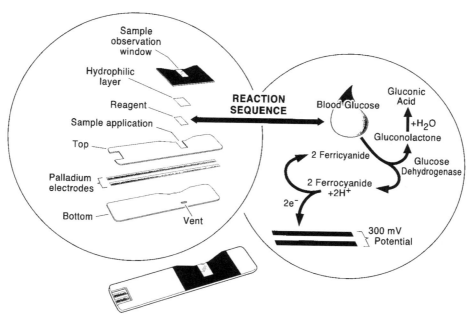

FIGURE 6.1. Principle of a glucose dehydrogenase (GD)-based biosensor. The handheld glucose meter system uses a GD-impregnated test strip with layered reagent and electrode components (left). After insertion of the test strip into the meter and the addition of a drop of blood, GD catalyzes the conversion of glucose, in the reaction sequence (right), that generates a current proportional to the glucose level.

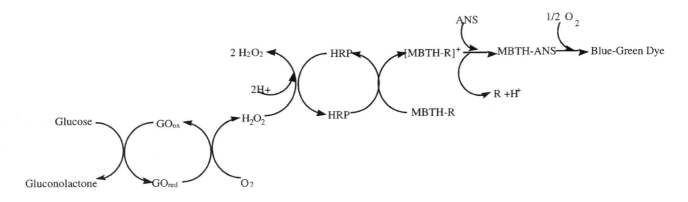

FIGURE 6.2. Principle of a glucose oxidase-based photometric biosensor. Glucose oxidase impregnated in the test strips catalyzes the oxidation of glucose into gluconolactone and hydrogen peroxide (H_2O_2). H_2O_2 is oxidized by horseradish peroxidase (HRP). Electrons released in the reaction oxidizes MBTH-R into [MBTH-R]$^+$, then producing MBTH-ANS for the color development (blue–green dye). GO$_{ox}$, glucose oxidase/flavin adenine dinucleotide (oxidized); GO$_{red}$, glucose oxidase/flavin adenine dinucleotide (reduced); H_2O_2, hydrogen peroxide; MBTH-R, meta[3-methyl 2-benzothiazolinone hydrazone] N-sulfonyl benzenesulfonic acid; ANS, 8-anilino-1-napthalenesulfonic acid; and MBTH-ANS, dye couple.

Glucose oxidase catalyses glucose into gluconolactone. The oxidation–reduction reaction of glucose is coupled to a chemical dye development. The color intensity is measured by an optical reflectance method. A specific wavelength of light emitted from the meter is directed at the color developed on the test strip. The change in the wavelength of light reflected is detected. The difference in the wavelength between the initial incident light and the reflected light is used to calculate the glucose concentration. The color intensity is calibrated to a glucose concentration by the vendor (59). The calibration algorithms are designated by code numbers, which are manually selected based on specifications on the test-strip package.

Potential Error Sources in Glucose Meter Measurements

Table 6.7 summarizes the reaction steps in amperometric and optical glucose measurements. A potential source of error in the testing of glucose using amperometry is the oxygen effect on glucose oxidase-based test strips. Figure 6.3 illustrates the oxygen effects on amperometric glucose measurement with glucose oxidase- and glucose dehydrogenase–based test strips. Glucose dehydrogenase-based test strips show negligible oxygen effects. For the glucose oxidase–based test strips, oxygen present on the test strip can participate in a side reaction that competes with the electron mediator/shuttle for the reoxidation of enzyme complex (GO/FAD$^+$). The competition results in a lower observed current. Equation 20 in Table 6.7 shows the possible oxygen-dependent side reaction. Increases in oxygen tension in whole blood results in decreases in glucose meter measurements (58,60–62).

Some glucose test strips (e.g., SureStepPro) separate plasma to some degree from the whole-blood sample with the use of a hydrophilic mesh and a microporous membrane for glucose testing. Changes in hematocrit will change the constituents of the plasma fraction in the whole-blood sample. Therefore, changes in hematocrit can affect glucose meter measurements

TABLE 6.7. PRINCIPLES OF AMPEROMETRIC AND PHOTOMETRIC GLUCOSE TEST STRIPS

Advantage H, Comfort Curve	
Glucose + GD/PQQ → gluconic acid + GD/PQQH$_2$	[Eq. 1]
GD/PQQH$_2$ + ferricyanide → GD/PQQ + ferrocyanide	[Eq. 2]
Ferrocyanide → ferricyanide + e$^-$	[Eq. 3]
SureStepPro, SureStepFlexx	
Glucose + GO/FAD → gluconic acid + GO/FADH$_2$	[Eq. 4]
GO/FADH$_2$ + O$_2$ → GO/FAD + H$_2$O$_2$	[Eq. 5]
H$_2$O$_2$ + MBTH + HRP → MBTH-R$^+$	[Eq. 6]
MBTH-R$^+$ + ANS + ½ O$_2$ → blue-green dye	[Eq. 7]
Precision PCx, Precision QID	
Glucose + GO/FAD → gluconic acid + GO/FADH$_2$	[Eq. 8]
GO/FADH$_2$ + ferricinium → GO/FAD + ferrocene	[Eq. 9]
Ferrocene → ferricinium + e$^-$	[Eq. 10]
GO/FADH$_2$ + O$_2$ → GO/FAD + H$_2$O$_2$	[Eq. 11]
Glucometer Elite	
Glucose + GO/FAD → gluconic acid + GO/FADH$_2$	[Eq. 12]
GO/FADH$_2$ + ferricyanide → GO/FAD + ferrocene	[Eq. 13]
Ferrocyanide → ferricyanide + e$^-$	[Eq. 14]
GO/FADH$_2$ + O$_2$ → GO/FAD + H$_2$O$_2$	[Eq. 15]
HemoCue	
Glucose + GD/NAD → gluconolactone + NADH	[Eq. 16]
MTT + NADH + diaphorase → MTTH (blue) + NAD	[Eq. 17]
GlucoWatch	
Glucose + O$_2$ + GO/FAD → H$_2$O$_2$ + gluconic acid	[Eq. 18]
H$_2$O$_2$ (oxidized on the surface of platinum) → 2e$^-$ + O$_2$ + 2H$^+$	[Eq. 19]
Oxygen-dependent side reaction	
GO/FADH$_2$ + O$_2$ → GO/FAD + H$_2$O$_2$	[Eq. 20]

GO, glucose oxidase; GD, glucose dehydrogenase; PQQ, Pyrroloquinoline quinone; PQQH$_2$, reduced Pyrroloquinoline quinone; NAD, nicotinamide; NADH, reduced nicotinamide; FAD, flavin adenine dinucleotide; FADH$_2$, reduced flavin adenine dinucleotide; HRP, horseradish preoxidase; MBTH, Meta[3-methyl 2-benzothiazolinone hydrazone] N-sulfonyl benzenesulfonic acid; ANS, 8-anilino-1-napthalenesulfonic acid.

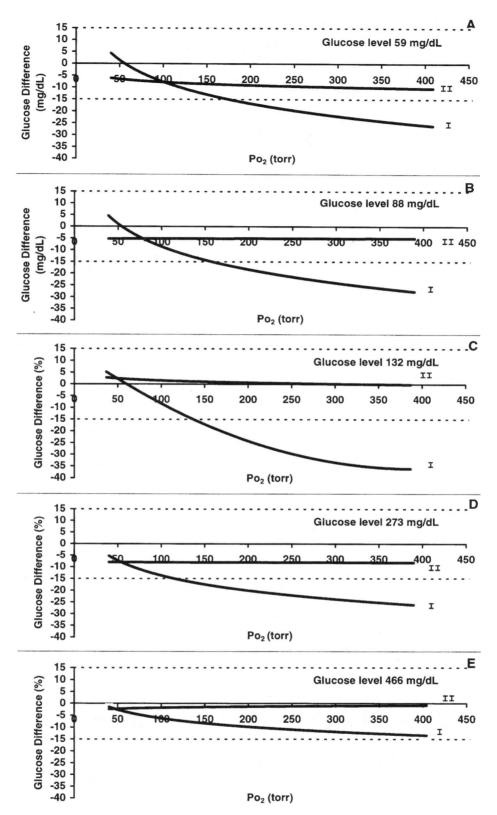

FIGURE 6.3. Oxygen effects on glucose meter measurements. High oxygen tension (>100 mm Hg) decreases glucose measurements on glucose oxidase-based test strips (line I). No apparent oxygen effects on glucose measurements with glucose dehydrogenase-based test strips (line II). The effects were evaluated at five different glucose levels: 59 mg per deciliter **(A)**, 88 **(B)**, 132 **(C)**, 273 **(D)**, and 466 **(E)**. The oxygen levels at each glucose concentrations were 40 to 400 mm Hg. The dashed lines represent the error criteria for 15 mg per deciliter at glucose levels of 100 mg per deciliter or lower and 15% at glucose levels greater than 100 mg per deciliter.

(59,63–65). To minimize the hematocrit effect on whole-blood glucose measurements, one portable device, the HemoCue B-Glucose analyzer (see Table 6.3), lyses RBCs with saponin in the test cuvette prior to testing. The lysed sample is more homogenous for glucose measurement with an absorbance photometry method. Clinical studies (66–70) showed minimal hematocrit effect on glucose measurement with the HemoCue analyzer. Current glucose meter systems are referenced to whole-blood reference methods (62), plasma methods (63), or deproteinized whole-blood methods (58). Differences in the reference methods may result in different glucose meter readings. Glucose meter measurements that are referenced to whole blood (e.g., One Touch, Bioscanner 2000, and Prestige Smart System) may be 10% to 15% lower than plasma-referenced glucose meter measurements (e.g., SureStepPro, FreeStyle, and In Charge). This is because plasma glucose levels are typically 10% to 15% higher than whole-blood glucose levels (71–73).

Immunoassay

The basic principle of an immunoassay is the use of an antibody and antigen to create a complex that can be measured (74). A secondary labeled antibody for the antigen can and often is used to form a sandwich complex to increase the specificity and sensitivity of the test. The amount of labeled antibody combined in the sandwich complex is proportional to the antigen in the samples. To quantitate the amount of antigen bound to the labeled antibody, a variety of labeling and detecting technologies are used.

Construction

The construction of immunoassay cassettes or test strips is based on dry-reagent technology. Typical construction of a lateral-flow test strip consists of five components: sample pad, conjugate pad, capture membrane, absorbent pad, and plastic backing with pressure-sensitive adhesive. Figure 6.4 shows the basic construction of the ACON HIV 1/2 test strips (Table 6.5). The sample pad contains chemicals such as buffers, salts, releasing agents, blocking agents, viscosity enhancers, or RBC separation agents. The purpose of the chemicals, when reconstituted, is to optimize the sample for the subsequent reactions. Glass fiber

and nonwoven polyester fibers are the most commonly used materials for the sample pad.

The conjugate pad contains the conjugate (labeled antibody), buffers, salts, stabilizer, and blocking agents. The conjugate, one of the most critical active reagents in the strip, is made by coupling the antibody or antigen of interest to the colloidal-colored latex or gold particles via physical adsorption, chemical bonding, or biotin–streptavidin reaction. The latex particle offers a much wider range of selections than the gold particle does in terms of functional groups for the coupling reaction. Glass fiber and nonwoven polyester fibers are the most commonly used materials for the conjugate pad. It is very important that the conjugate solution be uniformly distributed in and released from the pad to ensure a good reaction.

The substrate membrane is made of nitrocellulose or a similar material. The membrane provides the testing zones. The test-line and control-line solutions are deposited as narrow bands on the membrane and then dried. The important properties of the membrane include pore size, flow time, wettability, thickness, and protein-binding capacity. The absorbent pad functions to absorb the overflow of the sample. The plastic backing with the pressure-sensitive adhesive serves as a structural support for the layers above.

The solid-phase component of an immunoassay is associated with the immobilized antibodies that serve to capture the antigen bound to labeled antibody for quantitative or qualitative analysis. The immobilized antibodies may be situated as a narrow band along the membrane surface of the detection zone in a cassette-based immunoassay unit. The antigen–antibody complex can accumulate on this narrow band for qualitative or quantitative assessment (i.e., color or fluorescence intensity).

Various media have been used for the immobilizing of the antibodies. The materials used to mobilize the antibodies include coated tube/membrane surface and the coated bead. The coated-bead technology has the advantage of increasing the surface area where antibodies can attach, and it allows for more efficient mixing of antibodies and antigens.

Label and Testing

The common labeling technology used in POC immunoassay tests includes gold or latex label, fluorescent label, and enzyme-

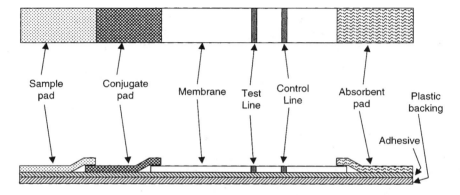

FIGURE 6.4. Schematic showing the construction of ACON HIV 1/2 immunoassay test strip. Top view (top) and side view (bottom). Please see the text for explanation.

linked labels. The benefit of direct-reading labels in immunoassay tests is that it allows visual interpretation of the results. This is a feature of many stand-alone immunodetection units. A gold-labeled immunoassay is used for cardiac troponin T (cTnT) detection in the Cardiac T Rapid Assay (Roche Diagnostic) (75,76). A cardiospecific anti-human cTnT antibody is labeled with gold particles. cTnT is bound to various epitopes using a biotin-labeled antibody and a gold-labeled antibody. When a test sample is introduced to the test cassette, cTnT in blood combines with the high-affinity biotinylated antibody and the cardiospecific gold-labeled antibody to form a sandwich complex, which consists of gold-labeled antibody, cTnT and biotin-labeled antibody immobilized in a solid phase. The antibody–antigen gold particle complex migrates by capillary action to the reading zone and appears as a purple ban. The purple color is because of the absorption property of gold nanoparticles, which is different from the yellow in regular gold. Unreacted gold-labeled antibody thereafter may combine with bovine cTnT immobilized distally to streptavidin band on the cellulose nitrate membrane. The formation of this second band, the control line, indicates that the test is valid and that the flow of plasma was unimpeded through the device. Without a detector/reader, quantitative results are not available; however, visual inspection of the lines provides a qualitative (positive or negative) result.

Competitive immunoassays with gold conjugates are used for testing for drugs of abuse. For example (77), the Triage Panel for Drugs of Abuse (Biosite Diagnostics, San Diego, CA) test cassette contains gold-conjugated drugs and their specific antibody. With a urine drug assay, drugs present in patient urine samples compete with the gold-conjugated drugs for the antibodies to form a complex. The complex is transferred to the detection zone. Any unbound gold-conjugated drugs are transferred to the detection zone, where they combine with immobilized antibodies. The combination of unbound gold-conjugated drugs and the antibodies produce a colored line, indicating a positive result. A negative specimen is indicated by the lack of a line because the gold-conjugated drug is not available to bind with the immobilized antibodies in the detect zone.

Fluorescent-labeled immunoassay is used to test the cardiac injury panel: myoglobin, CK mass, CK-MB mass, and cardiac troponin I (cTnI). The Alpha Dx Point-Of-Need system (Table 6.5) is one such device that incorporates a sandwich fluorescent immunoassay methodology for cardiac injury marker testing (78,79). In this system, fluorescein- and fluorescent-labeled antibodies and a solid-phase antibody are used. The fluorescence intensity is proportional to the amount of bound label, which in turn is proportional to the concentration of analyte in the sample. To obtain a reading, the fluorescence label is excited with a 640-nm diode laser. The resulting fluorescence is filtered and focused through a photomultiplier tube detector and converted into an electrical signal, which is related to the specific analyte concentration present.

The enzyme-linked color labeled technology, immunochromatography, has been used to test troponin I, myoglobin, and CK-MB (80–82). Each of these tests utilizes two gold-labeled monoclonal mouse antibodies and a biotinylated polyclonal goat capture antibody. Troponin I, myoglobin, and CK-MB

contained in the sample bind to their respective antibody to form a complex. This complex then migrates and adheres to the streptavidin immobilized in the detection zone. A positive result is indicated by a color line. For many immunodetection systems, the operator is required to interpret a color result. Therefore, it is important that all operators be tested for color blindness to ensure the quality of the results.

Noninvasive Technologies

Noninvasive instruments have received much attention in POCT. These instruments detect analytes without phlebotomy or fingerstick. For example, the GlucoWatch Biographer (Cygnus, Redwood City, CA) (Table 6.6) is a transcutaneous glucose monitor that is worn around the wrist like a watch and measures glucose extracted transcutaneously using a reverse iontophoresis method. In reverse iontophoresis, a low-level electrical current is passed through the skin between an anode and cathode. The current is carried by the migration of sodium ions to the cathode. Uncharged molecules such as glucose are carried along by convective transport (electroosmosis) and brought to the surface of the skin. Once glucose is extracted, it is measured using an amperometric biosensor. The device automatically takes intermittent (every 20 minutes) readings, thereby allowing the user to monitor his or her blood glucose levels at a nearly continuous state.

Another noninvasive clinical device is the Bispectral monitor (Aspect Medical, Natick, MA) which monitors the patient's degree of consciousness. The Bispectral processes the electroencephalography (EEG) signals from the patient using multivariate statistical methods. The responsiveness of the patient is scaled from 0 to 100, based on the different degrees of responsiveness of a patient under anesthesia, sedative agents, or comatose state. This monitor has been used in the OR (83,84), ICUs (85,86), and other clinical departments (87). Other noninvasive devices include the monitoring for bilirubin levels in neonates, pulse oximetry, and sublingual P_{CO_2}.

Chip-based Technologies

Chip-based technology uses microfabrication technology for the construction of biosensor chips. The dimension of the chips can be the size of a nickel or smaller, with a thickness of a few millimeters. Different materials and synthesizing techniques are applied to create these biosensor chips. The biosensor chips contain two main components, the sensors/electrodes and the channels. The channels are molded or etched with photolithography (88) onto the surface of materials, such as silicon, quartz, and plastic. The channels serve to direct the flow of the test sample to the site where sensors/electrodes are present. One of the advantages to chip-based technology is that it allows for the miniaturization of analytical instruments.

The i-STAT blood gas analyzer is an example of a POCT instrument that integrates this chip-based technology into its test cartridge. The sensors are microfabricated thin-film electrodes, which are created with the semiconductor manufacturing process technology. Depending on the cartridge model, different sensors, such as ISE electrodes, SSE electrodes, and conductometric sensors are configured to perform specific tests with chemistry-sensitive membranes and films containing reagent chemicals (www.istat.com). Once the sample is introduced to the sampling port, the capillary pump draws the sample through plastic tubing and to the microchannels, which then direct the blood sample to the test electrodes (i.e., pH, Na$^+$, Po$_2$, urea, hematocrit). The chip-based technology miniaturizes the analyzer, making this device handheld.

Chip-based technology can be integrated for immunoassay testing. Hundreds or thousands of spots can be deposited precisely on the chip for immunoassays or molecular diagnostics tests. Each spot of the capture molecule is matched with a complementary tagged conjugate that binds with the analyte of interest in the sample. For example, ThauMDx (Santa Barbara, CA, U.S.A.) has applied Evanescent Planar Waveguide™ (EPW™) technology to develop the LifeLite™ Cardiac Panel test, a multiplexing immunoassay that simultaneously measures three cardiac markers (troponin, CK-MB, and myoglobin) plus three integral controls in 5 minutes, using whole blood. Figure 6.5 illustrates the basic construction and test principles of the EPW™ technology.

The sample collection tube supplied with each cartridge on the LifeLite™ system contains fluorophore-tagged conjugates directed against each cardiac marker. When the sample is collected, the conjugates immediately dissolve and begin to bind and tag the analytes in the patient sample. When the sample passes over the surface of the EPW™ biochip housed inside the cartridge, the fluorophore-tagged conjugate–analyte complexes are bound to specific capture antibodies on biochip. The laser source and lens system directs light into the precision-molded plastic biochip. As light passes down the length of the biochip, differences in the indices of refraction between the plastic and adjacent sample cause total internal reflectance of the light, pro-

ducing an evanescent field in the sample immediately above the waveguide. The evanescent field excites the fluorophores that are bound to the biochip, and a charge-coupled device (CCD) camera/optics system precisely records the intensity of light emitted. Because the light signal intensity is proportional to the amount of analyte bound, quantitative measurements of analytes are generated using mathematic functions encoded by the software.

Chip-based technology is currently used in the research laboratory for polymerase chain reaction (PCR)-based nucleic acid analysis (89,90), genotyping (91,92), DNA sequencing (93,94), peptides (95), and proteins (96,97). Chip-based technology holds promise for the next generation of clinical instruments for the diagnoses of gene mutations, genetically inherited diseases, tumor markers, and immunodysfunction diseases.

ANALYTICAL ERRORS AND PERFORMANCE CRITERIA FOR POINT-OF-CARE TESTING INSTRUMENTS

Currently, no performance criteria have been established specifically for POCT instruments. All POCT instruments should follow the performance criteria used by the main laboratory instruments regardless of the instrument format and the analytic principles used. This is to ensure the quality of the measurements. Instrument performance can be compromised by errors introduced in the preanalytic, analytic, and postanalytic phases of the testing process.

Potential Errors in Point-of-Care Testing

Table 6.8 summaries potential preanalytic, analytic, and postan-

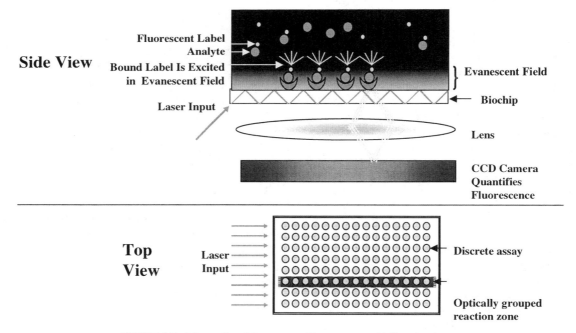

FIGURE 6.5. Schematics of Evanescent Planar Waveguide™ technology.

TABLE 6.8. POTENTIAL SOURCES OF ERRORS IN POCT

Preanalytic

Patient identity, record number, time, or date incorrect or missing

Specimen collection protocol not known, followed, or timed, or improper collection site

Wrong specimen source (i.e., capillary, venous, or arterial; *in vitro, ex vivo,* or *in vivo*)

Inconsistent or incorrect specimen handling, application, dosing, or volume

Absent or wrong anticoagulant (if required)

Inappropriate sample icing, instability, delay, dilution, contaminants, or storage

Hemolysis, erythrocyte settling, poor mixing, microclots, or degradation (e.g., metabolism)

Incorrect, mishandled, expired, unlabeled or unstable test strips, cartridges, cassettes, or reagents

Indwelling sensor artifacts (e.g., $\downarrow Po_2$, $\uparrow Pco_2$, $\downarrow pH$, $\downarrow\uparrow$temperature, or clotting around probe)

Leukocytosis (>50,000/μL), thrombocytosis (>600,000/ μL), or anemia (Hgb <7.5 g/dL)

Clinical contraindications (e.g., digit capillary in shock or poor peripheral perfusion)

Direct or indirect effects of transfused blood products or additives

Analytic

Physical perturbations (e.g., temperature, altitude, vibration, or humidity)

Extrinsic or intrinsic sample or aspiration anomalies (e.g., bubbles, viscosity, or thrombi)

Confounding variables (e.g., Po_2, Pco_2, pH, hematocrit, or osmolality) high, low, or changed

Matrix effects (e.g., proteins, lipids, dyes, cryoglobulins, or radiocontrast agents)

Native interferents (e.g., heterophile antibodies or autoimmune biproducts)

Interfering diluents, contaminants, preservatives, or drugs (pharmacologic or substance abuse)

Clotting/anti-clotting activators (e.g., coumadin, heparin, hirudin, or thrombolytic)

Method not calibrated, calibration protocol not followed, or calibration code wrong

Ex vivo blood cycling, calibration, or measurement problems

Calibration interval expired (e.g., *in vivo* sensor calibrated periodically to *in vitro* measurement)

Linear or reportable range exceeded, nonlinearity, drift, or sensor aging

Licensed (vendor-specified) range violated (e.g., newborn glucose limits or hematocrit)

Fundamental method or instrument inaccuracy, imprecision, or inconsistency

Lack of quality control (QC), proficiency testing, or performance monitors

QC or PT not performed by the correct person or no follow-up of problems

QC reagents unstable, volatile, expired, undated, contaminated, or mislabeled

QC inappropriate for the clinical decision thresholds (e.g., cTnI low control too high)

Test performed despite QC out of range or without periodic linearity check

Operator not educated, experienced, qualified, certified, or validated in testing or maintenance

Lack of recognition of instrument defect, malfunction, failure, or abnormality

Unstable power source (e.g., surges) or power interruption (e.g., blackout)

Postanalytical

Critical values omitted, not recognized, or not alerted

Incomplete test cluster from selection, deletion, or suppression error

Results not communicated to the physician, or communication lost, misplaced, or delayed

Instrument or data station memory, power, or battery failure

Transcription mistake, wrong units, no reference interval, or garbled data on print-out

Software delays, errors, bugs, or failures

No results documentation or transfer of data to the electronic medical record

Test results or quality monitors not reviewed (if statutes or accreditation requires)

Lack of bidirectional exchange of demographics, test results, quality data, or errors

POCT, point-of-care testing; PT, prothrombin time.

---

alytic error sources in POCT. An error in any one of these steps potentially could compromise the entire testing cycle and possibly affect physician decisions or patient outcomes. Clinicians and laboratorians should be aware of these potential error sources. The National Committee for Clinical Laboratory Standards (NCCLS) document EP18-P (98) provides a quality management guide for the potential error sources in the preanalytic, analytic, and postanalytic phases with single-use or unit-use devices (98). The document provides a table with a comprehensive list of potential failure modes for single-use devices. The table allows manufacturers and test sites to describe and document the potential errors in the devices. This guideline may be applicable to POCT instruments.

Glucose Testing Performance

Table 6.9 (58,99–106) shows the performance criteria for glucose meter measurements as recommended by several indepen-

dent professional organizations and experts in the field. The errors account for the operator performance, instrument performance (e.g., variations between test strip lots) (61,107), and interferences in the blood sample. No uniform consensus exists, however, on the error criteria that have been proposed. A few criteria appear too flexible (e.g., ±20% for the minimum acceptable clinical performance required for clinical effectiveness as recommended by the International Standards Organization) (106), whereas others are too demanding for the current technology (e.g., ±5% total error recommended by the American Diabetes Association) (102). We recommend the use of ±15 mg per deciliter for glucose levels below 100 mg per deciliter and ±15% of reference measurements for glucose levels greater than 100 mg per deciliter for the glucose error tolerance. The criteria avoid the discontinuity in the allowable error at glucose levels lower or higher than 100 mg per deciliter observed in the NCCLS criteria. The criteria we recommend are also suitable for the current technology. These criteria, however, should be tight-

TABLE 6.9. PERFORMANCE CRITERIA FOR HANDHELD GLUCOSE METERS

Error Tolerance Approach or Standard	Year	Source / Author (ref)
Glucose ≥100 mg/dL ± 15%	1998	POCT·CTR (58)
Glucose <100 mg/dL ± 15 mg/dL		
Glucose ≥100 mg/dL ± 20%	1998	FDA (103)
Glucose <100 mg/dL ± 20 mg/dL		
Glucose 30–400 mg/dL ± 5%	1996	ADA (102)
Glucose >100 mg/dL ± 20%	1994	NCCLS (99)
Glucose ≤100 mg/dL ± 15 mg/dL		
Glucose >70 mg/dL ± 15%	1994	Weiss et al. (100)
Glucose ≤70 mg/dL ± 20%		
Error grid analysis for neonates glucose monitoring	1994	Leroux et al. (105)
Glucose 30–400 mg/dL ± 10%	1992	ADA (101)
Glucose ≥70 mg/dL ± 20% (multidimensional grid)	1987	Clarke et al. (104)
See ISO/TC 212 document for additional standards	1999	ISO (106)

POCT•CTR, Point-of-Care Testing Center for Teaching and Research; FDA, U.S. Food and Drug Administration; ADA, American Diabetes Association; NCCLS, National Committee for Clinical Laboratory Standards; ISO, International Standards Organization.

ened to a ±10% error tolerance to encourage progressive improvement in clinical performance. The tightening of the error criteria is especially important to prevent devastating measurement errors in the monitoring of the hypoglycemic patient population, such as neonates, who typically have a glucose level at about 50 mg per deciliter (108–110). Recently, a working group on selective electrodes (WGSE) of the International Federation of Clinical Chemistry Scientific Division (IFCC-SD) proposed a recommendation for reporting blood glucose results (111). The recommendation suggests harmonizing to the concentration of glucose in plasma (with the unit mmol/L), irrespective of the sample type or technology. The group recommends using 1.11 for the conversion between the glucose concentration in blood to plasma when water and hematocrit levels are normal. This recommendation includes POC devices and methods that measure glucose concentration in whole blood.

Glucose meters can be used in the hospital and in patients' homes. The use of the glucose meter for critical care is controversial. In critically ill patients, changes in pH (112,113), hematocrit (59,63,114,115), oxygen tension (58,59,62,116), and medications (48,66,117,118) in whole-blood samples could falsely increase or decrease glucose measurements with handheld glucose meter systems. Clinical practitioners should understand the error sources in POCT.

Cardiac Injury Marker Testing Performance

Cardiac injury markers, such as cTnI, cTnT, CK-MB, and myoglobin, are extremely useful in the evaluation of acute coronary syndrome when the electrocardiogram (ECG) fails to provide definite diagnostic information. The diagnosis of acute myocardial infarction (AMI) and unstable angina is based on patient symptoms and signs, ECG monitoring, and cardiac injury markers. Recent guidelines (119–121) for the use of cardiac injury markers recommend that cTnI and myoglobin be used within 6 hours after the onset of chest pain for early diagnosis and that POCT be used if laboratory turnaround time is greater than 1 hour and immediate therapy is available.

The upper reference limit for the diagnosis of AMI using cardiac injury markers has been proposed. The diagnostic concentration cutoff for troponin is the 97.5th percentile of normal population as recommended by the National Academy of Clinical Biochemistry (NACB) and the International Federation of Clinical Chemistry (IFCC) (119,122). The 99th percentile (120) was recommended by the American College of Cardiology/American Heart Association (ACC/AHA). Recently, the European Society of Cardiology (ESC), NACB/IFCC, and ACC/AHA reached a consensus on a 99th percentile (123) for the cutoff level and an acceptable imprecision of ≤10% at the 99th percentile level.

The manufacturers of POCT instruments establish their own cutoff for the sensitivity and specificity of an instrument. The cutoff refers to a concentration at which the instruments show a positive result; however, the positive results may not represent a positive clinical diagnosis for AMI or unstable angina. There is no consensus on the performance (accuracy criteria) for POC cardiac injury marker (e.g., cTnI, cTnT, CK-MB, or myoglobin) testing. Also, there is a lack of a uniform reference method for comparing cTnI testing with the testing method of a hospital laboratory. The lack of a comparison method may hinder the setup of accuracy criteria and the implementation of the instrument for hospital use; it also may limit the use of the POC cTnI test to the ED. For clinical staff to integrate cardiac injury marker POCT for diagnosis purposes, one should consider (a) the clinical significance of instrument cutoff levels; (b) the present cutoff levels used in the health care system; (c) precision at those thresholds, and (d) published literature on the clinical evaluations of instrument sensitivity, specificity, and predictive value.

SELECTION AND EVALUATION OF POINT-OF-CARE TESTING INSTRUMENTS

Selection

Table 6.10 summarizes the criteria for the selection and evaluation of POCT instruments. To select a new instrument, one must consider the instrument characteristics, such as test clus-

TABLE 6.10. CRITERIA FOR THE SELECTION AND EVALUATION OF POINT-OF-CARE TESTING SYSTEMS

Medical efficacy in diagnosis, treatment, and management
Improved decision making and patient outcomes
Critical care profile, test clusters, patient-focusing, and indications
Therapeutic turnaround time for temporal optimization
Care path readiness for optimization of diagnostic–therapeutic strategies
Suitability for resuscitations, emergencies, peak workflow, and bursts in test volume

Economic efficacy
Professional productivity and satisfaction
Impact on length of stay
Cost-effectiveness by site, diagnosis, or outcome
Flexibility, modularity, exchangeability, expandability, and upgrade capability
Costs of instruments, consumables, and maintenance

Conservation of patient blood volume
Specimen volume, type, and matrix (e.g., whole blood, plasma, or serum) accepted
Medically useful half-life of test results
Elimination of unnecessary transfusions and their risks

Safety, ergonomics, security, and risk
Biohazard control, containment, and disposal
Speed, ease, simplicity, and user friendly operation
Identification, validation, notification, and security for operator and patient
Risk reduction features and on-site error minimization

Technical and quality features
Throughput, automated calibration, interrupt capability, and duration of analysis cycle
Compact, reliable, durable, lightweight, mobile, and power efficient with battery operation
Reagent stability, shelf life, lot size, and variability (biosensor, calibrant, cartridge)

Continuous quality improvement (quality control, quality monitors, proficiency testing)
Number and efficiency of preanalytical and postanalytical process steps
Analytical performance with whole-blood and other sample types (e.g., CSF and body fluids)
Compliance with federal, state, and accreditation regulations and training requirements

System performance
Accuracy, precision, bias, resolution, reproducibility, stability (biosensor drift), and response time
Linearity and performance in the high and low extremes of measurements, including critical limits
Consistency and relationship to tests performed in the parent (main) laboratory
Compatibility with other *in vitro,* and with *ex vivo* and *in vivo* whole-blood systems
Artifact elimination, error detection, interferences warning, and specimen flagging

Information interpretation and integration
Remote review, remote control, robotics, and data management system
Networking, interfacing (bidirectional), and wireless communications
Pattern recognition, alarms, and critical results notification
Information systems, data storage, and archiving capabilities
Communication of critical patient results from point-of-care locations
Interfacing with physiological patient monitors in critical care areas

Qualification of new devices and tests
Protocols for evaluation and method comparisons (NCCLS) to initiate new devices and tests
Instructions for meeting the requirements of federal, state, and voluntary accreditation agencies
Resources for training and education (interactive, video, CD-ROM, virtual, Internet, or other)

CSF, cerebrospinal fluid; NCCLS, National Committee for Clinical Laboratory Standards.

ters (test menu); the accuracy and precision, sample type (whole-blood, serum, plasma, or others), and test-volume requirements; operation, mobility, database connection, and cost. These selection factors are equally important; however, the sample size is crucial in anemic patients and in neonates, who have small blood volume. The frequency of blood drawing for laboratory testing could create unforeseen health complications (e.g., transfusion-acquired illness, infections, iatrogenic anemia). Minimizing blood loss is of utmost importance (124–126). Therefore, how one chooses a device requires a comprehensive investigation of product literature and specifications as well as an on-site demonstration and evaluation. A comparison evaluation overseen by the POCT coordinator or quality assurance manager is necessary.

Evaluation

Instruments should be evaluated under conditions of planned use. For example, if intended for use in the OR, a glucose meter should be evaluated for sensitivity to changes in oxygen tension because increased PO_2 levels (>100 mm Hg) can lower glucose meter measurements (58,61,62,127). Glucose meters chosen for use with neonates should provide acceptable glucose measurements with a high hematocrit level because increases in hemat-

ocrit could decrease glucose meter measurements (59,63–65). Table 6.11 summarizes the limitations of glucose meter systems. Glucose meter systems have a wide analytic (0–600 mg/dL) and hematocrit range (20%–70%). Generally, glucose meter measurements are accurate at normal physiologic glucose and hematocrit levels. At extreme low or high glucose and hematocrit levels, the meter performance needs to be to verified to determine the error levels because the extreme levels are important in demonstrating the meter use in critically ill patients. Clinical and laboratory studies show that changes in hematocrit can affect meter measurements (61,63,114,128).

Manufacturers of glucose meters may not state the effects of oxygen tension on glucose meter measurements. Studies have shown that high PO_2 can interfere with glucose measurements on glucose oxidase(GO)-based electrochemical test strips (58,60,62,116). Patient conditions, such as dehydration, shock (129), and medications (e.g., ascorbic acid, acetaminophen) (48,117), also can affect glucose meter measurements. In evaluation studies, measurements from the glucose meters should be compared with the manufacturer's specified reference method. Differences in the reference methods could result in significant differences in glucose evaluations (59).

When evaluating the performance of two instruments, it is important that the instruments tested be compared in parallel.

TABLE 6.11. CHARACTERISTICS OF GLUCOSE MONITORING SYSTEMS[a]

Test Strip	Instrument / Manufacturer	Linearity (mg/dL)	Enzyme	Test limitation		
				Hematocrit (%)	Po$_2$(mmHg)	Vendor-stated Interferences
HemoCue Cuvette[c]	HemoCue B-Glucose (HemoCue, Mission Viejo, CA, U.S.A.)	0–400	GO	None	Not applicable	Metabolites, (triglyceride and cholesterol)
Precison PCx Precison Xtra[d]	Precison PCx, Precison G, Precison Xtra (Abbott Diagnostics, Bedford, MA, U.S.A.)	20–600 20–600	GO GO	20–70 20–70	Not applicable Not applicable	Sample type, temperature and relative humidity, altitude, medications (acetaminophen and ascorbic acid), metabolites (uric acid, unconjugated bilirubin, cholesterol, and triglyceride), and patient condition (dehydration, hyperosmolar state, and shock)
SureStep	SureStep	0–500	GO	25–60	Not applicable	Patient condition (dehydration), medications (ascorbic acid, vasoactive agents), preservative (fluoride), altitude
SureStepPro	SureStepPro, SureStepFlexx, SureStep	0–500	GO	25–60, nonneonatal 25–65, neonates	Not applicable	As above
One Touch	One Touch Basic, One Touch Profile	0–600	GO	25–60	<45, [Glu] >150 mg/dL	Sample type, medication (ascorbic acid), metabolite (triglyceride), patient condition (hyperglycemic-hyperosmolar state)
One Touch Hospital	One Touch II Hospital	0–600	GO	25–6 , nonneonatal, 25–76, neonates 25–76, [Glu] ≤ 150 mg/dL[b] >60, [Glu] < 150 mg/dL[b]	<45, [Glu]>150mg/dL	As above
One Touch Ultra	One Touch Ultra	20–600	GO	30–55	Not applicable	Sample type, altitude, medications (acetaminophen, salicylates, uric acid, ascorbic acid), patient condition (receving oxygen therapy), metabolites (triglyceride and cholesterol)
One Touch FastTake	One Touch FastTake (LifeScan, Milpitas, CA, U.S.A.)	20–600	GO	30–55	Not applicable	As above
Glucometer Elite	Glucometer Elite XL (Bayer Diagnostics, Elkhart, IN, U.S.A.)	20–600	GO	20–60 >55, [Glu] <300 mg/dL	Not applicable	Sample type (neonatal blood), preservatives (fluoride and lodacetic acid), metabolites (cholesterol, triglyceride, uric acid), medication (ascorbic acid), patient condition (terminal malignant neoplasia, severe life-threatening infection, generalized massive edema, acute respiratory failure, and dehydrated/shock)
Advantage H	Accu-Chek Advantage H	10–600	GD	20–65, [Glu] <200 mg/dL 20–55, [Glu] >200 mg/dL	Not applicable	Sample type (neonatal blood), clinical test (xylose absorption testing), medical procedure (peritoneal dialysis solution containing icodextrin), altitude, patient conditions (dehydration, hypotension, hyperglycemic hyperosmolar nonketoic state, shock, metabolites (unconjugated bilirubin, triglyceride and cholesterol, uric acid, medication (acetaminophen), and carbohydrates (galactose and maltose), preservative (iodoacetate))

Comfort Curve	Accu-Chek Comfort Curve (Roche Diagnostics, Indianapolis, IN, U.S.A.)	10–600	GD	20–65, [Glu] <200 mg/dL 20–55, [Glu] >200 mg/dL	Not applicable	As above
In Charge	In Charge	20–600	GO	30–60	Not applicable	Sample type (neonatal blood), medication (ascorbic acid), metabolites (cholesterol, triglyceride, and uric acid), patient condition (pregnant diabetics, severely ill patients)
ExpressView	ExpressView (LXN, San Diego, CA, U.S.A.)	20–600	GO	30–60	Not applicable	As above
At Last	At Last System (Amira Medical, Scotts Valley, CA, U.S.A.)	40–400	GO	35–55	Not applicable	Medication (ascorbic acid), metabolite (triglyceride), preservatives (sodium fluoride)
Bioscanner	BioScanner (Polymer Technology System, Indianapolis, IN, U.S.A.)	20–600	GO	30–55	Not applicable	Preservatives (fluoride and oxalate), sample type (neonatal blood), medication (ascorbic acid), altitude, patient condition (dehydration)
Prestige	Prestige Smart System (Home Diagnostics, Fort Lauderdale, FL, U.S.A.)	25–600	GO	30–55	Not applicable	Preservatives (fluoride), medication (L-dopa), patient condition (hyperglycemia with hyperosmolarity, with or without ketosis, and dehydration)
FreeStyle	FreeStyle (TheraSense, Alameda, CA, U.S.A.)	20–500	GD	20–60	Not applicable	Sample type, metabolites (cholesterol, triglyceride), peritoneal dialysis solutions (containing icodextrin), clinical test (xylose absorption test), carbohydrates (galactose and maltose)

GO, glucose oxidase; GD, glucose dehydrogenase.
[a]Data in table were compiled in September 2001. Please refer to vendor for latest information.
[b]Hematocrit limits apply to neonate samples only.
[c]HemoCue test cuvettes require storage at 2° to 8°C. All other glucose monitoring systems listed in the table require room temperature storage.
[d]Glucose dehydrogenase (GD)-based Precision Xtra test strips are currently available.

TABLE 6.12. PRACTICE GUIDELINES FOR WHOLE-BLOOD ANALYSIS SPECIMEN PROCESSING

Time Limit	Container	Temperature	Measurement(s)
Immediate	Glass syringe	Room temperature	Po_2 when > 200 mm Hg
15 min	Plastic syringe	Room temperature	Po_2, O_2 Saturation, lactate
30 min	Plastic syringe	Room temperature	Glucose
30 min	Plastic syringe	Ice slush	Acid-base (pH, Pco_2, HCO_3^-), electrolytes (Na^+, K^+, Cl^-, Ca^{++})
1 h	Glass syringe or capillary	Ice slush	K^+ (plus the analytes below)
2 h	Glass syringe or capillary	Ice slush	pH, Pco_2, Po_2, O_2 saturation, hemoglobin, hematocrit, Ca^{2+}, and other electrolytes (except K^+)

Delays in the testing between instruments or changes in specimen temperature can introduce discrepancies, which may compromise the instruments' evaluation (130,131). Table 6.12 provides practice guidelines for testing time limits for whole-blood specimen analysis and processing for specific analytic measurements under different testing conditions and collection methods. The guidelines in Table 6.12 are from Burnet and colleagues (132), with the exception of glucose and lactate, for which the guidelines for sample processing are based on the results reported in Kost and colleagues (133). *Immediate* means as soon as possible, ideally within 5 minutes. Caution is advised when potassium measurements from samples stored in ice slush are delayed more than 30 minutes. Laboratory studies allow the evaluators to control and manipulate different variables in a test sample; this enables one to create test levels observed in critically ill patients for evaluation. Clinical studies can provide a "real world" instrument performance evaluation. Combination of clinical and laboratory evaluation models (61,134) may provide complete assessment information on instrument performance.

The error tolerance for differences between two instruments should focus on the level of inaccuracy, imprecision, linearity, or test range. An instrument could be accepted in one hospital (135–141), but it may not be accepted in another (142,143). Bland-Altman (59,144) analysis is used for assessing the measurement agreement between a chosen analyzer and an existing analyzer. The measurement differences are calculated by subtracting the measurements of the chosen and the existing analyzer. The differences are then compared with the mean of the measurements from the two analyzers. The degree of the differences from the chosen instrument measurement away from the mean may determine the instrument's acceptability. The NCCLS also provides a guideline for method comparison and bias estimation using patient samples (145).

CONCLUSIONS AND FUTURE PROJECTIONS

Point-of-care testing instruments have emerged as an important medical diagnostic tool, providing rapid, near real-time testing to improve patient outcomes. The availability of POCT instruments has revolutionized the way patient testing is performed, bringing laboratory testing to patients and, in the future, perhaps bringing more hospital services to patients. POCT instruments reduce test sample volume, enable testing with whole-blood specimens, and operate easily. The added mobility and stand-alone features of point-of-care devices facilitate the distribution of patient testing to match the evolution in modern health care systems.

Table 6.13 lists future challenges for POCT. The challenges include improvement of instrument design, development of

TABLE 6.13. FUTURE CHALLENGES FOR POINT-OF-CARE TESTING

Instrument design	Instrument mobility to patient sites and smaller instrument size
	Larger test menus, especially on smaller handheld devices
	Integration of microfabrication and nanofabrication technology
Noninvasive technology	Facilitation of patient compliance, self-monitoring, and management with less invasive and less painful approaches
	Elimination and minimization of potential infection from fingersticks and phlebotomy
Performance criteria	Universal performance criteria
	Evidence-based error tolerances
	Standardized reference methods
Informatics	Improvement in communication and networking between POCT devices and electronic databases
	Improvement or creation of universal interfacing between instrument and docking stations
	Development of wireless communication technology for downloading patient results into hospital databases from remote locations
Quality assurance	Integration of automated quality assessment features, such as intelligent and automatic quality control
	Educating and implementing personnel training and recertification programs for instrument operators
	Adding security features to POCT instruments
Clinical applications	Novel and fast detection methods to replace slow immunoassays
	On-site genetic and molecular diagnostic testing
	Application to microbiologic detection (e.g., in sepsis)

noninvasive technology, enhanced performance criteria, instrument connectivity, integrated quality assurance, and advanced clinical applications.

Instrument Design

Instrument size can limit access to where patient testing is performed, that is, in the OR, ICU, and neonatal ICU. There is a need for smaller, compact, portable, or handheld devices to improve access. The reduction in instrument size usually results in a decrease in the test menu. This limitation may be improved by the use of chip-based technology. Expanded test menus can improve information access in chemistry, hematology, hemostasis, microbiology, and genetics.

Noninvasive Technology

Noninvasive technology eliminates the need for fingerstick testing or phlebotomy, which may cause patient psychological distress (e.g., pain-related anxiety, fear, or panic), infection, and biocontamination. This technology can improve patient compliance and hence, improve patient self-monitoring and self-management. Noninvasive technology can be integrated into clinical devices for continuous patient monitoring.

Performance Criteria

The universal performance criteria comprise instrument inaccuracy, imprecision, and clinical error tolerance. Transportable and portable POCT instruments should be referenced to the same criteria. Handheld and immunoassay POCT instruments may need separate universal performance criteria. For example, a certain standard must be met for all glucose meters, hemostasis monitors, or immunoassay units (e.g., cTnI, hCG). Universal performance criteria promote comparability of POCT instrument performance and facilitate clinical evaluation and instrument selection.

Informatics

Integration and documentation of POCT results into hospital databases or patient electronic medical records is important for bidirectional flow (patient-to-physician and physician-to-patient flow) of information for patient management. To improve the documentation of patient test results on POCT instruments, there is a need for accessible docking or workstations with compatible data management software and "plug-and-play" interfaces so that results can be downloaded and recorded in the hospital database. Wireless bidirectional communication between instrument and the hospital database or workstation may eliminate the need for a physical docking system and may save valuable space in critical care areas.

Quality Assurance

Quality assurance should include instrument QC (i.e., intelligent, electronic), automatic QC, personnel training, and information processing to ensure consistent and reliable testing. Omitting QC

testing for expeditious testing is not recommended. One could override QC or the calibration cycle for emergency testing, however.

Personnel training enables the staff to understand the basic principles of the instrument, such as possible error sources, operating limitations, and the ability to troubleshoot. Training can reduce procedural errors in the preanalytic, analytic, and postanalytic steps.

Security is lacking on many handheld and portable devices. A personal identification number (PIN) or password is needed on handheld and portable devices to ensure the integrity (quality and confidentiality) of patient test results. The password feature would ensure that only qualified and trained persons can operate the instrument, hence ensuring the quality of the testing.

Clinical Application

Advanced POCT instruments can facilitate immunoassay detection with single-step whole-blood samples. Novel and fast detection methods can replace the slower manually operated immunoassay tests. The development of a direct whole-blood point-of-care system for diagnosis of bacteremia patients could replace time-consuming bacteria culturing. Integration of chip-based technology and PCR technology allows for on-site genetic and molecular diagnostic testing.

ACKNOWLEDGMENTS

We thank student researchers Sean Burgess and Nam Tran at the POCT·CTR. Valuable information was supplied by Ronald Blasig, Andrew Broderick, John Ellison, Chris Jarvinen, Debra M. Lee, Judith H. Lee, Phillip Y. Lee, Jinn-nan Lin, Jixun Lin, Joe Matolo, Carrie Mulherin, and David Shelby. We also thank the vendors for instrument technical information.

We also thank the following persons for their critique, review, and suggestions regarding this chapter: John Ellison, Frederick L. Kiechle, Larry J. Kricka, Lasse Larsson, Debra M. Lee, Judith H. Lee, Philip Lee, Jinn-nan Lin, Terry Shirey, and Alan Wu.

REFERENCES

1. Pelegri MD, Garcia-Beltran L, Pascual C. Improvement of emergency and routine turnaround time by data processing and instrumentation changes. *Clin Chim Acta* 1996;248:65–72.
2. Steindel SJ, Howanitz PJ. Changes in emergency department turnaround time performance from 1990 to 1993: a comparison of two College of American Pathologists Q-Probes Studies. *Arch Pathol Lab Med* 1997;121:1031–1041.
3. Becker RC, Cyr J, Corrao JM, et al. Bedside coagulation monitoring in heparin-treated patients with active thromboembolic disease: a coronary care unit experience. *Am Heart J* 1994;128:719–723.
4. Murray RP, Leroux M, Sabga E, et al. Effect of point of care testing on the length of stay in an adult emergency department. *J Emerg Med* 1999;17:811–814.
5. Collinson PO. The need for a point of care testing: an evidence-based appraisal. *Scand J Clin Lab Invest* 1999;59(Suppl 230):67–73.
6. Wu AHB, Clive JM. Impact of CK-MB testing policies on hospital length of stay and laboratory costs for patients with myocardial infarction or chest pain. *Clin Chem* 1997;43:326–332.
7. Zaloga GP. Monitoring versus testing technologies: present and

future. *Med Lab Observer* 1991;23:20–31.

8. Sands VM, Auerbach PS, Birnbaum J, et al. Evaluation of a portable clinical blood analyzer in the emergency department. *Acad Emerg Med* 1995;2:172–178.

9. Goodwin SA. Point-of-care testing in a post anesthesia care unit. *Med Lab Observer* 1994;26(Suppl 9):15–18.

10. McErlean ES, Deluca SA, Brown K, et al. Point of care testing for aPTT improves cost outcomes following coronary intervention. *J Am Coll Cardiol* 1998;31(Suppl 2):49A.

11. Kost GJ. Point-of-care testing in intensive care. In: Tobin MJ, ed. *Principles and practice of intensive care monitoring.* New York: McGraw-Hill, 1998:1267–1296.

12. Kost GJ. Point-of-care testing. In: Meyers RA, ed. *Encyclopedia of analytical chemistry.* New York: John Wiley and Sons, 2000:1603–1625.

13. Fuhrman SA, Travers EM, Handorf CR. The mobile laboratory in alternative site testing. *Arch Pathol Lab Med* 1995;119:939–942.

14. Kiechle FL, Ingram R, Karcher R, et al. Transfer of glucose measurements outside the laboratory. *Lab Med* 1990;21:504–511.

15. Frischauf P, Larsson L, Krarup T. New QC process validates new blood gas technology at each measurement. *Clin Chim Acta* 2001;307:75–85.

16. Louie RF, Tang Z, Shelby DG, et al. Point-of-care testing: millennium technology for critical care. *Lab Med* 2000;31:402–408.

17. Ehrmeyer SS, Laessig RH. Electronic "quality control" (EQC): is it just for unit use devices? *Clin Chim Acta* 2001;307:95–99.

18. Westgard JO. Electronic quality control, the total testing process, and the total quality control system. *Clin Chim Acta* 2001;307:45–48.

19. Meyerhoff ME. New *in vitro* analytical approaches for clinical chemistry measurements in critical care. *Clin Chem* 1990;36:1567–1572.

20. Zoppi F, Cristalli C. Ionized magnesium in serum and ultrafiltrate: pH and biocarbone effect on measurements with AVL 988-4 electrolyte analyzer. *Clin Chem* 1998;44:668–671.

21. Ising H, Bertschat F, Günther T, et al. Measurement of free magnesium in blood, serum and plasma with an ion-sensitive electrode. *Eur J Clin Chem Clin Biochem* 1995;33:365–371.

22. Huijgen HK, Sanders R, Cecco SA, et al. Serum ionized magnesium: comparison of results obtained with three ion-selective analyzers. *Clin Chem Lab Med* 1999;37:465–470.

23. Siggaard-Andersen O, Thode J, Wandrup J. The concentration of free calcium ions in the blood plasma: "ionized calcium." In: Siggaard-Andersen I, ed. *Blood pH, carbon dioxide, oxygen and calcium-ion.* Copenhagen: Private Press, 1981:163–190.

24. Rehak NN, Cecco SA, Niemela JE, et al. Linearity and stability of the AVL and Nova magnesium and calcium ion-selective electrodes. *Clin Chem* 1996;42:880–887.

25. Ritter C, Ghahramani M, Marsoner HJ. More on the measurement of ionized magnesium in whole blood. *Scand J Clin Lab Invest* 1996;56(Suppl 224):275–280.

26. Forrest ARW, Shenkin A. Dangerous pseudohyponatremia. *Lancet* 1980;2:1256.

27. Frier BM, Steer CR, Baird JD, et al. Misleading plasma electrolytes in diabetic children with severe hyperlipidemia. *Arch Dis Child* 1980;55:771–775.

28. Nabji AA, Blank DW. Pseudohyponatremia and hyperviscosity. *J Clin Pathol* 1983;36:834–835.

29. Pain RW. Test and teach (41). Diagnosis: hypertriglyceridemia with pseudohyponatremia in acute and chronic alcoholism. *Pathology* 1983;15:233, 331–334.

30. Howard JM, Reed J. Pseudohyponatremia in acute hyperlipemic pancreatitis: a potential pitfall in therapy. *Arch Surg* 1985;120:1053–1055.

31. Weisberg LS. Pseudohyponatremia: a reappraisal. *Am J Med* 1989;86:315–318.

32. Kost GJ. Accurate and efficient diagnosis of hyperosmolar coma. *Audio-Digest Internal Med* 1991;38.

33. Grateau G, Bachmeyer C, Taulera O, et al. Pseudohyponatremia and pseudohyperphosphatemia in a patient with human immunodeficiency virus infection. *Nephron* 1993;46:640.

34. Vaswani SK, Sprague R. Pseudohyponatremia in multiple myeloma. *South Med J* 1993;86:251–252.

35. Olivero JJ. Case in point: pseudohyponatremia due to hyperproteinemia in multiple myeloma. *Hosp Pract* 1994;29:61.

36. Sachs C, Levillain P. The real cause of discrepancy between plasma sodium results obtained by ISE and "dilution" techniques: an error in the dilution factor. *AACC Electrolyte/blood gas division newsletter* 1994;9:2–4.

37. Lawn N, Wijdicks EF, Burritt MF. Intravenous immune globulin and pseudohyponatremia. *N Engl J Med* 1998;339:632.

38. Ng SK. Intravenous immunoglobulin infusion causing pseudohyponatremia. *Lupus* 1999;8:488–490.

39. Rosenthal R, Koelz A, Vogelbach P. Pseudohyponatremia. *Schweiz Med Wochenschr* 2000;130:161.

40. Aw TC, Kiechle FL. Pseudohyponatremia. *Am J Emerg Med* 1985;3:236–239.

41. Durst RA, Siggaard-Andersen O. Electrochemistry. In: Burtis CA, Ashwood ER, eds. *Tietz textbook of clinical chemistry,* 3rd ed. Philadelphia, WB Saunders, 1999:133–149.

42. Bindra DS, Zhang Y, Wilson GS. Design and *in vitro* studies of a needle-type glucose sensor for subcutaneous monitoring. *Anal Chem* 1991;63:1692–1696.

43. Harrison DJ, Turner RF, Baltes HP. Characterization of perfluorosulfonic acid polymer coated enzyme electrodes and a miniaturized integrated potentiostat for glucose analysis in whole blood. *Anal Chem* 1988;60:2002–2007.

44. Moussy F, Jakeway S, Harrison DJ, et al. *In vitro* and *in vivo* performance and lifetime of perfluorinated ionomer-coated glucose sensors after high-temperature curing. *Anal Chem* 1994;66:3882–3888.

45. Lindh M, Lindgren K, Carlström A, et al. Electrochemical interferences with the YSI glucose analyzer [Letter]. *Clin Chem*1982;28:726.

46. Kaufmann-Raab I, Jonen HG, Jähnchen E, et al. Interference by acetaminophen in the glucose oxidase-peroxidase method for blood glucose determination. *Clin Chem* 1976;22:1729–1731.

47. Cartier L-J, Leclerc P, Pouliot M, et al. Toxic levels of acetaminophen produce a major positive interference on Glucometer Elite and Accuchek Advantage glucose meters [Letter]. *Clin Chem* 1998;44:893–894.

48. Tang ZP, Du XG, Louie RF, et al. Effects of drugs on glucose measurements with handheld glucose meters and a portable glucose analyzer for point-of-care testing. *Am J Clin Pathol* 2000;113:75–86.

49. Moatti-Sirat D, Velho G, Reach G. Evaluating *in vitro* and *in vivo* the interference of ascorbate and acetaminophen on glucose detection by a needle-type glucose sensor. *Biosens Bioelectron* 1992;7:345–352.

50. Scott MG, Heusel JW, LeGrys VA. Electrolytes and blood gases. In: Burtis CA, Ashwood ER, eds. *Tietz textbook of clinical chemistry,* 3rd ed. Philadelphia: WB Saunders, 1999:1056–1124.

51. McMahon DJ, Carpenter RL. A comparison of conductivity-based hematocrit determinations with conventional laboratory methods in autologous blood transfusions. *Anesth Analg* 1990;71:541–544.

52. Stott RAW, Hortin GL, Wilhite TR, et al. Analytical artifacts in hematocrit measurements by whole-blood chemistry analyzers. *Clin Chem* 1995;41:306–311.

53. Olthof CG, Kouw PM, Donker AJM., et al. Non-invasive conductivity technique to detect changes in haematocrit: *in vitro* validation. *Med Biol Eng Comput* 1994;32:495–500.

54. Lübbers DW, Opitz N. Die pCO2- / pO2-Optode: eine neue pCO2- bzw. pO2-Messonde zur Messung des pCO2 oder pO2 von Gasen und Flüssigkeiten. *Z Naturforsch C* 1975;30:532–533.

55. Gehrich JL, Lubbers DW, Opitz N, et al. Optical fluorescence and its application to an intravascular blood gas monitoring system. *IEEE Trans Biomed Eng* 1986;33:117–132.

56. Boalth N, Wandrup J, Larsson L, et al. Blood gases and oximetry: calibration-free new dry chemistry and optical technology for near-patient testing. *Clin Chim Acta* 2001;307:225–233.

57. Evenson MA. Spectrophotometric techniques. In: Burtis CA, Ashwood ER, eds. *Tietz textbook of clinical chemistry,* 3rd ed. Philadelphia: WB Saunders, 1999:75–93.

58. Kost GJ, Vu H, Lee JH, et al. Multicenter study of oxygen-insensitive handheld glucose point-of-care testing in critical care/hospital/ambulatory patients in the United States and Canada. *Crit Care Med* 1998;26:581–590.

59. Louie RF, Tang Z, Sutton DV, et al. Point-of-care glucose testing:

effects of critical care variables, influence of reference instruments, and a modular glucose meter design. *Arch Pathol Lab Med* 2000;124: 257–266.

60. Cross MH, Brown DG. Blood glucose reagent strip tests in the operating room: Influence of hematocrit, partial pressure of oxygen, and blood glucose level–a comparison of the BM-Test 1-44, BM-Accutest, and Satellite G reagent strip systems. *J Clin Monit* 1996;12:27–33.

61. Tang Z, Louie RF, Lee JH, et al. Oxygen effects on glucose meter measurements with glucose dehydrogenase- and oxidase-based test strips for point-of-care testing. *Crit Care Med* 2001;307:1062–1070.

62. Tang Z, Louie RF, Payes M, et al. Oxygen effects on glucose measurements with a reference analyzer and three handheld meters. *Diabetes Technology & Therapeutics* 2000;2:349–362.

63. Tang Z, Lee JH, Louie RF, et al Effects of different hematocrit levels on glucose measurements with handheld meters for point-of-care testing. *Arch Pathol Lab Med* 2000;124:1135–1140.

64. Hussain K, Sharief N. The inaccuracy of venous and capillary blood glucose measurement using reagent strips in the newborn period and the effect of hematocrit. *Early Human Development* 2000;57:111–121.

65. Hameed M, Pollard R, Sharief N. Bedside assessment of blood glucose in the neonatal period – an ongoing problem. *Br J Intensive Care* 1996;6114–6118.

66. Ashworth L, Gibb I, Alberti KG. Hemocue: evaluation of a portable photometric system for determining glucose in whole blood. *Clin Chem* 1992;38:1479–1482.

67. Vadasdi E, Jacobs E. HemoCue β-glucose photometer evaluated for use in a neonatal intensive care unit. *Clin Chem* 1993;39:2329–2332.

68. Wiener K. An assessment of the effect of haematocrit on the Hemo-Cue blood glucose analyzer. *Ann Clin Biochem* 1993;30(part 1): 90–93.

69. Nichols JH, Howard C, Loman K, et al. Laboratory and bedside evaluation of portable glucose meters. *Am J Clin Pathol* 1995;103: 244–251.

70. Karcher RE, Ingram RL, Kiechle FL, et al. Comparison of the Hemo-Cue β-Glucose photometer and Reflotron for open heart surgery. *Am J Clin Pathol* 1993;100:130–134.

71. Kempe KC, Czeschin LI, Yates KH, et al. A hospital system glucose meter that produces plasma-equivalent values from capillary, venous, and arterial blood. *Clin Chem* 1997;43;1803–1804.

72. Kost GJ, Bowen, T.P. New whole blood methods and instruments: glucose measurements and test menus for critical care. *J Intl Fed Clin Chem* 1992;3:160–172.

73. Fogh-Andersen N, D'Orazio P. Proposal for standardizing direct-reading biosensors for blood glucose. *Clin Chem* 1998;44:655–659.

74. Jefferis R, Deverill I. The antigen antibody reaction. In: Price CP, Newman DJ, eds. Principles and practice of immunoassay. New York: Stockton Press, Macmillan Publishers, 1991:1–18.

75. Muller-Bardorff M. Freitag H, Scheffold T, et al. Development and characterization of a rapid assay for bedside determination of cardiac troponin T. *Circulation* 1995;92:2869–2875.

76. Collinson PO, Gerhardt W, Katus HA, et al. Multicenter evaluation of an immunological rapid test for the detection of troponin T in whole blood sample. *Eur J Clin Chem Biochem* 1996;34:591–598.

77. Peace MR, Tarnai LD, Poklis A. Performance evaluation of four onside drug-testing devices for detection of drugs of abuse in urine. *J Anal Toxicol* 2000;24:589–594.

78. Apple FS, Anderson FP, Collinson P, et al. Clinical evaluation of the first medical whole blood, point-of-care testing device for detection of myocardial infarction. *Clin Chem* 2000;46:1604–1609.

79. Pierce JA, Ellsworth S. Triaging chest pain: point-of-need decision support using a cardiac panel. *Am Clin Lab* 2000;18–20.

80. Heeschen C, Goldmann BU, Moeller RH, et al. Analytical performance and clinical application of a new rapid beside assay for the detection of serum cardiac troponin I. *Clin Chem* 1998;44:1925–1930.

81. Hamm CW, Goldmann BU, Heeschen C, et al. Emergency room triage of patients with acute chest pain by means of rapid testing for cardiac troponin T or Troponin I. *N Engl J Med* 1997;337:1648–1653.

82. Brogan GX, McCuskey CF, Thode H Jr, et al. Evaluation of cardiac STATus CK-MB/myoglobin device for rapidly ruling out acute myocardial infarction. *Clin Lab Med* 1997;17:655–668.

83. Tufano R, Palomba R, Lambiase G, et al. The utility of bispectral index monitoring in general anesthesia. *Minerva Anestesiol* 2000;66: 389–393. [in Italian]

84. Johansen JW, Sebel PS, Sigl JC. Clinical impact of hypnotic-titration guidelines based on EEG bispectral index (BIS) monitoring during routine anesthetic care. *J Clin Anesth* 2000;12:433–443.

85. Simmons LE, Riker RR, Prato BS, et al. Assessing sedation during intensive care unit mechanical ventilation with the bispectral index and the sedation-agitation scale. *Crit Care Med* 1999;27: 1499–1504.

86. De Deyne C, Struys M, Decruyennaere J, et al. Use of continuous bispectral EEG monitoring to assess depth of sedation in ICU patients. *Intensive Care Med* 1998;24:1294–1298.

87. Bower AL, Ripepi A, Dilger J, et al. Bispectral index monitoring of sedation during endoscopy. *Gastrointest Endosc* 2000;52:192–196.

88. Dolnik V, Liu S, Jovanovich S. Capillary electrophoresis on microchip. *Electrophoresis* 2000;21:41–45.

89. Khandurina J, Mcknight TE, Jacobson SC, et al. Integrated system for rapid PCR-based DNA analysis in microfluidic devices. *Anal Chem* 2000;72:2995–3000.

90. Woolley AT, Hadley D, Landre P, et al. Functional integration of PCR amplification and capillary electrophoresis in a microfabricated DNA analysis device. *Anal Chem* 1996;68:4081–4086.

91. Hofgartner WT, Huhmer AFR, Landers JP, et al. Rapid diagnosis of herpes simplex encephalitis using microchip electrophoresis of PCR products. *Clin Chem* 1999;45:2120–2128.

92. Livache T, Fouque B, Roget A, et al. Polypyrrole DNA chip on a silicon device: example of hepatitis C virus genotyping. *Anal Biochem* 1998;255:188–194.

93. Chen YH, Wang WC, Young KC, et al. Plastic microchip electrophoresis for analysis of PCR products of hepatitis C virus. *Clin Chem* 1999;45:1938–1943.

94. Ueda M, Kiba Y, Abe H, et al. Fast separation of oligonucleotide and triplet repeat DNA on a microfabricated capillary electrophoresis device and capillary electrophoresis. *Electrophoresis* 2000;21:176–180.

95. Xue QF, Dunayevskiy YM, Foret F, et al. Integrated multichannel microchip electrospray ionization mass spectrometry: analysis of peptides from on-chip tryptic digestion of melittin. *Rapid Commun Mass Spectrom* 1997;11:1253–1256.

96. Figeys D, Aebersold R. Nanoflow solvent gradient delivery from a microfabricated device for protein identifications by electrospray ionization mass spectrometry. *Anal Chem* 1998;70:3721–3727.

97. Figeys D, Ning YB, Aebersold R. A microfabricated device for rapid protein identification by microelectrospray ion trap mass spectrometry. *Anal Chem* 1997;69:3153–3160.

98. National Committee on Clinical Laboratory Standards (NCCLS). Quality management for unit-use testing, vol 19. Document EP18-P. Wayne, PA: NCCLS, 1999, no. 24.

99. Barr JT, Betschart J, Bracey A, et al. Ancillary (bedside) blood glucose testing in acute and chronic care facilities. Villanova, PA: National Committee for Clinical Laboratory Standards, vol 14. Document C30-A, 1994:1–14.

100. Weiss SL, Cembrowski GS, Mazze RL. Patient and physician goals for self-monitoring blood glucose instruments. *Am J Clin Pathol* 1994; 102:611–615.

101. American Diabetes Association. Self-monitoring of blood glucose. *Diabetes Care* 1992;15(suppl 2):56–61.

102. American Diabetes Association. Self-monitoring of blood glucose. *Diabetes Care* 1996;19 (Suppl 1): S62–S66.

103. United States Food and Drug Administration (FDA), Division of Clinical Laboratory Devices. Review criteria for assessment of portable invasive blood glucose monitoring in vitro diagnostic devices which use glucose oxidase, dehydrogenase, or hexokinase mythology. Rockville, MD: FDA, March 1998.

104. Clarke WL, Cox D, Gonder-Frederick LA, et al. Evaluating clinical accuracy of systems for self-monitoring of blood glucose. *Diabetes Care* 1987;10:622–628.

105. Leroux M, Seshia MMK. Glucose meter use in nurseries: error grid evaluates clinical accuracy. *Lab Med* 1994;25:592–595.

106. International Standards Organization. Requirements for *in vitro*

blood glucose monitoring systems for self-testing in managing diabetes mellitus. ISO/TC 212 (Annex A)1999;21–23.

107. Louie RF, Tang Z, Chang K-CJ, et al. Measurement variability between test strip lots on five handheld glucose meter systems. *Clin Chem* 2000; 46(Suppl):6,A15.

108. Cole MD, Peevy K. Hypoglycemia in normal neonates appropriate for gestational age. *J Perinatol* 1994;14:118–120.

109. Halamek LP, Benaron DA, Stevenson DK. Neonatal hypoglycemia, Part I: background and definition. *Clin Pediatr* 1997;36:675–680.

110. Aynsley-Green A, Hawdon JM. Hypoglycemia in the neonate: current controversies. *Acta Paediatr Jpn* 1997;39(Suppl 1):S12–S16.

111. Burnett RW, D'Orazio P, Fogh-Andersen N, et al. International Federation of Clinical Chemistry and Laboratory Medicine: IFCC recommendation on reporting results for blood glucose. *Clin Chim Acta* 2001;307:205–209.

112. Kilpatrick ES, Rumley AG, Smith EA. Variations in sample pH and pO₂ affect ExacTech meter glucose measurements. *Diabetes Medicine* 1994;11:506–509.

113. Tang Z, Du X, Louie RF, et al. Effects of pH on glucose measurements with handheld glucose meters and a portable glucose analyzer for point-of-care testing. *Arch Pathol Lab Med* 2000;124:577–582.

114. Chance JJ, Li DJ, Jones KA, et al. Technical evaluation of five glucose meters with data management capabilities. *Am J Clin Pathol* 1999;111: 547–556.

115. Cross MH, Brown DG. Blood glucose reagent strip tests in the operating room: influence of hematocrit, partial pressure of oxygen, and blood glucose level—a comparison of the BM-Test 1-44, BM-Accutest, and Satellite G reagent strip systems. *J Clin Monit* 1996;12:27–33.

116. Kurahashi K, Maruta H, Usuka Y, et al. Influence of blood sample oxygen tension on blood glucose concentration measured using an enzyme-electrode method. *Crit Care Med* 1997;25:231–235.

117. Rice GK, Galt KA. *In vitro* drug interference with home blood-glucose-measurement systems. *Am J Hosp Pharm* 1985;42:2202–2207.

118. Lewis BD. Laboratory evaluation of the Glucocard blood glucose test meter. *Clin Chem* 1992;38:2093–2095.

119. Wu AHB, Apple FS, Brian Gibler W, et al. National Academy of Clinical Biochemistry Standards of Laboratory Practice: recommendations for the use of cardiac markers in coronary artery diseases. *Clin Chem* 1999;1104–1121.

120. Braunwald E, Antman EM, Beasley JW, et al. ACC/AHA guidelines for the management of patients with unstable angina and non-ST-segment elevation myocardial infarction: executive summary and recommendations. *Circulation* 2000;102:1193–1209.

121. Jaffe AS, Ravkilde J, Roberts R, et al. It's time for a change to troponin standard. *Circulation* 2000;102:1216–1220.

122. Panteghini M, Apple FS, Christenson RH, et al. Use of biochemical markers in acute coronary syndromes: IFCC Scientific Division, Committee on Standardization of Markers of Cardiac Damage. *Clin Chem Lab Med* 1999;37:687–693.

123. Joint European Society of Cardiology/American College of Cardiology Committee. Myocardial infarction redefined—a consensus document of the joint European Society of Cardiology/American College of Cardiology Committee for the Redefinition of myocardial infarction. *Eur Heart J* 2000;21:1502–1513.

124. Peruzzi WT, Parker MA, Lichtenthal PR, et al. A clinical evaluation of a blood conservation device in medical intensive care unit patients. *Crit Care Med* 1993;21:501–506.

125. Chernow B. Blood conservation in critical care: the evidence accumulates. *Crit Care Med* 1993;21:481–482.

126. Salem M, Chernow B, Burke R, et al. Bedside diagnostic testing: its accuracy, rapidity, and utility in blood conservation. *JAMA* 1991;266: 382–389.

127. Kilpatrick ES, Rumley AG, Smith EA. Variations in sample pH and pO₂ affect ExacTech meter glucose measurements. *Diabetes Medicine* 1994;11:506–509.

128. Tang Z, Louie RF, Kost GJ. Effects of changes in hematocrit and glucose levels on glucose meter measurements for point-of-care testing. *Lab Med Int* 2001;18(5):13–15.

129. Atkin SH, Dasmahapatra A, Jaker MA, et al Fingerstick glucose determination in shock. *Ann Intern Med* 1991;114:1020–1024.

130. Herr DM, Newton NC, Santrach PJ, et al. Airborne and rescue point-of-care testing. *Am J Clin Pathol* 1995;104(4 Suppl 1):S54–S58.

131. King JM, Eigenmann CA, Colagiuri S. Effect of ambient temperature and humidity on performance of blood glucose meters. *Diabetes Med* 1995;12:337–340.

132. Burnet RW, Covington AK, Fogh-Anderson N, et al. Recommendations on whole blood sampling, transport, and storage for simultaneous determination of pH, blood gases, and electrolytes *J Int Fed Clin Chem* 1994;6:115–120.

133. Kost GJ, Nguyen TH, Tang Z. Whole-blood glucose and lactate: Trilayer biosensors, drug interference, metabolism, and practice guidelines. *Arch Pathol Lab Med* 2000;124:1128–1134.

134. St-Louis P. Point-of-care blood gas analyzers: a performance evaluation. *Clin Chim Acta* 2001;307:139–144.

135. Murthy JN, Hicks JM, Soldin SJ. Evaluation of I-STAT portable clinical analyzer in neonatal and pediatric intensive care unit. *Clin Biochem* 1997;385–389.

136. Gault MH, Harding CE. Evaluation of i-STAT portable clinical analyzer in a hemodialysis unit. *Clin Biochem* 1996;29:117–124.

137. Burritt MF, Santrach PJ, Hankins DG, et al. Evaluation of the i-STAT portable clinical analyzer for use in a helicopter. *Scand J Clin Lab Invest* 1996;56:121–128.

138. Mock T, Morrison D, Yatscoff R. Evaluation of the i-SATA system: a portable chemistry analyzer for the measurement of sodium, potassium, chloride, urea, glucose, and hematocrit. *Clin Chem* 1995;187–192.

139. Prause G, Kaltenböck F, Doppler R. Die präklinische Blutgasanalyse. *Anaesthesist* 1998;47:490–495.

140. Pidetcha P, Ornvichian S, Chalachiva S. Accuracy and precision of the I-STAT portable clinical analyzer: an analytical point of view. *Journal of the Medical Association of Thailand* 2000;83:445–450.

141. Zaloga GP, Roberts PR, Black K, et al. Hand-held blood gas analyzer is accurate in the critical care setting. *Crit Care Med* 1996;24:957–962.

142. Ng VL, Kraemer R, Hogan C, et al. The rise and fall of I-STAT point-of-care blood gas testing in an acute care hospital. *Am J Clin Pathol* 2000;114:128–138.

143. Porath M, Sinha P, Dudenhausen JW, et al. Systemic instrumental errors between oxygen saturation analyzers in fetal blood during deep hypoxemia. *Clin Chim Acta* 2001;307:151–157.

144. Bland JM, Altman DG. Statistical methods for assessing agreement between two methods of clinical measurement. *Lancet* 1986;1: 307–310.

145. Kennedy JW, Carey RN, Coolen CC, et al. *Method comparison and bias estimation using patient samples.* Villanova, PA: National Committee for Clinical Laboratory Standards. Document EP9-A, 1995.

STANDARDIZATION OF POCT IN AN INTEGRATED HEALTH CARE SYSTEM

LOU ANN WYER
STEPHANIE SPINGARN

In 1996, Sentara hospital laboratories integrated their four hospital laboratories, with their separate management and test menus, to form one system of laboratories that would provide the same high-quality testing to the entire region. The task of integrating the laboratories initially was charged to its own leaders and management team. After 18 months with no decisions, the project ultimately was assigned to a multidisciplinary team of employees, with representatives from laboratory administration, finance, pharmacy, nursing, quality management, materials management, human resources, information technology, and the medical staff. Their job was to "reinvent" laboratory services with the following charter: reduce expenses significantly and maintain or improve quality, service, and cycle time measurements. Standardization and expansion of the point-of-care testing (POCT) program were two important components involved in reaching these goals.

The "reinventing team" addressed both processes and systems to ensure that a total cultural change could be implemented successfully. Laboratory management, test menus, methodologies, and visions were integrated into a single system approach. Staff members were reassigned to meet best the needs of the organization as services were centralized. From this new organizational structure, the role of clinical specialist for each technical discipline, including POCT/quality management, was developed. POCT staff members also were assigned to each facility, and a medical director was named to oversee technical discipline.

The reinventing team had done their homework. The organization wanted to eliminate sample transport times, decrease cycle times and handoffs, and decrease sample sizes, and POCT was emerging as an option to enhance patient care services. We were confident that this would result in positive patient outcomes and possibly contribute to a decreased length of stay. The first assignment for the new POCT clinical specialist and staff was to have all blood-gas testing performed at the patient's bedside. This was no easy task, but after 6 months of planning, the largest Sentara hospital successfully implemented bedside blood-gas testing. Over the next 11 months, the remaining three hospitals and an outpatient facility followed suit.

The planning stage for this implementation was enormous. Whereas use of the new technology was a cultural change for most, to some it was culture shock! After evaluating existing practices and identifying baseline measures, the process was redesigned. It also was necessary to redesign the support systems. Champions were identified from each of the patient care units to help move the staff through this change process. The champions consisted of nurses, laboratorians, and respiratory care practitioners who supported the vision of POCT and realized the benefits of providing test results at the bedside. We also had a physician to act as the spokesperson to other physician groups. The entire group worked with the POCT clinical specialist and staff to identify the steps along the journey to a successful implementation. This group helped to integrate the new process into their routines. They ensured that policies and procedures were user friendly and helped to develop training materials and training schedules for identified users. This core group of champions also developed an ongoing competency program and performance improvement monitors before the project was launched. The central blood gas laboratories were closed, and all testing was moved under the direction of the POCT section of the clinical laboratory. Throughout the entire planning stage, we realized that relationships were being built. These relationships still hold strong today. Some of the greatest resistors became our strongest supporters.

Communication throughout the course of this project was a key factor in establishing an effective and successful POCT program. Senior administration was kept updated on the progress of the project. Updates also were provided at staff meetings, both on the patient care units and in the clinical laboratory. Different types of communication tools were used to promote the same message. Both the laboratory and patient care groups had concerns about their future roles. The laboratory staff thought their jobs were being given to nonlaboratory staff, who were not necessarily qualified to perform the testing, and the patient care staff thought one more thing was being added to their already very busy routines. What everyone discovered was that we have redefined the way we provide patient care, and it is working with amazing efficiency.

Although this journey to reinvent laboratory services was long and tedious, the benefits have been enormous. An actual reduction in total efforts has been realized. Results are now available at the bedside within minutes. Physicians and respiratory practitioners can make treatment decisions immediately. Along with a rapid wean protocol, patients can now be extubated sooner. Information technology systems allow for data transfer to the laboratory and hospital information systems, eliminating several steps required by the nursing units with previous processes. Because the implementation team had an active role in the form of the final product, a win–win situation has become a reality.

Standardization efforts were continued when the glucose meters were updated with data management and connectivity. A committee of POCT staff, nurses, diabetes educators, materials, and information technology representatives was formed to develop a very detailed project plan. Elements of the plan included the request for proposals, contract negotiations, conducting pilots, training, implementation, and follow-up. The planning stages took a year and a half, and yet implementation at all four hospitals took only 3 weeks. Again, selecting the right people to work together to achieve a common goal was key.

The POCT program at Sentara has continued to grow as we have expanded services and added another hospital to our organization. Today, the POCT program has more than 3,000 users and is coordinated by a dedicated staff of 7.5 full-time employees across five hospitals. The Sentara POCT menu consists of glucose, blood gas, activated clotting time, prothrombin time, chemistries, urine dipstick, platelet function testing, hemoccult, gastroccult, hematocrit, hemoglobin, strep screen, pH and pregnancy testing. More than 125 nursing units perform tests that meet their specific patient and service needs. For example, all the outpatient surgery areas perform chemistry testing at the bedside. Warfarin clinics provide prothrombin time results immediately so that warfarin adjustments can be made before patients leave the clinic. This has resulted in decreased wait times for both patients and physicians, and it has improved customer satisfaction rates.

Currently, 185 glucose meters with barcode scanning capabilities and 106 bedside analyzers for blood gas and chemistry testing, both with data management functionality and connectivity, allow for an efficient flow of information. Program oversight by the clinical laboratory has been an integral component to keeping standardization intact. The POCT program is accredited by both the College of American Pathologists (CAP) and the Joint Commission on Accreditation of Healthcare Organizations (JCAHO) and the clinical laboratory holds the CLIA (Clinical Laboratory Improvement Amendment of 1988) license.

The POCT staff monitors daily performance of testing from each patient care unit. Electronic or liquid quality control is performed at defined intervals. POCT blood gas, chemistry, and glucose results are uploaded to the laboratory information system and flow into the hospital information system for retrieval anywhere in the system, a significant benefit since all hospitals share a common information system. The POCT staff performs all linearity and calibration verification procedures, establishes in-house quality control ranges and works with each patient care unit to ensure ongoing compliance. In conjunction with the users, the POCT section of the laboratory is constantly evaluating innovative testing methods and new procedures.

The POCT team approves procedures for standardization and ensures that the users are competent to perform each test. They perform a minimum of weekly inspections of all POCT units. Their high visibility on the patient care units has resulted in their becoming a reliable resource for any laboratory issue. Ongoing recognition of the work effort involved in maintaining this type of system has become standard for the POCT work group. Sentara management continues to reward laboratory POCT staff and users for their achievements.

Materials management also assists with the oversight of POCT supply ordering. An approved list of POCT supplies is available for order by the patient care units. This control point ensures that the patient care units do not randomly order new products. This process has been critical to maintaining the initial standardization effort.

Maintaining knowledge of the accreditation standards and ensuring overall program compliance are important aspects of the POCT staff educators' role. They prepare all patient care units for regulatory agency inspections. Although this can be challenging with so many users, we have been able to achieve high standards through team efforts. At the most recent CAP inspection both the quality management and POCT programs of Sentara Laboratory Services were applauded for their outstanding results and the interdepartmental collaborations.

Standardized competencies are developed each year for recertification of POCT procedures. A variety of teaching methods are used to facilitate the adult learner. Unique themes are used to reinforce skills while also having fun. The education and research department provides new employee orientation of POCT waived procedures, and the POCT staff provides orientation of the moderately complex procedures. The two groups collaboratively develop the new employee orientation schedules to provide frequent and timely training opportunities for new employees. Enrollment is done on-line so that schedules can be planned in advance, and training is provided away from the patient care unit.

How does one maintain such a high level of standardization in an integrated health system? Just managing the data is an enormous job. A calendar of systemwide POCT activities is mapped out annually. The calendar outlines the tasks assigned for each month, such as calibration verifications, linearities, maintenance schedules, and proficiency surveys. As these tasks are completed for each facility, they are signed off. A standard template is used for all quality-control activities and statistical analysis. This template builds in efficiency for the staff, especially as they work in other facilities. Nurse managers receive daily, weekly, or monthly reports for each test performed on their unit. A POCT compliance report details at a glance the compliance rates in each patient care unit at each facility. Standardized performance improvement reports are submitted monthly for systemwide reporting.

The success of Sentara's POCT program is the result of a collaborative effort by the entire health care professional team, whose ultimate goal has been to improve patient outcomes. As the technology becomes available, new procedures are investigated and implemented. For example, the recent initiative from the Connectivity Industry Consortium (CIC) to standardize the connectivity of POCT devices presents an opportunity to improve data management. Each implementation presents a challenge from which we learn. In the process, we also strengthen relationships with other health care professionals and with patients.

What have we learned? Support from administration is crucial. Strong commitment and involvement at such levels guarantee success. We have learned the importance of consolidating and changing the structures before changing the people. With-out support systems, changes cannot be maintained. We have learned that having the right people on the POCT team matters immensely. The administrative board and medical professionals must be involved, and focus is on progress. Communicate, communicate, communicate. Finally, we have learned to enjoy what we do and to be proud of what we accomplish.

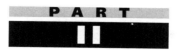

POINT-OF-CARE TESTING IN THE HOSPITAL AND CLINICAL PRACTICE

7

POINT-OF-CARE TESTING IN EMERGENCY MEDICINE

SEAN E. BOURKE
J. DOUGLAS KIRK
GERALD J. KOST

Since the advent of whole-blood biosensors, a wave of new technology has emerged that will have far-reaching implications for emergency medicine (1,2). This technology, known as *point-of-care testing* (POCT), is defined as testing at or near the site of patient care (3). Such devices promise to provide on-site accurate diagnostic results within 5 minutes of a physician's order. In doing so, they may expedite therapeutic turnaround time (TTAT), the time from ordering a test to delivering appropriate treatment. By expediting clinical decision making, POCT aims to improve patient outcomes and reduce patient acuity, morbidity, and mortality, especially during emergency resuscitations and critical care. Furthermore, for the fast-paced emergency department (ED), POCT offers the opportunity to improve efficiency and, therefore, improve patient throughput and quality of care.

The goal of this chapter is to identify how and why POCT technologies would benefit emergency medicine. For both emergency physicians and nonclinicians, this chapter describes the impact of rapid diagnostic data gathering on patient diagnosis, treatment, outcome, satisfaction, and ED disposition. The first section discusses the integration of POCT into the medical arena and its potential use in the ED. The second describes the unique ED environment and its suitability for POCT. The third discusses diagnoses commonly considered in the ED and illustrates how patient flow and appropriate treatment depend on diagnostic data collection. The last section highlights the value of rapid POCT and recommends strategies for optimal integration of POCT in the ED.

HISTORICAL BACKGROUND

The number of patients seeking care in EDs in the United States doubled between 1960 and 1979 (4), to a total of 81,244,699 visits annually (5). By 1995, nearly 100 million persons sought care in EDs each year (6). From 1997 to 1999, visits grew by 3% annually. In 1999, visits grew by between 6% and 8%, a figure that is expected to continue. This growth has increased further the pressure on emergency physicians to expedite patient flow. Although definitely not alone in culpability, conventional laboratory turnaround time (TAT), often prolonged beyond 1.5 hours (7) and, rarely, up to 4 hours (8), has emerged as one of the sources of patient delay (9–14) and patient and physician discontent (15). In 1988, more than 80% of clinical laboratories received complaints about test TAT (16). Laboratories could not keep pace with clinician demand or self-expectations.

In 1990, laboratories failed to meet clinicians' or laboratories' external TAT expectations 90% of the time and failed to meet internal goals 70% of the time (17,18). Increasingly, clinicians wanted faster results than the laboratory was prepared to provide (19), prompting one pathologist to ask, "Can we satisfy clinicians' demands for faster service? Should we try?" (20). For emergency physicians struggling to provide the highest quality of patient care possible, the answer is a resounding "Yes!" for the simple reason that faster service improves quality of care and patient satisfaction and also potentially increases revenue by expanding patient volume. Delayed test reporting promoted duplicate test (21) and statim test requests (22) as well as delayed hospital discharge (15). Long waits for laboratory testing correlated with prolonged length of stay (23) and reduced patient satisfaction in the ED (24) and acute care clinic (25).

One of the frustrations of emergency physicians is that the vast majority of laboratory TAT will involve sample collection and transport, not analysis. POCT devices offered the chance to remove that inefficiency and translate the expedited diagnostic results into improved clinical outcomes (26), prompt service, and decreased cost (26–31). Following in the footsteps of their surgical and intense care colleagues, emergency physicians thus began conducting pilot studies previewing the potential of POCT to expedite ED patient care.

In 1995, Sands and colleagues (32) observed that a POCT device with six measured analytes reported results sooner by 31 minutes for hematocrit, 43 minutes for electrolytes, and 44 minutes for blood urea nitrogen and glucose. Surveyed physicians reported that earlier laboratory values would have expedited therapy in 9.5% of cases. Results affected discharge or admission decisions 10.7% of the time. The study concluded that earlier laboratory results using a POCT device might have reduced ED length of stay for 17.3% of patients.

In 1996, however, Parvin and colleagues (23) conducted a study using a device similar to that used by Sands and colleagues. Parvin's group found that the POCT device failed to shorten ED length of stay regardless of final disposition, presenting symptom, or presence or absence of central laboratory testing. This study was flawed, however, in that it tested only five analytes and only 5% of the experimental group and 1% of the controls did not have analytes tested in the central laboratory as well as by POCT, thus making longer central laboratory TATs rate limiting. Additionally, the study failed to address or isolate other rate-limiting steps or performance issues that might have affected ED length of stay.

In 1998, Kendall and colleagues (33) tested the same device to see whether more rapid results might affect outcome. The device helped decisions to be made 74 minutes earlier for hematology tests, 86 minutes earlier for biochemical tests, and 21 minutes earlier for arterial blood gases. In 7% of cases, POCT results led to management changes considered critical. Nonetheless, they did not find that rapid POCT results decreased intradepartmental length of stay, mortality, or clinical outcome. Interestingly, however, 85% of the patients presenting to the ED in the hospital studied were admitted. Rate-limiting steps in intradepartmental length of stay in this case may have been bed availability or transfer efficiency. Unfortunately, for the 15% of people who were discharged home, it cannot be determined from the data whether they were discharged sooner given the faster diagnostic results. In any event, the investigators concluded that laboratory testing was not the rate-limiting step in ED flow or outcomes.

A more recent study by Murray and colleagues (34) looked at ED length of stay in a subgroup of patients whose laboratory evaluation could be done entirely by a POCT device. Patients were randomized and controlled by comparing the length of stay of patients whose diagnostic evaluation was made by the POCT devices compared with those whose evaluation was done by the central laboratory. In this case, patients who were discharged home after being diagnosed by a POCT device left 1 hour and 12 minutes sooner than the control group. Patients who were admitted showed no difference, but the primary outcome was not the time from ordering a test to the emergency physician interpreting the result; instead, it was the time between triage and the time the decision to admit was made by the consulting physician, not the emergency physician. For the admitted patients, this outcome measure, unfortunately, includes multiple confounding variables. Importantly, however, patients who went home did so significantly sooner in the POCT group.

To understand better how near-patient, rapid diagnostic testing can improve ED efficiency and patient outcomes, one needs a greater appreciation of the complexities of ED care and patient flow.

THE UNIQUE ENVIRONMENT OF EMERGENCY MEDICINE

Emergency departments service an acutely unpredictable number of patients with a wide range of medical conditions. The population evaluated spans from neonate to octogenarian. Generally, the doctor is meeting the patient for the first time. Emergency physicians make decisions by gathering data, developing diagnostic hypotheses, and testing the hypotheses through pertinent diagnostic tests (Table 7.1). The objectives of diagnostic

testing are to confirm a diagnosis, rule out life-threatening emergencies, monitor patient therapy, or initiate a diagnostic algorithm that may require further testing, depending on initial results. Appropriately considered, diagnostic tests should specifically test hypotheses that either impact care in or after the visit to the ED. Because confirmation of hypotheses is dependent on diagnostic test results, any ability to expedite diagnostic data

---

TABLE 7.1. PRIORITY EMERGENCY DEPARTMENT TESTS

Arterial blood gas: pH, Po$_2$, Pco$_2$, O$_2$Hb, COHb, met Hb
Cardiac markers: CK$_T$, CK-MB, relative index, cTnI or cTnT, myoglobin, BNP
Chemistry: Na$^+$, K$^+$, Cl$^-$, HCO$_3^-$, BUN, creatinine, glucose, Ca^{2+}, Mg^{2+}, phosphorous, lactate
   AST, ALT, total bilirubin, ALP, amylase, albumin
   Ketones, lipase, direct bilirubin
   Measured serum and urine osmolarity
   CSF and synovial fluid protein, glucose
   Peritoneal fluid albumin and total protein
Coagulation: PT with INR, aPTT, D-dimer
   Fibrinogen, thrombin time, fibrinogen degradation products
Drug test systems
   Ethanol level, qualitative tricyclic antidepressant screen
   Qualitative drugs of abuse screen: cocaine, amphetamines, barbiturates, benzodiazepine, PCP, opiates
   Acetaminophen, salicylate levels
   Antiepileptic levels: valproate, phenytoin, carbamazepine, phenobarbital
   Digoxin, iron, lithium, theophylline, ethylene glycol, methanol levels
Endocrine: Thyroid function (TSH, free T$_4$) and cortisol levels
Hematology
   CBC with differential and indices
   Serum Rh type and cross match
   ESR, CRP
   Cerebrospinal, peritoneal, or synovial fluid cell count and Gram's stain
Microbiology
   Infectious diarrhea screen: *Campylobacter, Salmonella, Shigella, Yersinia, Giardia,* amoeba, rotavirus, *E. coli* (toxigenic or H:0157), *C. Diff.* toxin
   Cerebrospinal fluid screen: meningococcus, pneumococcus, herpes
   Nasopharyngeal screen: group A β-hemolytic streptococcus, *B. pertussis,* RSV, influenzae, adenovirus, mononucleosis
   Skin assay: herpes simplex, herpes virus 6, varicella zoster
   Sputum assay: tuberculosis, pneumocystis
   Sexually transmitted disease assay: *Chlamydia,* gonococcus, trichomonas
   Vaginal assay: *Gardnerella* and *Candida*
Orthopedics: Synovial fluid assay for uric acid or calcium pyrophosphate
Pregnancy tests: Urine or serum qualitative β-hCG
   Serum quantitative β-hCG
Urinalysis: pH, specific gravity, protein, glucose, blood, LE, nitrites, urobilinogen
   Microscopic: RBC and WBC count and bacterial count

Po$_2$, partial pressure of oxygen; Pco$_2$, partial pressure of carbon dioxide; O$_2$Hb, oxygenated hemoglobin; COHb, carboxyhemoglobin; met Hb, methemoglobin; Hb, hemoglobin; CK$_T$, creatinine kinase total; cTnI, cardiac troponin I; cTnT, cardiac troponin T; BUN, blood urea nitrogen; HCO$_3^-$, bicarbonate; AST, aspartate aminotransferase; ALT, alanine aminotransferase; ALP, alkaline phosphatase; CSF, cerebrospinal fluid; PT, prothrombin time; INR, international normalized ratio; aPTT, activated partial thromboplastin time; PCP, phencyclidine; TSH, thyrotropin stimulating hormone; T$_4$, thyroxine; CBC, complete blood count; ESR, erythrocyte sedimentation rate; CRP, C-reactive protein; RSV, respiratory syncytial virus; β-hCG, beta human chorionic gonadotropin; LE, leukocyte esterase; RBC, red blood cell; WBC, white blood cell; BNP, B-type natriaretic peptide.

gathering should facilitate patient care, throughput, and therapeutic interventions. Several studies deciphered the intricacies of ED patient flow to reveal sources of patient delay (7–15,33–36). Numerous common themes emerge from these studies.

First, ED flow is divided into five main stages. The first stage is registration and triage. From here, they will be placed immediately in a patient bed (stage 2) or placed later, depending on patient acuity and current bed availability. The third stage, initial evaluation, also includes a variable wait time, which depends on patient acuity and the physician's current task load. In the fourth stage, the physician orders pertinent diagnostic studies, and the patient waits for these results. Generally, pending these results, some patients may require specialty consultation, which also takes variable amounts of time. The last stage entails disposition, namely, admission, transfer, or discharge home. Transfer to an outside hospital may be required if the patient needs specialty care (e.g., referral to a burn center), because of a request by the patient or an insurance company or health maintenance organization request, or when the current hospital has no bed availability. In the most common ED scenario, patients are sent home with appropriate follow-up care. Each stage contains rate-limiting steps and inefficiencies.

Second, ED patient care is treatment and disposition driven. Emergency physicians aim to confirm or exclude (life-threatening) diagnoses and treat with medication when indicated while concomitantly organizing the patient for discharge, transfer, or admission. Depending on patient diagnosis, between 30% and 94% of patients (11,12) require diagnostic tests. Because bed space and turnover determine patient flow, expediting this process facilitates ED efficiency.

Third, patient and physician satisfaction and patient outcome may be directly proportional to delays. Delayed diagnostic results waste time in several ways (Table 7.2) and may contribute to delays (Table 7.3). Such delays are frustrating for patients and emergency physicians, who are eager to gather requisite data, deliver treatment, and organize appropriate consultation or disposition. Rapid patient turnover is essential to minimize unnecessary waiting-room delays for patients, who may or may not have life-threatening disease. Rapid disposition is also

TABLE 7.2. RATE-LIMITING STEPS IN DIAGNOSTIC TESTING[a]

Test ordered
Test documented by clerk
Phlebotomy
Biohazard packaging
Transport
Blood sample received by laboratory
Accessioning
Transport for centrifugation and analysis
Centrifugation and analysis
Data entry into laboratory information system
Data reported
Data received by physician
Therapy ordered
Therapy received by patient

[a]The above steps combined constitute the therapeutic turnaround time (TTAT).

TABLE 7.3. DELAYED LABORATORY RESULTS: SOURCES OF PHYSICIAN INEFFICIENCY

Recheck for incomplete lab results
Call lab to inquire about delays
Explain to patients the reason for the delay
Reacquaint oneself with a case after a prolonged delay
Redraw after original samples found contaminated or hemolyzed
Redraw because of time obsolescence of lab results
Redraw for new tests because status of patient changed suddenly
Redraw because treatment affected analytes before test results were available
Call lab for results when the computer system is down
Check that lab samples were sent
Check that lab orders were entered

important to keep nursing and physician staff relatively free in anticipation of the unpredictable arrival of one or more critical care, labor-intensive patients.

Several studies have correlated diagnostic testing with prolonged ED length of stay. In 1978, Cue and Inglis (12) observed an average time for complete blood counts and urinalyses of 55 minutes, but they found only a minimally increased length of stay for patients undergoing such testing. Saunder's (13) 1987 study noted that laboratory delays increased treatment time from 31 to 126 minutes. In 1984, Heckerling (7) found that one-fourth of blood counts, three-eighths of urinalyses, and more than half of chemistry tests were not available after 1.5 hours in the laboratory.

To appreciate the frustration evoked by delayed results, however, one must look not only at mean laboratory TAT but also at the frequency and magnitude of upper limits of variance. In the ED, McConnell and Writtenberr-Loy (8) showed that urinalyses and prothrombin time (PT) or activated partial thromboplastin time (aPTT) averaged 70 minutes from laboratory clock-in to clock-out. Both had ranges, however, extending over 4 hours. Chemistry panels had an average and range just short of 1.5 and 3 hours, respectively. In a critical care facility at Memorial Sloan-Kettering Hospital, Fleisher and Schwartz (37) compared centralized laboratory equipment with a rapid-transport system. They concluded that the rapid transport system was more efficient but did so, however, based on mean TAT, ignoring the significant fraction of delayed outlying results. Whether because of inefficient transport, preanalytic sample deterioration, computer down time, or system overload, such delays cause tremendous frustration because they lead to delays and poor time management in an environment where time efficiency is critical to medical outcomes and effective, considerate patient care. Let us take a closer look at the value of attenuating diagnostic turnaround times using POCT devices.

THE VALUE OF SPEED, INTEGRATION, AND OPTIMIZATION

Emergency physicians are strongly drawn to improvements in diagnostic testing because diagnostic testing is central to emergency medicine efficiency, cost effectiveness, and patient care. Appropriate diagnostic testing guides clinical judgment and, when used rationally, promotes the cost-effective use of resources and optimization of patient care. The American College of Emergency Physicians (38) and others (39–41) have formed guidelines that provide an outline for cost-effective and appropriate diagnostic testing for arterial blood gas, complete blood count, and electrolyte testing. The pertinent results of this work are summarized in Table 7.4. Importantly, each of these frequently ordered diagnostic tests now can be completed at the point of care.

The opportunity for POCT exists because analytic time for diagnostic test analysis involves only 5% of TTAT, the time from a physician ordering a test to initiating therapy based on the test result. As a result, reduction of analytic time to 2 minutes and TTAT to 5 minutes using POCT technology should greatly improve ED efficiency, flow, and patient care. At this point, however, no definitive ED studies have demonstrated convincingly the potential benefits of POCT devices. Nonetheless, it seems intuitive to most emergency physicians that future studies will reveal that, when it is properly integrated and targeted to analyze critical diagnostic test clusters, POCT will prove a powerful tool that can facilitate patient flow (23,33), decrease cost (27,31), improve clinical outcomes (26,32), and improve ED patient (24) and physician satisfaction.

Currently, POCT clusters are too limited to manage the scope and variability of ED care. Optimization of efficiency, as a result, is not yet obtainable, and outcome studies (23,33) have therefore decried POCT as unable to affect critical endpoints,

TABLE 7.4. GUIDELINES FOR APPROPRIATE DIAGNOSTIC TESTING IN THE ED

Arterial blood gases and pH
  Cyanosis or symptomatic or significant smoke inhalation
  Significant dyspnea with or without suspected pulmonary pathology
  Significant respiratory distress: markedly impaired speech, fatigued asthmatic/COPD
  Perfusion failure, clinical "shock"
  Unexplained altered mental status and behavior (somnolence, agitation)
  Diabetic ketoacidosis
Electrolytes: Criteria for ordering Na, K, Cl, CO_2, BUN, glucose
  Persistent poor oral intake
  Vomiting for prolonged period
  Chronic hypertension
  Chronic diuretic use
  Recent seizure of unclear etiology
  Muscle weakness
  Age 65 years or older
  Alcoholism
  Altered mental status
  Recent history of electrolyte abnormality
  Diabetes
  Renal dysfunction
  ±Seizures
  ±Dizziness
Complete blood count (CBC)
  Pediatric fever of unknown origin
  Abdominal pain
  Suspected hemoglobin, hematocrit, platelet abnormality
  Immunocompromised patients

ED, emergency department; COPD, chronic obstructive pulmonary disease; BUN, blood urea nitrogen.

such as length of stay and mortality. Initial attempts to show the beneficial potential of POCT in the ED failed because devices were limited in their capability (23,32,33). For example, the referenced studies all tested the same POCT instrument with a test menu composed of a small fraction of diagnostic tests ordered from the ED. Nonetheless, critics used these conclusions to generalize about the inability of POCT instruments to effect critical outcomes. The summary of clinical strategies (42–74) (Table 7.5) illustrates why studies analyzing limited test menus would not show a greater benefit to rapid diagnostic testing. First, the range of required tests is significant (Table 7.1). Second, complete clusters of diagnostic and therapeutic tests are required to diagnose or exclude a given disease (Table 7.5). Testing two or three isolated analytes at the point of care is unlikely to have any effect on function or flow in emergency medicine unless the results include all the critical analytes required to confirm a diagnosis. Otherwise, analyte gaps are rate limiting.

As demonstrated through treatment of acute coronary syndromes (75,76), complete panels of requisite results available at the point of care can facilitate rapid diagnosis, risk stratification, and treatment. For acute myocardial infarction, the use of rapid POCT devices decreases cost and improves outcomes (75). As design and range of available POCT devices continue to improve, further studies will unveil potential clinical benefit in a variety of other common and critical clinical scenarios (Tables 7.6 and 7.7). Importantly, estimates predict that within 5 years several key ED test clusters will be available at the point of care.

Furthermore, to exploit the potential of this new technology and demonstrate it in controlled studies, other rate-limiting aspects of ED care need improvement, namely, institution-dependent delays external to diagnostic testing (77). For example, whereas Parvin and colleagues (23) failed to decrease ED length of stay by using a POCT device, their study also failed to address other workflow process issues. Similarly, Kendall and colleagues (33) showed that rapid POCT results greatly expedited decision-making, but they were not able to take advantage of the time saved by decreasing length of stay or clinical outcome. Conclusive studies evaluating POCT need to control for external delays. By addressing rate-limiting ED inefficiencies, one could convert the time saved using POCT devices into economic, clinical, and workflow improvements. Nonetheless, rapid POCT is not a panacea for delays in ED care because inefficiencies exist at each stage of care. These limitations uniformly need improvement to optimize patient safety and satisfaction and to allow rapid POCT to develop its yet unrealized potential.

For example, the fraction of patients requiring diagnostic laboratory testing in addition to radiologic studies might gain no benefit in disposition by using POCT unless EDs concurrently expedite obtaining radiographic films. By the same token, the patient who is rapidly diagnosed with an acute myocardial infarction but is delayed going to cardiac catheterization or receiving thrombolytic therapy has lost an opportunity to optimize care. As another example, picture a patient diagnosed within minutes with diabetic ketoacidosis. Using rapid POCT, therapy is initiated within minutes and disposition to the intensive care unit or medicine ward is known. The patient waits in the ED for 2 hours to be transferred, however, because cuts in housecleaning staff have delayed room preparation. Meanwhile,

TABLE 7.5. CLINICAL DIAGNOSTIC STRATEGIES

Diagnoses (Ref. No.)	Test Clusters Recommended in References	Effect on ED Diagnosis, Disposition, and Treatment
Cardiovascular		
Suspected myocardial infarction (42,43)	CK, CK-MB, cTnI or T, myoglobin	1
	CBC with differential	1
	Prothrombin time (PT)	2
	Activated partial thromboplastin time (aPTT)	2
	Consider toxicology screen for cocaine and amphetamine	2
Syncope (44)	CBC	2
	Na, K, Cl, T_{CO_2}	2
	CK, CK-MB, cTnI or T, myoglobin	2
	Blood urea nitrogen (BUN) and creatinine	2
	Glucose	2
Congestive heart failure—see chapter 38		
Central nervous system		
Cerebrovascular accident / ischemic stroke (45)	CBC	2
	PT, aPTT	1
	Toxicology screen for cocaine, amphetamine	2
	CK-MB, cTnI or T, myoglobin	2
Delirium (46,47)	Na, K, Cl, T_{CO_2} with anion gap	1
	BUN and creatinine	1
	Glucose	1
	Calcium or ionized calcium	1
	Arterial P_{O_2}, P_{CO_2}, pH, O_2 sat	2
	AST, ALT, ALP, total bilirubin	2
	Urinalysis	1
	Toxicology screen	1
	Thyroid function tests	2
	Carboxyhemoglobin	2
	CSF cytology, protein, glucose, Gram's stain	1
	CBC with differential and MCV	1
	Magnesium	2
Seizure not otherwise specified (NOS) (48)	Anticonvulsant medication levels	1
	Urinalysis with ketones	2
	Glucose	1
	Na, Cl, K, T_{CO_2} with anion gap	2
	Arterial P_{O_2}, O_2 sat, pH, P_{CO_2}	2
	Calcium or ionized calcium	2
	Drugs of abuse screen	2
	Qualitative β-hCG	2
	Thyroid function tests (hypothyroidism)	1
	CSF cytology, glucose, protein, Gram's stain	2
	BUN	2
	AST, ALT, total bilirubin, ALP	2
	CBC with differential	2
	Magnesium	2
	Erythrocyte sedimentation rate	2
Endocrinology		
Diabetic ketoacidosis (49,50)	Urine glucose and ketones	1
	Arterial O_2 sat, pH, P_{O_2}, P_{CO_2}	1
	Na, K, Cl, T_{CO_2} with anion gap	1
	Glucose	1
	Ketones	1
	CBC with differential	2
	Urinalysis	2
	Amylase	2
	CK-MB, cTnI or T, myoglobin	2
	Magnesium	1
	Calcium or ionized calcium	1
	Phosphorous	1
	Lactate	1

(continued)

TABLE 7.5. *(continued)*

Diagnoses (Ref. No.)	Test Clusters Recommended in References	Effect on ED Diagnosis, Disposition, and Treatment
Gastrointestinal		
Abdominal pain (NOS) (51)	Urinalysis	1
	CBC with differential	1
	Glucose	2
	Total bilirubin	2
	Amylase	1
	Stool occult blood	1
	Qualitative β-hCG (for women)	2
	BUN	2
Acute cholecystitis or ascending cholangitis (52)	CBC with differential	1
	AST, ALT, ALP, total bilirubin	1
	Amylase	1
	Lactate dehydrogenase (LDH)	3
Appendicitis (53)	CBC with differential	1
	Urinalysis	2
	Qualitative β-hCG (for women)	2
Diarrhea (54)	Stool occult blood	1
	Fecal leukocytes	2
	Stool ova and parasites	2
	Clostridium difficile toxin	2
	Albumin, calcium, phosphorous	3
	Peripheral blood smear	2
	Na, Cl, K, T_{CO_2}	2
	CBC with differential	2
	Stool bacterial culture	2
Pancreatitis (55)	Amylase	1
	Glucose	1
	AST	1
	CBC	1
	BUN and creatinine	1
	P_{O_2}, T_{CO_2}	2
	Calcium	1
	LDH	3
Spontaneous bacterial peritonitis (56,57)	Peritoneal fluid:	
	Cell count with differential	1
	Albumin	1
	Total protein	1
	Culture and sensitivity	1
	pH	3
	Glucose	3
	Amylase	3
	Gram's stain	3
	LDH	3
	Cytology	3
	Tuberculosis smear and culture	3
	Blood tests:	
	Albumin	1
	CBC	2
	AST, ALT, ALP, total bilirubin	2
	PT	1
Vomiting (NOS) (58)	CBC with differential	2
	Na, K, Cl, T_{CO_2}	1
	BUN and creatinine	1
	Glucose	1
	AST, ALT, ALP, total bilirubin	2
	Qualitative β-hCG (for women)	2
	Erythrocyte sedimentation rate	3

(continued)

TABLE 7.5. *(continued)*

Diagnoses (Ref. No.)	Test Clusters Recommended in References	Effect on ED Diagnosis, Disposition, and Treatment
Infectious disease		
Osteomyelitis (59)	Erythrocyte sedimentation rate	1
	CBC with differential	1
	Blood and wound cultures	1
	Urine culture	3
	CSF culture	3
Pediatric fever of unknown origin (60)	CBC with differential	1
	CSF cell count, glucose, protein	2
	CSF Gram's stain, culture, sensitivity	2
	Urinalysis with culture and sensitivity	1
	Fecal leukocytes	1
	Blood culture	1
	Additional tests for neonates:	
	Nasopharyngeal swabs for respiratory syncytial virus assay and viral cultures	2
	CSF polymerase chain reaction for herpes simplex virus	2
	Erythrocyte sedimentation rate	2
	C-reactive protein	2
	CSF viral cultures	2
Pelvic inflammatory disease (61)	Cervical wet mount and Gram's stain	1
	CBC with differential	1
	Erythrocyte sedimentation rate	2
	Cervical culture for *N. gonorrhea* and *Chlamydia*	1
Pneumonia (62)	Arterial P_{O_2}, P_{CO_2}, pH	2
	CBC with differential	2
	Sputum Gram's stain and culture	1
	Blood cultures	1
	Creatinine and BUN	2
	Immunocompromised hosts:	
	Lactate dehydrogenase	1
	Erythrocyte sedimentation rate	2
	Sputum smear for *Pneumocystis carinii*	2
	Sputum acid fast bacillus smears	2
Necrotizing fasciitis (63)	Gram's stain and culture of wound	1
	CBC with differential	1
Pyelonephritis (64)	Urinalysis	1
	Na, K, Cl, T_{CO_2}	1
	BUN and creatinine	1
	CBC with differential	2
	Blood culture	3
	Urine culture	1
Sepsis (65,66)	CBC with differential	1
	Urinalysis	1
	Glucose	1
	BUN and creatinine	1
	AST, ALT, ALP, total bilirubin	1
	PT	1
	aPTT	1
	Fibrinogen	1
	Fibrin degradation products	1
	Blood culture	1
Nephrology		
Acute renal failure (67,68)	Urinalysis, dipstick and microscopic	1
	Na, K, Cl, T_{CO_2} with anion gap	1
	BUN and creatinine	1
	Calcium	2
	Phosphorous	2
	Urinary sodium	3
	Fractional excretion of sodium	3
	Magnesium	3
	CBC	1
	Glucose	1

(continued)

TABLE 7.5. *(continued)*

Diagnoses (Ref. No.)	Test Clusters Recommended in References	Effect on ED Diagnosis, Disposition, and Treatment
Nephrolithiasis with renal colic (69)	Urinalysis	1
	BUN and creatinine	2
	CBC with differential	2
	Qualitative β-hCG	2
	Uric acid	2
	Calcium	3
	Phosphorous	3
Obstetrics and gynecology		
Ectopic pregnancy (70)	Hemoglobin and hematocrit	1
	Qualitative β-hCG (initial confirmation)	1
	Quantitative β-hCG	1
	Rh blood type	1
	Progesterone	2
	Type and cross match	1
Preeclampsia, eclampsia, or HELLP syndrome (70,71)	Urinalysis	1
	CBC	1
	AST, ALT, total bilirubin	1
	BUN and creatinine	1
	PT	1
	aPTT	1
	Glucose if seizing	1
	Magnesium	2
Pulmonary		
Pulmonary embolus (72)	D-Dimer	2
	Arterial P_{O_2}, P_{CO_2}, O_2 sat	2
Toxicology		
Acute acetaminophen overdose (73)	Acetaminophen level	1
	AST, ALT, ALP, total bilirubin	1
	PT, aPTT	2
	Na, K, Cl, T_{CO_2} with anion gap	3
	BUN and creatinine	3
	Glucose	3
	CBC with differential	3
Carbon monoxide poisoning (74)	OxyHb, DeoxyHb, COHb, MetHb	1
	Arterial pH, P_{CO_2}, P_{O_2}, O_2 sat	1
Trauma		
Blunt trauma	CBC	1
	Urinalysis	1
	Qualitative β-hCG (for women)	1
	Toxicology screen	2
	Lactate	2
	T_{CO_2}	2
	pH	2
	PT, aPTT	2
	Amylase	2
	AST, ALT, ALP, total bilirubin	2
	Creatinine	2
	CK total	2
	CK, CK-MB, cTnI or T, myoglobin	2
	Type and cross match	2

ED, emergency department; CK, creatine kinase; CK-MB, myocardial muscle creatine kinase isoenzyme; cTnI, cardiac troponin I; cTnT, cardiac troponin T; CBC, complete blood cell count; AST, aspartate aminotransferase; ALT, alanine aminotransferase; ALP, alkaline phosphatase; CSF, cerebrospinal fluid; MCV, mean corpuscular volume; β-hCG, beta human chorionic gonadotropin; HELLP, hemolysis, elevated liver enzymes, and low platelet count; T_{CO_2}, total carbon dioxide content. Note: Tests listed are from cited references, except cardiac injury markers, for which the tests listed have been clustered uniformly.
Scale:
One: Diagnostic tests generally required for appropriate diagnosis, disposition, and treatment.
Two: Diagnostic test results may effect diagnosis, disposition, and treatment under certain circumstances but these tests are not generally ordered.
Three: Diagnostic test result is unlikely to affect diagnosis, disposition, and treatment and tests are not generally considered.

TABLE 7.6. DIAGNOSES IN WHICH RAPID POCT MIGHT AFFECT OUTCOMES

Myocardial infarction and cardiac arrest: cardiac test clusters
Congestive heart failure: BNP, pro-BNP
Respiratory extremis: arterial blood gas
Altered mental status, unclear etiology: arterial blood gas
Ectopic pregnancy: CBC and quantitative β-hCG level
Diabetic ketoacidosis: arterial blood gas, glucose, and ketones
Hemorrhage secondary to trauma or gastrointestinal bleeding: hemoglobin/hematocrit
Overdose with specific treatment: acetaminophen, aspirin, digoxin, carboxyhemoglobin, ethylene glycol, methanol, iron, lithium, or theophylline levels
Pediatric fever of unknown origin: CBC, urinalysis, and cerebrospinal fluid cell count, glucose, and protein
Ascending cholangitis: CBC, total bilirubin, alkaline phosphatase, AST, and ALT
Occult subdural hematoma in presumed alcoholic: blood alcohol level
Hypoglycemia with altered mental status or seizures: blood glucose
Acute renal failure with hyperkalemia: potassium level
Meningitis: cerebrospinal fluid cell count, glucose, and protein
Sepsis: immediate pathogen identification

POCT, point-of-care testing; CBC, complete blood cell count; β-hCG, beta human chorionic gonadotropin; AST, aspartate aminotransferase; ALT, alanine aminotransferase; BNP, B-type natriuretic peptide.

waiting-room time increases when bed turnover is stagnant. Parallel delays need to be addressed and improved.

Unless it can be shown to reduce cost, POCT technology cannot succeed in modern emergency medicine. Cost in medical care, however, is a complex subject. It involves fixed costs (for salaried labor, buildings, and equipment), which are estimated to constitute 84% of hospital budgets (78) and variable costs (for medication and supplies), which are estimated to constitute 16% of hospital budgets. In regard to POCT, one could argue that institution of POCT devices in the ED would increase expense by adding fixed costs to the ED (by increasing equipment purchases and, potentially, labor required to operate the new devices) while traditional laboratory costs remained fixed at their usual level. At one institution, for example, the chief financial officer estimated that only by decreasing central laboratory volume by 50% could ED

TABLE 7.7. COMMON DIAGNOSES IN WHICH POCT COULD INCREASE ED THROUGHPUT

Ectopic pregnancy: CBC and qualitative β-hCG
Nontoxic acetaminophen ingestion: acetaminophen level
Seizure in known epileptic: anti-convulsant level
Pediatric fever of unknown origin: CBC with differential, urinalysis, cerebrospinal fluid cell count, glucose, and protein
Suspected but low clinical risk for deep vein thrombosis or pulmonary embolus: D-dimer
Uncomplicated renal colic secondary to nephrolithiasis: urinalysis
Spontaneous bacterial peritonitis: peritoneal fluid cell count with differential
Pancreatitis: amylase
Acute myocardial infarction and cardiac arrest: cardiac test clusters
Generalized weakness of unclear etiology: electrolyte panel
Tetany: ionized calcium

POCT, point-of-care testing; ED, emergency department; CBC, complete blood cell count; β-hCG, beta human chorionic gonadotropin.

POCT devices save the hospital money because only then could fixed costs be lowered by reducing infrastructure and labor in the central laboratory.

The benefit of any added cost of integrating POCT into emergency medicine is being shown in certain cases to outweigh any extra expense. For example, studies have demonstrated that accelerated ED-based diagnostic algorithms using a POCT device to expedite the rate of ruling in or ruling out patients as having acute myocardial infarction could have a significant impact on overall hospital and health care expenditures (75,79,80). In a capitated health care system where health care plans compete to provide quality service at the lowest possible cost, it could be argued that only systems poised to take advantage of such overall cost-saving systems would prosper.

Those who believe POCT might incur additional expense should also weigh the investment against the benefit of increasing the efficiency of patient care and patient consumption. For example, consider a city with multiple EDs competing to offer services to the local population. The emergency physician groups using POCT devices to minimize patient waiting times may attract a greater number of patients to their EDs. Less labor per patient seen in the ED may be required if throughput improves because each individual visit will consume less time and overall resources. Additionally, revenues might be incrementally augmented by decreasing the small percentage of patients who, frustrated by prolonged waiting times, leave before being seen by a physician.

Point-of-care testing has the potential to accelerate patient throughput in the ED. Such a goal is commendable for a number of reasons. First, by decreasing waiting times, the quality of service provided to patients could be improved by minimizing frustrating, inconvenient, and inefficient delays. Second, by expediting throughput, waiting patients with potentially life-threatening illnesses could be seen and treated sooner. Additionally, rapid patient disposition would decrease patient load per physician at a given time by decreasing individual patient length of stay. Accelerating patient disposition could free emergency physicians and nurses to focus on life-threatening problems when they arise. Implied herein, rapid POCT is not only an important means of improving outcomes in critical patients but also a means of expediting throughput of all patients, whether their diagnosis is benign or critical. An efficient ED is safer and offers patients better service.

To illustrate the central importance of diagnostic testing in emergency medicine, the following section will show how the treatment and disposition of various diagnoses commonly considered in emergency medicine hinge on receipt of diagnostic test results.

CLINICAL DIAGNOSES MADE AT THE POINT OF CARE

Table 7.5 lists the cluster of tests recommended when considering diagnoses commonly considered in emergency medicine. These diagnoses reflect the breadth of clinical conditions presenting to the ED and highlight the limited number of tests required to diagnose these conditions in the ED. Foremost, they illustrate how expedited test results using POCT devices could significantly accelerate the time in which diagnoses are made and treatment and disposition can begin. Several examples follow.

Pulmonary Embolus

No blood test can unequivocally identify or exclude the diagnosis of pulmonary embolism (Table 7.5) (81,82). Often suspected and potentially lethal, confirmation of pulmonary embolism remains very difficult without expensive and time-consuming studies, namely, compression ultrasonography, ventilation–perfusion (V/Q) pulmonary scan, computerized tomography (CT) scan, or pulmonary angiography. Each study has limitations. Compression ultrasonography is indirect and not definitive. V/Q scan is time and labor intensive and has variable sensitivity, depending on clinical suspicion. V/Q scans often produce indeterminate results in patients with pulmonary disease (i.e., 60% indeterminate results in chronic obstructive pulmonary disease). Whereas spiral CT may replace V/Q scanning in the future for initial evaluation, currently it, too, has variable sensitivity and a tendency to miss peripheral emboli. Like V/Q scanning, even with an inconclusive CT, a patient with a high clinical index of suspicion requires either admission for anticoagulation or definitive exclusion of embolic disease. The gold standard test, pulmonary angiography, has a death rate of 0.5% (83) and a risk of major nonfatal complications of 1%.

Patients in the ED at low risk for pulmonary embolism would benefit from a sensitive, specific, and rapid screening test. The purpose of the test would be to exclude low-risk patients clinically suspected of having a pulmonary embolus; this could be done without undertaking the aforementioned studies. Recently, clinicians developed interest in whole-blood D-dimer assays (84). D-dimer is a degradation product of circulating cross-linked fibrin. In the ED, it could screen low-risk patients to exclude pulmonary embolism (85). A whole-blood agglutination assay described by Wells and colleagues (86) and Turkstra and co-workers (87) has a sensitivity of 90% to 100% for pulmonary embolus or proximal deep-vein thrombosis, takes several minutes to perform, and may be done at the bedside. Recently, whole-blood assays with bedside capabilities were developed with sensitivity and specificity approaching the D-dimer's gold standard, the enzyme-linked immunosorbent assay (ELISA) (88,89). Wildberger and associates (90), for example, tested a bedside D-dimer assay that they found correctly identified all thrombotic disorders in the lower extremities that required further treatment. Whereas Wildberger and co-workers' results have since been questioned (91) and further studies will need to confirm the efficacy and safety of POCT devices able to screen for thrombotic disease, the benefit of a highly specific and sensitive screening assay remains. If a successful, rapid bedside assay were produced, more invasive, costly, and time-consuming diagnostics (V/Q, spiral CT, ultrasonography) could be reserved for patients with an abnormal screening test. Given that the vast majority of patients currently undergoing invasive diagnostic studies lack thrombotic pathology, such an assay could increase productivity by increasing bed turnover while saving patients time and money and minimizing their exposure to potential procedural complications.

Trauma

Initial trauma evaluations depend on few diagnostic assays (Table 7.5). Rapid results of the requisite tests could improve clinical and economic outcomes. In 1994, Frankel and colleagues (92) used a transportable microanalyzer at the bedside during ED trauma resuscitations. Using the bedside microanalyzer decreased iatrogenic blood loss, saved $160 for each patient tested, and decreased laboratory turnaround time from 64 to 6 minutes. They found the instrument accurate, expedient, and adequate. Asimos and associates (93) found that rapid results for hemoglobin, lactate, blood gases, and glucose using a POCT device during emergent trauma management occasionally led to changes in patient management that reduced morbidity or conserved resources. In another study, Herr and colleagues (94) used a POCT device in a prehospital helicopter system. On several occasions, test results led to prehospital resuscitation with blood products.

By measuring serum lactate levels, POCT devices could aid trauma resuscitation (95–99). Serial near-patient lactate levels would facilitate "real-time" assessment of patient resuscitation and severity of injury. Physicians could tailor therapy accordingly. Patients who are initially inadequately resuscitated are predisposed to ensuing life-threatening multiorgan dysfunction that requires costly intensive care. Using serial near-patient lactate levels, physicians could optimize effective resuscitation and in so doing may improve outcomes and decrease cost. For patients with traumatic brain injury, recent data suggest that prompt availability of serum protein S100β, a marker of brain damage, leads to improved clinical outcomes (100).

Vaginal Bleeding

Vaginal bleeding in women of childbearing age is a common ED presentation. Following the history and physical examination, diagnostic workup requires several studies (Table 7.5). First, a urine qualitative human chorionic gonadotropin (β-hCG) test to verify pregnancy and hematocrit level to assess potential blood loss. A positive urine pregnancy test (TAT estimated at 1 hour) obligates the physician to determine the Rhesus (Rh) type and to obtain a quantitative β-hCG. Depending on clinical suspicion with or without level of quantitative β-hCG, a pelvic ultrasound may be ordered to exclude ectopic pregnancy. What usually presents as a threatened miscarriage becomes unduly time consuming waiting for diagnostic test results, first for the qualitative urine pregnancy test with or without the quantitative β-hCG test and, second, the Rh type after confirmation of pregnancy. At certain institutions, the Rh type is not carried out by the central laboratory and is not reported on the central computer. Verification of that result requires an additional phone call.

Using POCT technology, the scenario could be different. One could have definitive results of hematocrit and of qualitative and quantitative β-hCG within 5 minutes. Patients with significantly decreased hematocrit could be rapidly transfused and triaged to surgery, potentially improving outcomes. Rapid Rh typing could facilitate administration of Rhogam and patient throughput. Ultrasound could be initiated sooner if diagnostic tests were expedited. Life-threatening hemorrhage or future infertility might be prevented in a patient with an ectopic pregnancy. Cost could be reduced by preventing unnecessary testing or admission. For example, in 1988 Gennis and colleagues (101) showed that a bedside qualitative β-hCG test was associated with decreased numbers of culdocentesis, ultrasound examinations, and hospital admissions. They projected that this bedside test decreased damage to fallopian tubes and future infertility. They calculated cost savings to their institution at $123,000 compared with traditional central laboratory testing.

To reiterate, most women of childbearing age with vaginal bleeding have either dysfunctional uterine bleeding (a diagnosis of exclusion), menorrhagia, or, if pregnant, medically uncomplicated threatened miscarriage. Following history and physical examination, their ED time is spent waiting for diagnostic data that help to risk stratify patients into those who can be safely discharged for follow-up, those who need further evaluation, and those who need admission with or without emergent surgery. Any ability to compress the time waiting for these diagnostic results will serve to facilitate patient throughput, expedite patient therapy, and optimize outcomes. POCT devices with rapid results offer that possibility.

Asthma

In 1988, Shier and colleagues (102) used a bedside POCT device that measures quantitative theophylline levels to reduce ED length of stay in asthmatics. The POCT instrument decreased time to reach a therapeutic drug concentration, thus shortening treatment time and attenuating ED length of stay compared with traditional therapy. Today in the United States, theophylline is rarely used to treat asthma, but the principles remain that bedside monitoring of therapeutic drug levels offers the possibility of optimizing ED patient care and reducing length of stay, and that POCT is valuable in respiratory distress.

Toxicology

Most patients with toxicologic ingestions enter the health care system through the ED. The patients then undergo evaluation and toxicologic screening tests to determine morbidity of ingestion. Patients with ingestions whose toxicity can be predicted from quantitative blood drug levels merit diagnostic laboratory tests because the need for treatment depends on toxin concentration. Examples include acetaminophen, aspirin, carbon monoxide, lithium, iron, methanol, digoxin, theophylline, ethylene glycol, and methanol.

For patients who present with severe or confusing symptoms but have ingested agents without specific therapy, levels may be indicated only if the patient is severely symptomatic or has a confusing clinical picture. Examples include ethanol, phenytoin, phenobarbital, and valproic acid. Diagnostic testing is not indicated, however, when there is a known ingestion, toxicity is determined clinically, and therapy is instituted based on the clinical picture instead of a specific drug level. Examples include tricyclic antidepressants, opiates, benzodiazepines, cyanides, and organophosphates.

Lastly, in patients with ingestions where toxicity does not correlate with levels and no specific treatment is needed, qualitative testing might help establish a diagnosis, but is not absolutely indicated. Examples include phencyclidine (PCP), hallucinogens, neuroleptics, cocaine, and amphetamines. Accordingly, diagnostic testing is also inappropriate when patients have minimal symptoms and physical examination findings with no history of ingestion or with ingestion of an unknown agent. An exception to the latter might be acetaminophen screening in potential suicidal ingestion, but more on this follows later. Of note, diagnostic screening tests are generally expensive, hampered by delayed results, and not always correlated with the substance ingested. An effective diagnostic algorithm combined with rapid point-of-care diagnostic testing might significantly expedite the rapidity with which a patient might be diagnosed and treated or excluded for a serious ingestion. Let us look at several examples.

In 1996, Sporer and Khayam-Bashi (103) formulated recommendations for selective screening of suicidal or suspected ingestions. This group recommended universal screening for acetaminophen levels because they found that 3% of patients had an occult or accidental ingestion and that 0.3% of patients with occult ingestions had levels toxic enough potentially to require liver transplantation (104). Overall, however, 80% of these ingestions had trivial acetaminophen levels not warranting treatment. These investigators found screening for salicylate overdoses using salicylate levels ineffective but instead recommended use of the anion gap and clinical picture as indicators of potentially significant salicylate toxicity. A POCT device with a 5-minute TTAT providing levels of acetaminophen and anion gap could screen for patients who either need potentially lifesaving treatment with charcoal and N-acetylcysteine (acetaminophen toxicity) or charcoal and bicarbonate with or without dialysis (salicylate toxicity). For most patients with nontoxic ingestions, however, patients with negative screening examinations could be discharged home or to psychiatric care in a fraction of the time currently required for trivial ingestions.

The Drug Abuse Warning Network (DAWN) reports estimates that 2.7% of ED visits are alcohol related and 1.1% illicit drug-related (105). Alcohol overdose is an example of an ingestion with no specific treatment. Levels, however, may be appropriate when the patient is unconscious or when the cause of the patient's alteration in consciousness is not entirely clear (e.g., polysubstance abuse or an alcoholic patient with underlying head trauma). In these situations, a POCT breathalyzer or blood or saliva alcohol tests (106) may guide the emergency physician in avoiding expensive additional workups, such as brain CT. On the other hand, the unconscious patient assumed to be intoxicated who actually has an underlying subdural hematoma from a drunken fall may easily and rapidly reveal his or her current state of sobriety with use of a POCT device. With the assumed source of the patient's altered state thus excluded, he or she could then undergo an immediate brain CT scan or lifesaving surgery if indicated.

Cocaine, the most frequently abused illicit drug with dangerous side effects, can cause myocardial infarction and dysrhythmias, cerebrovascular accidents, and rhabdomyolysis. To prevent these events and initiate treatment, rapid bedside results could benefit patient care. Of note, the treatment commonly given for acute myocardial infarction, that is, β-blockers, is contraindicated in cocaine toxicity because they exacerbate coronary vasospasm and lead to paradoxical hypertension through unopposed α-receptor agonism. For this reason, it would be beneficial to know in "real time," which patients with chest pain are suffering from cocaine-induced coronary vasospasm instead of thrombotic cardiac ischemia.

Overdoses with specific therapy that cause cardiovascular compromise are currently diagnosed clinically, partly because delays in diagnostic test results are too long to alter patient outcomes. Examples of such overdoses (and their therapy) include tricyclic antidepressants (sodium bicarbonate, crystalloids, and ventilatory support), digoxin (Fab fragments ± dialysis), β-blockers (glucagon and high-dose pressor therapy), and calcium channel blockers (calcium and pressors). An experienced clinician may be able to assess clinically such critical patients and rapidly initiate lifesaving therapy. Because clinical presentations of patients are frequently atypical, because not all clinicians are equally astute or experienced, and because emergency physicians often make critical decisions with limited information, a POCT device able to screen for such ingestions might help to guide therapy rapidly and optimize patient outcomes.

Further examples include opiates and benzodiazepines. Commonly abused, both substances can lead to respiratory failure in addition to pulmonary edema in the former and hypotension in the latter. These potential hazards, however, can be antagonized by appropriate reversal agents: Narcan (naloxone HCl) for opiates and flumazenil for benzodiazepines. Diagnosis of either of these overdoses could generally be made clinically, based on physical examination and response to reversal agents. Diagnostic tests, therefore, may be generally inappropriate. Situations arise, however, when screening for these two agents is warranted. Additionally, for the patient with chronic benzodiazepine use, treatment with flumazenil may initiate intractable status epilepticus and, as a result, diagnostic rapid POCT screening tests may at times avoid complications caused by diagnostic flumazenil.

Acute Renal Failure

Patients in acute renal failure may need immediate therapy with or without dialysis for a number of indications. Among them are severe hyperkalemia, other severe electrolyte imbalances, or acid–base disturbances. Patients with renal failure may present with hyperkalemia, which predisposes them to life-threatening cardiac arrhythmias. In light of the standard waiting time for diagnostic tests, hyperkalemia is generally diagnosed by electrocardiogram and therapy is instituted depending on the findings. Using a POCT device, however, one could know within minutes whether a patient was severely hyperkalemic, whether a patient's arrhythmia was being induced by hyperkalemia, or whether a nephrologist should be consulted immediately to arrange for dialysis. The same argument could be made for acute renal failure patients with severe hypocalcemia, hypermagnesemia, or metabolic acidosis. All these conditions can be life-threatening and stabilized with pharmacologic therapy prior to dialysis when needed. The sooner one can ascertain data to determine the severity of the imbalance, the sooner therapy can be started, morbidity prevented, and disposition of the patient appropriately enacted.

Diabetic Ketoacidosis

Patients with diabetic ketoacidosis (DKA) are initially screened with POCT glucose analyzers. For patients with hyperglycemia, however, the diagnosis of DKA requires confirmation of acidosis and ketonemia (Table 7.5). Both these results could be confirmed by using POCT devices. Acidosis or pH can be measured by using a POCT arterial (or venous) (107) blood gas device, and ketonemia can be measured or estimated using a blood or urine analyzer measuring ketonemia or ketonuria. Once the diagnosis of DKA is confirmed, potentially lifesaving therapy can be instituted and arrangements made for admission to medical intensive care units if necessary.

Of note, patients with DKA are total-body potassium depleted. Potassium replacement is indicated, but patients may be hyperkalemic or hypokalemic. Therapy with insulin, however, drives potassium into the intracellular space, which can exacerbate hypokalemia and predispose patients to arrhythmias. Treatment with potassium, on the other hand, can exacerbate hyperkalemia. As a result, insulin infusions and potassium replacement are often withheld until patients have urinated. With a rapid POCT device, electrolyte status, including potassium and anion gap, could be rapidly available and expedite diagnosis, treatment, and disposition.

Respiratory Failure

Patients in extreme respiratory distress often present initially to the ED. For these patients, endotracheal intubation may be lifesaving. Frequently, the decision to intubate is guided clinically by patient examination and bedside oxygen saturation. Rapid POCT arterial blood gas results could help guide intervention. For example, for chronic carbon dioxide (CO_2) retaining patients with chronic obstructive pulmonary disease or fatiguing asthmatics, rapid POCT analysis of the change from baseline of a patient's presenting CO_2 level might affect the decision to intubate or continue with less invasive therapy. In a similar way, by serial evaluations of patient hypercarbia, the relative effectiveness of current therapeutic interventions and the need for immediate intubation if faced with worsening respiratory failure could be assessed. Rapid arterial blood gas results would be useful in numerous other areas of resuscitation (Table 7.5) which call for critical test clusters that include additional analytes, such as K^+, Ca^{2+}, and other electrolytes.

Focus on Chest Pain Evaluation

Background

The evaluation of chest pain warrants a focused strategy and is addressed in detail because of its volume and the potential consequences to the patient, liability for the physician, and fiscal burden for the payer. This year, 2002, an estimated 1.2 million Americans will have a new or recurrent coronary attack (defined as acute myocardial infarction or fatal coronary heart disease) (108). Over 650,000 of these attacks will be first attacks, and 450,000 will be recurrent. Over 45% of people who experience a coronary attack in a given year will die from it. More than five million patients present each year to the ED with complaints of chest pain suggestive of myocardial ischemia and more than 40% of these visits lead to costly hospital admissions (109–111). Only a minority of the admitted patients ultimately will be diagnosed with acute coronary syndromes, however (112,113).

The inadequacy of current management strategies has led to a practice in which approximately 4% of patients with AMI or unstable angina are inadvertently discharged from the ED (114,115). These patients have a mortality rate nearly twice that of those correctly recognized on the initial visit (112,115,116). The failure to diagnose AMI accounts for the single greatest cause of dollars lost in malpractice claims against emergency physicians (117). This strategy has created an environment of significant legal risk that drives a liberal admission policy, resulting in an estimated cost of $10 billion annually to rule out AMI (111,118). There is a clear need for an accurate, efficient means of reducing unnecessary admission of patients who do not have acute coronary syndromes without compromising the care of those who do. The ability to recognize patients at low risk for acute coronary syndromes who present to the ED with chest pain led to alternatives to conventional coronary care for this group, including management in a chest pain center (113,119). This potentially more efficient approach to evaluating these low-risk patients can reduce unnecessary admissions, lower cost, and improve utilization of telemetry beds, all of which are essential to cost-effective care.

Chest pain centers are an organizational innovation intended to meet these challenges. They may be physical or virtual units. Their mission is to utilize an observation program or accelerated diagnostic protocol to improve the detection of patients with acute coronary syndromes and reduce the incidence of inappropriate discharge. Likewise, they may better identify chest pain patients without cardiovascular disease and reduce unnecessary hospital admissions.

A chest pain center–based strategy can solve most problems associated with an inpatient approach to rule out AMI. It selectively utilizes a greater number of diagnostic modalities, such as serial electrocardiograms (ECG) and cardiac injury markers, nuclear imaging, echocardiography, and ECG stress testing to avoid discharging patients with AMI (120), while reducing cost by avoiding unnecessary hospital admissions. Recent reports from institutions using a chest pain center or observation unit strategy have demonstrated an AMI missed rate from 0% to 0.4% (121,122) compared with a 2% rate with traditional inpatient evaluation (114). Chest pain centers have evolved from concept to fully operational clinical models that provide optimal efficiency in evaluating patients with chest pain (123).

Initial Risk Stratification

Studies during the past two decades demonstrated that low-risk patients with chest pain can be recognized by assessment of the ECG and clinical status at presentation (116,124–129). Brush and colleagues reported that the initial ECG can discriminate between high and low risk in these patients (127). Among patients hospitalized for AMI, a subgroup with a coronary event rate of less than 5% could be identified by the history, symptoms, and ECG (9). Furthermore, it was shown that in patients hospitalized for chest pain, a group with less than a 1% probability of developing complications could be distinguished by the initial clinical evaluation

(128). Evidence of low clinical risk in patients presenting with chest pain includes a normal or near-normal initial ECG, no signs of left ventricular dysfunction, stable cardiac rhythm, and a normal chest radiograph. For the purpose of initial risk stratification, based largely on Goldman's protocol, *low risk* is defined as a 7% or less risk of AMI (130). *Moderate risk* would include patients with a greater than 7% risk of AMI but an ECG that is not diagnostic of ischemia or infarction. Any patient with an ECG diagnostic of ischemia or infarction is clearly at *high risk*.

Although use of the ECG and clinical data has considerable value in triaging patients into low-, moderate-, and high-risk groups for acute coronary syndromes, it has limited ability to identify specific patients who have myocardial ischemia from those who do not (112). Symptoms of ischemia are often variable and the ECG is nondiagnostic in about half of patients with AMI (131). Therefore, more accurate methods, both traditional and innovative, have been applied to achieve further risk stratification in these patients. These include serial measurement of cardiac injury markers, immediate exercise treadmill testing, nuclear scintigraphy, and echocardiography. All these diagnostic modalities contribute to the accurate assessment of patients, each modality having advantages and disadvantages.

Cardiac Injury Markers

Whereas decision-making for patients with suspected myocardial ischemia in the ED has been based historically on the history and resting 12-lead ECG, there is significant evidence that cardiac injury marker testing can impact management. It addresses both the time-dependent process of myocardial necrosis and the potential benefit of intervention. POCT is performed at the bedside, and this technology's greatest potential to enhance care and reduce cost is in the evaluation of patients with chest pain in the ED or chest pain center. In this setting, POCT may allow more rapid clinical decision-making by reducing TTAT. This would facilitate earlier diagnosis and intervention, leading to improved triage, disposition, resource utilization, and clinical outcome. Recognition of AMI by any cardiac injury marker is dependent, however, on a lapse of time after symptom onset. Although POCT may provide more rapid results, it cannot obviate this diagnostic limitation (132).

The role of cardiac injury markers in the ED recently expanded to (a) confirming the diagnosis of AMI, (b) identification of patients with acute coronary syndromes who are at risk for adverse events, and (c) identifying patients who can be evaluated in the ED or chest pain center and safely discharged home versus those in need of hospitalization. Most recently, assays such as cardiac troponin provided physicians with extremely sensitive markers of injury that are highly cardiac specific (133). These markers have a lesser role in the management of patients with ECGs diagnostic of infarction, but in patients with nondiagnostic ECGs, they have had considerable value. Despite the recent addition of numerous promising injury markers, such as cardiac troponin I (cTnI), cardiac troponin T (cTnT), myocardial muscle creatine kinase isoenzyme (CK-MB) isoforms, and the resurgence of myoglobin use, there currently is no "single marker" that can accomplish all these goals. Combinations of various markers used in a diagnostic algorithm, however, may enable us to distinguish patients with myocardial injury from those without.

Several studies have evaluated the use of cardiac injury markers for the diagnosis of AMI. Myoglobin becomes elevated as early as 1 to 2 hours after symptom onset, making it particularly well suited for diagnosis of AMI in the first few hours after patient presentation. Additionally, the doubling of myoglobin values on successive samples drawn 2 hours apart has demonstrated superior sensitivity compared with using a single measurement that exceeds the reference range for normal (75,134–136). CK-MB remains a current standard for the diagnosis of AMI and, as such, provides comparative data for assessment of other injury markers. Unfortunately, it is also found in noncardiac tissues, thereby limiting its specificity. Several studies have shown that the overall sensitivity and specificity of detecting AMI is improved by serial evaluations of multiple cardiac injury markers (131,137–143). This practice allows for the combination of a marker that is very sensitive for injury during the first few hours after symptom onset, such as myoglobin, with markers such as CK-MB, cTnT, or cTnI, which are more cardiac specific and remain elevated longer. These studies suggest that patients with AMI can be effectively identified using an accelerated protocol in the ED or chest pain center, a strategy that is supported by a recent consensus statement (144). It is important to note that the sensitivity of each of these markers is affected by the time from symptom onset to sampling.

The cardiac troponins are more sensitive than CK-MB for myocardial necrosis and are a more useful prognostic tool in patients with acute coronary syndromes (145–151). They are challenging CK-MB as the preferred biomarker to identify myocardial injury, and likely will become the future gold standard for the diagnosis of AMI. Because of the use of CK-MB as a benchmark for the diagnosis of AMI, the specificity of the cardiac troponins as reported in several articles varies from 46% to 96% (152–154). Numerous studies suggest that approximately a third of patients with unstable angina have positive troponins (146,149,155,156). When these troponin elevations occur in the face of a normal CK-MB, patients should be classified as having minor or minimal myocardial injury. Compared with patients without troponin elevations, these patients have an increased risk of death, AMI, and need for revascularization (148,149,157,158). A consensus document of the Joint European Society of Cardiology/American College of Cardiology Committee for the Redefinition of Myocardial Infarction suggests that any amount of myocardial necrosis caused by ischemia should be labeled as AMI (159). This would include a cTnI, cTnT, or CK-MB value that exceeds the 99th percentile of a reference control group on at least one occasion for the troponins or successive samples for CK-MB.

At present, POCT is available for myoglobin, CK-MB, cTnI, and cTnT. Desirable characteristics of a POCT assay to detect these cardiac proteins include the following: (a) agreement with accepted assays (validity), (b) minimal variation of test results (reliability), (c) rapid therapeutic turnaround time, (d) minimal technical expertise or calibration demands, (e) disposable or low maintenance device, and (f) low cost (132). Several studies of POCT for AMI in the ED or chest pain center warrant review. The Rapid Evaluation by Assay of Cardiac Troponin T (REACTT) trial evaluated the utility of a qualitative cTnT

device in 721 patients, 102 with AMI (160). Testing at 0, 3, and 6 hours from presentation demonstrated a sensitivity of 70% and a specificity of 97%. The sensitivity of a laboratory-measured quantitative cTnT was only slightly better at 80%. Brogan and colleagues (161) studied a CK-MB/myoglobin POCT device in 277 ED chest pain patients and compared the results with quantitative central laboratory testing at 0, 1, and 3 hours after presentation. The sensitivity at 3 hours for the POCT device was 96%.

Hamm and colleagues (155) evaluated POCT devices for both cTnI and cTnT in 773 patients with chest pain and nondiagnostic ECGs. Testing was performed at 0 and 4 hours, with the second sample at least 6 hours after symptom onset. Cardiac event rates for negative tests were 1.1% for cTnT and 0.3% for cTnI. The odds ratio for a positive result in predicting a cardiac event was 25.8 for cTnT and 61.4 for cTnI. A recently completed trial, CHECKMATE evaluated the utility of a POCT multimarker strategy (MMS) in chest pain units. This study prospectively compared two POCT panels—CK-MB, cTnI, and myoglobin (MMS-1) versus CK-MB and cTnI (MMS-2)—with local laboratory testing. The primary endpoint was death or MI at 30 days. The POCT devices identified more positive patients (MMS-1 = 24% and MMS-2 = 19%) compared with 9% for the local laboratory. The time to positive test results was also 30 minutes faster in the POCT groups (162). Although a strategy of selecting POCT devices to create a panel of markers may be appealing, further investigation into their impact on real-time decision making and on costs is warranted.

Measuring cardiac troponin and myoglobin at 0, 2 to 4, and 6 to 9 hours after arrival is a very reasonable approach. Additional serial markers at 12 and 24 hours may be performed in selected cases but should be considered optional. In EDs that do not have the resources for 6 to 12 hours of observation in a chest pain center, testing for myoglobin may not be clinically useful because one of its primary benefits is the rapid identification of patients without AMI (144). This strategy is based on time of ED blood draw and is meant to encompass all patients regardless of time of chest pain onset. Although the sensitivity of cardiac injury marker testing is excellent, it is not sufficient to stand alone in stratifying patients' risk for AMI or adverse events. The results should gateway patients into diagnostic algorithms that utilize functional testing or cardiac imaging to complete the risk stratification process.

Cardiac Imaging and Functional Testing

The safety and utility of exercise testing for risk stratification of patients with chest pain who have stable anginal symptoms have been well established (163). Immediate exercise treadmill testing is a novel concept to risk stratify patients who present to the ED with chest pain suspicious of AMI who are considered to be at low risk based on clinical and ECG data. A study of 950 patients who underwent graded exercise testing after a 9-hour observation period showed patients with positive, nondiagnostic, and normal exercise tests had subsequent cardiac event rates of 26%, 3%, and 0.9%, respectively, during 1-year follow-up (164). Although there has been concern regarding the potential hazards of stress testing patients with possible AMI, the aforementioned data on initial risk stratification support the utility of the ECG and clinical assessment in recognizing chest pain patients at low risk for a coronary event and its complications.

Kirk and colleagues used immediate exercise treadmill testing in selected patients to identify those requiring admission and those who could undergo further evaluation on an outpatient basis (165). A preliminary report from this group in a limited number of patients with no history of coronary artery disease suggested that this strategy, as implemented by cardiologists, was practical and safe with a potential for major cost savings (166). In the former report (165), 212 underwent exercise testing with no adverse events, 13% of whom had positive results. Further evaluation revealed unstable angina in ten and AMI in three. This study suggested that immediate exercise treadmill testing in selected patients with acute chest pain was safe despite the possibility of testing patients with unrecognized AMI or unstable angina. All patients with negative tests and most with nondiagnostic tests were discharged immediately from the ED and managed as outpatients. Follow-up at 30 days revealed no ischemic complications. The University of California, Davis Medical Center now regularly utilizes immediate exercise treadmill testing in low-risk patients with chest pain (165–168). This method has been used safely and successfully thus far in more than 3,000 patients.

Radionuclide imaging has been established as a safe and accurate method to identify patients with coronary artery disease (169). Areas of decreased thallium or technetium-99m sestamibi uptake by the myocardium are seen as a negative scintigraphic image, indicating regions of ischemic or infarcted myocardium. These changes can be detected during the first 6 hours after symptom onset. Radionuclide testing in the ED is most useful as a diagnostic and prognostic tool when the ECG is nondiagnostic or has changes that preclude accurate interpretation (170). Some studies suggest it is a better prognostic indicator of future cardiac events than traditional biochemical markers of cardiac injury (171).

Sestamibi is superior to thallium in identifying acutely ischemic myocardium because it has a slow redistribution to ischemic myocardium that can allow for a several-hour delay prior to cardiac imaging. In low-risk patients, resting sestamibi perfusion imaging has been shown to identify accurately patients with acute coronary syndrome who are at risk for cardiac complications (122,172). The sensitivity of sestamibi perfusion imaging to identify acute coronary syndromes may be significantly higher than that of biochemical markers of cardiac injury obtained at presentation, such as cTnI (173). This finding has led to increased use of resting sestamibi scans in patients who present to the ED within 4 hours of chest pain onset who may not be candidates for other testing strategies.

Myocardial ischemia produces regional impairment of left ventricular wall motion, and this impairment may manifest before ECG alterations (174). Transthoracic echocardiography is a sensitive method for detection of these abnormalities and therefore has been used in the ED to detect ischemia in patients presenting with chest pain (175–180). Optimal utility of echocardiography for these purposes requires its immediate availability in the ED 24 hours a day because its sensitivity for diagnosing transient contractile abnormalities is highest during or shortly after ischemic pain. Echocardiography also may be helpful in its ability to detect some patients with aortic dissection, pulmonary embolus, peri-

cardial effusion, and complications of AMI, such as mural thrombi, ventricular septal defect, and papillary muscle rupture. Limitations of cardiac imaging and functional testing include the need for specialized equipment and personnel to perform and interpret the test. In addition, resting perfusion imaging and echocardiography may be insensitive in some patients with small zones of ischemia and cannot easily differentiate between acute infarction, previous infarction, and acute ischemia. This may limit its use in ED patients, especially those with prior AMI (181). In conjunction with biochemical markers, these diagnostic testing strategies provide an accurate and efficient method for early diagnosis of patients with acute coronary syndromes in the ED.

Temporal Management Optimization

Evaluation of patients with chest pain suspicious of AMI continues to be a challenge. It is now apparent that routine hospital admission is not indicated in patients without obvious acute coronary syndromes. The ability to stratify reliably patients into different levels of risk (low, moderate, high) has led to a more cost-effective approach in which an accelerated diagnostic protocol that is risk driven can be used in the ED or chest pain center. An algorithm that incorporates serial cardiac injury marker testing, exercise testing, radionuclide imaging, and echocardiography to stratify patients risk for acute coronary syndrome is effective in managing these patients, providing safe and accurate disposition from the ED. POCT for cardiac injury markers may be particularly well suited for this approach. Implementation of these strategies affords timeliness and potential for vital cost savings while maintaining sound patient care.

OVERVIEW OF CLINICAL STRATEGIES

Whereas this section highlighted diagnoses in which rapid POCT might optimize patient care and flow in the ED, evaluation strategies in other commonly encountered conditions (see Table 7.5) require highly ranked test clusters for evidence-based management and treatment of critically ill patients. In each of these diagnoses, one could argue that rapid POCT results might benefit ED patient care by expediting patient diagnosis and, in so doing, accelerate therapeutic interventions and patient disposition. Additionally, Table 7.6 lists diagnoses in which rapid POCT is likely to affect clinical outcomes, although these predictions have yet to be proven through controlled clinical studies. Table 7.7 lists common diagnoses in which POCT, if available, would likely expedite patient disposition through rapid confirmation or exclusion of diagnostic hypotheses.

Conclusions and Recommendations for Point-of-Care Testing in Emergency Medicine

POCT, properly exploited, offers emergency medicine an opportunity to advance patient care in terms of efficiency, overall cost savings, and clinical outcomes (182–184). To succeed, manufacturers need to produce simple-to-use devices with internally calibrated quality control that will provide a comprehensive cluster of requisite test results and transmit them to a centralized repository for permanent storage and physician access. As chaperones in a new age of decentralized testing, laboratory personnel should schedule visits to monitor device proficiency; those providing patient care will focus on medical strategies. Nursing staff needs proper device orientation and training, education about potential benefits, and adequate manpower to complete this additional mission. Lastly, physicians need to act on results quickly to expedite dispositions and optimize outcomes. The following list summarizes key elements of a successful POCT program in the ED.

Create complete diagnostic clusters of critical analytes.

Integrate data real time into centralized databases.

Coordinate systematic quality control monitoring.

Educate nurses about potential benefits and free them to complete required tests.

Train operators to ensure quality use.

Promote further investigation of impact of POCT on real-time decision-making and cost savings compared with traditional models.

Incorporate POCT into prehospital care where it may improve patient outcomes or expedite disposition, triage, and safety of patients.

Act on results promptly; otherwise, efficiency and improved outcomes may not occur.

Exploit expedited therapeutic TAT by identifying and improving external delays.

Foster coordination and assistance from fellow departments, particularly the laboratory but also trauma, cardiology, and others.

Hold high the principle of optimization of patient care as the driving force for continuous quality improvement tailored for the needs of each individual institution.

Coordination with involved departments is essential, most notably the clinical laboratory, but also other specialties whose patients stand to gain the most from optimal exploitation of POCT technologies in emergency medicine. These specialties include cardiology, trauma, general surgery, internal medicine, pediatrics, obstetrics, and emergency medical service (EMS). Additionally, when beneficial, these groups should be involved in studies aimed at uncovering the value of POCT in real-time decision making (improvement in ED TTAT, clinical outcomes, and length of stay) and cost savings compared with traditional models. External delays that inhibit the integration and exploitation of rapid diagnostic testing should be sought and removed.

Much inertia and collective resistance exists that would leave POCT in the ED unemployed. For those of us involved in the day-to-day challenges of acute emergency medical care, we urge those opposing integration to consider the potential benefits of POCT to emergency medical physicians and, most importantly, to the patients they serve. With patient care at the forefront of our interests, we oppose the status quo and strive to optimize health care delivery through the rapid integration of POCT technologies into the service of emergency medicine.

ACKNOWLEDGMENTS

We thank many individuals for editorial guidance and support in completing this chapter. For their invaluable comments and dedication, we would especially like to thank Paul Auerbach, M.D., Gus Garmel, M.D., Ed Klofas, M.D., and George Sternbach, M.D.

DISCLAIMER

REFERENCES

1. Kost GJ. New whole blood analyzers and their impact on cardiac and critical care. *Crit Rev Clin Lab Sci* 1993;30:153–202.
2. Marks V. Clinical biochemistry nearer the patient. *BMJ* 1983;286:1166–1167.
3. Kost GJ. Guidelines for point-of-care testing: improving patient outcomes. *Am J Clin Pathol* 1995;104:S111–S127.
4. Riggs LM. Emergency medicine: a vigorous new specialty. *N Engl J Med* 1981;304:480–483.
5. American Hospital Association. *Hospital statistics.* Chicago IL, 1980, p. 20.
6. American Hospital Association. *Hospital statistics,* Chicago, IL, 1996, p. 6.
7. Heckerling PS. Time study of an emergency room: identification of sources of patient delay. *Ill Med J* 1984;155:437–440.
8. McConnell TS, Writtenberr-Loy C. Whither waiting: turnaround times of laboratory tests for emergency room patients. *Lab Med* 1983;14:644–647.
9. Reiber NH. Survey of emergency room usage gives guidelines for improvement. *Hospital Topics* 1965;43:69–73.
10. Thorpe DP. A "time study" approach to the evaluation of emergency room activities. *J Maine Med Assoc* 1972;63:197–199.
11. Reilly TA, Stewart MM, Metsch JM, et al. Medical admission from an emergency room: factors associated with long delays. *Mt Sinai J Med* 1977;44:544–550.
12. Cue F, Inglis R. Improving the operations of the emergency department. *Hospitals* 1978;52:110–19.
13. Saunders CE. Time study of patient movement through the emergency department: sources of delay in relation to patient acuity. *Ann Emerg Med* 1987;16:1244–1248.
14. Saunders CE, Makens PK, Leblanc LJ. Modeling emergency department operations using advanced computer simulation systems. *Ann Emerg Med* 1989;18:134–141.
15. Selker HP, Beshansky JR, Pauker SG, et al. The epidemiology of delays in a teaching hospital. *Med Care* 1989;27:112–129.
16. Hallam K. Turnaround time: speeding up, but is it fast enough? *Med Lab Observer* 1988;20:28–34.
17. Howanitz PJ, Cembrowski GS, Steindel SJ, et al. Physician goals and laboratory test turnaround times: a College of American Pathologists Q-Probes study of 2673 clinicians and 722 institutions. *Arch Pathol Lab Med* 1993;117:22–28.
18. Hilborne LE, Oye R, McArdle JE, et al. Use of specimen turnaround time as a component of laboratory quality: a comparison of clinician expectations with laboratory performance. *Am J Clin Pathol* 1989;92:613–618.
19. Steindel, SJ. Timeliness of clinical laboratory tests: a discussion based on five College of American Pathologists Q-Probe studies. *Arch Pathol Lab Med* 1995;119:918–925.
20. Valenstein P. Can we satisfy clinicians' demands for faster service? Should we try? *Am J Clin Pathol* 1989;92(5):705–706.
21. Wilson GA, McDonald CJ, McCabe GP. The effect of immediate access to a computerized medical record on physician test ordering: a controlled clinical trial in the emergency room. *Am J Public Health* 1982;72:698–702.
22. Cole GW. Biochemical test profiles and laboratory system design. *Hum Pathol* 1980; 11:424–434.

23. Parvin CA, Lo SF, Deuser SM, et al. Impact of point-of-care testing on patients' length of stay in a large emergency department. *Clin Chem* 1996;42:711–717.

24. McMillan JR, Younger MS, DeWine LC. Satisfaction with hospital emergency department as a function of patient triage. *Health Care Manage Rev* 1986;11:21–27.

25. Chesteen SA, Warren SE, Woolley FR. A comparison of family practice clinics and free-standing emergency centers: organizational characteristics, process of care, and patient satisfaction. *J Fam Pract* 1986;23:377–382.

26. Halpern MT, Palmer CS, Simpson KN, et al. The economic and clinical efficiency of point-of-care testing for critically ill patients: a decision-analysis model. *Am J Med Qual* 1998;13:3–12.

27. Bailey TM, Topham TM, Wantz S, et al. Laboratory process improvement through point-of-care testing. *Journal of Quality Improvement* 1997;23:362–380.

28. Innanen VT, Barqueira-de Campos F. Point-of-care glucose testing: cost savings and ease of use with the ames glucometer elite. *Clin Chem* 1995;41:1537–1540.

29. Zaloga GP. Evaluation of bedside testing options for the critical care unit. *Chest* 1990;5:185S–90S.

30. Statland BE, Brzys K. Evaluating STAT testing alternatives by calculating annual laboratory costs. *Chest* 1990;5:198S–203S.

31. Tsai WW, Nash DB, Seamonds B, et al. Point-of-care versus central laboratory testing: an economic analysis in an academic medical center. *Clin Ther* 1994;16:898–910.

32. Sands VM, Auerbach PS, Birnbaum J, et al. Evaluation of a portable clinical blood analyzer in the emergency department. *Acad Emerg Med* 1995;2:172–178.

33. Kendall J, Reeves B, Clancy M. Point-of-care testing: randomised controlled trial of clinical outcome. *BMJ* 1998;316:1052–1057.

34. Murray RP, Leroux M, Sabga E, et al. Effect of point of care testing on length of stay in an adult emergency department. *J Emerg Med* 1999;17:811–814.

35. Goss ME, Reed JI, Reader GG. Time spent by patients in emergency room: survey at the New York Hospital. *New York State J Med* 1971; 71:1243–1246.

36. Fineberg, DA, Stewart MM. Analysis of patient flow in the emergency room. *Mount Sinai J Med* 1977;44:551–559.

37. Fleisher M, Schwartz, MK. Automated approaches to rapid-response testing: a comparative evaluation of point-of-care and centralized laboratory testing. *Am J Clin Pathol* 1975;104:S18–S25.

38. Cantrill SV, Karas S. *Cost effective diagnostic testing in emergency medicine.* Texas: American College of Emergency Physicians, 2000, 49–60, 89–92.

39. Lowe RA, Wood AB, Burney RE, et al. Rational ordering of serum electrolytes: development of clinical criteria. *Ann Emerg Med* 1987; 15:260–268.

40. Lowe RA, Arst HF, Ellis BK. Rational ordering of electrolytes in the emergency department. *Ann Emerg Med* 1991;20:16–21.

41. Singal BM, Hedges R, Succop PA. Prediction of electrolyte abnormalities in elderly emergency patients. *Ann Emerg Med* 1991;20:964–968.

42. Antman E, Braunwald E. Acute myocardial infarction. In: Braunwald E, ed. *A textbook of cardiovascular medicine.* Philadelphia: WB Saunders, 1998:1202–1204.

43. Aufderheide TP, Gibler WB. Acute ischemic coronary syndromes. In: Rosen P, ed. *Emergency medicine.* St. Louis: Mosby, 1998:1655–1716.

44. Hunt M. Syncope. In: Rosen P, ed. *Emergency medicine.* St. Louis: Mosby, 1998:1570–1582.

45. Barsan WG, Kothari R. Stroke. In: Rosen P, ed. *Emergency medicine.* St. Louis: Mosby, 1998:2184–2198.

46. Mendez MF. Delirium. In: Bradley W, Daroff R, Fenichel G, et al., eds. *Neurology in clinical practice.* Boston: Butterworth-Heinemann 1996:34–36.

47. Smith J. Organic brain syndrome. In: Rosen P, ed. *Emergency medicine.* St. Louis: Mosby, 1998:2132–2150.

48. Pollack CV, Pollack ES. Seizures. In: Rosen P, ed. *Emergency medicine.* St. Louis: Mosby, 1998:2150–2165.

49. Unger R, Foster D. Diabetes mellitus. In: Wilson J, Foster D, Kronenberg H, et al., eds. *Williams textbook of endocrinology.* Philadelphia: WB Saunders, 1998:1010–1012.

50. Cydulka R. Diabetes mellitus and disorders of glucose homeostasis. In: Rosen P, ed. *Emergency medicine.* St. Louis: Mosby, 1998:2456–2478.

51. Silen W. Abdominal pain. In: Braunwald E, Fauci AS, Isselbacher KJ, et al., eds. *Harrison's principles of internal medicine.* New York: McGraw-Hill, 1994:61–64.

52. Guss DA. Disorders of the liver, biliary tract, and pancreas. In: Rosen P, ed. *Emergency medicine.* St. Louis: Mosby, 1998:1981–2005.

53. Greenfield RH, Henneman PL. Disorders of the small intestine. In: Rosen P, ed. *Emergency medicine.* St. Louis: Mosby, 1998:2005–2022.

54. Friedman L, Isselbacher K. Diarrhea and constipation. In: Braunwald E, Fauci A, Hauser S, et al., eds. *Harrison's principles of internal medicine.* New York: McGraw-Hill; 1998:239–241.

55. Guss DA. Disorders of the liver, biliary tract, and pancreas. In: Rosen P, ed. *Emergency medicine.* St. Louis: Mosby, 1998:1981–2005.

56. Lewis TH, Schmidt GA. Acute and chronic hepatic disease. In: Hall JB, Schmidt GA, Wood LDH, eds. *Principles of critical care.* New York: McGraw-Hill, 1998:1253–1268.

57. Runyon BA. Care of patient with ascites. *N Engl J Med* 1994;330: 337–342.

58. Friedman L, Isselbacher K. Nausea, vomiting, and indigestion. In: Braunwald E, Fauci A, Hauser S, et al., eds. *Harrison's principles of internal medicine.* New York: McGraw-Hill, 1998:231–232.

59. Zink BJ. Bone and joint infections. In: Rosen P, ed. *Emergency medicine.* St. Louis: Mosby, 1998:2651–2669.

60. Zukin DD, Grisham JE, Saulys A. Fever in children. In: Rosen P, ed. *Emergency medicine.* St. Louis: Mosby, 1998:1088–1101.

61. Pointer JE, Mulligan-Smith DA. Genital infections. In: Rosen P, ed. *Emergency medicine.* St. Louis: Mosby, 1998:2310–2319.

62. Moran GJ, Talan DA. Pneumonia. In: Rosen P, ed. *Emergency medicine.* St. Louis: Mosby, 1998:1553–1569.

63. Guisto JA, Meislin HW. Soft-tissue infections. In: Rosen P, ed. *Emergency medicine.* St. Louis: Mosby; 1998:2669–2680.

64. Harwood-Nuss AL, Etheredge W, McKenna I. Urologic emergencies. In: Rosen P, ed. *Emergency medicine.* St. Louis: Mosby, 1998: 2227–2261.

65. Hines D, Lisowski J, Bone R. Sepsis. In: Gorbach S, Bartlett J, Blacklow N, eds. *Infectious diseases.* Philadelphia: WB Saunders, 1992: 655–658.

66. Munford RS. Sepsis and septic shock. In: Braunwald E, Fauci A, Hauser S, et al., eds. *Harrison's principles of internal medicine.* New York: McGraw-Hill, 1998:778–779.

67. Brady HR, Brenner BM. Acute renal failure. In: Braunwald E, Fauci A, Hauser S, et al., eds. *Harrison's principles of internal medicine.* New York: McGraw-Hill, 1998:1508–1510.

68. Wolfson AB, Israel RS. Renal function evaluation and the approach to the patient with acute renal failure. In: Rosen P, ed. *Emergency medicine.* St. Louis: Mosby, 1998:2261–2277.

69. Harwood-Nuss AL, Etheredge W, McKenna I. Urologic emergencies. In: Rosen P, ed. *Emergency medicine.* St. Louis: Mosby, 1998: 2227–2261.

70. Abbott JT. Acute complications related to pregnancy. In: Rosen P, ed. *Emergency medicine.* St. Louis: Mosby, 1998:2343–2363.

71. Strek ME, O'Connor M, Hall J. Critical illness in pregnancy. In: Hall JB, Schmidt GA, Wood LDH, eds. *Principles of critical care.* New York: McGraw-Hill, 1998:1571–1593.

72. Feied C. Pulmonary embolism. In: Rosen P, ed. *Emergency medicine.* St. Louis: Mosby, 1998:1770–1805.

73. Seger CL, Murray L. Aspirin, acetaminophen, and nonsteroidal agents. In: Rosen P, ed. *Emergency medicine.* St. Louis: Mosby, 1998: 1250–1263.

74. Nelson L, Hoffman R. Toxic inhalations. In: Rosen P, ed. *Emergency medicine.* St. Louis: Mosby, 1998:1443–1452.

75. Ng SM, Krishnaswamy P, Morissey R, et al. Ninety minute accelerated critical pathway for chest pain evaluation. *Am J Cardiol* 2001; 88:611-617.

76. Cardiology Preeminence Roundtable. *Perfecting MI rule out: best practices for emergency evaluation of chest pain.* Washington, DC: The Advisory Board Company, 1994.

77. Auerbach PS. Impact of point-of-care testing on healthcare delivery. *Clin Chem* 1996;42:2052–2053.

78. Roberts RR, Frutos PW, Ciavarella GG, et al. Distribution of variable vs fixed costs of hospital care. *JAMA* 1999;281:644–649.

79. Gomez MA, Anderson JL, Karagounis LA, et al. An emergency department-based protocol for rapidly ruling out myocardial ischemia reduces hospital time and expense: results of a randomized study (ROMIO). *J Am Coll Cardiol* 1996;28:25–33.

80. Wu AH, Clive JM. Impact of CK-MB testing policies on hospital length of stay and laboratory costs for patients with myocardial infarction or chest pain. *Clin Chem* 1997;43:326–332.

81. Bell WR, et al. Pulmonary thromboembolic disease. *Curr Probl Cardiol* 1985;10:1.

82. Schnonell ME. Failure to differentiate pulmonary infarction from pneumonia by biochemical test. *BMJ* 1966;1:1146.

83. Stein PD, Athanasoulis C, Alavi A, et al. Complications and validity of pulmonary angiography in acute pulmonary embolism. *Circulation* 1992;85:462–468.

84. Ginsberg JS, Wells PS, Kearon C, et al. Sensitivity and specificity of a rapid whole-blood assay for D-dimer in the diagnosis of pulmonary embolism. *Ann Intern Med* 1998;129:1006–1011.

85. Ginsberg JS, Wells PS, Brill-Edwards, et al. Application of a novel and rapid whole blood assay for D-dimer in patients with clinically suspected pulmonary embolism. *Thromb Haemost* 1995;73:35–38.

86. Wells PS, Brill-Edwards P, Panju SP, et al. A novel and rapid whole-blood assay for D-dimer in patients with clinically suspected deep vein thrombosis. *Circulation* 1995;91:2184–2187.

87. Turkstra F, Van Beek EJ, Ten Cate JW, et al. Reliable rapid blood test for the exclusion of venous thromboembolism in symptomatic outpatients. *Thromb Haemost* 1996;76:9–11.

88. Duet M, Benelhadj S, Kedra W, et al. A new quantitative D-dimer assay appropriate in emergency: reliability of the assay for pulmonary embolism exclusion diagnosis. *Thromb Res* 1998;91:1–5.

89. Oger E, Leroyer C, Bressollette L, et al. Evaluation of a new, rapid, and quantitative D-Dimer test in patients with suspected pulmonary embolism. *Am J Respir Crit Care Med* 1998;158:65–70.

90. Wildberger JE, Vorwerk D, Kilbinger M, et al. Bedside testing (SimpliRED) in the diagnosis of deep vein thrombosis. Evaluation of 250 patients. *Invest Radiol* 1998;33:232–235.

91. Farrell S, Hayes T, Shaw M. A negative SimpliRED D-dimer assay result does not exclude the diagnosis of deep vein thrombosis or pulmonary embolus in emergency department patients. *Ann Emerg Med* 2000;35:121–125.

92. Frankel HL, Rozycki GS, Ochsner MG, et al. Minimizing admission laboratory testing in trauma patients: use of a microanalyzer. *J Trauma* 1994;37:728–736.

93. Asimos AW, Gibbs MA, Marx JA, et al. Value of point-of-care blood testing in emergent trauma management. *J Trauma* 2000;48:1101–1108.

94. Herr DM, Newton NC, Santrach PJ, et al. Airborne and rescue point-of-care testing. *Am J Clin Pathol* 1995;104:S54–S58.

95. Broder G, Weil MH. Excess lactate: an index of reversibility of shock in human patients. *Science* 1994;143:1457–1459.

96. Shirey TS. *Stat lactate: the earliest indicator of oxygen deficiency and circulatory shock.* Waltham, MA: NOVA Biomedical, 1991.

97. Milzman D, Boulanger B, Wiles C, et al. Admission lactate predicts fluid requirements for trauma victims during the initial 24 hours. *Crit Care Med* 1994;22:A73.

98. Milzman D, Manning D, Presman D, et al. Rapid lactate can impact outcome prediction for geriatric patients in the emergency department. *Crit Care Med* 1995;23:A32.

99. Slomovitz BM, Lavery RF, Tortella BJ, et al. Validation of a hand-held lactate device in determination of blood lactate in critically injured patients. *Crit Care Med* 1998;26:1523–1528.

100. Jackson RGM, Samra GS, Radcliffe J, et al. Early falls in levels of S100 β in traumatic brain injury. *Clin Chem Lab Med* 2000;38:1165–1167.

101. Gennis P, Gallagher EJ, Andersen F, et al. Cost effectiveness of an accurate and rapid assay for serum human chorionic gonadotropin in suspected ectopic pregnancy. *Am J Emerg Med* 1988;6:4–6.

102. Shier JM, Sly RM, Boeckx RL, et al. Impact of AccuLevel on treatment of acute asthma. *Ann Allergy* 1988;60:523–526.

103. Sporer KA, Khayam-bashi H. Acetaminophen and salicylate serum levels in patients with suicidal ingestion or altered mental status. *Am J Emerg Med* 1996;14:443–446.

104. Sporer KA. Lecture to Stanford-Kaiser emergency medicine residency program. January 1999, Stanford, CA.

105. Office of Applied Studies, Substance Abuse and Mental Health Administration. Rockville, MD:1993.

106. Christopher TA, Zeccardi JA. Evaluation of the Q.E.D. saliva alcohol test: a new rapid accurate device for measuring ethanol in saliva. *Ann Emerg Med* 1992;21:1135–1137.

107. Brandenburg MA, Dire DJ. Comparison of arterial and venous blood gas values in the initial emergency department evaluation of patients with diabetic ketoacidosis. *Ann Emerg Med* 1998;31:459–465.

108. Heart and Stroke Statistical Update 2002. American Heart Association, Dallas, Texas 2001.

109. Selker HP. Coronary care unit triage decision aids: how do we know when they work? *Am J Med* 1989;87:491–493.

110. Weingarten SR, Riedinger MS, Conner L, et al. Practice guidelines and reminders to reduce duration of hospital stay for patients with chest pain: an interventional trial. *Ann Intern Med* 1994;120:257–263.

111. Weingarten SR, Ermann B, Riedinger MS, et al. Selecting the best triage rule for patients hospitalized with chest pain. *Am J Med* 1989;87:494–500.

112. Lee TH, Juarez G, Cook EF, et al. Ruling out acute myocardial infarction: a prospective multicenter validation of a 12-hour strategy for patients at low risk. *N Engl J Med* 1991;324:1239–1246.

113. Gibler WB, Runyon JP, Levy RC, et al. A rapid diagnostic and treatment center for patients with chest pain in the emergency department. *Ann Emerg Med* 1995;25:1–8.

114. Pope JH, Aufderheide TP, Ruthzaer R, et al. Missed diagnosis of acute cardiac ischemia in the emergency department. *N Engl J Med* 2000;342:1163–1170.

115. McCarthy BD, Beshansky JR, D'Agostino RB, et al. Missed diagnoses of acute myocardial infarction in the emergency department: results from a multicenter study. *Ann Emerg Med* 1993;22:579–582.

116. Lee TH, Cook EF, Weisberg M, et al. Acute chest pain in the emergency room. Identification and examination of low-risk patients. *Arch Intern Med* 1985;145:65–69.

117. Burke V, Onneil B, Gawad Y. Undiagnosed myocardial infarction: liability before and after thrombolytic therapy. *Academic Emergency Medicine* 1996;3:489(abst).

118. Roberts R, Kleiman NS. Earlier diagnosis and treatment of acute myocardial infarction necessitates the need for a 'new diagnostic mind-set.' *Circulation* 1994;89:872–881.

119. Gaspoz JM, Lee TH, Weinstein MC, et al. Cost-effectiveness of a new short-stay unit to "rule out" acute myocardial infarction in low risk patients. *J Am Coll Cardiol* 1994;24:1249–1259.

120. Zalenski RJ, Rydman RJ, Ting S, et al. A national survey of emergency department chest pain centers in the United States. *Am J Cardiol* 1998;81:1305–1309.

121. Graff L, Joseph T, Andelman R, et al. American College of Emergency Physicians information paper: chest pain units in emergency departments—a report from the Short-Term Observation Services Section. *Am J Cardiol* 1995;76:1036–1039.

122. Tatum JL, Jesse RL, Kontos MC, et al. Comprehensive strategy for the evaluation and triage of the chest pain patient. *Ann Emerg Med* 1997;29:116–125.

123. Kirk JD, Diercks DB, Turnipseed SD, et al. Evaluation of chest pain suspicious for acute coronary syndrome: Use of an accelerated diagnostic protocol in a chest pain evaluation unit. *Am J Cardiol* 2000;85:40B–48B.

124. Murata GH. Evaluating chest pain in the emergency department. *West J Med* 1993;159:61–68.

125. Lewis WR, Amsterdam EA. Evaluation of the patient with 'rule out myocardial infarction. *Arch Intern Med* 1996;156:41–45.

126. Lee TH, Rouan GW, Weisberg MC, et al. Sensitivity of routine clinical criteria for diagnosing myocardial infarction within 24 hours of hospitalization. *Ann Intern Med* 1987;106:181–186.

127. Brush JE Jr, Brand DA, Acampora D, et al. Use of the initial ECG to predict in-hospital complications of acute myocardial infarction. *N Engl J Med* 1985;312:137–141.

128. Goldman L, Cook EF, Johnson PA, et al. Prediction of the need for intensive care in patients who come to emergency departments with acute chest pain. *N Engl J Med* 1996;334:1498–1504.

129. Mulley AG, Thibault GE, Hughes RA, et al. The course of patients with suspected myocardial infarction: the identification of low-risk patients for early transfer from intensive care. *N Engl J Med* 1980;302:943–948.

130. Goldman L, Cook EF, Brand DA, et al. A computer protocol to predict myocardial infarction in emergency department patients with chest pain. *N Engl J Med* 1988;318:797–803.

131. Gibler WB, Lewis LM, Erb RE, et al. Early detection of acute myocardial infarction in patients presenting with chest pain and non-diagnostic ECGs: serial CK-MB sampling in the emergency department. *Ann Emerg Med* 1990;19:1359–1366.

132. Hudson MP, Christenson RH, Newby LK, et al. Cardiac markers: point of care testing. *Clin Chim Acta* 1999;284:223–237.

133. Kost GJ, Omand K, Kirk JD. A strategy for the use of cardiac injury markers (troponin I and T, creatine kinase-MB and mass, and myoglobin) in the diagnosis of acute myocardial infarction. *Arch Pathol Lab Med* 1998;122:245–251.

134. Vaidya HC. Myoglobin. *Lab Med* 1992;23:306–310.

135. Tucker JF, Collins RA, Anderson AJ, et al. Value of serial myoglobin levels in the early diagnosis of patients admitted for acute myocardial infarction. *Ann Emerg Med* 1994;24:704–708.

136. Brogan GX, Friedman S, McCuskey C, et al. Evaluation of a new rapid quantitative immunoassay for serum myoglobin versus CK-MB for ruling out myocardial infarction. *Ann Emerg Med* 1994;24:665–671.

137. Kontos MC, Anderson FP, Schmidt KA, et al. Early diagnosis of acute myocardial infarction in patients without ST-segment elevation. *Am J Cardiol* 1999;83:155–158.

138. Kontos MC, Anderson FP, Hanbury CM, et al. Use of the combination of myoglobin and CK-MB mass for the rapid diagnosis of acute myocardial infarction. *Am J Emerg Med* 1997;15:14–19.

139. Brogan GX, Bock JL, Hollander JE, et al. Evaluation of a multiple cardiac marker and electrocardiographic strategy for ruling out acute myocardial infarction in the emergency department. *Acad Emerg Med* 1998;5:464(abst).

140. Storrow AB, Liu T, Gibler WB, et al. Multiple early cardiac serum markers improve the detection of acute myocardial infarction within the first six hours after emergency department presentation. *Acad Emerg Med* 1999;6:445(abst).

141. Mikhail MG, Frederiksen S. The utility of a combined myoglobin and creatine kinase-MB rule-out protocol for acute myocardial infarction in a chest pain center. *Acad Emerg Med* 1998;5:520(abst).

142. Fesmire FM, Percy RF, Bardoner JB, et al. Serial creatine kinase (CK)-MB testing during the emergency department evaluation of chest pain: utility of a 2-hour CK-MB of +1.6 ng/ml. *Am Heart J* 1998;136:237–244.

143. DeWinter RJ, Koster RW, Sturk A, et al. Value of myoglobin, troponin T, and CK-MB$_{mass}$ in ruling out an acute myocardial infarction in the emergency room. *Circulation* 1995;92:3401–3407.

144. Wu AHB, Apple FS, Gibler WB, et al. National Academy of Clinical Biochemistry Standards of Laboratory Practice: recommendations for the use of cardiac markers in coronary artery diseases. *Clin Chem* 1999;45:1104–1121.

145. Hamm CW, Ravkilde J, Gerhardt W, et al. The prognostic value of serum troponin T in unstable angina. *N Engl J Med* 1992;327:146–150.

146. Lindahl B, Venge P, Wallentin L. Relation between troponin T and the risk of subsequent cardiac events in unstable coronary artery disease. *Circulation* 1996;93:1651–1657.

147. Ravkilde J, Nissen H, Horder M, et al. Independent prognostic value of serum creatine kinase isoenzyme MB mass, cardiac troponin T and myosin light chain levels in suspected acute myocardial infarction: analysis of 28 months of follow-up in 196 patients. *J Am Coll Cardiol* 1995;25:574–581.

148. Ohman EM, Armstrong PW, Christenson RH, et al. Cardiac troponin T levels for risk stratification in acute myocardial ischemia. *N Engl J Med* 1996;335:1333–1341.

149. Antman EM, Tanasijevic MJ, Thompson B, et al. Cardiac troponin I levels to predict the risk of mortality in patients with acute coronary syndromes. *N Engl J Med* 1996;335:1342–1349.

150. Polanczyk CA, Lee TH, Cook EFD et al. Cardiac troponin I as a predictor of major cardiac events in emergency department patients with acute chest pain. *J Am Coll Cardiol* 1998;32:8–14.

151. Antman EM, Sacks DB, Rifai N, et al. Time to positivity of a rapid bedside assay for cardiac-specific troponin T predicts prognosis in acute coronary syndromes: a thrombolysis in myocardial (TIMI) IIA substudy. *J Am Coll Cardiol* 1998;31:326–330.

152. Mair J, Artner-Dworzak E, Lechleitner P, et al. Cardiac troponin T for the differential diagnosis of ischemic myocardial damage. *Clin Chem* 1991;37:845–852.

153. Collinson PO, Moseley D, Stubbs PJ, et al. Troponin T for the differentiated diagnosis of ischemic myocardial damage. *Ann Clin Biochem* 1993;30:11–16.

154. Wu AHB, Valdes R, Apple FS, et al. Cardiac troponin T immunoassay for diagnosis of acute myocardial infarction. *Clin Chem* 1994;40:900–907.

155. Hamm CW, Goldmann BU, Heesheen C, et al. Emergency room triage of patients with acute chest pain by means of rapid testing for cardiac troponin T or troponin I. *N Engl J Med* 1997;337:1648–1653.

156. Katus HA, Remppis A. Diagnostic efficiency of troponin T in acute myocardial infarction. *Circulation* 1991;83:902–912.

157. Pettijohn TL, Spiekerman MAS, Watson LE, et al. Usefulness of positive troponin T and negative creatine kinase levels in identifying high-risk patients with unstable angina pectoris. *Am J Cardiol* 1997;80:510–511.

158. Galvani M, Ottani F, Ferrini D. Prognostic influence of elevated values of cardiac troponin I in patients with unstable angina. *Circulation* 1997;95:2053–2059.

159. Thygesen K, Alpert JS. Myocardial infarction redefined—a consensus document of the Joint European Society of Cardiology/American College of Cardiology Committee for the Redefinition of Myocardial Infarction. *J Am Coll Cardiol* 2000;36:959–969.

160. Baxter MS, Brogan GX, Harchelroad FP, et al. Evaluation of a bedside whole-blood rapid troponin T assay in the emergency department: rapid evaluation by assay of cardiac troponin T. REACTT Investigators Study Group. *Acad Emerg Med* 1997;4:1018–1024.

161. Brogan GX, Bock JL, McCuskey CF, et al. Evaluation of cardiac STA-Tus CK-MB/myoglobin device for rapidly ruling out acute myocardial infarction. *Clin Lab Med* 1997;17:655–668.

162. Newby LK, Storrow AB, Gibler WB, et al. Bedside multimarker testing for risk stratification in chest pain units: the chest pain evaluation by CK-MB, myoglobin, and troponin-I (CHECKMATE) study. *Circulation* 2001;103:1832–1837.

163. Lewis WR, Amsterdam EA. Chest pain emergency units. *Current Opinion in Cardiol* 1999;4:321–328.

164. Diercks DB, Storrow AB, Sayre MR, Liu T, Gibler WB. The prognostic effect of graded exercise testing in an emergency department chest pain diagnostic unit. *Am J Cardiol* 2000;86:289–292.

165. Kirk, JD, Turnipseed S, Lewis WR, Amsterdam EA. Evaluation of chest pain in low-risk patients presenting to the emergency department: the role of immediate exercise testing. *Ann Emerg Med* 1998;32:1–7.

166. Lewis WR, Amsterdam EA. Utility and safety of immediate exercise testing of low-risk patients admitted to the hospital for suspected acute myocardial infarction. *Am J Cardiol* 1994;74:987–990.

167. Lewis WR, Amsterdam EA, Turnipseed S, et al. Immediate exercise testing of low risk patients with known coronary artery disease presenting to the emergency department with chest pain. *J Am Coll Cardiol* 1999;33:1843–1847.

168. Amsterdam EA, Kirk JD, Turnipseed SD, et al. Immediate exercise testing for assessment of clinical risk in patients presenting to the emergency department with chest pain: Results in over 1000 patients. *Circulation* 1998;17:I774(abst).

169. Radensky PW, Hilton TC, Fulmer H, et al. Potential cost effectiveness of initial myocardial perfusion imaging for assessment of emergency department patients with chest pain. *Am J Cardiol* 1997;79:595–599.

170. Mace SE. Thallium myocardial scanning in the emergency department evaluation of chest pain. *Am J Emerg Med* 1989;7:321–328.

171. Silverman KJ, Becker LC, Bulkley BH, et al. Value of early thallium-

201 scintigraphy for predicting mortality in patients with acute myocardial infarction. *Circulation* 1980;61:996–1003.

172. Kontos MC, Jesse RL, Schmidt KL, et al. Value of acute rest sestamibi perfusion imaging for evaluation of patients admitted to the emergency department with chest pain. *J Am Coll Cardiol* 1997;30:976–982.

173. Kontos MC, Jesse RL, Anderson FP, et al. Comparison of myocardial perfusion imaging and cardiac troponin I in patients admitted to the emergency department with chest pain. *Circulation* 1999;99:2073–2078.

174. Hauser AM, Gangadharan V, Ramos RG, et al. Sequence of mechanical, electrocardiographic and clinical effects of repeated coronary artery occlusion in human beings: echocardiographic observations during coronary angioplasty. *J Am Coll Cardiol* 1985;5:193–197.

175. Peels CH, Visser CA, Kupper AJ, et al. Usefulness of two-dimensional echocardiography for immediate detection of myocardial ischemia in the emergency room. *Am J Cardiol* 1990;65:687–691.

176. Sabia P, Abbott RD, Afrookteh A, et al. Importance of two-dimensional echocardiographic assessment of left ventricular systolic function in patients presenting to the emergency room with cardiac-related symptoms. *Circulation* 1991;84:1615–1624.

177. Sabia P, Afrookteh A, Touchstone DA, et al. Value of regional wall motion abnormality in the emergency room diagnosis of acute myocardial infarction: a prospective study using two-dimensional echocardiography. *Circulation* 1991;84:185–192.

178. Kontos MC, Arrowood JA, Paulsen WH, et al. Early echocardiography can predict cardiac events in emergency department patients with chest pain. *Ann Emerg Med* 1998;31:550–557.

179. Mohler ER, Ryan T, Segar DS, et al. Clinical utility of troponin T levels and echocardiography in the emergency department. *Am Heart J* 1998;135:253–260.

180. Colon PJ, Guarisco JS, Murgo J, et al. Utility of stress echocardiography in the triage of patients with atypical chest pain from the emergency department. *Am J Cardiol* 1998;2:1282–1284.

181. Kjoller E, Nielsen SL, Carlsen J, et al. Impact of immediate and delayed myocardial scintigraphy on therapeutic decisions in suspected acute myocardial infarction. *Eur Heart J* 1995;16:909–913.

182. Hutsko GM, Jones JB, Danielson L. Using point-of-care testing to speed patient care: one emergency department's experience. *J Emer Nursing* 1995;21:408–412.

183. Price C. Point-of-care testing. *BMJ* 2001;322:1285–1288.

184. Steindel SJ, Howanitz PJ. Physician satisfaction and emergency department laboratory test turnaround time: observations based on College of American Pathologists Q-Probes Studies. *Arch Pathol Lab Med* 2001;125:863–871.

8

ON-SITE AND NEAR-PATIENT TESTING IN THE OPERATING ROOM

GERALD J. KOST
JOAN BULLOCK
GEORGE J. DESPOTIS

OBJECTIVES

The goal of this chapter is to present adaptive systems optimization (1) of point-of-care testing (POCT) in the operating room (OR) setting. Our guiding philosophy centers on accuracy, speed, simplicity, relevancy, and efficacy. The chapter begins with a discussion of practical POCT operations in the OR at the University Hospital, a regional health system hub, level I trauma center that handles more than 10,000 surgical cases per year and referral center of the University of California, Davis, Health System (UCDHS). The first case describes ionized calcium testing and performance mapping from the University Hospital OR. The second case presents on-site hemostasis testing and algorithmic treatment based on POC practices in the OR at Washington University in St. Louis. We conclude with recommendations for future needs of POCT in the OR environment.

POINT-OF-CARE TESTING OPERATIONS

This section describes the practical approach to POCT employed in the primary OR area in the University Hospital of the UCDHS. POCT in the OR started in the 1960s with the local invention of the activated clotting time (ACT) test (2), followed by near-patient satellite laboratory testing for blood gases and pH and then, in the early 1980s, the addition of simultaneous whole-blood biosensor-based analysis of electrolytes and metabolites (3).

Background, Staff, and Facilities

Currently, an authorized team consisting of perfusionists, certified anesthesia technicians, a medical technologist, and physicians performs on-site testing, including the ACT test. The licensed medical technologist performs near-patient testing in a 100-square-foot satellite laboratory located within the main OR area. This near-patient laboratory serves all surgical suites (16 suites), a postanesthesia care unit (22 beds), a preoperative holding area (six beds), a surgery center (four rooms), interventional radiology (two rooms), and obstetrics (two suites). In the absence of the medical technologist and as required by California statutes, certified anesthesia technicians and residents perform near-patient testing under the guidance of licensed physician anesthesiologists, who collaboratively direct POCT in the OR. POCT is part of the general OR disaster plan.

Therapeutic Turnaround Time

The medical technologist carries a pager for immediate response to test orders emanating from any of the OR suites or associated areas. The measurement cycle time for bench-top whole-blood analysis in the near-patient laboratory is about 2 minutes. The time from test ordering to appropriate treatment (TTAT) is less than 5 minutes. During brief periods, response time may approach 10 minutes because of increased testing volume, but direct local control of testing allows OR staff to adjust the order of testing to fulfill critical TTAT priorities. TTAT for bedside testing is less than 2 minutes.

Fast TTAT is maintained by backup consisting of (a) a second whole-blood analyzer in the near-patient OR laboratory, (b) specimen transport via pneumatic tube for whole-blood testing in a nearby satellite laboratory that serves hospital intensive care areas, and (c) delivery via courier to non-OR laboratories. Backup rarely is used, although routine specimens are transported from the recovery area as an expedient. Results reporting is via delivery of hard copy and connectivity to the laboratory information system. Planned computer workstations will display test results in the OR suites. In cardiac rooms, test results will appear in conjunction with overhead display of physiologic data.

Test Clusters

Testing is designed to meet the most critical needs of faculty attendings and surgical procedures and purposefully is limited to just a few analytes. The test menu for whole-blood analysis (4) performed with transportable bench-top instruments includes Na^+, Ca^{2+}, K^+, Cl^-, glucose, lactate, pH, PO_2, O_2 saturation, PCO_2, and hematocrit (by conductivity). Anesthesiologists order tests in various clusters, including full profiles and partial subsets, such as (a) electrolytes, glucose, lactate, and hematocrit; (b) arterial blood gases and pH; (c) venous electrolytes and hematorcrit; and (d) single analytes (e.g., glucose or hematocrit).

A microcentrifuge is used to check for hemolysis in specimens with greatly elevated K$^+$. Rarely, the microcentrifuge is used to perform spun hematocrits. There is potential for measurement artifacts in conductivity-based hematocrit measurements (5,6). An independent instrument will be introduced for on-site measurement of hemoglobin. Patient temperature is recorded. When needed, co-oximetry is performed in the backup satellite laboratory with immediate results reporting to the OR.

If there is no indwelling vascular access line but adequate peripheral vascular flow, adequate temperature, and no interfering factors (see Chapter 6), capillary samples may be used for handheld glucose testing between definitive whole-blood analyzer measurements of glucose in diabetic patients. Nursing staff, who are properly trained and understand the limitations of glucose meters, will perform this type of handheld POCT primarily in the recovery area.

The annual volume of near-patient testing is 10,000 to 12,000 specimens. About 50% are performed on the day shift, 40% on evenings, and 10% on nights. Generally, blood is drawn in a 3-mL heparinized syringe or, when necessary, a 1-mL heparinized syringe, which must be filled adequately. Whole-blood analysis is performed immediately. Research staff from the Point-of-Care Testing Center for Teaching and Research (POCT.CTR, www.poctctr.ucdavis.edu) and OR staff perform collaborative studies of new tests, instruments, and POC strategies in the OR (7).

Perfusionists monitor venous and arterial O$_2$ saturation and hematocrit, calibrated to baseline whole-blood analyzer measurements *in vitro*. Various *ex vivo* and *in vivo* monitoring devices, such as pulse oximetry, catheter-based recording, transesophageal echo (cardiac function), and *in vivo* probes (e.g., Paratrend, Agilent Technologies, Palo Alto, CA, U.S.A.), are used on a case-by-case and research basis. Tests not performed directly in the OR are performed in the clinical laboratory and may be moved on site (e.g., POC platelet count and function) (8–13). The availability of POCT in the OR has decreased the stat testing burden in the clinical laboratory and has improved the efficiency of both testing sites.

Accreditation, Competency, and Quality

In the OR, POCT is included under the Clinical Laboratories Improvement ACT (CLIA) certificate and College of American Pathologists (CAP) accreditation of the clinical laboratory. There have been no deficiencies on recent inspections. All personnel are trained and certified. Initial training is broad and covers topics such as universal precautions, specimen handling (including clots, dilution, and insufficient sample volume), calibration, linearity, software, quality control, corrective actions, documentation, proficiency testing, instrument maintenance (including deproteinization, electrode re-membraning, and line replacement), and technical assistance (on-site and off-site).

Personnel are tested for competency using a written checklist, and are recertified annually, with written documentation of continuing proficiency in POCT operations, instrument skills, and general knowledge, such as medical indications, transfusions, critical values, and drug interference. Scheduled retraining workshops and written protocols are used for positive reinforcement of skills. There is separate computer training and annual training in instrument troubleshooting. Only validated operators perform POCT in the OR.

Quality control testing is performed three times daily and includes (a) three levels of control for blood gases, electrolytes, and glucose; (b) a high-level (> 500 mg/dL) glucose control; (c) two levels of control for O$_2$ saturation and hematocrit; and (d) hematocrit controls on an as-needed basis when heparinized capillary hematocrits are performed. Operators log on using individual passwords. Quality control results are reviewed periodically and independently by a clinical laboratory supervisor to maintain objectivity and validity of the performance improvement program.

The OR near-patient laboratory subscribes to the CAP critical care/blood gas survey for proficiency testing, which is performed three times per year. OR whole-blood test results are compared quarterly with satellite blood gas laboratory results. As necessary, corrections are made for consistency. Hematocrit results also are verified internally. Instruments are interfaced with the laboratory information system. Critical values are flagged and reported immediately. OR staff manages the quality of patient monitoring equipment according to vendor specifications for clinical and investigational use.

Leadership and Mission

The OR laboratory supervisor, a medical technologist, is the POCT coordinator who reviews patient test and quality control results daily. Test results, along with billing codes, are verified for submission to medical records. A daily printout of testing is created for permanent nonvolatile archiving. When not performing POCT, the supervisor performs other oversight tasks, such as linearity studies, new control lot evaluations, preparation of educational resources, personnel training, continuing education, proficiency testing, accreditation self-inspections, budgetary management, supplies procurement, new test development, and creation or revision of procedures.

The most important leadership function of the supervisor is to ensure that fast and accurate test results are available for critical informed decisions that improve patient outcomes, particularly for prevention of surgical blood loss and maintenance of appropriate oxygenation and acid–base balance. Thus, the supervisor provides essential team coordination for responsive patient care. High-priority conditions for outcomes management and optimization include organ transplantation, cardiopulmonary bypass, massive trauma, vascular procedures, and other critical challenges.

SYSTEMS OPTIMIZATION

Table 8.1 presents a general toolbox of useful strategies for POCT in the OR. This section presents two specific examples of adaptive systems optimization for POCT in this setting.

TABLE 8.1. ADAPTIVE SYSTEMS OPTIMIZATION FOR POCT IN THE OR

Continuity of coverage for surgical suites, recovery, and preoperative and postoperative areas

Optimal therapeutic turnaround time (≤5 min), decision-making, and intervention

Continuous testing services as necessary 24 h/day and 7 days/wk

Availability of instrument backup and trained backup staff to minimize external failures

Consistency of specimens, analysis, and processing with POCT sites elsewhere

Conjoint method development, test implementation, and monitoring design

Appropriate and complete analytes, test clusters, and calculated parameters

Compatibility of *in vitro, ex vivo,* and *in vivo* testing modalities

Continuous monitoring synchronized with physiological observations

Physiological systems optimization through adequate immediate POCT information

Adaptation for premature infants, neonates, and complex patients with special needs

Coverage for extracorporeal circulation and special procedures (e.g., ECMO)

Anticipation of massive transfusion and its adverse effects on analyte measurements

Connectivity with computerized databases and visual display of test results

Capture of bedside test results in the patient's medical electronic record

Biohazard containment and disaster preparedness

Cohesive education, certification, and performance improvement

Strict fulfillment of legal, accreditation, and security requirements

Integrated trauma, surgery, and anesthesia strategies (e.g., algorithms and care paths)

Strong team leadership for synthesis of multifaceted POCT requirements

Collaborative optimization of temporal, fiscal, and medical resources

POCT, point-of-care testing; OR, operating room; ECMO, extracorporeal membrane oxygenation.

Example I: Ionized Calcium and Performance Mapping

Systems optimization represents an opportunity to improve outcomes in the OR. Calcium circulates in the blood in three primary forms: 42% to 47% protein bound, 46% to 52% free ("ionized"), and 4% to 8% chelated by small ligands such as lactate (3,4). Ionized calcium (Ca^{2+}) is the physiologically relevant fraction. Ca^{2+} is (a) critical for proper function of the heart, brain, and other organs; (b) important in myocardial contraction and conduction, in the maintenance of vascular smooth muscle tone, and in the normal function of metabolic systems; and (c) an essential intracellular messenger and biochemical modulator that can activate both beneficial and harmful processes.

During massive transfusion, citrate in transfused blood products binds Ca^{2+} and may elevate total calcium levels (3,4) (Fig. 8.1). Hence, total calcium may not correlate with Ca^{2+} levels or their rate of change, and only Ca^{2+} is meaningful for acute patient management. Direct whole-blood analysis of Ca^{2+} at the point of care achieves a TTAT of 5 minutes for rapid decision cycles needed to optimize therapy. In the early 1980s, this logic motivated placement of whole-blood analyzers in the OR at heart and liver transplant centers (14), including our own,

where early in the history of the POCT paradigm shift, key analytes such as K^+, Na^+, Ca^{2+}, glucose, hematocrit (or hemoglobin), blood gases, and pH were provided on site.

Whole-blood analysis and POCT contributed to the discovery of the clinical pathophysiology of Ca^{2+} and to the characterization of therapeutic levels and critical limits (15–21). Figure 8.2 presents a diagnostic-therapeutic (Dx-Rx) pattern for Ca^{2+} and illustrates clinical thresholds, pathophysiology events, treatment levels, critical limits, and the normal reference interval. There are significant risks if calcium treatment is given when not indicated. Additionally, severe ionized hypocalcemia may be associated with cardiac arrest that becomes refractory to resuscitation despite the restoration of Ca^{2+} levels to normal (3).

The explanation of the Dx-Rx pattern (Fig. 8.2) that follows starts at the top and works down the cascade of Ca^{2+} levels shown by the solid bars. Sanchez and colleagues (22) observed that Ca^{2+} levels of acutely ill children in the pediatric intensive care unit averaged 1.11 mmol per liter. Broner and colleagues (23) found that Ca^{2+} levels averaged 1.05 mmol per liter in nonsurviving critically ill pediatric patients, 46.2% of whom had ionized hypocalcemia. Cardenas-Rivero and co-workers (24) found that Ca^{2+} levels ranged from 0.88 to 1.04 mmol per liter in septic children and that mortality was 31% in those with ionized hypocalcemia.

Desai and colleagues (25) observed Ca^{2+} levels averaging 1.04 mmol per liter among critically ill medical intensive care unit adult patients with sepsis, cardiogenic shock, or cardiopulmonary arrest. Ca^{2+} levels were significantly lower in hypotensive patients than in normotensive patients (26). Lind and Carlstedt and their co-workers (27,28) found a mean Ca^{2+} level of 1.03 mmol per liter in septic patients during the first day in intensive care. Ca^{2+} and parathyroid hormone (PTH) levels were uncoupled at admission, possibly as a result of elevated cytokines, and were related to the inflammatory response, procalcitonin, and severity of disease. At the fourth day, Ca^{2+} levels were significantly lower in nonsurvivors than in survivors.

Taylor et al. (29) found that levels of Ca^{2+} in adult intensive care unit patients with sepsis averaged 0.91 mmol per liter. Zaloga and Chernow (30) reported a mortality rate of 50% for adult patients with the combination of sepsis and ionized hypocalcemia, with Ca^{2+} levels averaging 0.88 mmol per liter. Woo and colleagues (31) observed 100% mortality rates in adult patients with septic shock and levels of Ca^{2+} below 0.8 mmol per liter. In sepsis, both the total calcium and Ca^{2+} levels may be depressed, the latter disproportionately and unpredictably. The mortality rate was 71% in massively transfused adult patients with Ca^{2+} levels less than 0.70 mmol per liter (32).

In critical illness, ionized hypocalcemia is multifactorial and may result from hypomagnesemia, elevated circulating cytokines, transient hypoparathyroidism, vitamin D deficiency (poor absorption or activation), resistance to PTH or vitamin D, calcium binding, chelation, or cellular redistribution and sequestration. When the level of Ca^{2+} decreases below 1.0 mmol per liter, neurologic and cardiovascular signs, including dysrhythmias and hypotension, appear (3,33), as shown under "Pathophysiology" in Figure 8.2. Cardiac arrest has been reported when values of 0.47 to 0.60 mmol per liter occur, although the rate of change and clinical circumstances can produce fatal outcomes at other

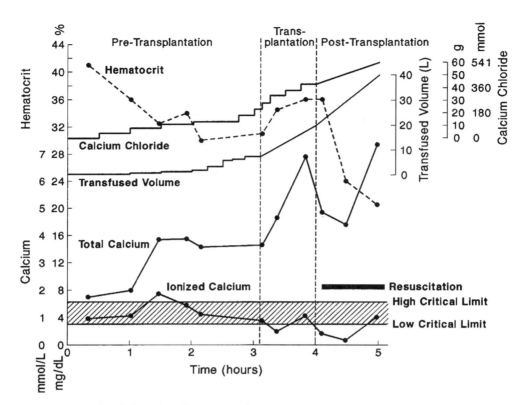

FIGURE 8.1. Rationale for point-of-care testing (POCT) in the operating room (OR): liver transplant case example. Changes in ionized calcium (Ca^{2+}) versus total calcium during massive transfusion illustrate the lack of correlation between the two analytes in the presence of chelators such as exogenous citrate from transfused blood products and endogenous small ligands, such as lactate, which accumulate during the anhepatic (transplantation) phase, bind Ca^{2+}, and remove it from the physiologic active pool needed for normal cardiac function. Cardiac function failed during the posttransplantation phase. Ionized calcium mean high and low critical limits (not known at the time of the case in the early 1980s) were based on data from a later U.S. national survey (17). For details of the case, please refer to Kost GJ, Jammal MA, Ward RE, et al. Monitoring of ionized calcium during human hepatic transplantation: critical values and their relevance to cardiac and hemodynamic management. *Am J Clin Pathol* 1986;86:61–70; Kost GJ. New whole blood analyzers and their impact on cardiac and critical care. *Crit Rev Clin Lab Sci* 1993;30:153–202.

levels (3,33,34). A low level of Ca^{2+} is an early predictor of mortality in critically ill surgical patients (35). Hence, frequent monitoring of Ca^{2+} is essential in the OR setting.

Figure 8.2 also shows that the adult (0.82 mmol/L) and pediatric (0.85 mmol/L) mean critical limits for ionized hypocalcemia correspond well to the critical clinical phenomena and the acute treatment thresholds. Therefore, the critical limits, which are from a 1992 national survey of United States medical centers and children's hospitals (17), represent sound thresholds for emergency notification of clinicians. A Ca^{2+} threshold level of 0.70 mmol per liter is a reasonable level at which to consider initiating calcium repletion in acutely ill patients with symptoms or signs of ionized hypocalcemia, especially low cardiac output and hypotension refractory to volume replacement or catecholamines (36).

Treatment of ionized hypocalcemia may not be beneficial in sepsis, however, where low Ca^{2+} possibly is a protective mechanism that limits injury from cellular overload and mitochondrial damage during the acute inflammatory response (37). Calcium treatment typically is not necessary when the Ca^{2+} level is 0.80 mmol per liter or higher (38), although a more conservative threshold may be necessary for the unconscious patient, in whom

anesthesia obscures symptoms and signs such as spasms (muscles, airways), tetany, and psychiatric impairment (3). Hence, frequent measurement of Ca^{2+} levels must be combined with careful observation of the patient's status, and treatment must be tempered in the presence of sepsis or potential sepsis.

Figure 8.3 illustrates a performance map for Ca^{2+} in a feedback system for patient monitoring. The goals of POCT systems optimization for Ca^{2+} in the OR are (a) to establish a feedback system with a rapid process cycle time; (b) to provide adequate physiologic information for fast diagnosis and therapy; (c) to conserve patient blood volume and scarce resources; and (d) to detect abnormalities in other important contextual analytes, such as potassium, that may change unexpectedly during surgical and transplant procedures. POCT provides rapid Ca^{2+} results for medial decision-making. Direct whole-blood measurements eliminate the need for total calcium measurement. Simultaneously, whole-blood cluster analysis facilitates temporal and Dx-Rx process optimization.

The "cluster analysis" node in the center of the performance map (Fig. 8.3) could include PTH (27,28,39), lactate, ionized magnesium, calcitonin precursors (40), or possibly other closely

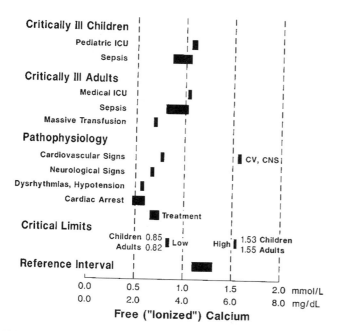

FIGURE 8.2. Diagnostic-therapeutic (Dx-Rx) pattern: the ionized calcium cascade. Clinical outcomes depend on critical pathophysiologic events associated with the cascade of ionized calcium levels. As ionized calcium decreases, morbidity and mortality rates increase. Point-of-care testing (POCT) is fast enough to enable optimization of Dx-Rx processes associated with the correction of ionized hypocalcemia. The treatment threshold is 0.70 to 0.80 mmol per liter. Please see text for details.

related or critical contextual analytes. For example, Johnson and co-authors (41) describe improved medical and economic outcomes resulting from on-site measurement of PTH in the context of parathyroid surgery. Please refer to Chapter 40 and Case Study D for additional information. Knowledge of trends in lac-

tate, which may bind Ca^{2+}, is useful in maintaining hemodynamic stability during extracorporeal membrane oxygenation (42–44). Confounding simultaneous abnormalities in ionized magnesium may contribute to coronary or cerebral vasospasm. The adaptive systems optimization approach integrates analyte measurements and synthesizes outcomes events in Dx-Rx patterns for cost-effective care.

By increasing knowledge of pathophysiologic events, POCT accelerates diagnosis and treatment, but completely optimized adaptive systems are not yet commonly available in OR settings. Like the migration of Ca^{2+} whole-blood analysis, other cluster tests will shift to the point of care. Simultaneous measurements, minimum TTAT, and cluster analysis facilitate a principle-centered approach that (a) integrates the Ca^{2+}-PTH physiologic feedback system into patient-specific Dx-Rx process optimization; (b) links process and temporal optimization; (c) prognosticates the severity of illness and survival in critically ill patients (35); and (d) maximizes the efficiency and efficacy of critical therapy, especially for maintenance of optimal cardiac function, whether or not the patient has heart disease (3). Therefore, adaptive systems optimization for Ca^{2+} and, by analogy, for other contextual analytes will help to reduce morbidity and mortality in the OR.

Example II: On-Site Hemostasis Testing and Algorithmic Treatment

The second example of adaptive systems optimization illustrates how POCT can be integrated with treatment algorithms to improve intermediate outcomes. The clinical problem is management of excessive bleeding in the setting of cardiac surgery. To understand the relative importance of optimizing management strategies for potentially life-threatening bleeding, the complex nature of this problem and setting need to be

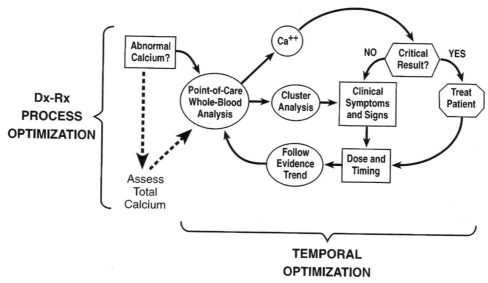

FIGURE 8.3. Ionized calcium performance map. This map is used in conjunction with the diagnostic-therapeutic pattern shown in Figure 8.2.

described. Therefore, we present a brief overview of this clinical problem and the pathophysiology of hemostatic system derangement related to this setting (45–177).

Patients undergoing cardiac surgery with cardiopulmonary bypass (CPB) are at risk for microvascular bleeding. The frequency of excessive bleeding with CPB can vary based on the definition used. For instance, 5% to 7% of patients have more than 2 L of blood loss within the first postoperative day (45), whereas 3.6% (46) to 4.2% (47) will require reexploration either to correct a potential surgical source of excessive bleeding or to evacuate a hemodynamically compromising accumulation of blood. The vast majority of these patients require red cell and hemostatic transfusion support. When patients undergo reoperation for excessive bleeding, more than 50% bleed secondary to various acquired hemostatic defects (discussed later) (48,49), whereas the remaining patients exhibit surgical sources for bleeding (46,47).

Excessive bleeding can result in one or more negative outcomes. Two large studies demonstrated that reexploration can be associated with a variety of negative outcomes, such as increased mortality, renal failure, sepsis, atrial arrhythmias, prolonged requirement for mechanical ventilatory support, and longer length of stay (46,47). Transfusion of allogenic blood or blood components is potentially associated with a number of adverse events, such as blood-borne disease transmission, increased incidence of wound infections, hemolytic and nonhemolytic transfusion reactions, increased mortality (47,50–53), and increased operative time (54) as well as increased cost. Based on a national annual frequency of 500,000 adult cardiac surgical procedures per year, an average cost of $250 per unit of blood, and an average transfusion rate of four units per patient (3.9 ± 5.9 U per patient) (45), costs related to red cell and non–red cell transfusions approximate $500 million annually.

Although preexisting hemostatic abnormalities occasionally cause excessive perioperative bleeding, more often exposure of blood to the extracorporeal circuit leads to impairment of the hemostatic system and excessive bleeding (49,54,55). Significant hemodilution related to the administration of crystalloid or colloid solution (e.g., CPB prime or cardioplegia), as well as to loss of platelets or coagulation factors via excessive use of cell salvage systems (45) may in part account for the decline of coagulation factors and platelets demonstrated with CPB (54,56).

Additionally, activation results from stimulation of both intrinsic (57) and extrinsic (58,59) pathways when blood interfaces with extracorporeal and pericardial surfaces as well as from the negative pressure of cardiotomy suction. This activation results in generation of thrombin (58,60–63) and excessive fibrinolysis (64–70), which can lead to consumption of platelets and labile coagulation factors (61,62,71), even in the presence of standard high-dose heparin-induced anticoagulation. Elastase release from polymorphonuclear leukocytes (72,73), tumor necrosis factor (74,75), complement activation (76–82), or white cell–platelet interactions (83–85) may impair hemostasis.

Whereas therapeutic heparin during bypass preserves the hemostatic system (71,86), residual heparin after protamine reversal can inhibit coagulation (predominantly factors Xa and IIa) (87) and platelet function (88,89). Heparin rebound can occur postoperatively and is secondary to release of heparin from

one of several heparin-binding sites (e.g., endothelial cells, histidine-rich glycoprotein) and may be precipitated by transfusion of plasma. Similarly, excess protamine can inhibit coagulation (90) and affect platelet function (91–93). In fact, several studies demonstrated improved bleeding or transfusion outcomes when protamine doses were reduced by approximately 50% or greater and when the protamine to total heparin ratio was reduced below 1 (94–97). Finally, systemic hypothermia used for myocardial and central nervous system protection also may increase perioperative blood loss (45), possibly related to its effect on platelet function (55,98,99) or to inhibition of temperature-dependent enzymatic steps within the coagulation cascade (48,68,100).

Excessive bleeding may be related to one or more of several acquired hemostatic defects (Table 8.2) (48,49). Excluding patients with incomplete surgical hemostasis (47), patients bleed excessively because of various acquired hemostatic defects, such as reductions in platelet number, size, and mass, acquired platelet dysfunction, reduction in plasma clotting factors, increased fibrinolytic activity, and inadequate heparin neutralization or excessive protamine (Table 8.2). Platelet-related abnormalities now are considered to be the most important defect in hemostasis in the early postoperative period following the use of extracorporeal circulation (49,55,101–104). Use of new platelet inhibitors for acute coronary syndromes may be associated with hemorrhagic complications in patients who subsequently undergo cardiac surgical procedures (105,106). These agents may be beneficial, however, if they reduce the incidence of urgent revascularization procedures or myocardial infarction (107,108), or are short acting and preserve platelets during CPB (109).

Plasma coagulation factors have been observed to decrease during and after CPB (54,56,64,110–113), with factors V and VIII being reduced to the greatest extent (54,56,111,113–115). During CPB, von Willebrand factor (vWF) levels generally decrease, whereas after CPB the plasma concentration of vWF may increase, characteristic of the acute-phase reactant nature of this molecule. A recent study indicates that reductions in factor XIII during cardiac surgery may be more important than once thought, based on an inverse relationship between blood loss and factor XIII levels (110). Decreases in fibrinogen levels during CPB generally remain within the normal range during CPB

TABLE 8.2. HEMOSTATIC ABNORMALITIES ASSOCIATED WITH CARDIAC SURGERY INVOLVING EXTRACORPOREAL CIRCULATION

Decreased or denatured coagulation factors
Decreased physiologic inhibitors (ATIII, protein C, protein S)
Decreased fibrinolysis inhibitors (PAI1, α–2 antiplasmin)
Disseminated intravascular coagulation (i.e., excessive thrombin activity)
Primary fibrinolysis
Platelet related:
    Thrombocytopenia
    Platelet activation, desensitization, or dysfunction
Hypothermia-related effects
Heparin-related
Protamine-related

ATIII, antithrombin III; PAI1, plasminogen activator inhibitor 1.

(54,113,114,116,117). On occasion, however, they can decrease substantially (71,115) secondary to hemodilution (49), disseminated intravascular coagulation, or excessive fibrinolysis. Increased fibrinolytic activity accompanying CPB (64,101) may be due either to increased activation of plasminogen via tissue plasminogen activator or to a decreased level of plasmin inhibitors such as type 1 plasminogen activator inhibitor (PAI-1) (118), in part related to hemodilution. Excessive fibrinolysis may occur in certain patients (119) and can lead to both fibrinogen depletion and elevated fibrinogen/fibrin split products, which may interfere with platelet function. Finally, excessive mediastinal fibrinolytic activity may result in excessive bleeding (120). This is supported by two studies that demonstrated reduced chest tube drainage when aprotinin has been topically applied to the heart, mediastinum, and pericardium (121,122).

Blood component administration in patients with excessive bleeding after CPB and heparin neutralization is generally empiric. Thus, transfusion of packed red blood cells (RBC), platelets, and fresh frozen plasma (FFP) to cardiac surgical patients requiring CPB varies considerably among institutions, in part as a result of prophylactic administration of FFP and platelets (123–126), despite evidence that this practice is unwarranted (116,127). This variability has been attributed to the empiric use of blood components such as FFP and platelets, which are administered in an attempt to distinguish between excessive microvascular bleeding resulting from hemostatic system impairment or surgical bleeding (128,129). Neither approach appears to be an appropriate strategy for patient management. Although a panel of laboratory-based screening tests may be useful in the differential diagnosis of intraoperative disorders of hemostasis (130), the clinical utility of laboratory tests is often limited by long TTAT (1,131). Waiting for laboratory coagulation results can potentially prolong operative time and increase blood loss. Prolonged TTAT has lead many investigators to study the role of POC coagulation tests in this setting with respect to optimizing management of the bleeding patient.

Despotis and colleagues (54,132–134) studied adult patients undergoing cardiac procedures with CPB. Subjects were selected from a large series of eligible patients (n = 362) if they had evidence of microvascular bleeding; patients were divided into two groups. A standard therapy group (n = 30 patients) supported with conventional laboratory testing was compared with an algorithmic treatment group (n = 36 patients) supported with on-site hemostasis testing. An algorithm was used to guide therapy and to divert unwarranted transfusions. Platelet count, prothrombin time (PT), and activated partial thromboplastin time (aPTT) pivoted decision pathways in the algorithmic sequence leading to treatment. The algorithm can be found in references 54 and 132, and, as modified, in references 135, 136, and 177, which also describe specific POCT instruments and methods. Table 8.3 provides a general list of devices used to assess nonplatelet hemostatic abnormalities. Despotis and colleagues (54) stated that "use of an on-site laboratory facilitated timely treatment of microvascular bleeding with specific hemostatic therapy."

It seems obvious that hemostatic transfusion should be initiated (a) if a clinical bleeding problem is present (e.g., excessive bleeding at the surgical site after protamine without an identifi-

TABLE 8.3. POINT-OF-CARE TESTS/INSTRUMENTS USED TO ASSESS NONPLATELET HEMOSTATIC ABNORMALITIES ASSOCIATED WITH CARDIAC SURGERY

Unneutralized heparin or heparin-rebound
  ACT-based tests
    Celite or kaolin ACT (Hemochron series instruments)
    Kaolin ACT heparinase test cartridge (ACT II or Hepcon instruments)
    SonACT (Sonoclot instrument)
    ICHOR ACT
  Non-ACT tests
    Heparin management test (HMT: TAS system)
    Whole-blood heparin concentration
      Theracon cartridge (Hepcon instrument)
      Synthetic fluorogenic substrate test (PROTOPATH system)
    Thrombin time/ heparin neutralized thrombin time (Hemochron series instruments)
    Heptest anti-IIa/Xa activity
Coagulation factor levels
  Whole-blood PT/aPTT instruments
    CoaguChek Plus and Pro DM
    ACT II, Hepcon
    Hemochron series
    Thrombolytic assessment system (TAS)
    MCA 210 (automated plasma-based PT/aPTT using whole blood)
  Fibrinogen concentration instruments
    Hemochron or Hemochron Jr.
    MCA 210
    TAS system
Fibrinolysis
  Thromboelastography (MA/M60 ratio)
  TAS system
  The SimpliRED D-dimer test

ACT, activated coagulation time; HMT, heparin management test; TAS, thrombolytic assessment system; PT, prothrombin time; aPTT, activated partial thromboplastin time; MCA, microsample coagulation analyzer. Notes: 1. Check with FDA and manufacturer for status of test approval and for recent modifications. 2. See also Chapter 6.

able surgical source or excessive postoperative chest tube drainage such as more than 100—200 mL/hour); or (b) when indicated by evidence of significant test abnormalities to prevent adverse outcomes (e.g., to decrease the risk of spontaneous intracranial hemorrhage in the cardiac surgery patient or to reduce postoperative bleeding/transfusion when using a test that has been shown to identify accurately patients with excessive bleeding). In a study of 47 consecutive patients (46 men, 1 woman) undergoing coronary artery bypass grafting with CPB, Gelb and associates (113) found that bleeding did not correlate with changes in routine coagulation parameters during and following surgery and advised that laboratory measurements "should not be used in isolation to guide the use of blood components."

These findings support the notion that platelet-related abnormalities and possibly technical factors, which were not assessed in this study, are the most likely causes of excessive bleeding after cardiac surgery. The observations of Gelb's group also are supported by several studies that have demonstrated that routine coagulation tests (PT, aPTT, and platelet count) have not been able to identify consistently patients with excessive blood loss after cardiac surgery (137–141). In contrast to the study of Gelb and co-workers, which did not utilize on-site testing or algorithm-based management, Despotis and colleagues combined on-site testing and algorithmic treatment to promote evidence-based patient care in the OR, as described in several publications (54,132–136,177).

On-site testing with algorithmic treatment (54,132) yielded statistically significant improvements in intermediate outcomes. Figure 8.4 shows reduced use of FFP, platelet, and RBC transfusions. Microvascular bleeding decreased from 326 to 158 mL, despite the more efficient use of blood products. Operative time decreased from 108 to 69 minutes. On-site testing provided a consistent TTAT of 4 minutes with a 95th percentile of only 6 minutes. In contrast, the response time for the standard laboratory approach averaged 44 minutes with a 90th percentile of 77 minutes. Although not statistically significant, there was a trend toward fewer reexplorations in the algorithmic treatment group (54). In this trial, use of POC diagnostics enabled physicians to differentiate microvascular bleeding from surgical bleeding and to change initial therapy in a substantial fraction of patients.

A transfusion algorithm alone will generally streamline blood product utilization. Nonetheless, on-site testing plus algorithmic treatment significantly improved intermediate outcomes, decreased blood donor exposures (132), and generated a financial savings of $1,504 per patient (133). According to Despotis and colleagues (136), identification of specific hemostasis defects optimizes transfusion- and pharmacologic-based therapy in patients with nonsurgical coagulaopathic bleeding, whereas identification of patients with surgical sources of bleeding is expedited when coagulation test results are relatively normal in the presence of excessive bleeding. Nuttall and colleagues (142) demonstrated that the POCT algorithmic systems approach is successful in reducing nonerythrocyte allogenic transfusion in the OR and blood loss in the intensive care unit.

Point-of-care assessment of heparin levels (for more effective suppression of hemostatic system activation (71,143)) and other test parameters, such as platelet function (Table 8.4), an important area of research, may also be beneficial to outcomes as

TABLE 8.4. POINT-OF-CARE TESTS/INSTRUMENTS USED TO ASSESS PLATELET-RELATED ABNORMALITIES ASSOCIATED WITH CARDIAC SURGERY

Simplate bleeding time
Tests based on response to platelet agonists
  Rapid platelet function assay (RPFA)/Ultegra instrument
    (aggregation of fibrinogen-coated beads)
  Chronolog whole blood aggregometer (electrical impedence)
  PFA-100 or Thrombostat (aperture closure time/flow rate)
  ICHOR (reduction in platelet count)
  HemoSTATUS/Hepcon (PAF-mediated acceleration of clot times
    expressed as clot ratio values)
Viscoelastic tests
  Thromboelastograph
  Sonoclot
  Hemodyne (platelet-mediated force transduction or clot retraction)
Miscellaneous
  Hemostatometry (pressure normalization time)
  Glass bead platelet retention method (degree of platelet retention
    within glass column)
  Flow cytometry (antibody-mediated fluorescence)

Notes: 1. Brief descriptions of the measurement parameters are contained within parentheses.
2. Check with FDA and manufacturer for the status of test approval and for recent modifications.

recently addressed in several studies (71,97,140,142–156). The findings of improved transfusion and bleeding outcomes as related to use of algorithms coupled to POC tests described by Despotis and associates (54,132) and Nuttall's group (142) have been confirmed by other studies. Use of transfusion algorithms based on thromboelastographic and, in some cases, laboratory-based test parameters reduced transfusion requirements and, in some cases, reexploration rates in patients undergoing cardiac surgery (Fig. 8.5) (152–154).

The POCT that assesses platelet function also may be helpful when identifying patients at risk for excessive bleeding who may also benefit from pharmacologic agents such as 1-deamino-8-D-arginine vasopressin (DDAVP). Although the findings of an early randomized study that demonstrated a significant reduction in perioperative blood loss by DDAVP (157) have been supported by several subsequent studies (158–163), several other studies could not confirm these findings (164–169). More recently, studies revealed that certain patient subsets may benefit from desmopressin, such as those requiring prolonged use of CPB (157), patients with excessive postoperative bleeding (e.g. >1,180 mL/24 hours) (170), patients on platelet-inhibiting drugs (158,160,161,171), or patients at high risk for excessive bleeding as identified by tests of hemostatic function (150,163,172). The first study by Czer and colleagues (163) demonstrated that desmopressin is beneficial when administered to patients with excessive bleeding and prolonged bleeding times.

Mongan and Hosking (172) studied the use of the thromboelastograph (TEG) for risk stratification of patients when evaluating post-CPB coagulation status. Hematocrit, platelet counts, PT, aPTT, and fibrinogen measurements were obtained in addition to TEG measurements after neutralization of heparin and discontinuation of bypass. Patients also were randomly assigned to receive either normal saline (placebo) or 0.3 μg of DDAVP per kilogram of body weight. A post-hoc analysis divided the patients into nor-

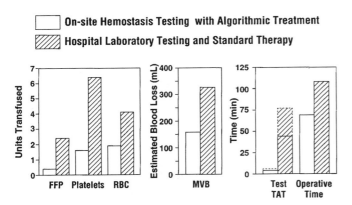

FIGURE 8.4. Effects of point-of-care hemostasis testing on intermediate outcomes. On-site hemostasis testing and a treatment algorithm in the operating room decreased fresh-frozen plasma (FFP), platelet, and red blood cell (RBC) transfusions. Estimated blood loss, turnaround time (TAT), and operative time also decreased. Changes were statistically significant ($p < 0.05$). The dashed lines show the 95th percentile for on-site turnaround time and the 90th percentile for laboratory turnaround time. (Drawn from data published in the study by Despotis GJ, Santoro SA, Spitznagel E, et al. Prospective evaluation and clinical utility of on-site monitoring of coagulation in patients undergoing cardiac operation. *J Thorac Cardiovasc Surg* 1994;107:271–279.)

On-site Hemostasis Testing with Algorithmic Treatment
Hospital Laboratory Testing and Standard Therapy

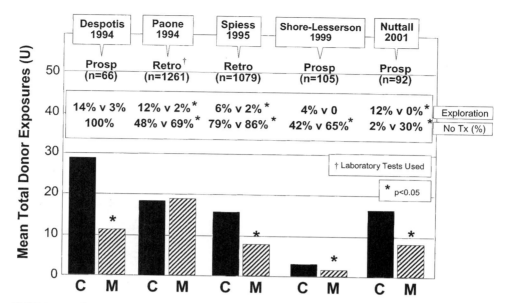

FIGURE 8.5. Effect of algorithm-based management of bleeding on clinical outcomes. The plot compares the results from studies by the groups of Despotis (54), Paone (51), Spiess (152), Shore-Lesserson (153), and Nuttall (142). Clinical outcomes include total donor exposures in units transfused (vertical axis), exploration rates, and the percentage of patients not requiring transfusion. The bars compare control (C) and monitored (M) cohorts in each study; the latter refers to the use of an algorithmic treatment protocol and point-of-care testing (POCT), except Paone and colleagues, who used laboratory-based testing. Prosp, prospective; Retro, retrospective; n, number of patients; U, units; and No Tx, no transfusion. Asterisk indicates significant difference.

mal or abnormal TEG groups based on TEG maximum amplitude (MA) measurements. The mediastinal chest tube drainage in the placebo-treated, abnormal MA (>50 mm) patients was substantially greater compared with normal (< 50 mm) MA patients, indicating that TEG could identify patients at risk for excessive bleeding. Of interest, the blood loss was similar in both DDAVP-treated patients with abnormal TEG values and placebo-treated patients who had normal TEG values. These findings indicate that DDAVP can improve hemostasis in patients who have abnormal TEG and who are at risk for increased blood loss. DDAVP also appeared to be effective in reducing blood loss and blood component administration in the early postoperative period in patients at risk for increased blood loss (TEG:MA <50).

These findings were confirmed in another recent trial that utilized the hemoSTATUS method (150). Two hundred and three patients scheduled for elective cardiac surgical procedures were enrolled in this prospective, double-blinded, placebo-controlled trial. After exclusion of 30 patients who required intraoperative management of microvascular bleeding with hemostatic blood products and 72 patients with normal clot ratio values, 101 patients with abnormal clot ratio values (i.e. % maximal < 60 in channel 5) after administration of protamine were randomly assigned to either placebo (n = 51) or DDAVP (n = 50) treatment arms. Desmopressin-treated patients had a 50% reduction in red cell (1.1 vs. 2.2 U), a 95% reduction in platelet (0.1 vs. 1.9 U), and 87% reduction in FFP (0.1 vs. 0.8 U) units transfused with an overall 69% reduction in total donor exposures (1.6 vs. 5.2 U) compared with patients who received placebo. Compared with placebo-treated patients, patients who received desmopressin also had a 39% (182 vs. 297 mL), 42% (299 vs. 513 mL), and 39%

(624 vs. 1028 mL) reduction in blood loss in the first 4, 8, and 24 postoperative hours, respectively (150). These studies (150,172) indicate that POC platelet function test systems may be useful in the identification of patients at risk for excessive bleeding and who may benefit from administration of pharmacologic agents (e.g., desmopressin) or in directing administration of hemostatic blood products.

Extension, with possible exceptions (173) to other problems in preoperative, postoperative, and intensive care may generate equivalent medical benefits and financial savings. In this second example, systems optimization of hemostasis POCT successfully guided therapeutic management (136,174–177). Important principles identified in this example and other hemostasis POCT studies (97,142,153) include (a) hematology–hemostasis testing performed at the POC enhances management of excessive perioperative bleeding, (b) integration of POCT into a problem-focused treatment algorithm is clinically effective, (c) rapid synthesis of test cluster results and clinical observations is practical and efficient in the OR setting, (d) timely evidence-based decision-making is both efficacious and cost-effective, and (e) optimization of hemostasis Dx-Rx processes improves intermediate outcomes. For additional information about general POC hemostasis testing, see Chapter 10.

CONCLUSIONS AND RECOMMENDATIONS

Adaptive POCT Systems Optimization

With the guidance of the POCT coordinator and well-trained personnel, POCT in the OR delivers prime advantages, such as early detection, correction, prevention, and optimization, which help avoid sublethal and lethal events that cumulatively affect morbidity and mortality rates. POCT would benefit from more complete and better-directed test clusters that assess the status of physiologic control systems and reveal the details of pathophysiologic mechanisms. This higher conceptual level would allow more extensive use of Dx-Rx feedback systems (e.g., Ca^{2+} homeostasis) and treatment algorithms (e.g., hemostasis). POCT instruments should display not only test results but also physiologic states and decision points graphically in flow charts to coordinate vital information at the bedside. *Adaptive POCT systems* solve problems where the goal of POCT is to enhance performance *and* to do it quickly.

Integrative Strategies

Integrative strategies that embed POCT in OR protocols have high probability of success. Fast TTAT and focused test clusters produce efficient and efficacious information, satisfy surgical needs, and spare scarce resources. Collaborative teamwork ensures timely and accurate test results that support evidence-based decisions. Cost effectiveness and improved medical outcomes result from this integrated approach to diagnosis, monitoring, and treatment. Each health system has unique needs. Additional clinical research is necessary to discover how POCT can improve outcomes in the OR environment for other institutions. Clever integration of bedside, near-patient, satellite (178–183), and mobile (184) testing, with dynamic custom tailoring to match local priorities, will fulfill important patient care goals.

Rapid Synthesis

Emerging technologies will shift the spectrum of POCT from *in vitro* testing without blood replacement to *ex vivo* testing with blood replacement and, ultimately, to noninvasive *in vivo* monitoring. Monitoring in the OR facilitates simultaneous biochemical and physiologic observations that keep pace with Dx-Rx processes, sudden changes, and unexpected crises. With a few exceptions, *ex vivo* and invasive and noninvasive *in vivo* monitoring have been slow to overcome hurdles associated with accuracy, precision, calibration, stability, localization, interference, miniaturization, and biocompatibility (185–187). Basic science research is needed to determine practical solutions to the clinical problems facing noninvasive *in vivo* monitoring.

Improved Medical and Economic Outcomes

Not just the results of tests count. Where and how they are performed must be integrated with patient care. Fast TTAT, POCT-driven Dx-Rx patterns, performance maps, and treatment algorithms with on-site testing represent integrated adaptive systems optimization for efficient and efficacious patient care. Transplant, cardiac, and other surgical procedures, with associated transfusion support, rank among the most expensive medical services (188–190). The evidence for cost effectiveness and improved outcomes of POCT in this critical setting is strong. Increasingly, POCT will be of major benefit in the OR in the future.

ACKNOWLEDGMENT

Figures 8.1–8.3 and Table 8.1 concepts used courtesy of Knowledge Optimization, Davis, CA, USA. Tables 8.2–8.4 used with permission from the Society of Thoracic Surgeons (177) and revised. Figure 8.2 revised with permission of the AMA (17).

REFERENCES

1. Kost GJ. The clinical systems manager: optimizing point-of-care testing. *Clinical Laboratory Management Review* 1998;12:353–363.
2. Hattersley PG. Activated coagulation time of whole blood. *JAMA* 1996;196:436–440.
3. Kost GJ, Jammal MA, Ward RE, et al. Monitoring of ionized calcium during human hepatic transplantation: critical values and their relevance to cardiac and hemodynamic management. *Am J Clin Pathol* 1986;86:61–70.
4. Kost GJ. New whole blood analyzers and their impact on cardiac and critical care. *Crit Rev Clin Lab Sci* 1993;30:153–202.
5. McMahon DJ, Carpenter RL. A comparison of conductivity-based hematocrit determinations with conventional laboratory methods in autologous blood transfusions. *Anesth Analg* 1990;71:541–544.
6. Stott RA, Hortin GL, White TR, et al. Analytical artifacts in hematocrit measurements by whole-blood chemistry analyzers. *Clin Chem* 1995;41:306–311.
7. Kost GJ, Vu HT, Inn M, et al. Multicenter study of whole-blood creatinine, total carbon dioxide content, and chemistry profiling for laboratory and point-of-care testing in critical care in the United States. *Crit Care Med* 2000;28:2379–2389.
8. Osende JI, Fuster V, Lev EI, et al. Testing platelet activation with a shear-dependent platelet function test versus aggregation-based tests: relevance for monitoring long-term glycoprotein IIb/IIIa inhibition. *Circulation* 2001;103:1488–1491.
9. Kereiakes DJ. Oral blockade of the platelet glycoprotein IIb/IIIa receptor: fact or fancy? *Am Heart J* 1999;138:S39–46.
10. Berkowitz SD, Frelinger AL, Hillman RS. Progress in point-of-care laboratory testing for assessing platelet function. *Am Heart J* 1998; 136:S51–S65.
11. Carville DGM, Schleckser PA, Guyer KE, et al. Whole blood platelet function assay on the ICHOR point-of-care analyzer. *Journal of Extra-Corporeal Technology* 1998;30:171–177.
12. Harrington RA, Kleiman NS, Granger CB, et al. Relation between inhibition of platelet aggregation and clinical outcomes. *Am Heart J* 1998;136:S43–S50.
13. Rinder HM. Platelet function testing by flow cytometry. *Clin Lab Sci* 1998;11:365–372.
14. Kost GJ, Shirey TL. New whole-blood testing for laboratory support of critical care at cardiac transplant centers and US hospitals. *Arch Pathol Lab Med* 1990;114:865–868.
15. Kost GJ. The challenges of ionized calcium: cardiovascular management and critical limits. *Arch Pathol Lab Med* 1987;111:932–934.
16. Kost GJ. Ionized calcium: cardiac significance, critical limits and clinical challenges. *Clin Chem* 1992;38:926–927.
17. Kost GJ. The significance of ionized calcium in cardiac and critical care: availability and critical limits at US medical centers and children's hospitals. *Arch Pathol Lab Med* 1993;117:890–896.
18. Kost GJ. Critical limits for urgent clinician notification at US medical centers. *JAMA* 1990;263:704–707.
19. Kost GJ. Critical limits for emergency clinician notification at United States children's hospitals. *Pediatrics* 1991;88:597–603.
20. Kost GJ. Using critical limits to improve patient outcome. *Medical Laboratory Observer* 1993;25:22–27.
21. Kost GJ. Designing critical limit systems for knowledge optimization. *Arch Pathol Lab Med* 1996;120:616–618.
22. Sanchez GJ, Venkataraman PS, Pryor RW, et al. Hypercalcitonemia

and hypocalcemia in acutely ill children: studies in serum calcium, blood ionized calcium, and calcium-regulating hormones. *J Pediatr* 1989;114:952–956.

23. Broner CW, Stidham GL, Westenkirchner DF, et al. Hypermagnesemia and hypocalcemia as predictors of high mortality in critically ill pediatric patients. *Crit Care Med* 1990;18:921–928.

24. Cardenas-Rivero N, Chernow B, Stoiko MA, et al. Hypocalcemia in critically ill children. *J Pediatr* 1989;114:946–951.

25. Desai TK, Carlson RW, Geheb MA. Prevalence and clinical implications of hypocalcemia in acutely ill patients in a medical intensive care setting. *Am J Med* 1988;84:209–214.

26. Desai TK, Carlson RW, Thill-Baharozian M, et al. A direct relationship between ionized calcium and arterial pressure among patients in an intensive care unit. *Crit Care Med* 1988;16:578–582.

27. Lind L, Carlstedt F, Rastad J, et al. Hypocalcemia and parathyroid hormone secretion in critically ill patients. *Crit Care Med* 2000;28:93–99.

28. Carlstedt F, Lind L, Rastad J, et al. Parathyroid hormone and ionized calcium levels are related to the severity of illness and survival in critically ill patients. *Eur J Clin Invest* 2001;28:898–903.

29. Taylor B, Sibbald WJ, Edmonds MW, et al. Ionized hypocalcemia in critically ill patients with sepsis. *Can J Surg* 1978;21:429–433.

30. Zaloga GP, Chernow B. The multifactorial basis for hypocalcemia during sepsis: Studies of the parathyroid hormone-vitamin D axis. *Ann Intern Med* 1987;107:36–41.

31. Woo P, Carpenter MA, Trunkey D. Ionized calcium: the effect of septic shock in the human. *J Surg Res* 1979;26:605–610.

32. Wilson RF, Binkley LE, Sabo FM, et al. Electrolyte and acid-base changes with massive blood transfusions. *Am Surg* 1992;58:535–545.

33. Drop LJ. Ionized calcium, the heart, and hemodynamic function. *Anesth Analg* 1985;64:432–451.

34. Urban P, Scheidegger D, Buchmann B, et al. Cardiac arrest and blood ionized calcium levels. *Ann Intern Med* 1988;109:110–113.

35. Burchard KW, Gann DS, Colliton J, et al. Ionized calcium, parathormone, and mortality in critically ill surgical patients. *Ann Surg* 1990; 212:543–550.

36. Zaloga GP. Hypocalcemic crisis. *Crit Care Clin* 1991;7:191–200.

37. Zaloga GP. Ionized calcium during sepsis. *Crit Care Med* 2000;28: 266–268.

38. Zaloga GP. Hypocalcemia in critically ill patients. *Crit Care Med* 1992;20:251–262.

39. Carlstedt F, Lind L, Wide L, et al. Serum levels of parathyroid hormone are related to mortality and severity of illness in patients in the emergency department. *Eur J Clin Invest* 1997;27:977–981.

40. Muller B, Becker KL, Kranzlin M, et al. Disordered calcium homeostasis of sepsis: association with calcitonin precursors. *Eur J Clin Invest* 2000;30:823–831.

41. Johnson LR, Doherty G, Lairmore T, et al. Evaluation of the performance and clinical impact of a rapid intraoperative parathyroid hormone assay in conjunction with preoperative imaging and concise parathyroidectomy. *Clin Chem* 2001;47:919–925.

42. Meliones JN, Moler FW, Custer JR, et al. Normalization of priming solution ionized calcium concentration improves hemodynamic stability of neonates receiving venovenous ECMO. *ASAIO J* 1995;41:884–888.

43. Toffaletti J, Hansell D. Interpretation of blood lactate measurements in paediatric open-heart surgery and in extracorporeal membrane oxygenation. *Scand J Clin Lab Invest* 1995;55:301–307.

44. Toffaletti J. Elevations in blood lactate: overview of use in critical care. *Scand J Clin Lab Invest* 1996;224(Suppl):107–110.

45. Despotis GJ, Filos KS, Zoys TN, et al. Factors associated with excessive postoperative blood loss and hemostatic transfusion requirements: a multivariate analysis in cardiac surgical patients. *Anesth Analg* 1996;82:13–21.

46. Dacey LJ, Munoz JJ, Baribeau YR, et al. Reexploration for hemorrhage following coronary artery bypass grafting: incidence and risk factors: Northern New England Cardiovascular Disease Study Group. *Arch Surg* 1998;133:442–447.

47. Moulton MJ, Creswell LL, Mackey ME, et al. Reexploration for bleeding is a risk factor for adverse outcomes after cardiac operations. *J Thorac Cardiovasc Surg* 1996;111:1037–1046.

48. Valeri CR, Khabbaz K, Khuri SF, et al. Effect of skin temperature on

platelet function in patients undergoing extracorporeal bypass. *J Thorac Cardiovasc Surg* 1992;104:108–116.

49. Woodman RC, Harker LA. Bleeding complications associated with cardiopulmonary bypass. *Blood* 1990;76:1680–1697.

50. Gravlee GP, Haddon WS, Rothberger HK, et al. Heparin dosing and monitoring for cardiopulmonary bypass. a comparison of techniques with measurement of subclinical plasma coagulation. *J Thorac Cardiovasc Surg* 1990;99:518–527.

51. Paone G, Spencer T, Silverman NA. Blood conservation in coronary artery surgery. *Surgery* 1994;116:672–677.

52. van de Watering LM, Hermans J, Houbiers JG, et al. Beneficial effects of leukocyte depletion of transfused blood on postoperative complications in patients undergoing cardiac surgery: a randomized clinical trial. *Circulation* 1998;97:562–568.

53. Goodnough LT, Brecher MG, Kanter MH, et al. Medical progress: transfusion medicine–blood transfusion. *N Engl J Med* 1999;340: 438–447.

54. Despotis GJ, Santoro SA, Spitznagel E, et al. Prospective evaluation and clinical utility of on-site monitoring of coagulation in patients undergoing cardiac operation. *J Thorac Cardiovasc Surg* 1994;107:271–279.

55. Khuri SF, Wolfe JA, Josa M, et al. Hematologic changes during and after cardiopulmonary bypass and their relationship to the bleeding time and nonsurgical blood loss. *J Thorac Cardiovasc Surg* 1992;104:94–107.

56. Kalter RD, Saul CM, Wetstein L, et al. Cardiopulmonary bypass: associated hemostatic abnormalities. *J Thorac Cardiovasc Surg* 1979; 77:427–435.

57. Heimark RL, Kurachi K, Fujikawa K, et al. Surface activation of blood coagulation, fibrinolysis and kinin formation. *Nature* 1980; 286:456–460.

58. Boisclair MD, Lane DA, Philippou H, et al. Mechanisms of thrombin generation during surgery and cardiopulmonary bypass. *Blood* 1993;82:3350–3357.

59. de Haan J, Boonstra PW, Monnink SH, et al. Retransfusion of suctioned blood during cardiopulmonary bypass impairs hemostasis. *Ann Thorac Surg* 1995;59:901–907.

60. Boisclair MD, Lane DA, Philippou H, et al. Thrombin production, inactivation and expression during open heart surgery measured by assays for activation fragments including a new ELISA for prothrombin fragment F1 + 2. *Thromb Haemost* 1993;70:253–258.

61. Menges T, Wagner RM, Welters I, et al. The role of the protein C-thrombomodulin system and fibrinolysis during cardiovascular surgery: influence of acute preoperative plasmapheresis. *J Cardiothorac Vasc Anesth* 1996;10:482–489.

62. Hunt BJ, Parratt RN, Segal HC, et al. Activation of coagulation and fibrinolysis during cardiothoracic operations. *Ann Thorac Surg* 1998; 65:712–718

63. Slaughter TF, LeBleu TH, Douglas JM Jr, et al. Characterization of prothrombin activation during cardiac surgery by hemostatic molecular markers. *Anesthesiology* 1994;80:520–526.

64. Holloway DS, Summaria L, Sandesara J, et al. Decreased platelet number and function and increased fibrinolysis contribute to postoperative bleeding in cardiopulmonary bypass patients. *Thromb Haemost* 1988;59:62–67.

65. Yoshihara H, Yamamoto T, Mihara H. Changes in coagulation and fibrinolysis occurring in dogs during hypothermia. *Thromb Res* 1985; 37:503–512.

66. Tabuchi N, de Haan J, Boonstra PW, et al. Activation of fibrinolysis in the pericardial cavity during cardiopulmonary bypass. *J Thorac Cardiovasc Surg* 1993;106:828–833.

67. Stibbe J, Kluft C, Brommer EJ, et al. Enhanced fibrinolytic activity during cardiopulmonary bypass in open-heart surgery in man is caused by extrinsic (tissue-type) plasminogen activator. *Eur J Clin Invest* 1984;14:375–382.

68. Lu H, Soria C, Cramer EM, et al. Temperature dependence of plasmin-induced activation or inhibition of human platelets. *Blood* 1991; 77:996–1005.

69. Cramer EM, Lu H, Caen JP, et al. Differential redistribution of platelet glycoproteins Ib and IIb-IIIa after plasmin stimulation. *Blood* 1991;77:694–699.

70. Adelman B, Michelson AD, Loscalzo J, et al. Plasmin effect on

platelet glycoprotein Ib-von Willebrand factor interactions. *Blood* 1985;65:32–40.

71. Despotis GJ, Joist JH, Hogue CW, et al. More effective suppression of hemostatic system activation in patients undergoing cardiac surgery by heparin dosing based on heparin blood concentrations rather than ACT. *Thromb Haemost* 1996;76:902–908.

72. Wachtfogel YT, Kucich U, Greenplate J, et al. Human neutrophil degranulation during extracorporeal circulation. *Blood* 1987;69:324–330.

73. Riegel W, Spillner G, Schlosser V, et al. Plasma levels of main granulocyte components during cardiopulmonary bypass. *J Thorac Cardiovasc Surg* 1988;95:1014–1019.

74. Clauss M, Grell M, Fangmann C, et al. Synergistic induction of endothelial tissue factor by tumor necrosis factor and vascular endothelial growth factor: functional analysis of the tumor necrosis factor receptors. *FEBS Lett* 1996;390:334–338.

75. van der Poll T, Jansen PM, Van Zee KJ, et al. Tumor necrosis factor-alpha induces activation of coagulation and fibrinolysis in baboons through an exclusive effect on the p55 receptor. *Blood* 1996;88:922–927.

76. Kirklin JK, Chenoweth DE, Naftel DC, et al. Effects of protamine administration after cardiopulmonary bypass on complement, blood elements, and the hemodynamic state. *Ann Thorac Surg* 1986;41:193–199.

77. Ferrer-Lopez P, Renesto P, Schattner M, et al. Activation of human platelets by C5a-stimulated neutrophils: a role for cathepsin G. *Am J Physiol* 1990;258:C1100–1107.

78. Kirklin JK, Westaby S, Blackstone EH, et al. Complement and the damaging effects of cardiopulmonary bypass. *J Thorac Cardiovasc Surg* 1983;86:845–857.

79. Taggart DP, Sundaram S, McCartney C, et al. Endotoxemia, complement, and white blood cell activation in cardiac surgery: a randomized trial of laxatives and pulsatile perfusion. *Ann Thoracic Surg* 1994;57:376–382.

80. Andreasson S, Gothberg S, Berggren H, et al. Hemofiltration modifies complement activation after extracorporeal circulation in infants. *Ann Thorac Surg* 1993;56:1515–1517.

81. Rinder CS, Rinder HM, Smith BR, et al. Blockade of C5a and C5b-9 generation inhibits leukocyte and platelet activation during extracorporeal circulation. *J Clin Invest* 1995;96:1564–1572.

82. Ovrum E, Mollnes TE, Fosse E, et al. Complement and granulocyte activation in two different types of heparinized extracorporeal circuits. *J Thorac Cardiovasc Surg* 1995;110:1623–1632.

83. Rinder HM, Bonan JL, Rinder CS, et al. Activated and unactivated platelet adhesion to monocytes and neutrophils. *Blood* 1991;78:1760–1769.

84. Rinder HM, Bonan JL, Rinder CS, et al. Dynamics of leukocyte-platelet adhesion in whole blood. *Blood* 1991;78:1730–1737.

85. Rinder CS, Bonan JL, Rinder HM, et al. Cardiopulmonary bypass induces leukocyte-platelet adhesion. *Blood* 1992;79:1201–1205.

86. Okita YO, Takamoto S, Ando M, et al. Coagulation and fibrinolysis system in aortic surgery under deep hypothermic circulatory arrest with aprotinin: the importance of adequate heparinization. *Circulation* 1997;96:376–381.

87. Hirsh J. Heparin. *N Engl J Med* 1991;324:1565–1574.

88. Khuri SF, Valeri CR, Loscalzo J, et al. Heparin causes platelet dysfunction and induces fibrinolysis before cardiopulmonary bypass. *Ann Thorac Surg* 1995;60:1008–1014.

89. John LC, Rees GM, Kovacs IB. Inhibition of platelet function by heparin: an etiologic factor in postbypass hemorrhage. *J Thorac Cardiovasc Surg* 1993;105:816–822.

90. Cobel-Geard RJ, Hassouna HI. Interaction of protamine sulfate with thrombin. *Am J Hematol* 1983;14:227–233.

91. Shigeta O, Kojima H, Hiramatsu Y, et al. Low dose protamine based on heparin-protamine titration method reduces platelet dysfunction after cardiopulmonary bypass. *J Thorac Cardiovasc Surg* 1999;118:354-360.

92. Mochizuki T, Olson PJ, Ramsay JG, et al. Does protamine reversal of heparin affect platelet function? *Anesth Analg* 1997;84:35.

93. Ammar T, Fisher CF. The effects of heparinase 1 and protamine on platelet reactivity. *Anesthesiology* 1997;86:1382–1386.

94. Berger RL, Ramaswamy K, Ryan TJ. Reduced protamine dosage for heparin neutralization in open-heart operations. *Circulation* 1968;37:II154–II157.

95. Guffin AV, Dunbar RW, Kaplan JA, et al. Successful use of a reduced dose of protamine after cardiopulmonary bypass. *Anesth Anal* 1976;55:110–113.

96. Moriau M, Masure R, Hurlet A, et al. Haemostasis disorders in open heart surgery with extracorporeal circulation: importance of the platelet function and the heparin neutralization. *Vox Sang* 1977;32:41–51.

97. Jobes DR, Aitken GL, Shaffer GW. Increased accuracy and precision of heparin and protamine dosing reduces blood loss and transfusion in patient undergoing primary cardiac operations. *J Thorac Cardiovasc Surg* 1995;110:36–45.

98. Valeri CR, Feingold H, Cassidy G, et al. Hypothermia-induced reversible platelet dysfunction. *Ann Surg* 1987;205:175–181.

99. Faraday N, Rosenfeld BA. *In vitro* hypothermia enhances platelet GPIIb-IIIa activation and P-selectin expression. *Anesthesiology* 1998;88:1579–1585.

100. Michelson AD, MacGregor H, Barnard MR, et al. Reversible inhibition of human platelet activation by hypothermia in vivo and in vitro. *Thromb Haemost* 1994;71:633–640.

101. Tanaka K, Takao M, Yada I, et al. Alterations in coagulation and fibrinolysis associated with cardiopulmonary bypass during open heart surgery. *J Cardiothorac Anesth* 1989;3:181–188.

102. Czer LS. Mediastinal bleeding after cardiac surgery: etiologies, diagnostic considerations, and blood conservation methods. *J Cardiothorac Anesth* 1989;3:760–775.

103. Harker LA. Bleeding after cardiopulmonary bypass. *N Engl J Med* 1986;314:1446–1448.

104. George JN, Shattil SJ. The clinical importance of acquired abnormalities of platelet function. *N Engl J Med* 1991;324:27–39.

105. Gammie JS, Zenati M, Kormos RL, et al. Abciximab and excessive bleeding in patients undergoing emergency cardiac operations. *Ann Thorac Surg* 1998;65:465–469.

106. Tardiff BE, Tcheng JE, Peck S, et al. Bleeding with coronary artery bypass surgery (CABG) in patients treated with a platelet glycoprotein IIb/IIIa inhibitor. *J Am Coll Cardiol* 1997;29:5212B–5212B.

107. Boehrer JD, Kereiakes DJ, Navetta FI, et al. Effects of profound platelet inhibition with c7E3 before coronary angioplasty on complications of coronary bypass surgery. EPIC Investigators: evaluation prevention of ischemic complications. *Am J Cardiol* 1994;74:1166–1170.

108. Raymond RE, Lincoff AM, Booth JE, et al. Coronary bypass surgery within 12 hours of administration of abciximab remains safe despite an increased risk of perioperative bleeding. *Eur Heart J* 1998;19:238.

109. Suzuki Y, Miyamoto S, Niewiarowski S, et al. Integrelin prevents prolonged bleeding times after cardiopulmonary bypass. *Ann Thorac Surg* 1998;66:373–381.

110. Shainoff JR, Estafanous FG, Yared JP, et al. Low factor XIIIA levels are associated with increased blood loss after coronary artery bypass grafting. *J Thorac Cardiovasc Surg* 1994;108:437–445.

111. Mammen EF, Koets MH, Washington BC, et al. Hemostasis changes during cardiopulmonary bypass surgery. *Semin Thromb Hemost* 1985;11:281–292.

112. Bick RL. Alterations of hemostasis associated with malignancy: etiology, pathophysiology, diagnosis and management. *Semin Thromb Hemost* 1978;5:1–26.

113. Gelb AB, Roth RI, Levin J, et al. Changes in blood coagulation during and following cardiopulmonary bypass: lack of correlation with clinical bleeding. *Am J Clin Pathol* 1996;106:87–99.

114. Gralnick HR, Fischer RD. The hemostatic response to open-heart operations. *J Thorac Cardiovasc Surg* 1971;61:909–915.

115. Despotis GJ, Goodnough LT, Joist JH. Monitoring coagulation in the perioperative cardiac surgical period: emerging strategies for prevention and treatment of microvascular bleeding. *Semin Thromb Hemostas* 2002 (*in press*).

116. Milam JD, Austin SF, Martin RF, et al. Alteration of coagulation and selected clinical chemistry parameters in patients undergoing open heart surgery without transfusions. *Am J Clin Pathol* 1981;76:155–162.

117. Harker LA, Malpass TW, Branson HE, et al. Mechanism of abnormal bleeding in patients undergoing cardiopulmonary bypass: acquired

transient platelet dysfunction associated with selective alpha-granule release. *Blood* 1980;56:824–834.

118. Teufelsbauer H, Proidl S, Havel M, et al. Early activation of hemostasis during cardiopulmonary bypass: evidence for thrombin mediated hyperfibrinolysis. *Thromb Haemost* 1992;68:250–252.

119. Chandler WL, Fitch JCK, Wall MH, et al. Individual variations in the fibrinolytic response during and after cardiopulmonary bypass. *Thromb Haemost* 1995;74:1293–1297.

120. Pelletier MP, Solymoss S, Lee A, et al. Negative reexploration for cardiac postoperative bleeding: can it be therapeutic? *Ann Thorac Surg* 1998;65:999–1002.

121. O'Regan DJ, Giannopoulos N, Mediratta N, et al. Topical aprotinin in cardiac operations. *Ann Thoracic Surg* 1994;58:778–781.

122. Tatar H, Cicek S, Demirkilic U, et al. Topical use of aprotinin in open heart operations. *Ann Thoracic Surg* 1993;55:659–661.

123. Goodnough LT, Johnston MF, Toy PT. The variability of transfusion practice in coronary artery bypass surgery: Transfusion Medicine Academic Award Group. *JAMA* 1991;265:86–90.

124. Goodnough LT, Soegiarso RW, Birkmeyer JD, et al. Economic impact of inappropriate blood transfusions in coronary artery bypass graft surgery. *Am J Med* 1993;94:509–514.

125. Surgenor DM, Wallace EL, Churchill WH, et al. Red cell transfusions in coronary artery bypass surgery (DRGs 106 and 107) [Erratum: *Transfusion* 1992;32:876]. *Transfusion* 1992;32:458–464.

126. Stover EP, Siegel LC, Parks R, et al. Variability in transfusion practice for coronary artery bypass surgery persists despite national consensus guidelines: a 24-institution study: Institutions of the Multicenter Study of Perioperative Ischemia Research Group. *Anesthesiology* 1998;88:327–333.

127. Simon TL, Akl BF, Murphy W. Controlled trial of routine administration of platelet concentrates in cardiopulmonary bypass surgery. *Ann Thorac Surg* 1984;37:359–364.

128. National Institutes of Health (NIH). Consensus conference: platelet transfusion therapy. *JAMA* 1987;257:1777–1780.

129. National Institutes of Health (NIH). Consensus conference: fresh-frozen plasma. Indications and risks. *JAMA* 1985;253:551–553.

130. Counts RB. *Transfusion practice in cardiac surgery: causes of bleeding in open-heart surgery.* Arlington, VA: American Association of Blood Banks, 1991:1–10.

131. Ellison N, Jobes DR. Effective hemostasis in the cardiac surgical patient: current status. In: Ellison N, Jobes DR, eds. *Effective hemostasis in cardiac surgery.* Philadelphia: WB Saunders, 1988:200.

132. Despotis GJ, Grishaber JE, Goodnough LT. The effect of an intraoperative treatment algorithm on physicians' transfusion practice in cardiac surgery. *Transfusion* 1994;34:290–296.

133. Despotis GJ, Santoro SA, Spitznagel E, et al. On-site prothrombin time, activated partial thromboplastin time, and platelet count: a comparison between whole blood and laboratory assays with coagulation factor analysis in patients presenting for cardiac surgery. *Anesthesiology* 1994;80:338–351.

134. Goodnough LT, Despotis GJ, Hogue CW, et al. On the need for improved transfusion indicators in cardiac surgery. *Ann Thorac Surg* 1995;60:473–480.

135. Despotis GJ, Joist JH, Goodnough LT. Monitoring of hemostasis in cardiac surgical patients: impact of point-of-care testing on blood loss and transfusion outcomes. *Clin Chem* 1997;43:1684–1696.

136. Despotis GJ, Skubas NJ, Goodnough LT. Optimal management of bleeding and transfusion in patients undergoing cardiac surgery. *Semin Thorac Cardiovasc Surg* 1999;11:84–104.

137. Gravlee GP, Arora S, Lavender SW, et al. Predictive value of blood clotting tests in cardiac surgical patients. *Ann Thorac Surg* 1994;58:216–221.

138. Essell JH, Martin TJ, Salinas J, et al. Comparison of thromboelastography to bleeding time and standard coagulation tests in patients after cardiopulmonary bypass. *J Cardiothorac Vasc Anesth* 1993;7:410–415.

139. Fassin W, Himpe D, Alexander JP, et al. Predictive value of coagulation testing in cardiopulmonary bypass surgery. *Acta Anaesthesiol Belg* 1991;42:191–198.

140. Despotis GJ, Levine V, Filos KS, et al. Evaluation of a new point-of-care test that measures PAF-mediated acceleration of coagulation in cardiac surgical patients. *Anesthesiology* 1996;85:1311–1323.

141. Murray D, Pennell B, Olson J. Variability of prothrombin time and activated partial thromboplastin time in the diagnosis of increased surgical bleeding. *Transfusion* 1999;39:56–62.

142. Nuttall GA, Oliver WC, Santrach PJ, et al. Efficacy of a simple intraoperative transfusion algorithm for nonerythrocyte component utilization after cardiopulmonary bypass. *Anesthesiology* 2001 94;773–781.

143. Codispoti M, Ludlam CA, Simpson D, et al. Individualized heparin and protamine management in infants and children undergoing cardiac operations. *Ann Thorac Surg* 2001;71:922–927.

144. Despotis GJ, Hogue CW, Santoro SA, et al. Effect of heparin on whole blood activated partial thromboplastin time using a portable, whole blood coagulation monitor. *Crit Care Med* 1995;23:1674–1679.

145. Despotis GJ, Joist JH, Hogue CW, et al. The impact of heparin concentration and activated clotting time monitoring on blood conservation: a prospective, randomized evaluation in patients undergoing cardiac operation. *J Thorac Cardiovasc Surg* 1995;110:46–54.

146. Despotis GJ, Alsoufiev A, Hogue CW, et al. Evaluation of complete blood count results from a new, on-site hemocytometer compared with a laboratory-based hemocytometer. *Crit Care Med* 1996;24:1163–1167.

147. Despotis GJ, Alsoufiev AL, Spitznagel E, et al. Response of kaolin ACT to heparin: evaluation with an automated assay and higher heparin doses. *Ann Thorac Surg* 1996;61:795–799.

148. Despotis GJ, Levine V, Goodnough LT. Relationship between leukocyte count and patient risk for excessive blood loss after cardiac surgery. *Crit Care Med* 1997;25:1338–1346.

149. Despotis GJ, Joist JH. Anticoagulation and anticoagulation reversal with cardiac surgery involving cardiopulmonary bypass: an update. *J Cardiothorac Vasc Anesth* 1999;13(Suppl 4):18–29,36–37.

150. Despotis GJ, Levine V, Saleem R, et al. Use of point-of-care test in identification of patients who can benefit from desmopressin during cardiac surgery: a randomised controlled trial. *Lancet* 1999;354:106–110.

151. Despotis GJ, Saleem R, Bigham M, et al. Clinical evaluation of a new, point-of-care hemocytometer. *Crit Care Med* 2000;28:1185–1190.

152. Spiess BD, Gillies BSA, Chandler W, et al. Changes in transfusion therapy and reexploration rate after institution of a blood management program in cardiac surgical patients. *J Cardiothorac Vasc Anesth* 1995;9:168–173.

153. Shore-Lesserson L, Manspeizer HE, DePerio M, et al. Thromboelastography-guided transfusion algorithm reduces transfusions in complex cardiac surgery. *Anesth Analg* 1999;88:312–319.

154. Royston D, von Kier S. Reduced hemostatic factor transfusion using heparinase-modified thromboelastography during cardiopulmonary bypass. *Br J Anaesthes* 2001;86:575–578.

155. Ereth MH, Nuttall GA, Santrach PJ, et al. The relation between the platelet-activated clotting test (HemoSTATUS) and blood loss after cardiopulmonary bypass. *Anesthesiology* 1998;88:962–969.

156. von Kier S, Smith A. Hemostatis product transfusions and adverse outcomes: focus on point-of-care testing to reduce transfusion need. *J Cardiothorac Vasc Anesth* 2000;14(Suppl 1):15–21.

157. Salzman EW, Weinstein MJ, Weintraub RM, et al. Treatment with desmopressin acetate to reduce blood loss after cardiac surgery: a double-blind randomized trial. *N Engl J Med* 1986;314:1402–1406.

158. Dilthey G, Dietrich W, Spannagl M, et al. Influence of desmopressin acetate on homologous blood requirements in cardiac surgical patients pretreated with aspirin. *J Cardiothorac Vasc Anesth* 1993;7:425–430.

159. Salzman EW, Weinstein MJ, Reilly D, et al. Adventures in hemostasis. Desmopressin in cardiac surgery. *Arch Surg* 1993;128:212–217.

160. Sheridan DP, Card RT, Pinilla JC, et al. Use of desmopressin acetate to reduce blood transfusion requirements during cardiac surgery in patients with acetylsalicylic-acid-induced platelet dysfunction. *Can J Surg* 1994;37:33–36.

161. Gratz I, Koehler J, Olsen D, et al. The effect of desmopressin acetate on postoperative hemorrhage in patients receiving aspirin therapy before coronary artery bypass operations. *J Thorac Cardiovasc Surg* 1992;104:1417–1422.

162. Fremes SE, Wong BI, Lee E, et al. Metaanalysis of prophylactic drug treatment in the prevention of postoperative bleeding. *Ann Thorac Surg* 1994;58:1580–1588.

163. Czer LS, Bateman TM, Gray RJ, et al. Treatment of severe platelet dysfunction and hemorrhage after cardiopulmonary bypass: reduction in blood product usage with desmopressin. *J Am Coll Cardiol* 1987; 9:1139–1147.

164. Hackmann T, Gascoyne RD, Naiman SC, et al. A trial of desmopressin (1-desamino-8-D-arginine vasopressin) to reduce blood loss in uncomplicated cardiac surgery. *N Engl J Med* 1989;321: 1437–1443.

165. Lazenby WD, Russo I, Zadeh BJ, et al. Treatment with desmopressin acetate in routine coronary artery bypass surgery to improve postoperative hemostasis. *Circulation* 1990;82:IV413–419.

166. Ansell J, Klassen V, Lew R, et al. Does desmopressin acetate prophylaxis reduce blood loss after valvular heart operations? A randomized, double-blind study. *J Thorac Cardiovasc Surg* 1992;104: 117–123.

167. Casas JI, Zuazu-Jausoro I, Mateo J, et al. Aprotinin versus desmopressin for patients undergoing operations with cardiopulmonary bypass: a double-blind placebo-controlled study. J *Thorac Cardiovasc Surg* 1995;110:1107–1117.

168. Temeck BK, Bachenheimer LC, Katz NM, et al. Desmopressin acetate in cardiac surgery: a double-blind, randomized study. *South Med J* 1994;87:611–615.

169. de Prost D, Barbier-Boehm G, Hazebroucq J, et al. Desmopressin has no beneficial effect on excessive postoperative bleeding or blood product requirements associated with cardiopulmonary bypass. *Thromb Haemost* 1992;68:106–110.

170. Cattaneo M, Harris AS, Stromber U, et al. The effect of desmopressin on reducing blood loss in cardiac surgery: a meta-analysis of double-blind, placebo-controlled trials. *Thromb Hemostas* 1995;74: 1064–1070.

171. Laupacis A, Fergusson D. Drugs to minimize perioperative blood loss in cardiac surgery: meta-analyses using perioperative blood transfusion as the outcome: the International Study of Perioperative Transfusion (ISPOT) Investigators. *Anesth Analg* 1997;85:1258–1267.

172. Mongan PD, Hosking MP. The role of desmopressin acetate in patients undergoing coronary artery bypass surgery: a controlled clinical trial with thromboelastographic risk stratification. *Anesthesiology* 1992;77:38–46.

173. Capraro L, Kuitunen A, Salmenpera M, et al. On-site coagulation monitoring does not affect hemostatic outcome after cardiac surgery. *Acta Anesthesiol Scand* 2001;45:200–206.

174. Goodnough LT, Despotis GJ. Establishing practice guidelines for surgical blood management. *Am J Surg* 1995;170(Suppl 6A):16S–20S.

175. Goodnough LT, Despotis GJ. Future directions in utilization review: the role of transfusion algorithms. *Transfus Sci* 1998;19:97–105.

176. Despotis GJ, Gravlee G, Filos K, et al. Anticoagulation monitoring during cardiac surgery: a review of current and emerging techniques. *Anesthesiology* 1999;91:1122–1151.

177. Despotis GJ, Goodnough LT. Management approaches to platelet-related microvascular bleeding in cardiothoracic surgery. *Ann Thorac Surg* 2000;70(Suppl 2):S20–S32.

178. Weil MH, Michaels S, Puri VK, et al. The stat laboratory: facilitating blood gas and biochemical measurements for the critically ill and injured. *Am J Clin Pathol* 1981;76:34–42.

179. Strickland RA, Hill TR, Zaloga GP. Bedside analysis of arterial blood gases and electrolytes during and after cardiac surgery. *J Clin Anesth* 1989;1:248–252.

180. Stewart FC, Morana NJ, Sears JJ, et al. Anesthesia laboratory for the pediatric operating room. *Int Anesthesiol Clin* 1992;30:177–188.

181. Goodwin SA. Point-of-care testing in a post anesthesia care unit. *Medical Laboratory Observer* 1994;26(9S):15–18.

182. Johnson KF. Does an on-site satellite laboratory reduce surgical delays? A study of delays in a same day surgical center. *AORN J* 1994;59:1275–1276,1279–1282,1285–1290.

183. McPeck M. A BG & E program for cardiac surgery. *Medical Laboratory Observer* 1994;26(9S):20–25.

184. Luckey L, Carey S, Hathorn G. POCT for coronary bypass patients: fast results without bypassing quality. *Medical Laboratory Observer* 1994;26:31–35.

185. Kost GJ, Hague C. The current and future status of critical care testing and patient monitoring: pathology patterns. *Am J Clin Pathol* 1995;104:S2–S17.

186. Kost GJ, Hague C. *In vitro, ex vivo,* and *in vivo* biosensor systems. In: Kost GJ, ed., *Handbook of clinical automation, robotics, and optimization.* New York: John Wiley and Sons, 1996:648–753.

187. Kost GJ. Point-of-care testing. In: Meyers RA, ed. *Encyclopedia of analytical chemistry: instrumentation and applications.* New York: John Wiley and Sons, 2000:540,1603–1625.

188. Young DS, Sachais BS, Jefferies LC. The costs of disease. *Clin Chem* 2000;46:955–966.

189. Young DS, Sachais BS, Jeffries LC. Laboratory costs in the context of disease. *Clin Chem* 2000;46:967–975.

190. Jefferies LC, Sachais BS, Young DS. Blood transfusion costs by diagnosis-related groups in 60 university hospitals in 1995. *Transfusion* 2001;41:522–529.

9

POINT-OF-CARE TESTING IN INTENSIVE CARE

PAUL A. H. HOLLOWAY

The definition of intensive care varies, depending on clinical setting and healthcare system. Common themes persist in terms of diagnostic testing in these units, whether supporting specialized or general facilities, and the nature of the clinical activity is predominantly organ system support requiring maximum efficiency in diagnostic and monitoring procedures. This section is aimed at broadbased point-of-care (POC) processes in intensive care units (ICUs) with adequate resources to allow at least optimal testing with good data transfer and recording systems.

Intensive care provides the ultimate forum for point-of-care testing (POCT) as the range of analyses, speed of turnaround, and speed of response to data retrieval are all critical to patient management, outcome, and throughput. It is the setting where the system is maximally tested and as such requires the highest level of technical and practical support both for analytical systems and for the users in order to provide optimal safety and efficiency. In Britain and other countries with developed national healthcare systems the process could currently be described as progressing from late childhood to early pubescence, with the clinical service benefiting in some ways from the advantages of late development imposed to a certain extent by the financial constraints of a public service industry. Such fiscal constraints impact inevitably on the severity of illness of the patients for whom limited intensive care resources are available to support, thus rendering POCT even more potentially cost effective. Where greater resources are provided for health care, definition of the intensive care patient may be broader with more varied needs for diagnostic testing, but there will always be a core patient population with multisystem failure and, as this often occurs with rapid onset, clinical management would be expected to benefit from effective POCT. The public profile and high costs of intensive care will ensure that it remains a well-audited activity and this should level the quality of the service across differing healthcare systems. For those who have watched the progression thus far, the forthcoming adolescence and early adulthood of POCT are intriguing and exciting prospects on the near horizon. This maturation process must, however, meet optimum quality standards, be supported by convincing cost-benefit analysis, and coincide with evolving clinical requirements (1–4).

For the purposes of this chapter, I am restricting the range of POCT to bedside and adjacent laboratory analysis of blood gases, metabolites, co-oximetry, and coagulation in support of existing monitoring of physiological parameters. These will be discussed largely in the context of a teaching hospital using a system in place that is representative of ICUs in most developed countries. The chapter concludes with hypotheses for the future direction of POCT in ICUs in the context of clinical demand, and current concepts in the interplay of molecular and metabolic medical science.

THE INTENSIVE CARE UNIT

The representative ICU is a general adult unit supporting the activities of a busy regional center providing all major clinical services, including a large renal unit (Table 9.1). ICU staff responsibilities are not limited to the ICU as clinical staff often have responsibility for patients in other locations, such as accident and emergency, hematology, infectious diseases, renal unit, and cardiac recovery wards.

Responsibility for direct patient care is structured to allow an independently supervised team of highly skilled and motivated nurses to manage the majority of day-to-day technical and pastoral care. Admission to the ICU and subsequent diagnostic and therapeutic decisions are made, in close liaison with nurses, by the medical team who also carries out most of the invasive procedures. In the context of diagnostic testing, a routine central-

TABLE 9.1. REPRESENTATIVE INTENSIVE CARE UNIT

The unit
  Adult medical and surgical ICU serving large teaching hospital, 12 beds, approximately 850 patients/year: 40% surgery, 30% general medicine, 30% A&E, cardiac center, outside referrals
Clinical team
  Medical—consultant medical staff: 2 physicians, 3 anaesthetists, 1 joint anaesthetist/physician; consultant medical support: 2 visiting anaesthetists, 1 microbiologist, 1 chemical pathologist (academic in dept medicine); junior medical staff: 10 specialist registrars, 6 anaesthetics, 4 medicine
  Nursing—1 nurse consultant, 80 senior specialist ICU nurses (14 on unit at any one time)
  Other dedicated ICU staff—1 pharmacist, 1 dietician, 8 physiotherapists, 2 information technologists (1 also a senior ICU nurse), administrative staff

TABLE 9.2. QUESTIONS ASKED IN AUDITS OF ICU BLOOD GAS MEASUREMENT IN 1997 AND 2001

Reasons for Performing ABG,1997	Reasons for Performing ABG, 2001	Changes to Patient Management Resulting from ABG
New admission	New admission	No change
After change in ventilation	After change in ventilation	Intubated
Before change in ventilation	Before change in ventilation	Extubated
Change in saturation	Change in saturation	Re-intubated
pH estimation	pH estimation	Increased ventilation
Potassium estimation	Potassium estimation	Decreased ventilation
Hb estimation	Hb estimation	Increased F_1O_2
Pre-extubation	Pre-extubation	Decreased F_1O_2
Post-extubation	Post-extubation	Potassium given
Change in respiratory pattern	Change in respiratory pattern	Blood given
No information	Glucose estimation	Hemofiltration
Other	Lactate estimation	Other
—	Chloride or calcium	—
—	Base excess or anion gap	—
—	Hemofiltration assessment	—
—	Co-oximetry	—
—	No information	—
—	Other	—

ABG, arterial blood gas analysis.

ized laboratory profile is performed early each morning with additional testing depending on organ system reviews in ward rounds. Arterial blood gas (ABG) analysis is carried out during the day (on average seven ABGs per patient per day) by the nursing staff and is usually prompted by the need to decide on changes in respiratory support, which are often triggered by alterations in data from pulse oximetry. Audit results appear in Tables 9.2 through 9.4.

Clinical management in this ICU is heavily supported by a bedside computer data system that coordinates data from bedside monitoring, an ICU laboratory, a central laboratory, and also manual input. There is a terminal located at each bed with several additional terminals in the unit and adjacent offices. The

bedside terminals are the central focus for patient management and ward round discussions; the system records all nursing procedures, pharmacy and physiotherapy input, as well as demographic data. The terminals have replaced the large A2-size paper records that still feature widely in ICUs. Bedside monitors evaluate physiological parameters (Table 9.5), and data are downloaded automatically and manually. The existing bedside monitors provide essential continuous monitoring of hemodynamic, respiratory, and cardiac physiological parameters that are supported by POC and central laboratory testing.

A small satellite laboratory located next to the unit houses two blood gas analyzers, glucose meters, and coagulation analyzers. Samples drawn from patients by the nursing staff are brought immediately to the analyzers where, following identification and analysis, data are directly downloaded from the analyzers to the clinical data system where further derived parameters are calcu-

TABLE 9.3 REASONS FOR ABG

Indication	1997 (%)	2001 (%)
New admission	3	1
After change in ventilation	29	34
Before change in ventilation	16	15
Change in saturation	11	13
pH estimation	8	3
Potassium estimation	19	11
Hb estimation	1	2
Pre-extubation	1	1
Post-extubation	1	0
Change in respiratory pattern	1	2
No information	1	0
Other	9	8
Glucose estimation	—	4
Lactate estimation	—	0
Chloride or calcium	—	0
Base excess or anion gap	—	3
Hemofiltration assessment	—	1
Co-oximetry	—	1

Note: Percentage total for 2001 does not equal 100 due to rounding.
ABG, arterial blood gas analysis.

TABLE 9.4. CHANGES TO PATIENT MANAGEMENT AS A CONSEQUENCE OF ABG RESULT

Result	1997 (%)	2001 (%)
No change	26	38
Intubated	0	0
Extubated	2	0
Re-intubated	0	1
Increased ventilation	4	9
Decreased ventilation	18	8
Increased F_1O_2	9	9
Decreased F_1O_2	19	18
Potassium given	16	7
Blood given	2	1
Hemofiltration	1	2
Other	1	9
No information	3	0

Note: Percentage totals do not equal 100 due to rounding.
ABG, arterial blood gas analysis.

TABLE 9.5. BEDSIDE PHYSIOLOGICAL PARAMETERS

Hemodynamic observations
Heart rate
Heart rhythm
Arterial blood pressure (BP)
Mean arterial BP (MAP)
Central venous pressure
Noninvasive BP
Temperature
Respiratory observations
Oxygen saturation (pulse oximetry)
Inspired oxygen (F_IO_2)
Respiratory rate
Ventilation mode (e.g., spontaneous ventilation, CPAP)
Peak inspiratory pressure (PIP)
Peak end expiratory pressure (PEEP)
Continuous positive airways pressure (CPAP)
Auto PEEP (actual)
Total PEEP
Pressure support
Ventilator respiratory rate
Total respiratory rate
Inspired tidal volume
Expired tidal volume
Spontaneous minute volume
Dynamic compliance
Inspiratory:expiratory ratio (I:E ratio)
Flow by
Humidifier temperature
Cardiac function measurements and calculations
Pulmonary artery pressure (PAP)
Mean pulmonary artery pressure (MPAP)
Pulmonary artery wedge pressure (PAWP)
Right atrial pressure
Right ventricular pressure
Mixed venous oxygen saturation
Cardiac output (CO)
Cardiac index (CI)
Stroke volume (SV)
Systemic vascular resistance (SVR)
SVR index (SVRI)
Pulmonary vascular resistance (PVR)
PVR index (PRVI)
Left ventricular stroke work (LVSW)
LVSW index (LVSWI)
Right ventricular stroke work (RVSW)
RVSW index (RVSWI)
Oxygen delivery
Oxygen consumption
Oxygen extraction ratio
Intracranial pressure monitoring
Intracranial pressure (ICP)
Cerebral perfusion pressure (CPP) (difference between MAP and mean ICP)

TABLE 9.6. POINT-OF-CARE LABORATORY TESTING IN INTENSIVE CARE

Measured	Calculated
Blood gases	
Po_2	Base excess (actual and standard)
pH	Bicarbonate
Pco_2	Total CO_2
Electrolytes	
Sodium	Anion gap
Potassium	Strong ion difference
Chloride	Osmolarity
Calcium, ionized	—
(Magnesium, ionized)	—
Metabolites	
Glucose	—
Lactate	—
(Urea)	—
(Creatinine)	—
Co-oximetry	
Oxyhemoglobin	Hematocrit (conductivity)
Carboxy hemoglobin	—
Methemoglobin	—
Deoxy hemoglobin	—
Sulphhemoglobin	—
Fetal hemoglobin	—
Total hemoglobin	—

The central clinical biochemistry laboratory provides all routine organ-specific biochemical analyses and is able to offer parameters to support the metabolic investigations provided by the blood gas analyzers, such as glucose, lactate, bicarbonate, and chloride. Because the latter metabolic analyses are organized predominantly for general ward and outpatient use, a turnaround time of several hours may be required for some assays. The medical staff in the ICU uses the central laboratory serum/plasma electrolytes as a reference for POCT electrolytes.

POC analyses currently carried out in the side laboratory are listed in Table 9.6. Most analyses are instigated by the nursing staff who, while using blood gas analyses in conjunction with the data from bedside pulse oximetry monitoring, will seek advice and direction on these from the unit's permanent medical staff.

INTENSIVE CARE—A SPECIAL CASE FOR POCT

Special Clinical Requirements

Maximum Focus on Clinical Physiology and Biochemistry

The efforts of the clinical team managing patients in intensive care concentrate predominantly on organ support, which requires regular and often constant monitoring of organ function through physiological parameters from direct and indirect clinical assessments as well as support from pathology and radiology. Much of the training in intensive care nursing and medicine centers on the interpretation of the patient's physiology, particularly in relation to respiratory and cardiac function, but most other organ function is best monitored by changes in biochemical profiles. These are not restricted to the refinements of blood gas, electrolyte, and metabolites but also include the bio-

lated. In this hospital, central biochemistry and hematology laboratories are situated three floors above the ICU and have an organized process for fast tracking and batching the ICU specimens and for directly downloading data to the ICU clinical data system. Neither laboratory has the resources to provide a direct interpretative component to the automated processing involved, but the consultant chemical pathologist in the ICU reviews biochemistry and ABG data each morning and is available to interpret metabolic data from the POC analysis and to instigate further requests as required.

chemical components in hematology, microbiology, and immunology investigations. The degree of interest in POC analysis of some parameters or components of organ function profiles largely depends on the potential rate of change in minutes rather than hours or days. For example, parameters of the liver function profile, such as serum albumin, alkaline phosphatase, bilirubin, alanine transaminase, gamma glutamyl transferase, or prothrombin time, may change relatively slowly during a 24-hour period (slow responders). Parameters of renal function or markers of inflammation, such as C-reactive protein (CRP) or procalcitonin (PCT) (fast responders), may change more rapidly and thus require more frequent testing.

Therapeutic Turnaround Time

Pressure resulting from the rapidly changing clinical course of many acutely ill patients, as well as from the evaluation and allocation of resources—and thus the need to relocate patients as soon as they no longer require intensive care management—all contribute to the need for minimum delay in clinical decision-making in response to diagnostic and monitor testing (5). Turnaround times of 2 hours or more from centralized laboratory services may be acceptable for some tests, but in most circumstances the average turnaround for intensive care investigations should be measurable in minutes (6,7). The concept of therapeutic turnaround time was conceived in a recent study comparing the clinical impact and staff satisfaction of bedside, satellite, and central laboratory analytical processes in critical care (8). Clinical decision-making delays will inevitably compromise clinical management and are often reasons for delays in relocation or discharge of patients, the "freeing up" of beds for others' use (9). Another pertinent issue relates to blood conservation, particularly bedside analysis with reduced sample volumes (10), although it would be relatively unusual for blood loss from routine testing to cause transfusion-dependent anemia (11). Extended therapeutic turnaround time for certain factors—such as clotting parameters, acute phase markers, or results of microbiological cultures—could lead to real inefficiencies. Delays may be entirely explicable at the laboratory end. An example may be a need for a repeat test due to a failure in a quality control process or the sample may have missed the fast-tracking line. Unfortunately, those working in the ICU are rarely able to track the analytical process and thus plan for such delays. Recent studies of the comparison of laboratory and POCT (8,12) included an evaluation of therapeutic turnaround times and confirmed the significance of this factor in critical care.

Metabolic "Awareness"

The complexities of modern clinical management and assessment may give the clinical team little time to reflect and focus on the patient's broader metabolic status. Current profiling allows restricted "snapshot" views confined to the measurement of blood glucose and gases with some support, when available, from electrolyte and metabolite measurements. Ideally, metabolic assessment should extend beyond these measurements in order to rationalize appropriate functional support for cardiac, renal, and gastrointestinal systems as well as general nutrition

and immuno-nutrition. The prime example of metabolic upheaval is diabetic ketoacidosis and yet this life-threatening medical emergency may not be adequately assessed in critical care or in the ICU. The blood glucose result will usually be the critical POC beacon signaling routine evaluation. Electrolyte and blood gas analyses (again, at POC) should follow, initializing the diagnostic and management algorithms that are well-worn paths for clinical management of most cases. There is, however, a risk of complacency when dealing with these conditions, as complications arise during management that need to be anticipated and corrected when they appear. The best example is hypokalemia as a result of potassium shifts during the correction of the acidosis, usually on top of preexisting depleted body potassium stores. Other examples include the development of hyperchloremic acidosis, lactic acidosis, and renal tubular acidosis. The first two are recognized complications that prolong, sometimes quite significantly, the recovery period of diabetic ketoacidosis and may indeed be the reason(s) for admission to the ICU. Most high-end blood gas analyzers now offer whole-blood chloride measurement, and this will, of course, allow the calculation of derivatives such as anion gap and strong ion difference (for the definition of strong ion difference, see "Metabolic Monitoring" subsection under "Future Developments" in this chapter). While clinicians may note the anion gap, the chloride result itself may be largely ignored and even a significant rise may go unnoticed by the medical and nursing staff. The unmeasured anion responsible for the high anion gap may be assumed to be lactate, but unless there is POC analysis of this parameter the assumption is often incorrect and thus potentially dangerous. Likewise, coincidental lactic acidosis on admission or during subsequent therapy of ketoacidosis is a serious complication and requires identification and correction when necessary (13). POCT during diabetic ketoacidosis has been shown to enhance metabolic awareness sufficiently to reduce length of stay in the ICU and thus costs per patient (9).

Metabolic awareness is a real pilgrimage that most of us assisting in the teaching and management of critical and intensive care medicine see as a valuable component resulting from the developments in POCT. The term "critical care profiling" has emerged, although for many clinical practices profiling may prove too costly and impractical (14). There are many other examples of the value of such metabolic assessment in critical care patients but the value of electrolyte and metabolite measurements in the management of endocrine, renal, and hepatic failure patients cannot be over emphasized.

Metabolic Management

There is a significant role in intensive care for the clinical management of metabolic syndromes and assisting the patient's metabolic response to respiratory disturbances. In certain circumstances, the metabolic response to a significant respiratory defect such as alkalosis may become inadequate and require metabolic support in addition to that for the respiratory component. Similar support may be required in respiratory acidosis, although metabolic interference can seldom contribute significantly in severe respiratory failure. In contrast, correction of metabolic disturbances can be achieved to a limited extent by the respiratory manipulation afforded to a ventilated patient, but in these circumstances when life-threatening metabolic acidosis develops, there is usually a need for direct active intervention in the metabolic process. The most striking, life-threatening, common acid-base condition is lactic acidosis where the prognosis is often very poor (more than 50%) and where metabolic salvage, although problematic, is essential and can be very rewarding (15–17). The causes are multiple, including cardiovascular shock and severe sepsis. Although the primary cause needs to be treated, the acidosis itself may require urgent correction. The need for metabolic monitoring of blood gases, lactate, and chloride during this treatment is critical to ensure optimal treatment and to anticipate and correct any overtreatment.

Most units now provide renal support in some form such as continuous veno-venous hemofiltration. This valuable process, used also for correction of fluid overload and removal of toxins and excess cations and anions, involves replacement of fluid using a buffered salt solution that usually enhances the alkalinizing component of the exercise. The selection of the correct type of replacement fluid is essential, as several studies have demonstrated the risks from use of the standard sodium lactate-based fluid in certain cases (18–22). All patients requiring hemofiltration or a similar type of renal support process need a metabolic workup before treatment and at regular intervals during treatment. Metabolic alkalosis is a common complication in intensive care patients, often secondary to significant renal or gastrointestinal chloride loss, and although often self-limiting it will frequently require active treatment usually with saline to provide the acid source. The treatment requires careful monitoring of blood gases and electrolytes and derived parameters such as strong ion difference.

Other contributions of POCT in metabolic management include the regular monitoring of ionized calcium in patients following thyroid and parathyroid surgery or during urgent treatment for hyper- and hypo-calcemia, and measurement of ionized magnesium in severe hypomagnesemia. Next is the obvious role of sodium and potassium measurements in the treatment of disturbances of these electrolytes (see "Special Metabolic Requirements" section). There is also a strong argument for the availability of facilities for POC urine electrolyte and osmolality measurements to complement those in blood.

Prognostication

Prognostication is a routine component of intensive–care patient management because it helps to focus treatment and resources for each individual and prepare nurses and visiting relatives for treatments as well as adverse consequences. Intensive care clinicians have developed several systems aimed at improving the prediction of severe complications or adverse outcomes. Although most involve assessment during the first 24 hours of admission, many will continue throughout the patient's stay in the unit (23–32). The scoring systems are all dependent on the accurate recording of physiological and pathological data collected for the patient during timed intervals and most of the data are obtained from bedside monitors or POC diagnostic systems. Not only are the POC biochemical markers such as PO_2, PCO_2, pH, base excess, lactate, and clotting indices essential

components of these systems, valuable prognostic information can be derived from individual markers. The calculation of base excess/deficit—and particularly the base deficit in a metabolic acidosis—is recognized as a marker of severity for an inadequately compensated metabolic acid-base disturbance, and extra weight is given to this marker by further characterization of the major anion in an acidosis such as lactate (33–35). Indeed, an increased blood lactate level has been reported by several studies to be a valuable independent predictor of a poor outcome in severe sepsis (36–39), falciparum malaria (40–42), and in triage following trauma (16,43). Markers of cardiac ischemia such as troponins are now recognized as valuable independent markers of severity allowing risk stratification and thus more focused clinical management. A POC system troponin analysis has yet to be evaluated in intensive care, but in certain settings it may prove to be of value (44–47).

POCT Criteria for ICU Admission and Discharge

Admission

Prior to admission to the ICU, most patients have been assessed by clinical staff members, who are often specialists from the ICU, to evaluate their requirements for intensive care. Some use criteria for admission guidelines that have been evolving over the past decade (48–51). Often decisions need to be taken very rapidly as the window of opportunity for filling a place in the unit may be limited and the state of ICU bed occupancy may, for instance, determine the timing of another patient's elective operation. ICU admission requirements usually depend on the degree and extent of organ dysfunction, and for this procedure to be effective the clinical assessment would ideally be supported by rapid diagnostic testing (31,43). The extent and scope of POCT outside the ICU are often very limited, but in centers where there is a regular flow of patients from distant wards to the ICU, provision of POCT is essential and would also complement the needs of acute care medical wards. For this to be optimal, the POCT remote from the ICU should ideally be interfaced to a laboratory or hospital computer information system.

Discharge

Likewise, effective POCT in the ICU is frequently required for discharge evaluation and this is an area where the extended scope of POCT would be valuable, again to support emerging guidelines to aid in these decisions (51,52). For example, a 2-hour wait for results of coagulation or cardiac markers would now be unacceptable, particularly when patient discharge, and therefore bed availability for another sick patient, is seriously delayed. The extension of the standard range for POCT in the ICU may thus include troponins, liver and renal function tests, and acute–phase inflammatory and coagulation markers.

Special Metabolic Requirements

The "Blood Gas" Profile

Two Surveys of "Blood Gas" Requests in ICUs

There is limited evidence in the literature defining the optimum frequency and scope of blood gas testing in ICU patients (53).

As part of the process of evaluating technology suitable for upgrading the POCT in the ICU, an audit was carried out in 1997 using a questionnaire completed by the unit nursing staff to establish testing relevance. Part of the aim of the audit derived from anticipation of a possible reduction in the number of tests to allow the introduction of bedside dry chemistry analyses directly inputted to the bedside monitors. The audit, carried out over a 1-week period, required completion of a questionnaire before and after performing blood gas analyses (Table 9.2), which requested details on the reason(s) for requesting blood gas analysis and the subsequent action, if any, as a result of the analysis. The results of the audit, while providing interesting and valuable insights into the process, failed to provide convincing rationales to reduce or restrict the number of daily blood gas analyses (an average of seven per patient). This first audit was carried out prior to the installation of the new analyzer with its additional metabolite and co-oximetry functions, and a second audit was carried out after the introduction of the enhanced repertoire. The results of the second audit, which used an identical format apart from extra questions relating to the additional parameters of lactate, glucose, chloride, and co-oximetry, revealed a very similar pattern apart from a decrease in requests for potassium (from 19% to 11%) and some new requests for anion gap and base excess. Blood lactate measurements, particularly trends, that are performed with most blood gases are valued by clinicians on the unit, but were not initiated specifically by the nurses. The most surprising features of the first audit included the high percentage (19%) of whole-blood potassium estimations performed as the primary reason for the "gas" and the relatively infrequent (8%) demand for the pH value as the primary reason. The requirement for blood gas values before and after changes in ventilation is linked to the bedside data from pulse oximetry monitoring, and it is significant that blood gas estimations brought about changes (usually a reduction) in FiO_2. The incidence of requesting POCT primarily for potassium estimation is a reflection of the concern for tight control of potassium in vulnerable intensive care patients. A concern that highlights a fundamental part of training in the use of POCT is that potassium in whole-blood analysis is potentially misleading when compared to its measurement in serum or plasma. The nursing staff is aware of this problem and initiates support of abnormal POC potassium results with central laboratory analyses when relevant, a reliable practice that should prevent potentially life-threatening, inappropriate treatment.

Electrolytes

During ICU ward rounds, probably the most complex and time consuming of the organ system reviews at bedside is renal, and particularly electrolyte, physiology. Underlying disease and secondary endocrine disease, as well as therapeutic interventions, significantly affect this assessment. The management of fluid balance (hydration state) requires regular blood *sodium* estimation. Sodium and water movement across cell membranes is influenced by alterations in vasopressin release or renal tubular aquaporin response as well as by changing renal, cardiac respiratory, and hepatic pathology, and also by drug regimens, and thus must be assessed at least three or four times a day in most ICU

patients. The role of the sodium ion in the corrective process of metabolic acidosis may also necessitate regular monitoring of sodium along with chloride. The demand for regular POC assessment of *potassium*, based essentially on the well-established and understood risks to myocardial function of significant extremes of serum potassium, was illustrated in the POCT audit. Potassium measurements by POCT analyzers need particularly rigorous quality assessment, as the degree of sensitivity required is high and clinical management demands optimal precision (10,54). *Chloride* measurements are now available in most POCT blood gas analyzers. The slow change to the use of these analyzers means that for many ICUs chloride measurement is still only available from the central laboratory (usually in a venous sample), which is assessed once a day and not matched directly to an arterial gas result (55). The anion gap is a valuable calculated parameter in ICU patients and chloride measurements are required for this parameter (56,57). As discussed later in the context of strong ion difference, the role of chloride derived from sodium chloride infusions in regular use following surgical procedures or in the treatment of metabolic alkalosis requires that this ion be monitored regularly in ICU patients.

Most efficient POCT systems in ICUs include ionized *calcium* and some also include ionized magnesium. Ionized calcium is measured in every blood gas analysis in most ICUs, and there is a strong argument against centralized laboratory measurement of total calcium for ICU patients, even if the laboratory issues a "corrected" calcium result. A number of factors—including therapeutic interventions such as giving citrated blood products, electrolyte, colloid, and drug therapy, as well as renal, gastrointestinal, nutritional, metabolic, and endocrine changes—are likely to significantly affect calcium homeostasis (58). The most significant clinical effect of hypocalcemia is cardiac dysrhythmia and risk of cardiac arrest, and this is easily treatable once diagnosed (59,60). Other effects of hypocalcemia yet to be evaluated clinically include the role in modulating cytokine activation (61). A large proportion of ICU patients at some stage in their stay require renal replacement therapy, usually hemofiltration. The assessment of ionized calcium is of paramount importance for this process, particularly in the assessment of buffer correction and when citrate is used as an anticoagulant. The calculation of "corrected" calcium, on the traditional basis of adjustment for changes in serum albumin concentration, is likely to be unreliable in ICU patients who will invariably have serum albumin concentrations in the range where analytical precision is poor and when other calcium-binding proteins such as globulins may be abnormal. In addition, the effects of acid-base disturbance are not taken into account in the routine laboratory measurement of total calcium. In hospitals that use "care maps" to assist junior staff in clinical management, ionized calcium requests may become routine specific analyses and the results regularly noted by clinical and nursing staff (62).

Serum *magnesium* declines by up to 65% in critical illness as a result of high metabolic demand, decreased absorption, and renal and gastrointestinal loss (62–64). The most common cause of hypomagnesemia in the ICU is from renal loss, magnesuria enhanced in metabolic acidosis, diuresis, and drug therapy affecting renal tubular function such as amphotericin and cyclosporin. Traditionally, serum total magnesium is measured daily and low levels are considered a sufficient marker of depleted total body magnesium to initiate magnesium replacement. In general, this practice probably suffices, as there are no convincing studies to show that hypomagnesemia causes major complications in the ICU although it must be assumed at the least to compromise electrical conduction and contractility in cardiac muscle. The most practical method of assessing total body magnesium status is measuring the excretion of a magnesium load, which can be achieved in ICU patients providing they have adequate renal function. The hypoproteinemia present almost universally in ICU patients adds a further complication and, if profound, may lead to misinterpretation of the serum total magnesium level, as approximately 30% of serum magnesium is albumin bound with 10% complexed to anions. Recent developments have led to the introduction of ionized magnesium measurements in some POCT systems but the clinical value of this measurement is yet to be determined (65,66). The most likely value of ionized magnesium assessment will be for patients with renal failure requiring hemofiltration or dialysis (67). However, there is no evidence to suggest that the measurement of serum ionized magnesium is a better reflection of total body levels because less than 1% is in extracellular fluids.

Metabolites

Blood Lactate

A detailed discussion of the arguments for and against POC analysis of blood lactate in the ICU (15,36,38,68) is beyond the scope of this chapter. That blood or serum lactate measurements are of value in the management of conditions such as congenital organic acidemias, some toxic states, and some infective conditions—most notably severe falciparum malaria (40,42)—cannot be questioned. The argument that the knowledge of an elevated blood lactate level may not directly influence general patient management has been promoted for many years, but in the ICU the need for focused informed management weakens this argument considerably. Recent studies have highlighted the prognostic value of elevated lactate in a variety of critical care situations (36,69–72), most notably severe sepsis and poor tissue oxygenation (73,74). The implication of the lactate ion in the generation of a significant base deficit, with its recognized poor prognosis, may lead to an acceleration in therapy of the acid-base defect in many circumstances. Part of the reason why lactic acidosis—defined here as any metabolic acidosis with an elevated blood lactate concentration—carries such a stigma is that the condition arises when production exceeds clearance, which occurs mainly in the later stages of multiorgan failure where other treatment regimes may be of limited benefit. In conditions where lactate defines the degree of decreased oxygen delivery, it must be understood that in most circumstances the decline is global rather than local. Attempts to assess local hypoxia, such as that of the splanchnic bed that preempts the onset of multiorgan failure and lactic acidosis, have included much recent work from measurements of gastric tonometry measuring the relative (lactic) acidosis of the splanchnic vascular bed (72). Lactic acidosis is a severe condition, as there is limited specific therapy for the condition, and the strong acidosis itself is responsible for cardiac dysfunction and is putatively the ultimate cause of death.

In my clinical experience, the introduction of regular blood lactate measurements in the ICU, particularly in any patient with a metabolic acidosis and significant base deficit, leads to a surprising change in insight of the pathophysiology of many conditions encountered in the ICU. Lactate is often hypothesized as the offending anion in unexplained metabolic acidosis, but just as often other anions, usually related to unrecognized renal dysfunction (i.e., phosphate, sulphate, and hippurate) or to fasting (i.e., ketones), are implicated. Similarly, significant blood lactate elevation is found in many conditions where the acid-base disturbance is not clearly apparent due to compensatory mechanisms and interference in the respiratory component. In other words, the clinician needs to be wary of interpreting elevated blood lactate unless a condition, such as severe cardiovascular shock, sepsis, or severe malaria, is the main clinical presentation. Interpretation has to be carried out by computing the available information on oxygen delivery; cardiac, respiratory, and hepatic function; and clinical variables. Even in sepsis, the interpretation of elevated blood lactate is compromised by a lack of understanding of the mechanisms responsible for the elevation (70,75), and is further complicated by the metabolic effects of inotrope therapy, as in septic shock (76–80). The effects of epinephrine and norepinephrine can be profound in certain circumstances (81), and are probably mediated by effects on hepatic gluconeogenesis rather than via tissue hypoperfusion (82). Traditional teaching has been based on studies demonstrating the mechanism of lactic acidosis in sepsis as secondary to an increased metabolic rate and decreased peripheral oxygen delivery. Recent work has suggested that peripheral oxygen consumption is relatively normal and that lactate metabolism balance is disturbed by increased lactate production in tissues, such as the lung, particularly when heavily infiltrated by lymphocytes that have a high capacity for lactate production (83–88). This is further compromised by a decrease in liver lactate clearance as a result of the effects on intermediary metabolism by the mediators of the inflammatory response, which may themselves be influenced by tissue hypoxia or washout following reperfusion.

The ICU in the John Radcliffe Hospital at Oxford is currently studying the role of sodium lactate as a buffer in the replacement fluid in hemofiltration (HF). This subject has received attention from others in recent years (19,21,89); a recent observational study of ICU patients suggested that sodium lactate should be substituted with a bicarbonate buffer in all HF patients with lactic acidosis or in those who develop significant hyperlactatemia during the procedure (18). The rationale for this is based on the concern that there may be a risk of developing lactic acidemia from the use of a lactate salt by saturating the lactate metabolism mechanisms of the liver, leading to an accumulation of endogenous lactic acid. The use of sodium lactate is usually accompanied by an alkalinizing effect. The only likely situation where lactic acidosis might be provoked or worsened is when lactate clearance significantly declines, such as in end-stage hepatic failure accompanied by an overproduction of lactate. Analysis of results from 27 patients revealed that the worst outcome occurred in patients with blood lactates more than 5 mmol/L and an increasing base deficit during HF. This study adds support to the view that regular monitoring of blood gases and metabolites is essential throughout HF in order to evaluate correct buffer replacement (90), although further studies including crossover interventions are required and are in progress (Fig. 9.1).

Blood Glucose

Blood glucose has featured in POCT for over 2 decades, although recent refinements have improved reliability in such areas as the ICU where extremes of blood oxygenation and hematocrit have interfered with some previously employed methods (91–95). The need for glucose testing extends well beyond the relatively infrequent requirements of closely monitoring the treatment of diabetic ketoacidosis, when in fact other parameters such as gases, electrolytes, and lactate claim higher priority. The innate stress of ICU admission and treatment with typically high doses of catecholamine inotropes or steroids induces significant hyperglycemia. Specific therapy, usually insulin infusion, is often considered appropriate to control the hyperglycemia. High metabolic rate, undernutrition, hypoadrenalism (primary or secondary), and hepatic dysfunction in multiorgan failure all compromise energy metabolism and thus require regular glucose monitoring. In practice, most ICUs test blood glucose with each blood gas measurement (therefore, approximately seven times per day). Other dedicated POC glucose analyzers are available, and will be advantageous if the unit regularly uses integrated metabolite analysis and direct downloading to clinical databases. Critical factors for POCT glucose are the sensitivity and accuracy at the low end of the range, which are required for critical diagnosis and management of hypoglycemia.

POC analysis to date has offered little in the way of blood *ketone* analysis. Diabetic ketoacidosis is assumed in diabetic patients admitted with metabolic acidosis, in the absence of a high blood lactate level or other measured anion to explain it. This assumption may be supported by urine analysis for ketonuria, but there are flaws in this process and many mixed-cause metabolic acidoses will not be properly documented. Another problem with relying on dry chemistry urinalysis (the strips can be used also for qualitative plasma analysis) for ketones is reliance on the acetoacetate measurement: the ketone represents only 10% or less of the total ketone concentration. The sensitivity of these analyses may not always be adequate when there is an elevated hydroxybutyrate/acetoacetate ratio such as occurs in severe acidoses. Recent work in ICU patients suggests that the mitochondrial redox state inferred from this ratio could prove to be of prognostic value in sepsis, although the instability of acetoacetate might make such an assessment impractical (79,96).

The level of ketosis may not directly influence clinical management, but an indication of the relative contribution of ketones to a mixed acidosis would be helpful in many cases. This is particularly important in starvation ketosis, which can be very severe and life threatening and not so readily recognized where there is no profound hypoglycemia (97–100). Alcohol toxicity is an increasing contributor to hospital admissions and can present with profound metabolic acidosis, predominantly a metabolic starvation ketosis that may be complicated by an underlying lactic acidosis compromised by hepatic insufficiency and thiamine deficiency (101,102). Nutritional assessment does not include monitoring the development of ketosis, but because nutritional support, and particularly the timing of onset following surgery, plays a significant role in ICU management, the role of POCT ketone analysis needs investigating (103).

Renal Function

For most purposes, routine central laboratory analysis of renal function performed by daily serum electrolyte, urea, and creatinine measurements, provide adequate assessment of renal function and of fluid management for ICU patients. Changes in glomerular function may be monitored in this forum as in any other in medicine, as long as the limitations of the parameters are accepted. More regular assessment of glomerular function could be promoted in patients with multiorgan failure (MOF), particularly as part of the assessment and monitoring of renal replacement therapies. Prediction of acute renal failure and tubular necrosis is required early, and assessment of free water clearance, fractional excretion of sodium, and urine/serum osmolality should be considered regularly and would be carried out if the process were managed by POCT. Many POCT analyzers now measure urea (urea nitrogen), and some measure creatinine also. Although there have been stringent technical assessments, studies are needed to evaluate clinical effectiveness (104). Of particular interest would be using POCT of renal function as part of the monitoring process during renal replacement therapies. Urine markers of vascular permeability, such as albu-

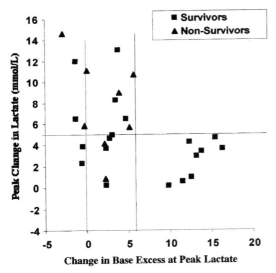

FIGURE 9.1. Observational study in 27 hemofiltration patients in ICU. All patients received lactate-buffered replacement fluid, and lactate tolerance was monitored by peak changes in blood lactate and base excess. All had starting base deficits of τ5 mmol/L and 14 (52%) had blood lactates τ3.5 mmol/L. Deteriorating base deficit and rising blood lactate to τ10 mmol was associated with worst outcome, while significant improvement in base deficit was best in patients with lactate tolerance and associated with survival (From Holloway P, Benham S, St John A. The value of blood lactate measurements in ICU: an evaluation of the role in the management of patients on haemofiltration, *Clin Chim Acta* 2001;307(1–2):9–13, with permission.)

min/creatinine ratio and colloid oncotic pressure, are discussed in the "Future Developments" section.

Hematology

Abnormalities in blood count and coagulation are the two most common hematology complications requiring investigation and monitoring in ICU patients, although increasingly patients may also need assessment of fibrinolysis (105,106). For the average nonhematologic patient, the abnormalities are secondary to the underlying disease or one of the disease processes such as sepsis, or in the case of coagulation, may also be due to an aspect of the patient's treatment. Assessment of the full blood count is a daily routine and in most instances can be carried out in the central laboratory where differential counts are provided and blood films can be prepared using reflex protocols. Although use of the white count is a crude but widely used marker of infection, there is seldom a requirement for more frequent testing, and thus rare indications for POCT. There are similar requirements for the use of ESR as a marker of inflammation and infection. For platelet measurements and d-dimers in the context of disseminated intravascular coagulation (DIC), there is a strong case for providing them at POC as there may be a need for frequent monitoring (e.g., every 2 hours) and for rapid change in management (i.e., a short therapeutic turnaround time) (107–110). Fibrinogen degradation products (FDP) measurement has been a traditional adjunct to DIC monitoring, and a recent study suggests that rapid and less expensive FDP testing would be adequate for this purpose once a diagnosis of DIC is made (111). Frequent analysis of coagulation parameters is appropriate in this context and POCT methods are now available for prothrombin time, activated partial prothrombin time, and activated clotting time, as well as d-dimers, although this area of POCT has had many technical difficulties and has a disadvantage in not being fully integrated into blood gas analyzers (112). Assessment of coagulation parameters on a regular basis is now considered valuable for most patients in the ICU, whether as a marker for DIC, hepatic dysfunction, or drug interactions, or for the management and prevention of thrombotic embolic (105, 110). In ICUs, regular hemoglobin measurements and hematocrit calculations are being provided by co-oximetry using existing equipment. Increasing use of POC hematology is anticipated as technology advances. Understanding of the pathophysiology of DIC and other coagulation complications associated with sepsis is gradually unfolding, and the role of investigations to complement possible therapies such as protein C and antithrombin III replacement awaits the results of clinical trials (113–117). D-dimer assessment on admission to the ICU has been suggested as a valuable marker of underlying microvascular pathology (118). Relatively well-established technology for thromboelastography (TEG) has been evaluated in cardiac surgery (119), and has been proposed as a valuable adjunct to POCT in critical care for platelet and fibrinolysis evaluation as well as coagulation (120). It is uncertain whether there is a role for TEG in monitoring coagulation during HF (121,122). Further studies of TEG in the ICU are needed.

Derived Parameters

The POCT processes available in the ICU are capable of calculating a variety of derived parameters, the most commonly required being bicarbonate, base excess, total CO_2, $p50$, anion gap, and osmolality. Bicarbonate, base excess, and total CO_2 can be further standardized for certain conditions and different fluid compartments. Until blood lactate and chloride measurements were routinely available from POCT, the base excess provided the most valuable marker of metabolic acid-base disturbance and it is still widely used in the rapid assessment of the sick patient (34,123–125).

The anion gap has fluctuated in popularity as a means of assessing metabolic acidoses. Despite the enhancement of the metabolic profile with the availability of lactate measurements, this estimate of unmeasured anions in combination with the base excess is still valuable (126,127). However, in the absence of blood lactate measurements, the anion gap cannot be relied upon as an indicator of lactate (128,129). For the assessment and management of metabolic alkaloses, a new derived parameter—strong ion difference (SID)—has been proposed (see "Metabolic Monitoring" subsection under "Future Developments"). Clinical studies are needed on this as well as the clinical value of some of the other derived parameters available in the ICU. Clinical examples tracking the changes in certain measured and derived parameters are shown in case examples (Figs. 9.2, 9.3, and 9.4).

The Testing Process

Benchtop versus Bedside

The selection of equipment for POC testing in intensive care is inevitably influenced by factors such as bed capacity; patient case mix; and the relative interest, organization, and turnaround times provided by the established diagnostic facilities on site. The rapidly evolving technology in this field not only provides a wide choice of equipment but also opportunities for weighing the many factors in selecting between benchtop and bedside analysis. The traditional process for POC testing in the ICU has involved the use of one or more dedicated benchtop analyzers situated at some distance from the patients, either at the nursing workstation or more typically in a side room or small laboratory. This arrangement may originally have evolved from practical considerations such as lack of space in the patient clinical area for blood gas analysis; convenience of access for all users, including non-ICU users; health and safety factors; noise; and ease of access for maintenance and servicing. Most of these considerations will continue to prevail, although most new analyzers are comparatively smaller and almost silent, and much of the routine quality control and troubleshooting can be carried out automatically and even remotely. The availability of bedside analyzers provides some opportunities for improving ICU clinical management, but there are many practical considerations that impact on the decision of which system to implement (Table 9.7).

Bedside POC analysis, provided either by handheld or by portable or mobile "benchtop" equipment, would appear to confer obvious advantages with respect to therapeutic turnaround time. For practical purposes, there should be a sufficient

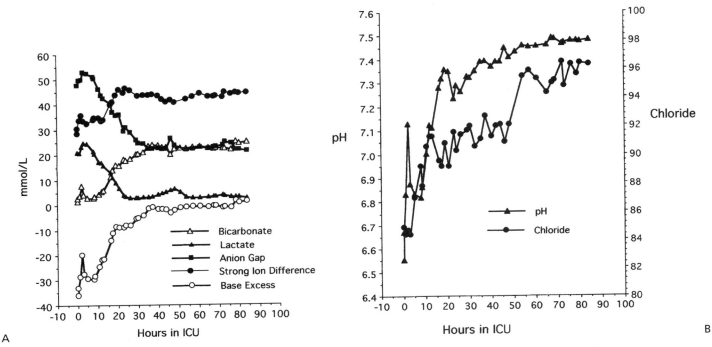

FIGURE 9.2. A, B: Metformin–lactic acidosis. A type-2 diabetic patient admitted to the accident and emergency ward with severe lactic acidosis secondary to a combination of metformin therapy and deteriorating renal function. Fundamental treatment included hemofiltration using a lactate-free replacement fluid buffered with bicarbonate. Note the 24-hour delay to achieve a normal blood lactate and thus strong ion difference (SID), and a delay of another 12 hours before bicarbonate, chloride, anion gap, and pH returned to normal. The SID proved of little value in this context.

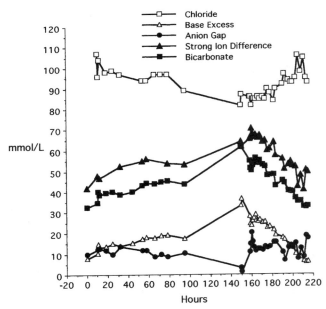

FIGURE 9.3. Metabolic alkalosis. A 10-day period during a 3-month stay in the intensive care unit by a woman recovering from extensive bowel surgery. A gradual loss of acid from the gastrointestinal tract deteriorated during a period (100 to 144 hours) when clinicians were unable to monitor blood gases. The fall in chloride was accompanied by significant increases in bicarbonate, base excess, strong ion difference (SID), and an expected fall in the anion gap. Chloride replacement coincided with a slow correction of the alkalosis traced clearly by the return of SID to normal. Note the lack of sensitivity of the changes in the anion gap.

number of bedside analyzers to ensure availability, and for the most extreme levels of intensive care an analyzer should be provided for each bed. The nurse is not required to leave the bedside to perform the analysis; for some tests and certain equipment, less than 2 minutes are necessary, compared to an average of 7 minutes using the more distant benchtop. In order to perform conventional benchtop analysis, a nurse from an adjacent bed or area is required to provide nursing "cover" for the duration. Protagonists of bedside analysis will argue that this requirement impacts on the nursing complement, a major factor in intensive care costs. There is little evidence, however, to support this argument, and performing POC analysis is only one of several reasons why the nurse may need to leave the bedside during a shift. Handheld devices and most portable equipment for bedside analysis use cartridge-based technology, with a limited range of analyses per cartridge. For a quick assessment of arterial gases prior to or after changes in ventilation, use of a single cartridge at the bedside would appear to be ideal. However, incorporating regular metabolic monitoring with these assessments of ventilation status may be more useful. Thus, whereas a sample taken to a benchtop multichannel analyzer requires only a single maneuver for all available tests, which are usually analyzed simultaneously, the bedside process may require the sequential use of three or more cartridges to acquire the same data. This may not only result in a longer therapeutic turnaround, but is also likely to distract the nurse from clinical observation and management, thus negating any advantage from performing the analyses at bedside. In a study comparing

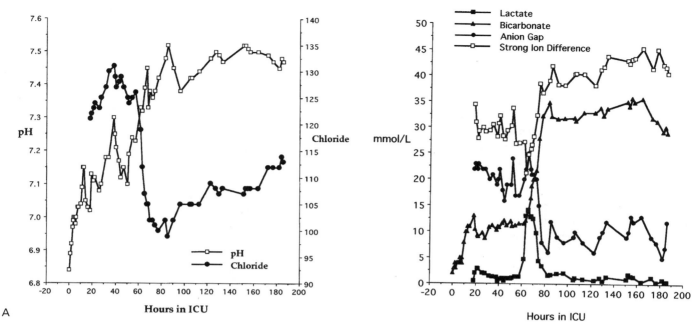

FIGURE 9.4. A, B: Hyperchloraemic acidosis. A type-1 diabetic patient presented with what appeared to be uncomplicated but severe ketoacidosis, but failed to respond rapidly to routine treatment. Admission to the intensive care unit coincided with improved point-of-care monitoring with the benefit of chloride and lactate measurements and thus anion gap and strong ion difference (SID) calculations. The severe hyperchloraemic acidosis, which was possibly due to a renal tubular acidosis or to saline treatment, improved with hemofiltration (HF) with lactate-buffered replacement fluid. The correction in bicarbonate and anion gap heralded the improvement in the acidosis, while the changes in SID were nonphysiological, as they reflected in part the changes in blood lactate resulting from the lactate load from the HF treatment.

TABLE 9.7. BENCHTOP VERSUS BEDSIDE ADVANTAGES AND DISADVANTAGES

	Advantages	Disadvantages
Benchtop	Greater range of analyzers	Transport requirements
	Greater range of tests and derivatives	Larger sample volumes
	Easier access for maintenance, etc.	Longer therapeutic TAT
	Simultaneous assays of full range	Too much data, too often
	Single QA process	Downtime for calibration
	Easy interface to computer systems	Downtime for maintenance
	May provide service to non-ICU units	Downtime for breakdown
	Remote QA and troubleshooting	Damage risk by non-ICU staff
	Low cost per test	High equipment cost
	Password protection	—
Bedside	Shorter therapeutic TAT	
	Potential saving of nurse time	Limited range of tests
	Almost zero maintenance	Limited range per cartridge
	Less downtime	Need for multiple cartridges
	Quick measurement of ventilator gases	QA performed by users
	Low equipment cost	Cartridge storage and preparation
	Value for low-volume users	High cost per test
	Value of mobility in ICU	Risk from mobility (e.g., theft)
	Ease of user training (mobility)	More complex interfacing
	Low sample volumes	—

ICU, intensive care unit; QA, quality assurance; TAT, turnaround time.

staff satisfaction with bedside, benchtop, and central laboratory analyses of blood gases, glucose, and electrolytes, the benchtop was preferred, followed by bedside (8).

Concerns about monitoring quality control (QC) of bedside equipment are only likely to emerge in large ICUs where QC would require prolonged daily input by dedicated personnel and when this activity would compromise constant availability of the devices. Nurses will usually be prepared to perform the minimum QC, providing the rest of the calibration process is simple and quick. Nonclinical personnel involved in this would spend more time in the unit's clinical area and would probably be disadvantaged by bedside analysis. This may add to concerns about infection control.

The main concern when considering bedside analysis for a large ICU is balancing benefits from shorter therapeutic turnaround times against higher running costs. Most handheld devices and portable analyzers have been designed for relatively low usage and are most efficient and economical when less than 20 samples are analyzed per day. For the small two- to three-bed ICU and the average high dependency unit, such throughput is likely and this process could be effective, particularly when the unit is not providing analyses for other clinical areas. Costs of bedside analysis may be 3 to 10 times higher than benchtop analysis. For an average ICU, bedside analysis is not likely cost effective. Another important factor to consider is that the apparent faster therapeutic turnaround from bedside analysis is reduced to a practical minimum by the interfacing of benchtop analysis with clinical computer data systems. This reduces the processes at the benchtop to simple sample introduction and PID, which should not take more than 25 seconds. The instrument can then be left to complete the analyses, the results of which would be downloaded instantly to the database and be accessible at the bedside by the time the nurse has returned there.

Available Technologies

The current range of technology available in Europe that is appropriate for use in the ICU appears in Table 9.8. The basic framework for all has been the blood gas analyzer with electrolyte and metabolite channels added as technology and demand have dictated. While these technologies have been developed with some guidance from the understanding of the physiological processes that need to be monitored in critically ill patients, certain areas, such as acid-base status, have been subject to changes in fashion. These changes, such as the use of base excess and/or anion gap, have not been driven by POCT technological developments. Assessment of acid-base status is the most vital marker of respiratory and metabolic function, and there can be little argument for excluding any of the vital parameters for this assessment in the ICU. Thus, equipment that does not incorporate a chloride channel, or only at the expense of another parameter such as calcium or glucose, may be a disadvantage in this setting. It is worth pointing out that for some measured and derived parameters, changes in the trend provide the most useful information at the bedside and regular recording of all necessary components is essential. This is particularly significant for analyzers that do not incorporate lactate measurement in cases where the calculation of anion gap becomes more significant.

TABLE 9.8. CURRENT AVAILABLE TECHNOLOGY FOR POCT IN INTENSIVE CARE IN EUROPE

Manufacturer	Model(s)
Benchtop	
AVL-Roche (Roche Diagnostics GnbH, D-628298 Mannheim, Germany)	Omni series
Bayer (Bayer House, Strawberry Hill, Newbury, Berkshire, RG14 1JA, UK)	RapidPoint, RapidLab series
Instrumentation Laboratories (IL (Europe), Viale Monza, 338-20128 Milan, Italy)	Synthesis
Nova Biomedical (Biomen Diagnostics, Pentos House, Falcon Business Park, Ivanhoe Road, Finchampstead, Berkshire RG40 1QQ, UK)	Stat Profile series
Radiometer (Radiometer Ltd, Manor Court, Manor Royal, Crawley, West Sussex RH10 2PY, UK)	700 series
Bedside	
AVL-Roche	OPTI CCA, OPTI R
Abbott Laboratories (Abbot Laboratories Ltd, MediSense Products, Abbot House, Norden Road, Maidenhead, Berkshire SL6 4XF, UK)	I-stat
Instrumentation Laboratories	GEM Premier 3000
Radiometer	ABL77

POCT, point-of-care testing.

Quality Assurance Process

The concept of quality assurance (QA), the entire quality process that includes QC, has now become accepted by the majority of those involved in providing health care, although it has been well entrenched in pathology laboratories for decades. Just a few years ago, a suggestion to nursing or medical staff that they would be required to undertake QC measurements on the analytical equipment they were entrusted to use to support their clinical management would have been met in most settings by firm resistance if not apathy or, even worse, derision. The most that would be considered would be correlation, usually in an informal way, with simultaneous results from the central laboratory. Modern methods of risk management and clinical governance have prepared the way for QA and this is as vital in POCT as it is in any other area in medicine. In most settings, QA is—and indeed should be—supervised by the central laboratories that will retain ultimate responsibility for the use of POC analyses. For the use of bedside POCT in the ICU, it is likely more practical that regular QA measurements would be carried out by users, who are predominantly nurses. This process requires appropriate documentation so that the POCT system can be included in accreditation schemes in place at the site. For many POCT devices, this process is supported by the equipment manufacturers, which allows for more centralized documentation of QA. It should be realized that QA covers preanalytical, analytical, and postanalytical phases. Several published guidelines are available and most countries now insist on regulation for POCT (130,131).

Equipment manufacturers provide internal QC material for use on their equipment, and in most countries external QA schemes are available for blood gas analysis, electrolytes, metabolites, and coagulation parameters. For blood gases, the best control material is a tonometered blood-based product, which can be prepared in a central laboratory and used for most if not all of the hospital's blood gas analyzers. This system works well in practice.

Maintenance

While most bedside POCT equipment is virtually maintenance free, benchtop analyzers require regular maintenance for system cleaning and for checking and changing consumables and sensors. Most sensors have a limited life span and variable stability, and require changing on a regular basis, depending on type and on rate of usage. Many systems now provide at extra cost remote access to allow checking of fluid levels, electrode status, calibration and QC, and other critical maintenance parameters, thus reducing the time required for on-site technical support. POCT equipment placed in busy clinical areas may not be easily accessible to laboratory technicians, and it is for this reason that siting of equipment in side rooms is often preferable. Despite the opportunity provided by remote access for monitoring equipment performance, benchtop analyzers still require daily cleaning and reagent changing, among other procedures.

Training of ICU Personnel

Current and future procedures for POCT in the ICU will only be acceptable and successful in clinical management if the users are given appropriate training. Facets of training include sampling, analysis, data processing, essential maintenance of equipment, interpretation of results, and management of unexpected results.

Training in the analytical process from obtaining fluid samples from the patient to sample handling and introduction to the analyzer, patient identification, and following the analytical pathway and processing of the data, should be carried out for each user individually. This should be coordinated by laboratory staff responsible for the hospital's POCT quality assurance and may be carried out by those involved in POCT equipment maintenance as well as by representatives of equipment manufacturers. Guidelines produced by laboratory accreditation authorities outline how training should be performed and documented (132,133). Requirements are becoming increasingly stringent and are incorporated into risk management policies. The ICU should appoint an individual responsible for overseeing initial and continuing training as well as liaison with laboratory technologists. The training of individuals can now be linked with user passwords, and most units find that this is a valuable means of both ensuring enforcement of training and preventing access to equipment by unauthorized and thereby reducing the attendant risk of abuse of the equipment. Such a policy will inevitably compromise the non-ICU use of POCT equipment, but should be invoked to enable adequate funding for POCT at other sites.

Although training in the use of POCT equipment is essential, of greater significance is training in the use of POC diagnostics in clinical management. The widespread practice of skill and responsibility transfer to lower-grade staff includes interpreting the management of some diagnostic tests and subsequent clinical actions. This practice has many benefits, including lower costs and greater job satisfaction for the individuals involved, but for the use of POCT, and particularly that in the ICU, such transfers must be very carefully assessed and carry some very high risks. Important concepts in clinical diagnostics relate to analytical precision and accuracy and to assay interferences, as well as differences between serum and whole blood analyses. These concepts should have been incorporated into training in medical school, and their significance is learned in the early years of clinical practice. However excellent the performance of a POCT analyzer may be, there will be occasions when results do not match clinical expectations and are inaccurate, perhaps for no identifiable reason. This is an accepted component and limitation of any clinical diagnostic process, and the clinician is trained to question anything that is unexpected or does not fit clinical assessments. This is a fundamental concept and must be transferred to those who adopt the management of POCT diagnostics. A prime example of a risk might evolve from a protocol for the management of serum potassium where nursing staff use POC whole blood potassium analysis for guidance on when to institute replacement or commence hypokalemic therapy. While such a protocol may be very valuable and practical, the system has to allow for the understanding of the physiological processes involved, the interaction of multiple pathological systems, the friability of the critically ill patient, assay interferences such as hemolysis, and for the unexpected "flyer" (134). Coping with unexpected results—knowing when to repeat analysis and/or send another sample for urgent analysis in the laboratory before taking what may be life-threatening action—becomes the responsibility of the transferee of these skills, and must be included in training. Such training will already be in place for much of the existing equipment in the ICU and would be expected for non-POCT analysis. This training can best be achieved by joint involvement of ICU clinicians and critical care clinical pathologists.

Connectivity

The users and manufacturers of POCT equipment in the ICU are now aware of the huge benefits to this process from efficient connectivity to clinical data systems that are increasingly used in ICU clinical management. Benchtop and bedside analytical equipment can now be interfaced with a large variety of clinical and laboratory data systems, and there is an impressive array of software available for remote access to POCT equipment for maintenance, QC, and patient data access. Not only does connectivity provide greater efficiency, but also compared to paper records, it adds extra security to, and an audit trail for, data transfer. Paper records are sometimes misplaced or are not immediately incorporated into the patient's clinical notes, and their absence may seriously compromise subsequent clinical management. There are, of course, medico-legal pressures to push this recording process to a more secure setting. For patient data to be usable, the user of the devices must enter patient details accurately, and this is becoming easier with the availability of barcode devices, which requires hospital admission barcode labeling, preferably using unique personal national health codes. Web-based software systems are available for localized use, but with the facility to use data for large-scale auditing of POCT activity, which is valuable for resourcing and epidemiological studies.

Security and Data Protection

The use of POCT equipment in the ICU could be secured by the use of passwords for trained users while the security of the equipment would be determined by appropriate siting surveillance and whether the unit uses immobile benchtop or portable bedside analysis. Reagent storage may be critical, particularly for hand-held bedside devices, and these facilities need to be adequately secure together with system power supplies. Security also covers the provision of adequate backup facilities, which may mean standby analyzers or availability of central laboratory analysis.

In most countries, the information transferred and stored by analytical equipment that contains patient medical histories is controlled by data protection laws that restrict access to authorized users. Although this may be easier to manage using simple systems without connectivity, the institution of the latter will ensure strict compliance, further enhanced by the use of password protection. This will extend beyond the ICU clinical data system if POCT equipment is connected to laboratory and/or hospital information systems to allow for wider data distribution, billing, and other accounting and audit processes.

FUTURE DEVELOPMENTS

The pace of change of technological developments in POC clinical diagnostics makes particularly relevant an attempt to project forward the direction that POCT in the ICU is likely to take in the next few years. It is difficult, and would be unwise, however, to speculate beyond the most realistic areas. Both technologists and clinical users will influence those involved in assessing the most productive routes for technological developments, but there is a unique role for the informed clinical pathologist who has an understanding of the clinical diagnostic process and for the stance that ICU clinicians and nurses will take with new developments. Changes will take place in this field and the pathologist should assume leadership in supporting the scientific rationale and to ensure that developments reach the standard of quality available in central laboratories and that they remain cost effective.

This section focuses on likely changes in the current repertoire but also projects in a limited way to new technologies that may emerge as a result of the molecular revolution from functional genomics to proteomics. ICU service providers are already aware that there is a finite capacity for those directly involved in patient care to perform diagnostic tests unless the process is integrated into bedside automated monitoring systems. The refinements in clinical diagnostics intimated here will almost definitely require a dedicated POC laboratory that might support all critical care areas and be sited in close proximity to them. This will be clear if the advances in science reveal a practical clinical physiological role for rapid assessment of proteome and genome snapshots. Studies will inevitably be needed to demonstrate that this would be cost

effective, but there is a real hope that critical care treatment will become far better targeted with more focused diagnostics.

Metabolic Monitoring

Extensions to Blood Gas and Electrolyte Profile and Acid-base Assessment

The existing electrolyte profile of POCT satisfies most common demands for clinical assessment of fluid balance, acid-base status, and extracellular ion distribution, and thus for membrane conductance and stability. The range is determined by the scope of available ion-specific electrodes that have been evaluated for whole-blood analysis. The most recent introduction to the scope of electrodes has been magnesium, although, as has already been discussed, the clinical value of ionized magnesium measurements in ICU patients remains to be established. In my experience, the learning curve for assessment and management of magnesium status can be long and intensive care clinicians are loath to instigate the relatively minor intervention of magnesium replacement when clinical benefits may be unclear.

Among the ions of potential value for clinical purposes, the phosphate anion, with its prime involvement in acid-base balance and cellular energetics, would seem to be a prime candidate for development as a POC analyte. Phosphorylation is such a key component of cell signaling and metabolic processes that it would not be unreasonable to assume it important, if not essential, that the blood's inorganic phosphorus concentration should be maintained within normal limits. Serum "phosphate" measurements are made routinely as part of the daily biochemistry profile but little is often done in response to the significant declines observed during the ICU stay. One significant reason for this reticence is that interpretation of serum phosphate levels in ICU patients is not straightforward. Most patients, particularly in the early postoperative phase, remain on limited nutritional support for the first few days in the ICU. During this period, there may be a considerable increase in metabolic demands. Apart from gastrointestinal losses and renal proximal tubular losses in some patients, there is a recognized disturbance in calcium homeostasis in many ICU patients—in part stimulated by the increased production of calcitonin precursors, such as procalcitonin in severe inflammation and particularly sepsis—which affects phosphate turnover (135). Other factors influencing serum phosphate in this situation are likely to include cytokines and other inflammatory mediators (136). Recent work has suggested that high ventilatory rates might play a significant role in inducing hypophosphatemia in ICU patients (137). Drug treatments and fluid replacement regimes will also influence serum phosphate, and increased metabolic phosphorylation requirements may mask the ensuing phosphate retention in patients with severe renal failure. Hypophosphatemia is a recognized complication during the management of diabetic ketoacidosis, and although there is limited literature to support phosphate replacement, it is usually given in this situation (138). Critical illness has profound effects on muscle bulk and activity, reflected in serum phosphate changes (139).

The relevant question for phosphate, as for other potential POC analytes in the ICU, is whether a clinical need exists for regular and fast-turnaround measurements of body fluid phosphate concentration that cannot be adequately provided by a central laboratory. The ICU dietician will note the serum phosphate in the daily profile as part of the nutritional assessment, but will not usually be involved in the management of severe hypophosphatemia in acute situations. The ideal in many situations would be to evaluate noninvasively phosphate metabolism and turnover in key tissues that may be compromised by circulatory failure or hypoxia (e.g., brain in stroke, myocardium in cardiac ischemia, liver in liver failure, or the kidney in acute renal failure). Nuclear magnetic resonance spectroscopy techniques have been developed for this, but they require movement of the patient to the equipment under strict conditions and this process is impractical and may in most cases be unethical. Thus, there are no clinical studies to support this procedure in ICU patients. An invasive technique for assessing muscle interstitial phosphate as well as pH, K^+, and lactate, involving microdialysis has been developed but there are no reports of its value in muscle and other tissues in clinical situations (140). The metabolic physician would reasonably argue that phosphate measurements should coincide in real time with blood gas and other electrolyte and metabolite concentrations as part of the metabolic profile, and thus would need to be available at POC. Clearly, studies are needed to evaluate this concept before such an inclusion in the POCT repertoire could be contemplated.

The use of the electrolyte panel in POCT has been confined largely to whole-blood analysis. Analysis of other fluids, particularly urine but also wound drainage fluid and pleural or peritoneal fluid, is not widely practiced, as most POC devices are not calibrated for analysis in these matrices. Urine assessment of pH, sodium, potassium, and chloride are indicated in vulnerable ICU patients where renal function needs to be protected and evaluated on a regular basis. Clinicians do not consider this assessment adequately, probably because the turnaround time from a distant central laboratory is usually unsatisfactory and there may be little if any expertise available when needed to help interpret the results. Thus, assessment of fractional excretion of sodium, serum and urine osmolality ratios, urine pH, and urine anion gap is usually problematic. POCT of the relevant parameters, particularly if linked to appropriate software for calculation, would be an advantage and aid in clinical management.

Regarding the use of electrolyte panels in its broadest sense, mention should be made here of colloid oncotic pressure (COP) measurement as an alternative to serum albumin and total protein in evaluating the risk of interstitial odema, which can significantly compromise the ICU patient and delay recovery. Significant changes to plasma COP ensue inevitably as part of the response to critical injury as a result of increases in capillary and glomerular permeability and the acute phase response on hepatic protein synthesis. The measurement of albumin, with or without total protein, fails to adequately reflect plasma COP as current clinical management of plasma volume expansion eschews albumin and other plasma protein replacement in favor of synthetic colloids. There are several products in use with differing molecular weights, and there is considerable patient variation in response, such that the rate and degree of replacement becomes largely empirical with the use of a loose protocol if any. The effect of inadequate treatment may be assessable clinically,

but there is concern that continuing and excessive colloid replacement may cause damage to capillaries and particularly glomeruli (141–143). POC measurement of plasma COP has been in sporadic use for some time and although measurement is inexpensive and would inevitably be cost effective as a bedside test, the techniques to date favor measurement in a side laboratory by dedicated staff.

The role of capillary leakage, particularly as a predictor of renal dysfunction and other organ failure, has been demonstrated by regular assessment of urine albumin excretion (144–147). Microalbuminuria, best assessed by urine albumin/creatinine ratios, could be measured at POC at intervals. This may prove to be of considerable value but further studies are needed on what would be a very manageable POCT process.

Recent reappraisals of the control mechanisms involved in determining acid base have highlighted a dilemma in using traditional parameters such as anion gap and base deficit, particularly in critical care (148–150). Known as the Stewart or Fencl-Stewart approach, this method recognizes that the independent variables determining the dissociation of weak electrolytes (H^+ and HCO^{3-}) and protein are PCO_2, the total concentration of weak acids, and the charge difference between the sum of strong cations and strong anions. The latter component, termed the strong ion difference (SID), can be derived by subtracting the sum of the measured strong anions (chloride and lactate) from the sum of strong cations (sodium, potassium, calcium, and magnesium) resulting in a "strong ion gap" (SIG) (151–153). The quoted reference intervals for this parameter are 40 to 42 mmol/L, and the SIG in most circumstances mirrors the anion gap with a rise in metabolic alkaloses (more than 45) and a fall in acidoses (less than 35). The concept here is to allow for the contribution of weak protein anions and focus on the powerful influence of sodium and chloride in the assessment of acid-base status, but this method's value in clinical management has yet to be proven (154). However, in one study the method has been shown to allow better prediction of mortality compared with base excess, anion gap, and lactate (126). Very high SIG values are seen in severe metabolic alkaloses with low serum chloride concentration, and the management of these conditions with sodium chloride replacement can be monitored more effectively using changes in SIG (155). SIGs can be measured at POC using most current equipment, and the clinical value of this measurement derived in the ICU needs to be evaluated.

Gastric tonometry is a relatively simple procedure that has been developed with the aim of providing earlier evidence of compromised splanchnic circulation or oxygen delivery (156). Based on the indirect measurement of intracellular pH from direct measurement of PCO_2 in adjacent tissues and of contiguous arterial gas (PCO_2 gap), the inference—which is supported by many studies—is that if the technique accurately measures local perfusion changes, these will occur before other more systemic markers of organ failure, such as hyperlactatemia, are manifest (157,158). Gastrointestinal mucosa has very high cell turnover and is highly susceptible to hypoperfusion, so subsequent mucosal necrosis is considered the herald of multiorgan failure, particularly in septic shock (159). Although new devices are relatively easy to insert and calibrate, they are semiinvasive, take time to equilibrate, and need frequent measurements.

There are as many skeptics as there are disciples of this technique, so it remains firmly in the research arena at present (160). A recent study in acute canine endotoxemia concluded that this measurement lacks adequate sensitivity and specificity at portal blood flow reductions of more than 50% (161). The most convincing evidence has come recently from duodenal and ileal sampling, but this type of sampling is technically more difficult. Less invasive and problematic is sublingual tonometry, but this too has yet to have proven clinical benefit (162).

Extensions to Metabolite Profile and to Cardiac Dysfunction Markers

The metabolite profile of POCT in the ICU is limited to glucose, lactate, urea, and creatinine, although few analyzers are available that measure all four. Separate analysis of bilirubin is also available but has very limited utility in adult units. There is currently much interest in assessment of mitochondrial function in ICU patients (96,163). Coincidental with this is a revival of the concept of assessing cytosolic and mitochondrial redox states in critical illness (79). In research laboratories and some clinical environments, these were inferred by lactate/pyruvate and 3-hydroxybutyrate/acetoacetate (ketone) ratio measurements as the latter are predominantly determined by the reduced nictotinamide adenine dinucleotide/nictotinamide adenine dinucleotide (NADH/NAD) ratios at respective cytosolic and mitochondrial intracellular sites. The normal ratio for both is approximately 10, but enzymatic analysis has limited sensitivity for pyruvate and acetoacetate at normal concentrations. Because the instability of the latter metabolites also requires rapid analysis, the resurgence of interest in these metabolites for clinical evaluation would definitely justify POC analysis. As mentioned earlier, there would be a considerable advantage in measuring blood ketones in critically ill patients.

POC measurement of biochemical markers of cardiac ischemia, particularly the troponins, is discussed elsewhere as applicable to other clinical settings and may only have a limited role in the ICU (46). Changes in cardiac activity and performance from slight dysrhythmias to major infarcts are closely monitored in the ICU patient and most are detected within a short time interval from the event. Troponin measurements have very high specificity but sensitivity is relatively poor for ICU management. The main situations where they may be of use in ICU are in the assessment or exclusion of cardiac contusion in trauma or to help stratify a cardiac event (164). There may be a role for troponin in the management of ICU sepsis (165) and perhaps also in combination with myoglobin and troponin measurements as provided at the POC by the Cardiac Reader, particularly to help rule out cardiac ischemia, but studies are needed.

Much attention has recently centered on brain natriuretic peptide (BNP) as a potential marker for evaluating cardiac failure. Existing clinical diagnostic and evaluation criteria can be significantly enhanced by measurements of this peptide, which is produced by the cardiac atria, and the levels in serum correlate well with the degree of atrial dysfunction (166,167). While most of the attention has been in outpatient and acute clinical admission assessment, there is a putative role for this test in the management of the ICU patient, and a POC method for BNP

analysis is available that could be applied in the ICU (168). This test could also be applicable in the interpretation of data from assessments of pulmonary artery catheter wedge pressure (169). More studies are needed.

Markers of Sepsis and Inflammation

Sepsis is the most significant complication and cause of mortality in ICU patients. In a recent survey in the United States, sepsis occurred in 2.26 of 100 hospital admissions with 50.5% cared for in ICUs, which in turn accounted for 6% to 10% of ICU admissions (170). The hospital mortality rate was 28.6%, which increased to 34.1% in ICU patients. The projected total mortality rate attributable to sepsis in the United States was higher than for myocardial infarction. Also revealed were average costs of more than US$20,000 for a hospital stay of almost 20 days per case of sepsis. The awareness of the risk for poor outcome from sepsis makes the ICU clinician constantly vigilant for the evidence of infection, and monitoring systems are usually in place to pick up early clinical and physiological signs and symptoms. The clinician is aware that most of the traditional infection markers are predominantly markers of the host's inflammatory response and thus lack specificity and also sensitivity, particularly in the early phase. The clinician needs to distinguish between the systemic inflammatory response syndrome (SIRS) and sepsis, and would like markers to be effective as early as possible, particularly in susceptible patients.

Acute phase proteins in serum have been used for many years in general medicine and particularly in infectious disease units to aid in the diagnosis of infection; the most widely used is C-reactive protein (CRP) (Table 9.9). CRP is synthesized in the liver in rapid response to IL6 stimulation and increases, which are usually

TABLE 9.9. CURRENT AND PUTATIVE MARKERS OF SEPSIS AND SIRS

Marker	Change
Body temperature	↓or↑
Heart rate	↑
Blood pressure	↓
Serum albumin	↓
Serum C reactive protein (CRP)	↑
White blood count (wbc)	↓or↑
Serum procalcitonin (PCT)	↑
Serum complement factors	↓or↑
Endotoxinemia	↑
Serum interleukins (IL-1, 4, 6, 8, 10)	↑
Serum interleukin receptors (IL-1, 2, 6)	↑
Serum tumor necrosis factor (TNF) and receptors	↑
Serum phospholipase 2	↑
Serum elastase	↑
Serum adhesion molecules (VCAM-1, ICAM-1, ELAM-1)	↑
Serum selectins (p-selectin, E-selectin)	↑
Serum neopterin	↑
Serum brain natriuretic peptide (BNP)	↑
Blood platelets	↓
Serum plasminogen activator inhibitor (PAI)	↑
Blood lactate	↑
Bactericidal/permeability increasing protein (BPI)	↑

SIRS, systemic inflammatory response syndrome.

substantial, occur within 3 to 4 hours of the onset of infection. Like other acute phase proteins, it has limitations to specificity for infection, as CRP levels also increase in many noninfective inflammatory conditions, such as rheumatoid arthritis, inflammatory bowel disease, and also following myocardial infarction. These specificity limitations have restricted the use of CRP in the ICU, and many clinicians do not consider CRP to be a valuable sepsis marker in the context of very sick and often traumatized patients with SIRS. Existing physiological markers, such as temperature, heart rate, and respiratory rate, as well as white cell count, comprise the usual infection panel and are satisfactory as infection markers in many cases, but again there is an unacceptable lack of specificity for sepsis. Recently, the infection probability score (IPS) system has been suggested. The IPS combines all of these parameters plus CRP and the sepsis-related (or alternatively sequential) organ failure assessment (SOFA) score; all are separately weighted for severity. Preliminary results using the IPS suggest that it could be superior to the traditional panel with impressive receiver operator characteristics, although more refinements of this model are probably needed to enhance sensitivity. When used in the ICU, widely available standardized laboratory assays for CRP are interpreted in the same way as the IPS, usually without formal measurement of SOFA score. In hospitals that lack fast CRP therapeutic turnaround, POC analysis of CRP might be valuable used alone or with other markers, particularly in the monitoring of the response to a known infection and for early detection of recurrence (171).

Much recent attention has been centered on procalcitonin (PCT)—another serum sepsis marker, a small protein precursor of calcitonin—which may have independent immune function in bacterial sepsis (172). Studies of calcitonin levels in critical care demonstrated a rise in infection and sepsis and these levels were shown to be positive predictors of mortality (173). PCT has been shown in many studies to be elevated in patients with sepsis and infection (174). Serum PCT has a larger dynamic range than CRP and levels rise earlier in the inflammatory process by 6 to 8 hours with a half-life of approximately 1 day. One recent study suggested that PCT has good predictive value for sepsis and severe multiple organ dysfunction syndrome (MODS) in trauma patients (175). Other studies have highlighted that while there is an increase in PCT in noninfectious inflammatory conditions in the ICU, such as burns, cardiogenic shock, and necrotizing pancreatitis, it appears to be still a better discriminator of sepsis than CRP. Many other clinical studies compared PCT with existing markers (176–185), and not all reached the same conclusions about the superiority of PCT. Studies to date have used an immunoluminometric assay, which measures procalcitonin plus other calcitonin precursors in a minimum turnaround time of 3 hours. The recent introduction of POC analytical devices will enable more clinical studies and is likely to push this into prominence in the ICU arena. Incorporation of PCT instead of CRP in an IPS would be worth evaluating. At present, PCT is generally favored as a marker and predictor of severe sepsis.

Other putative sepsis markers with potential for clinical use at POC include serum amyloid A protein, which has similar characteristics to CRP, BNP, and interleukin 6 (IL-6). The latter, for which there is a qualitative POC test (SEPTEST™), increases from 2 to 8 hours from the onset of infection and is persistent

unlike most other proinflammatory cytokines (185a). Other markers listed in Table 9.9, particularly the inflammatory mediators, and also proteomic markers yet to be identified, may eventually be helpful as markers of the host-specific response and thus help target therapy. Factors such as renal and hemofiltration clearance will need to be factored into the analysis (186). There may also be a place for the measurement of markers to assist management of specific therapies, such as the recently reported positive benefit of recombinant human activated protein C [drotrecogin alfa (activated)] replacement in severe sepsis (187). All these as well as CRP and PCT would need to be measured serially.

Functional analysis of host immune response to specific infections—for example, suppression of monocyte HLA-DR expression or *ex vivo* analysis of monocyte function in response to endotoxins such as TNF production—have been studied in sepsis and the latter may become a practical tool suitable for analysis at POC (188–190).

Continuous Monitoring

Techniques involving immobilized enzymes were developed in the 1970s for continuous *ex vivo* monitoring of metabolites in a diluted heparinized blood flow, but never reached regular clinical use. More recently, biosensor technology has become available with the potential for use in continuous *in vivo* and *ex vivo* monitoring (191,192). Biosensors combine the use of biological recognition molecules, such as enzymes or antibodies, with transducers using physical (e.g., thermal or gravimetric), electrochemical (e.g., potentiometric or amperometric), or optical systems. There are still many development difficulties, particularly with selection of the polymeric interface membranes and data processing, but systems have been developed for monitoring blood pH, P_{CO_2} P_{O_2}, sodium, potassium, glucose, and hematocrit. A study using an in-line *ex vivo* monitoring system in neonates to assess bias, precision, and blood loss has been reported with encouraging results and further studies are needed (193). Other systems have been reported for blood gases and a range of metabolites (194–198).

Microdialysis techniques have been developed specifically for ICU use with the capability of measuring glucose, phosphate lactate, and other selected metabolites, such as pyruvate, glycerol, urea, and glutamate (199). Systems that are still in the research phase monitor brain metabolism, ischemia in microsurgical flaps, and tissue fluid changes to detect organ failure (200–206). Small vials containing reagents for metabolites equilibrate at the chosen insertion site and are then analyzed in a dedicated POC analyzer. Software has been developed for results of these analyses to be incorporated into bedside monitors. They are yet to reach widespread acceptance in the general ICU and further studies are needed in both general and neurosurgical ICUs.

The value of continuous monitoring of any parameter in medicine must be clearly defined as biological variation. Dynamics affecting body fluid concentrations of most analytes mean that trends or rate of change over several collection intervals will be the only valuable feedback for clinical management. This is the fundamental concern of the clinician when considering monitoring of any kind and, if one considers interpretation of pulse oximetry as an example, for each analyte the noise in the system needs to be understood and built into the clinical response. Concerns about the reliability of existing systems and misinterpretation of sudden and perhaps unsustained changes have thus far kept biochemical monitoring in the research environment for most clinical situations.

Molecular Testing

POCT Pathogen Diagnostics

Our understanding of the range of pathogenic microbes is limited, partly because diagnostic tests have until recently been restricted by reliance on culture techniques. The ICU clinician is aware that much of the pathology in sepsis, particularly the systemic pathology, relates to the host inflammatory response to the infection, which continues long after appropriate antibiotic therapy has neutralized or killed the invading pathogen. Identification of the pathogen(s) is, however, eagerly sought as early as possible after the onset of sepsis for validation and correction of antimicrobial therapy, and current management requires rapid diagnosis as well as drug sensitivity and resistance. Empiric antimicrobial therapy prior to sample collection usually limits the sensitivity of culture techniques. The emergence of full genome sequences of microbial pathogens has not only enhanced our understanding of many infectious diseases but has also provided a range of technologies for improving and speeding diagnosis. Thus, polymerase chain reaction (PCR) diagnostic methods, which use selected genome sequences as molecular signatures for a number of pathogens, are now in clinical use for identification, strain typing, and resistance characteristics, and are beginning to address the unmet needs in this field. New methods will be able to identify some of the putative pathogens that have been uncultivable to date. Other benefits from the understanding of infectious disease genomics will be identification of products of microbial ribosomal DNA for serological diagnosis as well as therapeutic targets (207). High-density DNA multiplex microarrays could allow rapid microbial and viral detection.

There is a burden of bacterial DNA in the blood of normal healthy individuals, and we will need to understand this as a confounding factor. Much more relevant is the emergence of information on variability in the nature and kinetics of the host response to different pathogens and at different doses. For many responses in cytokines, chemokines, transcription regulators, for example, there are large differences between Gram −ve and Gram +ve infections. Genetic variations in the host response will need to be identified. As this type of information is unraveled, it is possible that characterization of active infection could be achieved by a combination of selective assessment of host response and genomic pathogen diagnosis. This would be computer aided and the clinical value of rapid diagnosis would be the greatest from POC analysis of these parameters. Technological advances in this area will make this approach a practical consideration, but it will need to be reliable, cost effective, and meet all QA and security criteria.

Host Risk Factor Genotyping

As discussed previously, more detailed molecular characterization of host response to infections may help to identify and target

appropriate treatment. Our understanding of the processes involved in host inflammatory response has advanced considerably in recent years. The results from more than 20 failed clinical trials of immunomodulation therapy for severe sepsis have suggested that innate host variability, particularly in the generation of endogenous mediators, plays a significant role in determining a poor outcome (208). The basis of this variability appears to be differences in the cytokine production profile released from proinflammatory (TH1) and antiinflammatory (TH2) T cells, due in part to allelic polymorphism in promoter regions of certain genes. Several studies describe associations between single nucleotide polymorphisms (SNPs or SNIPs) for mediators and susceptibility for infection or poor outcome. These include SNPs in tumor necrosis factor (TNF) promoter genes for the risk of cerebral malaria and mortality from sepsis in the ICU, plasminogen activator inhibitor (PAI) and mannose binding lectin (MBL) for meningococcal disease, and interleukin 1 receptor antagonist (IL-1ra) for poor outcome from severe sepsis (209–215). Many other studies have reported SNP associations (focused mainly on proinflammatory mediators) with poor outcomes in critical illness; the clinical relevance of these associations is still not clear (Table 9.10) (216,217). In the postgenome era, large-scale SNP scans are now being planned and current evidence suggests approximately 4.8 million SNPs in the 26,000 genes, a third of which have no known role. It is likely that many more associations between SNPs and clinical syndromes will be found. It should be noted that knowledge of SNP variability and associations does not infer transcriptional and posttranslational differences in expression of gene products. In addition, SNP analysis for selected genes will be productive only for genes with identifiable functional associations. Various methods are available for SNP analysis, some in current clinical use to assess transplantation risk factors, and many will be applicable to rapid POCT if or when it becomes relevant. For a restricted range of SNP analysis, dipstick technology is very feasible, while scans of approxi-

TABLE 9.10. SELECTED PROCESSES OF HOST RESPONSE IN SIRS WITH KNOWN OR PUTATIVE SNPS ASSOCIATED WITH SEVERE SEPSIS

Process	Examples
Infection susceptibility	Mannose binding lectin (MBL)
	Vitamin D receptor
Cytokines	Tumor necrosis factor (TNF)
	Interleukin 1 (IL-1)
	Lymphotoxin alpha
Adhesion molecules/co-stimulation	ICAM-1
	L-selectin
Chemokine receptors	Duffy
	CC-CKR-5
Coagulation/fibrinolysis/ atherosclerosis	Plasminogen activator inhibitor (PAI)
	Apo-E
	ACE-1
Antigen presentation	Heat shock proteins (HSP)
	Transporter in antigen presentation (TAP) 1, 2

SIRS, systemic inflammatory response syndrome; SNP, single nucleotide polymorphism.

mately 100 SNPs could be achieved by sequence specific primer (SSP) PCR methods already in use in transplant tissue-typing laboratories. For large-scale rapid analysis of thousands of SNPs, the Invader™ (Third Wave Technologies, Madison, WI, USA) technology is the most applicable (218).

Novel Proteome Analysis

Knowledge of the human genome sequence leads systems biology to the next phase of mRNA expression, which includes protein synthesis, proteomics, and the regulatory (epigenetic) networks that convert the chromosomal digital information into four-dimensional functioning biological systems, sometimes referred to as the "interactome." Proteomics—the study of protein expression and function on a genome scale—is expected to lead to a greater understanding of the key roles of protein-protein, protein-glyco-protein, and other protein-substrate interactions. This research requires high throughput analysis to identify and characterize the enormously flexible and dynamic range of cellular proteins, and may, for instance, eventually identify the 100,000 or more serum proteins as yet unknown. Much of this work is expected to provide information on normal regulatory processes and those involved in disease and the response to disease. In turn, these results are likely to point more accurately to specific markers of dysregulation that could be measured in blood and other body fluids. Multiplex protein microarray ELISAs or similar assay systems could then be used for rapid POC analysis.

Pharmacogenomics

One clear pathway into the postgenome era that is already in use in the pharmaceutical industry is pharmacogenetics, a process designed to overcome individual variations in response to therapies. Part of the effort involved in mapping SNPs will be to identify genetic loci involved in these variations. SNPs associated with a number of drug metabolizing systems, such as the cytochrome p450 system, are already known (Table 9.11), but only a small proportion of the SNPs eventually identified will have sufficient

functionality to change clinical outcomes. These SNPs may be simple ones, such as those associated with inhibition of drug metabolism leading to prolonged serum half-life and drug effects. Other SNPs, however, may be more complex. For example, there may be a polymorphism associated with overexpression of a drug metabolizing enzyme pathway, which increases the production of an intermediate metabolite that could lead to toxic metabolites. However, the unwanted effect of this genotype would only be manifest if there was a second genotype that led to the inhibition of a second enzyme system that metabolized the intermediate to a third harmless metabolite. Such information will not only enhance effective drug development, but also provide opportunities for appropriate drug use in patients with particular genotypes. Thus, in ICU management, drug therapy in critical situations might be enhanced by improved knowledge of the patient's genotype, an extension of the existing mechanism for dealing with the cholinesterase genotypes. An example may be treating a patient with severe sepsis and with a TNF-overproducing genotype with an anti-TNF antibody. The SNP analysis for inflammatory mediator expression could be performed swiftly at the POC using similar systems.

CONCLUSIONS

POCT in the ICU has reached a critical stage. Advances in technology complement those in medical science that are beginning to unravel many of the processes that must be evaluated to help prevent and to manage the onset of multiple organ dysfunction. Cost-benefit analysis that incorporates the additional advantages from more targeted therapy and enhanced connectivity may encourage rapid developments in this field over the next decade. Both ICU clinicians and clinical pathologists will need to work closely to lead the developments projected in Table 9.12. However, considerable variability in the acceptance rate of POCT among ICUs will remain, even within the same clinical establishment. While cost-benefit analysis involving therapeutic turnaround times may convince hospital management of the viabil-

TABLE 9.11. SELECTED DRUG METABOLIC PATHWAYS WITH KNOWN OR PUTATIVE SNPs ASSOCIATED WITH ALTERED DRUG METABOLISM RELEVANT TO ICU

Metabolic Pathway	Examples
P 450 system	CYP1A1, CYP2D6
Glutathione S transferases	GSTM1, GSTT1, GSTM3, GSTP1
Paroxonase	—
N-acetyl transferases	—
M epoxide hydrolase	—
Extracellular superoxide dismutase	—
Manganese superoxide dismutase	—
Tryptophan dioxygenase 2	—
Serotonin 5HT2a receptor	—
β adrenergic receptor polymorphisms	—
ACE inhibitors	I/D polymorphisms
Cholinesterase inhibitors	ApoE genotypes
Muscarinic agonists	Apo E genotypes
Protease inhibitors	HIV genotypes

ICU, intensive care unit; SNP, single nucleotide polymorphism.

TABLE 9.12. FUTURE (LIKELY AND DESIRABLE) ADDITIONAL DEVELOPMENTS IN POCT IN ICU

Metabolite and electrolyte
  Procalcitonin
  Brain natriuretic peptide
  Ketones
  Pyruvate
  Phosphate
  Ionized magnesium
  Colloid oncotic pressure
  Urine albumin/creatinine
  Urine electrolytes
Molecular
  Pathogen diagnosis and drug sensitivity
  Pharmacogenetic
  Host risk factor genetic (SNPs and/or proteomic)
  Pathogen-host "interactome"

ICU, intensive care unit; POCT, point-of-care testing; SNP, single nucleotide polymorphism.

ity of POCT, the process needs to be complemented at each site by effective connectivity as well as simplicity and reliability, all of which will require a coordinated effort and flexibility of working practices. It is evident that the diagnostics industry will increasingly include developments in POCT in parallel with those for main laboratory systems, resulting in greater opportunities to evaluate the potential for improved clinical care from POCT in the ICU.

ACKNOWLEDGMENTS

I would like to thank Dr. Christopher Garrard and the staff of the intensive therapy unit at the John Radcliffe Hospital, Oxford. In particular, I thank Dr. Chris Cairns for organizing and analyzing the initial blood gas audit in 1997; Drs. Julian Millo and Stephan Holt for the repeat audit in 2001; and Drs. Stuart Benham and Andrew StJohn, my collaborators in the Oxford hemofiltration lactate study.

REFERENCES

1. Auerbach PS. Impact of point-of-care testing on healthcare delivery [Letter]. *Clin Chem* 1996;42:2052–2053.
2. Kost GJ, Ehrmeyer SS, Chernow B. The laboratory-clinical interface: point-of-care testing. *Chest* 1999;115:1140–1154.
3. Bayne CG. Point of care testing: testing the system? *Nurs Manage* 1997;28:34–36.
4. Kane B. Point-of-care testing: instant gratification? *Ann Intern Med* 1999;130:870–872.
5. Castro HJ, Oropello JM, Halpern N. Point-of-care testing in the intensive care unit: the intensive care physician's perspective. *Am J Clin Pathol* 1995;104[Suppl 1]:S95–S99.
6. Harvey MA. Point-of-care laboratory testing in critical care. *Am J Crit Care* 1999;8:72–83, 84–85.
7. Muller MM, Hackl W, Griesmacher A. Point-of-care-testing—the intensive care laboratory. *Anaesthesist* 1999;48:3–8.
8. Kilgore ML, Steindel SJ, Smith JA. Evaluating stat testing options in an academic health center: therapeutic turnaround time and staff satisfaction. *Clin Chem* 1998;44:1597–1603.
9. Zaloga GP. Evaluation of bedside testing options for the critical care unit. *Chest* 1990;97[Suppl 5]:185S–190S.
10. Salem M, Chernow B, Burke R. Bedside diagnostic blood testing: its accuracy, rapidity, and utility in blood conservation. *JAMA* 1991;266:382–389.
11. Alazia M, Colavolpe JC, Botti G. Blood loss from diagnostic laboratory tests performed in intensive care units: preliminary study. *Ann Fr Anesth Reanim* 1996;15:1004–1007.
12. Kendall J, Reeves B, Clancy M. Point of care testing: randomised controlled trial of clinical outcome. *BMJ* 1998;316:1052–1057.
13. Halperin ML, Kamel KS, Cheema-Dhadli S. Lactic acidosis, ketoacidosis, and energy turnover: "figure" you made the correct diagnosis only when you have "counted" on it—quantitative analysis based on principles of metabolism. *Mt Sinai J Med* 1992;59:1–12.
14. Shirey TL. Critical care profiling for informed treatment of severely ill patients. *Am J Clin Pathol* 1995;104[Suppl 1]:S79–S87.
15. Mizock BA. Lactate and point-of-care testing [Editorial, Comment]. *Crit Care Med* 1998;26:1474–1476.
16. Abramson D, Scalea TM, Hitchcock R. Lactate clearance and survival following injury. *J Trauma* 1993;35:584–588, 588–589.
17. Stacpoole PW, Wright EC, Baumgartner TG. Natural history and course of acquired lactic acidosis in adults. DCA-Lactic Acidosis Study Group. *Am J Med* 1994;97:47–54.
18. Hilton PJ, Taylor J, Forni LG, Treacher DF. Bicarbonate-based haemofiltration in the management of acute renal failure with lactic acidosis. *QJM* 1998;91:279–283.
19. Thomas AN, Guy JM, Kishen R. Comparison of lactate and bicarbonate buffered haemofiltration fluids: use in critically ill patients. *Nephrol Dial Transplant* 1997;12:1212–1217.
20. Wright DA, Forni LG, Carr P, et al. Use of continuous haemofiltration to assess the rate of lactate metabolism in acute renal failure. *Clin Sci (Colch)* 1996;90:507–510.
21. Davenport A, Will EJ, Davison AM. Hyperlactataemia and metabolic acidosis during haemofiltration using lactate-buffered fluids. *Nephron* 1991;59:461–465.
22. Davenport A, Will EJ, Davison AM. Paradoxical increase in arterial hydrogen ion concentration in patients with hepatorenal failure given lactate-based fluids. *Nephrol Dial Transplant* 1990;5:342–346.
23. Marshall JC. Charting the course of critical illness: prognostication and outcome description in the intensive care unit [Editorial, Comment]. *Crit Care Med* 1999;27:676–678.
24. Marshall JC, et al. Multiple organ dysfunction score: a reliable descriptor of a complex clinical outcome. *Crit Care Med* 1995;23:1638–1652.
25. Tuchschmidt JA, Mecher CE. Predictors of outcome from critical illness: shock and cardiopulmonary resuscitation. *Crit Care Clin* 1994;10:179–195.
26. Costa JI, et al. Severity and prognosis in intensive care: prospective application of the APACHE II index. *Sao Paulo Med J* 1999;117:205–214.
27. Wong LS, Young JD. A comparison of ICU mortality prediction using the APACHE II scoring system and artificial neural networks. *Anaesthesia* 1999;54:1048–1054.
28. Markgraf R, Deutschinoff G, Pientka L, Scholten T. Comparison of acute physiology and chronic health evaluations II and III and simplified acute physiology score II: a prospective cohort study evaluating these methods to predict outcome in a German interdisciplinary intensive care unit. *Crit Care Med* 2000;28:26–33.
29. Vincent JL, Moreno R, Takala J. The SOFA (Sepsis-related Organ Failure Assessment) score to describe organ dysfunction/failure. On behalf of the Working Group on Sepsis-Related Problems of the European Society of Intensive Care Medicine. *Intensive Care Med* 1996;22:707–710.
30. Vincent JL, Ferreira F, Moreno R. Scoring systems for assessing organ dysfunction and survival. *Crit Care Clin* 2000;16:353–366.
31. Marinac JS, Mesa L. Using a severity of illness scoring system to assess intensive care unit admissions for diabetic ketoacidosis. *Crit Care Med* 2000;28:2238–2241.
32. Gunning K, Rowan K. ABC of intensive care: outcome data and scoring systems. *BMJ* 1999;319:241–244.
33. Mizock BA. Utility of standard base excess in acid-base analysis [Editorial, Comment]. *Crit Care Med* 1998;26:1146–1147.
34. Schlichtig R, Grogono AQ, Severinghaus JW. Human P_aCO_2 and standard base excess compensation for acid-base imbalance. *Crit Care Med* 1998;26:1173–1179.
35. Rixen D, Siegel JH. Metabolic correlates of oxygen debt predict posttrauma early acute respiratory distress syndrome and the related cytokine response. *J Trauma* 2000;49:392–403.
36. Bakker J, Gris P, Coffernils M, et al. Serial blood lactate levels can predict the development of multiple organ failure following septic shock. *Am J Surg* 1996;171:221–226.
37. Bakker J, Coffernils M, Leon M, et al. Blood lactate levels are superior to oxygen-derived variables in predicting outcome in human septic shock. *Chest* 1991;99:956–962.
38. Bernardin G, Pradier C, Tiger F, et al. Blood pressure and arterial lactate level are early indicators of short-term survival in human septic shock. *Intensive Care Med* 1996;22:17–25.
39. Marecaux G, Pinsky MR, Dupont E, et al. Blood lactate levels are better prognostic indicators than TNF and IL-6 levels in patients with septic shock. *Intensive Care Med* 1996;22:404–408.
40. Day NP, Phu NH, Mai NT, et al. The pathophysiologic and prognostic significance of acidosis in severe adult malaria. *Crit Care Med* 2000;28:1833–1840.
41. Taylor TE, Borgstein A, Molyneux ME. Acid-base status in paediatric Plasmodium falciparum malaria. *QJM* 1993;86:99–109.

42. Krishna S, Waller DW, ter Kuile F, et al. Lactic acidosis and hypoglycaemia in children with severe malaria: pathophysiological and prognostic significance. *Trans R Soc Trop Med Hyg* 1994;88:67–73.

43. Lavery RF, Livingston DH, Tortella BJ. The utility of venous lactate to triage injured patients in the trauma center. *J Am Coll Surg* 2000; 190:656–664.

44. Hirschl MM, et al. Analytical and clinical performance of an improved qualitative troponin T rapid test in laboratories and critical care units. *Arch Pathol Lab Med* 2000;124:583–587.

45. Collinson PO. The need for a point of care testing: an evidence-based appraisal. *Scand J Clin Lab Invest Suppl* 1999;230:67–73.

46. Hudson MP, et al. Cardiac markers: point of care testing. *Clin Chim Acta* 1999;284:223–237.

47. Ohman EM, et al. Risk stratification with a point-of-care cardiac troponin T test in acute myocardial infarction. GUSTOIII Investigators. Global Use of Strategies to Open Occluded Coronary Arteries. *Am J Cardiol* 1999;84:1281–1286.

48. Smith G, Nielsen M. ABC of intensive care: criteria for admission. *BMJ* 1999;318:1544–1547.

49. Bone RC, McElwee NE, Eubanks DH, Gluck EH. Analysis of indications for intensive care unit admission. Clinical efficacy assessment project: American College of Physicians. *Chest* 1993;104:1806–1811.

50. Goldhill DR, Worthington L, Mulcahy A, et al. The patient-at-risk team: identifying and managing seriously ill ward patients. *Anaesthesia* 1999;54:853–860.

51. Task Force of the American College of Critical Care Medicine, Society of Critical Care Medicine. Guidelines for intensive care unit admission, discharge, and triage. *Crit Care Med* 1999;27:633–638.

52. Bone RC, McElwee NE, Eubanks DH, Gluck EH. Analysis of indications for early discharge from the intensive care unit. Clinical efficacy assessment project: American College of Physicians. *Chest* 1993; 104:1812–1817.

53. Zimmerman JE, Seneff MG, Sun X, et al. Evaluating laboratory usage in the intensive care unit: patient and institutional characteristics that influence frequency of blood sampling. *Crit Care Med* 1997;25:737–748.

54. Bishop MS, Husain L, Kost GJ, et al. Multisite point-of-care potassium testing for patient-focused care. *Arch Pathol Lab Med* 1994;118:797–800.

55. Koch SM, Taylor RW. Chloride ion in intensive care medicine. *Crit Care Med* 1992;20:227–240.

56. Ishihara K, Szerlip HM. Anion gap acidosis. *Semin Nephrol* 1998;18:83–97.

57. Oster JR, Singer I, Contreras GN, et al. Metabolic acidosis with extreme elevation of anion gap: case report and literature review. *Am J Med Sci* 1999;317:38–49.

58. Lind L, Carlstedt F, Rastad J, et al. Hypocalcemia and parathyroid hormone secretion in critically ill patients. *Crit Care Med* 2000;28:93–99.

59. Kost G. The significance of ionised calcium in cardiac and critical care. *Arch Pathol Lab Med* 1993;117:890–896.

60. Zaloga G. Hypocalcaemia in critically ill patients. *Crit Care Med* 1992; 20:251–262.

61. Lobo FM, Zanjani R, Ho N, et al. Calcium-dependent activation of TNF family gene expression by Ca2+/calmodulin kinase type IV/Gr and calcineurin. *J Immunol* 1999;162:2057–2063.

62. Toffaletti J. Physiology and regulation: ionized calcium, magnesium and lactate measurements in critical care settings. *Am J Clin Pathol* 1995;104[Suppl 1]:S88–S94.

63. Fiser R. Ionized magnesium concentrations in critically ill children. *Crit Care Med* 1998;26:2048–2050.

64. Chernow B, Bamberger S, Stoilco M, et al. Hypomagnesemia in patients in postoperative intensive care [published correction appears in 1362.] *Chest* 1989;95:391–397.

65. Sanders G. Magnesium in disease: a review with special emphasis on the serum ionized magnesium. *Clin Chem Lab Med* 1999;37:1011–1033.

66. Frankel H. Hypomagnesemia in trauma patients. *World J Surg* 1999; 23:966–969.

67. Pedrozzi NT, Faraone A, Descoeudres R, et al. Circulating ionised and total magnesium in end-stage kidney disease. *Nephron* 1998;79:288–292.

68. De Jonghe B, Cheval C, Misset B, et al. Relationship between blood lactate and early hepatic dysfunction in acute circulatory failure. *J Crit Care* 1999;14:7–11.

69. Moomey CB, Jr, et al. Prognostic value of blood lactate, base deficit, and oxygen-derived variables in an LD50 model of penetrating trauma. *Crit Care Med* 1999;27:154–161.

70. Vincent JL. Lactate levels in critically ill patients. *Acta Anaesthesiol Scand Suppl* 1995;107:261–266.

71. Pinder M, Lipman J. Interpretation of lactate levels in critical illness. *S Afr J Surg* 1998;36:93–96.

72. Joynt GM, Lipman J, Gomersall CD, et al. Gastric intramucosal pH and blood lactate in severe sepsis. *Anaesthesia* 1997;52:726–732.

73. Pittard A. Does blood lactate measurement have a role in the management of the critically ill patient? *Ann Clin Biochem* 1999;36:401–407.

74. Bakker J, Schieveld S, Brinkert W. Serum lactate level as a indicator of tissue hypoxia in severely ill patients. *Ned Tijdschr Geneeskd* 2000; 144:737–741.

75. Desai VS, et al. Hepatic, renal, and cerebral tissue hypercarbia during sepsis and shock in rats. *J Lab Clin Med* 1995;125:456–461.

76. Day NP, Phu NH, Bethell DP, et al. The effects of dopamine and adrenaline infusions on acid-base balance and systemic haemodynamics in severe infection. *Lancet* 1996;348:219–223.

77. Levy B, Bollaert PE, Charpentier C, et al. Comparison of norepinephrine and dobutamine to epinephrine for hemodynamics, lactate metabolism, and gastric tonometric variables in septic shock: a prospective, randomized study. *Intensive Care Med* 1997;23:282–287.

78. Levy B, Nace L, Bollaert PE, et al. Comparison of systemic and regional effects of dobutamine and dopexamine in norepinephrine-treated septic shock. *Intensive Care Med* 1999;25:942–948.

79. Levy B, Sadoune LO, Gelot AM, et al. Evolution of lactate/pyruvate and arterial ketone body ratios in the early course of catecholamine-treated septic shock. *Crit Care Med* 2000;28:114–119.

80. Luchette FA, Robinson BR, Friend LA, et al. Adrenergic antagonists reduce lactic acidosis in response to hemorrhagic shock. *J Trauma* 1999;46:873–880.

81. Totaro RJ, Raper RF. Epinephrine-induced lactic acidosis following cardiopulmonary bypass. *Crit Care Med* 1997;25:1693–1699.

82. Reinelt H, Radermacher P, Kiefer P, et al. Impact of exogenous beta-adrenergic receptor stimulation on hepatosplanchnic oxygen kinetics and metabolic activity in septic shock. *Crit Care Med* 1999;27:325–331.

83. Routsi C, Bardouniotou H, Delivoria-Ioannidou V, et al. Pulmonary lactate release in patients with acute lung injury is not attributable to lung tissue hypoxia. *Crit Care Med* 1999;27:2469–2473.

84. Mizock BA. Lung injury and lactate production: a hypoxic stimulus? [Editorial, Comment]. *Crit Care Med* 1999;27:2585–2586.

85. Kellum JA, Kramer DJ, Lee K, et al. Release of lactate by the lung in acute lung injury. *Chest* 1997;111:1301–1305.

86. Haji-Michael PG, Ladriere L, Sener A, et al. Leukocyte glycolysis and lactate output in animal sepsis and *ex vivo* human blood. *Metabolism* 1999;48:779–785.

87. Gil A, Carrizosa F, Herrero A, et al. Influence of mechanical ventilation on blood lactate in patients with acute respiratory failure. *Intensive Care Med* 1998;24:924–930.

88. De Backer D, Creteur J, Zhang H, et al. Lactate production by the lungs in acute lung injury. *Am J Respir Crit Care Med* 1997;156:1099–1104.

89. Nimmo GR, Mackenzie SJ, Walker S, et al. Acid-base responses to high-volume haemofiltration in the critically ill. *Nephrol Dial Transplant* 1993;8:854–857.

90. Holloway P, Benham S, StJohn A. The value of blood lactate measurements in ICU: an evaluation of the role in the management of patients on haemofiltration. *Clin Chim Acta* 2001;307:9–13.

91. Kost GJ, Vu HT, Lee JH, et al. Multicenter study of oxygen-insensitive handheld glucose point-of-care testing in critical care/hospital/ambulatory patients in the United States and Canada. *Crit Care Med* 1998;26:581–590.

92. Kost GJ, Nguyen TH, Tang Z. Whole-blood glucose and lactate. Trilayer biosensors, drug interference, metabolism, and practice guidelines. *Arch Pathol Lab Med* 2000;124:1128–1134.

93. Louie RF, Tang Z, Sutton DV, et al. Point-of-care glucose testing:

effects of critical care variables, influence of reference instruments, and a modular glucose meter design. *Arch Pathol Lab Med* 2000;124: 257–266.

94. Tang Z, Lee JH, Louie RF, Kost GJ. Effects of different hematocrit levels on glucose measurements with handheld meters for point-of-care testing. *Arch Pathol Lab Med* 2000;124:1135–1140.

95. Tang Z, Du X, Louie RF, Kost GJ. Effects of pH on glucose measurements with handheld glucose meters and a portable glucose analyzer for point-of-care testing. *Arch Pathol Lab Med* 2000;124:577–582.

96. Yassen KA, Galley HF, Lee A, Webster NR. Mitochondrial redox state in the critically ill. *Br J Anaesth* 1999;83:325–327.

97. Miaskiewicz S, Levey GS, Owen O. Severe metabolic ketoacidosis induced by starvation and exercise. *Am J Med Sci* 1989;297:178–180.

98. Owen OE, Caprio S, Reichard GA Jr., et al. Ketosis of starvation: a revisit and new perspectives. *Clin Endocrinol Metab* 1983;12:359–379.

99. Grey NJ, Karl I, Kipnis DM. Physiologic mechanisms in the development of starvation ketosis in man. *Diabetes* 1975;24:10–16.

100. Mitchell GA, Kassovska-Bratinova A, Boukaftane Y, et al. Medical aspects of ketone body metabolism. *Clin Invest Med* 1995;18:193–216.

101. Brinkmann B, Fechner G, Karger B, DuChesne A. Ketoacidosis and lactic acidosis—frequent causes of death in chronic alcoholics? *Int J Legal Med* 1998;111:115–119.

102. Umpierrez GE, DiGirokmo M, Tuvlin JA, et al. Differences in metabolic and hormonal milieu in diabetic- and alcohol-induced ketoacidosis. *J Crit Care* 2000;15:52–59.

103. Rich AJ, Wright PD. Ketosis and nitrogen excretion in undernourished surgical patients. *JPEN Parenter Enteral Nutr* 1979;3:350–354.

104. Kost GJ, Vu HT, Inn M, et al. Multicenter study of whole-blood creatinine, total carbon dioxide content, and chemistry profiling for laboratory and point-of-care testing in critical care in the United States. *Crit Care Med* 2000;28:2379–2389.

105. Vervloet MG, Thijs LG, Hack CE. Derangements of coagulation and fibrinolysis in critically ill patients with sepsis and septic shock. *Semin Thromb Hemost* 1998;24:33–44.

106. Abraham E. Coagulation abnormalities in acute lung injury and sepsis [Comment]. *Am J Respir Cell Mol Biol* 2000;22: 401–404.

107. Bateman SW, Mathews KA, Abrams-Ogg AC, et al. Evaluation of point-of-care tests for diagnosis of disseminated intravascular coagulation in dogs admitted to an intensive care unit. *J Am Vet Med Assoc* 1999;215:805–810.

108. Rose VL, Dermott SC, Murray BF, et al. Decentralized testing for prothrombin time and activated partial thromboplastin time using a dry chemistry portable analyzer. *Arch Pathol Lab Med* 1993;117:611–617.

109. Seitz R, Egbring R. Disorders of blood coagulation in the intensive care unit: what is important for diagnosis and therapy?. *Klin Wochenschr* 1991;26:143–149.

110. Staudinger T, Locker GJ, Frass M. Management of acquired coagulation disorders in emergency and intensive-care medicine. *Semin Thromb Hemost* 1996;22:93–104.

111. Yu M, Nardella A, Pechet L. Screening tests of disseminated intravascular coagulation: guidelines for rapid and specific laboratory diagnosis. *Crit Care Med* 2000;28:1777–1780.

112. Werner M, Gallagher JV, Ballo MS, Karcher DS. Effect of analytic uncertainty of conventional and point-of-care assays of activated partial thromboplastin time on clinical decisions in heparin therapy. *Am J Clin Pathol* 1994;102:237–241.

113. Dhainaut JF. Introduction to the Margaux Conference on Critical Illness: activation of the coagulation system in critical illnesses. *Crit Care Med* 2000;28[Suppl 9]:S1–S3.

114. Levi M, de Jonge E, ten Cate H. Disseminated intravascular coagulation. *Ned Tijdschr Geneeskd* 2000;144:470–475.

115. Mavrommatis AC, Theodoridis T, Orfanidou A, et al. Coagulation system and platelets are fully activated in uncomplicated sepsis. *Crit Care Med* 2000;28:451–457.

116. Thijs LG. Coagulation inhibitor replacement in sepsis is a potentially useful clinical approach. *Crit Care Med* 2000;28[Suppl 9]:S68–S73.

117. Vincent JL. New therapeutic implications of anticoagulation mediator replacement in sepsis and acute respiratory distress syndrome. *Crit Care Med* 2000;28[Suppl 9]:S83–S85.

118. Shorr AF, Trotta RF, Alkins SA. D-dimer assay predicts mortality in critically ill patients without disseminated intravascular coagulation or venous thromboembolic disease. *Intensive Care Med* 1999;25:207–210.

119. Shore-Lesserson L, Manspeizer HE, DePerio M, et al. Thromboelastography-guided transfusion algorithm reduces transfusions in complex cardiac surgery. *Anesth Analg* 1999;88:312–319.

120. Stammers AH, Bruda NC, Gonano C, Hartmann T. Point-of-care coagulation monitoring: applications of the thromboelastography. *Anaesthesia* 1998;2:58–59.

121. Baldwin I, Tan HK, Bridge N, Bellomo R. A prospective study of thromboelastography (TEG) and filter life during continuous veno-venous hemofiltration. *Ren Fail* 2000;22:297–306.

122. Derrier M, Jambou P, Kaidomar M, et al. Thromboelastography and monitoring of coagulation in patients undergoing continuous venovenous hemofiltration. *Contrib Nephrol* 1995;116:159–162.

123. Morgan TJ, Clark C, Endre ZH. Accuracy of base excess—an *in vitro* evaluation of the Van Slyke equation. *Crit Care Med* 2000;28: 2932–2936.

124. Siggaard-Andersen O, Fogh-Andersen N. Base excess or buffer base (strong ion difference) as measure of a non-respiratory acid-base disturbance. *Acta Anaesthesiol Scand Suppl* 1995;107:123–128.

125. Wooten EW. Analytic calculation of physiological acid-base parameters in plasma. *J Appl Physiol* 1999;86:326–334.

126. Balasubramanyan N, Havens PL, Hoffman GM. Unmeasured anions identified by the Fencl-Stewart method predict mortality better than base excess, anion gap, and lactate in patients in the pediatric intensive care unit. *Crit Care Med* 1999;27:1577–1581.

127. Gilfix BM, Bique M, Magder S. A physical chemical approach to the analysis of acid-base balance in the clinical setting. *J Crit Care* 1993;8:187–197.

128. Mikulaschek A, et al. Serum lactate is not predicted by anion gap or base excess after trauma resuscitation. *J Trauma* 1996;40:218–224.

129. Levraut J, Bounatirou T, Ichai C, et al. Reliability of anion gap as an indicator of blood lactate in critically ill patients. *Intensive Care Med* 1997;23:417–422.

130. Haeney M. Setting standards for pathology service support to emergency services. *J R Soc Med* 2001;94[Suppl 39]:26–30.

131. Freedman D. Guidelines on point-of-care testing. In: Price CP, Hicks JM, eds. *Point-of-care testing*. Washington, DC: American Association of Clinical Chemistry Press, 1999:197–212.

132. Kost GJ. Guidelines for point-of-care testing. Improving patient outcomes. *Am J Clin Pathol* 1995;104[Suppl 1]:S111–S127.

133. Briedigkeit L, Muller-Plathe O, Schlebusch H, Ziens J. Recommendations of the German Working Group on medical laboratory testing (AML) on the introduction and quality assurance of procedures for point-of-care testing (POCT) in hospitals. *Clin Chem Lab Med* 1999; 37:919–925.

134. Gosling P. Point-of-care testing in the intensive care unit. In: CP Price, Hicks JM, eds. *Point-of-care testing*. Washington, DC: American Association of Clinical Chemistry, 1999:359–385.

135. Muller B, Becker KL, Kranzlin M, et al. Disordered calcium homeostasis of sepsis: association with calcitonin precursors. *Eur J Clin Invest* 2000;30:823–831.

136. Barak V, et al. Prevalence of hypophosphatemia in sepsis and infection: the role of cytokines. *Am J Med* 1998;104:40–47.

137. Paleologos M, Stone E, Braude S. Persistent, progressive hypophosphataemia after voluntary hyperventilation. *Clin Sci (Colch)* 2000;98: 619–625.

138. Berger W, Keller U. Treatment of diabetic ketoacidosis and non-ketotic hyperosmolar diabetic coma. *Baillieres Clin Endocrinol Metab* 1992;6:1–22.

139. Gamrin L, Andersson K, Hultman E, et al. Longitudinal changes of biochemical parameters in muscle during critical illness. *Metabolism* 1997;46:756–762.

140. MacLean DA, Imadojemu VA, Sinoway LI. Interstitial pH, K(+), lactate, and phosphate determined with MSNA during exercise in humans. *Am J Physiol Regul Integr Comp Physiol* 2000;278:R563–R571.

141. Nielsen OM, Engell HC. Effects of maintaining normal plasma colloid osmotic pressure on renal function and excretion of sodium and water after major surgery: a randomized study. *Dan Med Bull* 1985; 32:182–185.

142. Weil MH. Crystalloids, colloids, and fluid compartments. *Crit Care Med* 1999;27:3.

143. Hauet T, Faure JP, Baumert H, et al. Influence of different colloids on hemodynamic and renal functions: comparative study in an isolated perfused pig kidney model. *Transplant Proc* 1998;30:2796–2797.

144. Gosling P. Microalbuminuria: a marker of systemic disease. *Br J Hosp Med* 1995;54:285–290.

145. Gosling P. Microalbuminuria: a sensitive indicator of non-renal disease? *Ann Clin Biochem* 1995;32:439–441.

146. Pallister I, Gosling P, Alpar K, Bradley J. Prediction of posttraumatic adult respiratory distress syndrome by albumin excretion rate eight hours after admission. *J Trauma* 1997;42:1056–1061.

147. Coritsidis GN, Guru K, Ward L, et al. Prediction of acute renal failure by "bedside formula" in medical and surgical intensive care patients. *Ren Fail* 2000;22:235–244.

148. Stewart PA. Independent and dependent variables of acid-base control. *Respir Physiol* 1978;33:9–26.

149. Figge J, Jabor A, Kazda A, Fencl V. Anion gap and hypoalbuminemia. *Crit Care Med* 1998;26:1807–1810.

150. Kellum JA. Metabolic acidosis in the critically ill: lessons from physical chemistry. *Kidney Int Suppl* 1998;66:S81–S86.

151. Kellum J, Kramer D, Pinsky M. Strong ion gap: a methodology for exploring unexplained anions. *J Crit Care* 1995;10: 51–55.

152. Constable P. Clinical assessment of acid-base status: strong ion difference theory. *Vet Clin North Am Food Anim Pract* 1999;15: 447–471.

153. Eicker SW. An introduction to strong ion difference. *Vet Clin North Am Food Anim Pract* 1990;6:45–49.

154. Schlichtig R. Base excess vs strong ion difference: which is more helpful? *Adv Exp Med Biol* 1997;411:91–95.

155. Dorje P, Bree SE, Adhikary G, Mclaren DI. Hyperchloraemia causes metabolic acidosis by reducing strong ion difference [Letter]. *Anaesthesia* 2000;55:94.

156. Maynard N, Bihari D, Beale R, et al. Assessment of splanchnic oxygenation by gastric tonometry in patients with acute circulatory failure. *JAMA* 1993;270:1203–1210.

157. Hatherill M, Tibby SM, Evans R, Murdoch IA. Gastric tonometry in septic shock. *Arch Dis Child* 1998;78:155–158.

158. Creteur J, De Backer D, Vincent JL. Does gastric tonometry monitor splanchnic perfusion? *Crit Care Med* 1999;27:2480–2484.

159. Rasmussen I, Haglund U. Early gut ischemia in experimental fecal peritonitis. *Circ Shock* 1992;38:22–28.

160. Bernardin G, et al. Influence of alveolar ventilation changes on calculated gastric intramucosal pH and gastric-arterial PCO_2 difference. *Intensive Care Med* 1999;25:269–273.

161. Kellum JA, Garuba AK, Pinsky MR, et al. Accuracy of mucosal pH and mucosal-arterial carbon dioxide tension for detecting mesenteric hypoperfusion in acute canine endotoxemia. *Crit Care Med* 2000;28: 462–466.

162. Weil MH, Nakagawa Y, Tang W, et al. Sublingual capnometry: a new noninvasive measurement for diagnosis and quantitation of severity of circulatory shock. *Crit Care Med* 1999;27:1225–1229.

163. Chandel NS, Schumacker PT. Cellular oxygen sensing by mitochondria: old questions, new insight. *J Appl Physiol* 2000;88: 1880–1889.

164. Edouard AEA. Circulating cardiac troponin I in trauma patients without cardiac contusion. *Intensive Care Med* 1998;24:569–573.

165. Fernandes CJ, Jr, Akamine N, Knobel E. Cardiac troponin: a new serum marker of myocardial injury in sepsis. *Intensive Care Med* 1999; 25:1165–1168.

166. Chen HH, Burnett JC, Jr. The natriuretic peptides in heart failure: diagnostic and therapeutic potentials. *Proc Assoc Am Physicians* 1999; 111:406–416.

167. Cowie MR. BNP: soon to become a routine measure in the care of patients with heart failure? [Editorial]. *Heart* 2000;83:617–618.

168. Maisel AS, Koon J, Krishnaswamy P, et al. Utility of B-natriuretic peptide as a rapid, point-of-care test for screening patients undergoing echocardiography to determine left ventricular dysfunction. *Am Heart J* 2001;141:367–374.

169. Kazanegra R, Cheng V, Garcia A, et al. A rapid test for B-type natriuretic peptide correlates with falling wedge pressures in patients treated for decompensated heart failure: a pilot study. *J Card Fail* 2001;7:21–29.

170. Angus DC. Advances in sepsis. Paper presented at 30th International Educational and Scientific Symposium of the Society of Critical Care Medicine, February 10–14, 2001, p. 79, San Francisco.

171. Yentis SM, Soni N, Sheldon J. C-reactive protein as an indicator of resolution of sepsis in the intensive care unit. *Intensive Care Med* 1995;21:602–605.

172. Vincent JL. Procalcitonin: the marker of sepsis? [Editorial, Comment]. *Crit Care Med* 2000;28:1226–1228.

173. Lind LB, Ljunghall S. Pronounced elevation in circulating calcitonin in critical care patients is related to the severity of illness and survival. *Intensive Care Med* 1995;21:63–66.

174. Assicot MG, Carsin H. High serum procalcitonin concentrations in patients with sepsis and infection. *Lancet* 1993;341:515–518.

175. Wanner GA, Keel M, Steckholzer U, et al. Relationship between procalcitonin plasma levels and severity of injury, sepsis, organ failure, and mortality in injured patients. *Crit Care Med* 2000;28:950–957.

176. Ugarte H, et al. Procalcitonin used as a marker of infection in the intensive care unit. *Crit Care Med* 1999;27:498–504.

177. Rothenburger M, Markewitz A, Lenz T, et al. Detection of acute phase response and infection. The role of procalcitonin and C-reactive protein. *Clin Chem Lab Med* 1999;37:275–279.

178. Nijsten MW, et al. Procalcitonin behaves as a fast responding acute phase protein *in vivo* and *in vitro*. *Crit Care Med* 2000;28:458–461.

179. Oberhoffer M, Vogelsang H, Russwurm S, et al. Outcome prediction by traditional and new markers of inflammation in patients with sepsis. *Clin Chem Lab Med* 1999;37:363–368.

180. Aouifi A, Piriou V, Bastien O, et al. Usefulness of procalcitonin for diagnosis of infection in cardiac surgical patients. *Crit Care Med* 2000;28:3171–3176.

181. Boucher BA. Procalcitonin: clinical tool or laboratory curiosity? [Editorial, Comment]. *Crit Care Med* 2000;28:1224–1225.

182. Carlet J. Rapid diagnostic methods in the detection of sepsis. *Infect Dis Clin North Am* 1999;13:483–494.

183. Hatherill M, et al. Diagnostic markers of infection: comparison of procalcitonin with C reactive protein and leucocyte count. *Arch Dis Child* 1999;81:417–421.

184. Viallon A, Zeni F, Lambert C, et al. High sensitivity and specificity of serum procalcitonin levels in adults with bacterial meningitis. *Clin Infect Dis* 1999;28:1313–1316.

185. Muller B, Becker KL, Schachinger H, et al. Calcitonin precursors are reliable markers of sepsis in a medical intensive care unit. *Crit Care Med* 2000;28:977–983.

185a. Panacek EA, Williams GR, Olladurf O, et al. Treatment with Afc in patients with severe sepsis is associated with improved ICU-free days. *Crit Care Med* 2000;28(12)suppl;A623.

186. van Bommel EF, Hesse CJ, Jutte NH, et al. Impact of continuous hemofiltration on cytokines and cytokine inhibitors in oliguric patients suffering from systemic inflammatory response syndrome. *Ren Fail* 1997;19:443–454.

187. Bernard GR, Vincent JL, Laterre PF, et al. Efficacy and safety of recombinant human activated protein C for severe sepsis. *N Engl J Med* 2001;344:699–709.

188. Denzel C, et al. Monitoring of immunotherapy by measuring monocyte HLA-DR expression and stimulated TNFalpha production during sepsis after liver transplantation [Letter]. *Intensive Care Med* 1998;24:1343–1344.

189. Payen D, Faivre V, Lukaszewicz AC, Losser MR. Assessment of immunological status in the critically ill. *Minerva Anestesiol* 2000;66: 757–763.

190. Volk HD, Reinke P, Docke WD. Immunological monitoring of the inflammatory process: Which variables? When to assess? *Eur J Surg Suppl* 1999;584:70–72.

191. Siggaard-Andersen O, Gothgen IH, Fogh-Andersen N. Biosensors and bioprobes in anaesthesia and intensive care: from *in vitro* to *in vivo* monitoring. *Acta Anaesthesiol Scand Suppl* 1995;104:7–13.

192. Rolfe P. *In vivo* chemical sensors for intensive-care monitoring. *Med Biol Eng Comput* 1990;28:B34–B47.

193. Widness JA, Kulhavy JC, Johnson KJ, et al. Clinical performance of

an in-line point-of-care monitor in neonates. *Pediatrics* 2000;106:497–504.

194. Gfrerer RJ, et al. Novel system for real-time *ex vivo* lactate monitoring in human whole blood. *Biosens Bioelectron* 1998;13:1271–1278.

195. Kilger E, Briegel J, Schelling G, et al. Long-term evaluation of a continuous intra-arterial blood gas monitoring system in patients with severe respiratory failure. *Infusionsther Transfusionsmed* 1995;22:98–104.

196. Szaflarski NL. Emerging technology in critical care: continuous intraarterial blood gas monitoring. *Am J Crit Care* 1996;5:55–65.

197. Tobias JD, Connors D, Strauser L, Johnson T. Continuous pH and PCO_2 monitoring during respiratory failure in children with the Paratrend 7 inserted into the peripheral venous system. *J Pediatr* 2000;136:623–627.

198. Morgan C, Newell SJ, Ducker DA, et al. Continuous neonatal blood gas monitoring using a multiparameter intra-arterial sensor. *Arch Dis Child Fetal Neonatal Ed* 1999;80:F93–F98.

199. De Boer J, Korf J, Plijter-Groendijk H. *In vivo* monitoring of lactate and glucose with microdialysis and enzyme reactors in intensive care medicine. *Int J Artif Organs* 1994;17:163–170.

200. Goodman JC, Valadka AB, Gopinath SP, et al. Extracellular lactate and glucose alterations in the brain after head injury measured by microdialysis. *Crit Care Med* 1999;27:1965–1973.

201. Kushi H, et al. Importance of metabolic monitoring systems as an early prognostic indicator in severe head injured patients. *Acta Neurochir Suppl* 1999;75:67–68.

202. Landolt H, et al. Neurochemical monitoring and on-line pH measurements using brain microdialysis in patients in intensive care. *Acta Neurochir Suppl* 1994;60:475–478.

203. Nilsson OG, Brandt L, Ungerstedt U, et al. Bedside detection of brain ischemia using intracerebral microdialysis: subarachnoid hemorrhage and delayed ischemic deterioration. *Neurosurgery* 1999;45:1176–1185.

204. Haller M, Kilger E, Briegel J, et al. Continuous intra-arterial blood gas and pH monitoring in critically ill patients with severe respiratory failure: a prospective, criterion standard study. *Crit Care Med* 1994;22:580–587.

205. Hutchinson PJ, O'Connell MT, Maskell CB, Pickard JD. Monitoring by subcutaneous microdialysis in neurosurgical intensive care. *Acta Neurochir Suppl* 1999;75:57–59.

206. Hutchinson PJ, O'Connell MT, Al-Rawi PG, et al. Clinical cerebral microdialysis: a methodological study. *J Neurosurg* 2000;93:37–43.

207. Kuroda MO, Uchiyama T, et al. Whole genome sequencing of meticillin-resistant staphylococcus aureus. *Lancet* 2001;357:1225–1240.

208. Kox WJ, Volk T, Kox SN, Volk HD. Immunomodulatory therapies in sepsis. *Intensive Care Med* 2000;26:S124–S128.

209. McGuire W, et al. Variation in the TNF-alpha promoter region associated with susceptibility to cerebral malaria. *Nature* 1994;371:508–510.

210. Stuber FU, Book I, et al.–308 Tumour necrosis factor (TNF) polymorphism is not associated with survival in severe sepsis and is unrelated to lipopolysaccharide inducibility of the human TNF promoter. *J Inflamm* 1995;46:42–50.

211. Stuber F, et al. A genomic polymorphism within the tumor necrosis factor locus influences plasma tumor necrosis factor-alpha concentrations and outcome of patients with severe sepsis. *Crit Care Med* 1996;24:381–384.

212. Summerfield JA, Sumiya M, Levin M, at el. Association of mutations in mannose binding protein gene with childhood infection in consecutive hospital series. *BMJ* 1997;314:1229–1232.

213. Hermans PW, Hibberd ML, Booy R, et al. 4G/5G promoter polymorphism in the plasminogen-activator-1 gene and outcome of meningococcal disease. *Lancet* 1999;354:556–561.

214. Menges TH, Little P, Langefeld S, et al. Plasminogen-activator-inhibitor-1 4G/5G promoter polymorphism and prognosis of severely injured patients. *Lancet* 2001;357:1096–1097.

215. McGuire W, Knight JC, Hill A, et al. Severe malarial anemia and cerebral malaria are associated with different tumor necrosis factor promoter alleles. *J Infect Dis* 1999;179:287–290.

216. Kwiatkowski D. Genetic dissection of the molecular pathogenesis of severe infection. *Intensive Care Med* 2000;26:S89–S97.

217. Udalova IA, et al. Direct evidence for involvement of NF-kappaB in transcriptional activation of tumor necrosis factor by a spirochetal lipoprotein. *Infect Immun* 2000;68:5447–5449.

218. Kwiatkowski RW, et al. Clinical, genetic, and pharmacogenetic applications of the Invader assay. *Mol Diagn* 1999;4:353–364.

10

POINT-OF-CARE HEMATOLOGY, HEMOSTASIS, AND THROMBOLYSIS TESTING

PAULA J. SANTRACH

Point-of-care (POC) testing in the hematology and hemostasis realms has a long history and is currently growing rapidly due to both clinical and technological advances. In a recent survey of members of the American Association of Critical Care Nurses, coagulation testing was the second most common type of analysis performed at the patient's bedside (1). The most widespread applications of POC coagulation testing are in cardiac surgical and catheterization procedures; monitoring of anticoagulation and guidance of transfusion therapy are typical goals. In fact, clinical outcome studies for this type of coagulation testing are probably the best-defined and most consistently successful of all the ones that have been done for point-of-care testing (POCT). Furthermore, hemoglobin/hematocrit determinations have a long history of use as indications for red blood cell transfusions in numerous settings. Various POC tests and devices in terms of test principles, assay performance, and clinical applications are discussed in this chapter.

HEMATOLOGY TESTS AT THE POINT OF CARE

Complete blood counts (white blood cells, platelets, hemoglobin, hematocrit, red blood cells, and red blood cell indices) and white blood cell differential counts are typically performed using automated cell counters. These same tests can now be performed at the POC with smaller tabletop versions of the cell counters. Such technology may be found in physician offices, emergency departments, and intensive care units; rapid triage, rapid treatment of patients, or both are the primary goals. The use of platelet counts to guide transfusion therapy has become more widespread, particularly during liver transplantation and after cardiopulmonary bypass procedures. In these situations, a rapid turnaround time is necessary so that transfusion occurs in a timely manner when patient conditions can change quickly. A recent evaluation of an on-site cell counter in a cardiac surgical intensive care unit demonstrated acceptable performance compared to the laboratory instrument (2). Another POC hemocytometer (Ichor, Array Medical, Somerville, NJ) provides a complete blood count without a WBC differential and shows comparable performance to other laboratory and POC automated cell counters (3).

A different POC method for providing a hematological profile (hematocrit, white blood cell count, platelet count, granulocyte, and mononuclear cell counts) involves quantitative buffy coat analysis. This approach uses centrifugation in a specially designed capillary tube to separate the various cellular fractions and staining with acridine orange to identify and quantitate the white blood cells and platelets (4). Three studies have examined the performance of this method in samples from hematology/ oncology patients (4), emergency room patients (5), and an unselected patient population (6). Generally, there was good correlation with standard cell counters and clinically insignificant bias; however, 5% to 23% of samples could not be analyzed due to poor separation or measurements outside of the reportable range. Nontechnical personnel could operate the device as successfully as laboratory staff, although imprecision was somewhat higher with the nontechnical operators (6). The turnaround time of results was significantly faster than the central laboratory (mean less than 20 minutes versus 40 to 70 minutes for the laboratory). In a survey of emergency room physicians, 20% felt that the rapid result would have decreased the patient's length of stay in the emergency room and 85% felt that the result confirmed their clinical impression, but 43% felt that the result had no impact on patient management (5).

Probably the most widely used hematological parameters at the POC are the hemoglobin concentration and hematocrit. There are many methodologies available to measure these parameters in the near-patient setting. The centrifuge-based hematocrit has been available for many years and has shown clinically acceptable agreement with standard cell counters (7–11). Hematocrit can also be measured with a conductivity method, which utilizes the resistance of red blood cells to electrical conduction in a sample. This conductivity hematocrit technique may be found in stand-alone hematocrit devices or in multiparameter devices, typically in combination with blood gas and/or electrolyte analysis. In patients with normal concentrations of protein and electrolytes in their blood, the accuracy of the hematocrit is good (7–9). However, in samples of intraoperatively salvaged autologous blood, the conductivity hematocrit is falsely decreased due to the extremely low levels of protein in this blood product (7,9). In patient samples, a similar effect of total protein is evident; elevated concentrations of sodium and chloride can also falsely decrease the conductivity hematocrit (8). Some devices have algorithms to make adjustments for these situations; however, compensation may be incomplete and care must be taken in interpreting the results (7).

In routine medical care, hemoglobin measurements are obtained from standard laboratory hemacytometers or from oximeters usually integrated with blood gas analyzers. At the POC, the HemoCue Hemoglobin Analyzer (HemoCue Diagnostics AB, Ängelholm, Sweden) provides rapid hemoglobin measurements using a modified methemoglobin reaction with photometric quantitation. Many evaluations of this device have shown acceptable clinical performance compared to standard hemacytometers. Mean bias has ranged from 0.1 to 0.6 g/dL in surgical, obstetrical, and pediatric patient populations (7,12–15). The method is not affected by protein or lipid levels (7,16,17); air bubbles in the measuring cuvette must be avoided to prevent erroneous results. The Hb-Quick Hemoglobinometer (Avox Systems, Fair Oaks, TX) measures total hemoglobin concentration of whole-blood samples using a spectrophotometric method. Compared with the cyanmethemoglobin technique, the Hb-Quick shows excellent accuracy with clinically insignificant bias, low imprecision, and good linearity (18).

The clinical applications of POC hemoglobin or hematocrit testing focus on transfusion therapy and acute hemodilution during surgery. The currently recommended hemoglobin level at which the transfusion of red blood cells is usually required, is 6 to 7 g per deciliter in adults (19); this decision point may be higher in patients with concurrent cardiac, vascular or pulmonary disease. In cardiac surgery, acute hemodilution typically occurs during cardiopulmonary bypass and the hematocrit is the primary indicator of red-blood-cell transfusion in this setting (20). In many types of surgery, acute normovolemic hemodilution may be performed as a blood conservation strategy (21). This technique involves the intraoperative collection of autologous whole blood from a patient at the beginning of the surgical procedure and subsequent reinfusion in an attempt to minimize or avoid allogeneic transfusion. The amount of blood collected depends on the patient's initial hemoglobin, underlying medical condition, and acceptable minimum hemoglobin. Ongoing hemoglobin monitoring is essential to this procedure.

HEMOSTASIS TESTS AT THE POINT OF CARE

Activated Clotting Time

The activated clotting time (ACT) is a whole-blood coagulation test that is similar to the activated partial thromboplastin time. In this test, coagulation is initiated by a contact activator such as celite or kaolin; thus the test is sensitive to deficiencies in the coagulation factors in the intrinsic pathway (XII, XI, IX, VII) and the final common pathway (X, V, II) as well as the presence of heparin. Fresh whole blood is typically added to the activator in a test tube or cartridge and a timer is begun; some assays use citrated whole blood. Timing continues until the instrument detects the presence of a clot. Clot detection methods include change in pump-driven blood movement through a capillary tube, resistance to the movement of a plunger through the sam-

ple, displacement of a magnet in the sample, and change in the oscillation of paramagnetic iron particles. The resulting clotting times are typically ≥100 seconds.

Most activated clotting time methods use a very strong activator, typically kaolin or celite, in order to make the assay able to detect large amounts of heparin in the patient's blood. Such high-dose heparin therapy, in the range of 1 to 6 units/ml, is used in cardiopulmonary bypass surgery, vascular surgery, cardiac catheterization, and interventional radiology studies. Other procedures such as hemodialysis may use lower heparin doses; treatment of venous thromboembolism requires low doses of heparin in the range of 0.2 to 0.8 units/ml. Some manufacturers provide activated clotting time reagents with different activators, such as glass beads, for monitoring this lower-dose heparin therapy, and these assays may have different reference range and therapeutic range results. Patient studies have demonstrated that the high-dose reagents are insensitive to low levels of circulating heparin; in vascular surgery patients with heparin levels from 0.18 to 0.85 units/ml, only 4 of 17 ACTs were considered abnormal (22). Thus, it is important to utilize the correct reagents for each therapeutic application.

Most of the instruments currently available for activated clotting time tests are POC devices with the ability to do multiple coagulation tests, depending on which cartridge or test tube is selected. Some of the instruments for use in high-dose heparin therapy settings are outlined in Table 10.1. Some of these devices are being incorporated into existing POC blood gas and electrolyte instruments in an effort to provide broader test menus; other manufacturers are developing new activated clotting time methods for their noncoagulation POC instruments.

The activated clotting time is designed primarily to monitor high-dose heparin therapy. *In vitro* studies have shown that the test is linearly responsive to heparin concentrations above 1 unit/ml. Although the linearity of the heparin response is fairly well maintained when blood from anticoagulated patients is analyzed, the degree of response in terms of prolongation of the ACT varies from patient to patient (23,24) (Fig. 10.1). Some patients exhibit resistance to heparin in that their ACTs are not very prolonged despite multiple doses, which may be due to low levels of antithrombin III in the patient's blood (25). This variability in patient response to fixed doses of heparin is the basis for ACT monitoring during therapy (26,27).

Not all activated clotting times are equivalent as activators exhibit varying responsiveness to heparin. This is particularly true for celite and kaolin, both of which are used to monitor high-dose therapy. Several studies (28–31) have shown that celite-based results tend to be significantly longer than kaolin-based results even in the same patient (Fig. 10.2). The ACT+ assay uses kaolin, silica, and phospholipid as activators; when compared to the celite ACT, the ACT+ results were 10% to 20% longer and the range of differences between the two tests was −100 to +150 seconds (32). The Heparin Management Test has been shown to correlate with the Hemochron ACT, although paired samples can differ by up to 80 seconds (33). The MAX-ACT test contains a cocktail of celite, kaolin, and glass beads designed to maximize activation of Factor XII. Although the MAX-ACT tends to parallel the ACT during cardiopulmonary bypass, its results tend to be shorter due to lower sensitivity to heparin and hypothermia (34). Therefore, identifi-

TABLE 10.1. ACTIVATED CLOTTING TIME INSTRUMENTS FOR HIGH-DOSE HEPARIN THERAPY

Instrument	Manufacturer	Assay	Activator(s)	Sample Size	Sample Type	Duplicate Testing Performed
Actalyke	Helena Point of Care Beaumont, TX	1. ACT 2. MAX-ACT	1. Celite or kaolin 2. Celite, kaolin, glass cocktail	1. 2.0 mL 2. 0.5 mL	Fresh whole blood	No
HemoTec Automated Coagulation Timer (ACT) II /Hepcon HMS	Medtronic Inc. Parker, CO	ACT	Kaolin	0.4 mL	Fresh whole blood	Yes
CoaguChek Pro DM	Roche Diagnostics Corp. Indianapolis, IN	ACT	Celite	1 drop	Fresh whole blood	No
GEM PCL	Instrumentation Laboratory Lexington, MA	ACT		1 drop	Fresh whole blood	No
Hemochron Jr Signature	International Technidyne Corp. Edison, NJ	ACT+	Kaolin with silica and phospholipid	1 drop	Fresh whole blood	No
Hemochron series (401, 801, 8000, Response)	International Technidyne Corp. Edison, NJ	ACT	Celite or kaolin	2.0 mL	Fresh whole blood	No
ISTAT	Abbott Laboratories Bedford, MA	ACT	Celite	40 uL	Fresh whole blood	No
Rapidpoint Coag / Thrombolytic Assessment System (TAS)	Bayer Diagnostics Tarrytown, NY	Heparin Management Test (HMT)	Celite	1 drop	Fresh or citrated whole blood	No

cation of the assay/device is very important in the establishment of patient monitoring protocols and in the interpretation of published research studies.

The difference in celite and kaolin assays is accentuated when patients are treated with aprotinin. Aprotinin is a serine protease inhibitor that has been shown to decrease blood loss and transfusion requirements in cardiopulmonary bypass surgery; proposed mechanisms of action include protection of platelets from activa-

tion by the extracorporeal circuit, inhibition of activation of the clotting cascade, and inhibition of fibrinolysis. Many studies have shown that aprotinin significantly prolongs the celite ACT in the presence of heparin, both *in vitro* and *ex vivo* (35–39) (Fig. 10.3). This effect is not evident when a kaolin ACT is used for monitoring. There is some controversy regarding the underlying reason for this effect. According to Dietrich (36), aprotinin itself has anticoagulant activity through the inhibition of kallikrein and the

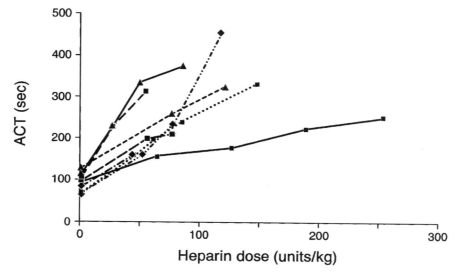

FIGURE 10.1. Heparin responsiveness of the activated clotting time, interpatient variability. (From Mulry CC, Le Veen RF, Sobel M, Lampe PJ, Burke DR. Assessment of heparin anticoagulation during peripheral angioplasty. *J Vasc Interv Radiol* 1991;2:133, with permission.)

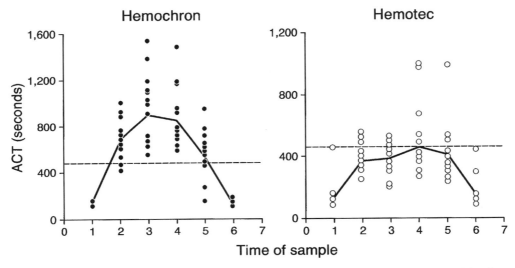

FIGURE 10.2. Comparison of activated clotting time results from celite (Hemochron) and kaolin (Hemotec) based assays. (From Andrew M, MacIntyre B, MacMillan J, et al. Heparin therapy during cardiopulmonary bypass in children requires ongoing quality control. *Thrombo Haemostas* 1993;70:937, with permission.)

prolongation of the celite ACT reflects this effect on the intrinsic pathway. In the kaolin ACT, aprotinin binds to the negatively charged kaolin, and thus cannot interact with the factors of the intrinsic pathway. Other investigators believe that the prolongation of the celite ACT is not indicative of the need for less heparin, because there is little effect when heparin is not present (38) and there is no effect on other heparin-sensitive tests (40).

Other patient factors may affect the activated clotting time. Owings et al. (41) have shown that the Heparin Management Test (HMT) correlates with the heparin concentration better than the ACT in children, who tend to have much lower levels of fibrinogen during cardiopulmonary bypass. Patients on warfarin therapy alone may have slightly longer ACTs, presumably due to warfarin's action on the vitamin K–dependent clotting factors (42). This effect may be important in monitoring low-dose heparin therapy, but is likely to be irrelevant during high-dose treatment. During percutaneous, transluminal coronary angioplasty, venous

ACTs were shown to be consistently longer than arterial ACTs, although there appeared to be no effect on patient treatment (43). The site of administration of the heparin bolus also appears to influence the prolongation of the ACT measured on a femoral vein sample. Central aorta administration of a 10,000-unit heparin bolus results in a relatively slow rise in the ACT to around 300 seconds, whereas the same amount given in the femoral artery produces a rapid rise to between 700 and 800 seconds followed by a decline to the 300-second range (44).

The manufacturer defines quality control for each activated clotting time device. The device typically performs a functional check. In order to meet regulatory requirements, many manufacturers provide electronic monitors that simulate testing when inserted into the instrument. Test cartridges or tubes can also be periodically evaluated with liquid control material in order to assess both the ongoing integrity of the reagents and the precision of the assay. In general, coefficients of variation generated

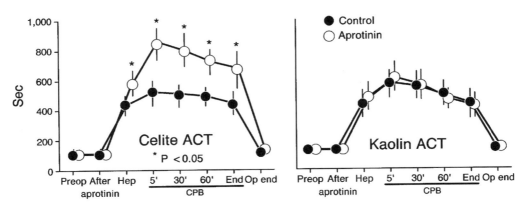

FIGURE 10.3. Effect of aprotinin on the celite- and kaolin-activated clotting times. (From Dietrich W, Dilthey G, Spannagl M, et al. Influence of high-dose aprotinin on anticoagulation, heparin requirement, and celite- and kaolin-activated clotting time in heparin-treated patients undergoing open-heart surgery. *Anesthesiology* 1995;83:679, with permission.)

from control material analyses vary from 3% to 10% for the ACT assays (P.J. Santrach, *unpublished data*, 1995).

Most ACT devices do not test duplicate patient samples on a regular basis. Studies of duplicate samples demonstrate that there is good agreement on the average (32,45). However, the differences can be significant (50 to 100 seconds) in individual cases (32) and the mean differences become greater during heparinization (58.7±57.7 seconds) (45). Thus, when a single ACT does not seem to match the clinical condition of the patient, the test should be repeated.

Method validation of ACT assays is challenging because there is no "gold standard" for comparison and fresh whole-blood samples are required. The high-dose ACT cannot be compared to the activated partial thromboplastin time due to diverse heparin sensitivities. Known amounts of heparin can be added to whole-blood samples to evaluate assay linearity. At best, any new method could be run in parallel with an existing assay in order to understand the heparin responsiveness in patient samples. With low-dose therapy, comparison to the activated partial thromboplastin time (APTT) could be considered mostly as a way to evaluate therapeutic ranges; at least one study has shown a good correlation between the two tests (24).

Heparin Assays

An alternative approach to monitoring heparin therapy involves the determination of heparin levels in the patient's blood. Previous data have shown the variability of the heparin dose response, the variability in heparin half-life, and the lack of correlation between the activated clotting time and plasma heparin levels during cardiopulmonary bypass (22,26,27,46). Studies (31,47) have demonstrated that although the ACTs (both celite and kaolin based) decline only gradually after the initial heparin bolus, the heparin levels exhibit a rapid initial drop followed by a more gradual one (Fig. 10.4). The continued high level of anticoagulation suggested by the ACT during bypass may reflect, in part, the effect of the concurrent hemodilution and hypother-

mia on the ACT rather than heparin function (47,48). Thus, there has been significant interest in better heparin monitoring protocols and two POC systems have been developed: the Hepcon HMS (Medtronic HemoTec, Parker, CO) and the Hemochron RxDx (International Technidyne, Edison, NJ).

The Hepcon HMS is a portable device for coagulation testing that uses the same principles of clot detection as the HemoTec ACT II. Up to six channels are available for testing along with an automated sample delivery system and an onboard computer. Four different types of assays can be performed as part of the heparin management protocol: heparin dose-response test, heparin test, high-range ACT, and heparinase ACT. The heparin dose-response cartridge contains six channels; each channel contains the kaolin activator and enough heparin to produce either a concentration of 2.5 units/ml, 1.5 units/ml, or no heparin (two channels each). A fresh whole-blood sample collected prior to heparinization is added and the clotting times are measured. A dose-response slope is calculated from the results; the heparin concentration needed to achieve an ACT of more than 480 seconds is extrapolated. If patient-specific information regarding height, weight, and extracorporeal volume are entered into the instrument, it will also calculate the bolus dose of heparin to be administered to the patient.

The heparin assay cartridge provides a semiquantitative measurement of the circulating heparin level using a protamine titration method. Each channel contains identical amounts of a dilute thromboplastin and varying amounts of protamine. Fresh whole blood is added to each channel. Protamine is known to neutralize heparin at a ratio of 1.3 mg per 100 units of heparin. Either excess protamine in the channel or excess heparin in the sample will prolong the clotting time; the channel with the shortest clotting time contains the amount of protamine that most closely matches the amount of heparin in the patient sample. Eleven different cartridges are available that span the range of 0 to 6.0 mg/kg or 0 to 8.2 units/ml of heparin. If the measured heparin concentration is less than that projected by the heparin dose-response assay, the device will calculate the amount

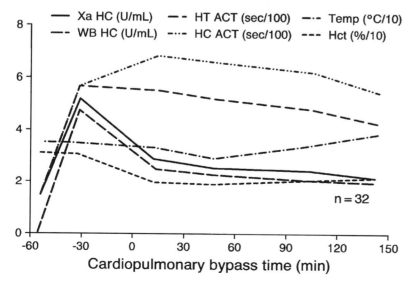

FIGURE 10.4. Comparison of activated clotting times and heparin levels during cardiopulmonary bypass. (XaHC, heparin concentration by anti-Xa method; WB HC, heparin concentration by whole blood protamine titration method; HT ACT, Hemotec activated clotting time; HC ACT, Hemochron activated clotting time.) (From Despotis GJ, Summerfield AL, Joist JH, et al. Comparison of activated coagulation time and whole blood heparin measurements with laboratory plasma anti-Xa heparin concentration in patients having cardiac operations. *J Thorac Cardiovasc Surg* 1994;108: 1076, with permission.)

of additional heparin that should be administered to the patient. The device also calculates the dose of protamine that should be administered to the patient to reverse heparinization.

The high-range ACT is a kaolin-based ACT identical to that performed in the HemoTec ACT II device previously described. It can be performed concurrently with a heparin cartridge so that the heparin level and heparin effect can be assessed together.

The heparinase ACT is designed to detect residual heparin following protamine reversal. This two-channel cartridge contains kaolin activator with a bacterial heparinase in one channel and kaolin activator alone in the other channel. If the fresh whole-blood sample contains residual heparin, the heparinase will eliminate its functional activity, resulting in a shorter ACT than measured in the channel without heparinase. Similar clotting times from both channels suggest that significant amounts of residual heparin are not present.

The Hemochron RxDx is an integrated drug and monitoring system using the Hemochron ACT devices (401, 801, or 8000). The heparin and protamine used in the test system is matched to the injectable heparin and protamine administered to the patient. The heparin response test consists of two ACTs: One uses celite activator alone, and the other contains celite activator and six units of heparin. The results of the two tests are used to determine a heparin dose-response curve and calculate the amount of heparin to be infused to achieve an ACT higher than 480 seconds (cardiopulmonary bypass application). Other reagents are also available to estimate dosing to achieve an ACT of at least 300 seconds (percutaneous transluminal coronary angioplasty application). The protamine response test also consists of two ACTs: One uses celite activator alone, and the other contains celite activator and 40 micrograms of protamine sulfate. The results of the two tests are used to determine a protamine dose-response curve and calculate the amount of protamine to be administered in order to neutralize the circulating heparin. Heparin neutralization can be confirmed with the protamine dose assay. This test consists of a standard celite ACT and a celite ACT with added protamine (10 micrograms). Comparison of the two ACTs should determine whether residual heparin is present and allow calculation of any additional protamine doses that should be given. The calculations can be performed either manually with tools provided by the manufacturer or using the computerized Hemochron 8000.

Heparin concentrations as measured by the Hepcon HMS have been compared to plasma antifactor Xa results in at least three studies. Despotis et al. (47,49) demonstrated excellent correlation between the two assays; bias analysis showed a mean difference of 0.002±0.53 units/ml, although the range of differences was generally ±1 unit/ml. In contrast, Hardy et al. (50) found a greater degree of difference between paired samples, particularly in samples obtained during cardiopulmonary bypass. Only 35% of the data points fell within their predetermined acceptance parameter of ±0.7 units/ml. Similar comparisons were performed by Schlueter et al. (51) at the heparin range of 0 to 1.6 units/ml. These *in vitro* studies showed good linearity over the tested range, excellent precision, and a slight underestimation of the heparin level. In general, the heparin assay performance appears excellent at low concentrations with increasing variability at higher concentrations. This may be related to the different types of assays that are being compared; the results of protamine titration and chromogenic assays are not always equivalent (52). The whole-blood heparin measurements are not affected by aprotinin (53).

Study of the heparin dose-response assay in normal individuals showed very good performance; the measured peak ACT was within 20% of the desired peak in 9 of 10 subjects who received a heparin dose based on the results of the heparin dose-response test (54). In cardiopulmonary bypass patients, Despotis et al. (55) confirmed the interpatient variability of the heparin response and found that the automated assay on the Hepcon tended to overestimate the heparin dose that was required compared to a manual method.

The heparinase ACT was evaluated in 19 cardiac bypass patients before, during, and after heparinization (56). Test results were as predicted when heparin was or was not present.

Lyophilized control material is available from the manufacturer for the heparin assay and the ACT; there is no commercial quality control for the heparin dose-response assay. The precision of the assays is 5% to 12% according to the manufacturer. Method validation for the heparin and heparinase tests can be performed by adding heparin to whole-blood samples.

Performance data on the RxDx system are not available in peer-reviewed journal articles. There are two studies on the clinical performance of these assays discussed in a later section. One disadvantage of this system is the use of celite as the activator in the tests; the effect of aprotinin on the celite ACT may significantly impact these tests as well. Easy-to-use control material is not available for these tests—heparin or protamine must be manually added to commercial control plasma for testing.

Prothrombin Time

The prothrombin time (PT) is a measure of the function of the extrinsic pathway of the coagulation cascade (Fig. 10.5). A blood specimen, typically citrated plasma, is mixed with a thromboplastin reagent and the time to clotting is determined. The thromboplastins are highly variable in terms of tissue source (brain, placenta, or lung), species source (human or animal), and preparation. As a result, they have different sensitivities to decreases in the concentrations of the coagulation factors, particularly the vitamin-K dependent ones (II, VII, IX, X). In fact, each combination of reagent and instrument produces variation in the test, making the interpretation of results from different laboratories problematic. The international normalized ratio (INR) system has been developed in an effort to standardize PT results (57). The INR is a prothrombin ratio that has been adjusted to represent a result that would have been obtained if an international reference reagent had been used to perform the test. The formula for calculating the INR is:

$$INR = (patient\ PT/\ mean\ normal\ PT)^{ISI}$$

An international sensitivity index (ISI) is determined for each reagent, usually by the manufacturer. The ISI represents the sensitivity of the thromboplastin to changes in coagulation-factor concentration; the more sensitive the reagent, the lower the ISI. An ISI of 1.0 reflects sensitivity identical to the international reference reagent. Although use of the INR has improved the com-

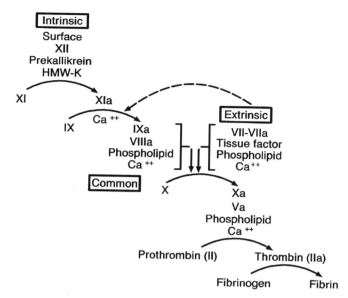

FIGURE 10.5. Coagulation cascade. Courtesy of the Mayo Clinic, Rochester Minnesota.

parability of results among laboratories, differences persist in some cases (58–60).

Various POCT systems for prothrombin time testing are available (Table 10.2). They consist of small, portable devices combined with single-use cartridges or strips containing various thromboplastin reagents. All of them utilize minute amounts of fresh whole blood as a sample; citrated blood specimens may be used in some cases. These samples may be obtained from capillary, arterial, or venous sources. Methodologies for clot detection include cessation of capillary or pump-induced movement, change in oscillation of paramagnetic particles, and alteration of fluorescence. Results are presented both in seconds and as INRs.

Evaluations of the POCT devices for PTs have been performed for the CoaguChek (61–71), CoaguChek Plus/Biotrack 512 Coagulation Monitor (62,72–79), Coumatrak (59,65,80–86), Hemochron Jr. (63,87), Thrombolytic Assessment System (TAS) (62,63,88,89), and ProTime (63,70,71,90–92). These evaluations typically consist of studies of both precision and accuracy. Precision can be assessed by repeated measurements of defined control materials. The coefficient of variation (CV) is the standard deviation divided by the mean of the repeated analyses, and is expressed as a percentage. Published reports indicate that the CVs for POC prothrombin time testing are usually in the range of 2% to 10% (64,67,74,78,83,88,89). Precision can also be examined by deter-

TABLE 10.2. POINT-OF-CARE INSTRUMENTS FOR PROTHROMBIN TIME TESTING

Instrument	Manufacturer	Sample Type			Sample Size	ISI of Thromboplastin
		Fresh Whole Blood	Citrated Whole Blood	Citrated Plasma		
CoaguChek	Roche Diagnostics Corp. Indianapolis, IN	Yes	No	No	10 μL	2.0
CoaguChek Pro DM / CoaguChek Plus / Biotrack / Coumatrak	Roche Diagnostics Corp. Indianapolis, IN	Yes	No	No	25 μL	2.0
GEM PCL	Instrumentation Laboratory Lexington, MA	Yes	No	No	25 μL	2.0
Hemochron Jr Signature	International Technidyne Corp. Edison, NJ	Yes	No	No	25 μL	2.0
ProTime Microcoagulation System	International Technidyne Corp. Edison, NJ	Yes	No	No	60 μL	1.0
Rapidpoint Coag / Thrombolytic Assessment System (TAS)	Bayer Diagnostics Tarrytown, NY	Yes	Yes	Yes	25 μL	1.0, 1.6

mining the differences between duplicate tests of patient samples. In one report, duplicate tests from capillary samples agreed within 0.25 INR units only 28% of the time (82).

Accuracy is usually assessed by comparing the results from the test system with a reference method using well-defined reference material. However, such an approach is problematic for prothrombin time testing due to the marked variation in performance among different thromboplastins and instruments. Therefore, the POC device is typically compared to the laboratory method in place at each institution by analyzing patient samples on both instruments. Most studies show good to excellent correlation (r value>0.8 in regression analysis) between POC and laboratory methods (62–64,66,67,69–71,73,75,76,78,83,86,89). However, the PT results in seconds are usually significantly different among methods unless the ISIs of the thromboplastins are very close. Comparison of the INR results shows better agreement in most cases.

It is important to examine the data using difference plots or Bland-Altman analysis. Difference plots can reveal both the magnitude of the method differences and any method bias, which can be either systematic (to the same degree throughout the range of measurement) or proportional (to varying degrees through the range of measurement). Many studies (61,62,66,72,75,81,82,88) have suggested that POC and laboratory methods agree well in the therapeutic range for oral anticoagulation (INR 2.0 to 3.0), but that POC tests tend to have a positive bias (overestimates the INR) below 2.0 and a negative bias (underestimates the INR) above 3.0. This negative bias also gets larger with higher INR values. Other studies show more consistent agreement with 90% of POC INRs within 0.5 units of the lab result (66) or a more consistent systematic bias (71,92). Additional factors that can contribute to differences between POC and laboratory tests include the use of capillary samples, which are more subject to technique variations during collection, and the use of whole-blood specimens, which may produce longer clotting times than plasma samples.

Another way to assess comparability of methods is to look for clinically important differences (different treatment decisions using POC and laboratory results). Recent studies have documented differences in clinical decision-making in 2% to 50% of paired results (70,71,90,92); the higher percentages were seen with POC devices exhibiting a significant positive bias (71,92).

Knowledge of the comparability of the POC and laboratory methods is important for the clinical user. POC prothrombin times or INRs that are significantly different from the lab results may still be used as long as the user can appropriately interpret them in terms of normal and abnormal; the comparative data can assist with this interpretation. If patient samples are going to be tested by the POC or the lab method at various times, the method comparison data again helps with the interpretation. Although comparison information can be obtained from the literature, facility-specific data are still critical because of the marked variation in reagents and instruments among institutions.

Activated Partial Thromboplastin Time

The APTT reflects the function of the intrinsic pathway of the coagulation cascade (Fig. 10.5). In the laboratory setting, citrated plasma is added to a reagent containing platelet phospholipid, calcium, and a surface activator for Factor XII, such as silica or kaolin. Deficiencies of the factors of both the intrinsic (XII, XI, IX, VIII) and final common pathways (X, V, II, fibrinogen) will produce prolongation of the APTT. The presence of heparin in the plasma sample will also result in an abnormal APTT. Manufactured APTT reagents vary in their sensitivity to both factor deficiency and heparin. Therefore, each institution should evaluate its test system to determine the normal range of values as well as the therapeutic range for heparin therapy. Inter-method differences can be significant and there is no standardization system for the APTT. The ratio of the patient's APTT to the mean normal APTT has been proposed as a way to interpret results, particularly as a guide to transfusion therapy. Recent work has suggested that the therapeutic range for heparin therapy should be determined by comparing the APTT results to actual heparin levels as measured by either anti-Xa or protamine titration methods.

POCT systems for APTTs are listed in Table 10.3. They consist of small, portable devices combined with single-use cartridges. All of them utilize minute amounts of fresh whole blood as a sample; citrated blood specimens may be used in some cases. These samples may be obtained from capillary, arterial, or venous sources. Methodologies for clot detection include cessation of capillary or pump-induced movement and change in oscillation of paramagnetic particles.

TABLE 10.3. POINT-OF-CARE INSTRUMENTS FOR ACTIVATED PARTIAL THROMBOPLASTIN TIME TESTING

Instrument	Manufacturer	Sample Type			Sample Size
		Fresh Whole Blood	Citrated Whole Blood	Citrated Plasma	
CoaguChek Pro DM / CoaguChek Plus / Biotrack 512	Roche Diagnostics Corp. Indianapolis, IN	Yes	No	No	25 ul
GEM PCL	Instrumentation Laboratory Lexington, MA	Yes	No	No	25 ul
Hemochron Jr. Signature	International Technidyne Corp. Edison, NJ	Yes	No	No	25 ul
Rapidpoint™ Coag / Thrombolytic Assessment System (TAS)	Bayer Diagnostics Tarrytown, NY	Yes	Yes	Yes	25 ul

Method evaluation studies involving POC-APTT devices demonstrate that precision based on repetitive testing of liquid control materials is in the range of 3% to 9% (78,89,93,94), which is very similar to that seen for prothrombin times. Despotis et al. (95) examined interinstrument precision with duplicate patient samples and found that the mean difference between the paired samples was +1.8 seconds (range of −4.4 to +8 seconds). Comparison of the POC and laboratory methods also shows good correlations (r >0.8) in most studies (76–78,89,93,95). However, these correlations can differ among hospitals (93) and among nursing units in the same hospital (89). These differences reflect the variable laboratory test systems and test operators used for comparison and emphasize the importance of evaluating the POC test system in the setting in which it will be used rather than just in the laboratory.

Studies also show that in many circumstances, the POC and lab APTT results in seconds do not match. The mean difference may be as much as 9 to 13 seconds (32,76,77,96,97), with the POC test typically longer. The clinical significance of this difference depends on the use of the POC APTT. Werner et al. (94) analyzed the decision-making agreement between POC and laboratory tests for heparin management. In a two-step nomogram for femoral sheath removal, the two methods resulted in the same clinical decision 93% of the time. However, in a six-step nomogram for heparin therapy following thrombolytic therapy, clinical agreement occurred only 53% of the time. A more recent study found that agreement on clinical decisions between the laboratory and the POC device occurred in 59% to 68% of cases (97). Therefore, as mentioned above for prothrombin time testing, each facility should evaluate the comparability of the two methods and may have to develop treatment nomograms specific for the APTT test method used.

Platelet Function Tests

Major developmental efforts have been focused on POCT for platelet function. One of the driving forces behind this activity is the known platelet function defect that occurs after cardiopulmonary bypass. If there was a reliable test for platelet dysfunction, the problem might be detected and treated before excessive bleeding developed. An understanding of the role of platelets in acute coronary syndromes has led to the use of platelet inhibitors; platelet function tests could shed more light on pathophysiology and treatment effectiveness. Labor-intensive platelet aggregation tests have been the gold standard, but their slow turnaround time does not allow them to be used to guide acute therapy. The bleeding time has also been a routine test for platelet dysfunction, but its use is problematic in terms of standardization and the practical inability to do multiple tests on the same patient in a relatively short period of time. The bleeding time is also not predictive of the risk of perioperative hemorrhage (98–100).

The platelet-activated clotting time (PACT) (HemoSTATUS, Medtronic HemoTec, Parker, CO) is designed to assess platelet function in terms of the ability of platelet activating factor (PAF) to shorten the kaolin-activated clotting time. The test is performed on the Hepcon HMS with a fresh whole-blood sample. The six-channel test cartridge contains kaolin, heparin, and varying concentrations of PAF (0 to 150 nM). The clotting

times are used to calculate clot ratios (1 − [ACT/control ACT]) and percent maximal responses (clot ratio/normal control clot ratio). Studies (101,102) have shown that the clot ratios at high PAF concentrations significantly decrease after cardiopulmonary bypass and significantly improve after the administration of platelets or desmopressin, consistent with the expected post-bypass platelet dysfunction. However, comparisons with standard platelet aggregation tests were not performed. Increasing amounts of abciximab, a glycoprotein IIb/IIIa inhibitor, cause dose-dependent decreases in the clot ratios *in vitro*, again suggesting that this test does reflect platelet function (103). However, the PACT is significantly affected by severe thrombocytopenia (less than 50,000/uL) and abnormal white blood cell counts (either low or high) (103).

The Platelet Function Analyzer (PFA-100, Dade Behring, Miami, FL) is designed to simulate primary hemostasis after injury to a small vessel (104–106). The test cartridges consist of a reservoir for citrated whole blood, a capillary tube and a collagen-coated membrane with a central aperture. An agonist [epinephrine or adenosine diphosphate (ADP)] present on the membrane and the high shear rates stimulate platelet activation, adhesion, and aggregation as the blood moves through the aperture under vacuum. The instrument measures the time to full closure of the aperture. Intrinsic platelet defects, von Willebrand disease, and platelet inhibition agents should cause prolongation of the closure time in the collagen/epinephrine cartridge (normal closure time less than 170 seconds). A prolonged closure time with the collagen/epinephrine cartridge but a normal closure time with the collagen/ADP cartridge (less than 114 seconds) may detect the effect of aspirin on platelets.

Comparison studies (106) with standard platelet aggregation testing have shown equivalent sensitivity (94.9%) and specificity (88.8%) in patients with a variety of platelet function defects. Other studies have demonstrated that the performance of the PFA-100 is superior to that of the bleeding time in identifying platelet-related defects in primary hemostasis, particularly von Willebrand disease (105,107–109). The therapeutic effect of desmopressin in von Willebrand disease may also be discerned (107–110). The ability of the device to detect aspirin effect appears to be good (106,111–114). Abciximab, a platelet glycoprotein IIb/IIIa blocking agent, produces dose-dependent prolongation of the closure time (112). Imprecision has been below 15% (105,106,111).

The Clot Signature Analyzer (CSA, Xylum, San Diego, CA) evaluates hemostatic function by subjecting untreated whole blood to physiologic flow and temperature conditions (115,116). Blood is perfused through a precision needle punch channel and a collagen reaction channel. In the punch channel, a needle pierces the perfusion tubing; blood flows out of the resultant holes (decreased luminal pressure) until occlusion occurs (recovery of luminal pressure). The time from the punch to recovery is the platelet hemostasis time (PHT). Eventually flow through the tubing ceases due to clotting. The time to total cessation of luminal flow is the clotting time (CT). In the collagen reaction channel, a type I bovine collagen fiber is set in the lumen along the direction of flow. As the blood moves past, platelets adhere to the fiber forming a thrombus that eventually completely occludes the lumen and drops the pressure to zero.

The time from the start of blood flow to a 50% drop in luminal pressure is named collagen-induced thrombus formation time (CITF). Preliminary studies (115,116) have demonstrated that the PHT and CITF are prolonged when blood contains antibodies to glycoprotein IIb/IIIa, glycoprotein Ib, and von Willebrand factor, consistent with a primary effect on platelet adhesion and aggregation. Prolongation of the CT is produced by heparin, indicating that this parameter reflects the activity of the coagulation factors.

The Rapid Platelet Function Assay (Ultegra, Accumetrics, San Diego, CA) is designed to measure the effect of glycoprotein IIb/IIIa inhibitors. The reagent cartridge for this device contains fibrinogen-coated polystyrene beads and a peptide that activates the thrombin receptor on platelets. When citrated whole blood is added to the two reaction chambers, the platelets in the sample and the beads agglutinate. Abciximab, which blocks glycoprotein IIb/IIIA, causes a dose-dependent inhibition of this agglutination. The results of this assay correlate highly with both standard platelet aggregation tests (r=0.98) and the percentage of unblocked glycoprotein IIb/IIIa (r=0.96) (116). Aspirin or heparin does not affect the results.

The Hemodyne clot retractometer (Hemodyne, Richmond, VA) evaluates platelet function based on the retraction and stability of a clot formed between the surfaces of a shallow cup and an overlying probe (117,118). A standardized platelet-rich plasma sample is placed in the cup and clot formation is allowed to proceed under controlled conditions. As the clot retracts, downward force is applied to the probe and measured. The clot modulus can also be calculated as a ratio of the downward force to the downward displacement. Preliminary studies suggest that the platelet force development is a linear function of the platelet concentration and is primarily dependent on platelet function, but independent of clot structure and fibrin concentration from 100 to 400 mg per deciliter (119,120). Clot modulus is significantly affected by both platelet function and fibrin structure. Glycoprotein IIb/IIIa blockade results in decreased platelet force development and clot modulus (121,122). In cardiac surgery patients, the platelet force development is not detectable during cardiopulmonary bypass and partially recovers after protamine administration, consistent with a defect in platelet function (123). Concurrent platelet aggregation testing showed a marked decrease in ADP- and ristocetin-induced aggregation during bypass that did not recover after protamine was given. Additional work suggests that heparin plays a major role in producing the bypass-induced platelet defects as measured by force development and clot modulus (124). Studies of platelet force development in other clinical situations have not been performed to date.

Plateletworks (Helena Laboratories, Beaumont, TX) is a POC whole-blood platelet aggregation assay. Two blood specimens are collected from the patient; one collection tube contains ethylenediaminetetraacetic acid (EDTA) and the other tube has a platelet agonist (ADP or collagen). The device is essentially a cell counter—a complete blood count is performed on both blood samples. In the EDTA tube, all of the patient's platelets should be in circulation and thus counted. In the agonist tube, the platelet aggregation should occur and thus the number of platelets counted should be less. The percent aggregation is calculated from the results of both samples. The manufacturer states that normal individuals will have 63% to 87% aggregation with collagen and 80% to 97% with ADP. Test results appear to correlate with traditional aggregometry using platelet-rich plasma (125).

Viscoelastic Tests of Clot Formation

Thromboelastography

Although originally developed by Hartert in 1948 (126), thromboelastography has only recently gained increasing application in clinical situations as a means of assessing multiple aspects of the hemostatic system. This device monitors the physical forces created by the coagulation and fibrinolysis of whole blood over time. A whole-blood specimen is placed into a heated sample cup; a piston is suspended in the sample and the cup rotates through a 4.45° angle. As coagulation progresses, fibrin strands form between the walls of the cup and the piston. This connection causes the piston to move with the cup and the movement is translated into a graphical tracing over time (Fig. 10.6). The sample cups were originally metal and had to be carefully cleaned between uses. Disposable plastic cups are now available. A delay of up to 3 minutes between the collection of a native whole-blood sample into a plastic syringe and the start of the thromboelastography (TEG) analysis does not appear to significantly alter the results (127). Citrated whole blood can also be used, provided that calcium is added at the beginning of the test; some differences in results may be seen depending on length and temperature of sample storage (128,129).

From the TEG tracing, the following parameters (see Fig. 10.7) may be measured, either manually or with computer software:

Reaction time (R time): the time from the start of the tracing to the onset of clot formation, which is defined as a 1-mm deflection

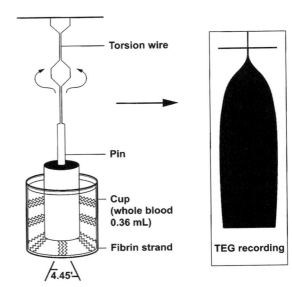

FIGURE 10.6. Thromboelastography: mechanism of action. (From Mallet SV, Cox DJA. Thromboelastography. *Br J Anaesth* 1992;69:307, with permission.) Courtesy of the Mayo Clinic, Rochester Minnesota.

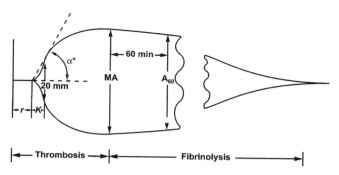

FIGURE 10.7. Thromboelastographic measurements. (From Mallet SV, Cox DJA. Thromboelastography. *Br J Anaesth* 1992;69:307, with permission.) Courtesy of the Mayo Clinic, Rochester Minnesota.

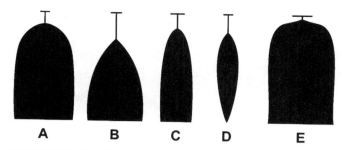

FIGURE 10.8. Thromboelastography: diagnostic patterns. **(A)** normal; **(B)** hemophilia; **(C)** thrombocytopenia; **(D)** fibrinolysis; **(E)** hypercoagulability. (From Mallet SV, Cox DJA. Thromboelastography. *Br J Anaesth* 1992;69:307, with permission.) Courtesy of the Mayo Clinic, Rochester Minnesota.

Clot formation time (K time): the time from initial clot formation to a fixed level of clot firmness, which is defined as a 20-mm deflection of the tracing

Angle (α): the maximum slope from initial clot formation to the shoulder of the tracing

Maximum amplitude (MA): the width of the tracing at its widest point

Clot lysis (Ly30): the rate of decrease in maximum amplitude 30 minutes after the MA. Other calculated values that also reflect the degree of clot lysis and have been used in the past include MA+30, MA+60, and A_{60}

What do these various TEG parameters represent in terms of coagulation function? Studies have tried to answer that question either directly or indirectly. The R time appears to reflect the function of the coagulation factors of the intrinsic pathway. Statistically significant correlations have been found between the R time and the APTT (130,131). Tuman et al. (132) also demonstrated that in cardiopulmonary bypass patients, the preoperative R time was not correlated with platelet aggregation studies but was shortened in the presence of celite activators, consistent with the suggested APTT relationship. Similar correlations are evident between the APTT and both the K time and the angle (131). Furthermore, the transfusion of cryoprecipitate, which contains factor VIII and fibrinogen, shortens the R time and the angle (130).

The MA is probably the most widely applied parameter of the TEG. Many studies have shown that the MA correlates with platelet count, platelet function (as determined by platelet aggregation studies), and fibrinogen concentration (130,132–136). Thrombocytopenia, decreased platelet function and/or hypofibrinogenemia produce decreased maximum amplitudes. Platelet transfusion increases the MA (reflecting the improvement in platelet count and/or function) as well as the angle and decreases the R time (reflecting the effect of the coagulation factors in the plasma of the platelet product) (130,137–139). The lysis time correlates with the euglobulin lysis time, which suggests that it represents the effect of fibrinolysis on the test system (130).

Although it is important to calculate and define the normal ranges for these parameters, clinical decisions are often made based on the characteristic pattern of the tracing as it develops (Fig. 10.8). In patients with coagulation factor deficiencies, such as hemophilia, or on anticoagulation therapy, the R and K times tend to be prolonged and the angle is decreased (Fig. 10.8B). Thrombocytopenia and platelet dysfunction produce a narrow tracing due to the predominant decrease in the maximum amplitude (Fig. 10.8C). Active fibrinolysis causes rapid tapering of the tracing, sometimes limiting the MA because clot lysis occurs so quickly (Fig. 10.8D). Patients with hypercoagulable states have TEG tracings with markedly shortened R and K times as well as a significantly increased angle (Fig. 10.8E).

Modifications of the standard TEG procedure have been proposed in some clinical situations as a means of gathering more useful data. Probably the most common modification is the addition of celite activator as a means of accelerating the test. Celite activation does provide faster results, but also changes the measured parameters; R and K times are decreased while the MA and clot lysis percent are increased (140). Heparinase has been added in an effort to detect the presence of heparin in the sample. In this case, the standard TEG is run in parallel with the heparinase TEG; similar results should be obtained if no heparin is present. This technique has been used to detect a heparin effect during the reperfusion stage of liver transplantation surgery (141,142), to detect residual heparin after protamine administration in cardiac surgery (143,144), and to investigate the effect of postoperative low-dose heparin in vascular surgery (145). Recently, a modified TEG procedure has also been developed in to monitor the use of platelet glycoprotein IIb/IIIa blockade therapy (122,146).

Sonoclot Coagulation and Platelet Function Analyzer

Another POC device that attempts to assess multiple aspects of the hemostatic system is the Sonoclot Coagulation and Platelet Function Analyzer (Sienco, Morrison, CO). Hemostatic function is interpreted from the mechanical impedance generated by the forming clot. A plastic probe is suspended in a fresh whole-blood sample contained in a heated plastic cuvette (Fig. 10.9). The probe oscillates through a defined amplitude at a defined frequency and is attached to a transducer. As the clot forms, more power is required to keep the probe oscillating at its set rate; these changes in impedance are translated into a tracing with a typical normal pattern (Fig. 10.9). The following parameters may be measured:

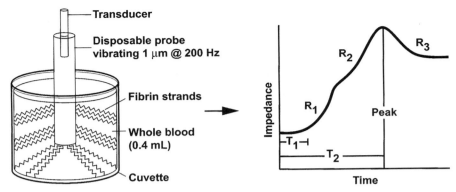

FIGURE 10.9. Principles of Sonoclot Coagulation and Platelet Function Analyzer. (From Tuman KJ, Spiess BD, McCarthy RJ, et al. Comparison of viscoelastic measures of coagulation after cardiopulmonary bypass. *Anesth Analg* 1989;69:69, with permission.)

SonACT (T1): The time from the onset of the test to the beginning of clot formation

Primary upward slope (R1): The rate of initial clot formation from baseline to the inflection point, which is considered to be initial clot retraction

Secondary upward slope (R2): The rate of clot formation from the inflection point to the peak

Time to peak (T2): The time from the onset of the test to the peak

Peak: The maximum amount of impedance developed during clot formation

Primary downward slope (R3): The rate of clot retraction

Direct correlations between Sonoclot parameters and common coagulation tests have not been documented. Much of the work on the Sonoclot has focused on its ability to represent platelet count and function. Early studies evaluating this device used recalcified platelet-rich plasma, platelet-poor plasma, or citrated whole blood as samples. Saleem et al. (147) demonstrated that the later slopes of clot formation (R2) and retraction (R3) were not seen in platelet-poor plasma; the tracing consisted only of the SonACT, R1, and inflection, which became a plateau. Platelet-rich plasma produced a more typical Sonoclot tracing; increasing platelet concentrations resulted in shortened SonACTs, increasing slopes (R1, R2, and R3), higher peaks, and shorter times to peak. In patients undergoing cardiopulmonary bypass, they found that abnormal tracings post-bypass could be returned to normal and bleeding decreased after platelet transfusion. In orthopedic patients, most of the Sonoclot parameters (R1, R2, R3, time to peak, etc.) were correlated with the platelet count (148). Some parameters were also correlated with age and gender in this study. The time to peak has been shown to have a significant negative correlation with collagen-induced platelet aggregation studies, fibrinogen concentrations, and platelet counts in cardiac surgery patients (149). The SonACT appears to reflect the activated clotting time and to be affected by heparin; prolongations after cardiopulmonary bypass can be normalized by administration of protamine (150). Inter- and intraindividual variability may be significant, particularly for the rate parameters—one study found coefficients of variation as high as 41% (151).

CLINICAL APPLICATIONS OF POINT-OF-CARE HEMATOLOGY/HEMOSTASIS TESTS

Cardiopulmonary Bypass Surgery

Heparin Monitoring

One of the earliest applications of POC coagulation testing is heparin monitoring during cardiopulmonary bypass surgery. The extracorporeal circuit requires extensive heparinization of the patient's blood in order to prevent clotting and rapid reversal at completion to minimize postoperative bleeding. The high heparin concentration (1 to 6 units/ml) is far beyond the sensitivity of the APTT and the clinical situation requires rapid assessment and treatment in order to prevent an adverse outcome. In 1966, Hattersley (152) described a whole-blood activated coagulation time, which has become the routine test for heparin monitoring. In 1975, Bull et al. (26) proposed a simplified monitoring protocol; variations of this approach have been used since then.

A typical heparin monitoring protocol for bypass includes:

A baseline ACT is performed. For bypass patients, this is usually less than 190 seconds for a celite ACT.

A weight-based dose of heparin is administered intravenously.

Another ACT is performed to determine if the goal of at least 480 seconds has been reached. If not, additional heparin is given. The extracorporeal circuit also contains 5000 units of heparin to minimize the drop in heparin concentration when bypass is begun.

During bypass, the ACT is performed every 30 to 60 minutes. Again, additional heparin is infused if the ACT is less than 480 seconds.

At the end of bypass, protamine sulfate is given in a dose based on the total amount of heparin administered (0.8 to 1.3 mg protamine per 100 units of heparin).

The ACT is performed to see if it has returned to the baseline result, indicating successful heparin neutralization. If not, additional protamine is infused.

As previously discussed, patients have varying heparin dose response and clearance. The threshold of 480 seconds has been set somewhat arbitrarily, as the only gold standard for adequacy of heparinization is the lack of clotting in the extracorporeal circuit. Animal studies have suggested that an ACT of at least 400 seconds will prevent the formation of fibrin monomers (153). The ACT does not correlate with heparin concentration during bypass, in part due to hemodilution and hypothermia. Questions remain about whether too little or too much heparin is being given and the role of excess protamine as well as excess heparin in post-bypass hemorrhage. As a result, investigators have studied the clinical performance of new monitoring protocols that involve the determination of heparin dose response for each patient, ongoing monitoring of heparin concentration during bypass, and a more specific determination of the postbypass protamine dose. Both the Hepcon HMS and Hemochron RxDx systems have been evaluated.

The standard monitoring protocol was compared to one using the Hepcon HMS by Despotis et al. (154). The study group patients had initial heparin doses determined by the results of the heparin dose-response test. Ongoing adequacy of heparinization was assessed by heparin concentration and additional doses were given if the level dropped below the optimal concentration identified by the dose-response test. Protamine doses were calculated based on the heparin concentration at the end of bypass. Adequacy of neutralization was assessed with the heparinase ACT. Postoperative bleeding was evaluated with POCT (prothrombin time, activated partial thromboplastin time, and platelet count); transfusions were given based on an algorithm. The study group received significantly more heparin than the control group (612±147 versus 462±114 units/kg); however, the post-bypass protamine doses were the same. In spite of the increased heparin administration, the post-bypass prothrombin time and activated partial thromboplastin time were significantly lower in the study group although 24-hour postoperative chest drainage was not significantly different. This group also received fewer platelet, plasma, and cryoprecipitate transfusions and had shorter operative times for closure. Further work (155) suggested that the improved outcome was due to better suppression of hemostatic activation as reflected by decreased consumption of coagulation factors and decreased production of fibrinopeptide A and D-dimers. Similar results have been demonstrated in a randomized trial of children (156) undergoing cardiopulmonary bypass.

DeLaria et al. (157) compared the Hemochron RxDx monitoring protocol to one using the Hepcon HMS (without the heparin dose-response test or the heparinase ACT). The RxDx protocol consisted of an initial dose determined by a heparin response test, ongoing maintenance of a heparin concentration of 3.0 to 3.5 mg per kilograms, and a protamine dose determined by a protamine response test (see previous section on heparin assays). Transfusions to both groups were given according to specific criteria. The average protamine dose for the RxDx group was significantly lower than the Hepcon group. The RxDx patients also had less chest tube drainage at 12 hours and transfusions; fewer RxDx patients required reexploration for postoperative hemorrhage. The improved outcome was attributed to the lower and presumably more correctly matched protamine doses that could be achieved using this integrated drug and testing system.

Jobes et al. (158) also studied the RxDx protocol in comparison to a conventional monitoring approach. An addition to the RxDx protocol involved assessment of the adequacy of neutralization. After the initial protamine dose, an ACT, thrombin time, and heparin-neutralized thrombin time were performed. If residual heparin of more than 0.05 unit/ml was present, the thrombin time should be prolonged and the heparin-neutralized thrombin time should be normal. As seen previously, the RxDx group received more heparin and less protamine, but exhibited less 24-hour chest tube drainage and was transfused less. In contrast, a later study found no improvement in postoperative bleeding and transfusion requirements with the use of the RxDx system (159).

The use of aprotinin to reduce blood loss in cardiopulmonary bypass surgery has introduced additional complexities into heparin monitoring due to its effect on the celite ACT as previously described. Three approaches have been suggested in these cases: (a) use a kaolin ACT in a conventional monitoring protocol, (b) use the celite ACT in a conventional monitoring protocol but keep the celite ACT at more than 750 seconds, or (c) use a kaolin-based heparin measurement system.

The conventional monitoring protocol is still the predominant one due to its long-standing success in cardiopulmonary bypass. However, these few studies on a heparin concentration approach are intriguing. Further clinical research should be performed to determine the optimal heparin management system.

Anticoagulation monitoring during cardiopulmonary bypass (CPB) is particularly problematic when patients have either a lupus anticoagulant or heparin-induced thrombocytopenia. Lupus anticoagulants prolong not only the APTT but also the ACT. Kaolin ACT tests are affected to a greater degree than celite-based tests. Although heparin can still be used as the anticoagulant, it may be necessary to use heparin measurements for monitoring (160). In contrast, patients with heparin-induced thrombocytopenia should not receive heparin during CPB. In such cases, hirudin may be used for anticoagulation; monitoring may be performed with the ecarin clotting time (161,162).

Post-Bypass Bleeding and Transfusion Therapy

A significant complication of cardiopulmonary bypass surgery is the development of excessive hemorrhage after bypass is completed. Such bleeding occurs in 5% to 25% of patients and predisposing risk factors appear to be repeat cardiac surgery, cyanotic heart disease, long bypass times, prior warfarin therapy, hypothermia, and fibrinolysis (163). The nature of the hemostatic defect produced by extracorporeal circulation is multifactorial and can include thrombocytopenia, platelet dysfunction, and coagulation factor deficiency. Thrombocytopenia, usually mild or moderate, typically occurs during surgery; both hemodilution (164,165) and platelet activation/adhesion (164) are thought to contribute to the lower platelet counts. The most consistent problem is alteration of platelet function as evidenced by prolonged bleeding times and abnormal platelet aggregation studies. The nature of this defect is not completely clear; hypothermia (164), platelet activation and degranulation (164,166), heparin (167,168), alterations in platelet membrane receptor molecules (169,170), and extrinsic inhibition (171) have all been suggested as causative factors. It is also known that coagulation factor concentrations significantly decrease during bypass related to both hemodilution and consumption. Dramatic fibrinolysis may also develop; however, in most cases, there is probably low-level fibrinolysis (172,173) that contributes to coagulation factor deficiency, particularly hypofibrinogenemia.

This complicated hemostatic picture has made the treatment of post-bypass bleeding challenging. In the past, the turnaround time of most laboratory tests were far too long to be of much use in the operating room; specific defects could not be easily identified and treated. Thus, cardiac surgeons and anesthesiologists had to use a generic approach to treatment: If bleeding occurred, a possible surgical source was evaluated and platelets and fresh frozen plasma were automatically transfused. If bleeding persisted, cryoprecipitate as well as additional platelet and plasma transfusions were administered. However, the availability of POCT in the operating room has significantly modified this treatment strategy.

Despotis et al. (73) evaluated the utility of POC coagulation studies and platelet counts on blood loss and transfusion requirements in CPB patients with post-bypass microvascular bleeding. The patients were randomized into either standard therapy or algorithm therapy groups. The algorithm therapy group had on-site prothrombin times, APTTs, and platelet counts available to them with a fast turnaround time; these results were used to guide transfusion therapy using a practice guideline. The standard group did not have rapid test results available and relied on the traditional practice for transfusion indications. Significant differences were seen in the algorithm group: fewer transfusions, shorter operative times, and less mediastinal chest tube drainage. Similar findings have been recently reported by Nuttall et al. (174) who used POC test results (platelet count, TEG, PT, and APTT) in an algorithm for intraoperative transfusions. They also found decreased postoperative blood loss, fewer transfusions of plasma and platelets, and a decreased incidence of surgical reoperation for bleeding in the algorithm group. These results suggest that the combination of transfusion guidelines and rapid testing can significantly improve the diagnosis and treatment of post-bypass hemorrhage.

However, differences in test methods (laboratory versus POC) and decision levels should be considered when designing such transfusion algorithms. In two different studies, Nuttall et al. (175,176) demonstrated that receiver-operator analysis could be used to determine the decision points for various coagulation-related tests that best predict the risk of ongoing hemorrhage. They have shown that abnormal PT and APTT results are common after bypass and that the most sensitive and specific decision points are higher than the upper limit of the reference range. Furthermore, the potential impact of other blood conservation strategies must be considered. For example, aprotinin can prolong the whole-blood APTT in a dose-dependent fashion (177).

The new POC platelet function tests are also being evaluated for their role in predicting and treating post-CPB hemorrhage. The platelet activated clotting time (PACT), when done upon arrival in the intensive care unit, has shown a significant correlation with the amount of postoperative mediastinal chest tube drainage at 4 hours (101). However, other studies have demonstrated only weak or no correlation with postoperative blood loss (102,178,179) with no improvement in prediction compared to routine coagulation tests. Other work suggests that the PACT

can identify a group of patients that would benefit, in terms of bleeding and transfusion needs, from the administration of desmopressin after CPB (180). Wahba et al. (181) found a moderate correlation between preoperative platelet function testing with the PFA-100 and total blood loss; however, the correlation was comparable to that seen with preoperative platelet count and duration of CPB. Other investigators have found no correlation of PFA-100 results with perioperative blood loss (182,183). A study (123) of the Hemodyne clot retractometer in cardiac surgery demonstrated that platelet force development (a measure of the clot retraction function of platelets) was abolished during bypass and recovered after administration of protamine. The percent recovery was inversely correlated with the amount of chest tube drainage at both 12 and 24 hours after surgery, but not with the ACT or the APTT.

The TEG has also been investigated as both a predictor of post-bypass hemorrhage and a guide to transfusion therapy. Tuman et al. (184) compared the TEG as well as the Sonoclot to routine coagulation tests (ACT, PT, APTT, platelet count, fibrinogen concentration) in terms of the ability to predict which of 42 CPB patients would experience significant hemorrhage. The mean values of all parameters were normal in these patients before heparinization, but nine patients had clinical bleeding post-bypass. After protamine administration, only the mean value of the maximum amplitude distinguished the group of bleeding patients from the group that did not bleed. For the Sonoclot, the distinguishing variables were the R2, peak, and R3. Overall, on an individual patient basis, the predictive accuracy of the routine coagulation tests was only 33% compared to 88% for the TEG and 74% for the Sonoclot; no patient with bleeding had a completely normal TEG or Sonoclot. This group had previously reported similar results (131). In contrast, two other studies (185,186) demonstrated no correlation between TEG results and postoperative blood loss, either preoperatively or post-bypass.

The TEG has also been used successfully to guide transfusion therapy perioperatively. A randomized placebo-controlled trial of desmopressin therapy after cardiopulmonary bypass (187) suggested that a maximum amplitude of less than 50 mm identifies patients who have an abnormality of platelet-fibrinogen interaction and benefit from desmopressin administration. Shore-Lesserson et al. (188) developed a post-bypass transfusion algorithm based on results from celite TEGs with and without heparinase, platelet counts, and fibrinogen concentrations. Compared to a different algorithm using routine coagulation tests (ACT, PT, APTT, fibrinogen, and platelet count), this randomized trial showed that the TEG-based algorithm resulted in significantly fewer patients receiving fresh frozen plasma and platelet transfusions. Royston and von Kier (189) used the R time and MA values from a heparinase-modified, celite-activated TEG performed during CPB in an algorithm for fresh frozen plasma and platelet transfusion. In their randomized trial of 60 patients, the algorithm group received significantly fewer transfusions although chest tube blood loss was not significantly different.

Liver Transplantation

Orthotopic liver transplantation is another clinical situation with a rapidly changing hemostatic picture that may benefit from the availability of POC coagulation tests. Preoperatively, these patients have multiple coagulation abnormalities due to their underlying liver disease. Coagulation factor deficiencies, thrombocytopenia, poor platelet function, and fibrinolysis may be seen. During transplantation, dramatic changes occur during the anhepatic stage with further decreases in platelet count and coagulation factor concentration as well as increasing fibrinolysis (190). Hemodilution, hypothermia, ionized hypocalcemia, and acidosis may compound these abnormalities. Coagulation status typically improves as the new liver becomes functional, although coagulopathy may persist postoperatively. Therefore, transfusion of multiple blood products is common and rapid test results may be beneficial in the selection of the appropriate blood component to treat specific abnormalities.

It is this clinical situation in which TEG became commonly applied in the 1980s. Kang et al. (130) studied the changes in the TEG patterns that occurred during transplantation and developed a transfusion algorithm using various TEG parameters as decision points. The relationship between TEG parameters and other coagulation tests is described earlier in this chapter. The algorithm indicated transfusion of fresh frozen plasma when the reaction time was more than 15 minutes, platelets when the maximum amplitude was less than 40 mm, and cryoprecipitate when the angle was less than 45 degrees. Compared to historical controls, the patients treated with the algorithm received fewer red blood cell and fresh frozen plasma transfusions, more platelet and cryoprecipitate transfusions, and less total fluids infused intraoperatively. The number of allogeneic donor exposures per patient was not significantly different. This approach has been extended to the postoperative period by Plevak et al. (191). This group compared a TEG-based algorithm to one using conventional coagulation tests. They found that when the TEG parameters were used, the patients received fewer fresh frozen plasma and cryoprecipitate transfusions, were exposed to fewer allogeneic blood donors, and incurred less cost. Other investigators compared the TEG, Sonoclot, and routine coagulation tests during the stages of the transplant procedure; in this study, the Sonoclot was not as sensitive as the TEG to coagulation abnormalities during surgery (192).

Cardiac Catheterization

Another clinical setting that utilizes high-dose heparin treatment is percutaneous, transluminal coronary angioplasty and other related cardiac catheterization procedures. Significant anticoagulation is required to prevent intracoronary thrombus secondary the presence of the catheter in the patient's circulation. POCT with the ACT has become routine for monitoring due to the need for rapid turnaround time during the procedure and the relatively high doses of heparin beyond the measuring range of the APTT.

The typical protocol in adults consists of either a single bolus of 10,000 units of heparin or a weight-adjusted heparin dose (100 units/kg); an activated clotting time of more than 300 to 400 seconds is often maintained with an intraprocedural heparin infusion (193,194). The optimal range for the ACT has not been well defined. A recent meta-analysis suggests that 350 to 375 seconds provides the best protection against ischemia at 7 days post-procedure without increasing the risk of hemorrhage

(195). However, some investigators have proposed that a 2,500-unit bolus of heparin with an average ACT of 185 seconds is sufficient (196). Differences among the various ACT assays are also evident in these patients and may necessitate the use of device-specific thresholds for the adequacy of anticoagulation (195,197,198). Protamine reversal is usually not performed. Patients may continue to receive low-dose heparin infusions after the procedure and the degree of anticoagulation is monitored with the activated partial thromboplastin rather than the ACT. Removal of the femoral sheath often depends on the ACT; it is removed when the ACT is less than 180 seconds.

Recently, platelet glycoprotein IIb/IIIa receptor blockade has become an accepted therapy to reduce the incidence of ischemic complications after percutaneous coronary revascularization (199,200). As a result of receptor blockade, fibrinogen cannot bind to the receptor and further platelet aggregation is prevented. The relationships among dosage, degree of platelet inhibition, and clinical outcome are not well defined (201). There is considerable interest in the use of POC platelet function tests to explore these correlations and to monitor such therapy in individual patients (201,202). However, the ideal assay has not yet been identified. The PFA-100 (203,204), the Rapid Platelet Function Assay (205,206), and the Clot Signature Analyzer (206) have been studied with mixed results. Furthermore, at least one of these agents, abciximab, appears to prolong the activated clotting time, which raises questions regarding possible anticoagulant as well as antiplatelet activity (207–209). Current studies suggest that the dose of heparin can be lowered and the ACT kept at a lower level to reduce the risk of bleeding complications while maintaining the reduction in risk (199).

Anticoagulation Monitoring

Heparin

Heparin is commonly used to provide rapid anticoagulation for the treatment of thromboembolism, unstable angina, and acute myocardial infarction. Peri-procedural heparin anticoagulation is also used in cardiac surgery (cardiopulmonary bypass), vascular surgery, and cardiac catheterization as previously described. Heparin, particularly subcutaneous preparations, may also be used for the prevention of thrombosis or embolism in selected patients at risk (52,210). Heparin exerts its anticoagulant effect by its ability to bind with antithrombin III and thereby increase the inactivation of thrombin, Factor IX, and Factor X.

Therapy with unfractionated heparin is challenging for a variety of reasons. The half-life of heparin is relatively short. There is a risk of thrombosis if too little heparin is given and a risk of bleeding if too much is administered; thus the therapeutic range is narrow. Heparin preparations vary in anticoagulant effect due to differences in molecular size, polysaccharide chain length, and bioavailability. Patients themselves also differ in their responsiveness to heparin as mentioned previously. Adding to the potential for confusion is the variable heparin responsiveness of APTT reagents (211), for which there is no available standardization scheme.

Typical heparin therapy consists of an initial intravenous bolus followed by a continuous infusion and periodic monitoring; standard doses of heparin are administered and subsequently adjusted based on the results of the APTT. The target for monitoring has been considered to be an APTT ratio (patient value/normal control value) of at least 1.5 in order to prevent thrombosis. Some studies (212,213) suggest that heparin measurements are a better monitor, but such assays are not in widespread use. Current recommendations are that the therapeutic range should be determined by each facility based on the APTT method used. Ideally, this range should correspond to heparin levels of 0.2 to 0.4 units/mL (protamine titration method) or 0.3 to 0.7 units/mL (anti-Xa method) (52).

Over the last few years, dose adjustments using weight-based nomograms (Table 10.4) have been proposed as an alternative strategy. A randomized trial of such a nomogram versus a fixed dosing schedule showed that the patients in the nomogram group reached the therapeutic range of APTT values faster than the control group, had a lower risk of recurrent thromboembolism, and had no increased risk of bleeding (214). Other studies have shown similar outcomes supporting this approach (215–222). The importance of rapid achievement of therapeutic levels of heparin was confirmed by a recent study by Hull et al. (223). They showed that patients who failed to achieve a therapeutic APTT by 24 hours after initiation of treatment had a much higher risk for recurrent thrombosis.

Although most of the previous work was performed using laboratory-based APTT methods, there have been some studies looking at these same questions with POC APTTs. In 1994, Becker et al. (224) demonstrated that the use of POCT significantly decreased the time from test performance to dose adjustment (mean 14.5 minutes versus 3.0 hours, p<0.001) and the time to achieve therapeutic APTTs (mean 8.2 versus 18.1 hours, p<0.005). A recent multicenter randomized trial compared weight-adjusted versus nonadjusted heparin dosing and laboratory versus POC APTT testing (225) confirming the improved intermediate outcomes for both the weight-adjusted protocol and for POCT. Similar results were seen as part of the Global Utilization of Streptokinase and TPA for Occluded Coronary Arteries (GUSTO-I) study (226).

Thus, POC-APTT testing may have an important role in improving outcomes for routine inpatient heparin monitoring. However, one must remember that POC APTT methods can give significantly different results from each other as well as from the laboratory methods (227). The POC method must be evaluated prior to implementation in order to verify the therapeutic APTT range. Using one APTT method consistently for monitoring is probably just as important in achieving good patient outcomes, particularly when multistep-dosing nomograms are employed (94,227).

Warfarin

Warfarin is the preferred agent for patients who require long-term anticoagulation therapy. Its anticoagulant effect is produced through antagonism of vitamin K, which ultimately decreases the coagulant activity of Factors II, VII, IX, and X. Thus, the prothrombin time is quite sensitive to warfarin's effect and is routinely used for monitoring. Regular monitoring is clinically important because intensity of therapy is a major risk factor for significant adverse events and outcomes are affected by specific patient characteristics/comorbidities (228). However, the variable responsiveness of diverse reagent-instrument combinations to factor deficiency requires that the prothrombin time be converted to the INR, as previously described. Table 10.5 contains current indications and therapeutic INR ranges for warfarin anticoagulation monitoring.

Traditionally, patients receiving oral anticoagulation therapy make periodic visits to their primary care provider, often monthly; laboratory testing is performed and advice is given regarding dosage adjustments. Because of long turnaround times for the laboratory tests, either the patient must wait at the provider's office for the results or the provider must try to contact the patient at a later time. As an alternative, specialized anticoagulation clinics have been developed with the goal of improving patient care and convenience (229–233). Nurses, pharmacists, and physicians with expertise in warfarin monitoring staff such clinics. Rapid return of test results is an important part of the clinic service, so that advice on dosage changes can be given directly to the patient and waiting time is minimized. Thus, in some anticoagulation clinics, prothrombin time testing is performed at the POC with a portable device (229,232). Patients followed with this practice model are more often within the therapeutic range and have fewer adverse thrombotic or hemorrhagic events according to recent studies (230–234). Investigators have also found significant cost savings either within the clinic visit itself (80) or as a result of the improved anticoagulant control (231–233).

The latest advance in oral anticoagulation monitoring is patient self-testing and management. In this model, patients measure their own INR using a POC device and either report their results to a healthcare provider for further advice or manage their own dosing based on an algorithm provided by their physician. Selected patients are capable of performing the test accurately

TABLE 10.4. AN EXAMPLE OF A WEIGHT-BASED NOMOGRAM FOR HEPARIN DOSING

Initial dose	80 units/kg bolus, then 18 units/kg/hour
APTT <35 s (<1.2 × control)	80 units/kg bolus, then 4 units/kg/hour
APTT 35–45 s (1.2–1.5 × control)	40 units/kg bolus, then 2 units/kg/hour
APTT 46–70 s (1.5–2.3 × control)	No change
APTT 71–90 s (2.3–3 × control)	Decrease infusion rate by 2 units/kg/hour
APTT >90 s (>3 × control)	Hold infusion 1 hour, then decrease infusion rate by 3 units/kg/hour

Raschke RA, Reilly BM, Guidry JR, et al. The weight-based heparin dosing nomogram compared with a "standard care" nomogram. A randomized controlled trial. *Ann Intern Med* 1993;119:874–881, with permission.

TABLE 10.5. RECOMMENDED THERAPEUTIC INR RANGES FOR WARFARIN ANTICOAGULATION

Medical Condition	Therapeutic Range (INR)
Treatment of venous thromboembolism	2.0–3.0
Prophylaxis of venous thrombosis	2.0–3.0
Prevention of systemic embolism (acute myocardial infarction, valvular heart disease, atrial fibrillation)	2.0–3.0
Tissue heart valves	2.0–3.0
Bileaflet mechanical valve in aortic position	2.0–3.0
Mechanical heart valves (high risk)	2.5–3.5

Hirsh J, Dalen JE, Anderson DR, et al. Oral anticoagulants: mechanism of action, clinical effectiveness, and optimal therapeutic range. *Chest* 2001;119: 8S–21S, with permission.

(235,236) and making good decisions with guidelines (237). Many studies have documented that better control of anticoagulation is achieved as measured by the time spent in the therapeutic range (237–241) and by the incidence of hemorrhage and recurrent thromboembolism (238,240). Patient satisfaction with this approach is high (235,236,239,242). Cost-effectiveness analysis suggests that although medical care costs are higher, the cost to the patient/caregiver is less and there is actual cost savings when the cost per avoided adverse event is considered (243).

Other Anticoagulants

Low molecular weight heparin preparations (enoxaparin, dalteparin, etc.) are becoming more commonly used for the prevention and treatment of acute thrombosis. A recent meta-analysis suggests that they are at least as safe and effective as unfractionated heparin (244). These compounds are derived from unfractionated heparin and are about one-third of its size. The anticoagulant effect is produced by the activation of antithrombin III. Because these compounds have longer plasma half-lives and more predictable responses to weight-adjusted doses, they typically have a daily dosing schedule and laboratory monitoring is not routinely done. In cases of renal failure, prolonged therapy, and pregnancy, periodic heparin determinations (anti-Xa method) are recommended (245).

Hirudin is a natural anticoagulant from the leech, *Hirudo medicinalis*. One preparation, lepirudin, is currently approved for anticoagulation in patients with heparin-induced thrombocytopenia (246). It binds directly to thrombin blocking both the catalytic and substrate-binding sites; thus it prevents the conversion of fibrinogen to fibrin and the activation of factors V, VIII, and XIII. Monitoring can be done with the APTT, using a target of 1.5 to 2.5 times the mean of the normal range (245). POC APTT testing has been shown to be responsive to the anticoagulant effect of hirudin (247).

Hirudin therapy may also be followed with the ecarin clotting time (ECT). Ecarin is a metalloproteinase from the venom of *Echis carinatus*; it activates prothrombin to form meizothrombin, which then converts fibrinogen to fibrin. Hirudin forms 1:1 complexes with meizothrombin, thereby inhibiting its effect on fibrinogen and prolonging the clotting time. Studies have shown that there is a good correlation between hirudin concentration

and lengthening of the ECT (248,249) and that the ECT can be used successfully for monitoring during cardiopulmonary bypass surgery (161). A POC-ECT is also available (162).

GUIDELINES FOR MANAGEMENT OF INTEGRATED TESTING PROGRAMS

Coagulation testing presents some unique challenges for POC programs. The major issue is the variation in test results based on the device used. Just as in the laboratory, different instrument-reagent combinations have different sensitivities to coagulation factor deficiencies and anticoagulant therapies. Although the International Normalized Ratio tries to correct for these differences with the prothrombin time, discrepancies continue to be seen, particularly when the INR is above the therapeutic range. Similar standardization schemes are not available for the APTT, ACT, or other functional tests. Therefore, the results of POC and laboratory tests may not be interchangeable and may cause considerable confusion among clinicians regarding interpretation. POC devices that give results close to the reference method should be selected and the number of different devices should be minimized. In some circumstances, device-specific therapeutic ranges may need to be instituted to appropriately guide treatment when POCT is utilized. Users need to then be educated regarding the nature of the differences in results, the importance of using the appropriate therapeutic range, and the avoidance of switching back and forth between the POC test and the lab tests. This may be easier to accomplish if the scope of the program is limited in terms of sites and operators.

Another important issue for a successful program is operator knowledge of the effect of preanalytical variables on test results. Sample type (capillary versus venous, fresh whole blood versus anticoagulated whole blood versus plasma), sample size, and timing of the collection may have significant impact on the accuracy of the results, particularly for coagulation testing. Test operators that do not have laboratory knowledge may be unaware of these concerns; the laboratory can play a significant role in providing this kind of expertise.

Fresh whole-blood samples must typically be analyzed immediately for the most accurate results. Although the coagulation system is activated once the sample is obtained, clotting does take some time, depending on the type of activator that is used. Some tests (e.g., the TEG) allow a limited time interval between collection and the start of the test even with fresh whole blood; however, the variability within this interval should be minimized. If anticoagulated whole blood is the specimen of choice, then the appropriate anticoagulant must be selected. Cell-counting devices typically use EDTA, coagulation tests require citrate, and platelet function tests may require specialty anticoagulants. Both the concentration of the anticoagulant solution and the ratio of anticoagulant solution to blood are critical determinants—this is particularly true for citrated specimens for coagulation testing. One of the common reasons to get inaccurate coagulation test results is over- or under-filling of the citrate-containing blood collection tube. Although laboratories typically can prevent these errors by rejecting obviously incorrectly collected samples, POC test operators may not be aware of the importance and potential impact of such an error.

For many tests, blood specimens may be capillary, venous, or arterial. With capillary samples, the collection technique is extremely important to ensure an accurate result. If excessive massaging is utilized to obtain capillary blood, the sample will be diluted with interstitial fluid resulting in incorrect cell counts and coagulation times. Similarly, venous and arterial punctures should be carried out with a minimum of trauma so that the coagulation system is not massively activated. If peripheral or central intravenous lines are utilized, 5 to 10 mL of "waste" blood is collected before a specimen for coagulation testing is obtained—this avoids contamination from the heparin used to keep the intravenous line patent.

Sample size is also critical for coagulation test accuracy. Reagent systems for these tests are designed for a specific activator to blood ratio. Samples that are too small will give shorter coagulation times; longer times may be obtained with samples that are too large. Fortunately, many of the POC test devices have systems to detect sample size abnormalities and prevent testing in such circumstances.

Given the above issues related to preanalytical variables and interpretation of results from various devices, training of test operators takes on major importance for a POCT program. Although device manufacturers often provide training, aspects that are specific to the site should also be included. Operator competency should be assessed at the conclusion of training and periodically thereafter through direct observation, written examination, and/or testing of unknown samples (patient or quality control).

Management of patient and quality assurance data is becoming an increasingly critical aspect of any POCT program. Records of training, competency assessment, operating procedures, patient testing, and quality control testing are required by regulatory and accrediting agencies. Patient test results, with the appropriate reference range, need to be documented in the patient's medical record in a consistent manner so that all healthcare personnel treating the patient have access to the information and that events can be reconstructed at a later time. As the number of operators, devices, and clinical sites increase, a manual record-keeping system becomes onerous. Automated data capture with downloading into data management systems and interfaces to electronic reporting and billing systems is becoming available for many POC tests; however, such systems are in their infancy for hematology and hemostasis tests.

CONCLUSIONS

POCT is an established and relatively common means of providing rapid results for hematological and hemostatic parameters. In general, this testing tends to have a focused application to particular settings (e.g., heparin monitoring during CPB surgery) rather than be widely available throughout inpatient or outpatient facilities. Specific outcomes studies have shown that improvements in both anticoagulation and transfusion therapy can be achieved with testing at the POC.

Assessment of platelet function is the current focus of intense research and clinical interest due to the introduction of new med-

ications to prevent postprocedural thrombosis. Numerous devices to assess platelet function are in development. Because of the complexity of the interaction among blood vessels, platelets, and coagulation factors in clot formation, the challenge is to find the right test that truly reflects the nature of the antithrombotic effect and that can guide both the application and intensity of the therapy. Since platelet function abnormalities may also contribute to hemorrhage, these devices may also be useful in platelet transfusion decisions. Major POCT advances are expected in these areas.

REFERENCES

1. Titus K. Nurses at the point of care whether or not labs are there. *CAP Today* 1996:25.
2. Despotis GJ, Alsoufiev A, Hogue CW, et al. Evaluation of complete blood count results from a new, on-site hemocytometer compared with a laboratory-based hemocytometer. *Crit Care Med* 1996;24: 1163–1167.
3. Despotis GJ, Saleem R, Bigham M, Barnes P. Clinical evaluation of a new, point-of-care hemocytometer. *Crit Care Med* 2000;28:1185–1190.
4. Riccardi A, Danuva M, Quartero L, et al. Hematological values from quantitative buffy coat analysis (QBC II) system: evaluation in a hematological/oncological outpatient section. *Haematologica* 1989;74: 375–378.
5. Paul RI, Badgett JT, Buchino JJ. Evaluation of QBC Autoread performance in an emergency department setting. *Pediatr Emerg Care* 1994;10:359–363.
6. Harrison RL, Birotte R, Harris L. A comparison between hemogram data as measured by technical and non-technical personnel using the QBC II. *Path Res Pract* 1990;186:391–394.
7. McNulty SE, Torjman M, Grodecki W, et al. A comparison of four bedside methods of hemoglobin assessment during cardiac surgery. *Anesth Analg* 1995;81:1197–1202.
8. McNulty SE, Sharkey SJ, Asam B, Lee JH. Evaluation of STAT-CRIT hematocrit determination in comparison to coulter and centrifuge: the effects of isotonic hemodilution and albumin administration. *Anesth Analg* 1993;76:830–834.
9. McMahon DJ, Carpenter RL. A comparison of conductivity-based hematocrit determinations with conventional laboratory methods in autologous blood transfusions. *Anesth Analg* 1990;71:541–544.
10. Weatherall MS, Sherry KM. An evaluation of the Spuncrit infra-red analyser for measurement of haematocrit. *Clin Lab Haem* 1997;19: 183–186.
11. Al-Odeh A, Varga ZA, Angelini GD. Haematocrit measurements during cardiopulmonary bypass surgery: comparison of three stat methods with a blood cell counter. *Perfusion* 1994;9:127–134.
12. Rippmann CE, Nett PC, Popovic D, et al. Hemocue, an accurate bedside method of hemoglobin measurement? *J Clin Monit* 1997; 13:373–377.
13. Laifer SA, Kuller JA, Hill LM. Rapid assessment of fetal hemoglobin concentration with the Hemocue system. *Obstet Gynecol* 1990;76: 723–724.
14. Cohen AR, Seidl-Friedman J. HemoCue system for hemoglobin measurement: evaluation in anemic and nonanemic children. *Am J Clin Pathol* 1988;90:302–305.
15. Berry SM, Dombrowski MP, Blessed WB, et al. Fetal hemoglobin quantitations using the Hemocue system are rapid and accurate. *Obstet Gynecol* 1993;81:417–420.
16. von Schenck H, Falkensson M, Lundberg B. Evaluation of "Hemo-Cue," a new device for determining hemoglobin. *Clin Chem* 1986;32: 526–529.
17. Marver CL, Smisek IM, Santrach PJ. Comparison of point of care methods for hemoglobin measurement during acute hemodilution in pediatric cardiopulmonary bypass. *Clin Chem* 1999;45:A33.
18. Gong A, Backenstose B. Evaluation of the Hb-Quick: a portable hemoglobinometer. *J Clin Monit* 1999;15:171–177.
19. Simon TL, Alverson DC, AuBuchon J, et al. Practice parameter for

the use of red blood cell transfusions. *Arch Pathol Lab Med* 1998;122: 130–138.

20. Utley JR, Gravlee GP. Special considerations in cardiopulmonary bypass. *Adv Cardiac Surg* 1996;7:87–100.
21. Kreimeier U, Messmer K. Hemodilution in clinical surgery: state of the art 1996. *World J Surg* 1996;20:1208–1217.
22. Murray DJ, Brosnahan WJ, Pennell B, et al. Heparin detection by the activated coagulation time: a comparison of the sensitivity of coagulation tests and heparin assays. *J Cardiothorac Vasc Anesth* 1997;11:24–28.
23. Mulry CC, Le Veen RF, Sobel M, et al. Assessment of heparin anticoagulation during peripheral angioplasty. *J Vasc Interv Radiol* 1991;2: 133–139.
24. Dougherty KG, Gaos CM, Bush HS, et al. Activated clotting times and activated partial thromboplastin times in patients undergoing coronary angioplasty who receive bolus doses of heparin. *Cathet Cardiovasc Diagn* 1992;26:260–263.
25. Despotis GJ, Levine V, Joist JH, et al. Antithrombin III during cardiac surgery: effect on response of activated clotting time to heparin and relationship to markers of hemostatic activation. *Anesth Analg* 1997;85:498–506.
26. Bull BS, Huse WM, Brauer FS, Korpman RA. Heparin therapy during extracorporeal circulation. II. The use of a dose-response curve to individualize heparin and protamine dosage. *J Thorac Cardiovasc Surg* 1975;69:685–689.
27. Bull BS, et al. Heparin therapy during extracorporeal circulation. I. Problems inherent in existing heparin protocols. *J Thorac Cardiovasc Surg* 1975;69:674–684.
28. Andrew M, MacIntyre B, MacMillan J, et al. Heparin therapy during cardiopulmonary bypass in children requires ongoing quality control. *Thromb Haemost* 1993;70:937–941.
29. Avendano A, Ferguson JJ. Comparison of Hemochron and HemoTec activated coagulation time target values during percutaneous transluminal coronary angioplasty. *J Am Coll Cardiol* 1994;23:907–910.
30. Hezard N, Metz D, Potron G, et al. Monitoring the effect of heparin bolus during percutaneous coronary angioplasty (PTCA): assessment of three bedside coagulation monitors. *Thromb Haemost* 1998;80: 865–866.
31. Horkay F, Martin P, Rajah SM, Walker DR. Response to heparinization in adults and children undergoing cardiac operations. *Ann Thorac Surg* 1992;53:822–826.
32. Carter AJ, et al. Clinical evaluation of a microsample coagulation analyzer, and comparison with existing techniques. *Cathet Cardiovasc Diagn* 1996;39:97–102.
33. Helft G, et al. Comparison of activated clotting times to heparin management test for adequacy of heparin anticoagulation in percutaneous transluminal coronary angioplasty. *Cathet Cardiovasc Diagn* 1998;45:329–331.
34. Leyvi G, Shore-Lesserson L, Harrington D, et al. An investigation of a new activated clotting time "MAX-ACT" in patients undergoing extracorporeal circulation. *Anesth Analg* 2001;92:578–583.
35. Despotis GJ, et al. Aprotinin prolongs activated and nonactivated whole blood clotting time and potentiates the effect of heparin in vitro. *Anesth Analg* 1996;82:1126–1131.
36. Dietrich W, et al. Influence of high-dose aprotinin on anticoagulation, heparin requirement, and celite- and kaolin-activated clotting time in heparin-pretreated patients undergoing open-heart surgery. *Anesthesiology* 1995;83:679–689.
37. Feindt P, Seyfert UT, Volkmer I, et al. Celite and kaolin produce differing activated clotting times during cardiopulmonary bypass under aprotinin therapy. *Thorac Cardiovasc Surgeon* 1994;42:218–221.
38. Wang JS, Lin CY, Hung WT, Karp RB. Monitoring of heparin-induced anticoagulation with kaolin-activated clotting time in cardiac surgical patients treated with aprotinin. *Anesthesiology* 1992;77:1080–1084.
39. Wendel HP, Heller W, Gallimore MJ, et al. The prolonged activated clotting time (ACT) with aprotinin depends on the type of activator used for measurement. *Blood Coagul Fibrinolysis* 1993;4:41–45.
40. Najman DM, Walenga JM, Fareed J, Pifarre R. Effects of aprotinin on anticoagulant monitoring: implications in cardiovascular surgery. *Ann Thorac Surg* 1993;55:662–666.
41. Owings JT, Pollock ME, Gosselin RC, et al. Anticoagulation of chil-

dren undergoing cardiopulmonary bypass is overestimated by current monitoring techniques. *Arch Surg* 2000;135:1042–1047.

42. Chang RJ, Doherty TM, Goldberg SL. How does warfarin affect the activated coagulation time? *Am Heart J* 1998;136:477–479.
43. Pesola GR, Johnson A, Pesola DA. Percutaneous transluminal coronary angioplasty: comparison of arterial vs. venous activated clotting time. *Cathet Cardiovasc Diagn* 1996;37:140–144.
44. Kerensky RA, Azar GJ Jr., Bertolet B, et al. Venous activated clotting time after intra-arterial heparin: effect of site of administration and timing of sampling. *Cathet Cardiovasc Diagn* 1996;37:151–153.
45. Gravlee G, Case LD, Angert KC, et al. Variability of the activated coagulation time. *Anesth Analg* 1988;67:469–472.
46. Esposito RA, Culliford AT, Colvin SB, et al. The role of the activated clotting time in heparin administration and neutralization for cardiopulmonary bypass. *J Thorac Cardiovasc Surg* 1983;85:174–185.
47. Despotis GJ, Summerfield AL, Hoist JH, et al. Comparison of activated coagulation time and whole blood heparin measurements with laboratory plasma anti-Xa heparin concentration in patients having cardiac operations. *J Thorac Cardiovasc Surg* 1994;108:1076–1082.
48. Huyzen RJ, van Oeveren W, Wei F, et al. In vitro effect of hemodilution on activated clotting time and high-dose thrombin time during cardiopulmonary bypass. *Ann Thorac Surg* 1996;62:533–537.
49. Despotis GJ, Joist JH, Goodnough LT, et al. Whole blood heparin concentration measurements by automated protamine titration agree with plasma anti-Xa measurements. *J Thorac Cardiovasc Surg* 1997; 113:611–613.
50. Hardy J-F, et al. Measurement of heparin concentration in whole blood with the Hepcon/HMS device does not agree with laboratory determination of plasma heparin concentration using a chromogenic substrate for activated factor X. *J Thorac Cardiovasc Surg* 1996;112:154–161.
51. Schlueter AJ, Pennell BJ, Olson JD. Evaluation of a new protamine titration method to assay heparin in whole blood and plasma. *Am J Clin Pathol* 1997;107:511–520.
52. Olson JD, Arkin CF, Brandt JT, et al. College of American Pathologists Conference XXXI on Laboratory Monitoring of Anticoagulant Therapy: laboratory monitoring of unfractionated heparin therapy. *Arch Pathol Lab Med* 1998;122:782–798.
53. Despotis GJ, Joist JH, Joiner-Maier D, et al. Effect of aprotinin on activated clotting time, whole blood and plasma heparin measurements. *Ann Thorac Surg* 1995;59:106–111.
54. Cipolle RJ, Uden DL, Gruber SA, et al. Evaluation of a rapid monitoring system to study heparin pharmacokinetics and pharmacodynamics. *Pharmacotherapy* 1990;10:367–372.
55. Despotis GJ, Alsoufiev AL, Spitznagel E, et al. Response of kaolin ACT to heparin: evaluation with an automated assay and higher heparin doses. *Ann Thorac Surg* 1996;61:795–799.
56. Baugh RF, Deemar KA, Zimmermann JJ. Heparinase in the activated clotting time assay: monitoring heparin-independent alterations in coagulation function. *Anesth Analg* 1994;74:201–205.
57. World Health Organization. *Standardisation, W.E.Co.B., 33rd Report.* WHO Technical Report Series. Geneva: World Health Organization, 1983:1–105.
58. Davis KD, Danielson CF, May LS, Han ZQ. Use of different thromboplastin reagents causes greater variability in International Normalized Ratio results than prolonged room temperature storage of specimens. *Arch Pathol Lab Med* 1998;122:972–977.
59. Le D, et al. The international normalized ratio (INR) for monitoring warfarin therapy: reliability and relation to other monitoring methods. *Ann Intern Med* 1994;120:552–558.
60. Ng VL, et al. Highly sensitive thromboplastins do not improve INR precision. *Am J Clin Pathol* 1998;109:338–346.
61. Douketis J, et al. Accuracy of a portable international normalization ratio monitor in outpatients receiving long-term oral anticoagulant therapy: comparison with a laboratory reference standard using clinically relevant criteria for agreement. *Thromb Res* 1998;92:11–17.
62. Gosselin RC, et al. Monitoring oral anticoagulant therapy with point-of-care devices: correlations and caveats. *Clin Chem* 1997;43:1785–1786.
63. Gosselin R, Owings JT, White RH, et al. A comparison of point-of-care instruments designed for monitoring oral anticoagulation with standard laboratory methods. *Thromb Haemost* 2000;83:698–703.

64. Hasenkam JM, Knudsen L, Kimose HH, et al. Practicability of patient self-testing of oral anticoagulant therapy by the International Normalized Ratio (INR) using a portable whole blood monitor: a pilot investigation. *Thromb Res* 1997;85(1):77–82.

65. Kaatz SS, White RH, Hill J, et al. Accuracy of laboratory and portable monitor International Normalized Ratio determinations: comparison with a criterion standard. *Arch Intern Med* 1995;155:1861–1867.

66. Koerner SD, Fuller RE. Comparison of a portable capillary whole blood coagulation monitor and standard laboratory methods for determining International Normalized Ratio. *Military Med* 1998; 163:820–825.

67. van den Besselaar AM, Breddin K, Lutze G, et al. Multicenter evaluation of a new capillary blood prothrombin time monitoring system. *Blood Coag Fibrinolysis* 1995;6:726–732.

68. van den Besselar AM. A comparison of INRs determined with a whole blood prothrombin time device and two international reference preparations for thromboplastin. *Thromb Haemost* 2000;84:410–412.

69. Marzinotto V, Monagle P, Chan A, et al. Capillary whole blood monitoring of oral anticoagulants in children in outpatient clinics and the home setting. *Pediatr Cardiol* 2000;21:347–352.

70. Murray ET, Fitzmaurice DA, Allen TF, Hobbs FD. A primary care evaluation of three near patient coagulometers. *J Clin Pathol* 1999;52: 842–845.

71. Chapman DC, et al. Accuracy, clinical correlation, and patient acceptance of two handheld prothrombin time monitoring devices in the ambulatory setting. *Ann Pharmacotherapy* 1999;33:775–780.

72. Anderson DR, Harrison L, Hirsh J. Evaluation of a portable prothrombin time monitor for home use by patients who require long-term oral anticoagulant therapy. *Arch Intern Med* 1993;153:1441–1447.

73. Despotis G, et al. Prospective evaluation and clinical utility of on-site monitoring of coagulation in patients undergoing cardiac operation. *J Thorac Cardiovasc Surg* 1994;107:271–279.

74. Jennings I, Luddington RJ, Baglin T. Evaluation of the Ciba Corning Biotrack 512 coagulation monitor for the control of oral anticoagulation. *J Clin Pathol* 1991;44:950–953.

75. Massicotte P, et al. Home monitoring of warfarin therapy in children with a whole blood prothrombin time monitor. *J Pediatr* 1995;127: 389–394.

76. McGlasson D, Paul J, Shaffer K. Whole blood coagulation testing in neonates. *Clin Lab Sci* 1993;6:76–77.

77. Nuttall GA, et al. Intraoperative measurement of activated partial thromboplastin time and prothrombin time by a portable laser photometer in patients following cardiopulmonary bypass. *J Cardiothorac Vasc Anesth* 1993;7:402–409.

78. Ruzicka K, et al. Evaluation of bedside prothrombin time and activated partial thromboplastin time measurement by coagulation analyzer Coaguchek Plus in various clinical settings. *Thromb Res* 1997; 87:431–440.

79. Samama CM, et al. Intraoperative measurement of activated partial thromboplastin time and prothrombin time with a new compact monitor. *Acta Anaesthesiol Scand* 1994;38:232–237.

80. Ansell J, Holden A, Knapic N. Patient self-management of oral anticoagulation guided by capillary (fingerstick) whole blood prothrombin times. *Arch Intern Med* 1989;149:2509–2511.

81. Bussey HI, Chiquette E, Bianco TM, et al. A statistical and clinical evaluation of fingerstick and routine laboratory prothrombin time measurements. *Pharmacotherapy* 1997;17:861–866.

82. Foulis PR, Wallach PM, Adelman HM, et al. Performance of the Coumatrak system in a large anticoagulation clinic. *Am J Clin Pathol* 1995;103:98–102.

83. Lucas F, et al. A novel whole blood capillary technique for measuring the prothrombin time. *Am J Clin Pathol* 1987;88:442–446.

84. Weibert RT, Adler DS. Evaluation of a capillary whole-blood prothrombin time measurement system. *Clin Pharm* 1989;8:864–867.

85. White RH, McCurdy SA, von Marensdorff H, et al. Home prothrombin time monitoring after the initiation of warfarin therapy. *Ann Intern Med* 1989;111:730–737.

86. Yamreudeewong W, Johnson JV, Cassidy TG, Berg JT. Comparison of two methods for INR determination in a pharmacist-based oral anticoagulation clinic. *Pharmacotherapy* 1996;16:1159–1165.

87. Quien E, Morales E, Cisar LA, et al. Plasma tissue factor antigen levels in capillary whole blood and venous blood: effect of tissue factor on prothrombin time. *Am J Hematol* 1997;55:193–198.

88. Kitchen S, Preston FE. Monitoring oral anticoagulant treatment with the TAS near-patient test system: comparison with conventional thromboplastins. *J Clin Pathol* 1997;50:951–956.

89. Rose VL, Dermott SC, Murray BF, et al. Decentralized testing for prothrombin time and activated partial thromboplastin time using a dry chemistry portable analyzer. *Arch Pathol Lab Med* 1993;117: 611–617.

90. Biasiolo A, Rampazzo P, Furnari O, et al. Comparison between routine laboratory prothrombin time measurements and fingerstick determinations using a near-patient testing device (Pro-Time). *Thromb Res* 2000;97:495–498.

91. Pierce MT, Crain L, Smith J, Mehta V. Point-of-care versus laboratory measurement of the International Normalized Ratio. *Am J Health-Syst Pharm* 2000;57:2271–2274.

92. Reed C, Rickman H. Accuracy of international normalized ratio determined by portable whole-blood coagulation monitor versus a central laboratory. *Am J Health-Syst Pharm* 1999;56:1619–1623.

93. Ansell J, et al. Measurement of the activated partial thromboplastin time from a capillary (fingerstick) sample of whole blood: a new method for monitoring heparin therapy. *Am J Clin Pathol* 1991;95: 222–227.

94. Werner M, Gallagher JV, Ballo MS, Karcher DS. Effect of analytic uncertainty of conventional and point-of-care assays of activated partial thromboplastin time on clinical decisions in heparin therapy. *Am J Clin Pathol* 1994;102:237–241.

95. Despotis GJ, Hogue CW Jr., Santoro SA, et al. Effect of heparin on whole blood activated partial thromboplastin time using a portable, whole blood coagulation monitor. *Crit Care Med* 1995;23:1674–1679.

96. Despotis GJ, et al. On-site prothrombin time, activated partial thromboplastin time, and platelet count. *Anesthesiology* 1994;80:338–351.

97. Smythe MA, Koerber JM, Westley SJ, et al. Use of the activated partial thromboplastin time for heparin monitoring. *Am J Clin Pathol* 2001;115:148–155.

98. Channing Rodgers RP, Levin J. A critical reappraisal of the bleeding time. *Sem Thromb Hemost* 1990;16:1–20.

99. Burns ER. Bleeding time: a guide to its diagnostic and clinical utility. *Arch Pathol Lab Med* 1989;113:1219–1224.

100. Gerwirtz AS, Miller ML, Keys TF. The clinical usefulness of the preoperative bleeding time. *Arch Pathol Lab Med* 1996;120:353–356.

101. Despotis GJ, Levine V, Filos KS, et al. Evaluation of a new point-of-care test that measures PAF-mediated acceleration of coagulation in cardiac surgical patients. *Anesthesiology* 1996;85:1311–1323.

102. Ereth MH, Nuttall GA, Klindowrth JT, et al. Does the platelet activated clotting test (HemoSTATUS) predict blood loss and platelet dysfunction associated with cardiopulmonary bypass? *Anesth Analg* 1997;85:259–64.

103. Despotis GJ, Ikonomakou S, Levine V, et al. Effects of platelets and white blood cells and antiplatelet agent C7E3 (Reopro) on a new test of PAF procoagulant activity of whole blood. *Thromb Res* 1997;86: 205–219.

104. Kundu SK, Heilmann EJ, Sio R, et al. Description of a in vitro platelet function analyzer—PFA-100. *Sem Thromb Hemost* 1995;21 [Suppl 2]:106–112.

105. Mammen EF, Alshameeri RS, Comp PC. Preliminary data from a field trial of the PFA-100 system. *Sem Thromb Hemost* 1995;21 (Suppl. 2):113–121.

106. Mammen EF, et al. PFA-100TM System: a new method for assessment of platelet dysfunction. *Semin Thromb Hemost* 1998;24:195–202.

107. Fressinaud E, et al. Screening for von Willebrand Disease with a new analyzer using high shear stress: a study of 60 cases. *Blood* 1998;91: 1325–1331.

108. Rand ML, Carcao MD, Blanchette VS. Use of the PFA-100 in the assessment of primary, platelet-related hemostasis in a pediatric setting. *Semin Thromb Hemost* 1998;24:523–529.

109. Cattaneo M, Frederici AB, Lecchi A, et al. Evaluation of the PFA-100 system in the diagnosis and therapeutic monitoring of patients with von Willebrand disease. *Thromb Haemost* 1999;182:35–39.

110. Fressinaud E, Veyradier A, Signaud M, et al. Therapeutic monitoring of von Willebrand disease: interest and limits of a platelet function analyser at high shear rates. *Br J Haematol* 1999;106:777–783.

111. Harrison P, et al. Performance of the platelet function analyzer PFA-100 in testing abnormalities of primary haemostasis. *Blood Coag Fibrinolysis* 1999;10:25–31.

112. Kottke-Marchant K, et al. The effect of antiplatelet drugs, heparin, and preanalytical variables on platelet function detected by the Platelet Function Analyzer (PFA-100). *Clin Appl Thromb Hemost* 1999;5:122–130.

113. Francis J et al. Can the Platelet Function Analyzer (PFA-100) test substitute for the template bleeding time in routine clinical practice? *Platelets* 1999;10:132–136.

114. Marshall PW, et al. A comparison of the effects of aspirin on bleeding time measured using the Simplate method and closure time measured using the PFA-100, in healthy volunteers. *Br J Clin Pharmacol* 1997; 44:151–155.

115. Li CKN et al. The Xylum Clot Signature Analyzer: a dynamic flow system that simulates vascular injury. *Thromb Res* 1998;92:S67–S77.

116. Li CKN, et al. Xylum CSA: automated system for assessing hemostasis in simulated vascular flow. *Clin Chem* 1997;43:1788–1790.

117. Carr ME, Measurement of platelet force: the Hemodyne hemostasis analyzer. *Clin Lab Manag Rev* 1995;9:312–320.

118. Carr ME. In vitro assessment of platelet function. *Transfus Med Rev* 1997;11:106–115.

119. Carr ME, Zekert SL. Measurement of platelet-mediated force development during plasma clot formation. *Am J Med Sci* 1991;302:13–18.

120. Carr ME, Carr SL. Fibrin structure and concentration alter clot elastic modulus but do not alter platelet mediated force development. *Blood Coag Fibrinolysis* 1995;6:79–86.

121. Carr ME Jr., Carr SL, Hantgan RR, Braaten J. Glycoprotein IIb/IIIa blockade inhibits platelet-mediated force development and reduces gel elastic modulus. *Thromb Haemost* 1995;73:499–505.

122. Greilich PE, Alving BM, Longnecker D, et al. Near-site monitoring of the antiplatelet drug abciximab using the Hemodyne analyzer and modified thromboelastograph. *J Cardiothorac Vasc Anesth* 1999;13:58–64.

123. Greilich PE, Carr ME Jr., Carr SL, Chang AS. Reductions in platelet force development by cardiopulmonary bypass are associated with hemorrhage. *Anesth Analg* 1995;80:459–465.

124. Carr ME, Carr SL, Greilich PE. Heparin ablates force development during platelet mediated clot retraction. *Thromb Haemost* 1996;75: 674–678.

125. Carville DG, Schleckser PA, Guyer KE, et al. Whole blood platelet function assay on the ICHOR point-of-care hematology analyzer. *J Extra Corpor Technol* 1998;30:171–177.

126. Hartert H. Blutgerinnung studien mit der thrombelastographie, einen neuen untersuchingsverfahren. *Klin Wochenschr* 1948. 26:577–583.

127. Orlikowski CEP, Murray WB, Rocke DA. Effect of delay and storage on whole blood clotting analysis as determined by thromboelastography. *J Clin Monit* 1993;9:5–8.

128. Bowbrick VA, Mikhailidis DP, Stansby G. The use of citrated whole blood in thromboelastography. *Anesth Analg* 2000;90(5):1086–1088.

129. Camenzind V, Bombeli T, Seifert B, et al. Citrate storage affects thromboelastograph analysis. *Anesthesiology* 2000;92(5):1242–1249.

130. Kang YG, Martin DJ, Marquez J, et al. Intraoperative changes in blood coagulation and thromboelastographic monitoring in liver transplantation. *Anesth Analg* 1985;64:888–896.

131. Spiess BD, Tuman KJ, McCarthy RJ, et al. Thromboelastography as an indicator of post-cardiopulmonary bypass coagulopathies. *J Clin Monit* 1987. 3:25–30.

132. Tuman KJ, et al. Comparison of thromboelastography and platelet aggregometry. *Anesthesiology* 1991;75:A433.

133. Chandler WL. The thromboelastograph and the thromboelastograph technique. *Semin Thromb Hemost* 1995;21:1–6.

134. Gottumukkala VN, Sharma SK, Philip J. Assessing platelet and fibrinogen contribution to clot strength using modified thromboelastography in pregnant women. *Anesth Analg* 1999;89:1453–1455.

135. Kettner SC, Panzer OP, Kozek SA, et al. Use of abciximab-modified thromboelastography in patients undergoing cardiac surgery. *Anesth Analg* 1999;89:580–584.

136. Oshita K, et al. Quantitative measurement of thromboelastography as a function of platelet count. *Anesth Analg* 1999;89:296–299.

137. McNulty SE, Sasso P, Vesci J, Schieren H. Platelet concentrate effects on thromboelastography. *J Cardiothorac Vasc Anesth* 1997;11:828–830.

138. Clayton DG, Miro AM, Kramer DJ, et al. Quantification of thromboelastographic changes after blood component transfusion in patients with liver disease in the intensive care unit. *Anesth Analg* 1995;81:272–278.

139. Tuman KJ, Spiess BD, McCarthy RJ, Ivankovich AD. Effects of progressive blood loss on coagulation as measured by thromboelastography. *Anesth Analg* 1987. 66:856–863.

140. Yamakage M, Tsujiguchi N, Kohro S, et al. The usefulness of celite-activated thromboelastography for evaluation of fibrinolysis. *Can J Anaesth* 1998;45:993–996.

141. Harding SA, Mallett SV, Peachey TD, Cox DJ. Use of heparinase modified thromboelastography in liver transplantation. *Br J Anaesth* 1997;78:175–179.

142. Pivalizza EG, Abramson DC, King FS. Thromboelastography with heparinase in orthotopic liver transplantation. *J Cardiothorac Vasc Anesth* 1998;12:305–308.

143. Spiess BD, Wall MH, Gillies BS, et al. A comparison of thromboelastography with heparinase or protamine sulfate added in vitro during heparinized cardiopulmonary bypass. *Thromb Haemost* 1997;78: 820–826.

144. Tuman KJ, et al. Evaluation of coagulation during cardiopulmonary bypass with a heparinase-modified thromboelastographic assay. *J Cardiothorac Vasc Anesth* 1994;8:144–149.

145. Gibbs NM, Bell R. The effect of low-dose heparin on hypercoagulability following abdominal aortic surgery. *Anaesth Intensive Care* 1998;26:503–508.

146. Greilich PE, Alving BM, O'Neill KL, et al. A modified thromboelastographic method for monitoring c7E3 Fab in heparinized patients. *Anesth Analg* 1997;84:31–38.

147. Saleem A, Blifeld C, Saleh SA, et al. Viscoelastic measurement of clot formation: a new test of platelet function. *Ann Clin Lab Sci* 1983. 13: 115–124.

148. Horlocker TT, Schroeder DR. Effect of age, gender, and platelet count on Sonoclot coagulation analysis in patients undergoing orthopedic operations. *Mayo Clin Proc* 1997;72:214–219.

149. Miyashita T, Kuro M. Evaluation of platelet function by Sonoclot analysis compared with other hemostatic variables in cardiac surgery. *Anesth Analg* 1998;87:1228–1233.

150. Stern MP, DeVos-Doyle K, Viguera MG, Lajos TZ. Evaluation of post-cardiopulmonary bypass Sonoclot signatures in patients taking nonsteroidal anti-inflammatory drugs. *J Cardiothorac Anesth* 1989;3: 730–733.

151. LaForce WR, Brudno DS, Kanto WP, Karp WB. Evaluation of the Sonoclot analyzer for the measurement of platelet function in whole blood. *Ann Clin Lab Sci* 1992;22:30–33.

152. Hattersley, PG. Activated coagulation time of whole blood. JAMA 1966;196:436.

153. Young J, Kisker T, Doty D. Adequate anticoagulation during cardiopulmonary bypass determined by activated clotting time and the appearance of fibrin monomer. *Ann Thorac Surg* 1978. 26:231–240.

154. Despotis GJ, Joist JH, Hogue CW Jr., et al. The impact of heparin concentration and activated clotting time monitoring on blood conservation: a prospective, randomized evaluation in patients undergoing cardiac operation. *J Thorac Cardiovasc Surg* 1995;110:46–54.

155. Despotis GJ, Joist JH, Hogue CW Jr., et al. More effective suppression of hemostatic system activation in patients undergoing cardiac surgery by heparin dosing based on heparin blood concentrations rather than ACT. *Thromb Haemost* 1996;76:902–908.

156. Codispoti M, Ludlam CA, Simpson D, Mankad PS. Individualized heparin and protamine management in infants and children undergoing cardiac operations. *Ann Thorac Surg* 2001;71:922–928.

157. DeLaria GA, et al. Heparin-protamine mismatch: a controllable factor in bleeding after open heart surgery. *Arch Surg* 1994;129: 945–951.

158. Jobes DR, Aitken GL, Shaffer GW. Increased accuracy and precision of heparin and protamine dosing reduces blood loss and transfusion

in patients undergoing primary cardiac operations. *J Thorac Cardiovasc Surg* 1995;110:36–45.

159. Shore-Lesserson L, Reich D, DePerio M. Heparin and protamine titration do not improve haemostasis in cardiac surgical patients. *Can J Anaesth* 1998;45:10–18.

160. Ducart AR, et al. Management of anticoagulation during cardiopulmonary bypass in a patient with a circulating lupus anticoagulant. *J Cardiothorac Vasc Anesth* 1997;11:878–879.

161. Potzsch B, Madlener K, Seelig C, et al. Monitoring of r-hirudin anticoagulation during cardiopulmonary bypass: assessment of the whole blood ecarin clotting time. *Thromb Haemost* 1997;75:920–925.

162. Koster A, Hansen R, Grauhan O, et al. Hirudin monitoring using the TAS ecarin clotting time in patients with heparin-induced thrombocytopenia type II. *J Cardiothorac Vasc Anesth* 2000;14:249–252.

163. Bick RL. Hemostasis defects associated with cardiac surgery, prosthetic devices, and other extracorporeal circuits. *Semin Thromb Hemost* 1985; 11:249–280.

164. Harker LA, Malpass TW, Branson HE, et al. Mechanism of abnormal bleeding in patients undergoing cardiopulmonary bypass: acquired transient platelet dysfunction associated with selective alpha-granule release. *Blood* 1980;56:824–834.

165. Mammen EF, et al. Hemostasis changes during cardiopulmonary bypass surgery. *Semin Thromb Hemost* 1985. 11:281–292.

166. Rinder CS, Bohnert J, Rinder HM, et al. Platelet activation and aggregation during cardiopulmonary bypass. *Anesthesiology* 1991;75:388–393.

167. John LCH, Rees GM, Kovacs IB. Inhibition of platelet function by heparin: an etiologic factor in postbypass hemorrhage. *J Thorac Cardiovasc Surg* 1993;105:816–822.

168. Khuri SF, Valeri CR, Loscalzo J, et al. Heparin causes platelet dysfunction and induces fibrinolysis before cardiopulmonary bypass. *Ann Thorac Surg* 1995;60:1008–1014.

169. Rinder CS, Mathew JP, Rinder HM. Modulation of platelet surface adhesion receptors during cardiopulmonary bypass. *Anesthesiology* 1991;75:563–570.

170. van Oeveren W, Harder MP, Roozendaal KJ. Aprotinin protects platelets against the initial effect of cardiopulmonary bypass. *J Thorac Cardiovasc Surg* 1990;99:788–797.

171. Kestin AS, Valeri CR, Khuri SF, et al. The platelet function defect of cardiopulmonary bypass. *Blood* 1993;82:107–117.

172. Hollaway DS, Summaria L, Sanesara J. Decreased platelet numbers and increased fibrinolysis contribute to postoperative bleeding in cardiopulmonary bypass patients. *Thromb Haemost* 1988. 59:62–67.

173. Hunt BJ, Paratt RN, Segal HC, et al. Activation of coagulation and fibrinolysis during cardiothoracic operations. *Ann Thorac Surg* 1998; 65:712–718.

174. Nuttall GA, Oliver WC, Santrach PJ, et al. Efficacy of a simple intraoperative transfusion algorithm for nonerythrocyte component utilization after cardiopulmonary bypass. *Anesthesiology* 2001;94:773–781.

175. Nuttall GA, Oliver WC, Beynen FM, et al. Determination of normal versus abnormal activated partial thromboplastin time and prothrombin time after cardiopulmonary bypass. *J Cardiothorac Vasc Anesth* 1995;9:355–361.

176. Nuttall GA, Oliver WC, Ereth MH, Santrach PJ. Coagulation tests predict bleeding after cardiopulmonary bypass. *J Cardiothorac Vasc Anesth* 1997;11:815–823.

177. Despotis GJ, et al. Aprotinin prolongs whole blood activated partial thromboplastin time but not whole blood prothrombin time in patients undergoing cardiac surgery. *Anesth Analg* 1995;81:919–924.

178. Ereth MH, Nuttall GA, Santrach PJ, et al. The relation between platelet-activated clotting test (HemoSTATUS) and blood loss after cardiopulmonary bypass. *Anesthesiology* 1998;88:962–969.

179. Shore-Lesserson L, et al. Platelet-activated clotting time does not measure platelet reactivity during cardiac surgery. *Anesthesiology* 1999; 91:362–368.

180. Despotis GJ, Levine V, Saleem R, et al. Use of point-of-care test in identification of patients who can benefit from desmopressin during cardiac surgery: a randomised controlled trial. *Lancet* 1999;354:106–110.

181. Wahba A, Sander S, Birnbaum E. Are in-vitro platelet function tests useful in predicting blood loss following open heart surgery? *Thorac Cardiovasc Surg* 1998;46:228–231.

182. Slaughter TF, Sreeram G, Sharma AD, et al. Reversible shear-mediated platelet dysfunction during cardiac surgery as assessed by the PFA-100 platelet function analyzer. *Blood Coagul Fibrinolysis* 2001; 12:85–93.

183. Lasne D, et al. A study of platelet functions with a new analyzer using high shear stress (PFA100) in patients undergoing coronary artery bypass graft. *Thromb Haemost* 2000;84:794–799.

184. Tuman KJ, Spiess BD, McCarthy RJ, Ivankovich AD. Comparison of viscoelastic measures of coagulation after cardiopulmonary bypass. *Anesth Analg* 1989;69:69–75.

185. Dorman BH, Spinale FG, Bailey MK, et al. Identification of patients at risk for excessive blood loss during coronary artery bypass surgery: thromboelastograph versus coagulation screen. *Anesth Analg* 1993;76: 694–700.

186. Wang JS, Lin CY, Hung WT, et al. Thromboelastogram fails to predict postoperative hemorrhage in cardiac patients. *Ann Thorac Surg* 1992;53:435–439.

187. Mongan PD, Hosking MP. The role of desmopressin acetate in patients undergoing coronary artery bypass surgery: a controlled clinical trial with thromboelastographic risk stratification. *Anesthesiology* 1992;77:38–46.

188. Shore-Lesserson L, Manspeizer HE, DePerio M, et al. Thromboelastography-guided transfusion algorithm reduces transfusions in complex cardiac surgery. *Anesth Analg* 1999;88:312–319.

189. Royston D, von Kier S. Reduced haemostatic factor transfusion using heparinase-modified thromboelastography during cardiopulmonary bypass. *Br J Anaesth* 2001;86:575–578.

190. Kang Y Coagulation and liver transplantation. *Transplant Proc* 1993; 25:2001.

191. Plevak D, Divertie G, Carton E, et al. Blood product transfusion therapy after liver transplantation: comparison of the thromboelastogram and conventional coagulation studies. *Transplant Proc* 1993;25:1838.

192. Goldman E, Yablok D, Tesi RJ, et al. Analysis of two thrombokinetic measurements (Thromboelastograph and Sonoclot) during liver transplantation. *Transplant Proc* 1993;25:1820.

193. Ferguson JJ, et al. Results of a national survey on anticoagulation for PTCA. *J Invas Cardiol* 1995;7:136–141.

194. Klein LW, Agarwal JB. When we "act" on ACT levels: activated clotting time measurements to guide heparin administration during and after interventional procedures. *Cathet Cardiovasc Diagn* 1996;37: 154–157.

195. Chew DP, Bhatt DL, Lincoff AM, et al. Defining the optimal activated clotting time during percutaneous coronary intervention. *Circulation* 2001;103:961–966.

196. Kaluski E, Krakover R, Cotter G, et al. Minimal heparinization in coronary angioplasty—how much heparin is really warranted? *Am J Cardiol* 2000;85:953–956.

197. Bowers J, Ferguson JJ. The use of activated clotting times to monitor heparin therapy during and after interventional procedures. *Clin Cardiol* 1994;17:357–361.

198. Popma JJ, et al. Heparin dosing in patients undergoing coronary intervention. *Am J Cardiol* 1998;82:19P–24P.

199. EPILOG Investigators. Platelet glycoprotein IIb/IIIa receptor blockade and low-dose heparin during percutaneous coronary revascularization. *N Engl J Med* 1997;336:1689–1696.

200. EPIC Investigators. Use of a monoclonal antibody directed against the platelet blycoprotein IIb/IIIa receptor in high-risk coronary angioplasty. *N Engl J Med* 1994;330:956–961.

201. Harrington RA, Kleiman NS, Granser CB, et al. Relation between inhibition of platelet aggregation and clinical outcomes. *Am Heart J* 1998;136:S43–S50.

202. Berkowitz SD, Frelinger AL, Hillman RS. Progress in point-of-care laboratory testing for assessing platelet function. *Am Heart J* 1998; 136:S51–S65.

203. Hezard N, et al. Use of the PFA-100 apparatus to assess platelet function in patients undergoing PTCA during and after infusion of c7E3

fab in the presence of other antiplatelet agents. *Thromb Haemost* 2000;83:540–544.

204. Madan M, Berkowitz SD, Christie DJ, et al. Rapid assessment of glycoprotein IIb/IIIa blockade with the platelet function analyzer (PFA-100) during percutaneous coronary intervention. *Am Heart J* 2001; 141:226–233.

205. Kereiakes DJ, Broderick TM, Roth EM, et al. Time course, magnitude, and consistency of platelet inhibition by abciximab, tirofiban, or eptifibatide in patients with unstable angina pectoris undergoing percutaneous coronary intervention. *Am J Cardiol* 1999;84:391–395.

206. Simon DL, Liu CB, Ganz P, et al. A comparative study of light transmission aggregometry and automated bedside platelet function assays in patients undergoing percutaneous coronary intervention and receiving abciximab, eptifibatide, or tirofiban. *Cathet Cardiovasc Intervent* 2001;52:425–432.

207. Ammar T, Scudder LE, Coller BS. In vitro effects of the platelet glycoprotein IIb/IIIa receptor antagonist c7E3 Fab on the activated clotting time. *Circulation* 1997;95:614–617.

208. Kereiakes DJ, Broderick TM, Chang DD, et al. Partial reversal of heparin anticoagulation by intravenous protamine in abciximab-treated patients undergoing percutaneous intervention. *Am J Cardiol* 1997;80:633–634.

209. Moliterno DJ, et al. Effects of glycoprotein IIb/IIIa endocrine blockade on activated clotting time during percutaneous transluminal coronary angioplasty or directional atherectomy (the EPIC trial). *Am J Cardiol* 1995;75:559–562.

210. Hirsh J, et al. Heparin and low-molecular weight heparin: mechanisms of action, pharmacokinetics, dosing considerations, monitoring, efficacy, and safety. *Chest* 1998;114:489S–510S.

211. Kitchen S, Preston FE. The therapeutic range for heparin therapy: relationship between six activated partial thromboplastin time reagents and two heparin assays. *Thromb Haemost* 1996;75:734–739.

212. Baker BA, Adelman MD, Smith PA, Osborn JC. Inability of the activated partial thromboplastin time to predict heparin levels. *Arch Intern Med* 1997;157:2475–2479.

213. Levine MN, Hirsh J, Gent M, et al. A randomized trial comparing activated thromboplastin time with heparin assay in patients with acute venous thromboembolism requiring large daily doses of heparin. *Arch Intern Med* 1994;154:49–56.

214. Raschke RA, Reilly BM, Guidry JR, et al. The weight-based heparin dosing nomogram compared with a "standard care" nomogram: a randomized controlled trial. *Ann Intern Med* 1993;119:874–881.

215. Shalansky KF, FitzGerald JM, Sanderji R, et al. Comparison of a weight-based heparin nomogram with traditional heparin dosing to achieve therapeutic anticoagulation. *Pharmacotherapy* 1996;16: 1076–1084.

216. Mungall D, Lord M, Cason S, et al. Developing and testing a system to improve the quality of heparin anticoagulation in patients with acute cardiac syndromes. *Am J Cardiol* 1998;82:574–579.

217. Brown G, Dodek P. An evaluation of empiric vs. nomogram-based dosing of heparin in an intensive care unit. *Crit Care Med* 1997;25: 1534–1538.

218. Cruickshank MK, Levine MN, Hirsh J, et al. A standard heparin nomogram for the management of heparin therapy. *Arch Intern Med* 1991;151:333–337.

219. Hollingsworth JA, Rowe BH, Brisebois FJ, et al. The successful application of a heparin nomogram in a community hospital. *Arch Intern Med* 1995;155:2095–2100.

220. Gunnarsson PS, Sawyer WT, Montague D, et al. Appropriate use of heparin: empiric vs nomogram-based dosing. *Arch Intern Med* 1995; 155:526–532.

221. Paradiso-Hardy FL, Cheung B, Geerts WH. Evaluation of an intravenous heparin nomogram in a coronary care unit. *Can J Cardiol* 1996;12:802–808.

222. Elliott CG, et al. Physician-guided treatment compared with a heparin protocol for deep venous thrombosis. *Arch Intern Med* 1994; 154:999–1004.

223. Hull RD, Raskob GE, Brant RF, et al. Relation between the time to achieve the lower limit of the APTT therapeutic range and recurrent

venous thromboembolism during heparin treatment for deep vein thrombosis. *Arch Intern Med* 1997;157:2562–2568.

224. Becker RC, Cyr J, Corrao JM, Ball SP. Bedside coagulation monitoring in heparin-treated patients with active thromboembolic disease: a coronary care unit experience. *Am Heart J* 1994;128:719–723.

225. Becker RC, Ball SP, Eisenberg P, et al. A randomized, multicenter trial of weight-adjusted intravenous heparin dose titration and point-of-care coagulation monitoring in hospitalized patients with active thromboembolic disease. *Am Heart J* 1999;137:59–71.

226. Zabel KM, Granger CB, Becker RC, et al. Use of bedside activated partial thromboplastin time monitor to adjust heparin dosing after thrombolysis for acute myocardial infarction: results of GUSTO-I. *Am Heart J* 1998;136:868–876.

227. Taylor CT, Petros WP, Ortel TL. Two instruments to determine activated partial thromboplastin time: implications for heparin monitoring. *Pharmacotherapy* 1999;19:383–387.

228. Ansell JE. Out-of-hospital coagulation monitoring and management. *J Thromb Thrombolys* 1999;7:191–194.

229. Ansell JE, Hamke AK, Holden A, Knapic N. Cost effectiveness of monitoring warfarin therapy using standard versus capillary prothrombin times. *Am J Clin Pathol* 1989;91:587–589.

230. Ansell JE, Hughes R. Evolving models of warfarin management: anticoagulation clinics, patient self-monitoring, and patient self-management. *Am Heart J* 1996;132:1095–1100.

231. Chiquette E, Amato MG, Bussey HI. Comparison of an anticoagulation clinic with usual medical care: anticoagulation control, patient outcomes, and health care costs. *Arch Intern Med* 1998;158: 1641–1647.

232. Fitzmaurice DA, Hobbs FDR, Murray ET. Primary care anticoagulant clinic management using computerized decision support and near patient International Normalized Ratio (INR) testing: routine data from a practice nurse-led clinic. *Fam Pract* 1998;15:144–146.

233. Gray DR, Garabedian-Ruffalo SM, Chretien SD. Cost-justification of a clinical pharmacist-managed anticoagulation clinic. *Drug Intell Clin Pharm* 1985;19:575–580.

234. Conte RR, et al. Nine-year experience with a pharmacist-managed anticoagulation clinic. *Am J Hosp Pharm* 1986;43:2460–2464.

235. OAMS Group. Point-of-care prothrombin time measurement for professional and patient self-testing. *Am J Clin Pathol* 2001;115: 288–296.

236. OAMS Group. Prothrombin measurement using a patient self-testing system. *Am J Clin Pathol* 2001;115:280–287.

237. Ansell JE, Patel N, Ostrovsky D, et al. Long-term patient self-management of oral anticoagulation. *Arch Intern Med* 1995;155: 2185–2189.

238. Beyth R, Quinn L, Landefeld C. A multicomponent intervention to prevent major bleeding complications in older patients receiving warfarin. *Ann Intern Med* 2000;133:687–695.

239. Cromheecke ME, et al. Oral anticoagulation self-management and management by a specialist anticoagulation clinic: a randomised cross-over comparison. *Lancet* 2000;356:97–102.

240. Koertke H, Minami K, Bairaktaris A, et al. INR self-management following mechanical heart valve replacement. *J Thromb Thrombolysis* 2000;9:S41–S45.

241. Watzke HH, Forberg E, Svolba G, et al. A prospective controlled trial comparing weekly self-testing and self-dosing with the standard management of patients on stable oral anticoagulation. *Thromb Haemost* 2000;83:661–665.

242. Kulinna W, Ney D, Wenzel T, et al. The effect of self-monitoring the INR on quality of anticoagulation and quality of life. *Sem Thromb Hemost* 1999;25:123–126.

243. Lafata JE, Martin SA, Kaatz S, Ward RE. Anticoagulation clinics and patient self-testing for patients on chronic warfarin therapy: a cost-effectiveness analysis. *J Thromb Thrombolysis* 2000;9:S13–S19.

244. Gould MK, Dembitzer AD, Doyle RL, et al. Low-molecular-weight heparins compared with unfractionated heparin for treatment of acute deep venous thrombosis: a meta-analysis of randomized, controlled trials. *Ann Intern Med* 1999;130:800–809.

245. Laposata M, Green D, Van Cott EM, et al. College of American

Pathologists Conference XXXI on Laboratory Monitoring of Anticoagulant Therapy: the clinical use and laboratory monitoring of low-molecular-weight heparin, danaparoid, hirudin and related compounds, and argatroban. *Arch Pathol Lab Med* 1998;122:799–807.

246. Greinacher A, Volpel H, Janssens U, et al. Recombinant hirudin (lepirudin) provides safe and effective anticoagulation in patients with heparin-induced thrombocytopenia: a prospective study. *Circulation* 1999;99:73–80.

247. Nurmohamed MT, Berckmans RJ, Morrien-Salmons WM, et al. Monitoring anticoagulant therapy by activated partial thromboplastin time: hirudin assessment. *Thromb Haemost* 1994;72:685–692.

248. Potzsch B, Hund S, Madlener K, et al. Monitoring of recombinant hirudin: assessment of a plasma-based ecarin clotting times assay. *Thromb Res* 1997;86:373–383.

249. Nowak G, Bucha E. Quantitative determination of hirudin in blood and body fluids. *Sem Thromb Hemost* 1996;22:197–202.

11

ON-SITE EVALUATION OF CHEST PAIN USING BIOMARKERS OF MYOCARDIAL INJURY

FRED S. APPLE

The assessment of patients with acute chest pain in emergency departments (EDs) is often a diagnostic challenge to physicians. Biochemical markers of myocardial injury have become extremely useful in assisting clinicians in confirming the diagnosis of acute myocardial infarction (AMI) in both patients with and without a diagnostic electrocardiogram (ECG) (1–3). In patients with unstable angina (UA) or acute coronary syndromes (ACSs) where the ECG often fails to provide conclusive diagnostic information, biochemical markers have also become reliable risk predictors of adverse short- and long-term outcomes (1–3). Improvements in technology and the implementation of monoclonal antibodies in immunoassays have led to an explosion of new instrumentation designated for rapid turnaround times (TATs). In addition, instrumentation has been developed that allows for both quantitative as well as qualitative detection of multiple markers of myocardial injury in whole blood, serum, or plasma. These new systems have been designed to provide testing capabilities in the central laboratory, in satellite laboratories, or closer to the bedside, and have been designated as point-of-care testing (POCT).

Several patient groups with varying clinical needs are optimal targets for implementation of POCT of myocardial injury markers. These patient groups include the following: (a) high-risk, ECG-diagnosed AMI patients qualifying for thrombolytic therapy; (b) high-risk, non-ST-segment elevation AMI patients; (c) moderate-risk ACS patients (UA patients with chest pain); and (d) low-risk, noncardiac, chest pain patients. In this chapter, clinical studies are reviewed that may or may not justify the use of POCT in each of these patient groups.

The goal of this chapter is to address the clinical and analytical aspects of POCT for the biochemical markers of myocardial injury. First, the pathophysiology of myocardial injury and implications of its diagnosis regarding use of markers is addressed. Second, the recently published guidelines and consensus documents that redefine AMI and reclassify ACS patients as either non-ST-segment myocardial infarction or UA (both heavily predicated on cardiac biomarkers) are discussed. Third, the goal and rationale for chest pain evaluation using clinical studies will address the role of POCT in myocardial injury markers. The urgency to obtain results and how results impact patient care, triage, management, and therapy are addressed. Clinical pathways are proposed that utilize multiple measurements of a single cardiac marker. The appropriate utilization of this pathway is discussed with regard to optimizing medical and economic outcomes. Fourth, specific POCT platform principles and instruments are reviewed, with a discussion of potential differences in standardization for measurement of selected markers between POCT devices and instrumentation used in the central laboratory.

PATHOPHYSIOLOGY OF MYOCARDIAL INJURY

The major course of AMI is atherosclerotic coronary artery disease (CAD), which contributes to narrowing of coronary arteries, plaque disruption, and thrombus formation (4–6). Myocardial ischemia and subsequent myocardial infarction usually begins in the endocardium and spreads to the epicardium. Irreversible injury has been documented if occlusion is complete for more than 15 to 20 minutes. However, restoration of blood flow within 6 hours is associated with myocardial salvage. A major determination of morbidity is the extent of myocardial damage.

The clinical history remains of substantial value in establishing an AMI diagnosis. The first symptom is usually angina at rest or with minimal activity and can be found in up to 50% of patients with AMI. Chest pain can be variable in intensity, is prolonged, and usually lasts for more than 30 minutes. In some patients, particularly the elderly, AMI is manifested not by chest pain but rather by chest tightness, weakness, congestion, nausea, or fainting. Studies show that between 40% and 50% of nonfatal AMIs are unrecognized by the patient and are found only on subsequent routine ECG.

The ECG changes of an AMI are those of ischemia. Myocardial cell injury and death are reflected by T-wave changes, ST segment changes, and the appearance of Q waves. The ST segment is elevated following myocardial injury. The diagnostic specificity of the ECG is 100%. If the ECG pattern is equivocal, then the clinician must depend on markers of myocardial injury. In about 15% to 20% of AMIs there are no changes on the initial ECG.

The ECG diagnosis of an old infarct is often difficult, especially without a tracing from the initial acute episode.

The precipitating factors in most patients are difficult to identify. The terminology of ACS has been defined to encompass a broad spectrum of ischemic heart disease symptoms including UA and non-ST-segment elevation AMI. Vascular injury and thrombus formation are key events in the initiation and progression of CAD and in the pathogenesis of ACS. Pathophysiologically, classification of vascular damage has been based on three stages: functional alterations of endothelial cells without substantial morphologic changes, endothelial denudation and critical damage with intact internal elastic lamina, and endothelial denudation with damage to both intima and media.

Most AMIs result from coronary atherosclerosis, which evolves from coronary thrombosis. Numerous factors contribute to the evaluation of atherosclerotic plaques that may rupture acutely, releasing thrombogenic substances that mediate platelet activation, thrombin generation, and fibrinolytic deficit. Newly formed thrombi interrupt blood flow and cause ischemic myocardial injury leading to myocardial necrosis. The process of plaque rupture has both immunologic and thrombotic activation. Enzymes such as collagenases and gelatinase, which mediate plasma disruption, usually are released by the intracellular components of the plaque. In AMI, the primary activation of the coagulation process is through the activation of factor VII, initiated by tissue factor from the ruptured plaque.

In patients with stable coronary artery disease, angina often results from increases in myocardial oxygen demands that overwhelm the ability of an occluded coronary artery to increase its delivery. In contrast, UA, non-ST-segment elevation AMI, and ST-segment elevation AMI present a continuation of the disease process characterized by abrupt decreases in coronary flow. In UA, episodes of thrombotic occlusion at a site of plaque disruption may lead to angina at rest. This labile thrombus may only occlude a vessel for 10 to 20 minutes. In non-ST-segment elevation AMI, the morphology of the lesion is often similar to that observed in UA, with one quarter of non-ST-segment elevation patients demonstrating a completely occluded artery at angiography. Often this complete coronary occlusion is followed by spontaneous reperfusion within the first 2 hours. In non-ST-segment elevation AMIs, the plaque damage is usually worse than in UA, resulting from a more persistent thrombotic occlusion, that is, more myocardial injury. In ST-segment elevation AMI, plaque disruption can be associated with ulceration, deep arterial damage, with high thrombogenic risk. This results in the formation of a fixed and persistent thrombus, which is occlusive, lead to abrupt cessation of myocardial perfusion, and necrosis of the involved myocardial tissue. Some thrombus formation appears to be an important factor in the progression of CAD and in the conversion of chronic to acute events after plaque disruption.

MYOCARDIAL INFARCTION REDEFINED

A consensus document authored by a joint committee of the European Society of Cardiology (ESC) and the American College of Cardiology (ACC) recently described that myocardial infarction (MI) should be redefined as any amount of myocardial necrosis, as indicated by an increase in cardiac biomarkers (cardiac troponin I or T or creatine kinase-MB [CK-MB]) in the setting of clinical ischemia (7,8). In addition, the ACC and American Heart Association (AHA) also recently published guidelines for the reclassification of patients with ACS, for which patients presenting with an increased cardiac marker (cardiac troponin) are classified as non-ST-segment elevation MI, and those with a normal troponin as UA (9). Both documents stress that a maximal concentration of cardiac troponin exceeding the decision limit (99th percentile of the values for a reference [normal] population) on at least one occasion during the first 24 hours after the index clinical event (ischemia) is defined as an MI. This redefinition is significant because an individual who was previously diagnosed as having UA would now be classified as an MI if positive for troponin. Several key issues regarding the document should be noted by both clinicians and laboratorians. First, the criteria for acute, evolving, or recent MI includes the typical rise and fall of cardiac troponin (or CK-MB) with at least one of the following: ischemia symptoms, development of Q waves on the ECG, ECG changes indicative of ischemia (ST-segment elevation or depression), or coronary artery intervention. Second, detectable increases in cardiac troponin (or CK-MB) are indicative of myocardial injury, but are not synonymous with an ischemic mechanism. Third, increases in cardiac troponin likely reflect irreversible injury. Fourth, the diversity of cardiac troponin assays, specifically for cardiac troponin-I (cTnI), has led to substantial confusion, mostly due to lack of standardization of assays. Therefore, clinical and analytical information for each cardiac troponin method should be validated through publication(s) in the peer-reviewed literature. Fifth, for patients with an ischemic mechanism of injury, serum cardiac troponin increases are related to prognosis. Sixth, blood sampling should be obtained up to 8 to 9 hours after onset of symptoms before a patient is ruled out for myocardial injury. Seventh, manufacturers of cardiac troponin assays should clarify potential sources of interferences, including heterophile antibodies, clot issues, serum versus plasma variability, and antibody-epitope recognition diversity for free, complex, degraded, phosphorylated, and oxidized forms of cardiac troponin I. Eighth, the acceptable imprecision at the 99th percentile of normal, the revised recommended medical decision cutpoint, should be less than 10% coefficient of variation (CV). Manufacturers need to document the concentrations at which both a 10% CV as well as a 20% CV are found. Finally, classification and care of patients with increases in cardiac troponins, who undergo interventional procedures such as angioplasty, should be individualized. No markers should be used to determine MI in cardiac surgery patients, such as in coronary artery bypass grafts.

CHEST PAIN EVALUATION—GOALS AND RATIONALE

Strategies for Ruling In and Ruling Out Acute Myocardial Infarction

The evaluation of patients presenting to the ED with chest pain continues to be a time-consuming and diagnostic challenge to clinicians. Over the past 5 years with the advances in technology, both new and traditional biochemical markers for myocardial cell injury have become more important in helping clinicians (a) avoid sending home non-diagnostic ECG AMIs (estimated to be 30,000 per year in the United States); (b) assist in the triage of both high-risk and moderate-risk ACS patients into appropriate levels of monitored and intensive care unit beds; and (c) confidently discharge patients with low risk of cardiac etiology. Further, new strategies of cardiac marker utilization have also provided clinicians with strong, independent information on short- and long-term risk of cardiac events both in the hospital and following hospital discharge.

Internationally, a large number of hospitals continue to use total creatine kinase (CK) (because of cost constraints) to rule in and rule out AMI in patients presenting with chest pain (10), despite the limitations presented by total CK and its isoenzyme CK-MB. These include lack of absolute myocardial specificity,

as well as the influence of muscle mass, exercise, sex, race, and age (11,12). Cost constraints often limit the use of the more expensive testing for CK-MB mass, cTnI, or cardiac troponin-T (cTnT). However, the new redefinition of MI (7,8) and reclassification of UA guidelines (9) heavily support the equivalence of cTnI and cTnT (with CK-MB mass as an acceptable alternative if troponin testing is not available) for the sensitive detection of AMI. The 100% cardiac specificity of cardiac troponins supports these conclusions (13,14). Since it is well recognized that CK-MB as well as both cardiac troponin I and T are not early markers of myocardial injury (it takes 3 to 8 hours following onset of chest pain to document increases above their respective upper reference limits) (15,16), early markers such as myoglobin and CK-MB isoforms have been investigated (and recommended in the new guidelines) to assist in the sensitive earlier detection and early triage of ACS patients. Fig. 11.1 demonstrates, using receiver operating characteristic (ROC)

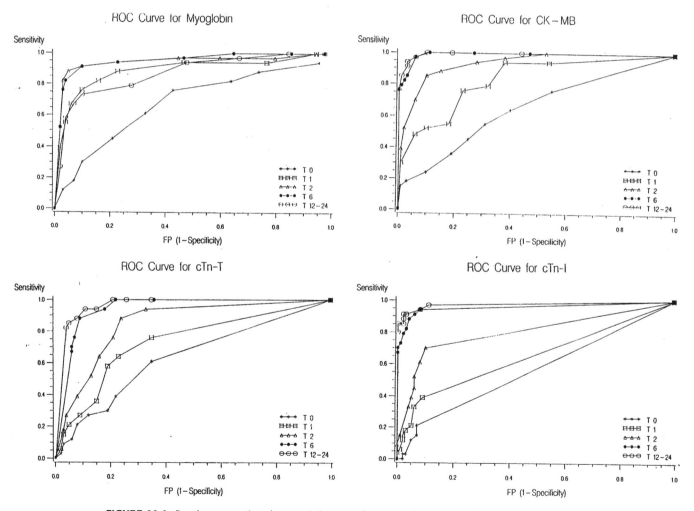

FIGURE 11.1. Receiver operating characteristic curves for myoglobin, creatine kinase-MB (CK-MB), cardiac troponin-T (cTnT), and cardiac troponin-I (cTnI) for detection of acute myocardial infarction. Curves represent times after presentation to emergency department at 0 hour, 1 hour, 2 hours, 6 hours, and 12 to 24 hours for each marker. Myoglobin, CK-MB, and cTnI were measured by the Dade Behring Stratus analyzer, and cTnT on the ES300 analyzer (Roche-BM). (Adapted from Tucker JF, Collins RA, Anderson AJ, et al., Early diagnostic efficiency of cardiac troponin I and troponin T for acute myocardial infarction, *Acad Emerg Med* 1997;4:13–21, with permission.)

curves, that both clinical sensitivity and specificity of myoglobin, CK-MB, cTnI, and cTnT improve over time following presentation to the ED (16). Further, the ROC curves graphically display myoglobin as the most sensitive early marker at less than 6 hours, with CK-MB, cTnI, and cTnT approaching greater than 90% sensitivity and specificity 6 to 12 hours after presentation. However, clinicians must acknowledge the lack of cardiac tissue specificity and lack of outcome studies regarding these early markers (17,18).

Numerous rule-in and rule-out AMI protocols have been published to assist clinicians in the triage of chest pain patients within 12 hours of presentation (19–27). It should be noted that throughout this discussion, the decision trees used for early diagnosis of AMI in the ED are based on the timing of presentation to the hospital being 0 hour, and not the onset of chest pain as 0 hour. It is so designated since the only reliable time is the time when the patient physically presents to the hospital. Unfortunately, the onset of chest pain taken during the patient's history is often unreliable, as more than 50% of chest pain onset times are inaccurate.

The program established by the Heart ER Program (27) for rapidly evaluating chest pain patients with low to intermediate probability of AMI (nondiagnostic ECG at presentation) appears to be the model most often used in clinical studies. Any patient with chest pain or discomfort clinically consistent with acute myocardial ischemia or AMI is evaluated over a 9- to 12-hour period. Based on the Heart ER Program findings, serial CK-MB mass monitoring every 3 hours up to 9 hours has consistently demonstrated greater than 98% sensitivity and greater than 98% specificity for ruling in and ruling out AMI at 9 hours following admission, compared to less than 50% sensitivity for serial ECG monitoring, echocardiography, and graded exercise testing.

Similar studies enrolling low to intermediate probability of AMI patients with nondiagnostic ECGs that have monitored cardiac troponins have also followed the guidelines established by the Heart ER protocol (monitoring markers of myocardial injury up to12 hours after presentation) (23, 26). Other studies have used the strategy of following markers up to 24 hours after presentation (16,22). For both cTnI and cTnT, the most widely cited study examined over 700 patients with acute chest pain for less than 12 hours presenting with a nondiagnostic (no ST-segment elevations) ECG (28). Blood was tested (qualitatively for both cTnI and cTnT) at admission (onset of chest pain was less than two hours after presentation) and at least 4 hours after admission so that at least one sample was taken at least six hours after the onset of chest pain. Of the 6% of patients with AMI, clinical sensitivity of a positive cTnT was 94% and sensitivity for cTnI was 100% (no statistical difference). Further, during 30 days of follow-up among more than 300 patients with UA, increases in cTnI or cTnT were shown to be strong, independent predictors of cardiac events, AMI, or cardiac-related death. Negative cTnI or cTnT test results were associated with low risk and allowed rapid and safe discharge of patients.

In chest pain evaluation protocols that have utilized quantitative cTnT and cTnI assays (either whole-blood POCT devices or central laboratory instruments that can provide rapid-result TATs), similar clinical sensitivities and specificities of more than

90% at more than 12 hours following presentation have been documented. One of several representative studies to compare cTnI and cTnT with CK-MB using serial 0-hour, 1-hour, 3-hour, 6-hour, 9-hour, and 12- to 24-hour sample draws, demonstrated that both cardiac troponins were equivalent to CK-MB mass at more than 6 hours; with sensitivities and specificities greater than 90% by 12 hours (16). Neither cardiac troponin assisted in the early (less than 2 hours) screening for AMI, as expected.

Studies have also used combined marker approaches, using both quantitative and qualitative POCT devices for cTnI, cTnT, myoglobin, and CK-MB mass measurements in chest pain evaluation protocols (16,20,22). Several trials have demonstrated that myoglobin is the most sensitive early marker of these, with greater than 90% sensitivity by 0 to 3 hours after presentation (29,30). No published study to date, however, has convincingly demonstrated that the added cost of testing for myoglobin assists in improving patient therapies or outcomes. However, it has been shown that myoglobin is an excellent negative predictor of muscle injury, as demonstrated by two early, successive (usually separated by 1 to 3 hours) negative results (whether qualitative or quantitative), with greater than 95% confidence for ruling out AMI (31). This type of testing approach may be beneficial in rural hospitals or clinics that may need to transport patients with more critical illnesses to larger medical complexes for appropriate care. However, at larger medical centers, an 8- to 12-hour blood-draw window, with monitoring of cardiac troponins, has gained considerable favor.

Using CK-MB isoforms as a proposed early marker, Puleo et al. (32) have shown that the CK-MB1/MB2 ratio could be used to diagnose or rule out AMI at 6 hours after presentation, with a sensitivity of 95.7% compared to a 48% sensitivity for CK-MB activity. A recent multicenter trial of patients who presented to the ED with chest pain, directly compared diagnostic sensitivity and specificity for CK-MB mass, CK-MB isoforms, cTnI, cTnT, and myoglobin (33). The findings suggested that CK-MB isoforms and myoglobin were more efficient for the early diagnosis (within 6 hours) of MI, whereas cTnI and cTnT were highly cardiac specific and particularly efficient after 6 hours. However, no statistical analysis of data at any time point was described. The Helena REP (electrophoresis) system (Helana Laboratories, Beaumont, TX) appears to be the only technology currently available for reliable isoform measurement, and has not been readily accepted by laboratories as a stat, 24-hour technology that could be adapted as a POCT device. This is especially true outside the central laboratory, which would require operation by nonlaboratory personnel.

Clinical studies that utilize quantitative and qualitative whole-blood POCT systems, which incorporate multiple markers in one device or side by side using multiple devices, have demonstrated consistent findings of clinical sensitivity and specificity for CK-MB mass, cTnI, and cTnT. Study results show more than 90% sensitivity and specificity 9 to 12 hours after admission in chest pain evaluation patients (34–39). A recent study (38) that evaluated one such quantitative system, the Biosite Triage (Biosite Diagnostics, San Diego, CA), however, demonstrated that combining multiple markers (CK-MB, cTnI, and myoglobin) did not improve the sensitivity or specificity for ruling in or ruling out AMI; single marker testing with cTnI was the most sensitive of the three markers. (Note that cTnT was not evaluated in this study.) In the study evaluating the Biosite Triage (38), cTnI demonstrated 93% sensitivity at 12 hours after presentation, which was comparable to parallel determinations of CK-MB, myoglobin, or cTnI, which demonstrated sensitivity levels of 97% (no statistical differences). Similar clinical sensitivities were demonstrated in the evaluation of the First Medical Alpha Dx (First Medical, Mountain View, CA)—a POCT system that simultaneously measures CK-MB, cTnI, myoglobin, and total CK (39)—which showed more than 90% sensitivity at 12 hours following admission using either cTnI or CK-MB. A multivariant-marker analysis of sensitivity or specificity, however, was not performed in the trial of the First Medical device (39). However, the Biosite and First Medical studies were not designed to appropriately address this issue; therefore, future studies need to address the role of multiple markers.

Several studies have now evaluated the Dade Behring Stratus CS (Dade Behring, Miami, FL) whole-blood POCT system for cTnI (CK-MB and myoglobin are also available on this platform) (40,41). Based on ROC curve analysis, a decision cutpoint of 0.15 µg/L was calculated for the detection of MI. In ACS patients 4 hours after arrival in the ED, at the 0.15 µg/L cutpoint, MI sensitivity was 98%, compared to the older generation Stratus II assay sensitivity of 85%. The 97.5% percentile in a healthy population was 0.08 µg/L. In 42% of patients with

UA, and cTnI was ≥0.08 µg/L. Performing a 30-day outcomes analysis, death or MI occurred in 25% of cTnI-positive patients versus 3% of cTnI-negative patients. Thus, this second-generation POCT system demonstrated accurate, analytically sensitive, and clinically reliable information.

A quantitative whole-blood bedside cTnT assay that complements the central laboratory Elecsys cTnT assay has recently been evaluated (42). In a method comparison of 140 samples, the cTnT POC test correlated well with the cTnT enzyme-linked immunosorbent assay (ELISA) (r=0.98). After 4 to 8 hours in patients with MI, 91% of all samples were positive. Areas under the ROC curves for detection of MI at the 0.1 µg/L cutpoint were comparable between the POCT and ELISA methods. The 99th percentile for 64 healthy individuals was less than 0.05 µg/L. Thus, accurate, analytically sensitive, and clinically reliable bedside cTnT testing, within 15 minutes, is now possible in suspected ACS patients.

In summary, the rapidly growing literature involving rapid evaluation protocols used in EDs that use markers of myocardial injury, one can conclude that a fast track protocol can assist in accurately triaging patients at high, intermediate, and low risk of cardiac pathology to appropriate levels of care and management by clinicians (43). However, an essential component of any protocol involves the timing of blood draws following presentation. Fig. 11.2 is a proposed schematic pertaining to how cardiac

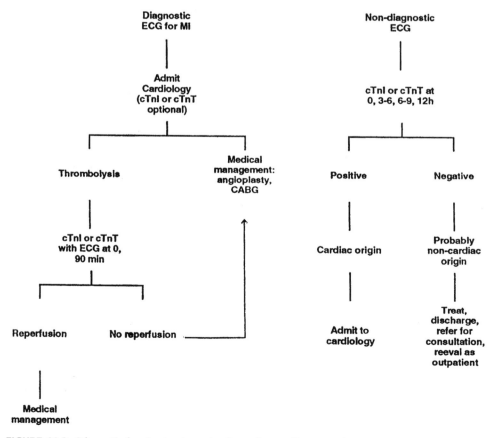

FIGURE 11.2. Schematic for chest pain evaluation using cardiac troponin-I or -T as a single marker to assist clinicians in ruling in and ruling out acute myocardial infarction.

markers could be utilized to assist in patient triage. Note that only cardiac troponin I or T is used instead of CK-MB mass and that myoglobin (as an early marker) is not recommended unless appropriate documentation becomes available to support the additional expense. Further, note that total CK, total LD, and LD isoenzymes (which are not discussed in this chapter) are never recommended as part of any strategy (44). This schematic supports the recently published ESC/ACC/AHA guidelines (7–9).

Strategies for the Role of Cardiac Markers for Risk Assessment

Numerous prospective and retrospective clinical studies have evaluated and compared the utility of measurements of cTnI, cTnT, and CK-MB for risk stratification or clinical outcomes assessment of ACS patients with possible myocardial ischemia in the ED (28,45–54). Patients presenting with a complaint of chest pain or other symptoms suggesting ACS have been assigned to blood sampling protocols including only a single draw at presentation to several serial draws over a 12- to 24-hour period following presentation. A large proportion of this heterogeneous ACS group is patients presenting with UA. In this

group, up to 50% progress to AMI or cardiac death within the first year.

Studies have demonstrated prognostic similarities between UA patients and those with ST-segment elevation infarction. The use of markers is not just simply one of rapidly ruling in or ruling out AMI, but also important for the medical management of patients with UA who are undergoing an acute coronary process (high to moderate risk) from those with chronic or stable coronary disease (low risk). Therefore, the goal of monitoring cardiac markers in ACS patients without AMI would be to identify possible unstable coronary disease and triage to an appropriate therapy regimen. This might allow the clinician to offer the patient, assuming an abnormal serum cardiac marker test is identified, alternative medical and procedural options such as antiplatelet or antithrombotic therapies, coronary angiogram, an echocardiography, a radionuclide scan, or exercise stress testing to possibly identify the pathologic etiology responsible for the tissue release of markers of myocardial injury.

One-quarter to one-third of patients with UA or chest pain patients in whom AMI has been ruled out have shown increased serum concentration of cTnI and or cTnT. Fig. 11.3 summarizes data from a recent meta-analysis on this subject (55). Clearly, increases in cTnT or cTnI are predicative of adverse

Study	Troponin +(ve)	Troponin -(ve)	Peto OR (95% CI Fixed)	
"ST elevation"				
Ohman, 1996	18 / 138	14 / 297		3.39 [1.56,7.33]
Stubbs, 1996	5 / 45	3 / 80		3.38 [0.77,14.96]
Gusto III, 1999	212 / 1127	1078 / 11539		2.82 [2.30,3.45]
Subtotal	235 / 1310	1095 / 11916		2.86 [2.35,3.47]
"no-ST elevation"				
Hamm,1992	10 / 33	1 / 51		11.71 [3.22,42.57]
Wu, 1995	8 / 27	3 / 104		31.52 [6.89,144.19]
Ohman, 1996	13 / 131	4 / 189		4.70 [1.74,12.67]
Cin, 1996	12 / 24	2 / 48		17.91 [5.24,61.25]
Stubbs, 1996	10 / 62	6 / 52		1.46 [0.51,4.19]
Antman, 1996	21 / 573	8 / 831		3.80 [1.80,8.03]
Galvani, 1997	5 / 22	4 / 69		6.55 [1.32,32.38]
Luscher, 1997	27 / 249	12 / 267		2.48 [1.28,4.76]
Solymoss, 1997	7 / 41	6 / 74		2.43 [0.73,8.05]
Ottani, 1997	11 / 47	1 / 47		6.62 [1.98,22.10]
Olatidoye, 1998	5 / 13	3 / 94		156.17 [17.39,1402.09]
Benamer, 1998	10 / 60	2 / 135		13.68 [3.87,48.33]
Rebuzzi, 1998	7 / 14	8 / 88		25.27 [5.18,123.23]
Brisics, 1998	3 / 22	2 / 70		7.96 [0.97,65.12]
Antman, 1998	4 / 116	15 / 481		1.11 [0.35,3.53]
Hamm, 1999	27 / 139	15 / 307		5.48 [2.76,10.87]
Subtotal	180 / 1573	92 / 2907		4.93 [3.77,6.45]
Total	415/2883	1187/14823		3.44 (2.94,4.03)

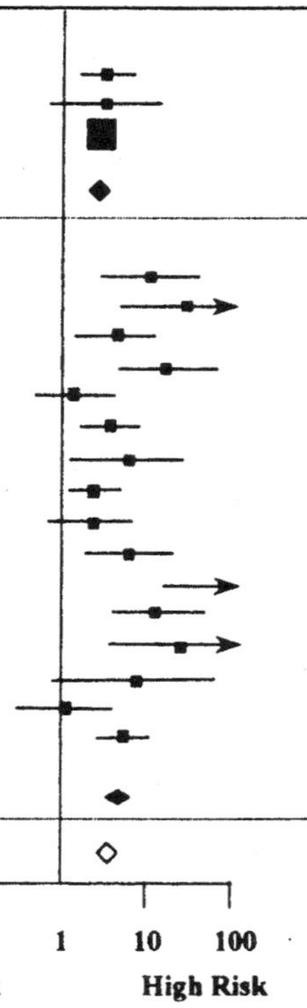

.01　.1　1　10　100

Low Risk　　**High Risk**

FIGURE 11.3. Odds ratios (ORs) and 95% confidence intervals (CIs) for risk of cardiac death and reinfarction at 30-day follow-up in patients with acute coronary syndromes (ACS). Pooled OR for ST↑ group is 2.86 (95% CI, 2.35–3.47; p<.0001). Pooled OR for no-ST↑ group is 4.93 (95% CI, 3.77–6.45; p<.0001). Pooled OR for overall group of patients with ACS is 3.44 (95% CI, 2.94–4.03; p<.00001). Troponin + (ve), troponin positive; troponin – (ve), troponin negative. (From Ottani F, Galvani M, Nicolini A, et al., Elevated cardiac troponin levels predict the risk of adverse outcome in patients with acute coronary syndromes, *Am Heart J* 2000;140:917–927, with permission.)

outcomes in ACS patients. Twenty-one studies were evaluated and odds ratios (ORs) (endpoint death or nonfatal MI) were calculated for both short-term (30 days) and long-term (5 months to 3 years) outcomes in patients with and without ST-segment elevation and in UA patients. Overall, in the approximately 18,000 patients included, at 30 days the OR for an adverse outcome was 3.4 for increased troponin. For patients with a positive troponin the OR to have an adverse outcome in patients with UA was higher (9.3) compared to patients with ST-segment elevation (4.9) for both short- and long-term outcomes. Therefore, both cTnT and cTnI offer the best risk assessment and their testing needs to be eased into current practice guidelines regarding diagnosis and management of ACS patients as useful risk stratification tools. This approach is supported in the new ESC/ACC/AHA guidelines. Care must be taken, however, when evaluating individual studies pertaining to prognostic significance. It is critical to determine the timing of sampling for cardiac marker measurements since results from a single draw at presentation may conflict with findings based on serial draws over a 24-hour period following presentation. It is recommended to draw two samples (for either cTnI or cTnT) on ACS patients who do not rule in for AMI; one at presentation and one at ≥ 9 hours following presentation. This will allow for an increase in either cardiac troponin to occur above baseline in a patient presenting with a very recent acute coronary lesion (54). It should not be overlooked, however, that a normal cardiac troponin does not remove all risk (55). It is highly recommended that cardiac marker results be provided to clinicians within 60 minutes, either using POCT or central laboratory instrumentation.

Strategies for Noninvasive Assessment of Reperfusion

Biochemical markers of myocardial injury are not routinely needed in patients with diagnostic ECG evidence of AMI but are useful for confirmatory reasons. Further, markers do not serve as an indication of which patients do or do not receive thrombolytic therapy. However, in patients that are indicated for and receive thrombolytic therapy, there is a growing body of evidence that early monitoring of markers may be useful in the noninvasive assessment of reperfusion success (56–59). Early and complete patency of infarct-related arteries is an important therapeutic goal during the early hours after the onset of AMI and markers may assist clinicians in patient management strategies. It is accepted that the kinetics of myocardial protein appearance in the circulation following AMI depends on the infarct area perfusion status. Early successful reperfusion is characterized by a rapid increase of markers and an early peak (Fig. 11.4). It is, however, difficult to assess the amount of irreversible injury by biochemical infarct sizing because of the variability in the amount of protein washout that appears in the circulation after reperfusion. The laboratory can best be used to assess reperfusion status following thrombolytic therapy when early, frequent blood sampling is combined with rapid analysis of a marker of myocardial injury. Several studies (56–59), all retrospective, have demonstrated that the use of one of three criteria, using the rate of increase of markers from pretherapy to 60 to 120 minutes posttherapy to determine the (a) slope, (b) an

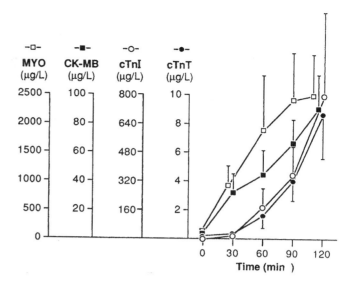

FIGURE 11.4. Time course of serum myoglobin (MYO), CK MB, cTnI and cTnT (mean with standard error) in acute myocardial infarction patients with complete reperfusion following thrombolytic therapy. (From Apple FS, Sharkey SW, Henry TD. Early serum cardiac troponin I and T concentrations after successful thrombosis for acute myocardial infarction. *Clin Chem* 1995;41:1197–1198, with permission.)

absolute increase, or (c) the ratio of the 90- to 0-minute values, will, with a high degree of accuracy, predict the success or failure of reperfusion. Studies that show the rapid increase of serum CK-MB, myoglobin, cTnT and cTnI have all demonstrated high sensitivities (more than 75%) to predict successful TIMI 3 reflow.

To summarize, AMI is now managed in a systemic, stepwise manner, where the use of anticoagulant, antiplatelet, and thrombolytic drugs all play pivotal roles. Thus, while the emphasis of this chapter is on the monitoring of biochemical markers of myocardial injury, such as cardiac troponins, CK-MB, and myoglobin, the profile of activation analytes of coagulation and platelets along with vascular distress markers may provide important information in the management of patients in the near future. Improvements in therapies for UA and non-ST-segment elevation MI are rapidly progressing. Glycoprotein IIb/IIIa platelet inhibitors have recently been shown in several clinical trials to improve outcomes in UA patients (60). Management has thus been directed at preventing progression of UA to AMI, because of the poorer prognosis such patients carry. However, thrombolytic therapy in UA is not indicated. Therefore, to be able to distinguish between UA and infarction in patients as soon possible after presentation to the ED becomes important. The clinical studies discussed in this chapter strongly support the utilization of cardiac troponins to assist clinicians with their differential diagnoses. However, clinicians continue to order multiple serial markers in AMI documented patients, with the explanation that they are looking for a peak concentration to occur or to assist in sizing the infarction. At present, it is not clear whether the expense of measuring several markers is justified based on whether patient management or therapy will be altered by the timing of the peak value of a biochemical marker.

POINT-OF-CARE ASSAYS FOR MYOCARDIAL INJURY MARKERS

As shown in Table 11.1, two qualitative and four quantitative rapid (less than 20 minutes TAT), whole-blood POCT devices have been evaluated and approved by the Food and Drug Administration (FDA) for one or more of the following markers (28,34–41): myoglobin, CK-MB mass, cardiac troponin I, cardiac troponin T, and total CK mass. In addition, three quantitative investigational devices are also noted. Numerous other platforms (normally found in the central laboratory) are also available for the (rapid) quantitative measurement of these markers in serum and plasma (3). Most of these also provide analytical TATs within 20 minutes of placing a specimen on the instrument. However, the focus of this section is mainly on the whole-blood devices. At present, approximately 10% of laboratories report using POCT devices, determined from the 2000 College of American Pathologists Survey CAR-C, as shown in Fig. 11.5. With the recent FDA approval and release of quantitative, whole-blood, POCT devices, it will be noteworthy to follow the changing trends.

With the development of rapid, whole-blood, POCT devices, for measurement of CK-MB mass, cTnT, cTnI and myoglobin, which have traditionally been performed on larger instruments in the central laboratory, it is important to briefly discuss how absolute concentrations from the same marker may or may not differ between instruments. Selection of antibodies for the epitopes they recognize as well as how an assay is standardized may affect results among assays from different manufacturers. Currently, there is not an internationally accepted standard reference material for myoglobin, CK-MB, or cTnI. Since only one manufacturer markets cTnT assays, independent of the qualitative or quantitative platform used, whole blood, serum, or plasma, within sample cTnT results should be highly concordant (42). For myoglobin, although there currently is no accepted reference standard material, concentrations among assays do not vary widely, likely because of common epitopes recognized by commercial antimyoglobin antibodies. The IFCC (International Federation of Clinical Chemistry) Markers of Cardiac Damage Scientific Committee is in the process of developing a standard material for myoglobin. For CK-MB mass, an AACC (American Association for Clinical Chemistry) standard subcommittee has been successful in developing a primary reference material that eliminates the 40% to 60% differences currently experienced among more than 10 commercial immunoassays (61). For cTnI, the AACC, with assistance from the IFCC committee, has established a standards subcommittee to develop a primary standard. Preliminary findings indicate that three materials (binary IC or tertiary TIC complexes) have been identified and round-robin validation studies are underway with the manufacturers of all cTnI immunoassays (62).

TABLE 11.1. WHOLE BLOOD POINT-OF-CARE TESTING PLATFORMS AND CARDIAC MARKER ASSAYS

Manufacturer	Platform	Markers	Volume (μL)	TAT (min)	Detection Limit (μg/L)	URL (μg/L)
Quantitative						
Dade-Behring	Stratus CS	Myoglobin	200	13	1.0	82.0
Glasgow, DE		CK MB	200		0.3	3.5
		cTnI	200		0.03	0.6
First Medical[a]	Alpha Dx	Myoglobin	250	20	5.0	180.0
Mountain View, CA		CK MB			0.5	7.0
		cTnI			0.09	0.4
		Total CK			10.0	190.0
Biosite[a]	Triage	Myoglobin	250	10	2.7	107.0
SanDiego, CA		CK MB			0.75	4.3
		cTnI			0.19	0.4
Roche	CARDIAC	cTnT	150	12	0.1	0.1
Indianapolis, IN	Reader	Myoglobin	150		30.0	70.0
Qualitative						
Spectral[a]	Cardiac	cTnI	200	15	1.5	1.5
Toronto, Canada	STATus	Myoglobin	200	15	100.0	100.0
		MB	200	15	5.0	5.0
Roche	Rapid Assay	cTnT	150	20	0.18	0.18
Indianapolis, IN		Myoglobin				
Qualitative-Investigational						
Thau MDx[a]	Lifelite	Myoglobin	not available			
Santa Barbara, CA		CK MB				
		cTnI				
Quantech[a]		Myoglobin	not available			
Eagen, MN		CK MB				
		cTnI				
Response Biomedical		Myoglobin	not available			
Vancouver, BC, Canada		CK MB				
		cTnI				

[a]Panel of tests obtained with each analysis; TAT, turnaround time; URL, upper reference limit.

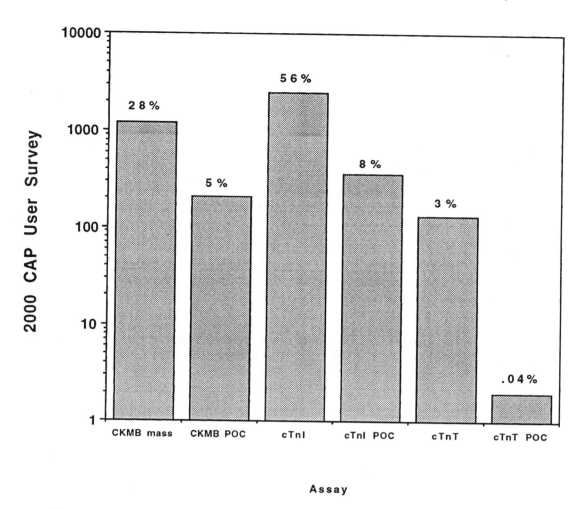

FIGURE 11.5. Number and percentages of laboratories using cardiac marker assays determined from a 2000 survey by the College of American Pathologists survey.

Currently, for cTnI, only Dade Behring has both a whole-blood POCT device (Stratus CS) and a central laboratory instrument (Dimension RxL) that measure cTnI and give equivalent results. Among all other cTnI methods, published slopes of regression equations compared against the Dade Behring Stratus II range from 0.10 to 3.50 (3,63). The wide variation in slopes is partially explained by the multiple forms of cTnI found in the blood and the multiple epitope regions recognized by the many different anti-cTnI-antibodies used, as well as the lack of standardization (64). Development of clinical databases for each cTnI assay becomes mandatory, although clinical trends among assays are comparable. For cTnT, Roche now has both an FDA-approved POCT method (Cardiac Reader) and a central laboratory method (Elecsys) that give equivalent results. A description of the whole-blood POCT devices follows.

Biosite Triage Cardiac Panel

The Triage Cardiac Panel is a fluorescence immunoassay used for the quantitative determination of CK-MB, myoglobin, and cTnI in heparinized whole blood and plasma. After addition of

the sample (several drops) to the sample port, cells are separated from plasma via a filter contained in the device. A predetermined quantity of plasma is allowed to react with fluorescent antibody conjugate within the chamber. After incubation and flow through a detection lane, complexes of the analytes and fluorescent antibody conjugates are captured on discrete zones resulting in binding assays specific for each analyte. The concentration of each analyte is directly proportional to the fluorescence detected. Mouse monoclonal and polyclonal antibodies against CK-MB, and myoglobin and mouse monoclonal and goat polyclonal antibodies against cTnI labeled with a fluorescent dye and immobilized on the solid phase are used. All results are available in 15 minutes. For bedside external quality control (QC), each Triage device contains two internal positive controls. The low control is set to approximately correspond to the signal one gets at the analyte medical decision cutoff. The high control corresponds to a signal at about 75% of the maximum signal of the dose-response curve. Further, the meter has the following capabilities: QC requirements programmed into the instrument, lockouts for unauthorized personnel, and a laboratory information system (LIS) interface. Imprecision for all three analytes at their respective decision cutoff concentrations are less than 13%. Calibration of the system is performed electronically and is lot specific. The manufacturer demonstrates that all forms of cTnI—free, complexed, oxidized, or reduced—are measured equivalently (64).

First Medical Alpha Dx System

The First Medical Inc. (FMI) Alpha Dx system is a fluorescence immunoassay platform that integrates automated solid-phase sandwich immunoassay capabilities with fluorescence detection. Quantitative measurement of a panel of four tests is performed on myoglobin, CK-MB mass, total CK mass, and cTnI. The system consists of an analyzer and test kits, with the kit containing test disks, Safe-T-Coupler unit, fluid cassette, and calibration diskette. The test disk contains all required test-specific reagents, along with bi-level quality controls for each test in stabilized dry form. The Safe-T-Coupler unit is used to load the blood collection tube into the analyzer. The fluid cassette contains a stabilized buffered detergent solution and is used to hydrate the dried reagents. The calibration diskette contains lot-specific calibration data and QC limits. The system is designed to automatically perform sample metering, reagent hydration, mixing, incubation, signal detection, and data management with results available in 20 minutes. Test results are available in both screen display and printout, and can be interfaced with a LIS. The Alpha Dx test utilizes three antibodies per assay: solid-phase monoclonal antibody, fluorescence-labeled antibody, and fluorescently labeled antifluorescence antibody, providing enhanced assay sensitivity. Fluorescent intensity is proportional to concentration of analyte. The test disk is also designed to measure the hematocrit or packed cell volume, which is used to convert the measured analyte concentration from a whole-blood sample into an equivalent serum sample. Imprecision of all four markers at their respective cutoff concentrations was less than 8.0%.

Dade Behring Stratus CS

The Stratus CS stat fluorometric analyzer is a fully automated system for the quantitative analysis of CK-MB, myoglobin, and cTnI. The system is designed to accept closed collection tubes of anticoagulated whole blood. The blood is separated into plasma and red cells on board via centrifugation. Tests to be performed are selected by introducing unitized TestPaks into the analyzer for the test method(s) of choice. The patient specimen may be identified via an internal bar-code reader while the TestPaks are identified as being for mass CK-MB, cTnI, or myoglobin via an internal bar-code reader. Up to four TestPaks may be introduced for each sample tested. All reagents required for specimen analysis are contained within the TestPaks. Dilutions may be automatically performed by including a test-specific DilPak with the appropriate TestPak in the test sequence. Results are available in 13 minutes.

All fluid transfers are accomplished using disposable tips. Radial partition immunoassay technology is utilized in a test format that incorporates antibodies linked to STARBURST dendrimers as the means of capturing the analyte of interest. Materials contained in the TestPaks include the dendrimer-anti-body reagent, an alkaline, phosphatase-labeled antibody reagent, a substrate-wash reagent, and a piece of glass-fiber filter paper. Lot-specific calibration parameters are provided as part of the bar-coded information on the TestPaks. A calibration curve is established for each new reagent lot and is updated periodically for a given method by introduction of a single CalPak and three TestPaks. Imprecision of all three markers at their respective cutoff concentrations is less than 7%.

Roche-Boehringer Mannheim Cardiac Reader System

The Roche Cardiac System analyzer can be used both for qualitative and quantitative measurement of cTnT. The test contains two monoclonal antibodies specific for cTnT, one gold labeled and the other biotinylated. The antibodies form a sandwich complex with any cTnT that is present in a whole-blood sample. Whole blood is dispensed into a sample well, red blood cells are removed from the sample as the specimen passes through a separation zone, and plasma passes through the detection zone in which the cTnT sandwich complexes accumulate along a line of streptavidin, appearing as a red streak (signal time). Excess gold-labeled antibodies gather along a control line signaling visually that the test was valid. The test signal increases in intensity in proportion to the cTnT concentration. The optical system of the Cardiac Reader recognizes two lines and measures the intensity of the signal line, which is integrated by internal software to a quantitative result. (Without the Reader, visual inspection of the lines serves as a positive/negative result.) A reading below the 0.1 μg/L detection limit is reported as low. Each test strip is calibrated against the second-generation quantitative cTnT assay. A coding chip programs the reader with calibration data unique to each lot of test strings. Qualitative and quantitative results are displayed within 15 minutes; however, as soon as the signal intensity exceeds the 0.1 μg/L cutoff, the Cardiac Reader signals a positive result through a red LED indicator. The indicator will go on in as little as 2 to 3 minutes when the cTnT concentration is high. Regarding QC, each new lot of devices should be tested with positive and negative cTnT controls, even though a control is included in each device to ensure proper technical performance. Imprecision at the decision cutoff concentration was less than 8.0%

Spectral Cardiac Status Rapid Tests

The Cardiac STATus Rapid Test assays provide qualitative test results for myoglobin, CK-MB, and cTnI. Assays employ solid-phase chromatographic immunoassay technology to detect, as in the case of cTnI, the presence of cTnI above an established cutoff in human blood, serum, and plasma samples. After a specimen is dispensed into a sample well, plasma or serum is transferred into a region containing monoclonal, anti-cTnI, antibody-dye conjugates and biotinylated, rabbit, polyclonal, anti-cTnI antibodies. These antibodies have cTnI in the sample to form complexes that migrate through the reaction strip. The antigen/antibody dye complexes are then captured by immobilized streptavidin in the TnI area. Additional protein dye conjugates not found in the TnI test area are later captured in the control (CON) area. Visible purplish horizontal bands will appear in the TnI and CON areas if the cTnI concentration is above the established cutoff. A visible purple band in the CON area indicates that the assay performed properly. If a band is only present in the CON area, the result is read as negative. If no band is present in the CON area, the test should be repeated regardless of the TnI band result. Results should be read at 15 minutes, since longer times could result in an inappropriate interpretation. Positive test results from high cTnI specimens may appear within 5 minutes. External QC testing is recommended at regular intervals, especially with each new lot of STATus test kits. The Cardiac STATus Troponin I has been calibrated against the Dade Behring Stratus cTnI assay, and the equivalent of a Stratus 1.5 µg/L concentration registers as a positive STATus result. Similar devices are available for myoglobin and CK-MB mass.

Point-of-Care Testing Assay Evaluation

The analytical and clinical evaluation of POCT assays and devices should be carried out by applying similar processes that have been used to evaluate instrumentation evaluated for the central laboratory. Precision and accuracy should be held to the same standards as central laboratory technology. Further, clinical sensitivity and specificity determinations should be assessed using appropriate patient populations needed to establish decision cutoffs for ruling in and ruling out AMI (using ROC curves over time following presentation to the hospital), as well as for establishing risk-stratification decision cutoffs in ACS patients. However, the new ESC/ACC/AHA guidelines support the use of the 99th percentile of a reference population as the desired upper cutpoint for detection of AMI. Both the laboratory and cardiology communities support this new cutpoint, emphasizing that the imprecision at this cutpoint be less than 10%. At present, few manufacturers' assays approach this imprecision goal. As an example, Fig. 11.6 demonstrates the type of data analysis that manufacturers should present regarding imprecision calculations at 20% CV, 10% CV, and where these imprecision values relate to the assay's 99th percentile cutpoint. Cur-

rent protocols used for submission to the FDA for 510K approval do not appear to satisfy these needs. Both the laboratory and clinical communities are lobbying the FDA to revise the imprecision standards required for troponin (and CK-MB mass) immunoassays prior to 510K approval.

Selection of the most appropriate POCT device for a specific hospital or clinic setting will highly depend on the numerous clinical and analytical issues addressed in this chapter; including need for rapid test TATs, cost issues, impact on clinicians' patient management, comparability of POCT results with central laboratory results, and so on. All issues essentially must be tied into the clinician's needs to evaluate AMI, risk assessments in ACS patients, reperfusion assessment, and laboratory and hospital economics. Two recent publications using POCT assays attempt to address the role of near-bedside testing using a single marker versus a multiple-marker strategy for ruling in or out AMI and risk assessment in ACS patients (Stratus CS (65); Biosite Triage (66)). Upon careful review of their methods, both reports (65,66) still fail to validate the analytical issues between central laboratory and POCT pertaining to assay imprecision at medical decision cutpoints as discussed and highlighted in this chapter.

CONCLUSIONS

- Advancements in technology and the incorporation of monoclonal antibodies into POCT and central laboratory instrumentation now allow for the detection of several biochemical markers of myocardial injury.
- The new ESC/ACC/AHA guidelines have redefined the definition of MI, and are predicated on increased cardiac troponin in the clinical setting of ischemic symptoms.
- POCT devices provide both whole-blood qualitative and quantitative results in less than 20 minutes, comparable to central laboratory systems that use serum and plasma. This alleviates lost time in specimen processing, transport, and result reporting, which in some situations may take as long as 2 to 4 hours, diminishing the value of the test in real-time decision-making.
- Rapid TATs of cardiac markers—within 30 to 60 minutes to clinicians—need to be the standard to allow for optimal patient care.
- In chest pain patients who present to the ED with an equivocal ECG for MI, markers of myocardial injury are critically important in the assessment of myocardial injury. Specifically, cTnI and cTnT, evaluated over a 12-hour period from presentation to the ED, demonstrate more than 90% clinical sensitivity and specificity for ruling in and ruling out an MI.
- Either cTnI or cTnT should replace CK-MB and total CK.
- An early marker, such as myoglobin, may not be necessary unless a rapid triage protocol (less than 6 hours) is implemented and demonstrated to improve patient management.
- Further, cardiac troponins provide information to clinicians that improves their ability to appropriately risk stratify (assist in predicting clinical outcomes) ACS patients, make therapeutic decisions, monitor reperfusion success, and differentiate skeletal muscle from heart muscle injury.

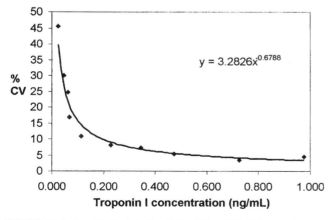

$$y = 3.2826x^{0.6788}$$

FIGURE 11.6. Sensitivity data for Ortho Vitros ECi cTnI assay for ten pools, ranging from 0.025 to 0.97 µg/L, analyzed over 28 days. The concentrations at 10% coefficient of variation (CV) and 20% CV were 0.194 µg/L and 0.070 µg/L, respectively.

Future studies are necessary to evaluate whether bedside POCT in the intensive care unit, ED, or ambulance actually provides diagnostic information in a more timely manner to the clinician that would allow for improvements in patient management and therapies. At present, no studies have adequately addressed the cost effectiveness of having POCT replace central laboratory testing, whether performed in the coronary intensive care unit or the ED.

REFERENCES

1. Wu AHB, ed. *Cardiac markers*, 1st ed. Totowa, NJ: Humana Press, 1998:300.
2. Kaski JC, Holt DW, eds. *Myocardial damage: early detection by novel biochemical markers*, 1st ed. London: Kluwer Academic Publishers, 1998:214.
3. Adams JEII, Apple FS, Jaffe A, Wu AHB, eds. *Markers in cardiology: current and future clinical applications*. AHA Monograph Series. Armonk, NY: Futura Publishing, 2001:272.
4. Apple FS, Henderson AR. Cardiac function. In: Burtis CA, Ashwood ER, eds. *Textbook of clinical chemistry*, 3rd ed. Philadelphia: WB Saunders, 1998:1178–1203.
5. Braunwald E. *Heart disease: a textbook of cardiovascular medicine*, 5th ed. Philadelphia: WB Saunders, 1997:1900.
6. Roberts R, Morris D, Pratt CM, et al. Pathophysiology, recognition, and treatment of acute myocardial infarction and its complications. In: Schlant RC, Alexander RW, eds. *The heart*. New York: McGraw-Hill, 1994:1107–1184.
7. Joint European Society of Cardiology/American College of Cardiology. Myocardial infarction redefined—a consensus document of the Joint European Society of Cardiology/American College of Cardiology Committee for the redefinition of myocardial infarction. *J Am Coll Cardiol* 2000;36:959–969.
8. Jaffe AS, Ravkilde J, Roberts R, et al. It's time for a change to troponin standard. *Circulation* 2000;102:1216–1220.
9. Braunwald E, Antman EM, Beasley JW, et al. ACC/AHA guidelines for the management of patients with unstable angina and non-ST-segment elevation myocardial infarction. *J Am Coll Cardiol* 2000;36:970–1062.
10. De Leon A, Farmer CA, King G, et al. Chest pain evaluation unit: a cost effective approach for ruling out acute myocardial infarction. *South Med J* 1989;82:1083–1089.
11. Silverman LM, Mendell JR, Sahenk Z, et al. Significance of creatine phosphokinase isoenzymes in Duchenne dystrophy. *Neurology* 1976;26:561–564.
12. Apple FS, Rogers MA, Casal D, et al. Creatine kinase MB isoenzyme adaptations in stressed human skeletal muscle obtained from marathon runners. *J Appl Physiol* 1985;59:149–53.
13. Bodor GS, Porterfield D, Voss EM, et al. Cardiac troponin I is not expressed in fetal and healthy or diseased adult human skeletal tissue. *Clin Chem* 1995;41:1710–1715.
14. Ricchiuti V, Voss EM, Ney A, et al. Cardiac troponin T isoforms expressed in renal diseased skeletal muscle will not cause false-positive results by the second generation cardiac troponin T assay by Boehringer Mannheim. *Clin Chem* 1998;44:1919–1924.
15. Wu AHB, Valdes R Jr, Apple FS, et al. Cardiac troponin T immunoassay for diagnosis of acute myocardial infarction and detection of minor myocardial injury. *Clin Chem* 1994;40:900–907.
16. Tucker JF, Collins RA, Anderson AJ, et al. Early diagnostic efficiency of cardiac troponin I and troponin T for acute myocardial infarction. *Acad Emerg Med* 1997;4:13–21.
17. Vaidya HC. Myoglobin: an early biochemical marker for the diagnosis of acute myocardial infarction. *J Clin Immunoassay* 1994;17:35–39.
18. Wu AHB, Wang XM, Gornet TG, et al. Creatine kinase MB isoforms in patients with myocardial infarction and skeletal muscle injury. *Clin Chem* 1992;38:2396–2400.
19. Lee TH, Juarex G, Cook EF, et al. Ruling out acute myocardial infarc-

tion: a prospective multicenter validation of a 12-hour strategy for patients at low risk. *N Engl J Med* 1991;324:1239–46.
20. Levitt MA, Promes SB, Bullock S, et al. Combined cardiac marker approach with adjunct two-dimensional echocardiography to diagnose acute myocardial infarction in the emergency department. *Ann Emerg Med* 1996;27:1–7.
21. Fesmire FM, Percy RF, Bardoner JB, et al. Serial creatine kinase MB testing during the emergency department evaluation of chest pain: utility of a 2-hour ΔCK MB of +1.6 ng/mL. *Am Heart J* 1998;136:237–44.
22. Kost GJ, Kirk JD, Omand K. A strategy for the use of cardiac injury markers (troponin I and T, creatine kinase MB mass and isoforms, and myoglobin) in the diagnosis of acute myocardial infarction. *Arch Pathol Lab Med* 1998;122:245–251.
23. D'Costa M, Fleming E, Patterson MC. Cardiac troponin I for the diagnosis of acute myocardial infarction in the emergency department. *Am J Clin Path* 1997;108:550–555.
24. Chang CC, Ip MPC, Hsu RM, et al. Evaluation of a proposed panel of cardiac markers for diagnosis of acute myocardial infarction in patients with atraumatic chest pain. *Arch Pathol Lab Med* 1998;122:320–324.
25. Gomez MA, Anderson JL, Karagounis LA, et al., for the ROMIO Study Group. An emergency department based protocol for rapidly ruling out myocardial ischemia reduces hospital time and expense: results of a randomized study (ROMIO). *J Am Coll Cardiol* 1996;28:25–33.
26. Pervaiz S, Anderson FP, Lohmann TP, et al. Comparative analysis of cardiac troponin I and creatine kinase MB as markers of acute myocardial infarction. *Clin Cardiol* 1997;20:269–271.
27. Gibler WB, Runyon JP, Levy RC, et al. A rapid diagnostic and treatment center for patients with chest pain in the emergency department. *Ann Emerg Med* 1995;25:1–8.
28. Hamm CW, Goldmann BU, Heeschen C, et al. Emergency room triage of patients with acute chest pain by means of rapid testing for cardiac troponin I or troponin T. *N Engl J Med* 1997;337:1648–1653.
29. Gibler WB, Gibler CD, Weinshenker E, et al. Myoglobin as an early indicator of acute myocardial infarction. *Ann Emerg Med* 1987;16:851–856.
30. Tucker JF, Collins RA, Anderson AJ, et al. Value of serial myoglobin levels in the early diagnosis of patients admitted for acute myocardial infarction. *Ann Emerg Med* 1994;24:704–708.
31. Montague C, Kircher T. Myoglobin on the early evaluation of acute chest pain. *Am J Clin Path* 1995;104:472–476.
32. Puleo PR, Meyer D, Wathen C, et al. Use of a rapid assay of subforms of creatine kinase MB to diagnose or rule out acute myocardial infarction. *N Engl J Med* 1994;331:561–566.
33. Zimmerman J, Fromm R, Meyer D, et. al. Diagnostic marker cooperative study for diagnosis of myocardial infarction. *Circulation* 1999;99:1671–1677.
34. Panteghini M, Cuccia C, Pagani F, et al. Comparison of the diagnostic performance of two rapid bedside biochemical assays on the early detection of acute myocardial infarction. *Clin Cardiol* 1998;21:394–398.
35. Sylven C, Lindahl S, Hellkvist K, et al. Excellent reliability of nurse-based bedside diagnosis of acute myocardial infarction by rapid dry-strip creatine kinase MB, myoglobin, and troponin T. *Am Heart J* 1998;135:677–683.
36. REACTT Investigators Study Group. Evaluation of a bedside whole blood rapid troponin T assay in the emergency department. *Acad Emerg Med* 1997;4:1083–1089.
37. Gerhardt W, Ljungdahl L, Collinson PO, et al. An improved rapid troponin T test with a decreased detection limit: a multicenter study of the analytical and clinical performance in suspected myocardial damage. *Scan J Clin Lab Invest* 1997;57:549–558.
38. Apple FS, Christenson RH, Valdes R, et al. Simultaneous rapid measurement of whole blood myoglobin, CK MB, and cardiac troponin I by the Triage Cardiac Panel for detection of myocardial infarction. *Clin Chem* 1999;45:199–205.
39. Apple FS, Anderson FP, Collinson P, et al. Clinical evaluation of the First Medical whole blood, point-of-care testing device for detection of myocardial infarction. *Clin Chem* 2000;46:1604–1609.

40. Heeschen C, Goldmann BV, Langenbrink L, et al. Evaluation of a rapid whole blood ELISA for quantification of troponin I in patients with acute chest pain. *Clin Chem* 1999;45:1789–1796.
41. Heeschen C, Deu A, Langenbrink L, et al. Analytical and diagnostic performance of troponin assays in patients suspicious of acute coronary syndromes. *Clin Biochem* 2000;33:359–368.
42. Muller-Bardoff M, Rauscher T, Kampmann M, et al. Quantitative bedside assay for cardiac troponin T: a complimentary method to centralized laboratory testing. *Clin Chem* 1999;45:1002–1008.
43. Selker HP, Zalenski RJ, Antman EM, et al. An evaluation of technologies for identifying acute cardiac ischemia in the emergency department: a report from a national heart attack alert program working group. *Ann Emerg Med* 1997;29:13–87.
44. Jaffe AS, Landt Y, Parvin CA, et al. Comparative sensitivity of cardiac troponin I and lactate dehydrogenase isoenzymes from diagnosis of acute myocardial infarction. *Clin Chem* 1996;42:1770–1776.
45. Green GB, Li DJ, Bessman ES, et al. Use of troponin T and creatine kinase MB subunit levels for risk stratification of emergency department patients with possible myocardial ischemia. *Ann Emerg Med* 1998;31:19–29.
46. Sayre MR, Kaufmann KH, Chen IW, et al. Measurement of cardiac troponin T is an effective method for predicting complications among emergency department patients with chest pain. *Ann Emerg Med* 1998;31:539–549.
47. Polanczyk CA, Lee TH, Cook EF, et al. Cardiac troponin I as a predictor of major cardiac events in emergency department patients with acute chest pain. *J Am Coll Cardiol* 1998;32:8–14.
48. Newby LK, Christenson RH, Ohman EM, et al. Value of serial troponin T measures for early and late risk stratification in patients with acute coronary syndromes. *Circulation* 1998;98:1853–1859.
49. Antman EM, Sacks DB, Rifai N, et al. Time to positivity of a rapid bedside assay for cardiac specific troponin T predicts prognosis in acute coronary syndromes: a thrombolysis in myocardial infarction IIAQ substudy. *J Am Coll Cardiol* 1998;31:326–330.
50. Galvani M, Ottani F, Ferrini D, et al. Prognostic influence of elevated values of cardiac troponin I in patients with unstable angina. *Circulation* 1997;95:2053–2059.
51. Wu AHB. Use of cardiac markers as assessed by outcomes analysis. *Clin Biochem* 1997;30:339–350.
52. Christenson RH, Duh SH, Newby LK, et al. Cardiac troponin T and cardiac troponin I: relative values in short term risk stratification of patients with acute coronary syndromes. *Clin Chem* 1998;44:494–501.
53. Olatidoye AG, Wu AHB, Feng YJ, et al. Prognostic role of troponin T versus troponin I in unstable angina pectoris for cardiac events with

meta-analysis comparing published studies. *Am J Cardiol* 1998;81:1405–1410.
54. Hamm CW, Ravkilde J, Gerhardt W, et al. The prognostic value of serum troponin T in unstable angina. *N Engl J Med* 1992;327:146–150.
55. Ottani F, Galvani M, Nicolini A, et al. Elevated cardiac troponin levels predict the risk of adverse outcome in patients with acute coronary syndromes. *Am Heart J* 2000;140:917–927.
56. Apple FS, Sharkey SW, Henry TD. Early serum cardiac troponin I and T concentrations after successful thrombolysis for acute myocardial infarction. *Clin Chem* 1995;1197–1198.
57. Christenson RH, Ohman EM, Topol EJ, et al. Assessment of coronary reperfusion after thrombolysis with a model combining myoglobin, creatine kinase MB and clinical variables. *Circulation* 1997;96:1776–1782.
58. Tanasijevic MJ, Cannon CP, Wybenga DR, et al. Myoglobin, creatine kinase MB, and cardiac troponin I to assess reperfusion after thrombolysis for acute myocardial infarction: results from TIMI 10A. *Am Heart J* 1997;134:622–630.
59. Laperche T, Steg PG, Dehoux M, et al. A study of biochemical markers of reperfusion early after thrombolysis for acute myocardial infarction. *Circulation* 1995;92:2079–2086.
60. The PURSUIT Trial Investigators. Inhibition of platelet glycoprotein IIb/IIIa with eptifibatide in patients with acute coronary syndromes. *N Engl J Med* 1998;339:436–443.
61. Christenson RH, Vaidya H, Landt Y, et al. Standardization of creatine kinase MB mass assays: the use of recombinant CK MB as reference material. *Clin Chem* 1999;45:1414–1423.
62. Christenson RH, Duh SH, Apple FS, et al. Standardization of cardiac troponin I assays: round robin of ten candidate reference materials. *Clin Chem* 2001;47:431–437.
63. Apple FS. Clinical and analytical standardization issues confronting cardiac troponin I. *Clin Chem* 1999;45:18–20.
64. Wu AHB, Feng YJ, Moore R, et al. Characterization of cardiac troponin subunit release into serum after acute myocardial infarction and comparison of assays for troponin T and I. *Clin Chem* 1998;44:1198–1208.
65. Newby LK, Storrow AB, Gibler WB, et al. Beside multimarker testing for risk stratification in chest pain units: the chest pain evaluation by creatine kinase-MB, myoglobin, and troponin I (CHECKMATE) study. *Circulation* 2001;103:1832–1837.
66. Ng SM, Krishnaswamy, Morrisey R, et al. Mitigation of the clinical significance of spurious elevations of cardiac troponin I in settings of coronary ischemia using serial testing of multiple cardiac markers. *Am J Cardiol* 2001;87:994–999.

12

BEDSIDE TESTING, GLUCOSE MONITORING, AND DIABETES MANAGEMENT

JAMES H. NICHOLS

BEDSIDE TESTING

Definition

Bedside testing encompasses a variety of patient-care scenarios. In the strictest definition of the term, the test is conducted at the patient's bedside in a hospital environment. The instrument and supplies or reagents are carried into the patient's room. Results from bedside testing are, thus, available faster than testing in a distant laboratory and have the potential to offer more rapid clinical treatment and intervention. In a physician's office or home-care setting, bedside testing can refer to instrumentation that is carried into the examination room or to the patient's side. Yet, bedside testing in a more general sense can also include testing conducted on the patient's nightstand, in the patient's bathroom, or on a portable cart moved into the patient's room. Even testing conducted in a spare room or utility closet down the hall from the patient is considered by some practitioners to be within the realm of bedside testing.

The various ways in which bedside testing is conducted can lead to technical differences in test results due to preanalytical, analytical, and postanalytical effects. Use of devices originally manufactured for home testing, for instance, can yield inaccurate results when utilized in a healthcare setting on acute or critically ill patients (1). Variations in clinical practice and the utilization of bedside tests can further generate differences in patient outcome and cost effectiveness. Even practice differences among sites within a single healthcare organization can create differences over a ten-fold range in cost (2). Optimization of testing at the bedside therefore requires expertise from multiple disciplines as well as a complete understanding of the patient-care environment and the manner in which the testing is performed.

Alternatives to Bedside Testing

Bedside testing is conducted to provide faster turnaround time (TAT) of results. By bringing the testing device closer to the patient, results are assumed to provide faster treatment of the patient (3). However, the TAT has multiple components (Fig. 12.1) (4,5). Although laboratorians often acknowledge TAT as

the intralaboratory time over which they have most control, clinicians consider laboratory TAT as the time from placing the test order to when the result is picked up by the clinician (the therapeutic TAT).

Delays in any step can prolong the entire process. For bedside testing, TAT is reduced by eliminating the transportation (transporting the sample to a distant laboratory) and processing (if whole-blood analysis) steps. Delays in collecting the specimen or acknowledgment of the result and institution of therapy can still prolong therapeutic TAT. Optimal TAT thus requires efficiency at each step in the testing process.

Alternatives to bedside testing focus on optimizing therapeutic TAT by either reducing the transportation delays or by bringing the laboratory closer to the patient (6). Messengers or transportation personnel dedicated to carry samples from the patient-care units to the laboratory have been the traditional method of getting samples to the laboratory. By scheduling defined pickup times or even on-demand service with radio pagers for stat samples, transport personnel are a low-technology means of solving transportation issues. This system is efficient in moving samples, but can create processing jams within the laboratory when large batches of stat samples arrive at the same time.

Newer pneumatic tubes offer the transportation of specimens across distances of several blocks in under a few minutes. A network of point-to-point tubes from patient-care units to the central laboratory promises to reduce delays in transportation. Brigham and Women's Hospital, Boston, was able to deliver stat test results from the central laboratory in 9.5 minutes by using pneumatic transport tubes in conjunction with whole-blood analysis as compared to 8.5 minutes at the bedside. This minimal difference in TAT did not justify the expense of bedside testing at nearly double the per-test cost of central laboratory testing at this location (7).

The University of Southern California Medical Center, Los Angeles, also evaluated their ability to deliver stat services to the emergency department by monitoring the components of TAT delays (8). By improving their laboratory information system and upgrading their pneumatic tube system, the central laboratory was able to save 3 minutes in the steps under the control of

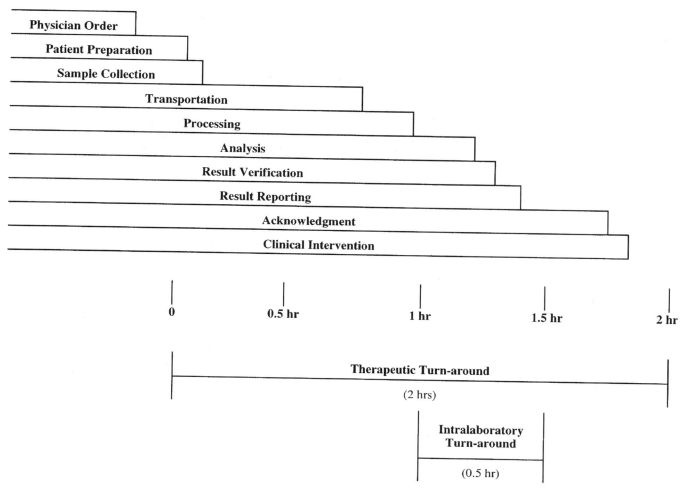

FIGURE 12.1. Turnaround times for a hypothetical laboratory test. Note that the difference between the therapeutic and intralaboratory time involves preanalytical and postanalytical delays outside the laboratory. In this example, by eliminating the transport and processing steps (whole-blood analysis), point-of-care testing would still have over a 1-hour therapeutic turnaround time unless delays in other steps are addressed (as in physician acknowledgment or patient preparation time).

the laboratory, primarily in transport of specimens to the central laboratory. The major delay of 41 to 45 minutes, however, was determined to be physician acknowledgment of the test result. This exemplifies the need to address the entire testing process when seeking faster laboratory results.

Other alternatives to bedside testing involve moving the analysis closer to the patient. While this may include opening a formal satellite laboratory adjacent to critical patient-care units, other options include on-demand or scheduled testing by a phlebotomy team, use of roving technologists, mobile carts, or even robotically controlled systems (9). Home healthcare and physicians office networks often utilize automobiles, shuttles, and sometimes taxis (for stat samples) in order to transport samples collected at ancillary sites to a central laboratory. The choice between testing alternatives—a central lab with transport services versus a rapid-response lab closer to the clinic or bedside testing—is determined by the particular factors acting at each patient-care site (10). Consideration of the technical, operational, and cost factors will assist in the optimization of testing

(11,12). While bedside testing can offer some efficiency, it cannot guarantee improved outcomes without analysis of the entire system and ongoing monitoring that actual TATs meet expectations.

BEDSIDE GLUCOSE TESTING

Since its inception over 20 years ago, capillary blood glucose testing has now become the standard of care for monitoring hyperglycemia and for controlling the long-term complications of diabetes. Although modern glucometers are smaller, simpler, and have enhanced data management, these devices are a source of continued concern over test result quality. The U.S. Food and Drug Administration has received more complaints about glucose monitoring devices than for any other medical device. By the end of 1992, there were over 3,200 incidents, including 16 reports of death, filed with the agency (13,14). With its prevalence as one of the most frequently performed bedside tests, blood glucose is an excellent place to begin an understanding of the technical and operational issues involved in bedside testing.

Continuity of Test Results

Bedside glucose testing is widely utilized in health care. For a clinician to be able to treat a patient, there must be a defined correlation or continuity between test results from different sites and analytical methods (1). A diabetic patient may enter the healthcare system through an emergency room, be transferred to an operating room, a postoperative recovery room, an intensive care unit (ICU), and finally end up in a general medical unit. After discharge, care may be delivered at home with visiting nurses or the patient may go to an outpatient clinic, or even begin self-monitoring of blood glucose. Bedside glucose results at these different locations could be conducted on different instruments by multiple operators. Glucose meter results could also be interspersed with results from the central laboratory and possibly other satellite laboratories (1). In order to effectively treat patients, results from each glucose meter must correlate with results from all laboratories within a health system; otherwise, separate reference ranges will need to be published in order to assist in result interpretation. If a known bias exists between the glucose meter and a central or satellite laboratory, then clinicians must offset their treatment based on the degree of analytical bias. Results must also be recorded in the patient's medical record in a manner that will allow the clinician to determine from which method (central, satellite, or bedside testing) the result was generated. Ensuring continuity of test results forms the basis of laboratory quality assurance (QA).

Use of bedside devices in a healthcare environment places additional burden on the technical performance of these devices (15–19). Unfortunately, the same technologies are often utilized in both home self-monitoring and hospital care (15) (Table 12.1). In the home environment, glucose meters are utilized by patients to monitor their own glucose levels and alter insulin therapy or diet based on the results. Most diabetics who self-monitor their blood glucose are generally healthy except for the complications of their diabetes. They are ambulant and active, have normal hematocrits, and utilize capillary blood to monitor their own levels (1). Hospitalized patients present with acute and chronic illnesses and tend to stay in bed. Nurses and clinicians perform the testing as opposed to patient self-testing. In a hospital environment, multiple glucose meters are used on different patients by a variety of staff. Samples other than capillary fingersticks (venous and arterial blood) are possible, and even preferred in the critical care units due to the presence of indwelling lines (1). Thus, home self-monitoring and hospital use are different. The patient populations are unique and have discrete characteristics.

Technical Considerations

Technical performance is a consideration given the variety of glucose meters that are available on the market and the diverse

TABLE 12.1. COMPARISON OF POINT-OF-CARE TESTING ENVIRONMENTS

Home Self-Monitoring	Bedside Hospital Testing
Single operator	Multiple operators
Single device	Multiple devices
Serial monitoring on one device interspersed with central lab results	Single points on multiple devices
Ambulant patient	Patients confined to bed
Patient generally healthy	Acute and chronic illnesses
Capillary samples only	Noncapillary samples possible

Reproduced from Nichols JH. Management of near-patient glucose testing. *Endocrinology and Metabolism In-Service Training and Continuing Education.* 1994;12(12):325–334, with permission from American Association for Clinical Chemistry Press.

patient populations and healthcare demands on these devices. Not every glucose meter will fit with every patient population. Analytical goals need to be defined and performance examined prior to implementing a device in a particular patient setting (19,20).

Common bedside glucose meters rely on enzyme-coupled reactions for the detection of glucose (Fig. 12.2). Although infrared devices are available, they are still largely experimental. The primary reaction is a quantitative, enzymatic consumption of β-D-glucose. The initial consumption of glucose can be detected and quantitated via the transfer of electrons to coupled reaction intermediates by spectrophotometry, reflectance spectrophotometry, or amperometry.

Glucose oxidase is a common enzymatic method on the bedside market, although newer meters utilize glucose dehydrogenase as well as hexokinase. Abbott/Medisense (Bedford, MA) Precision G (21) and PCX, Bayer (Tarrytown, NY) Glucometer Elite (22,23), and LifeScan (Milpitas, CA) OneTouch II (20–22,24,25) and SureStep meters (21) utilize glucose oxidase as their primary reaction. Blood gas analyzers also utilize glucose oxidase to sense glucose concentrations, such as the AVL (Roswell, GA), Chiron (Medfield, MA), Instrumentation Laboratory (Orangeburg, NY), Nova (Waltham, MA), and Radiometer (Westlake, OH) instruments that are frequently found in satellite, rapid response laboratories, or on portable carts at the bedside.

Glucose enzymes consume 1 mole of glucose to produce 1 mole of electrons. These electrons reduce molecular oxygen to hydrogen peroxide (LifeScan meters) or can be transferred to a coenzyme, FAD (Abbott/MediSense Precision G). Hydrogen peroxide can be further reduced to water using electrons donated from a chromogenic substrate in a reaction catalyzed by peroxidase (LifeScan). Oxidation of the chromogen produces a colored product with an intensity that is proportional to the amount of glucose in the specimen. This color can be measured visually (Roche/Boehringer-Mannheim Chemstrip BG test strips, Indianapolis, IN) or through reflectance spectrophotometry using a portable meter (LifeScan). Alternatively, an iron-containing intermediate or coenzyme can utilize a detecting electrode and constant voltage to quantify the current and

Glucose oxidase

<u>Reflectance spectrophotometry</u> (LifeScan One Touch II)

$$\text{Glucose} + O_2 \xrightarrow{\text{glucose oxidase}} \text{gluconic acid} + H_2O_2$$

$$H_2O_2 + \text{reduced chromogen} \xrightarrow{\text{peroxidase}} H_2O + \text{oxidized chromogen}$$
(colorless)   (colorless)

<u>Electrochemical</u> (Abbott, Medisense Precision G)

$$\text{Glucose} + FAD \xrightarrow{\text{glucose oxidase}} \text{gluconic acid} + FADH$$

$$FADH + 2\ MED_{ox} \xrightarrow[\searrow 2e^-]{\text{voltage}} FAD + 2\ MED_{red}$$

Hexokinase

<u>Reflectance Spectrophotometry</u> (Bayer Glucometer, Encore)

$$\text{Glucose} + ATP \xrightarrow{\text{hexokinase}} \text{glucose-6-phosphate} + ADP$$

$$\text{Glucose-6-Phosphate} + NAD \xrightarrow{\text{glucose-6-phosphate dehydrogenase}} \text{6-phosphogluconate} + NADH$$

$$NADH + \text{chromogen} \longrightarrow NAD + \text{chromogen}$$
(colorless)   (colored)

Glucose Dehydrogenase
<u>Spectrophotometric</u> (HemoCue Glucose)

$$\alpha\text{-D-glucose} \xleftrightarrow{\text{mutarotase}} \beta\text{-D-glucose}$$

$$\beta\text{-D=Glucose} + NAD \xrightarrow{\text{glucose dehydrogenase}} \text{D-gluconolactone NADH}$$

$$NADH + MTT \xrightarrow{\text{diaphorase}} NAD + MTTH$$
(colorless)   (colored)

<u>Electrochemical</u> (Roche Advantage)

$$\text{Glucose} + \text{HCF III} \xrightarrow{\text{glucose dehydrogenase}} \text{gluconolactone} + \text{HCF II}$$

$$\text{HCF II} \xrightarrow[\searrow e^-]{\text{voltage}} \text{HCF III}$$

FIGURE 12.2. Bedside glucose meter methodologies. Chemical reactions used by point-of-care glucose meters. (O_2, molecular oxygen; H_2O_2, hydrogen peroxide; H_2O, water; FAD and FADH, oxidized and reduced flavin adenine dinucleotide; MED_{ox} and MED_{red}, oxidized and reduced electrochemical mediator; ATP, adenosine triphospate; ADP, adenosine diphospate; NAD and NADH, oxidized and reduced nicotine adenine dinucleotide; MTT and MTTH, oxidized and reduced 3-(4,5-dimethylthiazol-2-yl)-2,5-diephenyl-2H-tetrazolium bromide; HCF II and HCF III, oxidized and reduced hexacyanoferrate.)

reducing equivalents of glucose (Abbott/Medisense Precision G, Bayer Glucometer Elite). Blood gas analyzers utilize a Clark oxygen-sensing electrode to determine the consumption of molecular oxygen, indirectly measuring glucose, as equimolar amounts of glucose and oxygen are consumed in the initial reaction with glucose oxidase.

Hexokinase is also utilized by some glucose meters (Miles Glucometer (24,26,27) and Encore (20) meters). Hexokinase phosphorylates glucose, which is then oxidized by glucose-6-phosphate dehydrogenase coupled with the reduction of nicotine adenine dinucleotide (NAD). The reduction of NAD to NADH can be followed photometrically at 340 nm on a chemistry analyzer like those found in many hospital laboratories, or NAD can be regenerated from NADH by reduction of a chromogenic compound, producing a color that is proportional to glucose in the specimen. The intensity of color can be quantitated by reflectance spectrophotometry.

Glucose dehydrogenase is a third enzyme used by bedside glucose meters. It is found on the Accuchek Advantage (21,23,26) (Roche/Boehringer-Mannheim, Indianapolis, IN) and HemoCue (20,22,28–30) (HemoCue A-B, Anelholm, Sweden; HemoCue, Mission Viejo, CA) glucose meters. Glucose is oxidized by reduction of NAD with glucose dehydrogenase and NAD is regenerated through reduction of a chromogenic compound. HemoCue is unique in the use of a fixed-volume, 5 μL cuvette, and the use of spectrophotometric optics (as opposed to reflectance spectrophotometry) in its device. HemoCue also adds a mutarotase to shift the anomeric equilibrium in order to enhance the detection of both α-D-glucose and β-D-glucose. Glucose dehydrogenase can also be linked to a detecting electrode to measure glucose electrochemically (Roche/Boehringer Mannheim Advantage).

With the variety of glucose methods available, an evaluation of technical performance should be conducted on the patient population for which the device is intended by the operators who will utilize the device in routine operation (20,21). In this manner, the evaluation can mimic actual use as closely as possible. Technical criteria that should be evaluated include (19):

■ Accuracy
■ Recovery
■ Linearity
■ Precision
■ Interferences (unique to the healthcare setting and patient population)

Result agreement is a major concern in a healthcare system with multiple glucose meters and glucose methodologies. Evaluation of accuracy can estimate the method agreement within an institution. Accuracy can be determined by comparison of the bedside glucose meter with a "gold standard" for glucose or more frequently by reference to a particular analytical methodology. As there is no single "reference" method for glucose, manufacturers utilize different reference methods that can lead to differences in results among glucose meters. In a clinical environment, it is more appropriate to reference glucose meters against the main clinical laboratory methodology within the institution in order to ensure agreement of glucose results across the healthcare system, independent of analyzing

method. This is problematic, since most laboratory methods analyze serum or plasma while glucose meters are designed to analyze whole blood. Accuracy is thus difficult to assess on glucose meters, as a whole blood matrix is unstable and most glucose meters are unable to analyze aqueous solutions or serum without erythrocytes. Stabilized whole-blood standards further show matrix effects and generate different results among glucose meters. Correlation of meter results to a laboratory method using patient specimens is technically easier and more meaningful, because it indicates method agreement using actual patient populations.

Accuracy evaluation must further consider the calibration of glucose meters. In order to produce a rapid result, portable glucose meters accept a whole-blood, unprocessed specimen, but the results may be reported as whole blood or converted to plasma/serum equivalents (1). Glucose can be assumed to diffuse freely in the water space of whole blood. Because erythrocytes contain less water per unit volume than plasma or serum, whole-blood results are less than plasma or serum at any glucose concentration. The exact difference will depend on the mass of erythrocytes (or hematocrit) and can be estimated at 11% for patients with a 45% hematocrit (1,31) (Table 12.2).

Although whole blood is applied to glucose test strips, the enzymatic reactions that occur are not equally exposed to the entire sample. Test-strip methods utilize multiple layers of absorbent material to filter out erythrocytes and other blood interferences, allowing the plasma or serum water to diffuse through to the enzyme reagents on the back of the strip (Fig. 12.3). The separation that occurs in the multiple layers of test strips makes this technology more susceptible to viscosity effects. Pure plasma or serum and high hematocrits (as in neonatal samples) present extremes of fluidity and viscosity that can lead to result bias. Differences in the manufacturing process and fragility in the patient's erythrocytes can further lead to varying amounts of erythrocyte lysis during analysis. The viscosity effects and variable cell lysis prohibit the transfer of test strips

TABLE 12.2. ESTIMATION OF DIFFERENCES BETWEEN WHOLE BLOOD AND PLASMA/SERUM

Assume the water content is:
  Plasma = 93%
  Erythrocytes (RBC) = 73%
Whole blood water content is:
  = [RBC contribution] + [Plasma contribution]
  = [hematocrit × RBC water (%)] + [(1-hematocrit) × plasma water (%)]
  = (0.45)(73) + (0.55)(93)
  = 84 mL of water per 100 mL of whole blood
Because glucose is equally distributed in blood water:
(Plasma water content) / (whole blood water content)
  = 93 / 84
  = 1.107
Plasma glucose is ~11% higher than whole blood glucose in a sample at 45% hematocrit.

Reproduced from Nichols JH. Management of near-patient glucose testing. *Endocrinology and Metabolism In-Service Training and Continuing Education.* 1994;12(12):325–34, with permission from the American Association for Chemistry Press.

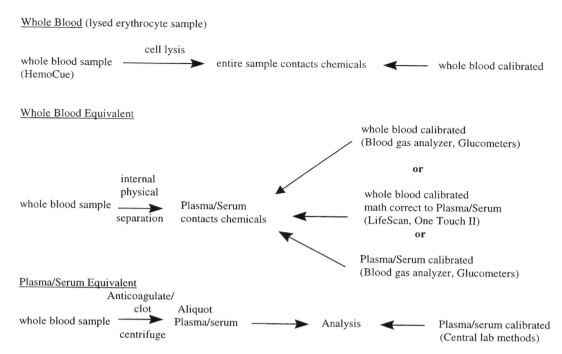

FIGURE 12.3. Analytical effect of device calibration. HemoCue offers a whole-blood lysate analysis, since the entire lysed sample senses the chemical reaction and the device is whole-blood calibrated. Other glucose meters and blood gas analyzers, while accepting a whole-blood sample, report a variety of values depending on calibration and/or postanalytical mathematical corrections (whole-blood equivalent). Central laboratory methods generally report plasma/serum equivalent values.

among manufacturers and lock consumers into a meter-test strip-control set.

Other devices, such as the HemoCue, utilize saponin in their cuvettes that result in total cell lysis prior to analysis. HemoCue thus reports a whole-blood value that is independent of sample hematocrit, since the entire lysate participates in the analytical reaction. Blood gas analyzers, on the other hand, accept whole-blood samples but do not lyse erythrocytes, since they also report electrolytes such as sodium and potassium. The glucose electrodes on these analyzers are exposed to only the plasma or serum portion of blood. The concentration of glucose is determined from the plasma or serum portion rather than the entire whole-blood specimen.

Despite differences in the technology, glucose meter calibrations further complicate the prediction of laboratory correlation (Fig. 12.3). Although glucose meters can accept a whole-blood specimen, a device can be calibrated to report either a whole-blood result (Roche/Boehringer Mannheim, HemoCue, and LifeScan meters) or the plasma or serum "equivalent" of whole blood (Bayer Encore, LifeScan SureStep (32), and Roche/Boehringer-Mannheim Accuchek Advantage (33)). Alternatively, a glucose meter can take the result and through a fixed internal offset, mathematically correct the whole-blood result to a plasma or serum "corrected" result (LifeScan One Touch II meter). These three methods of calibration—whole blood, plasma/serum equivalent, or plasma/serum corrected—can lead to different results on the same specimen, complicating the cor-

relation and interpretation of results when multiple meters are used in an institution.

These different methods of calibration are particularly sensitive to the hematocrit of the specimen and cause significant bias in samples with extremes of hematocrit. Since the glucose meter market is primarily driven by home–self-testing sales, glucose meters are generally calibrated using "normal" hematocrits in the range of 40% to 45%. However, most acutely ill oncology and postsurgical patients have much lower hematocrits (average of 30% to 35%), while neonates have higher than "normal" hematocrits (up to 70%). Significant errors can be introduced into results by assuming normal hematocrits in meter calibration (20,21,34) or during the meter conversion from whole blood to plasma/serum-corrected results. Evaluation of glucose meters on the patient population for which the device is intended is critical to determining whether the meter will fit into the patient-care setting.

Tolerance limits on acceptable glucose meter performance should be set prior to evaluating technical performance. The Association of Clinical Biochemistry (35) and the American Diabetes Association Consensus Conference (36–38) have made similar proposals for whole-blood, glucose self-monitoring. Accuracy should be within 15% of the reference method, and precision should have a coefficient of variation (CV) of less than 5% (Fig. 12.4). The main laboratory method is the recommended reference for determining meter accuracy in the clinical setting, as some of the "manufacturer's" reference methods are

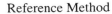
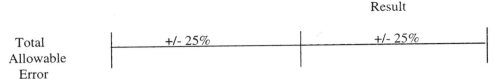
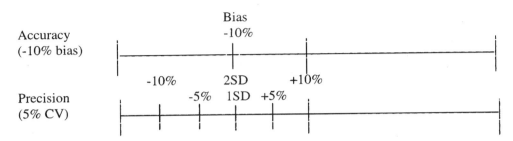
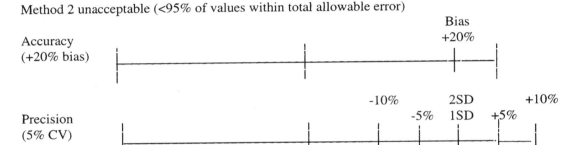

FIGURE 12.4. Analytical goals. In this example, the total allowable clinical bias is ±25%. Method 1 is acceptable, since the sum of bias and imprecision still allows for more than 95% of the values to fall within allowable error. Method 2 is unacceptable and extends outside the allowable error limits.

not commonly available (gas chromatography/mass spectrometry/mass spectrometry, which is expensive and labor intensive, or the Yellow Springs Instrument (Yellow Springs, OH) analyzer, for instance, which is rarely used clinically anymore). For a control range of two standard deviations, these limits would allow a total variance of 25% (15% accuracy error and 2 × 5 = 10% precision error). A total variability of 25% is similar to the maximum acceptable tolerance (22% total error or CV of less than 11%) for glucose determined by a survey of practicing physicians (39). Self-monitoring analytical goals with CVs of less than 7% are tighter than the current recommendations (40). Future goals for glucose meter tolerance have been proposed with accuracy to within 5% of the laboratory (36–38), which matches the clinical goal for CVs of less than 2.2% proposed earlier (41). Most glucose meters, however, are still not able to achieve these levels, particularly in the hypoglycemic range. Setting goals to this stringency would lead to a rejection of many devices currently being marketed (20–22, 42,43). With this realization in mind, the National Committee for Clinical Laboratory Standards (NCCLS) has recommended accuracy goals of ±15 mg/dL at glucose levels below 100 mg/dL and ±20% for levels above 100 mg/dL (19). This recommenda-

tion, however, results in a discontinuity in error tolerance in the middle of the preprandial range of glucose levels, and others have recommended ±15 mg/dL at glucose levels under 100 mg/dL and ±15% for levels over 100 mg/dL for more consistency throughout the range (44,37–39).

Once tolerance goals have been set, evaluation of accuracy can be conducted through comparison of clinical samples with other laboratory methods within a healthcare system. Whole-blood correlations, however, present problems with glucose stability, anticoagulation, and specimen type (45,46). Glucose meters and blood gas analyzers accept whole blood, whereas most laboratory methods prefer plasma or serum. Whole-blood results are immediately available at the bedside, while laboratory samples must be transported to another location for analysis. Glucose is continuously consumed by the cellular portions of blood during the time required for transportation and processing. Glycolysis can change the true glucose by an average of 5% to 7% an hour (47,48). Plasma is thus a better specimen than serum, because it can be immediately separated from cells without waiting for the sample to clot. Once separated from cells, plasma glucose is stable for several hours, provided there is no bacterial growth. However, plasma requires specimen additives or anticoagulants (heparin, citrate, and EDTA) that can affect the enzyme activity of glucometer technologies. Glycolysis inhibitors (fluoride, iodoacetate, and oxalate) can also affect glucometer reactions and bias test results. In addition, glycolysis inhibitors, being charged molecules, do not freely diffuse across cellular membranes and the total inhibition may take several hours to reach maximum effect. Glycolysis can continue during the time required to achieve inhibition leading to differences in glucose concentrations among split samples.

The choice of specimen type further complicates laboratory comparisons (20,49–51). Although optimal correlation is determined by splitting the same sample, capillary fingersticks often do not provide enough sample for both bedside and central laboratory testing. In addition, reagent strips using glucose oxidase are adversely affected by low oxygen tension, causing venous samples to be unacceptable on some glucometers (52,53). Compromises can be made by comparison of capillary blood analyzed by a bedside glucometer with a simultaneously collected venous or arterial specimen for central laboratory analysis (in an appropriate anticoagulant and glycolysis inhibitor) (50). This practice provides the ideal specimen for both analyses, but does not consider the physiologic differences between arterial, capillary, and venous blood. In the fasting state, normal arterial-venous concentration gradients are comparable, differing by only 7 to 10 mg/dL. Yet, postprandial differences due to the effects of insulin and cellular metabolism can increase this concentration gradient to more than 70 mg/dL (51,54). Method correlations must, therefore, consider the following in the experimental design:

- Type of specimen
- Transportation time
- Presence of glycolysis inhibitors
- Anticoagulants
- Metabolic state of the patient (fasting, postprandial, etc.)
- Analytical methodology and calibration (whole blood versus plasma)

Recovery, in contrast to accuracy, is evaluated by spiking known amounts of glucose into aliquots of a single blood specimen. Recovery is thus an indication of the effect of sample matrix on the method. Matrix effects contribute to the wide divergence among diverse glucose meters on interlaboratory proficiency surveys (55,56). Differences as much as two- to three-fold are noted among some manufacturers on the same proficiency sample.

Precision is a measure of the reproducibility of meter results. Precision, split into within-day and between-day (total) components, can be estimated by repeated measurement of a single sample in the same day or over several days. Precision is generally performed on artificial controls or stabilized whole-blood specimens, because these samples are stable over longer periods of time. However, control specimens do not always reflect actual patient performance. In some cases, control performance may be less or greater than with actual patient samples (20,45). Furthermore, patient whole-blood specimens are not stable over extended periods due to glycolysis and additionally, some meters (Abbott/MediSense Precision G) are adversely affected

by the age of the specimens or the presence of microclots on test strips.

Accuracy, recovery, and precision can all affect method linearity. Linearity samples can be prepared by splitting a patient sample into two aliquots, spiking one with glucose standards to elevate the glucose concentration and mixing the high and low samples in the appropriate proportions to achieve a set of increasing glucose specimens. This method, however, can introduce bias in some glucometer methods due to differences in oxygen, hematocrit, and age of the sample (21). Stabilizing glycolysis through the use of glycolysis inhibitors can also introduce method biases as mentioned earlier. For these reasons, some manufacturers now produce artificial linearity solutions for verifying the calibration of their devices. Due to the aqueous nature of these solutions, these linearity samples are not entirely interchangeable among glucose methods and matrix effects are evident on some methods. Verification of linearity is critical to determining the reportable range of glucose results, as some methods (blood gas analyzer electrodes) can drift over time, significantly affecting linearity at the high and low ends of the reportable range. In addition, meters are programmed to report results within a defined range, but they are not necessarily linear within the full extent of this range. Tolerance goals should be set so as to ensure that an acceptable percentage of point-of-care (POC) values fall within tolerance limits throughout the reportable range. Some meters are acceptable only within the range where most patients are encountered (75 to 400 mg/dL) (57), and problems can be seen at the high and low limits of the reportable range (22,58). Initial evaluation of ranges and routine verification of these limits allows confidence in the results in those areas of the reportable range.

Besides the technical criteria of accuracy, recovery, precision, and linearity, factors unique to the healthcare setting can also alter meter results (Table 12.3). Light, temperature (59,60), exposure to air (test strip vials left open), altitude (61,62), and humidity (59,62) can affect method stability due to the delicate nature of enzyme reagents. Heat from a radiator or freezing during shipment can damage test strips. Strips and meters exposed to the heat of summer or cold of winter in the trunk of the car of a home nurse or ambulance will adversely affect the stability

TABLE 12.3. POTENTIAL SOURCES OF TECHNICAL INTERFERENCES WITH POINT-OF-CARE TEST METHODS

Specimen	Technical Bias
Hematocrit	Reaction timing
Lipemia	Sample volume
Additives/glycolysis inhibitors	Incorrect application
Sampling artifacts (line draws, capillaries)	
Physiologic	**Reagent Stability**
Fasting state	Light
Specimen type (venous, arterial, capillary)	Temperature
Oxygen tension	Air exposure
Drug therapy	Humidity

Note: While not comprehensive, this list provides an example of the various sources of testing errors and the complexity of the technical considerations that need to be controlled when moving testing to the point of care.

of results. Delays in transporting unprocessed glucose samples and exposure to ambient temperatures can also affect the recovery of glucose (63). Patient factors, such as fasting status, and insulin can further alter normal arterial-capillary-venous glucose gradients (31,51). Oxygen therapy and extremes in pH can affect glucose methods (44,64,65). Lipemia and hematocrit (29,34,66) can interfere with the analysis as can the presence of hemolysis (67), anticoagulants, and glycolysis inhibitors. Metabolic byproducts such as uremia (34) in renal disease can be sources of potential errors. Reducing sugars and substances such as ascorbic acid can act as alternate electron carriers. Therapeutic agents such as salicylate can also interfere with some methods (68,69). Physiologic effects such as shock and vascular disease can alter peripheral circulation, leading to discrepancies between central and capillary glucose concentrations (70,71). Predicting all sources of error is often difficult, and ultimately the actual performance on the intended patient population is the best means of determining potential problems prior to implementation.

Operator Effects

Although the technical methodology is a major factor for bedside glucose meter performance, operational factors, operator technique, and the manner in which the meters are used equally affect meter performance. While newer generations of meters are more automated, former models required the operator to time the enzyme reactions and wipe blood off the test strip to stop the reaction before reading the results. These "time-and-wipe" systems, which are still widely marketed, demonstrate more operator-to-operator variance, because performance depends on:

- Volume of blood applied to the strip
- Method of wiping (blotting, forward, backward, or side to side)
- Depth of wiping
- Material used to wipe blood (facial tissue, Kimwipe, paper towel, napkin)

Timing is critical to wipe systems, as overexposure by only a few seconds can influence results (1,29).

Other operator criteria involve how easy the device is to use and maintain. Devices with multiple steps that require volumetric pipetting are inherently more complicated and less reliable than fully automated instrumentation (72,73). The educational level and specific training of the operator can affect the quality of test results. Most bedside glucose meters are now so simple to operate that there is little problem, provided that the operator—whether nurse, clinician, or patient—is provided with standardized training on the specific device in order to appreciate the sources of preanalytical, analytical, and postanalytical variability peculiar to that meter (74). The educational level and motivation of the operator is particularly problematic when utilizing instrumentation requiring frequent or complicated maintenance (as in blood gas analyzers) (73). Most nursing and clinical staff are not motivated by laboratory issues, as their primary directive is patient care (75,76). Laboratory testing and performance of maintenance on glucose meters are secondary concerns for

them. Devices with little to no maintenance will achieve better compliance than instrumentation requiring frequent, time-consuming maintenance and calibration. Volume effects are also important when considering use on neonates or patients with circulatory problems where adequate amounts of sample may be an issue (1,20,77). Portability of the instrument and the weight, size, and shape of the device must be considered in relation to the operator (77). Infection control is another issue, as devices that are difficult to clean or are poorly maintained can be sources of nosocomial, antibiotic-resistant infections (77,78).

Data management is a glucose meter feature in increasing demand. Agencies such as the Joint Commission on the Accreditation of Healthcare Organizations (JCAHO), College of American Pathologists (CAP), Commission on Office Laboratory Accreditation (COLA), and Centers for Medicare and Medicaid Services (CMS) through the Clinical Laboratory Improvement Amendments of 1988 (CLIA '88), and individual states have regulations requiring specific QA documentation (79). Glucose meters that can automatically capture, store, and manage required information through computerization offer advantages over devices without this capability (77,80).

Medical Indications

Limiting the use of bedside testing is foremost to the quality and cost effectiveness of bedside testing (81). Universal use of bedside testing is comparable to ordering every available laboratory test on a patient in the hope that something will be abnormal. Diagnostic laboratory testing should complement the clinical symptoms, and bedside testing as with any laboratory test should be incorporated into standard critical pathways of care for selected diseases only when clinical information or particular clinical questions need to be answered. In addition to clinical need for bedside testing, the timing of the result must also be important. The choice of using a central laboratory, bedside testing, or a rapid-response satellite laboratory should be justified by the critical need for test information and when the result will be acted on for the most cost-effective patient outcome. Technical performance differences among methodologies in each of these locations will also determine how the laboratories should be used—for diagnosis, screening, or management. Although recent advances in meter technology have greatly improved meter accuracy and precision, bedside glucose meters have still not achieved the 5% accuracy goals recommended by the American Diabetes Association (20–22,36–38,42,43). Until such time that glucose meters can achieve these standards 100% of the time, bedside glucose meters should not be used for the diagnosis of diabetes (i.e., to analyze samples from a glucose tolerance test). Appropriate clinical indications for glucose meters as outlined by the National Committee for Clinical Laboratory Standards would include (19):

- Continued management of blood glucose in diabetics and patients with unstable glucose who require rapid, frequent testing
- Rapid diagnosis of coma-of-unknown origin and detection of patients whose symptoms suggest abnormal glucose concentrations

- Perioperative management of surgical, obstetric, and postpartum diabetic mothers
- Monitoring patient receiving parenteral hyperalimentation and medications affecting glucose concentrations
- Inpatient and outpatient education

Cost Effectiveness and Outcomes

Despite the prevalence of glucose meters in healthcare settings today, there are no well-controlled, blinded crossover studies that demonstrate improved patient outcomes in a hospital setting. There are, however, several uncontrolled studies showing isolated cost savings. One study in a critical care unit has indicated the usefulness of bedside glucose testing and obtaining a rapid result in moving patients out of an ICU faster and saving overall healthcare costs (82). Bedside glucose monitoring was found to have a direct impact on the treatment of diabetic ketoacidosis. Although the total number of glucose tests remained the same (36 tests per patient), transferring glucose testing from the central laboratory to the bedside decreased the average ICU stay by 1 day and reduced overall hospital stays by 3 days (82). The faster TATs of bedside glucose testing also benefited patients outside of the ICUs at Morton Plant Hospital in Clearwater, Florida (83). Patients with a primary diagnosis of diabetes mellitus who received bedside capillary monitoring of blood glucose were discharged an average of 1.8 days sooner than those who did not. Overall volumes of central laboratory blood and urine glucose testing also decreased after hospital-wide implementation of bedside testing, with a savings of approximately $40 on glucose testing per admission (83). These two studies, however, were conducted prior to the implementation of CLIA '88 QA guidelines with enhanced documentation and supervision requirements (79), and were not conducted in a blinded, crossover fashion. With the current acceptance of bedside glucose testing as the "standard" in health care, few institutions for ethical reasons would now grant institutional research approval on human subjects for such crossover studies that involved a patient population left without glucose monitoring or as a control group to demonstrate differential outcomes.

In home self-monitoring, there are studies, such as the Diabetes Control and Complications Trial, that show significant improvement in the control of glucose levels through the use of glucose meters by insulin-dependent diabetics and delay of long-term vascular complications due to the enhanced control of glucose levels (84). Ongoing studies, however, have failed to demonstrate similar improvements in patient outcome from equivalent glucose control in noninsulin-dependent diabetics (85–87). While there is an association between elevated blood glucose levels and long-term microvascular and neurologic complications leading to morbidity and mortality in both insulin and noninsulin-dependent diabetics, control of glucose levels through diet, self-monitoring, exercise, or insulin has only been shown to improve outcome in insulin-dependent diabetics (88). A study involving home monitoring of blood glucose in 20 pregnant insulin-dependent diabetics resulted in 23.9 fewer days in the hospital and 4.2 more clinic visits. Thus, glucose monitoring in this patient population reduced hospitalizations and

improved outpatient follow-up without compromising outcome (89). Similar results in noninsulin-dependent populations have not been demonstrated.

Global, long-term patient outcome studies such as the Diabetes Control and Complications Trial, however, are difficult to conduct. Cost effectiveness of various laboratory delivery options is easier to study, and there are several reports that describe the effects of various operational factors on the cost of bedside glucose testing. The cost of bedside testing in general is characterized by high unit or variable costs for reagents and low fixed cost for instrumentation (12) (Table 12.4). Most glucose meters are provided by manufacturers at no cost or at minimal charge, since profits are generated primarily through the cost of each test strip. This is opposite the central laboratory, where glucose tests can be performed for pennies a test, but the fixed cost of instrumentation and hospital overhead for facility space, light, and water is in the hundreds of thousands of dollars. As test volume increases, the fixed costs in the central laboratory can be spread over more tests, making overall testing more cost effective. For bedside testing, the same is also true, but test costs drop less with increased volume than in the main laboratory due to the high initial costs of training multiple operators and ongoing costs of documenting their competency and supervising bedside quality.

This point was clarified at the Veterans Affairs (VA) Medical Center in New York. The cost per test of bedside glucose testing was compared with central laboratory testing. The VA medical center, with 660 beds, performs about 200 glucoses a month (2,250 per year) using 54 in-house, credentialed, registered nurses on glucose meters versus sending the specimens to a central laboratory. Although indirect overhead costs were comparable between bedside and centralized testing, the direct costs were considerably greater for bedside testing, particularly for labor and supplies. Education and competency had to be documented for a larger number of staff with bedside testing. Additional labor was required for nurse manager oversight and for laboratory staff to perform documentation inspection, instrument validation and maintenance, data entry into the computer, and annual analyst competency. Bedside testing was thus 3.6 times more expensive per test than central laboratory testing. If extrapolated to 172 VA hospitals across America, bedside testing could cost the VA Administration an additional $3 million a year (90).

TABLE 12.4. COST COMPARISON BETWEEN POINT-OF-CARE AND CENTRAL LABORATORY TESTING

Point of Care	Central Laboratory
High unit reagent cost	Low reagent cost
Low instrument cost	High instrument cost
Control cost dependent on patient volume	Low control cost (high patient volume)
Higher proficiency cost (more sites)	Lower proficiency cost (fewer sites)
Low facility cost (no fixed space requirement)	High facility cost (remodeling, space, light, electricity, etc.)
Higher training and competency costs (more operators)	Lower training and competency costs (limited operators)
High supervision cost (more operators/sites)	Lower supervision cost (fewer operators/sites)

The effect of test volume is exemplified at Massachusetts General Hospital. The cost of bedside glucose testing was compared among various nursing units. Massachusetts General performs 67,596 glucose tests a year with 54 glucose meters and 972 nurses. The hospital average cost for bedside glucose testing was $4.19 versus $3.84 for central laboratory testing. However, this cost was highly variable among nursing units, with a median of $5.52 and a range of $3.08 to $48.16 per test. This variability could be attributed to test volume differences among nursing units. In high-volume nursing units, the test cost was actually lower than central laboratory cost, whereas in low-volume nursing units the cost was significantly inflated (2).

Ensuring the quality of test results requires regular analysis of quality control (QC) samples. For sites with few patients, the ratio of nonpatient, QC testing will be much higher, resulting in higher cost for each patient test. Decreasing the amount of nonpatient testing is one way of minimizing test cost. Massachusetts General Hospital found that the percent-cost composition of bedside testing, labor (80%) and supplies (20%), differed from central laboratory costs: labor, 43%; supplies and instrumentation, 15%; and indirect costs, 42%. Patient testing represented only 49.2% of the bedside activities on the average nursing unit, and 50.8% of the activity was QA related. Massachusetts General Hospital further compared itself with an affiliate institution, McLean Hospital, which performed only 1,656 glucose tests on 16 glucose meters. At McLean, the cost of bedside glucose testing was much higher, $13.49 per test, and QA activities accounted for almost 82% of the testing activity. Bedside testing costs are thus dependent on testing volumes and the percentage of nonpatient testing activity (2).

Minimizing the number of bedside operators in a healthcare setting is another means of limiting the cost of testing. In order to be cost effective, a balance must be struck between maintaining a minimal number of staff to cover clinical needs without training a surplus. Winkelman et al. described two scenarios for bedside glucose testing: (a) bedside testing by a registered nurse or (b) specimen collection, transportation to a central laboratory, and analysis by laboratory technologists. The cost of using nursing staff more than doubled the per-test cost ($6.62 for bedside testing by nurses versus $3.30 per central laboratory test). The cost, however, could be lowered from $6.62 to $4.78 per test by transferring 55% of the bedside testing to the central laboratory ([0.45 × $6.62] + [0.55 × $3.30] = $4.78). Cost savings for bedside testing could thus be achieved by minimizing the number of trained staff performing testing and optimizing the volume of testing conducted at the bedside (7).

Limiting bedside testing to only those sites with critical medical need and using the laboratory for other routine testing is one way to minimize cost. Introduction of bedside testing does not necessarily result in an equal shifting of central laboratory test numbers to the bedside. Due to testing for operator training and QA, implementation of bedside testing can actually increase the number of glucose tests performed by a health system, particularly when considering the additional testing required from inappropriate performance or interpretation of the result (57,91). Implementation of glucose meters may increase utilization due to the convenience of having testing on the nursing unit.

While bedside glucose testing can be more expensive than testing in the central laboratory depending on volume, number of operators, and nonpatient activities, bedside testing generally costs less than operating a satellite, rapid-response laboratory. This makes intuitive sense, as a 24-hour satellite laboratory cannot utilize labor as efficiently as either a busy central laboratory or bedside testing where operators are caring for patients when they are not performing bedside tests. Staff in a satellite laboratory must stay on site in order to provide a rapid response for samples. Unless test volume is such that the staff is always busy, or there are other tasks that the staff can perform, there will be periods of time when staff do not have samples to analyze, resulting in lost productivity and higher test costs. Methodist Hospital of Indiana examined this option when considering stat testing alternatives and found the cost of performing blood gas, electrolyte, and hematocrit testing in a stat laboratory to be 1.7 times the cost of performing bedside testing on a GEM-STAT analyzer. The cost analysis assumed 50 panels per day (18,250 panels per year). Although bedside testing on a portable cart saved $8.40 per panel compared to a satellite stat laboratory, the cost of bedside testing, $211,385, was an additional hospital expense. If some savings could be achieved through labor and test reductions in the central (or stat) laboratory, then these savings could be used to offset the added bedside expenses (92).

In another bedside testing example (11), three delivery options were compared: (a) central laboratory testing with specimens collected and transported by phlebotomists, (b) bedside testing by registered nurses, and (c) on-demand bedside testing by a team of phlebotomists. With an annual central laboratory volume of 120,000 glucose tests, the hospital testing costs totaled $366,143. Performance of testing at the bedside by nursing resulted in about the same costs, $344,864, even with the inclusion of savings from fewer central laboratory stat requests (total of 144,000 tests per year = 60,000 central laboratory + 84,000 bedside tests). However, using a phlebotomy team, the authors were able to demonstrate a cost savings of approximately $100,000.

The main difference in this analysis was the inclusion of internal and external failure costs. Internal failure costs represented increased stat requests and repeat testing because of the delay in laboratory TAT under the central laboratory option. External failure costs included wasteful duplicative pharmacy and dietary services because of the slow turnaround of glucose test results for diabetic patients. Inclusion of costs associated with unnecessary test requests, medications, and therapeutic interventions because of delayed or incorrect test results addresses the overall hospital costs and shifts the cost analysis toward a patient outcome viewpoint (11).

The point of view is fundamental to the perspective of any cost analysis (Fig. 12.5). Laboratory administrators may only analyze the effects of bedside testing from the central laboratory perspective. This perspective focuses on the potential loss of central test numbers due to implementation of bedside testing and the need to maintain satellite and central laboratory services. Analysis from a nursing point of view would focus on the additional burden of laboratory testing on an already overburdened patient-care demand. Analysis from the perspective of a hospital administrator would incorporate the overall testing costs with

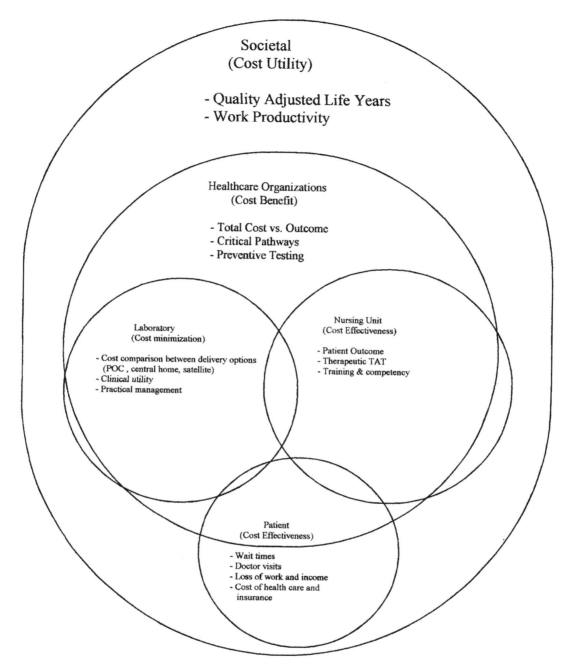

FIGURE 12.5. Effects of viewpoint on cost analysis. Testing options that may be more costly to the laboratory could be more effective when considering more global patient, healthcare organization, or societal outcomes.

the savings that could be achieved by discharging a patient earlier or by eliminating duplicative orders, delays in nutritional services, and increased stat laboratory requests due to slow laboratory TATs. The more global cost analyses are inherently different because they incorporate patient outcome to examine overall cost effectiveness or cost benefit as opposed to merely comparing costs among delivery options. Critical review of any

cost analysis must take into account the point of view of the authors and evaluate whether all patient factors and external and internal factors have been considered. Higher costs in laboratory testing can oftentimes be offset by improved patient satisfaction, movement through patient units, and other indicators of outcome. More research is needed in the area of bedside glucose testing to definitively prove its unique benefits to patient care.

Bedside Testing as a Transition to Patient Self-Management

Some benefits and outcomes, however, cannot be quantified. Morton Plant Hospital in Clearwater, Florida, demonstrated a hospital-wide savings in glucose testing per admission after implementation of bedside testing. Revenue generated was transferred to the Diabetes Education Center to cover the ongoing cost of nurse training and patient education. The gain in patient education and enhanced involvement of patients in self-management from the bedside testing program was unexpected. Inpatients could directly observe the results of their diabetes management protocols while in the hospital. Nurses performing the testing could emphasize how glucose levels relate to diabetes effects and reinforce the importance of self-testing once discharged. In addition, use of devices in the hospital that were popular in the home setting provided opportunities for patient education in the proper analytical technique and emphasis on preanalytic and postanalytical test variables. These important advantages to a bedside testing program cannot be quantified, and it is difficult to place a specific monetary value on such subjective outcomes for cost comparisons.

New data management capabilities of home testing meters that are currently under investigation allow the capture and storage of patient results for review by clinicians at their next office visit. Review of data from a glucose meter can indicate the compliance and motivational level of patients in their day-to-day routine, highlighting those patients that require more intensive intervention. Use of telephone modems and Internet connectivity offer time-saving advantages to the patient, allowing the remote review of their data and optimization of therapies without a physician office visit.

Bedside glucose testing can be viewed as a continuum of care. From the time that a patient is identified as a hospital in-patient, through their outpatient clinics, home-nursing settings and individual self-testing, data integration of test information offers the ability to track the success of therapy to normal patient glucose levels. In order to most fully utilize the available data, there must be comparability between results in all of these healthcare settings. Innovations in the QA and standardization of different glucose methods will enhance the value of such data tracking in the future.

Patient outcomes research regarding bedside testing has focused on devices and instrumentation for blood gas, glucose, electrolyte, coagulation, and hemoglobin testing. Manually interpreted methods such as urine dipsticks, and occult blood, pregnancy, and infectious disease tests have been relatively ignored. A recent survey (93) estimated that nine out of ten hospitals are increasing the use of bedside or POC testing, yet only 7% have conducted any cost study to justify the purchase, QC, calibration, and maintenance of the variety of bedside tests used. The primary reason for this growth in bedside testing is the need for faster TATs. While development efforts are improving the technical performance, QA, and management of bedside devices, manually interpreted tests remain a source of continued problems in health care today. In a recent survey of British physicians (94), blood glucose and urine dipstick testing were the most commonly performed bedside tests. TAT was the most frequent indication for bedside testing. Yet, while 85% of clinicians trusted central laboratory results, 38% did not trust bedside results, and 35% of physicians would not accept responsibility for results obtained at the bedside (94). The difficulty of supervising and managing manually interpreted tests contributes to this general distrust of bedside testing, and an understanding of the issues surrounding waived bedside testing is important when developing a total bedside testing QC program.

INTEGRATED BEDSIDE TESTING PROGRAMS

Accreditation Guidelines and Legal Constraints

Bedside testing in the United States is regulated by a hierarchy of federal, state, and private accreditation guidelines. Specific details of these guidelines is the focus of a separate chapter, and this discussion focuses only on those guidelines that cover waived testing under CLIA '88 (95–98). All laboratory testing in the United States that is utilized for patient diagnosis or management must meet at a minimum the federal guidelines of CLIA '88. These regulations do not, however apply to testing conducted for research, tests conducted by the federal government, or drugs of abuse testing, which have separate regulations specific to this testing. CLIA '88 guidelines outline the validation, QC, and documentation that must be met to perform laboratory analyses for patient care. Tests are separated by the technical difficulty of the methodology into waived, moderate, and high complexity categories. Monetary penalties for noncompliance with these guidelines are enforced through the CMS and Medicare reimbursement for laboratory services. Noncompliance carries risk of both fines and loss of federal reimbursement. States have additional laboratory regulations. Some have more stringent guidelines than CLIA '88.

Besides the federal and state regulations, there are a number of private accreditation agencies that inspect and certify laboratory testing. The CAP (99) and the JCAHO (100,101) certify hospitals and nursing homes, while the COLA (102) certifies physician office laboratories. These organizations have deemed status with the CMS/CLIA '88 (103) and with some states that allow inspection by the private accreditation agency to meet CLIA and state guidelines. Since the private accreditation agencies minimally match CLIA '88 regulations, and are more stringent in many instances, reinspection by the federal government or state is not necessarily required.

While the specific regulations of each accreditation agency vary, bedside testing should meet the minimal guidelines for CLIA '88 as interpreted by the JCAHO (100,101). These guidelines recommend that:

- The purpose of the testing; diagnosis, screening, or management, be defined for the healthcare institution or more specifically for the particular patient setting.
- The supervisory and testing personnel must be identified.
- The personnel must have initial training and orientation specific to the device adequate to meet laboratory needs, and personnel should demonstrate ongoing competency.
- Written policies and procedures should be readily available to all testing personnel.

- QC on samples of known concentration should be performed daily or at a frequency recommended by the manufacturer.
- There should be a documented result trail linking a patient's result to an individual operator, testing device, and the QC on that device.

Additional requirements for method validation, laboratory oversight, regular review of QC, proficiency testing, color blindness testing of operators, and integration of the bedside testing program within the institutional QA scheme are recommended by more stringent agencies such as CAP (99). All regulations are necessarily vague and only give general recommendations without specific ways in which to meet the requirements. Each organization is encouraged to structure its QA programs to meet the regulations while optimizing delivery of patient care. As there are multiple ways to interpret the guidelines, each organization will have different healthcare goals and views, and no single best way to meet regulations. What works in one institution may be too disruptive in another. Healthcare practice managers should weigh the options that work in other model healthcare systems in developing their own unique solution to meeting regulatory guidelines.

Organization and Strategies for Quality Assurance

The need for quality in bedside testing is illustrated by the numerous examples of outcomes from poorly supervised testing. In one U.S. location, unsupervised bedside glucose conducted by nonlaboratory staff differed by over 34% from the clinical laboratory at a mean glucose of 180 mg/dL and led to inappropriate categorization of hypoglycemic and normoglycemic patients. However, these same personnel, after implementation of a QA program involving standardized operator training, QC, and laboratory supervision, were able to reduce the CV of bedside glucose from 17% to 8% and improve results to clinically acceptable levels (72). In a more recent British study at ten health clinics, 21% of total cholesterol results differed by more than 1 mmol/L (37 mg/dL) with coefficients of variation of 18–20% due to lack of training (40%), inadequate maintenance (70%) and poor QC practices (50%) (104). Poorly maintained devices at the bedside have not only been the source of unreliable results but can be a reservoir of infectious organisms. Hospital *Enterobacter cloacae* infections in a neonatal ICU have been linked to a blood gas analyzer (78) and the spread of *Serratia marcescens* and *Pseudomonas aeruginosa* have been traced to dirty urinometers (105,106). Institution of a standardized training program increased the percentage of correctly interpreted hemoccult slides from 60% to 91% and continued at a level of 91% six to nine months after the training (107). For every type of bedside test, there are examples where unsupervised testing and variable operator technique have led to poor results and problems in patient care.

Studies like these have prompted the federal CLIA '88 regulations for stricter QA of bedside testing (95–98). Medical associations have also recommended institution of QA programs for selected analytes. The American Diabetes Association (36–38) and the Association of Clinical Biochemists (35), for example,

have recommended implementing a program to address the entire testing process from preanalytical sample collection to analysis to postanalytical result interpretation. The continuous quality improvement (CQI) model is an excellent foundation for bedside testing programs and is a recommendation of the JCAHO for all hospital QA programs (100,101). This model is based on a plan, design, measure, assess, and improve cycle. For bedside testing, planning can occur through discussion in a multidisciplinary task force. Designing a standardized program involves setting up policies and procedures. Measurement of quantitative quality monitors provides a means of statistically assessing ongoing quality. Assessing performance indicates areas for improvement. Improvement modifies the current program to address specific problem areas. The cycle can then start again with the planning stage for implementing changes to the program. Design allows for setting up new monitors of performance that can then be measured and assessed for further program improvement. Use of this CQI model will guarantee forward movement of a bedside QA program and continued improvement in quality.

Gaining control over bedside testing can be difficult given the inherent simplicity of the test kits and the many ways in which they can enter a healthcare institution. Forming a multidisciplinary task force to address bedside testing issues is a good means of getting a handle on an out-of-control problem. This task force should be composed of everyone who has a part in bedside testing. Representation should include central laboratory personnel, physicians, nurses, hospital administration, infection control, purchasing, and other involved disciplines. A multidisciplinary task force can provide a forum for resolving problems and discussing testing alternatives to best meet patient-care needs. Each member can bring his or her unique perspective on an issue to the table. Laboratory personnel can focus on the technical aspects of a given test and their understanding of the regulations that must be followed. Clinicians can discuss the TAT needs for their patient population, while nurses who frequently perform the testing can raise issues surrounding the balancing of test documentation and QC with their already overburdened schedules for patient care. Hospital administration representatives are important as liaisons to the governing medical board, and their understanding of the value of test QA is fundamental to resource allocation and budgeting for the program. Infection control should be involved to review maintenance aspects of test devices that will be carried from bed to bed, or from house to house in home healthcare settings, to ensure proper device cleaning and to prevent the spread of nosocomial infections. Purchasing is another key member to block the acquisition of unauthorized devices in the institution and to assist in the purchase of single lots of tests that will help minimize the ongoing validation of reagent shipments.

All of these disciplines must work in concert to provide an optimal outcome. When requests for new bedside tests are made or when issues with ongoing testing occur, this task force is the best resource to set policies regarding the use and QA of tests. Through discussion of testing alternatives, drawing on the expertise of the committee members, the task force can optimize the manner in which the testing is to be conducted. Solutions unique to an institution can thus be formed to best meet the needs of all parties, guaranteeing a successful initial implementation and ongoing compliance with the institutional policies. Such cooperation is a good example of crossdisciplinary institutional quality improvement to provide for accreditation inspectors.

Proficiency Testing

Bedside testing is part of a continuous spectrum of care that a healthcare organization can provide to its patients. Laboratory results conducted on hospitalized inpatients whether from bedside, rapid-response satellite, or central laboratories must agree with results from affiliated outpatient clinics and home health care. Since many physicians treat patients based on bedside tests without a full comprehension of their limitations with respect to central laboratory testing, bedside tests must give results of comparable accuracy to those of the central laboratory. Otherwise, separate reference ranges will need to be developed along with an education program for clinicians on the interpretive differences between bedside and central laboratory tests. Comparability between all testing conducted within an institution can be achieved through regular splitting of patient specimens (analyzing part of the sample on site and the other in a remote laboratory and then documenting the agreement) or through subscription to a proficiency survey program that provides blinded specimens for comparison with other external laboratories across the United States.

Matrix differences are an obvious concern with either split sampling or with proficiency testing. For blood testing, many bedside tests utilize whole blood in order to provide rapid results, while central laboratory testing prefers serum or plasma. In addition, some analytes are unstable, such as glucose, and will degrade over time (31). This limits the acceptability of split samples for bedside testing.

Proficiency programs have an equal problem with matrix effects. Processing of whole-blood or urine specimens to stabilize cells and analytes can actually bias the results of some devices (55,56). Evaluation against similar devices of identical technology provides a better means of scoring true performance, and in many cases reduces the effect of this matrix problem.

Future QA for accuracy will utilize the ability of bedside devices to capture data. By integrating bedside tests with central laboratory tests in the electronic medical record, true differences in routine practice can be more effectively monitored. Unfortunately, this alternative will have to wait for the conversion of health care to a full electronic medical record and for a means of capturing data from manual visually interpreted tests, such as occult blood, urine dipsticks, and pregnancy and rapid strep tests (80,108).

Personnel Training and Competency

Operator inconsistencies are a frequent source of problems with bedside testing quality. One common concern has involved the educational level of the operators, particularly if bedside test operators do not have a laboratory background (57,72–74). With standardized initial training that is specific to a simple bedside testing device, reliable results can be

obtained and there is no significant difference between nontechnical and technical operators (72,73). The simpler devices that have the least number of analytical steps have been found to generate the most reliable results in the hands of nontechnical staff. However, as the number of analytical steps and the difficulty increases (volumetric pipetting, for instance), statistical differences are noted between technical and nontechnical operators (72,73).

A recent survey of hospital-bedside glucose QA programs in the United States that demonstrated the most significant levels of continued improvement focused on operator training (42,109). The characteristics of these programs were:

- Involvement of the laboratory personnel in initial training of operators;
- Use of standardized training materials, such as videotapes, as part of the training;
- Repeat training and review of performance at scheduled intervals;
- Regular comparison of bedside results to the central clinical laboratory; and
- Use of the computerized data capture of devices for storing QC and patient data.

These programs standardized initial training and monitored ongoing competency through both performance reviews at scheduled intervals and by comparison of patient results obtained through routine use. Capturing data for review was an additional aspect that assisted in program supervision.

Initial training is often more easily standardized than documentation of ongoing competency. There are three common ways to document ongoing competency: visual inspection at regular intervals, routine performance of QC, and analysis of blind samples as with proficiency surveys (100,101). Large programs with many staff members can spend the equivalence of several technologists just inspecting the technique of bedside operators. Performance of split patient samples and distribution of a single proficiency survey to all operators can also be complicated. Analysis of routine QC, while a better alternative compared to the cost of labor and expense of additional testing, is not easy, given the limitations of most manufacturer data reduction software and the difficulty in interfacing bedside devices to hospital and laboratory information systems (12,110).

Supervision of routine test performance is a critical part of maintaining high quality testing. Experience from large academic institutions has determined that operators tend to fall back into their old patterns of behavior unless continuous oversight is maintained (110,111). Specific compliance problems were noted with maintenance of bedside devices and with the return of proficiency sample results (110,111). Only through continued monitoring can an assessment of overall quality be made for future educational intervention.

Documentation

Documentation is the key to regulatory compliance (79). When inspectors review a program, documentation provides the evidence for institutional compliance and improvement. However, supervision and monitoring of program quality require central collection and review of data, which can be time consuming. This oversight task is multiplied by the number of devices and operators in a healthcare system (12,110). Recent developments in automated data management of bedside devices through the capture of appropriate information, transmission of this information to a central database, and statistical reduction will assist in the future management of bedside testing (80,108). For institutions with dozens of devices and hundreds of operators, computerized data reduction is mandatory to being able to manage the program (110).

There are at least five areas of documentation that must be managed in order to meet regulatory guidelines (110):

- Device validation records of initial performance for future troubleshooting as well as documentation of device repair and technical maintenance. Validation records also provide documentation of initial control and reagent lot verifications.
- QC to document compliance with manufacturers' regulations and for use in proving operator competency.
- Proficiency samples to prove accuracy of bedside tests. Documentation of linearity sets of known concentration can verify the calibration over the reportable range.
- QA monitors can document the operator's compliance with institutional policy and provide a record for follow-up.
- Patient results can provide a result trail linking operator to device and QC on the device, but more globally when linked to electronic medical record data, can provide information on clinical necessity, test TATs, and patient outcomes.

Although modern devices are more sophisticated than in the past, data management of bedside testing is still limited, and there is currently no capacity for monitoring nursing unit compliance, deficiencies and their correction, initial device validation, maintenance, and ongoing lot verifications. Manufacturers differ widely in their ability to capture and statistically reduce data. There are currently no industry standards regarding the capture of data or its transmission to other databases. In addition, the data reduction software differs among manufacturers and is somewhat limited in functionality. While QC charts and operator or device means and standard deviations are generated, there are no current capabilities for comparative statistics.

Johns Hopkins University has over 1,800 glucose operators and 200 HemoCue operators. Despite differences in the software among manufacturers, we transfer data to a customized database in order to generate operator and meter comparative statistics (110) (Table 12.5). Routine QC data are utilized to generate hospital-wide means. The mean of each operator or device can then be compared to the hospital target and the differences graded by the standard deviation interval (SDI). Setting a fixed limit (more than two or three SDIs) identifies operators whose technique differs from other operators and meters generating different results in routine practice. Use of the SDI is advantageous, because it provides a quantitative comparison among operators and devices, removing the ambiguity of visual inspection. The SDI utilizes routine QC, so additional time, reagents, and testing are not required to prove competency. This method is biased against infrequent operators, since they contribute less to the group mean to which everyone is compared. However, this bias specifically targets infrequent operators,

TABLE 12.5. POINT-OF-CARE DATA MANAGEMENT REPORT SUMMARIZING OPERATOR STATISTICS

Name	Lot	Cuvette Type	Control Lot	Operator					Group			
				N	Mean	SD	CV	SDI	N	Mean	SD	CV
Angela Doctor	97762											
		QCC	—	1	12.70	—	—	−0.20	76	12.74	0.17	1.37%
		QCH	50	1	16.90	—	—	2.12	52	16.02	0.41	2.58%
		QCL	50	1	8.10	—	—	1.85	52	7.78	0.18	2.26%
Beverly Nurse	97762											
		QCC	—	4	12.65	0.06	0.46%	−0.49	76	12.74	0.17	1.37%
		QCH	50	3	16.20	0.56	3.44%	0.43	52	16.02	0.41	2.58%
		QCL	50	3	7.50	0.20	2.56%	0.14	52	7.78	0.18	2.26%
Debra Practitioner	97762											
		QCC	—	2	12.60	0.00	0.00%	−0.78	76	12.74	0.17	1.37%
		QCH	50	1	16.40	—	—	0.91	52	16.02	0.41	2.58%
		QCL	50	1	7.60	—	—	−1.00	52	7.78	0.18	2.26%
Felix Trainee	97762											
		QCC	—	2	12.85	0.07	0.55%	1.14	248	12.69	0.14	1.13%
		QCH	50	1	15.80	—	—	−0.52	164	16.00	0.39	2.41%
Elaine Worker	97762											
		QCC	—	1	12.60	—	—	−0.78	76	12.74	0.17	1.37%
		QCH	50	1	16.70	—	—	1.64	52	16.02	0.41	2.58%
		QCL	50	1	7.50	—	—	−1.56	52	7.78	0.18	2.26%

Note: The control performance of each operator is compared to other operators through the standard deviation interval (SDI). Those outside of defined criteria (2SD) are watched closely for further problems and/or retrained. CV, coefficient of variation; N, number; QCC, control cuvette; QCH and QCL, high and low controls; POCT, point-of-care testing; SD, standard deviation; SDI, standard deviation interval.
Taken from the Johns Hopkins Medical Institutions Department of Pathology, Core Lab POCT Program.

which is advantageous as these are the operators who should be identified for retraining. Use of a personal computer platform allows the capture and reduction of data from all devices in the same manner, standardizing our QA program. All this can be accomplished automatically and problem reports are generated that require follow-up, additional training, or nursing unit intervention. In this manner, we can save labor while still maintaining a high degree of laboratory oversight. Such programs, however, are limited by the ability of devices to capture data. More than 50% of all bedside testing currently involves visually interpreted tests that do not currently have any means of data capture, unless each test is manually entered into a computer for review.

Practical Considerations

The full impact of a bedside QA program is only realized in actual practice. Through detection and troubleshooting of unexpected problems, technical aspects of bedside tests can be revealed due to characteristics of particular patient populations or the manner in which the bedside tests are utilized. Johns Hopkins University noted a higher frequency of glucose meter breakage in the optical windows and a lack of correlation with the central laboratory on selected patients in one specific ICU. On follow-up, it was discovered that staff were drawing fingerstick blood into glass capillaries (previously banned by Johns Hopkins University for infection control reasons) and carrying the samples to a utility closet down the hall, where the glucose meters were stored, for analysis. The length of time to carry the specimens down the hall resulted in clotting of the blood sample prior to analysis. Staff members were, thus, having difficulty applying an adequate sample to the test strip. Tamping of the glass capillary on the optic window resulted in meter breakage. Laboratory evaluation of plastic capillary tubes with various anticoagulants proved to be inadequate in blocking the clotting cascade due to the difficulty of sufficiently mixing the small amount of sample in the capillary tube. The alternative was to reeducate the staff in the need for rapid sample analysis for fingersticks by bringing the glucose meters to the patient. This would also provide the opportunity to reinforce the requirement that line draws be collected in heparinized syringes. It was only through the continuous monitoring of the bedside testing process that we were able to resolve the issue and reeducate staff, as this problem was not predicted during initial implementation. This experience stresses the benefits of close supervision for the prompt, dynamic resolution of problems and the maintenance of the highest quality test results. Practical issues such as these examples are good topics for resolution by a multidisciplinary task force where the advantages and disadvantages of various options can be weighed.

CONCLUSIONS

Bedside testing promises improved patient care through faster turnaround of diagnostic results. The actual outcome, however, depends on the quality of the device, prompt acknowledgment of the result, and consideration of the limitations of the test for appropriate interpretation. Recent studies (112,113) further indicate the need for careful limitation and performance evaluation of POC testing instruments. Supervision of bedside testing is mandatory to obtaining quality results, but laboratory oversight requires significant labor for review and correction of compliance deficiencies. The future of bedside testing relies on the ability to manage the information provided by the test results and integrating this information with the patient's medical record to determine the best delivery options for effective patient outcomes.

Recommendations for bedside testing include:

- Forming a multidisciplinary task force as a forum for discussing bedside testing issues.
- Evaluation of bedside methods on the intended patient population by actual operators to ensure that the technology meets clinical expectations and needs.
- A QA program built on the CQI model is a basic step to guaranteeing ongoing improvement in bedside testing quality.
- The QA program should meet regulatory guidelines with minimal changes to current practice.
- The QA program should be realistic, so that institutional policies can be achieved.
- Data management is an essential aspect of enhancing bedside utility. Manufacturers need to follow connectivity standards for the automated capture, transmission, statistical reduction, and review of data to meet regulatory guidelines without labor input, and to provide institutions with the means to customize the data output as a management tool.
- Patient outcomes need to be monitored to determine if bedside testing is meeting expectations and if the testing is effective.

REFERENCES

1. Nichols JH. Management of near-patient glucose testing. *Endocrinology and Metabolism In-Service Training and Continuing Education* 1994;12:325–334.
2. Lee-Lewandrowski E, Laposata M, Eschenbach K, et al. Utilization and cost analysis of bedside capillary glucose testing in a large teaching hospital: implications for managing point of care testing. *Am J Med* 1994;97:222–230.
3. Goodwin SA. Point-of-care testing in a post anesthesia care unit. *MLO* 1994;26[Suppl]:15–18.
4. Zaloga GP. Monitoring versus testing technologies: present and future. *MLO* 1991;23[Suppl]:20–31.
5. Nichols JH. POCT: A viable solution to turnaround time delays. *MLO* 1998;30[Suppl]:4–5..
6. Seamonds B. Medical, economic and regulatory factors affecting point-of-care testing: a report of the conference on factors affecting point-of-care testing, Philadelphia, PA, 6–7 May 1994. *Clin Chim Acta* 1996;249:1–19.
7. Winkelman JW, Wybenga DR, Tanasijevic MJ. The fiscal consequences of central vs distributed testing of glucose. *Clin Chem* 1994;40:1628–1630.
8. Saxena S, Wong ET. Does the emergency department need a dedicated stat laboratory? Continuous quality improvement as a management tool for the clinical laboratory. *Am J Clin Pathol* 1993;100:606–610.
9. Felder RA. Robotics and automated workstations for rapid response testing. *Am J Clin Pathol* 1995;104[Suppl 1]:S26–S32.

10. Fleischer M, Schwartz MK. Automated approaches to rapid-response testing: A comparative evaluation of point-of-care and centralized laboratory testing. *Am J Clin Pathol* 1995;104[Suppl 1]:S18–S25.

11. Handorf CR. POC testing: must quality cost more? *MLO* 1993;25 [Suppl]:28–33.

12. Nichols JH. Cost analysis of point-of-care laboratory testing. In Weinstein RS, ed. *Advances in pathology and laboratory medicine* Mosby: Chicago, 1996;121–134.

13. Food and Drug Administration. Improving glucose monitoring for diabetics. *FDA Consumer* 1990 May :32–35.

14. Greyson J. Quality control in patient self-monitoring of blood glucose. *Diabetes Care* 1993;16:1306–1308.

15. ECRI. Portable blood glucose monitors. *Health Devices* 1994;23: 64–99.

16. Williams JR, Alling K. A program for normal glycemic control of insulin-dependent diabetes. *Diabetes Care* 1980;3:160–2.

17. Sonksen PH, Judd S, Lowy C. Home monitoring of blood glucose: new approach to management of insulin-dependent diabetic patients in Great Britain. *Diabetes Care* 1980;3:100–107.

18. Gifford-Jorgensen RA, Borchert J, Hassanein R, et al. Comparison of five glucose meters for self-monitoring of blood glucose by diabetic patients. *Diabetes Care* 1986;9:70–76.

19. Barr JT, Betschart J, Bracey A, et al. *Ancillary (bedside) blood glucose testing in acute and chronic care facilities.* Villanova, PA: National Committee for Clinical Laboratory Standards (Document C-30A), 1994;14(12):1–14.

20. Nichols JH, Howard C, Loman K, et al. Laboratory and bedside evaluation of portable glucose meters. *Am J Clin Pathol* 1995;103: 244–251.

21. Chance JJ, Li DJ, Jones KA, et al. Technical evaluation of five glucose meters with data management capabilities. *Am J Clin Pathol* 1999; 111(4):547–556.

22. Trajanoski Z, Brunner GA, Gfrerer RJ, et al. Accuracy of home blood glucose meters during hypoglycemia. *Diabetes Care* 1996;19: 1412–1415.

23. Moses R, Schier G, Matthews J, et al. The accuracy of home glucose meters for the glucose range anticipated in pregnancy. *Aust N Z J Obstet Gynaecol* 1997;37:282–286.

24. Kilpatrick ES, McLeod MJ, Rumley AG, et al. A ward comparison between the One Touch II and Glucometer II blood glucose meters. *Diabet Med* 1994;11:214–217.

25. Hunt JA, Alojado NC. A new, improved test system for rapid measurement of blood glucose. *Diabet Res Clin Prac* 1989;7:51–55.

26. Thai AC, Ng WY, Lui KF, et al. Three new glucose reflectance meters: Diascan, Glucometer II, and Reflolux II. *Diabet Res Clin Prac* 1989;7:75–81.

27. Rumley AG. Improving the quality of near-patient blood glucose measurement. *Ann Clin Biochem* 1997;34:281–286.

28. Phillipou G, Seaborn CJ, Hooper J, et al. Capillary blood glucose measurements in hospital inpatients using portable glucose meters. *Aust N Z J Med* 1993;23:667–671.

29. Devreese K, Leroux-Roels G. Laboratory assessment of five glucose meters designed for self-monitoring of blood glucose concentration. *Eur J Clin Chem Clin Biochem* 1993;31:829–837.

30. Ashworth L, Gibb I, Alberti KGMM. HemoCue: Evaluation of a portable photometric system for determining glucose in whole blood. *Clin Chem* 1992;38:1479–1482.

31. Tustison Wa, Bowen AJ, Crampton JH. Clinical interpretation of plasma glucose values. *Diabetes* 1966;15:775–777.

32. Kempe KC, Czeschin LI, Yates KH, et al. A hospital system glucose meter that produces plasma-equivalent values from capillary, venous, and arterial blood. *Clin Chem* 1997;43:1803–1804.

33. Lane A, Geadah D, Lagerriere M, et al. Performance of the new plasma-compatible Advantage blood glucose test strips. *Clin Biochem* 1997;30:465–468.

34. Jacobs E, Vadasdi E, Roman S, et al. The influence of hematocrit, uremia and hemodialysis on whole blood glucose analysis. *Lab Med* 1993;24:295–300.

35. Price CP, Burrin JM, Nattrass M. Extra-laboratory blood glucose measurement: a policy statement. *Diabet Med* 1988;5:705–709.

36. American Diabetes Association. Consensus statement on self-monitoring of blood glucose. *Diabetes Care* 1987;10:95–99.

37. American Diabetes Association. Self-monitoring of blood glucose. *Diabetes Care* 1994;17:81–86.

38. American Diabetes Association. Self-monitoring of blood glucose. *Diabetes Care* 1996;19:S62–S66.

39. Skendzel LP, Barnett RN, Platt R. Medically useful criteria for analytic performance of laboratory tests. *Am J Clin Pathol* 1985;83: 200–5.

40. Weiss SL, Cembrowski GS, Mazza RS. Patient and physician analytic goals for self-monitoring blood glucose instruments. *Am J Clin Pathol* 1994;102:611–615.

41. Fraser CG. Analytical goals for glucose analyses. *Ann Clin Biochem* 1986;23:379–389.

42. Howanitz PJ, Jones BA. Bedside glucose monitoring: Comparison of performance as studied by the College of American Pathologists Q-Probes Program. *Arch Pathol Lab Med* 1996;120:333–338.

43. Trinick TR, Duly E. Experience of a quality assessment scheme for non-laboratory glucose meters. *J Clin Pathol* 1992;45:77–78.

44. Kost GJ, Vu HT, Lee JH, et al. Multicenter study of oxygen-insensitive handheld glucose point-of-care testing in critical care/hospital/ ambulatory patients in the United States and Canada. *Crit Care Med* 1998;26:581–590.

45. Van't Sant P, Hovenier JT, Kreutzer HJ. Quality control of "one-touch" II blood glucose meters used by nurses in clinical departments. *Eur J Clin Chem Clin Biochem* 1994;32:723–725.

46. Meehan CD, Bove LA, Jennings AS. Comparison of first-generation and second-generation blood glucose meters for use in a hospital setting. *Diabetes Educator* 1992;18:228–231.

47. Weissman M, Klein B. Evaluation of glucose determinations in untreated serum samples. *Clin Chem* 1958;4:420–422.

48. Kost GJ, Nguyen TH, Tang Z. Whole-blood glucose and lactate: trilayer biosensors, drug interference, metabolism, and practice guidelines. *Arch Pathol Lab Med* 2000;1128–1134.

49. Chaisson KM. Comparison of arterial and capillary blood glucose with the use of the Accu-chek III. *Prog Cardiovasc Nurs* 1995;10: 27–30.

50. Carr SR, Slocum J, Tefft L, et al. Precision of office-based blood glucose meters in screening for gestational diabetes. *Am J Obstet Gynecol* 1996;173:1267–1272.

51. Vallera DA, Bissell MG, Barron W. Accuracy of portable blood glucose monitoring: effect of glucose level and prandial state. *Am J Clin Pathol* 1991;95:247–252.

52. Kilpatrick ES, Rumley AG, Smith EA. Variations in sample pH and pO2 affect ExacTech meter glucose measurements. *Diabet Med* 1994;11:506–509.

53. Halloran SP. Influence of blood oxygen tension on dipstick glucose determinations. *Clin Chem* 1989;35:1268–1269.

54. Larsson-Conn U. Differences between capillary and venous blood glucose during oral glucose tolerance tests. *Scand J Clin Lab Invest* 1976;36:805–808.

55. American Association of Bioanalysts. *Whole blood glucose survey.* Brownsville, TX: American Association of Bioanalysts, 1998.

56. College of American Pathologists. *Whole blood glucose survey.* Northfield, IL: College of American Pathologists, 1998.

57. Cohen FE, Sater B, Feingold KR. Potential danger of extending SMBG techniques to hospital wards. *Diabetes Care* 1986;9:320–322.

58. Bennett BD. Blood glucose determination: point-of-care testing. *South Med J* 1997;90;678–680.

59. King JM, Eigenmann CA, Colagiuri S. Effect of ambient temperature and humidity on performance of blood glucose meters. *Diabet Med* 1995;12:337–340.

60. Ridgewell P, Holmes J. effect of temperature on results obtained with the Reflolux II. *Clin Chem* 1990;36:1705–1706.

61. Gautier JF, Bigard AX, Douce P, et al. Influence of simulated altitude on the performance of five blood glucose meters. *Diabetes Care* 1996;19:1430–1433.

62. Gregory M, Ryan R, Barnett JC, et al. Altitude and relative humidity influence results produced by glucose meters using dry reagent strips. *Clin Chem* 1988;34:1312.

63. Lewis K, Joyce-Nagata B, Fite EG. The effect of time and temperature on blood glucose measurements. *Home Healthcare Nurse* 1992;10:56–61.

64. Louie RF, Tang Z, Sutton DV, et al. Point-of-care glucose testing: Effects of critical care variables, influence of reference instruments, and a modular glucose meter design. *Arch Pathol Lab Med* 2000;124:257–266.

65. Tang Z, Du X, Louie RF, et al. Effects of pH on glucose measurements with handheld glucose meters and a portable glucose analyzer for point-of-care testing. *Arch Pathol Lab Med* 2000;124:577–582.

66. Tang Z, Lee JH, Louie RF, et al. Effects of different hematocrit levels on glucose measurements with handheld meters for point-of-care testing. *Arch Pathol Lab Med* 2000;124:1135–1140.

67. Kilpatrick ES, Rumley AG, Rumley CN. The effect of haemolysis on blood glucose meter measurement. *Diabet Med* 1995;12:341–343.

68. Tang Z, Du X, Louie RF, et al. Effects of drugs on glucose measurements with handheld glucose meters and a portable glucose analyzer. *Am J Clin Pathol* 2000;113:75–86.

69. Sylvester ECJ, Price CP, Burrin JM. Investigation of the potential for interference with whole blood glucose strips. *Ann Clin Biochem* 1994;31:94–96.

70. Atkin SH, Dasmahapatra A, Jaker MA, et al. Fingerstick glucose determination in shock. *Ann Intern Med* 1991;114:1020–1024.

71. Walker EA. Quality assurance for blood glucose monitoring: the balance of feasibility and standards. *Nurs Clinic North Am* 1993;28:61–70.

72. Nanji AA, Poon R, Hinberg I. Comparison of hospital staff performance when using desk top analysers for "near patient" testing. *J Clin Pathol* 1988;41:223–225.

73. Nanji AA, Poon R, Hinberg I. Near-patient testing: quality of laboratory test results obtained by non-technical personnel in a decentralized setting. *Am J Clin Pathol* 1988;89:797–801.

74. Belsey R, Morrison JI, Whitlow KJ, et al. Managing bedside glucose testing in the hospital. *JAMA* 1987;12:1634–1638.

75. Hilton S, Rink E, Fletcher J, et al. Near patient testing in general practice: Attitudes of general practitioners and practice nurses, and quality assurance procedures carried out. *Br J Gen Pract* 1994;44:577–580.

76. Lamb LS, Parrish RS, Goran SF, et al. Current nursing practice of point-of-care laboratory diagnostic testing in critical care units. *Am J Crit Care* 1995;4:429–434.

77. Emergency Care Research Institute. Portable blood glucose monitors. *Health Devices* 1994;23:64–99.

78. Acolet D, Ahmet Z, Houang E, et al. Enterobacter cloacae in a neonatal intensive care unit: account of an outbreak and its relationship to use of third generation cephalosporins. *J Hosp Infect* 1994;28:273–286.

79. Ehrmeyer SS, Laessig RH. Regulatory requirements (CLIA '88, JCAHO, CAP) for decentralized testing. *Am J Clin Pathol* 1995;104[Suppl 1]:S40–S49.

80. Jacobs E, Laudin AG. The satellite laboratory and point-of-care testing: integration of information. *Am J Clin Pathol* 1995;104[Suppl 1]:S33–S39.

81. Wu AHB. Reducing the inappropriate utilization of clinical laboratory tests. *Conn Med* 1997;61:15–21.

82. Zaloga GP. Evaluation of bedside testing options for the critical care unit. *Chest* 1990;97:185S–190S.

83. Trundle DS, Weizenecker RA. Capillary glucose testing: a cost-saving bedside system. *Lab Manage* 1986;24:59–62.

84. The Diabetes Control and Complications Trial Research Group. The effect of intensive treatment of diabetes on the development and progression of long-term complications in insulin-dependent diabetes mellitus. *N Engl J Med* 1993;329:977–986.

85. Jarrett RJ, Shipley MJ. Type 2 (non-insulin-dependent) diabetes mellitus and cardiovascular disease—putative association via common antecedents: further evidence from the Whitehall Study. *Diabetologia* 1998;31:737–740.

86. Colwell JA. Intensive insulin therapy in type II diabetes: Rationale and collaborative clinical trial results. *Diabetes* 1996;45[Suppl 3]:S87–S90.

87. Allen BT, DeLong ER, Feussner JR. Impact of glucose self-monitoring on non-insulin treated patients with type II diabetes mellitus: Randomized controlled trial comparing blood and urine testing. *Diabetes Care* 1990;3:1044–1050.

88. Kennedy L. A clinical endocrinologist speaks about his diagnostic and management concerns. AACC Online Symposium—the new ADA diabetes guidelines: implications for the clinical laboratory, 1988.

89. Cox R, Scott RS, MacLean AB, et al. Home monitoring of blood glucose in diabetic pregnancy. *N Z Med J* 1981;94:371–373.

90. Greendyke RM, Cost analysis of bedside blood glucose testing. *Am J Clin Pathol* 1992;97:106–107.

91. Bell DSH. Hazards of inaccurate readings obtained by self-monitoring of blood glucose. *Diabetes Care* 1990;13:1131–1132.

92. Statland BE, Brzys K. Evaluating STAT testing alternatives by calculating annual laboratory costs. *Chest* 1990;97:198S–203S.

93. Bickford GR. Decentralized testing in the 1990s: a survey of United States hospitals. *Clin Lab Med* 1994;14:623–645.

94. Gray TA, Freedman DB, Burnett D, et al. Evidence based practice: clinician's use and attitudes to near patient testing in hospitals. *J Clin Pathol* 1996;49:903–908.

95. Department of Health and Human Services, Health Care Finance Administration. Clinical laboratory improvement amendments of 1988, final rule. *Federal Register* 1992 Feb 28;57:7001–7288.

96. Department of Health and Human Services, Health Care Finance Administration. Medicare, Medicaid and CLIA programs—CLIA program fee collection: correction and final rule. *Federal Register* 1993 Jan 19;58:5211–5237.

97. Department of Health and Human Services, Health Care Finance Administration. CLIA program: categorization of tests and personnel modifications. *Federal Register* 1995 Apr 24:20035–20051.

98. Department of Health and Human Services, Health Care Finance Administration. CLIA program: categorization of waived tests. *Federal Register* 1995 Sept 13:47534–47543.

99. CAP Laboratory Accreditation Program. *Inspection checklist: point-of-care testing.* Northfield, IL: College of American Pathologists, 2000:Section 30.

100. JCAHO. *Accreditation manual for pathology and laboratory services.* Oakbrook, IL: Joint Commission on Accreditation of Healthcare Organizations, 1998.

101. JCAHO. *CAMH comprehensive accreditation manual for hospitals.* Oakbrook Terrace, IL: Joint Commission on Accreditation of Healthcare Organizations, 2000.

102. COLA. *Laboratory accreditation manual.* Columbia, MD: Commission on Office Laboratory Accreditation, 2000.

103. Department of Health and Human Services, Health Care Finance Administration. Clinical laboratories improvement act program: accreditation and exemption rule. *Federal Register* 1992 July 31;57: 33991–34021.

104. Summerton AM, Summerton N. The use of desk-top cholesterol analysers in general practice. *Public Health* 1995;109:363–367.

105. Rutala WA, Kennedy VA, Loflin HB, et al. Serratia marcescens nosocomial infection of the urinary tract associated with urine measuring containers and urinometers. *Am J Med* 1981;70:659–663.

106. Kocka FE, Roemisch E, Causey WA, et al. The urinometer as a reservoir of infectious organisms. *Am J Clin Pathol* 1977;67:106–107.

107. Fleisher M, Winawer SJ, Zauber AG, et al., National Polyp Study Work Group. Accuracy of fecal occult blood test interpretation. *Ann Intern Med* 1991;114:875–876.

108. Elevitch FR. Multimedia communications networks: Patient care through interactive point-of-care testing. *Clin Lab Med* 1994;14: 559–567.

109. Jones BA, Howanitz PJ. Bedside glucose monitoring quality control practices: a College of American Pathologists Q-probes study of program quality control, documentation, program characteristics, and accuracy performance in 544 institutions. *Arch Pathol Lab Med* 1996; 120:339–345.

110. Nichols JH, Dyer K, Liszewski CA, et al. Standardizing the quality assurance of near-patient testing. The confluence of critical care analysis and near-patient testing. Proceedings of the 17th international symposium of the Electrolyte/Blood Gas Intercontinental

Working Group of the International Federation of Clinical Chemistry, Nice, France, June 4–7, 1998.

111. Lewandrowski K, Cheek R, Nathan DM, et al. Implementation of capillary blood glucose monitoring in a teaching hospital and determination of program requirements to maintain quality testing. *Am J Med* 1992;93:419–426.

112. Tang Z, Louie RF, Payes M, et al. Oxygen effects on glucose measurements with a reference analyzer and three handheld meters. *Diabetes Technology Therapeutics* 2000;2:349–362.

113. Tang Z, Louie RF, Lee JH, et al. Oxygen effects on glucose meter measurements with glucose dehydrogenase- and oxidase-based test strips for point-of-care testing. *Crit Care Med* 2001;29:1062–1070.

13

NURSING STRATEGIES FOR POINT-OF-CARE TESTING

STEPHANIE STORTO POE
DEBRA L. CASE-CROMER

POINT-OF-CARE TESTING: A NURSING PERSPECTIVE

Today's marketplace demands services that are not only efficient and cost effective, but that also have the added value of improving patient outcomes (1). Patient care is increasingly rendered by teams of healthcare providers and certain outcomes are relevant to a number of disciplines (2). The current trend of moving many laboratory tests closer to the point of patient care is part of a growing effort to shift the focus of care to the patient (3). By definition, point-of-care testing (POCT) refers to testing that occurs at or near the point of patient care. Bedside testing, generally performed by nursing staff, is the subset of POCT in which testing occurs at the point of patient care, usually in the patient's room or bathroom. The "real-time" capture of laboratory data afforded by POCT has the potential to facilitate rapid clinical decision making by the medical staff. It also has the potential to consume a significant amount of time on the part of nurses and the laboratory personnel dedicated to POCT. According to the Clinical Laboratory Improvement Amendment of 1988 (CLIA '88), the quality of provision of all laboratory testing is site neutral, that is, expectations for quality are the same no matter where the testing occurs (4). Regardless of whether a test is performed in the clinical laboratory, a satellite laboratory, or at the bedside, the unremitting definition of quality must be acceptable patient outcome.

Laboratory, nursing, and medical professionals are forging new relationships as they strive to clarify the role of POCT in the achievement of optimum patient outcomes. The objectives of this chapter are (a) to describe the ambivalence with which nursing views POCT; (b) to review the principles, responsibilities, ownership, accountability, and supervision of POCT in contemporary healthcare settings; (c) to present quality control (QC) and proficiency testing from a nursing perspective; (d) to describe the role of performance enhancement in POCT; (e) to describe POCT training issues and modalities; and (f) to suggest strategies that optimize implementation of POCT and evaluation of patient outcomes.

NURSING AND THE INTERDISCIPLINARY TEAM

The Art and Science of Nursing

This section presents a brief overview of the dichotomous nature of nursing, the dynamic role of the nurse, and the effects of each on nurses' perception of POCT. Nursing scholars have written extensively on the nature of nursing as both science and art. The classic book, *Nursing: The Finest Art, An Illustrated History* (5), describes in exquisite detail the profession's struggle to maintain a balance between the scientific aspects of nursing and the fine art of nursing. Nursing is defined as "not merely a technique but a process that incorporates the elements of soul, mind, and imagination" (5). As they enter the 21st century facing a growing nursing shortage of global proportions (6,7), nurses are confronted with the increasingly complex and challenging task of doing more with less, and find themselves striving ardently to hold on to the "art" of nursing.

New technologies are constantly flooding the healthcare market. Fueled by the debate over whether technology is at odds with nursing, two divergent viewpoints have emerged: technological optimism and technological romanticism (8). Optimistic nurses link technology to the science of nursing. These clinicians believe that POCT devices are beneficial to patients as well as staff and can be readily assimilated into or used as an adjunct to nursing practice. Several illustrations of this viewpoint are found in nursing publications. In a comparative study of bedside and laboratory measurements of hemoglobin, nurse researchers found that bedside measurement of hemoglobin increased efficiency in patient care, decreased risk of blood transmitted infection for staff, and decreased cost to the patient (9). In a report on the use of a portable, handheld, whole-blood analyzer in a 577-bed trauma center, nurses determined that the immediate availability of critical patient information aided in initial patient assessment and allowed for more rapid clinical decision-making (10). They also concluded that this time-saving technology enabled nursing staff to spend less time waiting for laboratory results and more time caring for patients. In an article enumerating the top 10 recent innovations in patient care in trauma critical care settings, nurses ranked the use of point-of-care (POC) arterial blood gas analyzers as "number one" (11). Use of such devices was felt to significantly improve quality of care for the most critical patients and reduce weaning times for recovering patients.

Conversely, nurses who subscribe to technological romanticism see technology as detracting from the art of nursing. They believe POC devices that had the potential to save time and labor have actually increased the amount of time and labor nurses expend. A survey of 197 acute care clinicians representing a wide range of clinical specialties revealed that clinicians felt POCT saved medical, but not nursing, time (12). This increased pressure on nurses' time was noted as a limiting factor in another study that evaluated POCT in the general practice setting (13).

More often than not, the relative merits of POCT are viewed with ambiguity. In a survey of critical care nurse consultants, investigators found that an overwhelming majority of respondents reported that patient-care needs and current staffing patterns made it difficult for nurses to assume responsibility for *in vitro* diagnostic procedures (14). This finding appeared to be true even when nurses saw POCT as necessary and helpful in patient management.

In addition to the philosophical "nursing science versus nursing art" dilemma, nurses are being faced with more tangible changes in their roles and practice patterns. Many contemporary nurses were reared on the principles of primary nursing and professional practice. Participative decision-making, peer review, and collaborative practice have been firmly ingrained in their culture. Reengineering, restructuring, and redesign initiatives have changed the way the work of nursing is organized and the manner in which care is delivered. Work environment changes that have emerged from these initiatives include: (a) cross-training of nursing personnel to achieve the flexibility of a more diverse, multiskilled workforce; (b) decentralizing services to patient-care units; and (c) increasing the use of unlicensed personnel (2). In addition, there has been an increased reliance on contracted personnel to fill vital nursing vacancies. It is within the context of these new patient-care delivery models that nursing accomplishes all of its functions, including POCT.

Nurses assume many roles in the course of rendering patient care, some of which may be transparent to the outside observer. As coordinators of care and case managers, they ensure consistency across the continuum of care. Nurses integrate knowledge of the social, behavioral, biological, and physical sciences into patient care. Registered nurses supervise care rendered by both licensed and unlicensed assistive personnel and delegate aspects of care to these personnel based on the level of skill and expertise of each job description.

The role of the nurse is constantly evolving. To meet the needs of a highly technological, complex, and dynamic society, new theories, techniques, skills, and tools are being used in practice (15). Nurses provide services to patients in a variety of settings (hospitals, clinics, physicians' offices, and community outreach centers) and subsettings (acute care, critical care, long-term care/rehabilitation, psychiatric care, and ambulatory care). Specific tasks and functions vary with the requirements of the diverse patient populations. Nurses may manage an elaborate array of invasive devices, provide group therapy, administer complex medication therapies, and/or provide a protective environment for patients at risk for injury or infection. They may also perform POCT or supervise assistive personnel who perform such tests.

Nurses influence patient outcomes. The degree of positive or negative impact that a nursing intervention has on patient outcomes is related to the appropriateness of the intervention for the particular patient as well as the skill and technique used in carrying out the intervention (15). When nurses accept responsibility for POCT, they should participate in a thorough assessment of whether the particular test to be performed is appropriate for the patient population served. Once clinical relevance at the POC has been determined, nurses should be as committed to developing and maintaining the appropriate skills and techniques necessary to perform the test as they are to maintaining competencies in other patient-care functions.

Principles, Responsibilities, Ownership, Accountability, and Supervision

This section presents a brief overview of the allocation of accountability and responsibility among the various disciplines with a vested interest in POCT. The interdisciplinary nature of POCT programs is emphasized and indications for testing in a variety of healthcare settings are outlined. Finally, the roles of laboratory professionals and medical staff as members of the interdisciplinary POCT team are delineated.

In the United States, all hospitals, clinics, and private diagnostic laboratories are mandated to follow Clinical Laboratory Improvement Amendments of 1988 (CLIA '88) regulations, which require that the Centers for Medicare and Medicaid Services (CMS) issue certificates for laboratory testing sites (16). POCT programs are often the responsibility of laboratory personnel because clinical laboratory staff are familiar with QC, proficiency testing, and related record keeping to meet regulatory requirements. When there is laboratory oversight of POCT, the hospital is only required to apply for a single CLIA certificate.

POCT occurs at or near the site where patient care is rendered. Testing at the POC in acute and long-term care settings is usually referred to as bedside testing. These tests are typically performed by nursing staff. In acute care hospitals, POCT may also be performed by respiratory therapists, especially in critical care areas. Diagnostic laboratory tests are also carried out at the POC in outpatient settings. In locations such as ambulatory surgery, screening centers, and specialty care centers, the analyst is most often a member of the nursing staff. Nurses and emergency medical technologists operate POCT devices in emergency transport vehicles. In physicians' offices, and other areas in which there may not be a consistent nursing presence, such testing is performed by the medical staff or medical assistive personnel.

Nurse executives are ultimately accountable for the quality of nursing practice. When POCT is integrated into the practice of nurses, nurse leaders share responsibility with laboratory leaders for the quality of testing. Regardless of which discipline is listed as the responsible party, QC, performance enhancement, and cooperation are critical to the success of POCT programs (1).

Comprehensive patient care requires an interdisciplinary approach. An interdisciplinary approach takes the concept of "multidisciplinary" one step further (17) (Fig. 13.1). In multidisciplinary approaches, although many disciplines take part in the patient's care, their efforts may not be coordinated in a well-documented way. By contrast, care planning and evaluation processes are highly integrated in interdisciplinary approaches and there is collective ownership of the outcomes of care.

The development of an interdisciplinary POCT team, committee, or task force has been widely recommended to manage POCT issues (1,18,19). This team should be charged with setting standards for appropriate use, monitoring, and evaluation of POCT. Active representation is essential from any department that has an interest in this diagnostic methodology. Primary stakeholders include nursing, medical, and laboratory staff. Although the standards set should be site neutral, specific testing needs for each setting are unique. Membership should include representatives from general, critical, and ambulatory care settings. At appropriate junctures in the decision-making process, other departments such as infection control, pharmacy, purchasing, and nutrition support should be consulted.

The shift of testing from the core laboratories to decentralized stat laboratories or to the bedside has, to a large extent, been motivated by demand for more rapid results (20). The process for meeting the demand for more rapid turnaround time (TAT) of laboratory results is unique to each organization's needs, facilities, traditions, and mission. While rapid-transport vacuum systems with well-staffed stat laboratories offer an option to POCT in some organizations, many others are relying on POCT in one form or another (1). Some facilities place strategically located satellite laboratories near or within critical care areas. POC devices may be dedicated to areas in which there is demonstrated need, such as patient-care units, procedure areas, clinics, physicians' offices, rescue vehicles, and patients' homes (14).

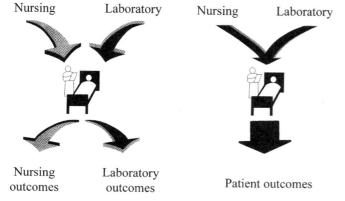

FIGURE 13.1. Schematic representation of interdisciplinary approaches as differentiated from multidisciplinary approaches. In multidisciplinary approaches, although many disciplines are involved in patient care, each discipline maintains responsibility for its own discipline-specific outcomes. In interdisciplinary approaches, the process of planning and evaluating care is highly integrated and there is collective ownership of the outcomes of that care.

Critical Care and Acute Care Settings

POCT is used to "facilitate immediate evidence-based medical decisions that improve[s] patient outcomes and reduce[s] patient acuity, criticality, morbidity, and mortality, especially during life-threatening crises and emergency resuscitations" (3). Nowhere is this a more appealing goal than in critical care areas (medical, surgical, neurotrauma, pediatric, and neonatal intensive care units; cardiothoracic surgical recovery units; postanesthesia care units; emergency departments; and operating rooms). A recent multicenter study found that performance of nonlaboratory personnel and medical technologists was equivalent for POCT in critical care settings (21).

Two primary benefits are gained by testing in or near critical care settings. First, the fast TAT afforded by POCT technology allows for more rapid and efficient clinical diagnosis, treatment, and management. The ability to generate diagnostic test results with enough speed to capture physicians' thoughts during critical moments at the bedside has been proposed as a practical optimizer for POCT (3). A rapid response time of 5 minutes or less is desirable during emergency resuscitations and life-threatening crises (22). In critical care areas, laboratory results that take longer than a few minutes to be reported may be obsolete (23). Second, the added value to patient care may not result from faster TAT, but rather from use of testing methods that require substantially less specimen (1). Depletion of blood volume is a serious problem in critical care, especially for neonates (22). Iatrogenic blood loss in critically ill patients has been estimated at 25 to 125 microliters/day (24). POCT methodologies offer the ability to use microsample technology, thereby reducing phlebotomy-related blood loss and promoting conservation of the patient's blood volume.

There are two potential benefits of POCT in critical care areas. First, POCT may reduce delays or cancellations of surgical procedures and may decrease time spent in the operating room due to unavailable laboratory results (24,25). Second, faster test results that stimulate diagnosis and therapeutic intervention could, conceivably, have significant economic benefits. In this era of climbing healthcare costs, managed care, an aging population, and more critically ill patients, the potential for POC technologies to decrease the length of stay and accelerate transfer from critical care to less costly acute-care settings is quite real (22). When weighing the cost of POCT against its potential benefit, institutions should conduct a multifaceted economic analysis that includes considerable attention to labor costs. These costs outweigh the costs of equipment and consumable materials for POCT and are of great concern to departments of nursing.

Costs associated with initial training, QC, proficiency testing, competency training, and test performance can be prohibitive in large teaching institutions. In such settings, there are many geographically distant sites staffed by a large number of nursing personnel who must rotate to cover patient-care requirements 24 hours a day, 7 days a week. By necessity, many of these nursing staff members must be trained and competent in POCT in order to ensure that proficient personnel are present at all times. Even in cases where other nursing personnel are certified to perform these tests, the registered nurses who supervise these workers must also maintain competency. Added costs are particularly high in critical care areas where patient-care needs are highly complex and variable and critical-care-unit staffing requirements are more expensive than in acute care areas.

Efforts are underway to study the workflow complexities associated with analysis of the cost effectiveness of POCT in critical care areas (26). These analyses take into consideration three factors that must coexist in order for cost-benefits to be achieved: (a) timely reporting of test results to the decision-making provider, (b) simultaneous availability of information gleaned from other vital diagnostic tests, and (c) efficient workflow processes, such as bed availability and patient transportation.

Bedside Testing

POCT occurs in satellite laboratories or at the bedside or other point of patient care. Although some critical care areas are serviced by satellite laboratories located either on or near the patient-care unit, tests performed in these "mini-labs" may be limited to a few critical tests. These limitations may be instituted due to space or resource constraints. As an adjunct to satellite laboratories, critical care nurses often perform bedside testing.

Acute care settings may not have access to critical care satellite laboratories, or the tests that are required in acute care settings may not be offered in the satellite sites. In the past decade, the clinical profile of hospitalized patients has been transformed to reflect a population with highly complex healthcare needs. The drive to diagnose and treat patients as quickly and efficiently as possible is almost as strong for acute-care patient populations as it is for critical care patients. Therefore, bedside testing is also common in acute care areas.

A variety of laboratory tests are performed at the bedside. These include, but are not limited to, tests listed in Table 13.1. An ever-expanding market of portable laboratory devices is generating an even broader range of bedside testing possibilities.

By far the most common test performed at the bedside is glucose monitoring. Approximately 16 million people, or 5.9% of the population of the United States, have diabetes (27). The incidence of diabetes in the general hospital population has been reported as approximately 10% (28). Bedside monitoring of capillary blood glucose enhances the management of hospital-

ized patients with diabetes (29). Immediate test results facilitate therapeutic decision making and, conceivably, can shorten hospital stays. Patient comfort is supported by avoiding the need for phlebotomy, and patient education is augmented by commencement of self-monitoring training during hospitalization.

Factors both intrinsic and extrinsic to the patient have been found to contribute to increased result variability with bedside operation of glucometers; hence, clinicians are cautioned to consider their sampling practices, patient characteristics, and meter limitations when interpreting results (30). Patient characteristics include disease state, hematocrit (31), and hydration status. Analyst factors include multiple operator techniques and use of noncapillary specimens. Standardization of procedures is vital to minimizing result variability in this patient population.

Arterial blood gas analysis has long been a standard practice in critical care units. In a study of critical care nursing practice, the second most commonly performed POC test was arterial blood gas analysis (14). A variety of instruments are available, such as those that involve placing an optical sensor either directly within the patient (*in vivo*) or in a tubing system that allows blood circulation to a sensor located outside the body (*ex vivo*) (32). These technologies are used to (a) evaluate adequacy of ventilation in patients with respiratory insufficiency, (b) determine optimal ventilator settings in patients with hypoxemia, (c) assess the efficacy of treatment for metabolic disorders, and (d) identify unstable cardiopulmonary status prior to the appearance of clinical symptoms (33).

Coagulation analyzers, although less common than glucose and arterial blood gas devices, are also used at the bedside in critical care and outpatient settings (14). Activated clotting time (ACT) and activated partial thromboplastin time (PTT) are frequently performed in these settings for monitoring of heparin anticoagulation and protamine neutralization (3). Nursing, medical technologist, and respiratory therapy staff perform coagulation testing on patients undergoing cardiac catheterization, coronary artery bypass graft surgery, organ transplantation, extracorporeal membrane oxygenation, and hemodialysis (34).

Potentially life-threatening electrolyte abnormalities commonly occur in critical care patients. Patient-care outcomes can be enhanced by bedside whole-blood analyzers that offer timely determination of electrolyte status (ionized calcium, potassium, sodium, chloride, and magnesium) in addition to oxygenation (PO_2, SO_2), ventilation (CO_2), perfusion (SvO_2, lactate), and acid-base balance (pH, bicarbonate) (32).

Measuring blood hemoglobin levels is a frequently performed clinical laboratory test and is an integral part of the nursing care of postoperative patients with volume deficits. Rapid detection of volume depletion in surgical intensive and intermediate care units may enable more timely administration of intravenous fluids or blood products. Concentration of blood hemoglobin is used to screen for anemia, polycythemia, hemolysis, and other altered hematologic states. Early intervention may facilitate attainment of discharge criteria of postanesthesia care units, resulting in a decrease in length and cost of hospitalization (9).

Testing of gastric contents often occurs on critical care as well as acute-care surgical units. The clinical utility of testing gastric pH and occult blood in critically ill patients is well established.

TABLE 13.1. TESTS COMMONLY PERFORMED AT THE BEDSIDE

Blood glucose monitoring
Arterial blood gas analysis
Hemoglobin monitoring
Coagulation studies
Electrolyte analysis
Fecal occult blood measurement
Gastric occult blood measurement
Gastric pH measurement
Urine dipstick analysis
Urine specific gravity measurement
Urine pregnancy testing
Urine drug testing
Use of nitrazine paper to test pH of other body fluids

Significant physiologic stress such as multiple trauma, prolonged artificial ventilation, gram-negative sepsis, and major surgery may precipitate upper gastrointestinal bleeding or ulcer formation (referred to as stress ulcer syndrome) (35). The ability to monitor gastric contents for pH and occult blood allows clinicians to define and prescribe optimal prophylactic therapy for patients at high risk for stress ulcer formation.

Other Situations

In ambulatory care settings, POCT offers more timely information to the healthcare provider as well as improved patient convenience. As patients are discharged earlier, assessment and detection of complex medical problems becomes even more critical in outpatient settings, such as clinics and specialty care centers, and in the home health arena. A recent study reported that nurse-led clinics could effectively use a combination of POCT and computerized decision-support software to manage patients on oral anticoagulation therapy (36).

Use of POCT in the interventional radiology and invasive cardiology setting has the potential to decrease waiting time for cardiovascular procedures. A recent study found that POCT decreased patient wait time for patients needing renal testing, while for patients needing coagulation testing, wait times only improved when systematic changes were made in workflow (37).

POCT also facilitates early diagnosis and intervention in emergency transport situations. Examples of rescue and other unique locations in which POCT is used include (a) space shuttles and space stations; (b) helicopter and fixed-wing aircraft for patient transport; (c) ships, submarines, and other nautical locales; (d) emergency ground vehicles such as ambulances; (e) disaster and emergency rescue situations; and (f) military field operations (3).

Role of Laboratory Professionals and Medical Staff

Responsibilities for POCT are distributed to reflect the training and expertise of each discipline, as well as organizational structures and processes. Laboratory personnel are knowledgeable about the preanalytical, analytical, and postanalytical limitations of POCT, and therefore, may assist in clinical interpretation of results (38). These professionals are experienced in such tasks as evaluating technology, correlating methods, defining normal ranges, writing protocols, managing instruments, coordinating supplies, providing backup, and overseeing and documenting training of clinicians who perform POC tests (39). Laboratory professionals have also assumed responsibility for QC checks, maintenance of logs, downloading of patient results, and preventive maintenance and troubleshooting of devices (10). In addition, when moderate- or high-complexity tests are performed at the POC, laboratory professionals are mandated by regulation to supervise the execution of these tests.

Medical staff must define situations for which POCT provides appropriate patient care, that is, which add value to patient services by improving patient outcome (1). According to C. Gresham Bayne (40), the "most important controversy surrounds what is least addressed—which tests are most critical to

the timely medical decisions of caregivers?" Physicians, as critical decision makers, should participate actively in the development of POC systems for their respective service areas. Furthermore, when medical staff are involved in the actual performance of the laboratory tests, they are responsible for test performance and all other POCT functions relegated to other disciplines that perform these diagnostic laboratory tests. Physicians who directly supervise medical assistive personnel who perform POC tests should also maintain competence in all aspects of the performance of those tests.

QUALITY CONTROL AND PROFICIENCY TESTING: THE NURSING PERSPECTIVE

This section presents a brief description of the principle of total quality management (TQM). A more detailed discussion of this principle is found in Chapter 26 of this text. There are five broad categories of POCT performance monitoring: (a) device validation, (b) QC, (c) proficiency testing, (d) compliance with institutional procedures, and (e) review of medical outcomes (38). Two of these approaches to monitoring the quality of laboratory testing (QC and proficiency testing) are described and the impact of these monitoring activities on nursing is discussed. Finally, recommendations are made to nurse leaders with respect to ensuring the success of quality assurance (QA) activities in maximizing quality patient outcomes.

Total Quality Management, Quality Control, and Proficiency Testing

Total quality management entails the critical review of all steps of the laboratory testing process: preanalytical (i.e., specimen collection, storage, and/or transport), analytical (i.e., competence of the analyst, and accuracy and reliability of analytic hardware and/or software used to perform the test), and postanalytical (i.e., documentation of patient results and integration of results into patient care) (41). Nurses are generally familiar with pre- and postanalytical steps, especially specimen collection and integration of results into patient care. They are less accustomed to analytical steps, which often occur in a laboratory distant to the point of patient care. When accepting the responsibility for bedside testing, nursing staff also accept responsibility for ensuring the quality of all steps of the laboratory testing process.

QC and proficiency testing are two well-established approaches to evaluate the quality of laboratory testing (41). QC uses pseudo specimens of known concentrations and composition to determine accuracy (relationship of a given result to the correct or true results) and precision (agreement between replicate analyses on the same sample). Proficiency testing employs the analysis of occasional specimens of unknown concentration or composition with the added feature of interlaboratory result comparison. Both QC and proficiency testing have also been used to assess the personal competence of analysts.

A regular schedule of inspections is necessary to maintain the high quality of device-dependent tests such as blood glucose monitoring. Many POCT programs rely on monthly inspections by laboratory personnel using a checklist of performance requirements. Such checklists include such activities as (a) daily QC within normal limits, or if not within normal limits, then with documented appropriate corrective action; (b) cleanliness of analytic hardware, such as glucose or hemoglobin meters; (c) proper storage of analytic software, such as test strips; (d) lots of test strips and control solutions properly labeled and within expiration date; (e) use of analytic hardware or software limited to certified analysts; and (f) performance of QC and proficiency testing by certified analysts (42). Recent technologic advances have resulted in analytic hardware with sophisticated data management capabilities that enable information such as performance of QC and proficiency testing by qualified analysts to be downloaded into a laboratory information system. This allows for data reduction and generation of reports, such as lists of unauthorized analysts and analysts who have not done QC within the specified time frame. Some items still require visual observation, such as cleanliness of meters; however, data management systems have allowed for streamlining this QA measure. In addition, many of these new devices are programmed to "lock out" the user if QC has not been performed (43).

Impact of Quality Assurance Activities on Nursing

The implementation of QA activities on busy patient-care units presents a formidable task to nursing staffs. Most laboratory professionals recommend rotating QC activities among staff, requiring analysts to document QC results and, when failures occur, to document corrective actions (42). The rotation of QC analysts is not easily accomplished on patient-care units. Laboratory personnel have restricted tasks in the testing cycle, whereas bedside caregivers have much broader responsibilities within the same cycle (4). Large test runs ("factory environments") in central laboratories contrast sharply with limited test runs ("boutique environments") on patient-care units.

The "24 hours a day, 7 days a week" nature of the typical nursing unit results in the need to train many nursing personnel to perform the desired POC test. Staffing mix (number of registered nurses and other licensed and unlicensed nursing staff) and shift rotation schedules vary from day to day. The opportunity to perform a particular test varies from moment to moment, depending upon the nature of the patient population on the unit and the assigned patient caseload. For tests that are performed with higher frequency, this tends to be less of a problem. However, for tests that are performed sporadically, the opportunity to perform QC or proficiency testing may be limited. It is the infrequent analyst who would potentially benefit most from proficiency testing. Therein lies the quandary. Proficiency testing provides an opportunity for nursing staff to exercise the skills required for maintenance of competency but also requires opportunity and time, an increasingly scarce commodity.

Cost analyses of POCT have revealed that costs are higher on units on which large numbers of nursing staff perform relatively fewer tests. This is in part due to the training and competency requirements of analysts. It has been recommended that organizations should limit the performance of bedside glucose testing to a limited number of analysts on clinical units where testing is

required more than five times per day (42). Unfortunately, with current staff mix and scheduling practices, this may not be possible. In addition, geographic distances between nursing units and minimum staffing levels may not allow for alternatives such as sharing of analytical hardware among units.

Laboratory professionals have a strong background in process QC. They are comfortable with such analytical concepts as calibration, accuracy, and precision (41). The same statement is not typically true of nurses and other nonlaboratory professionals who are more outcome oriented. Many nurses consider performance of QC a less than optimal use of their precious time—time that could be better spent at the bedside giving direct care to the patient. These same nurses are generally overconfident in the reliability of the devices, test strips, and reagents used in POCT. Once skeptics are convinced that instrumentation is not necessarily foolproof, they may concede the importance of QC, but would still prefer that the laboratory perform these procedures. Although some organizations have delegated QC checks to laboratory personnel (10), the HCFA expects that staff performing patient tests will also perform QC and proficiency testing (1). The HCFA also specifies that the function of the laboratory is to oversee and provide consultation for POC services.

Some clinicians that perform QC tasks do so for the wrong reasons. They may focus more on the regulatory aspect of the task and less on the clinical utility of these measurements. Since more importance is attached to patient outcomes than to processes defined by regulation, clinicians may tend to undervalue the benefits of QC.

The Role of Nursing Leadership in Total Quality Management

If nursing leaders do not create a vision for front-line staff of how POCT adds value to patient care, then any attempt at implementing such a program will surely fail. The importance and proper use of QC and proficiency testing should be reinforced as a vital tool for performance enhancement rather than as sheer drudgery or of negligible value (41). Nurse leaders should work with laboratory leaders in streamlining QC and proficiency testing requirements to achieve goals with the least possible consumption of resources. Training and education must include an emphasis on TQM, in which the entire cycle of the process is taken into consideration when seeking to enhance performance.

PERFORMANCE ENHANCEMENT

This section presents an overview of the nine dimensions of performance identified by the Joint Commission for Accreditation of Healthcare Organizations (JCAHO) and their application to POCT. Regulatory requirements are summarized and the use of TQM as a strategy to enhance performance is discussed.

The JCAHO suggests that the most important component of a solid POCT program is the integration of the program with the organization's performance improvement initiatives (44). The JCAHO has defined a host of requirements for POCT (all of which are equivalent to or exceed those of government regu-

TABLE 13.2. JCAHO DIMENSIONS OF PERFORMANCE AS APPLIED TO POINT-OF-CARE TESTING

Dimension	Goal	Goal-attainment Activities
Efficacy	Medical efficacy in diagnosis, treatment, and management	Medical effectiveness and outcomes studies Results reporting
Appropriateness	Appropriateness of particular tests for specific patient populations	Selection of test menu Choice of test method and/or instrumentation
Availability	The availability of the particular test to the patient who needs it	Selection of test menu Personnel selection
Effectiveness	The degree to which the test is done in the correct manner to achieve desired patient outcomes	Personnel training Instrument calibration Quality control Written procedures Test performance
Timeliness	The degree to which the test is performed at the necessary time during the patient's episode of care	Test performance Written procedures
Safety	The degree to which the risk posed by the test to patients and healthcare providers is minimized	Maintenance of equipment Specimen collection and handling Bloodborne pathogen training
Efficiency	The ratio of patient outcome to resources required to perform point-of-care testing	Cost-benefit analysis
Continuity	The continuity of testing over time	Proficiency testing Quality control Adherence to written procedures
Respect and caring	The degree to which use of these tests demonstrates respect and caring for the patient	Patient satisfaction

JCAHO, Joint Commission on Accreditation of Healthcare Organizations.

lations) and has outlined nine dimensions of performance to aid in meeting these requirements (45). By focusing on these dimensions, interdisciplinary POCT teams are able to measure compliance with regulatory requirements and track progress toward improvement. Quality is about choice—choice of test method and/or instrumentation, selection and training of personnel, written procedures, instrument calibration, equipment maintenance, QC, specimen collection/handling, and test performance (44). Each choice affects the quality of patient care and the achievement of desired outcomes. Table 13.2 outlines the JCAHO dimensions of performance as they can be applied to POCT goals and goal-attainment activities.

Doing the Right Thing

The first two dimensions revolve around what is done. The aim is simple—do the right thing. The JCAHO requires definition of medical use for all laboratory tests performed at the point of patient care. By looking at the efficacy and appropriateness of particular POC tests for specific patient populations, organizations can ensure that the test is relevant to the patient's clinical needs, given the current state of the art. To this end, clinicians are urged to define the medical situations for which POCT provides appropriate care. These definitions should include those situations for which POCT improves decision-making and patient outcomes.

Doing the Right Thing Well

The remaining dimensions revolve around how organizations do what they do. Once it has been determined that the right POC tests are being done, organizations need to ensure that the tests are done well. The appropriate test should be available to those patients who need it. The degree to which the test is done in the correct manner to achieve desired patient outcomes has an impact on the effectiveness of testing. The test should be provided at the necessary time during the patient's episode of care, resulting in therapeutic TAT for temporal optimization. In addition, the risk to patients and healthcare providers should be minimized, including biohazard control, containment, and disposal. Other dimensions of performance to be considered include (a) ratio of patient outcomes to resources required, or the efficiency of POCT; (b) continuity of testing over time; and (c) respect and caring with which testing is provided to patients, including the elimination of unnecessary duplicate testing.

Regulatory requirements help to ensure that tests are done in a consistent, appropriate manner. These requirements are discussed in greater detail in Chapter 27 of this text. These provisions include (a) written policies delegating responsibility and accountability for the various aspects of testing, including performance and supervision of performance; (b) written procedures describing how to correctly perform the patient test and QC procedures, as well as the appropriate documentation of both; (c) training and documentation of continued competence of analysts; (d) performance of QC checks that meet or exceed manufacturer's minimum requirements and review of such checks with documented remedial actions; and (e) surveillance of patient test results and quality monitors (39).

Analysis of common accreditation inspection deficiencies highlights the importance of the total quality principle and continuous performance improvement for POCT. The total quality principle for POCT uses the TQM strategy as operationalized through each organization's self-determined performance enhancement program to meet all patients' needs irrespective of where the diagnostic test is performed (34).

CASE STUDIES (THE JOHNS HOPKINS HOSPITAL AND HEALTH SYSTEM)

This section briefly describes the Johns Hopkins Hospital and the Johns Hopkins Health System, as well as the decentralized management system under which it operates. Three case studies are presented. The first is a description of how the development of a successful interdisciplinary POC team was accomplished in a decentralized management environment. This is followed by an illustration of nursing leadership in defining the role of bedside testing. The final case study presents a description of the implementation of bedside testing on a clinical nursing unit that has an integrated patient-care delivery system.

The Johns Hopkins Health System is comprised of two acute care hospitals, a chronic care hospital and nursing home, a 19-site ambulatory care practice, and a home health service. The 1,025-bed Johns Hopkins Hospital offers highly specialized care to patients from all over the world. The 678-bed Johns Hopkins Bayview Medical Center includes a 331-bed community teaching hospital and 347 nonacute beds.

The Johns Hopkins Hospital functions under a decentralized management system in which operating responsibilities and financial accountability are held by the clinical departments (referred to as functional units) (46). A physician chief is at the helm of each functional unit, with a nursing director and an administrator completing the management triad. There are 10 functional units that act as, in effect, specialty hospitals: emergency medicine, medicine, neurosciences, obstetrics and gynecology, ophthalmology, oncology, pediatrics, psychiatry, surgery, and outpatient center. In day-to-day operations, these functional units are serviced by numerous affiliate support departments, one of which is the department of pathology.

In 1993, the Laboratory Advisory Committee of the Medical Board decided to address the regulatory requirements specific to POCT as a joint initiative of the departments of pathology and nursing. A simultaneous decision was made that all systems, tests, kits, or reagents designed for use in POCT must be reviewed by the department of pathology prior to purchase. Developing a successful program in this highly decentralized environment presented a great challenge to the organization and to the disciplines involved. While the short-term goal has been to standardize POC instrumentation and processes across all functional units within the Johns Hopkins Hospital, the long-term goal is to do so throughout the entire Health System.

Team Building in a Decentralized Management Environment

The formidable task of building a successful interdisciplinary team was compounded by the fact that typical interactions between primary patient-care providers (nursing and medical staff) and the diagnostic support department (pathology staff) have been related to patient-specific laboratory transactions. The potential for nurses and physicians to view laboratory personnel

as attempting to "tread on their turf" was quite real. Fortunately, in its continual quest for service excellence, Johns Hopkins Medicine has defined service standards that form an integral part of the job descriptions of all employees. Familiar concepts such as customer relations, self-management, teamwork, communication, ownership/accountability, and continuous performance improvement have provided the framework through which the work of our team has been accomplished.

The value of customer relations cannot be underestimated. Patients and families are not the sole customers of healthcare providers. Relationships between and among internal customers are pivotal to the accomplishment of interdisciplinary goals. Basic practices such as treating each other with respect and courtesy and acknowledging different perspectives have been indispensable to the successful functioning of our team. It was made clear from the start that the pathologist would take a facilitating, rather than authoritarian, stance. Without a nursing co-chair, quality improvement efforts might have been seen as intrusive (47).

Each discipline has a unique worldview, and the nature of that paradigm colors how members interact with the rest of the world and with each other. The intangible notion of quality has been conceptualized in a variety of ways (4). Healthcare providers often define quality in subjective terms. The clinical utility of test results, the convenience of bedside testing, and the ability to achieve a "real-time" evaluation of the patient's status were seen by our nurses and physicians as valuable commodities. Laboratory personnel, on the other hand, are more objective, assigning value to that which is constant, measurable, and technically based. Because of these differences in perception, nursing and medical staff initially exhibited overconfidence in the reliability of POCT instruments. Likewise, laboratory personnel tended to underestimate the impact of QC requirements on the functioning of patient-care units. Recognition and acceptance of divergent viewpoints was essential to avoiding turf battles and finger-pointing.

A pivotal step in understanding the customer is defining each discipline's requirements for a POC system (19). A team evaluation of glucose meters provided the opportunity for representatives of each discipline to discuss their requirements. Nursing staff desired a system that was portable, durable, reliable, simple to operate, easy to learn to use, low maintenance, and that minimized infection control hazards. They also wanted a device that was operationally similar to devices that patients would use at home so that self-management training could occur during hospitalization. Laboratory staff desired an instrument that was accurate, precise, and that stored QC and patient test results that could be downloaded into a central data station in the laboratory to track QC compliance.

Teamwork and communication are basic concepts that go hand in hand. Offering advice to nurse executives about interdisciplinary teams, Kathy Sanford (48) wrote that teamwork "is work and people will not commit energy to it unless they see value in it." Early on, we obtained the necessary "buy-in" from each discipline, as each became acutely aware of the importance of the interdisciplinary team in assuring optimal patient outcomes. For teams to work as they are meant to work, team leaders and members must be able and willing to acknowledge the expertise of team members from each discipline and the valuable contributions each makes to the success of the venture (49). Representatives from nursing, medicine, and pathology recognize and support the skills and qualities that each discipline brings to our team. Team members (and leaders) willingly exchange information with each other, and defer to each other's authority in their respective fields. A spirit of collegiality, as evidenced by cooperation, trust, respect, and timely responsiveness to requests, has been critical to the success of our team.

Given the decentralized nature of our organization, it is even more important that each team member be committed to the principles of self-management and ownership/accountability. As role models in the clinical arena, nursing and medical staff representatives abide by institutional policies and procedures related to POCT and take ownership of the responsible use of equipment and resources. They also take on the responsibility for encouraging an ongoing assessment of the clinical relevance of POCT as well as the associated human and resource requirements. Laboratory representatives are responsible for assessing the impact of tests that could be moved back to the laboratories, as well as the supervisory needs related to moderately and highly complex tests that need to be performed at the bedside. Each team member is responsible for ensuring that all stakeholders are involved in any decisions that affect POCT.

Mutuality has been explored as an interaction style that encourages accountability. Henson (50) defines mutuality as "a dynamic process characterized by an exchange between people related to a common goal or shared purpose." Each member of our team believes the other can contribute in a manner conducive to decision making. Discussions reflect give-and-take, exchange of ideas, respect for all possibilities, creativity, and humor. We each have a stake in the common goal of improved patient outcomes.

Finally, the team is guided by the principles of continuous performance improvement. The organization's strategic initiatives as well as the quality initiatives of the JCAHO have ensured that continuous performance improvement has become ingrained in our culture. It is universally recognized that performance of important functions and processes (such as POCT) is reflected in patient outcomes, the cost or efficiency of services, and patients' and others' satisfaction. Each functional unit and each department (including nursing and pathology) have well-defined performance improvement programs that are based on the institution's model. The cycle for performance improvement in this model is composed of activities that include plan, design, measurement, assessment, improvement, communication, and monitoring improvement of new or current functions or processes of patient care (51). Interdisciplinary performance improvement activities are highly encouraged throughout the organization.

Nursing Leadership in Defining the Role of Point-of-Care Testing

The nursing clinical performance improvement program has three major intents: (a) to maximize the health of patients served, (b) to improve the processes of patient care, and (c) to

efficiently utilize the resources required to meet these objectives (52). Priorities are based on those activities that have the greatest potential to improve clinical processes and patient outcomes. The vice president for nursing and patient-care services has the authority and responsibility for establishing and maintaining nursing care and service standards and for routinely measuring performance and outcomes against these standards. Directors of nursing are responsible for the implementation of the program in their respective functional units and are accountable for the quality of nursing care in those units. They identify unit-specific competencies and hold all clinical nursing staff accountable for demonstrating individual competencies. The central department of nursing administration supports these efforts by coordinating professional practice, staff education, performance improvement, research, and clinical systems initiatives that cross the entire department of nursing.

One such initiative, born out of identified opportunities for performance improvement, is the POCT program. As the program was beginning to take shape, each director of nursing initiated discussions with the chiefs of service in their respective functional units regarding the clinical utility of bedside testing in each of the patient-care areas. Several factors were taken into consideration. First, the hospital has several satellite laboratories for the adult, pediatric, and neonatal critical care units, as well as the emergency department. The main purpose of these laboratories is to provide rapid turnover of a limited number of critical tests. Second, an extensive labor cost analysis of tests done at the bedside was completed for each clinical nursing unit. This included a detailed accounting of labor costs related to actual performance of patient tests, performance of QC, proficiency testing, and training and annual updates to maintain analyst competency. Finally, a review of the clinical pertinence of providing the test on the nursing unit, versus sending the test to the central or stat laboratories, was discussed. For most tests, the critical decision-making point revolved around whether the results of the tests were needed for clinical decision-making purposes in less than 1 hour (which is the current TAT for the stat laboratory).

Discussions of clinical pertinence went on over a period of months. Nurse managers within each functional unit shared their views on this issue and held discussions with the medical directors of their units relative to the needs of their particular patient populations. The ensuing intellectual discourse often resulted in consultation with key representatives of the department of pathology for their expertise in identifying laboratory resources and alternatives to POCT.

The culmination of this massive effort was the elimination of a variety of nondevice bedside tests from the patient-care units, with the retention of only those tests that were felt to be clinically necessary to remain at the bedside. Use of one device-dependent test (urine-specific gravity) was also reduced at the point of patient care. Use of other device-dependent tests has not changed as a result of this effort.

As seems to be the case in many comparable institutions, bedside glucose testing has remained at the POC and is performed on over 60 of the clinical nursing units. Internal laboratory and clinical unit evaluations have resulted in the selection of a single blood-glucose monitoring system that uses glucose biosensors (test strips) in conjunction with a handheld, digital, battery-powered device to be used throughout the institution. These devices were validated in both acute care and critical care sites. This practice is consistent with recommendations that use of glucose dehydrogenase-based biosensors to guide insulin therapy be validated in critical care settings for protocols for which accuracy requirements need to be carefully defined (53). Clinical effectiveness of such tests may be reduced by drugs, acid-base imbalances, hyperosmolality, hyperviscosity, and other potentially confounding variables.

Other device-dependent tests are used in selected areas only, for much smaller numbers of patients who would benefit from these tests being done at the bedside. For example, bedside hemoglobin measurements are done in only a few areas. Five of these are in the surgical functional unit (cardiac surgical intensive care unit, surgical intensive care unit, intermediate care unit, postanesthesia recovery unit, and the cardiac progressive care unit), and one is in the outpatient functional unit (again, on a postanesthesia recovery unit). Again, laboratory and clinical unit evaluations resulted in the selection of a single hemoglobin monitoring system.

ACT testing is done in the operating room (by cardiovascular perfusionists), on the renal dialysis unit (by nurses), in the cardiovascular diagnostic laboratory (by technologists and nurses), and in the pediatric intensive care unit (by respiratory therapists). Prothrombin time tests are performed by nurses in the outpatient cardiac clinic and in home health care. Activated PTT tests are done by nurses in home health care.

Before institutional reevaluation of POCT, many nursing units were sites for bedside urine-specific gravity testing. Some units used urometers to obtain these measurements and other units that required a more precise determination, such as pediatrics, used total solids refractometry. Laboratory evaluation determined that total solids refractometry is more precise, less costly to QC (due to the larger volume of solution needed for QC procedures on urometers), and less of an infection control hazard. Therefore, it was decided that all units performing this test would use total solids meters. In addition, urine-specific gravity testing is classified as a moderately complex test by CLIA '88, and, as such, is subject to more stringent regulations than waived testing. When the needs and resources of the units were reassessed, it was determined that there were only two sites in which it was necessary to perform urine-specific gravity testing at the point of patient care. These were clinical units on which chemotherapy is administered to children, and rapid determination of urine-specific gravity plays a critical role in the administration of these agents in pediatric populations. Other clinical units that require urine-specific gravity measurements with a 1-hour therapeutic TAT now send their patient specimens to the core laboratory via a STAT messenger.

In past years, a variety of both device- and nondevice-dependent tests "showed up" at the bedside and became a part of the nursing care of patients throughout the hospital. The velocity of the technologic revolution made it difficult for the government to keep pace with the influx of bedside laboratory tests (54). The government has made a concerted effort to rectify this problem, and regulations are now beginning to catch up with the technologic revolution. In efforts to protect the public, nondevice tests that used to be performed at the bedside without benefit of QC activities are now more tightly regulated. The increased QC requirements and the determination that many of these tests did not need to be done at every bedside resulted in decreased use of nondevice tests at the POC in our institution.

Although use of these tests at the bedside has decreased in our institution, measurements of gastric and/or fecal occult blood appear to be the most frequently performed nondevice-dependent laboratory tests at the POC. Laboratory and clinical unit evaluations resulted in the selection of a single product for fecal occult blood testing as well as a single product for testing of gastric contents for occult blood. These tests are done on most psychiatric, pediatric, medical, and surgical units, and a few oncology units. The adult emergency department sends gastric and fecal specimens to its satellite laboratory.

Gastric pH testing is done on many surgical units (including the cardiac surgical intensive care, surgical intensive care, and intermediate care units) using a standardized product. The test is also performed in the pediatric emergency room and the endoscopy suites.

Another manual test used on a much less frequent basis is urine dipstick testing. Laboratory and bedside evaluations resulted in the selection of two products for use throughout the institution. These include one test strip that allows testing of glucose, protein, pH, blood, ketones, and bilirubin, and a second test strip that allows testing for glucose and protein only. These tests have been determined to be clinically pertinent on most surgical and pediatric units.

Finally, urine pregnancy testing is performed in a limited number of settings throughout the institution. Again, laboratory and clinical unit evaluations allowed for selection of a single product. Early detection of pregnancy has been deemed important in the outpatient surgery recovery room, the women's health center, the diabetes center, and two medical clinics.

Nursing leadership has kept a close eye on the effect of recent changes in tests performed at the POC. For a few units that decided to send fecal and gastric occult blood tests to the core laboratories, an insufficient TAT due to transport difficulties in our large institution resulted in discussions regarding the return of these tests to the bedside. In response to laboratory and other turnaround concerns, the institution purchased a rapid-transport vacuum system. It has been recorded that institutions with appropriate placement of pneumatic tube stations, given adequate staffing, can provide essentially equivalent TATs for central laboratories to TATs from stat satellite laboratories (14). This has been our experience.

As new technologies are introduced, and requests are made to incorporate them into the POCT program, nursing leadership will be at the forefront of decision making. The unique relationship between the directors of nursing and the functional unit directors enables an ongoing and comprehensive assessment of the clinical value of tests approved for bedside use by the laboratory. The collaboration of nursing leadership and laboratory leadership has served to facilitate implementation of clinically pertinent tests at the POC.

Bedside Testing in an Integrated Patient-Care Delivery System

As is the case in many comparable institutions, dramatic changes in patient-care requirements and the societal mandate for stewardship of valuable healthcare resources have directly resulted in a reengineering of our patient-care delivery system. Many Hopkins nurses were reared on the principles of primary nursing and professional practice. Seeking to preserve these fundamental values, our nursing service department defined new structures and processes that would support the roles, functions, and relationships within the new care delivery model.

Within our system for patient-care delivery, the nurse manager is accountable for the overall direction of the clinical unit's model, and, as such, is accountable for POCT by nursing personnel on that unit. Nurse clinicians take a leadership role in the management of patient-care systems and resources. In our decentralized management system, while each job description is standardized, the focus of each role varies according to the unit's patient-care requirements. For clinical units that have defined a need for POCT, nurse clinicians are generally appointed to manage that testing. Responsibilities may include oversight of QC activities, ongoing training and education of analysts, and participation in new device trials.

A schematic representation of our model for patient-care delivery at the clinical unit level is depicted in Fig. 13.2. Membership of the model is comprised of a diverse, multiskilled workforce that is maximized to its fullest extent of competency, education, and licensure (55). For example, nurse clinicians (registered nurses), licensed practical nurses, and unlicensed trained assistive personnel (clinical nursing interns, clinical technicians, and clinical associates) perform the actual patient tests.

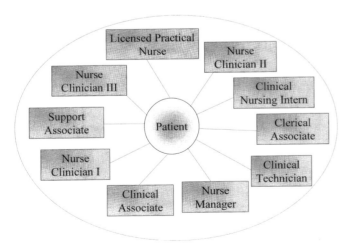

FIGURE 13.2. Schematic representation of The Johns Hopkins Patient Care Delivery Model. The focus of care delivered by this integrated multiskilled team is the patient. It is this structure that supports continuity of care in all aspects of nursing care, including point-of-care testing (POCT). The nurse manager is accountable for POCT on the unit. Nurse clinicians, licensed practical nurses, clinical nursing interns, clinical technicians, and clinical associates perform point-of-care tests. Support associates manage testing supplies and quality control materials and clerical associates ensure availability of appropriate documentation tools.

Support associates manage unit supplies of testing and QC materials and may also serve as "runners" to deliver specimens to the critical care or emergency department satellite laboratories. Clerical associates ensure the availability of documentation forms. Personal responsibility and teamwork are key to the success of POCT at the unit level.

TRAINING PROGRAMS AND MODALITIES

Overview of Training

Training is a critical component of the total quality program for POCT. Staff education related to bedside testing includes initial orientation, ongoing continuing education, and retraining/refreshers for users. Learning needs and educational program design are determined by test complexity, institutional needs, and the professional disciplines involved. These staff-training requirements are often cited as a disadvantage associated with POCT (38). The following sections examine educational design elements and strategies that may be used to minimize some of the obstacles associated with POCT training.

Goals of Training

The primary goal of POCT training programs is to assure that staff is competent in performing testing, thereby assuring accurate patient results. Since POCT is usually performed by nursing staff with limited technical expertise, adequate training is needed to improve test performance and to prevent errors (56). Nursing personnel sometimes make errors because of lack of understanding of test systems and the complex technology involved in producing a seemingly simple test result. More commonly, nursing personnel perform POCT procedures incorrectly because of distraction or inattention to details. In both of these scenarios, training may assist in pointing out the patient consequences of not following testing procedures carefully (56).

The secondary goal of training programs is compliance with hospital and laboratory regulatory agency standards (CLIA, JCAHO, and the College of American Pathologists [CAP]). The CAP requires that "(1) all personnel are knowledgeable about the contents of procedure manuals . . . relevant to the scope of their testing activities; (b) the person(s) performing the tests have adequate, specific training and orientation to perform the tests offered; and (c) there is a documented program to ensure that each person performing POCT maintains satisfactory levels of competence." The JCAHO requires that operators have "adequate, specific training," and that observation of technique, acceptable performance of QC procedures, or split sample unknowns be used to validate/document staff training and competence (39).

In order to achieve these two goals, POCT training programs should include content about the following:

- Appropriate uses and limitations of the test
- Specimen collection and handling procedures
- Patient test procedure
- Patient results reporting and documentation
- Importance of QC and QC procedures

- Safety measures (standard precautions, biohazard waste disposal, sharps handling)
- Maintenance of devices
- Troubleshooting and resources
- Follow-up for abnormal results

The JCAHO recommends the development and use of a training manual that includes a list of the training activities and materials to be used, and a checklist of the steps involved in performing the test (44).

Challenges of Point-of-Care Testing Training

There are major challenges related to POCT training for an institution. These challenges include training large numbers of users who have many competing patient-care responsibilities, limited time for training, widely varying educational levels, and dealing with staff resistance to POCT procedures. Strategies to overcome these barriers must be built into educational program design and instructional methodologies if training is to be effective.

Nursing staff members are responsible for many aspects of patient care, and very often nurses consider POCT "a secondary responsibility that is accorded lower priority than other patient-focused nursing responsibilities" (39). Restricting POCT to those tests for which immediate patient results are needed to guide decisions about clinical care is helpful in overcoming this problem. If nurses are performing laboratory testing only when it is genuinely needed for patient care, it is more likely to be viewed as an important activity.

In many institutions, time for staff education and training is not built into staffing models and the number of budgeted nursing positions. This factor, combined with increasing patient acuity, staffing shortages, and multiple competing patient-care priorities, makes time for training limited. Strategies to overcome this barrier include the following:

- Keeping training content concise and focused on just the "need to know"
- Using alternatives to classroom training, such as self-study packets, computer-based learning modules, and videotapes
- Scheduling class times during staff "downtimes" and in a nearby location

When institutions implement a new POC test, very often large numbers of employees with a wide range of educational levels must be trained. These individuals range from physicians with postdoctoral degrees to unlicensed assistive personnel with high school diplomas. In order to provide information at a level appropriate for the educational levels of the learners, it may be necessary to offer a variety of educational approaches and programs. For example, nurses and physicians may learn quite well by reading a printed self-learning packet; however, it may be more effective educationally to offer classes with the opportunity for hands-on practice for unlicensed assistive personnel.

Dealing with resistance against POCT procedures is one of the most challenging issues in POCT training (19). Nursing staff have limited technical laboratory expertise, and are often unfamiliar with issues such as QC and QA of laboratory testing. "Clinical staff simply do not have the 'cultural orientation' of the laboratorian to intuitively understand why we are compulsive about issues like calibrating instruments and quality control. . . . They [nurses] do not understand the need for QC; they view it as an unnecessary, nonpatient-care activity, and are passionately outspoken about their belief that patient test results are reliable without QC" (14). Nurses often believe that quality is in the device, and because of their lack of technical training, are often not aware of the test variability produced by operator technique (57). Education aimed at correcting these misconceptions and pointing out the potential impact of incorrect procedures or techniques on patient test results and clinical care is the most effective means of overcoming this barrier.

Who Is Responsible for Training?

The American Society for Clinical Laboratory Science (ASCLS) position paper on POCT finalized in 1996 (58) states, "The laboratory must maintain responsibility for the development of appropriate training programs for the nonlaboratory personnel in the use of ancillary testing equipment, test procedures, documentation, review of test results, performance and monitoring of QC, corrective action, proficiency testing, and equipment management. A review of personnel competency must be built into these programs." This position is based on the premise that clinical laboratory scientists have the expertise and experience in laboratory testing/technologies, and the ASCLS in this same document has gone so far as to say, "Training of nonlaboratory personnel must be done through a structured curriculum under the auspices of trained laboratory personnel."

However, most POCT is done by nursing personnel, and the nursing service is responsible for overseeing such testing, including direct supervision of operators, day-to-day operation of the nursing unit, unit staffing/budgeting, and overall patient-care quality. Laboratory personnel have a narrower scope of patient-care responsibilities, and often have difficulty understanding the impact of bedside testing procedures on the nursing unit. For these reasons, in many institutions, nursing departments take primary responsibility for POCT training (39). The most effective approach to this dilemma would be to develop and implement educational programs as a collaborative effort between laboratory and nursing services.

Adult Education Principles

In order to be effective, POCT training programs must be based on principles of adult learning and incorporate learner needs into program design and delivery. The literature describing the principles of adult learning is immense (59–63). Some of these principles with direct application to POCT training include:

- Adults must identify the need to learn.
- Adults prefer learning experiences that are problem centered, practical, immediately applicable, and not too theoretical.
- Adults come to learning situations with existing knowledge and prior experiences, which need to be recognized, built on, and sometimes unlearned.

- Adults have self-esteem needs that need to be protected/supported in learning experiences.
- Adults prefer learning situations that show respect for the individual, including not preaching to or "talking down" to them, showing respect for their time, and providing for their physical comfort.
- Adults learn best when they are active participants in the learning experience.

It is important that planning and implementation for the POCT training program incorporate these principles to enhance learning and retention.

Training Methodologies

There are a wide variety of instructional methods that may be used in POCT education, including classroom training (lecture/demonstration), on-the-job training, and self-study using printed materials, multimedia presentations, and/or computer-assisted instructional programs. The training methodology(ies) selected should be determined by the type of learning to be achieved (cognitive, psychomotor, or affective), staff time available/allocated for training, cost, learner preference, and institutional culture. Frequently, use of a combination of instructional methods is effective (64) (Table 13.3).

Classroom instruction, which includes both didactic information and demonstration with hands-on practice, is a very frequently used teaching modality for bedside testing. Taking employees off the job for instruction is costly, but it is the preferred method in many institutions. Instructors for POCT classes can be test manufacturer representatives, nursing service educators, and/or laboratory service employees. There are advantages and disadvantages associated with the employment of each type of instructor. The use of manufacturer representatives is cost saving for the institution, and these persons have advanced knowledge of the testing mechanism itself. However, they are often unfamiliar with the institution-specific procedures and QC program, and may not be able to teach that content effectively. In most institutions, nursing educators are able to teach POCT effectively; however, as with bedside nurses, they have many competing priorities, and may not have the time available to teach all of the classes needed. Laboratory service employees possess an in-depth knowledge of the testing devices and QC procedures, but often do not understand the overall picture of patient-care and unit operations. In many situations, laboratory employees are unable to present information at a level helpful to nursing personnel and in a style that communicates an understanding of the working environment and multiple priorities of the nurse. Ideally, classroom instruction should be a collaborative effort among the manufacturer, nursing service, and laboratory personnel, using the strengths inherent to each group. Having representatives from each of these parties may be quite time-consuming and costly, and an effective alternative would be to involve all three parties in the educational program planning and design.

Some institutions are now beginning to use new instructional technologies to enhance and improve training. Web-based instruction (WBI) over the Internet or an institution's intranet

TABLE 13.3. INSTRUCTIONAL METHODOLOGIES

Methodology	Type of Learning	Advantages	Disadvantages	Recommendations for Use
Classroom training Lecture Demonstration with return demonstration Discussion	Cognitive Psychomotor Affective	Preferred learning modality by many people; meets socialization needs of staff; resistance issues may be dealt with	Costly because of need to take employees off the job and reliance on "live" instructors; need to offer classes for off-shift and weekend employees; difficult to accommodate large groups of employees because of hands-on practice component; requires training equipment/supplies for classroom use	Schedule enough sessions to limit group size to 12 or less; offer classes geographically close and at staff "down times"
On-the-job training	Cognitive, psychomotor, affective	May be done in employee "down time"; cost effective; uses equipment/supplies available on nursing units	Uses unit-based trainers who need training; incorrect procedures or inappropriate shortcuts may be passed on	Provide good training for trainers; use standardized handouts, skill checklists to assure consistency of information
Self-study program Printed self-learning packet Multimedia presentations (videotape, slide/tape program, computer-assisted instruction)	Cognitive Cognitive, psychomotor	Cost effective; available to staff at any time; available when instructors may not be; allows self-paced learning; helpful for areas with high staff turnover rates and need for frequent orientation of new employees; videotapes often available from test vendors	Not a preferred learning method for many individuals; multimedia/computer-based programs require equipment, hardware/software, which may be costly; institution-specific multimedia presentations costly and time-consuming to produce	Use unit-based trainers to validate learning via written test and skill checklist

is one of these new approaches to staff education that may be an effective modality in bedside testing training. WBI is interactive, multimedia, computer-based instruction in which the learner is tested online and receives automatic, immediate feedback until an acceptable level of competence is detected. Test scores may be downloaded into databases, and reports for users, educators, and managers may be automatically generated and distributed (65,66). WBI is commonly said to provide "just enough, just in time" learning, merging staff training with performance support, and to provide training that is twice as effective, because of its highly interactive nature, in half of the time. New instructional technologies such as WBI may be extraordinarily helpful in overcoming some of the problems currently associated with POCT training.

Regardless of the instructional methodologies selected for POCT training, supplemental educational resources for users should be readily available on the nursing units. These include printed and/or online reference materials, procedure manuals, videotapes, posters/flyers, and telephone numbers and e-mail addresses of laboratory resource people, to which users may refer as needed.

Examples of Point-of-Care Testing Training Programs

The following examples describe POCT training programs recently implemented at The Johns Hopkins Hospital that used two very different approaches to educating users.

Multiple Bedside Test Training

In the fall of 1997, the interdisciplinary team identified a need to retrain all staff performing a number of near-patient tests in order to improve the accuracy of test results and to increase compliance with regulatory agency standards. The following bedside tests were targeted: gastric occult blood and pH, fecal occult blood, urine dipsticks, urine-specific gravity, and pH testing with nitrazine paper. Because of the need to complete this training quickly, the large number of employees needing training, and the wide scope of training content (multiple tests), it was decided that a printed self-study packet with accompanying written posttest would be the most effective educational strategy. The self-study packet was developed by the coordinator for nursing education, with input from laboratory personnel. Departmental nurse educators distributed the packet/test, collected/scored the completed tests, and maintained training records. The self-study packet was developed for use with nursing staff, but was also used by physicians who performed POCT. The first page of the packet and a sample instruction sheet are included as Figs. 13.3 and 13.4. Fig. 13.5 shows an example of a test-specific sheet included in the self-study packets of those staff members who perform gastric occult blood and pH testing.

Blood Glucose Meter Training

In the spring of 1998, The Johns Hopkins Hospital implemented new blood glucose meters. Representatives from nurs-

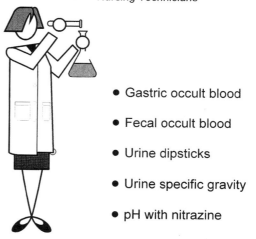

NEAR PATIENT TESTING

Self Study Packet for Nurses,
Clinical Associates, Clinical Nursing Interns,
Nursing Technicians

- Gastric occult blood
- Fecal occult blood
- Urine dipsticks
- Urine specific gravity
- pH with nitrazine

FIGURE 13.3. Cover page of near-patient testing self-study packet developed and used to train staff of The Johns Hopkins Hospital. (Produced with permission of The Johns Hopkins Hospital. Copyright 1997, The Johns Hopkins Hospital.)

ing service, laboratory service, and the meter manufacturer collaborated to develop a comprehensive program that included training of unit-based instructors, operators (nurses and unlicensed assistive personnel), new nursing employees, and staff requiring retraining (see Table 13.4). Because meter operation and maintenance, patient testing, and QC procedures for this device were fairly complex, it was determined that a multi-modal training approach would be used, with classroom training serving as the backbone. Classes for unit instructors and meter operators were done by vendor representatives, with nursing and laboratory staff giving input about content and instructional methods. Unit-based instructors provided training for staff members who were unable to attend a class (Table 13.4). Nursing educators instructed new employees about the meters. A self-study packet and vendor-provided videotapes supplemented the classes. A written test and a skill competency checklist were used to evaluate and document learning (see Figs. 13.6 and 13.7).

Evaluation of Learning

With POCT training, as with all education, it is important to evaluate the effectiveness of the program. There are four levels of educational program evaluation, each of which has implications for POCT training (67).

- *Did the employees like the training?* This level of evaluation is very subjective; however, it is important to assess learner reactions to the training since in many cases, if participants do not like a program, they often will not learn from it. Written participant evaluation forms are usually used to collect this information.

WE HAVE BEEN DOING BEDSIDE TESTING FOR YEARS --- WHY ALL OF THIS NOW?

Near patient tests (also referred to as bedside tests or waived tests) are laboratory tests performed on the nursing unit rather than in a laboratory setting. Testing methods classified as waived testing under federal law (Clinical Laboratory Improvement Amendments 1988, CLIA) and regulation are required to meet specific standards defined by JCAHO. Many of these standards were developed to improve and maintain the quality of testing for patients in virtually all settings.

These standards for waived testing relate to (1) training and skill validation for persons performing the tests; (2) quality control (QC) procedures to validate test accuracy and proper test performance; and, (3) documentation of test results and QC.

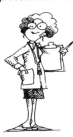

Since any laboratory analysis performed at the bedside is considered a "lab test," unit staff who perform bedside tests are required to comply with the standards for each test, and at JHH, all bedside testing is monitored by the Department of Pathology Performance Improvement Program.

The JCAHO survey of JHH laboratory services will be done in early August 1997. Before that survey, we must demonstrate/document that all bedside test operators have had training in both the patient testing and QC procedures for all tests done.

This packet provides you with needed information about bedside tests performed on your unit. If you have additional questions about any near patient test refer to (1) the green *Near Patient Testing Procedure Manual* on your nursing unit or (2) call the Pathology Performance Improvement Office, x5-2645.

FOR ALL TESTS:

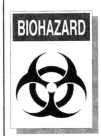

- Use Universal Precautions/wear gloves when doing bedside testing.
- Discard excess body fluids/wastes in toilet/hopper.
- Dispose of test slides, dipsticks, paper, etc., in red biohazard bag.

- Check expiration date on all test supplies/ reagents.
- Date all bottles of supplies & reagents when opened.
- Discard if expired or opened date is unrecorded.

- If testing is delayed/interrupted, label the specimen with the patient's name, history #, date/time.
- Record patient test results on the nursing flow sheet, including the date/time of testing, and the name or initials of the person performing the test.
- Document successful completion of QC by placing a ✔ next to the patient test result on the nursing flow sheet.

Please read this packet carefully, take the post test at the end, and turn your test in to _____ by _____.

FIGURE 13.4. Overview page of near-patient testing self-study packet developed and used to train staff of The Johns Hopkins Hospital. The information provided on this page applies to all point-of-care tests covered in the packet. (Produced with permission of The Johns Hopkins Hospital. Copyright 1997, The Johns Hopkins Hospital.)

GASTRIC OCCULT BLOOD AND pH
GASTROCCULT®

SPECIMEN COLLECTION

- Use only a fresh gastric sample, and test promptly. Do not test refrigerated samples, or those from other body sites.

- Some foods (uncooked meats, raw fruits and vegetables) and medications (ascorbic acid and antacids) may interfere with test accuracy. Refer to the *JHH Near Patient Testing Procedure Manual* for more information.

PATIENT TESTING

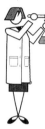

1. Wear protective gloves (biohazard precautions).
2. Check that the pH control has been run within the week.
3. Open the slide, and prepare to time the test for a 30 seconds reading.

4. Apply 1 drop of gastric sample to the pH test area and 1 drop to the Gastroccult® (occult blood) test area.

5. Within 30 seconds, read the pH by comparing the color of this spot with the pH color comparators on the slide.

6. Apply 2 drops of Gastroccult® developer to the occult blood test area. Read occult blood results within 60 seconds. The development of any blue color in the occult blood test area is regarded as a positive. Note: Some gastric samples may be highly colored and appear green or blue on the test slide. Only additional blue color is considered positive in such cases.

7. Record patient test results on nursing flow sheet, including date/time of testing, and name or initials of person doing test.

QUALITY CONTROL

Note --- Gastroccult® tests require 2 types of quality control.

FREQUENCY:
1. Occult blood QC (Performance monitor) - after each patient test.
2. pH - weekly or when opening new box of slides.

PROCEDURE:

1. Occult blood QC (Performance monitor):

    a. Place 1 drop of Gastroccult® developer between the positive and negative performance monitor areas on the Gastroccult® slide.

    b. Read within 10 seconds. No color should appear in the negative location; a blue color should appear in the positive location.

    c. Document Gastroccult® slide and developer lot numbers and lot changes in QC log.

    c. Note failures in QC log; discard the patient result, and repeat both the patient care test and the QC procedure on new slide.

2. pH QC

    a. Check the Gastroccult® QC log to ensure that the pH control buffers have been validated within the prior week.

    b. Check the pH of each buffer (one at pH 2.0; one at pH 7.0) on two separate Gastroccult® slides, using the patient test procedure.

Note: Stored at room temperature, Gastroccult® slides and developer will remain stable to the expiration date stamped on each slide and developer bottle.

FIGURE 13.5. Sample page of near-patient testing self-study packet developed and used to train staff of The Johns Hopkins Hospital. This page covers gastric occult blood and pH testing. (Produced with permission of The Johns Hopkins Hospital. Copyright 1999, The Johns Hopkins Hospital.)

TABLE 13.4. BLOOD GLUCOSE METER EDUCATIONAL PROGRAM

Component	Participants	Time Frame	Learning Objectives (Participant will be able to....)	Methodology	Evaluation of Learning	Faculty
Train-the-trainer sessions	Unit-based trainers, nurse educators, nurse managers	April 1– April 15, 1998	1. Perform patient test and QC with blood glucose meter 2. Describe appropriate uses/ limitations of meter, guidelines for patient results reporting and documentation, safety measures, meter maintenance, troubleshooting, and resources 3. Describe changes in JHH QC standards related to new meter 4. Identify role of unit-based trainer	Class (1 hr) Lecture/ discussion, demonstration Handouts: What's new? Trainer guidelines	Written test Return demonstration documented on skill checklist	Vendor representatives
Current user inservices	Nurses, clinical associates, technicians	April 15– May 15, 1998	1. Perform patient test and QC with blood glucose meter 2. Describe appropriate uses/ limitations of meter, guidelines for patient results reporting and documentation, safety measures, meter maintenance, troubleshooting, and resources 3. Describe changes in JHH QC standards related to new meter	Departmental/ unit classes (1/2 hr) Lecture/ discussion, demonstration Handout: What's new?	Written test Return demonstration, documented on skill checklist	Vendor representatives and/or unit based trainers
New user orientation	New nurses, clinical associates, technicians	During orientation	1. Perform patient test and QC with blood glucose meter 2. Describe appropriate uses/ limitations of meter, guidelines for patient results reporting and documentation, safety measures, meter maintenance, troubleshooting, and resources 3. Describe JHH QC standards related to bedside blood glucose testing	Determined by departmental educator Self-learning packet and videotape available	Written test Return demonstration, documented on skill checklist	Departmental educators and/or unit-based trainers

JHH, Johns Hopkins Hospital; QC, quality control.

- *Did participants learn from the training?* Employees may have liked the training, but did not learn from it. Cognitive learning may be evaluated through the use of written or verbal testing, and psychomotor skill development may be readily assessed via return demonstration and documented on skill checklists. Attitudinal or affective learning may be evaluated via discussion, employee feedback, and/or behavioral change.

- *Did employees use the new knowledge/skill on the job?* Participants may have learned, but did they actually use the new information/skill on the job? Behavior change is the ultimate goal of staff education, and it is important to evaluate the degree to which employee on-the-job performance was positively affected by the training. Aggregate data about staff compliance with and performance of tests and QC procedures may be helpful in identifying weaknesses and strengths in the training program (44).

- *Did the training make a difference to the organization?* What is the impact/effect on the institution's patient-care or business results? This is the highest level of evaluation and, with POCT, this level would assess its impact on patient clinical and financial outcomes, and compliance with regulatory agency requirements.

Cost of Training

POCT is sometimes reported as cost saving, but are the costs of training included in these analyses? Training "costs," but this cost is often hidden! Even if it doesn't show up on the budget, the institution pays. The most significant expense associated with training is staff time, both users' and instructors'. This includes time required for initial start-up education, ongoing updates, needed retraining, and quarterly competency demonstration (as required by the JCAHO). These salary costs are calculated using the average salary plus 22% for employee benefits. Additional costs include instructional equipment/ supplies, printed materials, and audiovisual aides. The cost of a bedside testing educational program varies depending on the device complexity and instructional methodologies used. Table 13.5 shows a cost comparison of the two educational programs described previously.

There are strategies for reducing the cost of training. These include the following:

- *Make sure training is the solution to problem.* The need for initial staff training is commonly accepted; however, continuing education is often erroneously identified as the solution to employee

NEAR PATIENT TESTING
SELF LEARNING PACKET POST TEST

➤ *Please use the answer sheet provided. Do not write on this test.*
➤ *Turn your completed answer sheet in to the person identified on the second page of the self learning packet.*
➤ *Remember to record this education activity on your Developmental Resume.*

ALL BEDSIDE TESTS:

True or false

1. Nursing staff performing bedside testing do not need to comply with JCAHO and other regulatory agency standards for laboratory testing.

2. Protective gloves should be worn when performing bedside testing.

3. All test slides, dipsticks, paper, etc., are disposed of in red biohazard bags.

4. Before using any bedside testing supplies/reagents, you need to check the expiration date on the container, and discard if expired or date opened is not indicated.

5. Patient test results and successful completion of QC are documented on the nursing flow sheet.

6. Quality control (QC) tests are done to validate test accuracy and proper test performance.

Short answer

7. List 2 resources you may use if you have questions about bedside testing.

    A. _____

    B. _____

GASTRIC OCCULT BLOOD (GASTROCCULT®):

True or false

1. Some food and medications may interfere with accurate Gastroccult® test results.

2. Gastroccult® may be used to test refrigerated gastric samples and body fluids other than gastric contents.

FIGURE 13.6. First page of post test of near-patient testing self-study packet developed and used to train staff of The Johns Hopkins Hospital. (Produced with permission of The Johns Hopkins Hospital. Copyright 1997, The Johns Hopkins Hospital.)

performance problems. If there is a performance problem, training is an expensive intervention, and may not be the real solution to the problem, and in reality, performance problems are seldom due to gaps in skill/knowledge. Other factors that lead to performance problems include lack of standards/expectations, incentives, and/or motivation (68). Training should not be used to solve these nontraining problems.

■ *Make sure only the people who need training get it.* If knowledge or skill deficits have been identified, educational interventions should be done only for those employees with these needs. Bedside testing devices that electronically download and analyze QC data are able to pinpoint employees in need of retraining, based on their failure to achieve acceptable test results. Massive educational programs targeting large groups of employees are very costly, and warranted only if knowledge and/or skill deficits are present in only a portion of individuals.

■ *Keep employees out of the classroom as much as possible.* The most costly educational program is any program that takes the

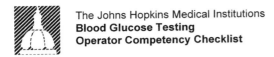

The Johns Hopkins Medical Institutions
Blood Glucose Testing
Operator Competency Checklist

Name (PRINT) _____ Title _____ Employee ID # _____

Date _____ Nursing unit _____ Dept _____ Written test (check one) ☐ PASS ☐ FAIL

Instructions: Instructor will supervise performance of skills by employee. All steps must be performed as indicated in order for competency to be determined adequate. Instructor will sign the form when all steps are performed correctly. Send both copies to the Pathology Core Lab - POCT Program (Nelson B-112). The yellow copy will be returned to the unit with the operator's bar coded ID. Upon return to the unit, the yellow copy will be placed in the operator's personnel file.

REQUIRED PERFORMANCE
QUALITY CONTROL PROCEDURE (Daily on each meter; quarterly for each operator)
1. Dates control solution vials when opening. States to discard after appropriate "opened" expiration date or on/after printed expiration date.
2. Presses CTRLS key.
3. Verifies strip code, presses YES.
4. Enters operator ID by scanning bar code or manually typing.
5. Presses LEVEL 1.
6. Verifies control solution lot number, presses YES.
7. Runs a control test for LEVEL 1.
8. Obtains result and removes strip. Enters comment code, if necessary.
9. Repeats steps 5 - 8 with LEVEL 2 solution.
PATIENT TEST PROCEDURE, using Universal/Standard Precautions
1. Puts on gloves; cleans site on patient's finger and allows to dry.
2. Prepares lancet device.
3. Turns GTS on by pressing blue button.
4. Presses PAT key.
5. Verifies strip code and presses YES.
6. Enters operator ID and patient ID (history #) by scanning bar code or manually typing.
7. After monitor initializes, Inserts strip into monitor.
8. Performs finger puncture and applies blood to strip.
9. Applies pressure to site to stop bleeding, and disposes of lancet in biohazard waste container.
10. Obtains result; disposes of strip in biohazard waste container.
11. Enters comment code, if necessary. If no comment required, presses ENTER.
12. Documents patient results on medical record flowsheet (result, date/time, meter ID #, operator initials).
13. States what findings to report to physician/nurse.
14. States where to find troubleshooting information and where to get additional assistance.

Instructor signature/title: _____

FIGURE 13.7. Operator skill checklist used to validate and document competency of the staff of The Johns Hopkins Hospital in performing bedside blood glucose testing. (Produced with permission of The Johns Hopkins Hospital. Copyright 1997, The Johns Hopkins Hospital.)

TABLE 13.5. COST COMPARISON OF TWO POINT-OF-CARE TESTING TRAINING PROGRAMS

	Multiple Test Training Using Self-Study Packet as Primary Training Modality	Blood Glucose Meter Training Using Classes as Primary Training Modality
Number of employees trained	1800	1800
Average training time/employee	.25 hour	.5 hour
Salary costs for users, unit-based trainers, nurse educators, education coordinator	$18,800	$33,400
Printing, materials, supply costs	$810	$1,082
Total cost	**$19,610**	**$34,482**

employee away from his or her job and into a classroom. Alternative instructional methodologies, used in a "just enough, just in time" mode, are significantly more cost effective, and when used appropriately, as effective as classroom training. These alternatives include videotapes, self-study packets, computer-based modules, job aids (written instructions employees refer to as needed), and on-the-job training.

CONCLUSIONS AND RECOMMENDATIONS

Peter Drucker (69) observed that knowledge "constantly makes itself obsolete, with the result that today's advanced knowledge is tomorrow's ignorance." POCT has been described as a "work in progress," affected by a multitude of regulatory, managerial, quality, and turf issues (70). Rapid knowledge of POC test results is valuable only to the extent that results are used for immediate diagnostic and therapeutic decision-making. The emphasis must be on clinical outcomes.

The analysis of outcomes of care is essential for guiding informed decision making in all aspects of health care (2), and is particularly relevant to POCT. Five reasons to analyze outcomes have been proposed: (a) payers are demanding information about the results of patient-care delivery, (b) outcomes are an integral part of accreditation, (c) consumers have a right to know about the outcomes of care, (d) regulatory agencies demand information on outcomes, and (e) outcomes represent the basic reason for administering care (71).

In an era where managed care companies seek out cost-effective, care-delivery systems and hospitals strive to reduce the cost of labor, newer "pocket-sized" POCT devices are flooding the market. Before these devices are automatically absorbed into the rapidly accelerating POCT expansion, their potential to enhance patient outcomes must be assessed.

Implementation of a POCT program is teeming with obstacles to be overcome. Barriers that have been identified as capable of stifling quality initiatives are (a) an organizational culture that is not amenable to change, (b) lack of perceived management support, (c) QA as an afterthought rather than a proactive stance, (d) lack of interdisciplinary teams, and (e) cost of education, training, technology, supplies, and QC (72). The latter part of the 20th century was punctuated by dramatic changes in patient-care requirements and the birth of a new breed of patient-consumer. A societal demand for stewardship of valuable healthcare resources generated reengineering, restructuring, and redesign

initiatives that continue today. The delivery of nursing care has been profoundly altered by these initiatives. Recommendations have been made regarding the need to assess short- and long-term impacts of regulatory requirements and standards on POCT, including training and competency evaluation, QC, proficiency testing, data management, and personnel standards (1). These recommendations become even more pressing as the resources available to render direct patient care are spread more thinly.

Nurses play an equivalent role with other stakeholders in setting standards for appropriate utilization, monitoring, and review of POCT. Despite the fact that nurses are the principal analysts in most POCT programs, the ultimate success of a truly effective program does not rest with nursing alone. POCT crosses organizational boundaries and presents unique challenges to the various disciplines (41). It represents a cross-disciplinary function best accomplished by teams of interdependent staff. As health care evolves, the lines among disciplines become more obscure and overlap, intermingling interventions and responsibilities among disciplines (15). There is a strong synergistic relationship between nursing service, the hospital laboratories, and the medical staff. In order for the common goal of quality patient care to be achieved, process and communication must freely cross intraorganizational boundaries.

The information provided in this chapter provides a springboard for creative dialogue among interdisciplinary POCT team members regarding how to minimize potential barriers and focus on enhancing patient outcomes. The skill with which nursing maintains its delicate balance between art and science is particularly helpful in facilitating the development of effective interdisciplinary programs. Nurse leaders can enhance the achievement of the mutual goal of improved patient outcomes through the following mechanisms:

- Active participation and co-leadership in decision making regarding which POC tests are appropriate for particular patient populations given the organization's climate, structure, and processes.
- Visible commitment to ensuring that the nursing workforce develops and maintains appropriate skills and techniques necessary to perform POCT.
- Collaboration with laboratory leaders to streamline QC and other performance monitoring requirements to achieve desired outcomes with the least possible consumption of resources (17).
- Collaboration with laboratory personnel in the structuring of training programs that assure competency with minimal interruption of other patient-care priorities.

- Advocacy of emphasizing patient outcomes during program evaluation initiatives.
- Knowledge of technological advances, health policy, marketplace, and political factors affecting the demand for POCT.

REFERENCES

1. Seamonds B. Medical, economic, and regulatory factors affecting point-of-care testing: a report of the conference on factors affecting point-of-care testing, Philadelphia, PA, 6–7 May 1994. *Clin Chem Act* 1996;249:1–19.
2. Jones KR, Jennings BM, Moritz P, Moss MT. Policy issues associated with analyzing outcomes of care. *Image: J Nurs Scholar* 1997;29: 261–267.
3. Kost GJ. Point-of-care testing in intensive care. In: Tobin MJ, ed. *Principles and practice of intensive care monitoring.* New York: McGraw-Hill, 1998:1267–1296.
4. Handorf CR. Quality control and quality management of alternate-site testing. *Clin Lab Med* 1994;14:539–557.
5. Donahue MP. *Nursing: the finest art, an illustrated history.* St. Louis: CV Mosby, 1995.
6. Health Care Advisory Board. Nursing Executive Watch. International nursing shortage triggers recruitment battle. January 2, 2001. Available at: *http:www.advisory.com.*
7. Stewart, M. New nursing shortage hits: causes complex. *American Nurse* March/April 1998. Available at: *http:www.nursingworld.org.*
8. Sandelowski M. (Ir)reconcilable differences? The debate concerning nursing and technology. *Image: J Nurs Scholar* 1997;29:169–172.
9. Krenzischek DA, Tanseco FV. Comparative study of bedside and laboratory measurements of hemoglobin. *Am J Crit Care* 1996;5:427–432.
10. Hutsko GM, Jones JB, Danielson L. Using point-of-care testing to speed patient care: one emergency department's" experience. *J Emerg Nurs* 1995;21:408–412.
11. Pierce B. The top 10 recent innovations in patient care in trauma ICU. *J Trauma Nurs* 1997;4:53–55.
12. Gray TA, Freedman DB, Burnett D, et al. Evidence-based practice: clinician's use and attitudes to near patient testing in hospitals. *J Clin Pathol* 1996;49:903–908.
13. Hilton S, Rink E, Fletcher J, et al. Near patient testing in general practice: attitudes of general practitioners and practice nurses and quality assurance procedures carried out. *Brit J Gen Prac* 1994;44:577–580.
14. Lamb LS, Parrish RS, Goran SF, et al. Current nursing practice of point-of-care laboratory diagnostic testing in critical care units. *Am J Crit Care* 1995;4:429–434.
15. Lamb-Havard, J. Nurses at the bedside influencing outcomes. *Nurs Clin North Am* 1997;32:579–587.
16. ECRI. Regulatory requirements for decentralized laboratory testing. *Health Devices* 1995;24:176–177.
17. Poe SS, Nichols JH. Quality assurance, practical management, and outcomes of point-of-care testing: nursing perspectives, Part II. *Clin Lab Manage Rev* 2000:14:12–18.
18. Miller KA, Miller NA. Joining forces to improve point-of-care testing. *Nurs Manage* 1997;28:34–37.
19. Bailey TM, Topham TM, Wantz S, et al. Laboratory process improvement through point-of-care testing. *J Qual Improv* 1997;23:362–380.
20. Valenstein P. Laboratory turnaround time. *Am J Clin Path* 1996;105: 676–688.
21. Kost GL, Vu HT, Inn M, et al. Multicenter study of whole-blood creatinine, total carbon dioxide content and chemistry profiling for laboratory and point-of-care testing in critical care in the United States. *Crit Care Med* 2000;28:2379–2389.
22. Kost GL. Guidelines for point-of-care testing: improving patient outcomes. *Am J Clin Path* 1995;104[Suppl 1]:S111–S127.
23. Castro HJ, Oropello JM, Halpern N. Point-of-care testing in the intensive care unit: the intensive care physician's perspective. *Am J Clin Path* 1995;104[Suppl 1]:S95–S99.
24. Harvey M. Point-of-care laboratory testing in critical care. *Am J Crit Care* 1999;8:72–83.
25. McConnel EA. Hold the lab in the palm of your hand. *Nurs Manage* 1999;30:57–59.
26. Auerbach PS. Impact of point-of-care testing on healthcare delivery. *Clin Chem* 1996;42:2052–2053.
27. American Diabetes Association. *Diabetes facts and figures.* Alexandria, VA: American Diabetes Association, 2000.
28. Lee-Lewandrowski E, Laposata M, Eschenbach K, et al. Utilization and cost analysis of bedside capillary glucose testing in a large teaching hospital: implications for managing point of care testing. *Am J Med* 1994;97:222–230.
29. American Diabetes Association. Position statement: bedside blood glucose monitoring in hospitals. In: *Clinical practice recommendations.* Alexandria, VA: American Diabetes Association, 2000;23(S1):1.
30. Nichols JH, Howard C, Loman K, et al. Laboratory and bedside evaluation of portable glucose meters. *Am J Clin Path* 1995;103:244–251.
31. Tang Z, Lee JH, Louie RF, et al. Effects of different hematocrit levels on glucose measurements with handheld meters for point of care testing. *Arch Path Lab Med* 2000;124(8):1135–40.
32. Dirks JL. Diagnostic blood analysis using point of care technology. *AACN Clin Issues* 1996;7:249–259.
33. Dirks JL. Innovations in technology: continuous intra-arterial blood gas monitoring. *Crit Care Nurs* 1995;15:19–27.
34. Oberhardt BJ. Thrombosis and hemostasis testing at the point-of-care. *Am J Clin Path* 1996;104[Suppl 1]:S72–S78.
35. Eisenberg P, Muhs MJ. QI study in the ICU: bedside testing of gastric contents. *Nurs Manage* 1996;27:48J–48M.
36. Fitzmaurice DA, Hobbs FD, Murray ET, et al. Oral anticoagulation management in primary care with the use of computerized decision support and near-patient testing: a randomized, controlled trial. *Arch Intern Med* 2000;160:2343–2348.
37. Nichols JH, Kickler TS, Dyer KL, et al. Clinical outcomes of point-of-care testing in the interventional radiology and invasive cardiology setting. *Clin Chem* 2000;46:543–550.
38. Nichols JH, Poe SS. Quality assurance, practical management, and outcomes of point-of-care testing: laboratory perspectives, part I. *Clin Lab Manage Rev* 1999;13:341–350.
39. Kost GJ. Planning and implementing point-of-care testing systems. In: Tobin MJ, ed. *Principles and practice of intensive care monitoring.* New York: McGraw-Hill, 1998:1297–1328.
40. Bayne CG. Point-of-care testing: testing the system? *Nurs Manage* 1997;28:34–36.
41. Handorf CR. Assuring quality in laboratory testing at the point of care. *Clin Chem Act* 1997;260:207–216.
42. Laposata M, Lewandrowski KB. Near patient blood glucose monitoring. *Arch Pathol Lab Med* 1995;119:926–928.
43. Sokoll LJ, Nichols JH. Evaluation of a HemoCue® blood hemoglobin photometer with data management functions. *Clin Chem* 1996; 42:S191.
44. JCAHO. *Quality point-of-care testing.* Oakbrook Terrace, IL: Joint Commission on Accreditation of Health Care Organizations, 1999.
45. JCAHO. *Framework for improving performance: from principles to practice.* Oakbrook Terrace, IL: Joint Commission on Accreditation of Health Care Organizations, 1994.
46. Heyssel RM, Gaintner JR, Kues IW, et al. Decentralized management in a teaching hospital. *New Eng J Med* 1984;310:1477–1480.
47. Boyce N. Making the transition from dictator to facilitator: lab leadership on a POCT team. *Clin Lab News* 1998;23(2):14–15.
48. Beyers M. About multidisciplinary teams. *Nurs Manage* 1998;29:56.
49. Curtin LL. Jonathan Livingston Seagull on teams. *Nurs Manage* 1998; 29:5–6.
50. Henson RH. Analysis of the concept of mutuality. *Image: J Nurs Scholar* 1997;29:77–81.
51. Johns Hopkins Hospital. *The seven steps to performance improvement.* Baltimore, MD: Johns Hopkins Hospital, 1998.
52. Johns Hopkins Hospital. *The nursing practice and organization manual, volume I.* Baltimore, MD: Johns Hopkins Hospital, 1998.
53. Kost GJ, Vu H-T, Lee JH, et al. Multicenter study of oxygen-insensitive handheld glucose point-of-care testing in critical care/hospital/ambulatory patients in the United States and Canada. *Crit Care Med* 1998;26:581–590.

54. Bayne CG. Pocket-sized medicine: new POC technologies. *Nurs Manage* 1997;28:30–32.

55. Johns Hopkins Hospital. *The PCDM implementation resource manual.* Baltimore, MD: Johns Hopkins Hospital, 1997.

56. Lamb LS. Responsibilities in point-of-care testing: an institutional perspective. *Arch Pathol Lab Med* 1995;119:886–889.

57. Baer DM, Belsey RE. Managing quality and risk of bedside testing. *Perspec in Healthcare Risk Manage* 1990;(Winter):3–7,P.235.

58. American Society for Clinical Laboratory Science. *Position paper: point of care testing.* Bethesda, MD: American Society for Clinical Laboratory Science, 1996.

59. Knowles M. *The adult learner: a neglected species.* Houston: Gulf Publishing, 1978.

60. Cross KP. *Adults as learners.* Washington, DC: Jossey-Bass Publishers, 1984.

61. Brookfield SD. *Understanding and facilitating adult learning.* San Francisco: Jossey-Bass Publishers, 1986.

62. Hiemstra R, ed. *Creating environments for effective adult learning.* New directions for adult and continuing education series. San Francisco: Jossey-Bass Publishers, 1991.

63. Cranton P. *Understanding and promoting transformative learning.* San Francisco: Jossey-Bass Publishers, 1991.

64. Geber B. Re-engineering the training department. *Training* 1994;5:27–34.

65. Filipczak B. Training on intranets: the hope and the hype. *Training* 1996;9:24–32.

66. Hibbard J. Learning revolution. *Information Week* 1998 March 9:44–60.

67. Geber B. Does your training make a difference? *Training* 1995;3:27–34.

68. Filipczak B. A manager's guide to training. *Training* 1997;7:35–40.

69. Drucker P. The future that has already happened. *Harv Bus Rev* 1997;75:18–32.

70. Kost GJ, Ehrmeyer SS, Chernow B, et al. The laboratory-clinician interface: point-of-care testing. *Chest* 1999;115:1140–1154.

71. Schlenker RE. *Outcomes across the care continuum: home health care.* Presented at the AAN Conference on Outcome Measures and Care Delivery Systems, American Academy of Nursing, June 1996, Washington, DC, 1996.

72. Messner K. Barriers to implementing a quality improvement program. *Nurs Manage* 1998:29:32–36.

14

POINT-OF-CARE TESTING FOR INFECTIOUS DISEASES

MICHAEL B. SMITH
GAIL L. WOODS

Laboratory testing in the diagnosis of infectious diseases has traditionally involved primarily the use of laboratory-centered tests such as culture or serology. The use of this type of testing strategy has an inherent time delay resulting from time required to transport the specimen to the laboratory, batch processing of numerous specimens, time for incubation, interpretation of results on a laboratory schedule, and batch reporting of results. In today's medical environment, which requires more rapid disposition of patients than ever before, point-of-care testing for infectious diseases can play an important role in evaluation, diagnosis, and disposition of patients in a more efficient manner. This involves the utilization of both traditional methodologies and new innovative tests based on molecular methods. In this chapter, these tests will be reviewed and discussed with respect to their applications and efficacy.

VIRAL INFECTIONS

Herpes Viruses

Herpes simplex virus (HSV), both HSV1 and HSV2, and varicella-zoster virus (VZV) can cause significant morbidity and mortality in neonates and immunocompromised patients. Thus, the ability to detect the virus rapidly and initiate acycolvir therapy, or in the case of a pregnant woman with herpes genitalis to proceed with a C-section, is of extreme importance. Of the methods available to detect HSV and VZV—cell culture, immunofluorescent antibody (FA), enzyme immunoassay (EIA), and the Tzanck smear—only the Tzanck smear is practical for near-patient testing. Preparing the smear involves scraping the base of the suspected herpetic lesion, smearing the cells on a glass slide, air drying, and staining with a Wright-Geimsa, methylene blue, or toluidine blue stain. The slide is then examined microscopically for characteristic multinucleated giant cells with molded nuclei and "ground glass" nuclear chromatin. Sensitivity of the Tzanck smear ranges from 23% to 70% and depends primarily on the type of lesion that is sampled. In one study (1,2), the sensitivity was 66.7% for vesicular lesions, 54.5% for pustules, and 16.7% percent for crusted lesions. With regard to specificity, the cytopathic changes induced by HSV1, HSV2, and varicella-zoster virus cannot be differentiated, and occasionally smears from lesions of diseases such as pem-

phigus or contact dermatitis have been incorrectly called positive (3). While a positive Tzanck smear can be useful in the proper clinical setting, its low sensitivity precludes a negative smear from being used to dictate therapy in critical situations. If time does not allow submitting a specimen to the laboratory for culture, FA testing, or EIA, sound clinical judgment probably is the most sensitive test available for diagnosing HSV.

Respiratory Syncytial Virus and Influenza Virus

Respiratory syncytial virus (RSV) and Influenza virus are considered together because they both cause respiratory infections that are difficult to distinguish clinically. Testing for one is often accompanied by testing for the other. RSV is the most common cause of respiratory infection in infancy and the most common virus causing pediatric hospitalization (4). In addition, RSV has been shown to be a significant cause of morbidity and mortality in the immunocompromised and elderly (5,6). Influenza A and B are the agents of epidemic flu, a significant cause of morbidity and mortality in the same age groups at risk for RSV. Rapid diagnosis of respiratory infections caused by RSV is important to allow the institution of ribavirin therapy in infants at high risk for poor outcome, cohorting of infected patients to prevent nosocomial spread, and curtailment of unnecessary antibiotic use (7). Similarly, rapid diagnosis of influenza allows the use of amantidine or ramantidine for Influenza A and initiation of infection control measures to limit nosocomial spread in chronic care facilities (8).

Cell culture has been considered the "gold standard" for the isolation of RSV; however, like serological studies, which are also sensitive and specific, results are not finalized in a clinically relevant period of time. FA testing for viral antigens in respiratory epithelial cells requires a fluorescent microscopic and is highly subjective. EIA has proven to be both sensitive and specific for the detection of viruses, and the solid-phase EIA, requiring neither equipment nor specialized training, has been adapted for the rapid testing environment and marketed commercially. Available products are the Directogen RSV (Becton-Dickinson, Sparks, MD) and the TestPack RSV (Abbott, Abbott Park, IL). In the TestPack, after the addition of buffer and filtering of the specimen, RSV antibody-coated microparticles and antibody are added to the specimen to form an antibody-antigen-antibody complex if RSV is present. The solution is transferred to a reaction disk and an enzyme-labeled antibody, a wash, and substrate (alkaline phosphatase) are added in sequence, producing a purple "+" if RSV is present and a "−" if absent. Results are available in 20 minutes. The Directogen differs slightly, in that viral antigen is nonspecifically bound to a membrane, followed by addition of antibody and substrate, and the formation of a purple triangle if RSV is present. The Directogen requires 15 minutes to perform.

In evaluations of the solid-phase EIA tests, sensitivity of the Directogen RSV has ranged from 61% to 100%, specificity from 80% to 100%, predictive value of a positive result (PPV) from 81% to 91%, and predictive value of a negative result (NPV) from 75% to 93%, when compared to culture and FA (9–13). The TestPack has shown a sensitivity of 57% to100%, a specificity of 84% to100%, a PPV of 91% to 100%, and a NPV of 85% to 96% (9,12–20). The lower sensitivity values seen with both systems were confined to one study (13) in which the authors suggested that the large volume they used for nasal washes (6 mL) might have reduced the sensitivity.

Specimen quality and type influence sensitivity, with nasal washes having been demonstrated to be superior to swabs. In one study, sensitivity of both the TestPack and the Directogen were reduced from 86.2% to 64.9 % and 83.5 to 43.6%, respectively, when nasal swabs rather than washes were used (9). Excess mucous in specimens can cause problems in filtration, rendering some specimens uninterpretable. Dilution of the specimen 1:3 or treatment with a mucolytic agent such as dithiothrietol and retesting will usually solve this problem (11,19). Timing of the specimen during the patient's course has also been shown to influence sensitivity. EIA is more likely to be positive in the first week after onset of symptoms, whereas culture and immunofluorescent antibody have a greater sensitivity after this period (10,20).

With respect to influenza, there has been a proliferation of rapid antigen tests in the last several years compatible with bedside testing (Table 14-1). As with the RSV assays, sensitivity is affected by specimen type and different manufacturers recommend certain specimen types for their assays. A novel rapid assay using the detection of neuraminidase activity is ZstatFlu (Zymetx, Oklahoma City, OK), which can detect both Influenza A and B (Table 14-1). Sensitivity for this assay is reduced for Influenza B relative to A (40.9% versus 76.4%, respectively) (23).

These rapid assays can be useful in making acute management decisions (25). Sensitivity appears to vary over a wide range for all tests from laboratory to laboratory; and because the consequence of a false negative may have important implications, these tests are best used as screening tests. Negative results should be confirmed by cell culture and/or fluorescent antibody testing, which have the added advantage of identifying other viral respiratory pathogens that may be present.

Rotavirus

Rotavirus, an RNA virus in the family Reoviridae, is an important cause of highly infectious epidemic gastroenteritis in children under 2 years of age worldwide, with epidemics occurring in winter months. In the United States, rotavirus is responsible for one-third to one-half of pediatric gastroenteritis hospitalizations (2,26). In addition, it may cause diarrhea in adults, particularly geriatric patients and those in chronic care settings (27–29). Rapid identification of rotavirus in either the hospital or chronic care setting is important in preventing nosocomial spread and excluding other potential causes of diarrhea.

Electron microscopy (EM) of stool is the reference method for detecting rotavirus; however, many facilities do not have access to EM and turnaround time is not clinically relevant. In most cases, rotavirus is detected by EIA, which has a sensitivity

TABLE 14.1. RAPID TESTS FOR DETECTION OF INFLUENZA A AND B

Test (Manufacturer)	Method	Sensitivity (%)	Specificity (%)
Directogen Flu A (Becton-Dickinson, Cockeysville, MD)[a]	EIA	75–100	96.3–100
Directogen Flu A/B (Becton-Dickinson, Cockeysville, MD)[b]	EIA	81–86	91–100
FluOIA A/B (Biostar, Inc., Boulder, CO)[c]	EIA	62–86	52–80
Quickview A/B (Quidel Corp., San Diego, CA)[b]	EIA	73–81	96–99
ZstatFlu (ZymeTx, Oklahoma City, OK)[d]	Neuraminidase activity	46–70	76–96

[a]Leonardi GP, Leib H, Birkhead GS, et al., Comparison of rapid detection methods for Influenza A and their value in health-care management of institutionalized geriatric patients. *J Clin Microbiol* 1994;32:70–74; Dominguez EA, Taber LH, Couch RB, Comparison of rapid diagnostic techniques for respiratory syncytial and Influenza A virus respiratory infections in young children. *J Clin Microbiol* 1993;31:2286–2290; Reina J, Munar M, Blanco I, Evaluation of a direct immunofluorescence assay, dot-blot enzyme immunoassay, and shell vial culture in the diagnosis of lower respiratory infections caused by Influenza A virus. *Diagn Microbiol Infect Dis* 1996;25:143–145; Waner JL, Todd SJ, Shalaby H, et al. Comparison of Directogen FLU-A with viral isolation and direct immunofluorescence for the rapid detection and identification of Influenza A virus. *J Clin Microbiol* 1991;29:479–482, with permission.
[b]Sensitivity and specificity are based on data provided by the manufacturer.
[c]Covalciuc KA, Webb KH, Carlson CA. Comparison of four clinical specimen types for detection of Influenza A and B viruses by optical immunoassay (FLU OIA Test) and cell culture methods. *J Clin Microbiol* 1999;37:3971–3974, with permission.
[d]Noyola DE, Clark B, O'Donnell FT, et al. Comparison of new neuraminidase detection assay with an enzyme immunoassay, immunofluorescence, and culture for rapid detection of Influenza A and B viruses in nasal wash specimens. *J Clin Microbiol* 2000;38:1161–1165, with permission.
EIA, enzyme immunoassay.

ranging from 88% to 100% and a specificity of 84% to 98%, depending on the commercial test used (2). However, EIA testing is usually performed in batches on a set schedule in the laboratory and requires several hours, making rapid results impossible. Latex agglutination testing is a commercially available format suitable for near-patient testing. A drop of either centrifuged or filtered stool and buffer solution is placed on a slide with a dark background and mixed with a suspension of latex particles that have been coated with rotavirus-specific antibody. Clumping of the latex particles visualized against the dark background indicates the presence of rotavirus. Results are available in 17 to 20 minutes, depending on the product used.

Several latex kits for rotavirus have been placed on the market, and performance in published evaluations has varied. Overall, when compared to EM and/or EIA, sensitivity has ranged from 61% to 95%, specificity from 80% to 100%, predictive value of a positive result from 76% to 100%, and predictive value of a negative result from 76% to 94% (30–36). In general, the sensitivity of the Meritic (Meridian Diagnostics, Cincinnati, OH) and Virogen Rotatest (Wampole, Cranbury, NJ) tests have been higher, at 71% to 95% and 86% to 95%, respectively, while sensitivity of the Rotalex (Orion Diagnostica, Somerset, NJ) and the Slidex Rota-Kit (bioMerieux Vitek, Hazelwood, MO) has been lower, 61% to 81% and 73% to 82%, respectively (30–36). The Virogen Rotatest (Wampole), however, does not detect one of the serotypes of rotavirus, and in one study (30,35,36), it had a higher incidence of false positives.

A solid-phase EIA using filtered stool, the TestPack Rotavirus (Abbott, Abbott Park, IL), is also available. The test is similar to the TestPack RSV and Flu-A. The test requires 10 minutes to perform. In comparisons with EM and EIA, the TestPack has shown sensitivity of 95% to 100% and a specificity of 83% to 99% (37–40). Lipson et al. (39) noted a high incidence of false positives—a reason for which they could not explain—resulting in a specificity of 83%, which is lower than the other studies cited.

The ImmunoCard STAT Rotavirus Assay (Meridian Diagnostics, Cincinnati, OH) is a new assay using an immunogold, horizontal-flow membrane platform. Using stool vortexed with a supplied diluent, a positive test is indicated by a red-purple line on the membrane after 10 minutes. In a recently published study (41), sensitivity, specificity, positive predictive value, and negative predictive value were 94%, 100%, 100%, and 93.4%, respectively.

Based on published evaluations, either the latex kits or the solid-phase EIA can serve as a rapid screening test for rotavirus in the near-patient environment. There appears to be variation in sensitivity among the latex products, and the solid-phase EIA has shown a higher sensitivity in some evaluations. Sensitivity is affected by the timing of specimen procurement, as a higher sensitivity for the latex tests have been demonstrated when testing is done during the first week of symptoms, when virus shedding is highest, than after (32,42). An additional consideration is cost; the solid-phase EIA is more expensive that the latex kits.

Human Immunodeficiency Virus

The detection of antibodies to the human immunodeficiency virus (HIV-1) in infected individuals is crucial for diagnosis of infection and for controlling its transmission. Most testing is accomplished through the use of EIA tests as an initial screen, followed by confirmatory testing with either FA or Western blot. While the sensitivity and specificity of these tests are high (greater than 99%), the required days to weeks to accomplish testing can result in difficult management decisions in situations where the need for prophylaxis is in question. These include after occupational exposure, pregnant women in labor, or the loss of opportunity for counseling when infected patients do not return for results. In an effort to reduce the time to obtain results, a few rapid assay systems have been developed, of which one is currently approved by the Food and Drug Administration for use in this country.

The SUDS HIV-1 Test (Single Use Diagnostic Systems, Abbott/Murex Diagnostics, Norcross, GA) is an EIA-based test. Plasma or serum is incubated in a sample cup with reaction diluent and latex particles coated with *gag* and a sequence from *env* (transmembrane glycoprotein) antigens. The mixture is transferred to the SUDS cartridge where latex particles with bound antibody are trapped in a fiberglass filter, the filter is washed to remove unbound conjugate, and substrate is added, followed by a stop solution. A blue color in the center of the cartridge device after 15 to 30 minutes indicates a positive test. The SUDS test has demonstrated a sensitivity of 99.3% to 100% and a specificity of 96.3% to 99.5% (43–45). In one study, it was noted that an increase of ambient temperature above the recommended temperature (20° to 25°C) by 3°C resulted in a seven-fold increase in false-positive results, so careful attention to environmental conditions appears to be important in the use of this test (43). In addition, although not currently approved for use with urine, the SUDS HIV-1 test has been shown in preliminary studies to detect HIV-1 antibody in urine (46). Both urine and oral mucosal transudate fluid have been demonstrated to be reliable specimen sources by conventional EIA, and the advantages offered by these sources (e.g., ease of procurement and reduced danger of transmission to healthcare personnel) suggest that further evaluation of their use in rapid testing may be beneficial (47,48).

Other causes of false positives include autoimmune disorders, hemodialysis, hemophilia, multiple myeloma, and human error (49). In addition, while the prevalence of HIV-1 infection in most patient populations in this country is low, the predictive value of a negative test is very high, and it is accepted that a negative EIA screening result can be reported without confirmation (48). In patient populations with low prevalence, however, the predictive value of a positive test will not have the same high value; and because of the significant medical, social, and psychological implications, a positive EIA test for HIV-1 antibody must be confirmed by an alternate testing method.

In certain environments, the Centers for Disease Control (CDC) and Association of State and Territorial Public Health Laboratory Directors support informing the patient of a positive rapid assay result, despite the risk that it may represent a false positive (50). These environments are primarily sexually transmitted disease clinics and HIV-1 testing clinics. Up to 40% of patients fail to return for results (51). In one study at a sexually transmitted disease clinic where the rapid test was used and positive results reported to the patient, 97% of HIV-1 positive individuals returned for the results of confirmatory testing, an increase of 23% over baseline (51). In addition, because the majority of those tested were not infected, testing and counseling were accomplished in a single visit, reducing psychological stress on those tested, reducing cost for the tested subject, and improving efficiency for the clinic (51). Similarly, rapid testing for HIV-1 facilitates administration of zidovudine to infants of HIV-1 infected mothers within the 12 to 24 hours recommended by the CDC (52). Although the SUDS test has demonstrated utility in this role, a high rate of false-positive tests in low-prevalence populations must be taken into consideration (53).

Varicella Zoster Virus (VZV) Antibodies

VZV is the etiologic agent of chicken pox and shingles. Prior to the availability of a vaccine, chicken pox was a common childhood illness with only rare fatalities; however, primary infection in adults is associated with more serious disease and a fifteen-fold increase in mortality (2). In addition, VZV can cause severe, potentially fatal, disseminated disease in immunocompromised patients. Infection during the first trimester of pregnancy or just prior to delivery can result in congenital or perinatal varicella, respectively, both of which are associated with significant morbidity and mortality in the newborn. Determination of immune status is important in assessing the need for prophylactic varicella immune globulin, which must be administered within 72 to 96 hours of exposure for maximum effectiveness, and to manage nosocomial exposures. Immune status is determined by detecting IgG antibodies, which appear 4 to 5 days after symptoms and persist for life.

Although serological testing is often performed by EIA or the fluorescent antibody to membrane assay (FAMA), individual or small numbers of specimens can be tested rapidly using commercially available latex agglutination assays, which use polystyrene particles coated with antigens to VZV. Doubling dilutions of sera (use of plasma has not been evaluated for use) are placed on a reaction card supplied by the manufacturer and a drop of the particle emulsion is added. The card is rotated for 10 minutes on a mechanical rotator at between 95 to 100 rpm under a humidity hood, and examined for visible clumping of the polystyrene particles by holding the card at 6 inches from a high-intensity incandescent lamp. A positive test is indicated by visible clumping. High reactive, low reactive, and negative controls are supplied by the manufacturer.

False-negative reactions may occur due to prozone phenomena; therefore to avoid this, testing two dilutions (1:2 or 1:4 and 1:64) of each patient sample simultaneously is recommended (54). If acute and convalescent sera are being tested, titers can be determined by carrying out doubling dilutions beyond 1:64. A four-fold rise in titer from acute to convalescent sera indicates recent infection. False-positive reactions, although unusual, can occur. They have been associated with performing the test outside the recommended temperature range (23° to 29°C) and holding the reaction card too close to the incandescent lamp source and thus drying the reaction mixture. When compared to the FAMA, the latex test has shown a sensitivity of 92% and a specificity of 93% (55). The advantages of the latex test are the rapidity with which results are obtained (15 to 30 minutes), low cost relative to the EIA and FAMA, and simplicity. The test is not efficient for testing large volumes of specimens and does not detect IgM antibodies.

Infectious Monoculeosis

Infectious monoculeosis (IM) is a common febrile lymphoproliferative disease caused by Epstein-Barr virus (EBV), a member of the herpesvirus family. Classic signs and symptoms are non-specific and include fever, pharyngitis, lymphadenopathy, and hepatosplenomegaly. Atypical lymphocytosis commonly occurs. These findings can all be caused by many other infectious agents, including cytomegalovirus (CMV), adenovirus, toxoplasma, hepatitis A and B viruses, rubella, HIV, and Group A *Streptococcus* (56). In addition, IM may have an atypical presentation, such as abdominal pain or cough due to mesenteric lymphadenopathy and hilar adenopathy (57). IM usually is self-limited; however, complications such as splenic rupture can occur, and precautions such as limitation of activity may be required. Exclusion of the other infections in the differential is important because some may require specific treatment and/or infection control measures.

Rapid differentiation of EBV-induced IM from other agents in the differential diagnosis involves the detection of heterophile antibodies, which are IgM antibodies that react with antigens on cells of various mammals, but not with antigens on EBV. Heterophile antibodies are present in approximately 60% to 70% of patients after the first week of illness and in 80% to 90% by the third to fourth week (2). However, 15% to 20% of adults with IM may not produce heterophile antibodies, and more than 50% of children under the age of 4 years will not produce them (57). No relationship between the titer of these antibodies and the severity of the illness exists (58). Heterophile antibodies are not specific for IM and can be seen in infections with other viruses such as CMV, hepatitis A virus, and parvovirus B19.

Rapid detection of heterophile antibodies involves one of three types of tests: a slide agglutination test with whole, red-blood-cell, heterophile antigen (horse), a latex slide agglutination test with purified heterophile antigen, or a solid-phase immunoassay with purified heterophile antigen. Agglutination tests using whole-red-blood-cell antigen, which were the first tests developed, require an adsorption step with antigen from guinea pig kidney (which adsorbs heterophile antibodies stimulated by antigens other than EBV). This is followed by the addition of horse red cells, which results in agglutination if EBV heterophile antibodies are present. The latex tests are simpler to perform, because they do not require the adsorption step; however, the overall time to perform the two types of tests is similar (5 to 10 minutes). Immunoassays involve a solid surface with immobilized heterophile antigen to which is added a mixture of patient serum and labeled anti-human globulin. If the serum contains heterophile antibodies, a sandwich of heterophile antigen (heterophile antibody) labeled anti-human globulin is present on the test surface, which is indicated by a color change with addition of substrate if the label is an enzyme, or by the presence of color if the label is colored latex. In evaluations, the sensitivity of these tests has ranged from 82% to 100% and specificity 93.3% to 100% (59–62). In a study by Linderholm et al. (63), in which all three testing methods were compared, sensitivity and specificity were similar for all three: 63% to 84% and 85% to 100%, respectively. The predictive value of a positive result was 80% to 92% for the whole red-blood-cell tests and 91% to 100% for the purified, heterophile, antigen agglutination and EIA tests, while the predictive value of a negative result did not exceed 85% for any of the tests. The lower sensitivity levels in the latter study were due to the inclusion of an equal number of children under the age of 12 years. In this group, the sensitivity did not exceed 50% for any of the tests, emphasizing important limitations of heterophile antibody testing in children. An EIA using EBV-specific antigens was also included in this study; however, performance was no different than the heterophile antibody tests.

Heterophile antibody testing by rapid methods is an important part of the evaluation of a patient with suspected IM. Many of the heterophile antibody tests have waived status under CLIA '88 (Clinical Laboratory Improvement Amendments 1988), making their use in the near-patient testing environment even more attractive. It should be remembered that the predictive value of a negative result, especially in young children, is not high. Therefore, when IM is suspected and the heterophile antibody test is negative, testing for antibodies to EBV-specific antigens is indicated.

BACTERIAL INFECTIONS

Lower Urinary Tract Infections

The lower urinary tract infections cystitis and urethritis are common throughout life. In all age groups, females have a higher incidence, except in the immediate period after birth. In addition, cystitis is a common nosocomial infection, primarily in patients with indwelling urinary catheters. Bacteria are the primary cause of these infections. Aerobic gram-negative bacteria are the most frequent pathogens, although some gram-positive bacteria comprise a significant portion of nosocomial infections. Patients with lower urinary tract infections often have dysuria, frequency, urgency, and occasionally fever and suprapubic tenderness. However, these symptoms can occur in genitourinary tract infections due to *Neisseria gonorrhoeae, Chlamydia trachomatis* in the presence of renal caluculi, or rarely in the presence of vaginitis.

Laboratory diagnosis of lower urinary tract infections involves culture of a mid-stream, clean-catch urine specimen. Since the initial article by Kass in 1956 (64), a urine culture comprised of a single species of bacteria in a concentration of at least 1×10^5 colony-forming units/milliliter (CFU/mL) has been accepted as an important laboratory criterion for the diagnosis of an acute cystitis. Other authors (65) have pointed out that concentrations of bacteria as low as 1×10^2 CFU/mL are significant in certain populations, most notably in women with the acute urethral syndrome (65). Growth of 1×10^2 to 1×10^4 CFU/mL can be significant in catheter-related infections and 1×10^3 CFU/mL can indicate infection in males.

Because quantitative urine cultures require 24 to 48 hours before a final result is available, attempts to develop rapid screens to identify patients with lower urinary tract infections

have been developed. The identification of bacteria in urine by light microscopy is a quick and economical method for rapid screening. Identification of bacteria in unstained uncentrifuged urine is the least sensitive method, whereas gram-stained and centrifuged urine is the most sensitive (66). Quantitative criteria have been determined for uncentrifuged, gram-stained urine: ≥1 bacteria per oil immersion field correlates with a bacterial concentration of 1×10^5 CFU/mL (66). Sensitivity in various studies using uncentrifuged urine has ranged from 72% to 97% using cultures with 1×10^5 CFU/mL as a standard, and while the specificity and predictive value of a positive result have been low, the predictive value of a negative result consistently has been higher than 99% (67). Both sensitivity and predictive value of a negative result of this method decrease as the culture colony count used for the reference method decrease, 78% and 81%, respectively, at 1×10^3 CFU/mL (67). Around 50% of acutely symptomatic females have colony counts of less than 1×10^5, limiting the usefulness of microscopy for bacteruria in this and other populations with low colony count infections (66). In addition, because bacteria in the urine can result from colonization or contamination, the false-positive rate with this test can be high. The presence of numerous epithelial cells, the presence of gram-positive bacilli or cocci, or a mixture of different types of bacteria suggests contamination.

Infection can be most effectively differentiated from colonization or contamination by the presence or absence of pyuria. Urinary excretion of more than 400,000 neutrophils per hour correlates with infection, and a concentration of more than 10 neutrophils/mm³ in urine correlates with this excretion rate (67). The most accurate and relatively simple method to determine leukocyte concentration in urine is examination of uncentrifuged urine in a hemocytometer. Determination of pyuria by microscopic examination of urinary sediment without the use of a hemocytometer is not accurate, because of variations in initial urine volumes, centrifugation speed and time, resuspension volume after centrifugation, and inconsistencies in counting because of lack of grid lines (66). Standardization of these variables makes results closer to those obtained with a hemocytometer (68).

The Greiss test, in which nitrate on an impregnated strip is reduced to nitrite by nitrate reductase in bacteria, has been used as a rapid urine screen. The test has poor sensitivity (35% to 85%) but high specificity (92% to 100%) (66). False negatives may occur if the infecting bacterium does not possess nitrate reductase (*Staphylococcus* sp., *Enterococcus* sp., and *Pseudomonas* sp.); the patient is on diuretics; or the urine has a pH of less than 6, high levels of urobilinogen, or contains ascorbic acid (66,67).

A similar concept is the use of substrate-impregnated strips that are acted upon by leukocyte esterase present in neutrophils to detect pyuria. The leukocyte esterase strip is more sensitive than the nitrate test, demonstrating a sensitivity of 75% to 96% and a specificity of 94% to 98% (66). The leukocyte esterase strip is prone to false-positive results, demonstrating a PPV around 50% (67). False-negative results may be caused by ascorbic acid and high levels of protein (67). Combination strips with both leukocyte esterase and nitrate are available; however, they have essentially the same performance characteristics as the leukocyte esterase test alone: sensitivity, 79% to 91%; specificity 60% to 79%; PPV, 23% to 66%; and NPV, 93% to 99% (70–78).

Rapid screens of urine may be useful in determining which patients require further assessment for the presence or absence of a lower urinary tract infection. Because the population of patients with lower urinary tract infections is heterogeneous and the effectiveness of each of the tests varies with bacterial concentration, type of infecting organism, and chemical composition of the urine, no one test will be adequate in all cases. For symptomatic individuals, direct microscopic examination of urine is superior, because a negative leukocyte esterase or nitrate test cannot exclude infection; leukocyte esterase, in contrast, may be used in asymptomatic patients (66). The nitrate reductase test has low sensitivity and is not recommended as a stand-alone test. Sound clinical judgment and confirmation of screening test results with quantitative culture should be used to assess patients with suspected lower urinary tract infection.

Streptococcus Pyogenes Pharyngitis

Pharyngitis is a common reason for physician office visits in this country with approximately 30% of pediatric and 5% of adult cases caused by *Streptococcus pyogenes* (Group A Streptococcus) (79). Because signs and symptoms of Group A Streptococcus pharyngitis (i.e., sore throat, dysphagia, fever, headache, abdominal pain, coryza, hoarseness, and tonsillar exudate) are nonspecific, diagnosis based on clinical findings alone is difficult. Throat culture has been the primary method of diagnosis; however, results take 24 to 72 hours. Although antibiotic therapy may be delayed for up to 9 days without compromising their effect in preventing rheumatic fever, up to 55% of family practitioners and 75% of pediatricians will begin therapy prior to obtaining culture results (79). Reasons for this are the inability to ensure that patients will return for culture results, the desire to alleviate the discomfort of the patient, and the importance of limiting spread of the bacteria. This practice exposes patients without Group A Streptococcus to needless antibiotic therapy and potential drug reactions.

In an attempt to enable physicians to determine in a timely fashion which patients require antibiotic treatment, rapid systems designed to detect Group A Streptococcus antigen have been developed. Latex agglutination tests in which beads coated with antibody to Group A polysaccharide were the first generation of rapid Group A Streptococcus tests. The latex tests were plagued by low sensitivity and subjectivity in assessing the presence or absence of agglutination (80). The rapid detection tests require an extraction step prior to running the assay, where the Group A carbohydrate is extracted by acid or cell wall active enzymes. The EIA format has been adapted for detection of Group A Streptococcus antigen. Most rapid EIA tests are membrane immunoassays in which Streptococcal antigen bound to antibody is immobilized on a membrane, and a detector enzyme acts upon an added substrate to produce a color change indicating a positive test. Several other formats are available, including an EIA test with antibodies conjugated to liposomes (Q Test Strep, Becton Dickinson, Franklin Lakes, NJ) and a sandwich EIA that uses a micro-well format, allowing multiple rapid tests to be run more efficiently (Visuwell Strep-A, ADI Diagnostics, Ontario, Canada).

While EIA-based tests have shown better performance than the latex tests in many evaluations, there does not appear to be one product that is superior to the others and none are as sensitive as cultures. Sensitivity has ranged from 39% to 95.8%, specificity from 79% to 100%, PPV of 65% to 100%, and NPV of 81% to 98.3% (80–85). Variation in performance of the same product from one testing site to another occurs, and has been attributed to the quality of specimen obtained, how the specimen is maintained prior to testing, and the training of the individuals performing the test (79,80,84). Collecting the specimen from both tonsils is more likely to capture Group A streptococci than from one tonsil. In two studies where each tonsil was sampled with a separate swab, one side was negative for Group A Streptococcus in 20% and 28.5% of cases (79,85). Swabs that have been moistened with transfer medium reduce the sensitivity of Group A Streptococcus EIA tests compared to dry swabs (83,86).

A recent innovative format in EIA-based, Group A Streptococcus rapid testing is the optical immunoassay Strep A OIA (Biostar, Boulder, CO). This test is comprised of a silicon wafer with anti–Group A polyclonal rabbit antibody on the surface. Reflected light on the surface creates a gold color. Extracted streptococcal antigen is mixed with a horseradish-peroxidase-labeled antibody and the resultant immune complex is allowed to bind to the antibody on the silicon wafer. Substrate is added, which reacts with the enzyme labeled antibody, creating a precipitate on the surface. The resultant change in thickness of layers causes a change in reflective properties of the surface, visualized as a purple color. A negative test is indicated by no change in color of the test surface. Initial evaluations of this test were very favorable, suggesting that the test was more sensitive than the routine culture of Group A Streptococcus and this could obviate the need for confirmatory cultures (87). Subsequent evaluations have shown a sensitivity of 81% to 92.3%, a specificity of 89% to 97.4%, PPV of 77% to 91.5%, and NPV of 93% to 95.8% (83,85,88). A culture is therefore required to confirm negative results. In addition, weak positive results can be difficult to detect, and less than thorough washing may lead to confusion of a negative with a weak positive (88).

While these rapid diagnostic tests for Group A Streptococcus pharyngitis allow administration of antibiotic therapy based on a positive result, the American Academy of Pediatrics recommends that all negative tests be confirmed by culture because these tests are not as sensitive as cultures (89). Therefore, since cultures will be done in a high proportion of cases, the added cost of doing the rapid test must be considered when deciding whether they should be used. In addition, because no one product is clearly superior to the others, and variability in performance occurs between testing sites and between individuals performing the test, careful attention to training is warranted, and correlation studies with culture prior to implementing a particular Group A Streptococcus direct antigen test are recommended (90). Many of the Group A Streptococcus direct antigen tests have waived status under CLIA '88.

Helicobacter Pylori

Helicobacter pylori is a gram-negative, spiral-shaped, microaerophilic bacterium that inhabits the mucous overlying the gastric mucosa and produces gastritis. Worldwide the rate of infection is high, occurring during childhood in underdeveloped countries and later in industrialized countries such as the United States (91). *H. pylori* causes peptic ulcer disease and is associated with gastric carcinoma and primary B cell lymphoma of the stomach. Detection of the organism in infected patients is important, since effective therapy is available. Numerous methods for detecting the presence of *H. pylori* exist, some of which require an invasive procedure and some of which do not. Diagnostic tests that can be done without an endoscopy-obtained biopsy include the ^{13}C and ^{14}C breath tests, serology, and an EIA stool antigen test. Methods requiring tissue biopsy include histology, smear/touch prep cytology, culture, polymerase chain reaction, and rapid urease testing. Of these, rapid urease testing, smear/touch prep cytology, and serology have been adapted to the near-patient testing environment.

Rapid urease testing is based on the production of the enzyme urease by *H. pylori*. The CLO test (Delta West, Australia) was the first of the rapid urease tests developed and is available worldwide. The test consists of a plastic slide with a cup containing urea agar with phenol red indicator and a bacteriostatic agent, into which is embedded a biopsy specimen. The slide is sealed with a plastic cover and incubated at 30° to 40°C (often the physician's pocket). If *H. pylori* is present, urease degrades urea, producing ammonia and causing an increase in pH, changing the phenol red from yellow to red. The test is read preliminarily at 1 hour and again at 24 hours. Besides agar-based tests, tests using reagent strips are available (PyloriTek, Serim Research, Elkhart, IN). The newer tests are read at 1 hour and do not require rereading at 24 hours. The diverse rapid urease tests appear to be essentially equivalent (91). Studies have demonstrated sensitivity ranging from 71% to 98%, specificity from 68% to 100%, PPV from 79% to 100%, and NPV 79% to 98% (91–95).

At least 100,000 bacteria are required to produce a positive rapid urease test (96). Therapy decreases the bacterial load, and H_2 receptor antagonists cause a shift of the primary site of infection from the antrum to the corpus/fundus (93). Sensitivity was reduced from 91% to 79% by prior treatment with H_2 receptor antagonists (93). As a result, the rapid urease tests are not recommended for evaluation of effect of therapy (97).

H. pylori infection elicits an immune response in almost all adults (96). Both IgA and IgG are produced, but IgG appears to correlate more closely with disease (97). Serum IgG antibodies can be used to confirm the presence of infection in some patients. Several membrane EIA and latex agglutination tests have been developed that allow serological assessment in the near-patient environment. An example of an EIA-based test in a card format is the FlexSure HP (Smith-Kline Diagnostics, San Jose, CA), which has a bacterial-associated protein, HM-CAP, bound to a blue pad. A second pad, pink in color, is moistened with buffer to reconstitute the conjugate. A drop of serum is added to the blue pad and if antibodies are present, they bind to a strip of immobilized HM-CAP. The card is folded so that the pink and blue pads touch. If antibodies have been bound to the HM-CAP strip, conjugate is bound to both the test line and a second control line, and two lines on the pad indicate a positive test after 4 minutes. A negative test is indicated by the appearance of the control line only. Latex agglutination tests consist of latex particles coated with extracted antigens of *H. pylori*. Addi-

tion of serum containing antibodies results in agglutination in 3 minutes. Loy et al. (98) reviewed the literature and used meta-analysis to compare performance of different serological tests for *H. pylori* antibodies, concluding that the different tests were essentially equivalent, with a mean sensitivity of 85% and mean specificity of 79%. The FlexSure test, which was not included in their review, has shown a sensitivity ranging from 62.5% to 93.3% and a specificity of 77% to 96% (97–101).

Several caveats exist for using serology to diagnose *H. pylori* infection. Antibodies persist even after eradication of the organism, and although titers decline in 50% of patients after 6 months, serology is of limited usefulness in assessing effect of therapy (96,97). In addition, detection of the antibody does not distinguish between current and past infection. This is a particular consideration when evaluating older patients, who may have had *H. pylori* infection in the past and no longer do, but have persistent IgG antibody. Younger patients can also present a problem due to an inconsistent immune response. Khana et al. (100) demonstrated that the sensitivity of serology for diagnosis of infection was lower in children (75%) than in adults (92%). These investigators also demonstrated that the performance of serological assays varied based on the geographic region of the world in which patients reside (100). Because of the antigenic variation among strains of *H. pylori* in different parts of the world, experts recommend validation of any serological test for *H. pylori* antibodies in the population in which it will be used (100,102).

A third method to detect *H. pylori* that can be utilized in a rapid manner is cytologic examination of smears, prepared either as touch imprints of biopsies or as brushing smears. Both have the advantage over histology of sampling the mucous layer on the surface of the mucosa, which may be lost during tissue processing. Brushing cytology has the added advantage of sampling a larger area. Smears may be either air dried or alcohol fixed, depending on the stain used. Various stains may be used, such as the gram stain, methylene blue, eosin and methylene blue, or modified Wright stain. In one study (103), the sensitivity and specificity, respectively, of brushing cytology were 100% and 92.5%, compared to 66.7% and 80% for histology. In a similar study using imprint cytology and a modified Geimsa stain, sensitivity and specificity were 100% (104).

Several tests for detecting *H. pylori* are available and the choice is influenced by the clinical situation because none of the tests is optimal in all cases. Using more than one test increases sensitivity, and many recommend using at least two different methodologies, particularly if the first test performed is negative (95,105). The rapid tests described here are suited to the near-patient environment, such as the endoscopy suite, and can be used to allow initiation of therapy prior to obtaining results from a more time-consuming test such as histology or culture. Many of the rapid urease tests and rapid serology tests have waived status under CLIA '88, adding to their convenience.

Mycoplasma Pneumoniae

Mycoplasma pneumoniae is a cell-wall-deficient bacterium that causes mild respiratory illness, tracheobronchitis, and pneumonia in humans. Disease occurs both endemically year-round and as epidemics every 3 to 7 years, usually in the fall. It is responsible for 10% to 20% of community-acquired pneumonias, with a higher incidence in children (106). Antibody prevalence studies have shown a 5.3% annual infection rate in adults and children, with an 8.8% rate in children aged 5 to 9 (106). Although infection with *M. pneumoniae* is self-limited, antibiotic treatment with a tetracycline or a macrolide will significantly shorten the illness. Identification of cases based on clinical manifestations alone is difficult, as there is overlap of signs and symptoms with other bacterial and viral causes of respiratory illness. In the laboratory, *M. pneumoniae* is difficult to culture; it requires specialized media and grows slowly, sometimes requiring several weeks to isolate. Despite the advent of newer methods of diagnosis such as the polymerase chain reaction and DNA hybridization, the primary method of diagnosis has been and continues to be serology. Complement fixation and most of the newer serological tests, based on EIA technology or FA, are laboratory tests, and thus not suitable for near-patient testing. Two methods of assessing the serological status of a patient with respect to *M. pneumoniae* are, however, rapid and potentially useful in a near-patient setting.

Cold agglutinins are detected in the serum of up to 75% of patients with *M. pneumoniae* pneumonia, and the amount present appears to correlate with the degree of pulmonary involvement (106). These autoantibodies directed against the I antigen on erythrocytes appear at the end of the first week or early in the second week of illness. Detection of these cold agglutinins in the laboratory involves mixing serial dilutions of the patient's serum with type O red cells. However, Garrow (107) described a rapid bedside screening test in 1958 that is clinically useful. Approximately 1 mL of blood is placed in a tube with sodium citrate anticoagulant, and the tube is allowed to cool at 0° to 4°C in ice water or in a refrigerator for 3 to 4 minutes. The tube is tilted to check for macroscopic agglutination, and if present, the tube is warmed to 37°C, usually in the hand or pocket of the person doing the test, and rechecked for agglutination after several minutes. If the agglutination disappears with warming, the test is positive for cold agglutinins. A positive rapid test correlates with a titer higher than 1:64, and a titer higher than 1:32 is accepted as strong evidence of *M. pneumoniae* infection (107,108). Cold agglutinins have also been demonstrated in adenovirus, influenza, RSV, CMV, and mumps infections, as well as in lymphoproliferative diseases (109).

The presence of antibodies specific to *M. pneumoniae* can be detected rapidly with the use of membrane EIA technology. The Immunocard Mycoplasma Kit (Meridian Diagnostics, Cincinnati, OH) and the *Mycoplasma pneumoniae* Immunoglobulin G (IgG/IgM) Antibody Test System (Remel, Lenexa, KS) are the two currently available tests for which evaluations have been published. Both involve the addition of patient serum to a card containing sample and control wells, followed by an enzyme-labeled antihuman antibody, and conjugate. A color change in the sample well indicates a positive test. Test results are obtained in about 7 to 10 minutes. The Meridian product detects only IgM, while the Remel EIA detects both IgG and IgM. Compared to other serological methods, sensitivity and specificity of the two membrane EIA products are higher than 90% (110–112).

Several latex agglutination products to detect antibodies to *M. pneumoniae* in serum are available in Europe, and evalua-

tions have demonstrated mixed results (113,114). No data concerning the single latex agglutination product (Meristar MP, Meridian Diagnostics, Cincinnati, OH) have been published in the United States; however, the manufacturer claims a sensitivity of 91% and specificity of 96% compared to complement fixation. The test detects both IgM and IgG.

Several problems exist in using serology as the sole laboratory method to diagnose *M. pneumoniae*. In the first 7 to 10 days of illness, no antibodies are present, causing the disease to be undiagnosed if a single serological test is performed early in the illness. Laboratory-based evaluation has traditionally used a four-fold increase in antibody titers in paired serum specimens drawn at least 4 weeks apart to detect such cases. Tests that detect only IgM may miss infection in patient groups in which an IgM response to infection occurs less frequently, that is, patients with re-infection or those aged over 40 years (112,115). While using tests that detect both IgM and IgG theoretically could detect cases in these groups, it must be remembered that detection of IgG in a single specimen does not reliably distinguish acute from past infection. Utilization of a test that detects IgM is the most specific; however, if it is early in a patient's illness and clinical suspicion is high, a negative IgM test result should be confirmed by respiratory culture or paired acute and convalescent serum for IgG titers.

Bacterial Enteritis

Diarrheal illnesses are common worldwide and can occur in both the outpatient and inpatient settings. They can be classified into two broad categories based on the general pathogenetic mechanism by which the diarrhea is produced by the infecting organism. Secretory or noninflammatory diarrheas result from an alteration in the absorptive ability of the gastrointestinal tract, and examples include diarrhea caused by rotavirus, Norwalk agent, *Cryptosiridium*, *Vibrio cholerae*, enterotoxigenic *Escherichia coli*, and *Cyclospora*. In contrast, inflammatory diarrheas result from destruction of the mucosal lining of the gastrointestinal tract, either by invasion by the organism or production of a cytotoxin. Examples include diarrhea due to *Shigella* sp., *Salmonella* sp., *Campylobacter jejuni*, and *Clostridium difficile*. Cultures of feces may identify the organism responsible for diarrhea, but the delay of 48 to 72 hours required for the culture impairs its utility in the immediate management of the illness. Rapid differentiation between the two types of diarrheal illnesses may be important for a number of reasons. Some inflammatory diarrheas require antibiotic treatment (e.g., *Campylobacter jejuni* or *Clostridium difficile)*, and knowing the general type of diarrhea a patient has can allow institution of appropriate public health measures prior to obtaining culture results. In addition, differentiation could result in cost savings by determining which patients may benefit from feces culture.

Destruction of the mucosal lining of the gastrointestinal tract by pathogenic bacteria results in dysenteric stools, feces containing neutrophils, mucous, and blood. Detection of these components has been proposed as a useful way to differentiate between the two general categories of diarrheal illnesses. The presence of neutrophils in inflammatory diarrhea has been recognized and utilized diagnostically since the early 1900s (116). A fresh specimen is required, and feces in a cup or container are superior to a swab or specimen obtained from a diaper (117). The most frequent method of detecting neutrophils is a wet prep prepared by mixing a small amount of feces on a clean slide with two drops of methylene blue dye, placing a cover slip over the mixture, and examining the smear under oil immersion (1000×). Other methods include staining air-dried or alcohol-fixed smears with a gram stain or modified Wright stain, or using an automatic stainer such as that used to stain peripheral blood smears (118,119). The number of neutrophils required for a positive result has not been standardized. Criteria that have been used include 1 neutrophil per 20 oil immersion fields, more than 2 neutrophils per 5 oil immersion fields, and more than 5 neutrophils per oil immersion field (116,120,121).

Microscopy for fecal neutrophils requires intact white cells, which may not always be present despite the fact the patient has an inflammatory diarrhea. Detection of lactoferrin, a glycoprotein in specific or secondary granules of neutrophils that chelates iron, thus preventing its use by bacteria, appears to be a sensitive surrogate marker for neutrophils (117). Commercially available (Leuko-Test, Techlab, Blacksburg, VA), the test consists of latex beads coated with rabbit antihuman, lactoferrin antibody, which is mixed in an equal volume of stool sample, resulting in agglutination within 3 minutes if lactoferrin is present. However, lactoferrin is found in colostrum, mature human milk, and blood, and false-positive reactions occur in infants who are breast fed (122).

Detection of blood in stool may help identify patients with dysenteric illnesses. Many tests for detecting blood are commercially available, all of which depend on the peroxidase or pseudo-peroxidase activity present in blood reacting with a chemical indicator such as guiac, benzidine, or orthotoluidine, to produce a color change upon the addition of hydrogen peroxide. These tests differ slightly in sensitivity, but given the amount of blood present in the feces with these illnesses, this is of little practical concern.

When used alone, tests for detecting neutrophils and blood are relatively insensitive and nonspecific. Sensitivity and specificity of microscopy for fecal leukocytes range from 31% to 89% and 60% to 94%, respectively, and for fecal occult blood, 31% to 87% and 50 to 94%, respectively (118–120,122–124). As a single test, fecal lactoferrin has the highest sensitivity, ranging from 85% to 97%, but its specificity is low (15% to 79%) (120,122,124). Two studies (122,124) reported improved sensitivity (84% to 100%), but not specificity, by using fecal lactoferrin in combination with fecal leukocytes or fecal occult blood, and requiring that either rather than both be detected for the evaluation to be considered positive. The PPV in evaluations of these tests, singly or in combination, has been low but the NPV has been relatively high (82% to 100%). If fecal lactoferrin in combination with either fecal leukocytes or fecal blood results in a negative test, fecal culture for bacterial pathogens may not be necessary. However, if clinical suspicion for bacterial enteritis is high, fecal culture should be performed regardless of the result of the rapid test.

Sepsis Due to Gram-Negative Bacteria

Sepsis is defined as the presence of the systemic inflammatory response syndrome (SIRS) in the face of a confirmed infectious process (125). SIRS is a constellation of clinical parameters associated with a systemic response to a severe assault on the physiological equilibrium of the human body, of which there are many causes, only one of which is sepsis. About one-half of cases of sepsis are due to gram-negative bacteria, and of these patients, about one-half develop septic shock (125). With progression along the spectrum of SIRS to septic shock, there is an increase in multiple-organ failure that can lead to death. Sepsis/septic shock is the most common cause of death in intensive care unit patients (125).

For patients at risk for sepsis, the ability to rapidly identify those with impending septic shock and multi-organ failure would allow specific therapy and may reduce morbidity and mortality. Because clinical parameters associated with SIRS are nonspecific and blood cultures may require days to become positive, a laboratory marker for the early diagnosis of sepsis would be valuable. Several substances have been evaluated, including cytokines, complement, phospholipids, and endotoxin, but only the latter has correlated with the development of multi-organ failure or mortality (126,127).

The *Limulus* amebocyte lysate assay (LAL) is based on the conversion of a lysate from the amebocyte of the horseshoe crab, *Limulus polyphemus*, to a clot in plasma, a process induced by the presence of endotoxin. The test is technically involved, rendering it unsuitable for the bedside testing environment. Its utility in detecting sepsis is currently controversial, with some studies finding good correlation and others finding only an association with fungal sepsis (126–129). Further, there are many inhibiting substances, its sensitivity is at the limit of the levels of endotoxin found in the blood, and false positives can be caused by endotoxin on testing materials (130,131).

Much of the endotoxin in blood of patients with endotoxemia is bound and cannot be detected by the LAL assay, which detects only free endotoxin. In an effort to make a more sensitive test and overcome many of the technical difficulties with the LAL assay, Rylatt et al. (132) developed an agglutination assay (SimpliRED Endotoxin Test, AGEN Biomedical, Brisbane, Australia), based on the ability of polymyxin B to bind endotoxin. Polymyxin B is bound to a monoclonal antibody that binds to glycophorin-A on red cell membranes, producing a hybrid molecule that will bind both red blood cells and endotoxin, resulting in crosslinking of red blood cells and visible agglutination of whole blood within 2 minutes. In the one published evaluation (127), the test detected 34 of 38 patients with culture-proven, gram-negative bacteremia with a false-positive rate of 1.5%. The authors of this study concluded that the assay was useful in detecting patients at risk for multi-organ failure.

D-dimer, a breakdown product of fibrin, has been proposed as a surrogate marker for sepsis and the same company that developed the SimpliRed Endotoxin Test has also developed a bedside agglutination assay to detect D-dimer (SimpliRed D-dimer, AGEN Biomedical, Brisbane, Australia). Based on a monoclonal antibody for D-dimer coupled to an antibody against a universal red cell antigen, whole-blood agglutinates in 2 minutes if D-dimer is present. The test showed a sensitivity of 66.7% for gram-positive bacteremia and 61.5% for gram-negative bacteremia, with a negative predictive value of 96% to 98% (133). The problem with this surrogate marker is the frequency that fibrinolysis occurs with other disorders or conditions, such as trauma, malignancy, burns, liver disease, cardiovascular disorders, autoimmune disorders, and deep venous thrombosis.

Currently, no reliable test for the rapid diagnosis of sepsis exists. Indeed, the clinical value of the one marker that has been extensively evaluated, endotoxin, as a diagnostic tool has been questioned, because not all patients with gram-negative sepsis have circulating endotoxin and not all patients with demonstrable endotoxin have sepsis (131,132). Endotoxin may have a role as a prognostic marker in those patients in whom it is identified, but a reliable early diagnostic marker for sepsis is not yet available (127,131).

Bacterial Vaginosis

Bacterial vaginosis is a polymicrobial infection in which the normal flora of the vagina (primarily lactobacilli) is replaced by a predominance of other bacteria, including *Gardnerella vaginalis*, *Mobiluncus* sp., *Prevotella* sp. and genital *Mycoplasma* sp. Approximately one-half of women with this infection experience symptoms such as pruritis, pain, odor, dysuria or frequency, and vaginal discharge; the remainder are asymptomatic. It is probably the most frequent vaginal infection in sexually active women, resulting in 5 million to 10 million patient visits annually (135). Bacterial vaginosis has been associated with an increased risk of preterm birth in pregnant patients and possibly with pelvic inflammatory disease and endometritis in nonpregnant women. Diagnosis is based on the presence of three of four criteria described by Amsel et al. (135): a vaginal pH higher than 4.5, a fishy odor of vaginal secretions on addition of potassium hydroxide (KOH), a thin watery discharge, and the presence of "clue" cells.

The vaginal pH increase to more than 4.5 is due to the lack of the normal lactic acid producing lactobacilli. Vaginal pH is assessed by placing a small amount of vaginal discharge on pH paper and comparing the resultant color change with color scales provided by the manufacturer. However, vaginal pH is affected by recent intercourse, menstruation, douching, or large quantities of cervical mucus, all of which can cause inaccurate results with pH paper (136).

The amine test, or "whiff" test, wherein the addition of 10% KOH to vaginal secretions results in volatization of amines (tetramethylamine, putrescine, cadaverine, and others) produced by the bacteria causing the infection, results in a "fishy" odor. It can be affected by the same factors as described for pH (136). The amine test is positive in 82% to 87% of patients with bacterial vaginosis (137). Specificity ranges from 82% to 97% (137). However, the test is subjective and dependent on the olfactory sensitivity of the observer.

Evaluation for clue cells is performed by a wet prep, in which material obtained by a vaginal wall scraping is added to a drop of 0.9% normal saline on a glass slide, a cover slip added, and the fluid is examined microscopically. Clue cells are squamous cells completely covered by small coccobacilli (morphology characteristic of *G. vaginalis*) with obscuring of the cell margins. Strict adherence to this definition is important in maintaining specificity. Clue cells indicate a high bacterial load and are found in more than 90% of patients with bacterial vaginosis (139). In the Amsel criteria, the presence of any clue cell is considered significant. Some authors have recommended that 20% of epithe-

lial cells present be clue cells; however, this results in a statistically significant reduction in sensitivity (139).

With the exception of the vaginal pH, the Amsel criteria are subjective and difficult to apply uniformly. In proficiency testing for diagnosing various types of vaginitis sponsored by the American Academy of Family Practice from 1990 to 1994, physician diagnostic accuracy was lowest for bacterial vaginosis (79%) (140). Attempts to identify a laboratory test that is objective and suited to a near-patient environment have centered on the use of gram-stained vaginal smears. This test has met with some success, and some consider it the reference method for diagnosing the disorder (141).

Several methods of standardizing evaluation of the gram-stained smears have been developed. These systems involve identifying and quantitating diverse bacterial morphotypes: large gram-positive rods (lactobacilli), small gram-negative rods (*Prevotella* sp. and *G. vaginalis*), and small curved gram-negative to gram-variable rods (*Mobiluncus sp.*). The system described by the Vaginal Infection and Prematurity Study Group entails determining the average number of the different morphotypes per oil immersion field, assigning this average a score, and adding the scores of the different morphotypes together to determine a total score from 0 to 10 (142). A score higher than 7 is diagnostic of bacterial vaginosis. This system is accurate and reproducible with good inter- and intra-observer agreement; however, it is relatively labor intensive (139,141–143). Other authors have advocated a more simplified system such as that of Thomason et al. (144), in which 400× fields are evaluated without counting, to determine if lactobacilli outnumber nonlactobacilli morphotypes and if clue cells are present. Vaginosis is diagnosed if nonlactobacilli outnumber lactobacilli in more than one-half of fields evaluated and if clue cells are seen in more than 2 of 20 fields (144). This method appears to be comparable to the previously described method of the Vaginal Infection Study Group (144).

Oligonucleotide probe technology has been applied to the diagnosis of bacterial vaginosis. The Affirm VP III System (Microprobe, Bothell, Washington) utilizes an automated processor to detect *G. vaginalis*, *Trichomonas vaginalis*, and *Candida albicans*. A vaginal swab specimen is incubated in lysis buffer for 5 minutes, buffer and substrate are added, and the solution is placed in a specimen caddy and placed on the processor. If specific nucleic acids are present, hybridization with a biotinylated probe occurs and streptavidin-horseradish peroxidase is bound to captured nucleic acid. Finally, indicator substrate is converted to a blue color if bound enzyme conjugate is present on beads on the specimen caddy. Results are available in 30 minutes. Compared to the gram stain, the sensitivity, specificity, PPV, and NPV of the Affirm are 94%, 81%, 80%, and 94%, respectively (134). This low specificity has been seen in other studies and probably is related to the detection of *G. vaginalis* in clinically insignificant amounts (140). One author (134) recommends using the Affirm in conjunction with at least one other test, such as the vaginal pH or whiff test.

Gonorrhea

Gonorrhea is a sexually or perinatally transmitted bacterial infection caused by *Neisseria gonorrhoeae*, a gram-negative coccus that grows in pairs with adjacent sides flattened (diplococci). It most commonly occurs as a purulent urethritis in men and endocervicitis in women, but can result in disseminated infection, anorectal or pharyngeal infection, peri-hepatitis, pelvic inflammatory disease, or conjunctival infections in infants (opthalmia neonatorum). Diagnosis is based on isolation of the bacteria from an infected site; however, a rapid presumptive diagnosis prior to obtaining culture results can be obtained in cases of urethritis/endocervicitis by using a smear of purulent exudate. This is particularly important in environments where immediate treatment is optimal because of concern that patients may not return for treatment when culture results are available, or to prevent spread of infection while awaiting culture results.

Identification of the characteristic gram-negative diplococci in neutrophils on a smear of exudate from the male urethra or endocervix stained with gram stain is the method used for rapid diagnosis. The sensitivity and specificity of this test for symptomatic males ranges from 89.1% to 98.6% and 94.9% to 98.7%, respectively (145–148). The PPV and NPV are approximately 95% and 93%, respectively (145,147). For women, the test is not as useful, with sensitivity and specificity ranging from 16% to 65.4% and 88.4% to 100%, respectively (145–147). The PPV and NPV for the endocervical smear are 97% and 51%, respectively (145,147). An endocervical smear positive for intracellular gram-negative diplococci can have diagnostic utility; however, a negative smear is unreliable. A gram-stained smear of material obtained from the pharynx or rectum is not useful diagnostically, due to the presence of many commensal bacterial species with an identical morphology.

Alternatively, a single stain can be utilized to detect the bacteria, rather than the two stains, and two reagents required in the gram stain. Oxtoby et al. (145) demonstrated no difference in sensitivity or specificity utilizing the safranin stain when compared to the gram stain. Other stains such as methylene blue or methyl green-pyronin can be used. While simpler to perform and more rapid, such stains may require more care and skill in interpreting, and strict attention must be paid to morphology of the bacteria to maintain specificity.

FUNGAL INFECTIONS

Superficial Mycoses

Dermatophytosis are infections caused by three genera of molds—*Epidermophyton*, *Trichophyton*, and *Microsporum*—and are among the most common infections in humans. Any portion of the skin may be involved, but the feet, groin, scalp, and nails are the most common sites. Although characteristic, the clinical appearance of the raised, annular, scaly patch seen in dermatophytosis is not pathognomonic and other skin disorders must be included in the differential diagnosis. In addition, depending on the infecting organism and the immune status of the patient, lesions can be pustular or altered by self-treatment with over-the-counter medications before the patient sees the physician. The fungi are keratinophilic and infect the stratum corneum of the skin, and so can be easily cultured; however, growth and identification requires from 1 to 3 weeks.

Although definitive identification of the fungus requires culture, microscopic examination of skin scrapings for hyphae can provide a rapid diagnosis of dermatophytosis. Scrapings can be obtained with a scalpel blade or a larger intact superficial biopsy of the stratum corneum can be obtained by placing two halves of a razor blade in opposition to one another and moving it over the stratum corneum parallel to the skin surface (149). Effective visualization of hyphae requires dissolving or clearing of the keratin on the slide. This is most commonly accomplished by adding the scrapings to 10% to 30% KOH on the slide, with resultant dissolving of the keratin in 10 to 15 minutes. The time required to clear the slide can be reduced to less than 1 minute by gently heating the slide; however, care must be taken not to dry the solution (150). Other solutions that have been used for clearing include 10% Na_2S (clears skin scrapings in 1 minute, nail scrapings in 5 to 10 minutes), 5% sodium larylsulfate (SDS; requires 10 to 20 minutes for clearing), and xylene (results in immediate clearing) (150). Na_2S has been cited as the most efficient solution for this purpose; however, the odor created by the resultant production of H_2S when it reacts with keratin may be offensive to some (150). Various stains have been used to enhance visualization of hyphae, including ink, chlorazol black E, lactophenol cotton-blue, and methylene blue, without significant improvement in sensitivity (150). Lowering the microscope condenser to the point where hyphae appear refractile may improve visualization somewhat.

Despite the popularity of the KOH prep, there are relatively few studies that address the diagnostic accuracy of this test in detecting dermatophytosis. Sensitivity has ranged from 77% to 88%, specificity 62% to 95%, PPV 59% to 73%, and NPV 79% to 98% (151,152). When detecting superficial yeast infections of the skin, sensitivity is only 25% to 50% (151,152).

An alternative to the KOH prep is a simple preparation, in which a segment of cellophane tape is placed over the lesion on the skin, and then removed and placed on a glass slide. Several drops of Albert's solution, a mixture of glacial acetic acid, toluidine blue, malachite green, ethanol, and water, are placed at the edge of the tape and allowed to run under it (153). Hyphae and yeast immediately stain purple in contrast to nonstaining keratin. The method is purported to have the same sensitivity as the KOH prep (153).

Candida Vaginitis

Vaginal infection with *Candida* species is an infection that almost all women suffer from at least once during their lifetime (141). Over 80% of infections are caused by *Candida albicans*, and most of the remainder by *C. tropicalis* and *C. glabrata* (141). Clinical signs and symptoms including a thick discharge, pruritis, vaginal and vulvar erythema, and the occasional presence of vulvar fissures are characteristic but not pathognomonic. Culture is not indicated, except in certain circumstances discussed below, because 15% to 20% of women are asymptomatically colonized with *C. albicans*, and isolation of the yeast does not necessarily indicate infection (141).

Diagnosis of *Candida* vaginitis is made by the demonstration of pseudo-hyphae and yeast on a KOH preparation. The smear is prepared in a fashion similar to that described in the "Superficial Mycoses" section; however, the specimen is most often obtained by rubbing a swab on the lateral vaginal wall, which is then rubbed onto a slide and mixed with 10% to 30% KOH. Sensitivity of the KOH prep for detecting *Candida* vaginitis varies from 19% to 91%, although in most studies it ranges from 70% to 85% (140,141,154–158). In the American Academy of Family Practice Proficiency Testing Program from 1990 to

1994, sensitivity of the KOH smear ranged from 82% to 97% (140). Specificity in these studies was 90% to 99%. If the KOH prep is negative and the suspicion for *Candida* vaginitis remains high, some recommend a vaginal culture for yeast; however, as previously mentioned, colonization with *Candida* is not uncommon and other causes of vaginitis must be ruled out (141).

TABLE 14.2. SUMMARY OF TESTS FOR INFECTIOUS DISEASE POINT-OF-CARE TESTING

Infection	Test Method	Comments
Viral infections		
Herpes simplex virus/Varicella-zoster virus	Tzanck smear	Sensitivity depends on stage of the lesion sampled
Respiratory syncytial virus	Solid/phase EIA	More sensitive early in infection; nasal washes superior to nasopharyngeal swabs
Influenza A/B	Solid/phase EIA	Throat and nasopharyngeal swabs equivalent to nasal wash (in adults)
Rotavirus	Latex agglutination	Sensitivity varies with manufacturer
	Solid/phase EIA	More sensitive than latex in some studies
HIV-1	Solid/phase EIA (SUDS)	FDA approval for serum or plasma only
Varicella-zoster antibody	Latex agglutination	Detects IgG only
Infectious mononucleosis (Heterophile antibody)	Whole RBC agglutination	Performance is similar for all three methods; predictive value of a negative result very low for children
	Latex agglutination	
	Solid/phase EIA	
Bacterial infections		
Urinary tract infections	Microscopy for bacteria in urine	Centrifugation and gram stain increase sensitivity
	Nitrate test	Low sensitivity
	Leukocyte esterase	More sensitive than nitrate
Group A streptococcus	Solid/phase EIA	No one product of the many available is superior; some have waived test status under CLIA 1988
Helicobacter pylori	Rapid urease	Not recommended for evaluation of therapy
	Solid phase EIA for IgG	Does not distinguish between current and past infection
	Imprint smears	More sensitive than histology
Mycoplasma pneumoniae	Cold agglutinins	Not all infected patients develop agglutinins; not specific
	Solid/phase EIA for antibody	Not as sensitive as laboratory-based EIA methods
	Latex agglutination for antibody	No published evaluations for product available in U.S.
Bacterial enteritis	Microscopy for white blood cells	Standardized criteria for positivity not established
	Lactoferrin	High sensitivity but low specificity
	Occult blood	Using a combination of these tests improves sensitivity, not specificity
Gram negative sepsis	Endotoxin agglutination test	Does not appear useful as a diagnostic test; may have prognostic value
Bacterial vaginosis	Vaginal pH testing	Affected by many factors leading to possible inaccuracy
	Amine ("whiff") test	Highly subjective
	Clue cells by wet prep	High sensitivity; requires microscopy skills
	Gram stain of vaginal smear	Considered reference method; requires microscopy skills
	Oligonucleotide probe (Affirm VP III)	High sensitivity, low specificity
Gonorrhea	Gram stain	Useful for urethral smears from males; unreliable for endocervix, pharynx, rectum
Fungal infections		
Dermatophytosis	KOH prep	Widely used; few studies addressing efficacy; poor for diagnosing yeast infections of the skin
Candida vaginitis	KOH prep	Widely used; dependence on culture for diagnosis in case a negative KOH not recommended; other causes of vaginitis must be excluded
	Oligonucleotide probe (Affirm VP III)	Higher sensitivity than KOH
Parasitic infections		
Trichomonas vaginalis	Saline wet prep	Widely used; requires immediate microscopic exam as motility lost with cooling
	Oligonucleotide probe (Affirm VP III)	More sensitive than wet prep; system most useful in women with infections caused by more than one species

EIA, enzyme immonoassay; KOH, potassium hydroxide.

The automated nucleic acid probe system (AffirmVP III, Microprobe, Bothell, WA) described in the "Bacterial Vaginosis" section appears to be more accurate than the KOH prep in diagnosing *Candida* vaginitis, with a sensitivity of 75%, specificity of 96%, PPV of 82%, and NPV of 94% (140). These same values for the KOH smear in this study were 40%, 90%, 51%, and 86%, respectively (140). The nucleic acid probe system was particularly useful in detecting infections with more than one organism, the incidence of which was 14% in this study. In these cases, sensitivity was 17.5% for the KOH prep compared to 55% for the Affirm VP III (140).

PARASITIC INFECTIONS

Trichomonas Vaginalis

The protozoan *Trichomonas vaginalis*, which is sexually transmitted, is a common cause of vaginitis and urethritis in women and urethritis in men. Classic symptoms such as a frothy malodorous discharge and "strawberry cervix" in women are seen in only a very small fraction of infected patients, and approximately 25% to 50% of women are asymptomatic (141,159). The most sensitive and specific method of diagnosing this disease is culture; however, this requires 2 to 7 days and is not always available. Trichomonads can be detected in routine pap smears, but the sensitivity of this method is questionable and results often are not available for many days (160).

The most frequently used rapid method for diagnosis of trichomoniasis is the wet prep, first described by Donne in 1836 (160). Vaginal discharge, obtained with a swab or loop, is mixed with normal saline and placed on a glass slide. After placement of a cover slip, the slide is examined microscopically for the presence of motile trichomonads. It is important to make and examine the prep immediately, or maintain the specimen at 37°C until it can be viewed, because the organisms lose motility on cooling. The sensitivity of this technique ranges from 57% to 83%, specificity from 97% to 100%, PPV from 64% to 100%, and NPV 94% to 99% (134,140,155,159,160). Various stains, such as methylene blue, have been utilized to attempt to improve sensitivity, but have not shown a significant improvement in detection rate (160,161). Sensitivity of the wet mount is adversely affected by prior douching in women, dropping from 57% to 21% in one study (159).

The Affirm VP III DNA probe system as described in the "Bacterial Vaginosis" section is more sensitive than the wet mount for detecting *Trichomonas*. Sensitivity of 83% to 87%, specificity of 99% to 100%, PPV of 82% to 100%, and NPV of 94% to 99% have been reported (134,140).

Neither the wet mount nor the DNA probe are sufficiently sensitive to exclude *Trichomonas* infection based on a negative result. Negative tests in the face of a high index of suspicion clinically should be followed by culture. A commercially available plastic pouch (InPouch, BIOMED Diagnostics, San Jose, CA) that is inoculated at the bedside, transported to the laboratory, incubated, and examined microscopically without opening, is convenient for both the caregiver and laboratory personnel.

CONCLUSIONS (TABLE 14.2)

- Use of rapid tests for infectious disease testing can allow earlier appropriate management and disposition of patients.
- These tests are for the most part relatively insensitive compared to laboratory-based tests and are often merely presumptive.
- Correlation with the clinical picture is mandatory.
- Negative tests frequently require follow-up with the appropriate laboratory-based tests.
- As the frequency of infectious diseases varies with the season or during epidemics, PPV and NPV will vary for a given test and thus the utility of the test in making management decisions may vary.
- Cost of many of the new molecular-based rapid tests for infectious diseases is high relative to laboratory-based tests, and this higher cost must be balanced against savings obtained in earlier management of the patient.

REFERENCES

1. Solomon AR, Rasmussen JE, et al. The Tzanck smear in the diagnosis of cutaneous herpes simplex. *JAMA* 1984;251:633–635.
2. Woods GL. Herpesviruses. In: Woods GL, Guiterrez. *Diagnostic Pathology of Infectious Diseases*. Malvern, PA: Lea and Feibiger, 1993: 46–64.
3. Nahass GT, Goldstein BA, Zhu WY, et al. Comparison of the Tzanck smear, viral culture, and DNA diagnostic methods in detection of herpes simplex and Varicella-Zoster infection. *JAMA* 1992;268: 2541–2544.
4. Mendoza J, Rojas A, Navarro JM, et al. Evaluation of three rapid enzyme immunoassays and cell culture for detection of respiratory syncytial virus. *Eur J Clin Microbiol Infect Dis* 1992;11:452–454.
5. Englund JA, Sullivan CJ, Jordan C, et al. Respiratory syncytial virus in immunocompromised adults. *Ann Intern Med* 1988;109:203–208.
6. Sorvillo FJ, Huie SF, Strassburg MA, et al. An outbreak of respiratory syncytial virus pneumonia in a nursing home for the elderly. *J Infect* 1983;9:252–256.
7. Adcock PM, Stout GG, Hauck MA, et al. Effect of rapid viral diagnosis on the management of children hospitalized with lower respiratory tract infection. *Pediatr Infect Dis J* 1997;16:842–846.
8. Leonardi GP, Leib H, Birkhead GS, et al. Comparison of rapid detection methods for Influenza A and their value in health-care management of institutionalized geriatric patients. *J Clin Microbiol* 1994;32: 70–74.
9. Michaels MG, Serdy C, Barbadora K, et al. Respiratory syncytial virus: a comparison of diagnostic modalities. *Pediatr Infec Dis J* 1992; 11:613–616.
10. Kok T, Barancek K, Burrell CJ. Evaluation of the Becton Dickinson Directogen Test for Respiratory Syncytial Virus in nasopharyngeal aspirates. *J Clin Microbiol* 1990;28:1458–1459.
11. Waner J, Whitehurst NJ, Todd SJ, et al. Comparison of Directogen RSV with viral isolation and direct immunofluorescence for the identification of Respiratory Syncytial Virus. *J Clin Microbiol* 1990;28: 480–483.
12. Halstead D, Todd S, Fritch G. Evaluation of five methods for respiratory syncytial virus detection. *J Clin Microbiol* 1990;28: 1021–1025.
13. Dominguez EA, Taber LH, Couch RB. Comparison of rapid diagnostic techniques for Respiratory Syncytial and Influenza A virus respiratory infections in young children. *J Clin Microbiol* 1993;31: 2286–2290.

14. Mendoza J, Rojas A, Navarro JM, et al. Evaluation of three rapid enzyme immunoassays and cell culture for detection of Respiratory Syncytial Virus. *Eur J Clin Microbiol Infect Dis* 1992;11:452–454.

15. Thomas EE, Book LE. Comparison of two rapid methods for detection of Respiratory Syncytial Virus (RSV) (TestPack RSV and Ortho RSV ELISA) with direct immunofluorescence and virus isolation for the diagnosis of pediatric RSV infection. *J Clin Microbiol* 1991;29: 632–635,

16. Wren CG, Bate BJ, Masters HB, et al. Detection of Respiratory Syncytial virus antigen in nasal washings by Abbott TestPack immunoassay. *J Clin Microbiol* 1990;28:1395–1397.

17. Miller H, Milk R, Diaz-Mitoma F. Comparison of the VIDAS RSV assay and the Abbott Testpack RSV with direct immunofluorescence for detection of Respiratory Syncytial Virus in nasopharyngeal aspirates. *J Clin Microbiol* 1993;31:1336–1338.

18. Sweirkosz EM, Flanders R, Melvin L, et al. Evaluation of the Abbott TESTPACK RSV enzyme immunoassay for detection of Respiratory Syncytial Virus in nasopharyngeal swab specimens. *J Clin Microbiol* 1989;27:1151–1154.

19. Olsen MA, Shuck KM, Sambol AR. Evaluation of Abbott TestPack RSV for the diagnosis of Respiratory Syncytial Virus infections. *Diagn Microbiol Infect Dis* 1993;16:105–109.

20. Garea MT, Lopez JM, Perez del Molino ML, et al. Comparison of a new commercial enzyme immunoassay for rapid detection of Respiratory Syncytial Virus. *Eur J Clin Microbiol Infect Dis* 1992;11: 175–177.

21. Reina J, Munar M, Blanco I. Evaluation of a direct immunofluorescence assay, dot-blot enzyme immunoassay, and shell vial culture in the diagnosis of lower respiratory infections caused by Influenza A virus. *Diagn Microbiol Infect Dis* 1996;25:143–145.

22. Waner JL, Todd SJ, Shalaby H, et al. Comparison of Directogen FLU-A with viral isolation and direct immunofluorescence for the rapid detection and identification of Influenza A virus. *J Clin Microbiol* 1991;29:479–482.

23. Noyola DE, Clark B, O'Donnell FT, et al. Comparison of new neuraminidase detection assay with an enzyme immunoassay, immunofluorescence, and culture for rapid detection of Influenza A and B viruses in nasal wash specimens. *J Clin Microbiol* 2000;38: 1161–1165.

24. Covalciuc KA, Webb KH, Carlson CA. Comparison of four clinical specimen types for detection of Influenza A and B viruses by optical immunoassay (FLU OIA Test) and cell culture methods. *J Clin Microbiol* 1999;37:3971–3974.

25. Adcock PM, Stout GG, Hauck MA, et al. Effect of rapid viral diagnosis on the management of children hospitalized with lower respiratory tract infection. *Pediatr Infect Dis J* 1997;16:842–846.

26. Brandt CD, Kim HW, Rodriguez WJ, et al. Pediatric viral gastroenteritis during eight years of study. *J Clin Microbiol* 1983;18:71–78.

27. Echeverria P, Blacklow NR, Cukor GG, et al. Rotavirus as a cause of severe gastroenteritis in adults. *J Clin Microbiol* 1983;18:663–667.

28. Marrie TJ, Spencer HS, Faulkner RS, et al. Rotavirus in a geriatric population. *Arch Intern Med* 1982;142:313–316.

29. Halvorsrud J, Orstavik I. An epidemic of rotavirus-associated gastroenteritis in a nursing home for the elderly. *Scand J Infect Dis* 1980; 12:161–164.

30. Mathewson JJ, Winsor DK, Dupont HL, et al. Evaluation of assay systems for the detection of rotavirus in stool specimens. *Diagn Microbiol Infect Dis* 1989;12:139–141.

31. Gilchrist MJR, Bretl TS, Moultney K, et al. Comparison of seven kits for detection of rotavirus in fecal specimens with a sensitive, specific enzyme immunoassay. *Diagn Microbiol Infect Dis* 1987;8:221–228.

32. Brandt CD, Arndt CW, Evans GL, et al. Evaluation of a latex test for rotavirus detection. *J Clin Microbiol* 1987;25:1800–1802.

33. Doern GV, Herrman JE, Henderson P, et al. Detection of rotavirus with a new polyclonal antibody enzyme immunoassay (Rotazyme II) and a commercial latex agglutination test (Rotalex): comparison with a monoclonal antibody enzyme immunoassay. *J Clin Microbiol* 1986; 23:226–229.

34. Knisley CV, Bednarz-Prashad AJ, Pickering LK. Detection of rotavirus in stool specimens with monoclonal and polyclonal antibody-based assay systems. *J Clin Microbiol* 1986;23:897–900.

35. Dennehy PH, Gauntlett DR, Tente WE. Comparison of nine commercial immunoassays for the detection of rotavirus in fecal specimens. *J Clin Microbiol* 1988;26:1630–1634.

36. Thomas EE, Puterman ML, Kawano E, et al. Evaluation of seven immunoassays for detection of rotavirus in pediatric stool samples. *J Clin Microbiol* 1988;26:1189–1193.

37. Marchlewicz B, Spiewak, Lampinen J. Evaluation of Abbott TestPack Rotavirus with clinical specimens. *J Clin Microbiol* 1988;26: 2456–2458.

38. Chernesky M, Castriciano S, Mahony J, et al. Ability of the TestPack Rotavirus enzyme immunoassay to diagnose rotavirus gastroenteritis. *J Clin Microbiol* 1988; 26:2459–2461.

39. Lipson SM, Leonardi GP, Salo RJ, et al. Occurrence of nonspecific reactions among stool specimens tested by the Abbott TestPack Rotavirus enzyme immunoassay. *J Clin Microbiol* 1990;28:1132–1134.

40. Brooks RG, Brown L, Franklin R. Comparison of a new rapid test (TestPack Rotavirus) with standard enzyme immunoassay and electron microscopy for the detection of rotavirus in symptomatic hospitalized children. *J Clin Microbiol* 1989; 27:775–777.

41. Dennehy PH, Hartin M, Nelson SM, et al. Evaluation of the ImmunoCardSTAT! Rotavirus Assay for detection of Group A rotavirus in fecal specimens. *J Clin Microbiol* 1999;37:1977–1979.

42. Pai CH, Shahrabadi MS, Ince B. Rapid diagnosis of rotavirus gastroenteritis by a commercial latex agglutination test. *J Clin Microbiol* 1985;22:846–850.

43. Kassler WJ, Haley C, Jones WK, et al. Performance of a rapid, on site human immunodeficiency virus antibody assay in a public health setting. *J Clin Microbiol* 1995;33:2899–2902.

44. Stetler HC, Granade TC, Nunez CA, et al. Field evaluation of rapid HIV serologic tests for screening and confirming HIV-1 infection in Honduras. *AIDS* 1997;11:369–375.

45. Tribble DR, Rodier GR, Saad MD, et al. Comparative field evaluation of HIV rapid assays using serum, urine, and oral mucosal transudate specimens. *Clin Diagn Virol* 1997;7:127–132.

46. Constantine NT, Zhang X, Li L, et al. Application of a rapid assay for detection of antibodies to human immunodeficiency virus in urine. *Am J Clin Path* 1994;101:157–161.

47. Gallo D, George JR, Fitchen JH, et al. Evaluation of a system using oral mucosal transudate for HIV-1 antibody screening and confirmatory testing. *JAMA* 1997;277: 254–258.

48. Berrios DC, Avins AL, Haynes-Sanstad K, et al. Screening for human immunodeficiency virus in urine. *Arch Pathol Lab Med* 1995;119: 139–141.

49. Bylund DJ, Ziegner UHM, and Hooper DG. Review of testing for human immunodeficiency virus. *Clin Lab Med* 1992;12:305–333.

50. Centers for Disease Control and Prevention. Update: HIV counseling and testing using rapid tests—United States, 1995. *MMWR* 1998;47: 1045–1051.

51. Kasler WJ, Dillon BA, Haley C, et al. On-site, rapid HIV testing with same-day results and counseling. *AIDS* 1997;11:1045–1051.

52. Centers for Disease Control and Prevention. Public Health Service Task Force recommendations for the use of antiretroviral drugs in pregnant women infected with HIV-1 for maternal health and reducing perinatal HIV-1 transmission in the United States. *MMWR* 1998; 47:1–30.

53. Rajegowda BK, Das BB, Lala R, et al. Expedited human immunodeficiency virus testing of mothers and newborns with unknown HIV status at time of labor and delivery. *J Perinat Med* 2000;28:458–463.

54. Unadkat P, Newman B, and Tedder RS. The detection of varicella zoster antibodies by simultaneous competitive EIA and its comparison with radioimmunoassay, latex agglutination, and antiglobulin type EIA. *J Virol Meth* 1995;51:145–152.

55. Steinberg SP, Gerson AA. Measurement of antibodies to Varicella-Zoster Virus by using a latex agglutination test. *J Clin Microbiol* 1991; 29:1527–1529.

56. Bailey RE. Diagnosis and treatment of infectious mononucleosis. *Am Fam Physician* 1994;49:879–885.

57. Hickey SM, Strasburger VC. What every pediatrician should know about infectious mononucleosis. *Pediatr Clin North Am* 1997;44: 1541–1556.

58. Lennette ET, Henle W. Epstein-Barr virus infections: clinical and serologic features. *Lab Manage* 1987;25:23–28.

59. Cook L, Midgett J, Willis D, et al. Evaluation of a latex-based heterophile antibody assay for diagnosis of acute infectious mononucleosis. *J Clin Microbiol* 1987;25:2391–2394.

60. Tilton RC, Dias F, Ryan R. Comparative evaluation of three commercial tests for detection of heterophile antibody in patients with infectious mononucleosis. *J Clin Microbiol* 1988;26:275–278.

61. Kim M, Wadke M. Comparative evaluation of two test methods (enzyme immunoassay and latex fixation) for the detection of heterophil antibodies in infectious mononucleosis. *J Clin Microbiol* 1990; 28:2511–2513.

62. Farhat S, Finn S, Chua R, et al. Rapid detection of infectious mononucleosis-associated heterophile antibodies by a novel immunochromatographic assay and a latex agglutination test. *J Clin Microbiol* 1993;31:1597–1600.

63. Linderholm M, Boman J, Juto P, et al. Comparative evaluation of nine kits for rapid diagnosis of infectious mononucleosis and Epstein-Barr Virus–specific serology. *J Clin Microbiol* 1994;32:259–261.

64. Kass E. Asymptomatic infections of the urinary tract. *Trans Assoc Am Physicians* 1956;69:56–64.

65. Stamm WE, Counts GW, Running KR, et al. Diagnosis of coliform infections in acutely dysuric women. *N Engl J Med* 1982;307:463–468.

66. Pappas PG. Laboratory in the diagnosis and management of urinary tract infections. *Med Clin N Am* 1991;75:313–325.

67. Pezzlo M. Detection of urinary tract infections by rapid methods. *Clin Microbiol Rev* 1988;1:268–280.

68. Alwall N. Pyuria: deposit in high-power microscopic field WBC/hpf versus WBC/mm^3 in counting chamber. *Acta Med Scand* 1973;194: 537–540.

69. Hurlbut TA, Littenberg B, et al. The diagnostic accuracy of rapid dipstick tests to predict urinary tract infection. *Am J Clin Pathol* 1991; 96:582–588.

70. Males BM, Bartholomew WR, Amsterdam D. Leukocyte esterase-nitrite and bioluminescence assays as urine screens. *J Clin Microbiol* 1986;22:531–534.

71. Jones C, MacPherson DW, Stevens DL. Inability of the Chemstrip LN compared with quantitative urine culture to predict significant bacteriuria. *J Clin Microbiol* 1986;23:160–162.

72. Bartlett RC, O'Neill D, McLaughlin JC. Detection of bacteriuria by leukocyte esterase, nitrite, and the Automicrobic System. *Am J Clin Pathol* 1984;82:683–687.

73. Pfaller MA, Scharnweber G, Stewart B, et al. Improved urine screening using a combination of leukocyte esterase and the Lumac System. *Diagn Microbiol Infect Dis* 1985;3:243–250.

74. Cannon HJ, Goetz ES, Hamoudi AC, et al. Rapid screening and microbiologic processing of pediatric urine specimens. *Diagn Microbiol Infect Dis* 1986;4:11–17.

75. Marsik FJ, Owens D, Lewandowski J. Use of the leukocyte esterase and nitrite tests to determine the need for culturing urine specimens from a pediatric and adolescent population. *Diagn Microbiol Infect Dis* 1986;4:181–183.

76. Ditchburn RK, Ditchburn JS. A study of microscopical and chemical tests for the rapid diagnosis of urinary tract infections in general practice. *Br J Gen Prac* 1990;40:406–408.

77. Gutman SI, Solomon RR. The clinical significance of dipstick-negative, culture positive urines in a veterans population. *Am J Clin Pathol* 1987;88:204–209.

78. Pezzlo MT, Wetkowski MA, Peterson EM, et al. Detection of bacteriuria and pyuria within two minutes. *J Clin Microbiol* 1985;21: 578–581.

79. Pichichero ME. Culture and antigen detection tests for streptococcal tonsillo-pharyngitis. *Am Fam Physician* 1992;45:199–205.

80. Donatelli J, Macone A, Goldman DA, et al. Rapid detection of group A streptococci: comparative performance by nurses and laboratory technologists in pediatric satellite laboratories using three test kits. *J Clin Microbiol* 1992;30:138–142.

81. Heiter BJ, Bourbeau PP. Comparison of two rapid streptococcal antigen detection assays with culture for diagnosis of streptococcal pharyngitis. *J Clin Microbiol* 1995; 33:1408–1410.

82. Drulak M, Bartholomew W, LaScolea L, et al. Evaluation of the modified Visuwell Strep-A Enzyme Immunoassay for the detection of group A-streptococcus from throat swabs. *Diagn Microbiol Infect Dis* 1991;14:281–285.

83. Dale JC, Vetter EA, Contezac JM, et al. Evaluation of two rapid antigen assays, Biostar Strep A OIA and Pacific Biotech CARDS O.S., and culture for detection of group A streptococci in throat swabs. *J Clin Microbiol* 1994;32:2698–2701.

84. Kellog JA, Bankert DA, Schonauer TD, et al. Detection of group A streptococci by aerobic culture and a new simplified immunoassay in three pediatric practices and a hospital laboratory. *J Clin Lab Anal* 1991;5:367–371.

85. Roe M, Kishiyama C, Davidson K, et al. Comparison of Biostar Strep A OIA Optical Immune Assay, Abbott Testpack Plus Strep A, and culture with selective media for diagnosis of group A streptococcal pharyngitis. *J Clin Microbiol* 1995; 33:1551–1553.

86. Drulak MT, Raybould TJG, Yong J, et al. Comparison of Visuwell enzyme immunoassay to culture for detection of group A *Streptococcus* in throat swab specimens. *Diagn Microbiol Infect Dis* 1988;11: 181–187.

87. Harbeck RJ, Teague J, Crossen GR, et al. Novel, rapid optical immunoassay technique for detection of group A streptococci from pharyngeal specimens: comparison with standard culture methods. *J Clin Microbiol* 1993;31:839–844.

88. Baker DM, Cooper RM, Rhodes C, et al. Superiority of conventional culture technique over rapid detection of group A *Streptococcus* by optical immunoassay. *Diagn Microbiol Infect Dis* 1995;21:61–64.

89. American Academy of Pediatrics. Group A Streptococcal Infections. In: *1994 Redbook: report of the Committee on Infectious Diseases.* Elk Grove Village, IL: American Academy of Pediatrics, 1994:430–439.

90. Radetsky M, Solomon JA, Todd JK. Identification of streptococcal pharyngitis in the office laboratory: reassessment of new technology. *Pediatr Infect Dis J* 1987;6:665.

91. Yousefi MM, El-Zimaity HMT, Cole R, et al. Comparison of agar gel (CLOtest) or reagent strip (Pyloritek) rapid urease tests for the detection of *Helicobacter pylori* infection. *Am J Gastroenterol* 1997;92: 997–999.

92. Elitsur Y, Hill I, Lichtman S, et al. Prospective comparison of rapid urease tests (PyloriTek, CLOtest) for the diagnosis of *Helicobacter pylori* infection in symptomatic children: a pediatric multicenter study. *Am J Gastroenterol* 1998;93:217–219.

93. Lerang F, Moum B, Mowinckel P, et al. Accuracy of seven different tests for the diagnosis of *Helicobacter pylori* infection and the impact of H$_2$-receptor antagonists on test results. *Scand J Gastroenterol* 1998; 33:364–369.

94. Thijs JC, van Zwet AA, Thijs WJ, et al. Diagnostic tests for *Helicobacter pylori*: prospective evaluation of their accuracy, without selecting a single test as the gold standard. *Am J Gastroenterol* 1996; 91:2125–2129.

95. De Boer WA. Diagnosis of *Helicobacter pylori* infection. Review of diagnostic techniques and recommendations for their use in different clinical settings. *Scand J Gastroenterol* 1997;32[Suppl 223]:35–42.

96. Megaud F. Advantages and disadvantages of current diagnostic tests for the detection of *Helicobacter pylori*. *Scand J Gastroenterol* 1996;31 [Suppl 215]:57–62.

97. Faigel DO, Childs M, Furth E, et al. New noninvasive test for *Helicobacter pylori* gastritis: comparison with tissue based gold standard. *Dig Dis Sci* 1996;41:740–748.

98. Loy CT, Irwig LM, Katelaris PH, et al. Do commercial serological kits for *Helicobacter pylori* infection differ in accuracy? A meta-analysis. *Am J Gastroenterol* 1996;91:1138–1144.

99. Graham DY, Evans DJ, Peacock J, et al. Comparison of rapid serological tests (Flexsure HP and Quickvue) with conventional ELISA for detection of *Helicobacter pylori* infection. *Am J Gastroenterol* 1996; 91:942–948.

100. Khana B, Cutler A, Israel N, et al. Use caution with serologic testing for *Helicobacter pylori* infection in children. *J Infect Dis* 1998;178:460–465.
101. Sharma TK, Young E, Miller S, et al. Evaluation of a rapid, new method for detecting serum IgG antibodies to *Helicobacter pylori*. *Clin Chem* 1997;43:832–836.
102. Jensen AK, Andersen LP, Wachman CH. Evaluation of eight commercial kits for *Helicobacter pylori* IgG antibody detection. *APMIS* 1993;101:795–801.
103. Libera MD, Pazzi P, Carli G, et al. Brush cytology: a reliable method to detect *Helicobacter pylori*. *J Clin Gastroenterol* 1996;22:317–321.
104. Misra SP, Dwivedi M, Misra V, et al. Imprint cytology—a cheap, rapid and effective method for diagnosing *Helicobacter pylori*. *Postgrad Med J* 1993;69:291–295.
105. Rune SJ. Diagnosis of *Helicobacter pylori* infection. When to use which test and why. *Scand J Gastroenterol* 1996;31[Suppl 215]:63–65.
106. Cherry JD. Mycoplasma and Ureaplasma infections. In: Cherry JD, ed. *Textbook of pediatric infectious diseases*. Philadelphia: WB Saunders, 1998:2259–2286.
107. Garrow DH. A rapid test for the presence of increased cold agglutinins. *BMJ* 1958;2:206–298.
108. Griffin JP. Rapid screening for cold agglutinins in pneumonia. *Ann Intern Med* 1969;70:701–705.
109. Jacobs E. Serological diagnosis of *Mycoplasma pneumoniae* infections: a critical review of current procedures. *Clin Infect Dis* 1993;17[Suppl 1]:S79–82.
110. Alexander T, Gray LD, Kraft JA, et al. Performance of Meridian Immunocard *Mycoplasma* Test in a multicenter clinical trial. *J Clin Microbiol* 1996;34:1180–1183.
111. Thacker WL, Talkington DF. Comparison of two rapid commercial tests with complement fixation for serologic diagnosis of *Mycoplasma pneumoniae* infections. *J Clin Microbiol* 1995;33:1212–1214.
112. Fedorko DP, Emery DD, Franklin SM, et al. Evaluation of a rapid enzyme immunoassay for serologic diagnosis of *Mycoplasma pneumoniae* infection. *Diagn Microbiol Infect Dis* 1995;23:85–88.
113. Liebermann D, Liebermann D, Horowitz O, et al. Microparticle agglutination versus antibody-capture enzyme immunoassay for diagnosis of community-acquired *Mycoplasma pneumoniae* pneumonia. *Eur J Clin Microbiol* 1995;14:577–584.
114. Karppelin M, Hakkarainen K, Kleemola M, et al. Comparison of three serological methods for diagnosing *Mycoplasma pneumoniae* infection. *J Clin Pathol* 1993;46:1120–1123.
115. Dorigo-Zetsma JW, Wertheim-van Dillen PME, Spanjaard L. Performance of Meridian Immunocard *Mycoplasma* Test in a multicenter clinical trial. *J Clin Microbiol* 1996;34:3249–3250.
116. Huicho L, Campos M, Rivera J, et al. Fecal screening tests in the approach to acute infectious diarrhea: a scientific overview. *Pediatr Infect Dis J* 1996;15:486–494.
117. Guerrant RL, Araujo V, Soares E, et al. Measurement of fecal lactoferrin as a marker of fecal leukocytes. *J Clin Microbiol* 1992;30:1238–1242.
118. Seigel D, Cohen P, Neighbor M, et al. Predictive value of stool examination in acute diarrhea. *Arch Pathol Lab Med* 1987;111:715–718.
119. DuBois D, Binder L, Nelson B. Usefulness of the stool Wright's stain in the emergency department. *J Emerg Med* 1988;6:483–486.
120. Yong W, Mattia AR, Ferraro MJ. Comparison of fecal lactoferrin latex agglutination assay and methylene blue microscopy for detection of fecal leukocytes in *Clostridium difficile*-associated disease. *J Clin Microbiol* 1994;32:1360–1361.
121. Pickering LK, DuPont HL, Olarte J, et al. Fecal leukocytes in enteric infections. *Am J Clin Path* 1977;68:562–565.
122. Huicho L, Garaycochea V, Uchima N, et al. Fecal lactoferrin, fecal leukocytes and occult blood in the diagnostic approach to childhood invasive diarrhea. *Pediatr Infect Dis J* 1997;16:644–647.
123. McNeely WS, DuPont HL, Mathewson JJ, et al. Occult blood versus fecal leukocytes in the diagnosis of bacterial diarrhea: a study of U.S. travelers to Mexico and Mexican children. *Am J Trop Med Hyg* 1996;55:430–433.
124. Silletti RP, Lee G, Ailey E. Role of stool screening tests in diagnosis of inflammatory bacterial enteritis and in selection of specimens likely to yield invasive enteric pathogens. *J Clin Microbiol* 1996;34:1161–1165.
125. Rangel-Frausto MS, Wenzel RP. The epidemiology and natural history of bacterial sepsis. In: Fein AM, Abraham EM, Balk RA, et al. *Sepsis and multiorgan failure.* Baltimore, MD: Williams & Wilkins, 1997:27–34.
126. Parsons PE, Moss M. Early detection and markers of sepsis. *Clin Chest Med* 1996;17:199–212.
127. Kollef MH, Eisenberg PR. A rapid qualitative assay to detect circulating endotoxin can predict the development of multiorgan dysfunction. *Chest* 1997;112:173–180.
128. Elin RJ, Hosseini J. Clinical utility of the limulus amebocyte lysate (LAL) test. In: ten Cate JW, Buller HR, Sturk A, eds. *Bacterial endotoxins: structure, biomedical significance, and detection with the limulus amebocyte lysate test.* New York: Alan R. Liss, 1985:307–324.
129. Bates DW, Parsonnet J, Ketchum A, et al. Limulus amebocyte assay for the detection of endotoxin in patients with sepsis syndrome. *Clin Infect Dis* 1998;27:582–591.
130. Hurley JC. Endotoxemia: methods of detection and clinical correlates. *Clin Microbiol Rev* 1995;8:268–292.
131. Bayston KF, Cohen J. Bacterial endotoxin and current concepts in the diagnosis and treatment of endotoxaemia. *J Med Microbiol* 1990;31:73–83.
132. Rylatt D, Wilson K, Kemp BE, et al. A rapid test for endotoxin in whole blood. *Prog Clin Biolog Res* 1995;392:273–284.
133. Quick G, Eisenberg P. Bedside measurement of D-dimer in the identification of bacteremia in the emergency department. *J Emerg Med* 2000;19:217–223.
134. Briselden AM, Hillier SL. Evaluation of Affirm VP Microbial Identification Test for *Gardnerella vaginalis* and *Trichomonas vaginalis*. *J Clin Microbiol* 1994;32:148–152.
135. Amsel R, Touton PA, Speigel CA, et al. Nonspecific vaginitis: diagnostic criteria and microbial and epidemiologic associations. *Am J Med* 1983;74:14–22.
136. Hillier SL. Diagnostic microbiology of bacterial vaginosis. *Am J Obstet Gynecol* 1993;169:455–459.
137. Sonnex C. The amine test: a simple, rapid, inexpensive method for diagnosing bacterial vaginosis. *Br J Obstet Gynaecol* 1995;102:160–161.
138. Martius J. Bacterial vaginosis. *Curr Prob Dermatol* 1996;24:34–39.
139. Schwebke JR, Hillier SL, Sobel JD, et al. Validity of the vaginal gram stain for the diagnosis of bacterial vaginosis. *Obstet Gynecol* 1996;88:573–576.
140. Ferris DG, Hendrich J, Payne PM, et al. Office laboratory diagnosis of vaginitis: clinician-performed tests compared with a rapid nucleic acid hybridization test. *J Fam Pract* 1995;41:575–581.
141. Carr PL, Felsenstein D, Freidman RH. Evaluation and management of vaginitis. *J Gen Intern Med* 1998;13:335–346.
142. Nugent RP, Krohn MA, Hillier SL. Reliability of diagnosing bacterial vaginosis is improved by a standardized method of gram stain interpretation. *J Clin Microbiol* 1991;29:297–301.
143. Joesoef MR, Hillier SL, Josodiwondo S, et al. Reproducibility of a scoring system for Gram stain diagnosis of bacterial vaginosis. *J Clin Microbiol* 1991;29:1730–1731.
144. Thomasen JL, Anderson RJ, Gelbart SM, et al. Simplified Gram stain interpretive method for diagnosis of bacterial vaginosis. *Am J Obstet Gynecol* 1992;167:16–19.
145. Oxtoby MJ, Arnold AJ, Zaidi AA, et al. Potential shortcuts in the laboratory diagnosis of gonorrhea: a single stain for smears and nonremoval of cervical secretions before obtaining test specimens. *Sex Transm Dis* 1982;9:59–62.
146. Goh BT, Varia KB, Ayliffe PF, et al. Diagnosis of gonorrhea by gram stained smears and cultures in men and women: role of the urethral smear. *Sex Transm Dis* 1985;12:135–139.
147. Goodhart ME, Ogden J, Zaidi A, et al. Factors affecting the performance of smear and culture tests for the detection of Neisseria gonorrhoeae. *Sex Transm Dis* 1982; 9:63–69.
148. Rothenberg RB, Simon R, Chipperfield E, et al. Efficacy of selected diagnostic tests for sexually transmitted diseases. *JAMA* 1976;235:49–51.

149. Shelley WB, Shelley ED. Surgical pearl: use of a double razor blade to obtain stratum corneum specimens for potassium hydroxide examination. *J Am Acad Dermatol* 1997;36:91.

150. Monod M, Baudraz-Rosselet F, Ramelet AA, et al. Direct mycological examination in dermatology: a comparison of different methods. *Dermatologica* 1989;179:183–186.

151. Haldane DJ, Robart E. A comparison of calcofluor white, potassium hydroxide, and culture for the laboratory diagnosis of superficial fungal infection. *Diagn Microbiol Infect Dis* 1990;13:337–339.

152. Miller MA, Hodgson Y. Sensitivity and specificity of potassium hydroxide smears of skin scrapings for the diagnosis of tinea pedis. *Arch Dermatol* 1993;129:510–511.

153. Serrano L, Bieley HC, Reyes BA. Albert's solution versus potassium hydroxide solution in the diagnosis of tinea versicolor. *Int J Dermatol* 1994;33:182–183.

154. Bergmann JJ, Berg AO, Schneeweiss R, et al. Clinical comparison of microscopic and culture techniques in the diagnosis of candida vaginitis. *J Fam Prac* 1984;18:549–552.

155. McLennan MT, Smith JM, McLennan CE. Diagnosis of vaginal mycosis and trichomoniasis. *Obstet Gynecol* 1972;40:231–234.

156. Sobel JD, Schmitt C, Meriwether C. A new slide latex agglutination test for the diagnosis of acute candida vaginitis. *Am J Clin Pathol* 1990;94:323–325.

157. Weissberg SM. Evaluation of a dipstick for Candida. *Obstet Gynecol* 1978;52:506–509.

158. Davies RR, Savage MA. Evaluation of a dehydrated test strip for the detection of yeasts. *J Clin Pathol* 1975;28:750–752.

159. Fouts AC, Kraus SJ. *Trichomonas vaginalis*: reevaluation of its clinical presentation and laboratory diagnosis. *J Infect Dis* 1980;141:137–143.

160. Krieger JN, Tam MR, Stevens CE, et al. Diagnosis of Trichomoniasis: comparison of conventional wet-mount examination with cytologic studies, cultures, and monoclonal antibody staining of direct specimens. *JAMA* 1988;259:1223–1227.

161. Eddie DAS. The laboratory diagnosis of vaginal infections caused by *Trichomonas* and *Candida* (*Monilia*) species. *J Med Microbiol* 1968;1:153–159.

15

POINT-OF-CARE DRUG TESTING

ALAN H. B. WU

Point-of-care testing (POCT) for selected analytes is performed in emergency departments (ED), critical care units, and other areas of the hospital to improve the turnaround time for receiving results of critical laboratory tests. These results are used to determine the need for initiating therapeutic measures (e.g., insulin for diabetic patients), for triaging patients to the appropriate level of care (e.g., cardiac markers to rule out acute myocardial infarction), and for monitoring important physiologic parameters of critically ill patients (e.g., blood gases, electrolytes, bleeding times). POCT is also important in providing laboratory data for physician offices in real time so that management decisions can be made while the patient is still in the office (e.g., measurement of glycosylated hemoglobin for diabetic patients). With POCT for drugs, these same reasons apply. The objectives of this chapter are to acquaint the reader with specific rationales for drug testing and how POC can provide an alternative to central laboratory- and instrument-based testing. It begins with a description of the scope of drug testing today. Each scenario has individual needs with regard to desired turnaround times, menu of analytes to be tested, cost of providing results, degree of regulatory control, and even the quality of the results obtained. The need for obtaining rapid drug testing is justified in the next section. POCT is not appropriate for every drug-testing arena. The focus is on testing in hospital EDs and forensic drug testing in the workplace. Specific POCT devices for alcohol and drugs of abuse are described in the next section. The number of commercially available test devices has exploded in recent years. Although the need for POCT for therapeutic drugs is not as great as for drugs of abuse, commercial POCT devices are available for theophylline and anticonvulsant drugs. POCT has a bright future as regulatory agencies begin to see the advantage of on-site testing with improved no-reagent assays. The abuse of novel drugs also will provide fuel for new drug testing markets.

THE SCOPE OF DRUGS OF ABUSE TESTING

Drug abuse continues to be a major problem in the United States and throughout the Western world, and it is a significant cause of morbidity and mortality. Drug testing in the workplace is used to identify exposed persons so that appropriate counseling or treatment or both can be arranged. In the ED, drug testing is used for diagnostic and therapeutic management purposes for patients who present with acute overdoses or drug-related problems. Specific antagonists and antidotes are available for many of the commonly abused drugs. Psychiatric in-patients are tested for drugs of abuse after returning from weekend or holiday furloughs. For medical compliance and probation programs, rehabilitated impaired professionals sign a consent form and undergo regular urine drug testing as a condition for allowing them to return to work. Convicts on parole may be subject to regular drug testing as a condition of parole. In athletic arenas, drug testing is conducted to detect persons who attempt to enhance their bodies or performance for a particular sporting event. Drugs for nonmedical use are banned by nearly all athletic organizations, such as the International Olympic Committee, National Collegiate Athletic Association, National Football League, and the Amateur Athletic Union. Such rules are not equally applied to all sports; Major League Baseball, for example, permits use of anabolic steroids.

It should be clear from the scope and diversity of the various applications that drug testing is a multibillion-dollar industry. Most drug testing is conducted in hospital laboratories or commercial reference laboratories. For forensic testing, samples must be delivered from the collection site to the laboratory under strict chain-of-custody conditions. The need for fast turnaround time of results has led to the development of POCT devices that can be performed at the site of specimen collection. The general advantages and disadvantages for POCT for drugs of abuse are summarized in Table 15.1.

TABLE 15.1. ADVANTAGES AND DISADVANTAGES FOR POCT FOR DRUGS OF ABUSE

Advantages
    Shorter turnaround time for results
    Reduces or eliminates chain-of-custody documentation
    Samples tested negative for drugs do not need to be delivered to the laboratory for confirmation analysis
Disadvantages
    Definitive confirmations not available on POCT platform
    Possible misinterpretation of results
    Currently not approved for federal drug testing programs
    Consumable costs higher

POCT, point-of-care testing.

Drugs of Abuse Testing in the Workplace

It has been well established that employees who regularly abuse drugs have lower productivity and higher absentee rates than their non–drug-abusing counterparts. Surveys conducted by the Substance Abuse and Mental Health Services Administration (SAMHSA), have shown that, relative to employees who do not abuse drugs, workers who report illicit drug use are more likely to have unexcused absences (12.1% vs. 6.1%), to be fired by employers (4.6% vs. 1.6%), to have voluntarily left an employer in the past year (25.8% vs. 13.6%), and to have been involved in a workplace accident in the past year (7.5% vs. 5.5%) (1). Considering the high costs of training new employees and the difficulty of finding qualified staff in today's economy, drug abuse is a major expense to all employers.

The medical costs incurred by drug-abusing employees are also substantially higher. In an effort to reduce the problem of drug abuse, U.S. President Ronald Reagan signed legislation in 1986 requiring that all federal employees undergo preemployment and random testing of urine for selected drugs of abuse. It was considered that linking a person's source of income was more likely to be effective in reducing the rate of drug abuse than to educate the public on the dangers of drug abuse on health. The signing of this executive order led to the development of federal guidelines that specify the conditions for the collection, analysis procedures, and reporting of results for drugs of abuse testing (2). Drug testing is now regulated by the Substance Abuse and Mental Health Services Administration (SAMHSA), a branch of the U.S. Health and Human Services (HHS). Table 15.2 lists the drugs and the screening and confirmation cutoff concentrations that are currently part of the SAMHSA program. This program has provided guidelines for testing *adulterants*, that is, substances intentionally added to urine in the attempt to

invalidate results. Laboratories are not permitted to test for drugs other than those listed. These guidelines apply to all federal employees and to those operating under the jurisdiction of the Department of Transportation (DOT), Department of Defense, and Nuclear Regulatory Commission (NRC). Whereas SAMHSA regulations currently do not permit use of POCT devices for on-site drug testing, the NRC has allowed use of POC screening tests. Pilot programs, such as that for the U.S. Post Office, also have been conducted (3).

The success of the mandatory federal programs led employers within private industry also to perform widespread employee drug testing. Because these employers are not subjected to SAMHSA guidelines, they are free to modify the drug testing conditions, such as lowering the cutoff concentrations. For example, SAMHSA recently raised the opiate cutoff concentrations to 2,000 ng per milliliter to minimize the number of employees who produce positive results from consumption of foods that contain poppy seeds. Most employers of unregulated testing, however, continue to use the 300 ng per milliliter opiate cutoff concentration. Private corporations also can choose to test other drugs that are not part of the SAMHSA guidelines, such as benzodiazepines, barbiturates, methadone, and propoxyphene. For drug testing of health care workers, specific drugs not readily available to the general public can be tested such as fentanyl, meperidine, oxycodone, hydromorphone, propoxyphene, and meprobamate.

The DOT also established regulations and procedures for the random testing for ethyl alcohol (4). Like testing for drugs of abuse, the alcohol testing process consists of screening, followed by confirmation of positive results. The screening test is conducted on breath or saliva and is considered positive when ethanol concentrations equal or exceed 0.020%. The confirmation test is conducted by breath 30 minutes after the screening test. This delay was added to protect against false-positive results that can occur if the subject uses alcohol-containing mouthwashes just prior to the screening test. Unless more mouthwash is used after the screening and before the retest procedure, a person who has not recently consumed alcohol will have negative results. The DOT also established minimum qualifications and training of personnel who conduct breath-alcohol tests (breath-alcohol technicians, or BATs).

Drugs of Abuse Testing for Clinical Toxicology

Statistics on the incidence of ED admissions where drugs were present as a cause of presenting symptoms, or as an incidental finding, are tabulated by the Drug Abuse Warning Network (DAWN) (5). Data from 1993 are shown in Table 15.3. For comparison purposes, this table also shows the incidence for the abuse of these drugs within the prior month of the survey from the general population as tabulated from the National Institute on Drug Abuse (NIDA) household survey, conducted the same year as the DAWN report (6). An index has been calculated in Table 15.3 as the ratio of reported ED drug incidence to the reported drug use within the general population. High relative values indicate that the drug is associated with ED visits and suggests a high potential of the drug for significant toxicity. A

TABLE 15.2. DRUGS AND CUTOFF CONCENTRATIONS FOR FEDERAL DRUG TESTING PROGRAMS[a]

Drug/ Adulterant	Screening Cutoff	Confirmation Cutoff
Amphetamines	1,000	
Amphetamine		500
Methamphetamine		500[b]
Cocaine	300	
Benzoylecgonine		150
Opiates	2,000	
Codeine		2,000
Morphine		2,000
6-Monoacetyl morphine		10
Phencyclidine	25	25
Tetrahydrocannabinol	50	
9-Carboxy-THC		15
Creatinine	<20 mg/dL[c]	<20 mg/dL
Specific gravity	<1.003[d]	<1.003
pH	≤3 or ≥11	≤3 or ≥11
Nitrites	≥500 µg/L	≥500 µg/L

THC, tetrahydrocannabinol.
[a]All cutoffs in ng/mL.
[b]Also requires the presence of amphetamine at ≥200 ng/mL.
[c]Urine with values below these limits is considered diluted. If the creatinine is ≤5 and the specific gravity ≤1.001 or ≥1.020, the specimen is considered substituted.

TABLE 15.3. INCIDENCE OF POSITIVE DRUG RESULTS FOR EMERGENCY VISITS AND THE GENERAL U.S. POPULATION[a]

Drug	ED Incidence (%)[b]	General Population (%)[c]	ED Drug Index[d]
Alcohol	2.7	49.6	5
Cocaine	0.14	0.6	23
Heroin/morphine	0.090	0.1	90
THC	0.032	4.3	0.7
Benzodiazepines	0.58	0.3	19
Analgesics	0.081	0.7	12
PCP	0.007	0.2	3
LSD	0.004	0.8[d]	5

ED, emergency department; THC, tetrahydrocannabinol; PCP, phencyclidine; LSD, lysergic acid diethylamide.
[a]Data given in percent of the adolescent and adult U.S. population (≥12 yr of age).
[b]From the Drug Abuse Warning Network. *Preliminary estimates from the Drug Abuse Warning Network.* Rockville, MD: Substance Abuse and Mental Health Administration, U.S. Dept. of Health and Human Services Advance Report no. 8, 1994.
[c]From the *National Institute on Drug Abuse (NIDA) Household Survey on Drug Abuse. Population estimates 1994.* Rockville, MD: Substance Abuse and Mental Health Services Administration, U.S. Dept. of Health and Human Services, 1995. Reported use over the previous month (indicating current user).
[d]Ratio of ED incidence of drug use to the general population ×100.

low ratio suggests that presence of the drug may have been an incidental finding to the presenting symptoms.

Excluding nicotine from tobacco (not tabulated by DAWN), alcohol is the most common finding at 2.7%. In many EDs, blood alcohol levels are determined routinely for medicolegal purposes in trauma cases caused by motor vehicle accidents. Alcohol has a low ED drug index, reflecting the lack of significant toxicities at "recreational" or social alcohol use (i.e., <100 mg/dL in blood). All other drugs of abuse collectively account for about 1% of ED admissions, with cocaine having the highest incidence of this group. Cocaine is a powerful vasoconstrictive drug that produces significant cardiac toxicities. As such, teenagers and young adults who normally have a low likelihood of coronary artery disease present to the ED with chest pain after intravenous or intranasal use or smoking "crack" cocaine. This drug has a high ED drug index (Table 15.3), demonstrating the dangers it carries. Cocaine metabolizes to benzoylecgonine and ecgonine methyl ester, which are detected in urine.

According to DAWN, opiates, most notably in the form of heroin, are the next most common type of drug associated with ED visits. Heroin is a very short-acting drug that is highly addictive. It metabolizes first to 6-monoacetyl morphine (6-MAM) and then to morphine. An opiate drug overdose in a patient produces respiratory depression, profound sedation, and coma. Morphine and codeine are also drugs abused in the general population. The opiate drugs as a group have a very high ED drug index.

The incidence of finding other drugs in connection with an ED visit (Table 15.3) is considerably lower, largely reflecting their low incidence of abuse within the general population. A notable exception is marijuana (tetrahydrocannabinol, THC), which has a high use in the general population and a low

reported incidence among ED patients. Marijuana does not produce significant acute toxic effects and therefore is not the cause of acute symptoms in patients presenting to the ED; it has a relatively low ED drug index (Table 15.3). Many hospital laboratories have stopped THC testing in their routine ED drug screens. Lysergic acid diethylamine (LSD) is a hallucinogenic drug that also has a low reported ED incidence. In this case, the low index might be caused by the lack of a convenient assay when the DAWN survey was conducted in 1993. Although nonisotopic urine drug tests for LSD are now available (7), there are no POC assays for LSD. The benzodiazepines have a fairly high ED drug index, suggesting a high potential for toxicity. Sedatives such as Valium do not contribute to significant morbidity or mortality. Only a few of the 721 deaths reported to the Toxic Exposure Surveillance System in 1996 involved benzodiazepines, despite the high incidence of these drugs (8). The high ED index might reflect the common practice of administering benzodiazepines for patients to control seizures.

Drugs of Abuse Testing in Other Environments

Medical Compliance Programs

Drug abuse among health care workers, such as doctors, nurses, and pharmacists, is a particular challenge for drug-testing laboratories because they have access to drugs not available to the general public. The narcotics are the most common drugs abused in this population. In a recent national survey of U.S. physicians, 39.9% and 7.5% responded that they had used minor opiates (including codeine and propoxyphene) and major opiates (including meperidine and fentanyl), respectively, on at least one occasion (9). The use of all prescription analgesics among physicians is some 5 to 20 times higher than use by the general population, as reported in the 1990 NIDA survey, in which groups were stratified according to age and sex (10). Drug treatment programs for physicians and nurses are now in place in most states. In some cases of narcotic abuse, opiate antagonists such as naltrexone are used as a deterrent to further abuse. A therapeutic drug concentration of these antagonists blocks the desired opiate drug effect. An essential part of any drug treatment program includes regular testing of urine for controlled substances. The analysis of prescription analgesics is particularly difficult because commercial assays for use in humans are not available for oxycodone, oxymorphone, hydrocodone, hydromorphone, meperidine, meprobamate, and fentanyl. In the specific case of fentanyl, urine concentrations are extremely low (<0.5 ng/mL), making analysis of the parent compound in urine very difficult. Fentanyl abuse is a very popular drug for abuse among anesthesiologists because it is widely used in their practice and because of its short duration of action (11). Unfortunately, it is also a highly addictive drug and has led to several fatalities (12).

Drug Testing for Criminal Justice

Illegal drug use and trafficking are major causes of criminal arrests. In a study conducted among arrestees in Baltimore, 69% to 75% had a positive urine test for drugs, including a cocaine incidence of 54% to 65%, heroin 40% to 46%, and marijuana 9% to 20% (13). In-prison drug treatment programs have been initiated and have reduced the incidence of recidivism in research studies within a year of release from jail (14). Drug testing of convicts on probation with revocation of parole privileges is also being evaluated to determine whether it reduces the rate of rearrest. The Justice Department has determined that on-site drug testing with POC devices is acceptable for this application (15), and various POC devices are in widespread use. Because of the costs of confirmation testing, these prisoners usually are not afforded the benefits of having their positive urine results retested by gas chromatography or mass spectrometry analysis. A positive screening result from an immunoassay may be sufficient presumptive evidence to confront parolees and possibly deny privileges. A false-positive immunoassay screening result caused by the use of over-the-counter medications is not a concern for parole officers because parolees are instructed to avoid any and all drug use.

Drug Testing in Sports

In addition to "recreational" drugs, such as cocaine, heroin, or THC, drugs and hormones also are used to improve athletic performances. Anabolic steroids and human growth hormones are used to increase strength and build muscle mass, which can create a competitive advantage for persons who participate in certain sports (e.g., football, wrestling, boxing, weight lifting, track and field, body building, cycling, crew) (16). Erythropoietin and other blood-doping techniques improve endurance by increasing red cell mass and are abused by athletes in highly aerobic sports such as swimming, cycling, track and field, and cross-country skiing. Diuretics are used in athletes that require rapid weight loss (e.g., boxers, wrestlers, and horse-racing jockeys). The use of β-blockers improves the rhythm of the heart and can improve competitive events that require a steady hand, such as archery and riflery. Puberty-delaying drugs and hormones can be especially useful for events that are dominated by teenaged girls, such as figure skating or gymnastics. Urine testing for drugs is currently conducted on a random basis and immediately before or after major competitive events (e.g., the Olympics).

Point-of-care testing devices are not available for performance drugs and hormones that are abused by athletes because of the large numbers of drugs that can be abused (notably the synthetic anabolic steroids) and the difficulty in obtaining accurate results. Moreover, the long turnaround time for reporting of results (days to weeks) does not appear to be a critical issue. This situation is not likely to change because the commercial market for such devices is currently too small (compared with workplace or ED toxicology) for manufacturers to justify the research and development effort needed. POCT for endogenous hormones would be further complicated by the need to have quantitative results to distinguish between native and exogenous hormone use. For example, a ratio of testosterone to epitestosterone exceeding 6:1 in urine is used to suggest exogenous testosterone use (17). Interpretation guidelines for determining the presence of exogenous substances such as growth hormone, erythropoietin, and creatine have not been established.

NEED FOR RAPID TESTING ASSAYS FOR DRUGS OF ABUSE

Workplace Drug Testing

For all testing for drugs of abuse in the workplace, SAMHSA requires strict documentation of chain of custody (COC). The COC includes signatures of all persons who have been involved with the testing process: sample collection, delivery to the testing laboratory, accessioning, processing aliquots, screening and confirmation analysis, and review of results by the certifying scientist and medical review officer (MRO). Breaks in the COC documentation can lead to invalidation of the result by an attorney. The analysis of urine by a POCT device should reduce the amount of COC documentation necessary, particularly if the collector performs the test itself. Negative results would obviate the costs associated with sending the sample to drug-testing laboratories. It also may be possible that the donor of the urine could witness the testing process, thus providing more assurance as to the accuracy of the process. A major disadvantage for POCT devices is that most of the current devices have not incorporated indicators of adulterant use (e.g., pH, specific gravity, creatinine) or for specific adulterants themselves (e.g., glutaraldehyde or nitrite). Moreover, the level of education and training required to be a collector is considerably less than for a medical technologist; therefore, errors in the interpretation of visual POCT endpoints are more likely. At present, SAMHSA does not permit use of POCT devices for mandated urine drug-screening tests.

Emergency Department Drug Testing

In the ED, statim drug testing can be very important in the management of the heavily intoxicated or overdosed patient. The presence of a collection of symptoms related to a particular drug intoxication is known by ED physicians as a *toxidrome*. Examples of toxidromes include cholinergic (e.g., organophosphates), anticholinergic (antidepressants), sympathetic (amphetamines, cocaine, phencyclidine), opioid (heroin, morphine), sedative–hypnotic (barbiturates, benzodiazepines), and hallucinogenic (marijuana, cocaine, amphetamines, phencyclidine, lysergic acid diethylamide) (18). The identification of specific drugs of abuse causing these symptoms can determine whether a specific antagonist or antidote is used. Table 15.4 lists some of these countermeasures to drugs frequently encountered in the ED. Some of these therapies, such as naloxone, are not particu-

TABLE 15.4. ACUTE THERAPEUTIC MANAGEMENT OF DRUG OVERDOSES

Drugs	Drug Management
Amphetamines	Opioid antagonist (naloxone)
Cocaine	Seizure and agitation control (benzodiazepines)
Marijuana	None (no acute clinical problems)
Benzodiazepines	Flunazemil
Barbiturates	Naloxone if ventilation is decreased
Phencyclidine	Seizure and agitation control (benzodiazepines)
Acetaminophen	N-acetylcysteine
Salicylates	Peritoneal or hemodialysis
Tricyclic antidep.	Physostigmine
Volatiles	Peritoneal or hemodialysis

larly harmful, and can be used even before a determination has been made by the laboratory in its search for opiates. Use of other antidotes, however, may have considerable side effects. Thus, results of urine drug-screening tests performed with a rapid turnaround time can be helpful in determining which patients warrant treatment with these antagonists.

Until recently, results of urine drug tests were not available to the ED in "real time" (i.e., within minutes of patient presentation), and therapeutic decisions were made based on clinical grounds alone. Treating physicians had to rely on their clinical judgment and previous experience. A well-trained medical specialist in clinical toxicology usually does not require real-time confirmation of drug exposure. Most overdose presentations, however, occur during the late evening hours or on weekends, when EDs are more likely to be staffed with inexperienced junior house officers (19), thus justifying the need for stat drug testing. Today, drug-screening assays are available on laboratory-based clinical chemistry analyzers. For hospitals with a rapid system for delivery of specimens from the ED to the laboratory (e.g., with a pneumatic tube), results can be reported to the ED staff within 1 hour. Although this may not be ideal, in many ED overdose situations, it suffices. For institutions without an efficient delivery system, or if a shorter testing turnaround time is necessary, satellite laboratory or bedside POCT for drugs of abuse may be the best alternative.

Of particular concern to ED physicians is the need to produce rapid results for patients with accidental or purposeful (suicidal) overdoses of analgesics. Before the development of safety caps for over-the-counter bottles, salicylates and acetaminophen were the most common drugs accidentally overdosed by small children. Although the incidence has reduced in recent years, more than 90,000 cases of acetaminophen and 20,000 salicylate ingestions were treated in the United States in 1993 (20), and 228 deaths from analgesic ingestion were reported in 1996 (8). Patients presenting with an acute salicylic acid poisoning present with a respiratory alkalosis within the first 12 hours followed by a metabolic acidosis (21). Those with acetaminophen overdoses develop a delayed onset of acute hepatic necrosis, as evidenced by increased activities of serum aspartate and alanine aminotransferases. Acute testing for these drugs facilitates early triage and management of poisonings. Nomograms that indicate toxicities and risks based on blood concentrations and time of ingestion are available for both drugs. Toxic concentrations of acetaminophen, for example, should be treated with N-acetylcysteine to replace hepatic glutathione levels (Table 15.4). Liver transplantation is a last resort therapeutic option for patients with severe hepatocellular injury.

Because of these toxic effects, the need for screening the blood of all ED patients who present with a suggestion of suicidal ideation or altered mental status has been considered by several investigators. Sporer and Khayam-Bashi found only a 0.16% and 0.30% incidence of salicylates and acetaminophen in patients without accompanying symptoms (22). Nevertheless, routine acetaminophen testing may be warranted because of the severe consequences and costs of liver transplantation even in a single missed case. POCT could be helpful if the central laboratory cannot deliver results with a reasonably short turnaround time (e.g., ≤1 hour).

POINT-OF-CARE DRUG TESTING PLATFORMS
Alcohol

Most clinical laboratories test alcohol in serum or plasma using the enzymatic alcohol dehydrogenase (ADH) assay:

$$\text{ethanol} + NAD^+ \xrightarrow{\text{ADH}} \text{acetaldehyde} + NADH + H^+$$

The product of this reaction, NADH, is measured at 340 nm using a spectrophotometer. The acetaldehyde produced by this reaction also can be coupled to an indicator reaction with diaphorase and a tetrazolium dye to form a blue color. This assay cannot be conveniently used to measure whole-blood alcohol because of the spectral interferences caused by the presence of erythrocyte hemoglobin. Because legal statutes for alcohol concentrations are written for whole blood, an estimate of the whole blood alcohol result can be obtained by multiplying the serum result by a factor to account for differences in the water content between these samples. A serum-to-whole blood ratio of 1.14:1 is sometimes used (23). Toxicology laboratories that report alcohol concentrations for forensic purposes generally use a gas chromatography (GC). The sampling of the head-space gas above a heated closed sample with a gas-tight syringe enables the direct GC analysis of whole blood samples.

Point-of-care testing for alcohol relies largely on the sampling of either saliva or breath. Mean saliva ethanol concentrations are about 9% higher than those in whole blood because of differences in the water content of these two specimens (24). Several POCT devices for saliva have been approved for use as screening devices for evidential alcohol testing by the DOT. The Alco screen device (Table 15.5) is a dipstick that samples oral fluids and tests for alcohol directly. This test makes use of alcohol oxidase coupled with an indicator reaction:

$$\text{ethanol} + O_2 \xrightarrow{\text{alcohol oxidase}} \text{acetaldehyde} + H_2O_2$$

$$H_2O_2 \xrightarrow{\text{peroxide}} \text{blue line} + H_2O$$

The presence of a blue line on the dipstick indicates a positive result. Two dipsticks are available: a qualitative 4-minute assay with a 0.02% cutoff (designed for use with DOT alcohol screening programs) and a semiquantitative 2-minute assay where the color of the pad is compared against a chart.

The QED device (Table 15.5) makes use of a swab to sample oral fluids from the mouth. It is then inserted into a POCT device. The ethanol concentration, corrected for the difference in water content between saliva and blood, is determined using the alcohol dehydrogenase assay with a visual "thermometer-like" calibrated scale. The assay has been validated against a GC assay on whole blood collected simultaneously, producing a slope of 1.0 and a correlation coefficient of 0.98 by linear regression analysis (25).

Breath-alcohol measurements for alcohol have been the benchmark for roadside traffic law enforcement for many years. By definition, all breath analysis is POCT (i.e., testing is done at the site of the subject/donor). Portable instruments are widely used by police officers because a breath sample is not collected and sent to a laboratory. These devices measure the breath concentration of

TABLE 15.5. REPRESENTATIVE COMMERCIAL POINT-OF-CARE TESTING DEVICES FOR DRUGS OF ABUSE

Manufacturer (Location)	Product	Type/Assay Principle
Portable alcohol analyzers		
Chematics (N. Webster, IN)	Alco screen	Saliva, alcohol oxidase
STC (Bethlehem, PA)	Q.E.D.	Saliva, alcohol dehydrogenase
Roche (Sommerville, NJ)	On-site	Saliva, alcohol dehydrogenase
Medi-Scan (Denver, CO)	BreathScan	Breath alcohol, colorimetric indicator
Guth (Harrisburg, PA)	Mark X	Breath alcohol, biosensor
Intoximeter (St. Louis, MO)	AlcoSensor III,IV	Breath alcohol, fuel cell
Breathalyzer	ABT100	Breath alcohol, electronic sensor
Repco (Raleigh, NC)	AlcoTec	Breath alcohol, electronic sensor
Drugs of abuse		
Editek (Burlington, NC)	Verdict	Single device, immunochromatography
Roche (Indianapolis, IN)	Frontline	Single dipstick device
Roche (Indianapolis, IN)	TesTstik	Single dipstick device
Avitar (Canton, MA)	Visualine II	Multidrug, immunochromatography
Bionike	Drugs of abuse	Multidrug, immunochromatography
Biosite (San Diego, CA)	Triage	Multidrug, immunochromatography
Dipro Diag (Louisville, KY)	Dipro 10 panel	Multidrug, immunochromatography
Forefront Diag (Laguna Hills, CA)	InstaCheck	Multidrug, immunochromatography
Jant Pharmacal (Encino, CA)	Accutest	Multidrug, immunochromatography
1-Step Direct (Large, PA)	DTx	Multidrug, immunochromatography
Orion (Sommerset, NJ)	Status DS	Multidrug, immunochromatography
PharmaTech (San Diego, CA)	QuickScreen	Multidrug, immunochromatography
PharmChem (Menlo Park, NY)	PharmScreen	Multidrug, immunochromatography
Rimstar (Denver, CO)	AccuSign	Multidrug, immunochromatography
Syva (Cupertino, CA)	RapidTest DAU	Multidrug, immunochromatography
Worldwide Medical (Irvine, CA)	First Check	Multidrug, immunochromatography
Accuracy-One, Inc. (Camarillo, CA)	Rapid Drug Screen Card	Multidrug, immunochromatography
Roche (Sommerville, NJ)	TesTcup	Multidrug, collection cup/analysis
Am. Biomedica (Ancramdale, NY)	Rapid drug screen	Multidrug, POC with slotted collection cup
Point of Care (Rockville, MD)	Genie Cup	Multidrug, collection cup/assay
Drug Free Enterprises	DrugCheck 5	Multidrug, collection cup/assay
Avitar (Canton, MA)	Oral Screen	Saliva, immunochromatography

alcohol, expressed in units of breath alcohol in grams per 210 L of expired breath (26). This result correlates to blood concentrations measured in grams per liter. In most U.S. states, the legal driving limit is 0.1%. Federal legislation, however, may lower the limit to 0.08%. If this legislation passes, states that do not adopt this standard by 2004 will begin to lose part of their federal funding for their highways. Intoxicated drivers are liable for criminal charges and drivers license revocation for driving while intoxicated (DWI). Bench (nonportable) breath analyzers measure alcohol concentrations using infrared (IR) absorption spectrophotometry. Alcohols have a characteristic IR absorption at 3.3 and 3.5 μm, corresponding to the stretching of the O-H and C-H bonds. Because all alcohols have these absorption bands, one advantage of breath-alcohol analyzers is that other alcohol intoxicants, such as methanol, isopropanol, and ethylene glycol, can be detected. Such information can be used in conjunction with the osmol and anion gap measurement (27).

Portable breath-alcohol measuring devices make use of electronic sensors (as listed in Table 15.5). The largest manufacturer of portable devices (Intoximeter, Inc., St. Louis, MO, U.S.A.) makes use of an amperometric "fuel" cell as a detector. The cell oxidizes ethanol to acetic acid with the resulting measurement of current. Another manufacturer has developed a solid-state biosensor designed for measurement of breath alcohol (Guth Laboratories, Harrisburg, PA, U.S.A.). The sensor is composed of a tin oxide ceramic semiconductor.

Breath analyzers also can be used as POC devices for testing in the ED. There are several advantages to performing breath testing in lieu of collecting and testing blood (Table 15.6). Breath testing is not subject to regulations by the Clinical Laboratory Improvement Act of 1988 (CLIA '88) because a sample is not separately collected. This situation is similar to the exempt status of pulse oximeter testing, which also does not involve the collection of a discreet sample. On the other hand, if a breath sample is collected and retained (e.g., in a balloon) and sent for analysis, this testing would be covered by CLIA. Because results of alcohol tests are sometimes used in civil or criminal cases, there are many other advantages in the elimination of blood alcohol measurements. Testing at bedside does not require COC documentation. Moreover, laboratory personnel are not subpoenaed into court for collecting, handling, transporting, or testing samples. The disadvantages of ED breath testing are shown in Table 15.6. Most notably, it may be difficult to obtain sufficient volumes of breath from obtunded or overdosed patients. A mask connected to the breath-alcohol device to the patient may be helpful in these cases. Highly agitated patients may also be unwilling to donate a breath sample for fear of future retribution by law enforcement officers. Because blood is invariably collected from these patients for routine laboratory tests, the patient is not likely to know that an ethanol test has been ordered.

Errors in breath-alcohol analysis can occur with breath-alcohol analysis relative to the actual blood-alcohol concentrations.

TABLE 15.6. ADVANTAGES AND DISADVANTAGES FOR BREATH-ALCOHOL POC ANALYSIS IN THE ED

Advantages	Disadvantages
Waived by CLIA '88	Devices have high theft potential
Fast turnaround time (<1 min)	Sampling of comatose or highly agitated patients difficult
Low instrument costs (<$1,000)	Difficult to bill patient
Negligible consumable expenses	Difficult to link results onto medical record
Minimal chain-of-custody documentation	
Lab personnel not subpoenaed in court	

POC, point of care; ED, emergency department; CLIA '88, Clinical Laboratory Improvement Act of 1988.

If the subject has alcohol in the mouth, falsely high values can occur. Falsely high values can also occur if alcohol is sampled during the preabsorptive state (28). On the other hand, if there is an insufficient amount of air sampled into the device, falsely low results can occur because the anatomic dead air space between the mouth and device chamber would contain little alcohol (29). Modern breath-alcohol meters do not produce falsely high results as a result of other volatiles, such as acetone produced in diabetic subjects (30).

Spot Tests

The first POCT assays for therapeutic drugs and drugs of abuse were spot tests. A *spot test* is a qualitative technique in which a reagent is added (sometimes by an eyedropper) to an aliquot of a patient's sample (usually urine). The presence of the target drug is determined by a change in the color caused by a reaction of the substance or its metabolite with the reagent. Spot tests are not as specific or sensitive as immunoassays. The major advantages are that they are inexpensive and require no instrumentation. Although spot-test kits have not been largely commercialized, they can be prepared easily from reagents typically available in clinical laboratories. Table 15.7 lists drugs and the reagents used in some spot tests that have been developed. A comprehensive listing has been prepared in early editions of clinical chemistry textbooks (31). The simplest spot tests require no sample preparation, incubation steps, or instrumentation and are ideal for ED POCT or bedside analysis. The most common example of

this test is the Trinder's reagent (ferric nitrate) for salicylates. A violet color suggests the presence of salicylates. Other spot tests require additional steps, which necessitates that they be performed in a clinical laboratory. An example is the test for halogenated hydrocarbons, in which a blood sample is extracted with ether, reacted with alkalinized pyridine, and placed into a boiling water bath. A red color indicates the presence of chloroform, chloral hydrate, or carbon tetrachloride. To meet regulations for biohazardous materials, this test would require a hood to be installed for ventilation of the organic solvents. A spot test for acetaminophen is available, but it is rarely used because of the steps involved. An immunochromatographic POC assay for acetaminophen may be of value for routine testing of suspected ED patients, but there are no commercially available assays as yet.

Drugs of Abuse in Urine

Antibodies for Immunoassays

All POC immunoassays for drugs of abuse require the use of antibodies directed against one or more of the drugs in a particular class. The following discussion describes the targeted drug for each POC analyte. Table 15.8 lists the other drug analogs and metabolites and the degree of cross-reactivity obtained from manufacturers' package inserts for selected commercial POC devices (32). Antibodies used in the amphetamine assay are targeted to either d-amphetamine or d-methamphetamine or both in a "cocktail" of two antibodies.

TABLE 15.7. POC SPOT TESTS FOR DRUGS OF ABUSE

Drug(s)	Reagent(s) and Procedure
Simple spot tests (bedside test)	
Acetone	Sodium nitroprusside (dipstick test)
Imipramine/desip.	Acid dichromate (Forrest reagent)
Paraquat	Sodium bicarbonate and sodium dithionite
Phenothiazines	Ferric chloride, perchloric, nitric acid
Salicylates	Ferric nitrite (Trinder reagent)
Complex spot tests (lab test)	
Acetaminophen	Cold acid, sodium nitrite, and α-naphthol reagent
Chloral hydrate	Ether extract, alkaline pyridine, and boil
Ethchlorvynol	Acidify, chloroform extraction, evaporation, reaction with $HgNO_3$
Heavy metals	Acidify and boil sample with copper wire (Reinsch test)
Volatiles	Conway microdiffusion dish

POC, point of care.

TABLE 15.8. CROSS-REACTIVITIES FOR POC DRUGS OF ABUSE ASSAYS

Drug	ONTRAK	Triage	First Check	AccuSign
Amphetamines				
1-Methamphetamine	<1	10	NA	NA
1-Amphetamine	NA	3	NA	14
3,4-Methylenedioxyamph.	NA	33	50	200
3,4-Methylenedioxymeth.	NA	33	NA	10
Cocaine				
Free cocaine	20	10	60	14
Ecgonine methylester	<1	NA	NA	NA
Opiates				
Morphine-3-glucuronide	75	61	100	100
Codeine	200	100	120	100
6-Monoacetylmorphine	NA	100	NA	NA
Oxycodone	<1	1	NA	1.5
Hydromorphone	100	75	43	NA
PCP				
Thienlcyclohexylpiperidine	100	100	1	1
Phencyclohexamine	17	5	NA	NA
THC				
Δ^8-THC	NA	17	<1	<1
11-OH-Δ^9-THC	>100	10	NA	NA
8-OH-Δ^9-THC	>100	NA	NA	NA
8,11-diOH-Δ^9-THC	>100	<1	50	NA
Barbiturates				
Amobarbital	100	100	15	NA
Barbital	200	33	15	NA
Butabarbital	80	100	60	
Butalbital	80	100	150	
Pentobarbital	40	100	30	
Phenobarbital	29	66	6	
Benzodiazepines				
Alprazolam	67	100	6,000	
Chlordiazepoxide	27	6	30	
Clonazepam	53	1	<1	
Diazepam	40	67	300	
Lorazepam	67	66	6	
Nitrazepam	NA	60	30	
Temazepam	68	100	600	

POC, point of care; NA, not available; PCP, phencyclidine; THC, tetrahydrocannabinol.
Some data were taken from O'Connor E, Ostheimer D, Wu HB, Limitations of forensic urine drug testing by methodology and adulteration. *AACC Ther Drug Monit-Toxicol Update* 1993;14:275–296.

In general, there is little cross-reactivity toward the L-forms, which are sympathomimetic amines found in over-the-counter cold medications and not illicit substances. In the cocaine assay, antibodies are raised against benzoylecgonine, the principal inactive urine metabolite, with little cross-reactivity toward free cocaine itself. For opiates, antibodies are directed against morphine because it is the principal metabolite for both heroin and codeine. Codeine often produces a higher degree of cross-reactivity than the targeted drug, as shown in Table 15.8. The target for phencyclidine (PCP) is the parent drug itself, although other analogs also can have significant cross-reactivities. For marijuana, the target is 11-nor-Δ^9-THC-9 carboxylic acid, although there is significant cross-reactivity toward many of the other THC metabolites. Secobarbital is the targeted drug for the barbiturates, with most assays having a significant cross-reactivity toward the other barbiturates. Oxazepam is principally the targeted analyte/metabolite drug for benzodiazepine immunoassays. Although oxazepam is itself a drug, it is the active metabolite for other benzodiazepines,

such as chlordiazepoxide, diazepam, halazepam, prazepam, and temazepam.

Commercial Devices

Most POC drug testing assays make use of the immunochromatography format (33) (Fig. 15.1A). A urine sample is added to a device containing a drug-specific mouse antibody conjugated to dye such as colloidal gold. If the urine sample is devoid of the targeted drug (Fig. 15.1B), the conjugated antibody from the device is free to react with immobilized analyte to produce a visible line. Excess conjugate also reacts with antimouse antibodies immobilized onto another position of the test area. This second line is the device's procedural control. A positive result indicates that there has been sufficient flow of urine to the test area. If the urine sample contains the targeted drug at a concentration that exceeds the preset cutoff limit of the device (Fig. 15.1C), the drug from the urine sample binds to the mouse conjugate, thereby prohibiting it from binding to the immobilized antibody. In this situation, no

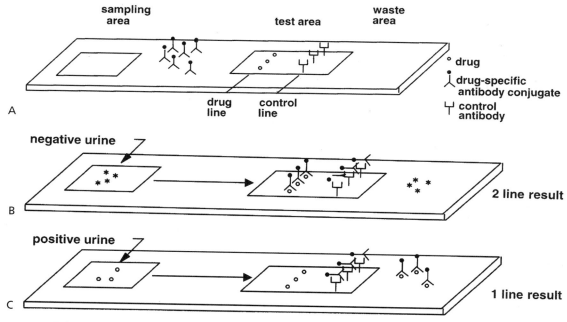

FIGURE 15.1. Schematic representation of a "negative indicating" point-of-care (POC) urine drug screen device. **A**: Diagram of device regions. **B**: Flow of urine containing no target analyte results in the binding of the drug conjugate to the drug line and control indicators to the control line. Two lines are produced. **C**: Flow of urine containing the target analyte exceeding the cutoff concentration results in the binding of the drug to the drug line and control indicators to the control line. One line is produced.

line is formed in the drug-detection area. Some of the conjugate does react with the immobilized antimouse antibodies to produce a positive result for the procedure control. This "negative logic" scheme whereby a positive result produces one line and a negative result produces two lines is contrary to many other (nontoxicology) POCT devices, such as qualitative assays for cardiac markers. The presence of the procedural control becomes essential for the correct interpretation of results.

Multianalyte devices constitute the next generation of POC drug testing assays. Table 15.5 lists many of the devices that are commercially available. The Triage Panel (Biosite Diagnostics, San Diego, CA, U.S.A.) was the first to offer a multianalyte POCT device. This device provides results on either seven or eight different classes of drugs of abuse (two product menus are available) and compares well against other immunoassays and gas chromatography/mass spectrometry (GC/MS) (34). For the benzodiazepines, the Triage Panel is superior to laboratory-based immunoassays because the antibodies used are directed toward glucuronide metabolites instead of parent benzodiazepine drugs (35). Unlike the testing scheme shown in Figure 15.1, the Triage device operates under "positive logic"; that is, a line is produced when the drug is present above the threshold limits. The procedure does require transfer of the sample and the antibody conjugate to the membrane surface and has a wash step.

Assays that do not require a transfer or washing step are more convenient. The Frontline assay (Roche, Indianapolis, IN, U.S.A.) is a dipstick test that produces a positive result in the presence of the drug and requires no pipetting of urine. In one comparative study, the correlation of results to other immunoassays was high (>90%) (36). The TesTstik (Roche, Indianapolis,

IN, U.S.A.) is very similar. The absence of a wash step also enables the direct testing of urine from the sample collection cup itself. In the TesTcup design (Roche, Sommerville, NJ, U.S.A.), the testing device is built into the urine collection cup (37). Turning the cap enables direct transfer of an aliquot of sample (metering) and analysis of the urine sample for multiple drugs. This device is currently being evaluated in a pilot study for preemployment drug testing for the U.S. Postal Service (3). If this program is successful, it may initiate more on-site POC drug testing.

Recently, the HHS conducted evaluations of 15 on-site drugs or POC devices for drugs mandated for testing of federal employees (38). A major objective of this ongoing study is to determine how the cutoff concentrations and the subjective ability of testers to read visually the endpoints of POC devices compare with objective laboratory-based analysis. Preliminary results show that there are differences in the rate of false-positives and false-negatives between devices.

Adulterants

The consequences for an employee with a confirmed positive urine drug test are significant in workplace testing programs, ranging from disciplinary action to job dismissal. Because of these penalties, many persons attempt to pass a drug test by adding foreign substances or "adulterants" to a collected urine sample prior to testing in an attempt to invalidate results (39). In the early years of the federal program, the common adulterants were items found in urine collection station bathrooms, for example, detergents, soaps, and bleach. These items are added to unwitnessed collections as a last-minute effort to spoil a test. Today, urine adulteration is more sophisticated; several commercial products are available. *In vivo* adulterants, such as osmotic diuretics, are consumed with copious amounts of water by the drug test donor before collection in an attempt to dilute urine drug concentrations to below cutoff limits. *In vitro* adulterants are clandestinely added to urine after collection and are designed to interfere with specific drug-screening and confirmation assays. An example of an *in vitro* adulterant is glutaraldehyde, sold under the label "Urinaid," which produces false-negative results for drug-screening enzyme immunoassays (37). Nitrites (sold as "Klear") interfere with the recovery of marijuana metabolites targeted in GC/MS confirmation assays (40). Pyridinium chlorochromate is the latest adulterant, which acts in a similar manner as Klear (41). A comprehensive list of *in vitro* adulterants and their effect on specific laboratory-based assays, such as the enzyme-multiplied immunoassay technique (EMIT), fluorescence polarization immunoassay, and radioimmunoassay is available (42,43).

For POC drugs-of-abuse testing devices, no systematic studies have been done on the effect of household or commercial adulterants. Because of differences in the measurement principles between POC and laboratory-based systems, it is unlikely that adulterants in POC devices will behave in exactly the same manner. Adulterants that retard or impede urine flow to the test areas will likely produce a negative interference for most POC devices that make use of immunochromatography. As shown in Figure 15.2, POC assays that produce no line for a positive result can be misinterpreted easily. These devices usually have a built-in procedural control that should signal to the analyst that an invalid result has been achieved. Unfortunately, POC devices are designed for testing by persons not trained in forensic toxicology and may overlook the importance of the procedural controls.

The SAMHSA drug-testing laboratories are required to perform basic tests to detect the presence of adulterated samples. Urine samples containing low-specific-gravity or creatinine concentrations suggest the presence of a dilutional adulterant. Alterations in urine pH may indicate household adulterant use, such as bleach, soap, detergent, vinegar, or lemon juice. There are also specific laboratory tests for the presence of glutaraldehyde and nitrite adulterants. One manufacturer produced a dipstick test panel for urine creatinine, nitrite, glutaraldehyde and pH (AdultaCheck 4, Chimera Research and Chemical, Inc., North Largo, FL). This dipstick differs from urinalysis dipsticks because cutoff concentrations are designed specifically to detect urine drug-testing adulterants rather than for concentrations observed in pathologic diseases. The use of this dipstick is ideal for off-site drug screenings by POCT devices. Because many adulterants act by oxidizing drugs to other compounds, the next generation of adulterant dipstick and laboratory-based tests will be able to indicate the presence of oxidizing agents.

Nontraditional Samples for Drug Testing

Although urine is the most widely used sample for drugs of abuse testing, there are limitations to this type of sample. For workplace toxicology, urine samples can be adulterated easily when the subject is left alone in the bathroom to donate the sample. In the ED, unconscious patients may require the insertion of a Foley catheter. Patients with acute or chronic renal failure may be unable to donate sufficient quantities of urine. Results of urine drug testing provide only information about recent drug use (e.g., within the past few days). For these reasons, toxicologists have sought other types of samples for drug testing. Hair testing has received a lot of interest because, depending on the length of the donor's hair, results can indicate exposures to drugs dating back several weeks or months (44). For newborns, the analysis of meconium for drugs of abuse can indicate in utero drug use by the mother dating back several months. Sweat is an attractive sample because patches can be worn for several days and can be used to monitor abstinence in compliance programs and in law enforcement (45). A commercial sweat collection patch is available (Pharmchem Laboratories, Menlo Park, NY, U.S.A.). Unfortunately, POCT devices are not available or likely to be in the near future because of the difficulty in extracting drugs from hair, meconium, or sweat. On the other hand, there is commercial interest in the development of POC devices for drug testing of oral fluids. One manufacturer (Avitar, Canton, MA, U.S.A.) developed a prototype assay for the screening analysis for morphine in saliva. In a study conducted by the manufacturer, the POC saliva test showed a 95% concordance with EMIT results of urine collected simultaneously (46), which is not a routine practice. With regard to adulteration, saliva testing may have an advantage over urine because collection is performed directly by the collector. A donor is not likely to introduce foreign solvents or substances into the mouth for purposes of invalidating drug test results. A disadvantage of oral fluids is that it is difficult to obtain large volumes of saliva needed for GC/MS confirmation (47). Several commercial saliva collection devices are available for collecting higher volumes (Salivette, Sarstedt, Newton NC, U.S.A.; Orasure, STC Technologies, Bethlehem PA, U.S.A.; and the Finger Collectur, Avitar, Cantun, MA). A study of these devices revealed differences in the recovery of drugs compared with collection by natural expectoration (48). Clearly, more studies of this type are needed before this alternate sample can be used routinely.

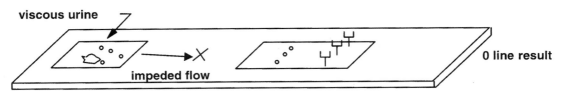

FIGURE 15.2. Interference of a point-of-care testing (POCT) device by a viscous adulterant.

At-home Drug Testing

The next generation of POC devices may be configured for at-home testing. This could aid parents who want to determine the presence of drug use by their children or employees who wish to determine whether their urine is positive before an "official" test conducted by an employer. Results of at-home testing are not reported to employers, law-enforcement agencies, or medical records; thus, they would not affect a person's ability to obtain life or medical insurance or a driver's license. The U.S. Food and Drug Administration (FDA) recently approved POCT devices for at-home use. The Pharmatech (San Diego, CA, U.S.A.) QuickScreen kit contains a test strip and a urine cup (49). Results are obtained in 10 minutes. Positive results may prompt the subject to try to postpone the test, to dilute urine with diuretics, or to adulterate the urine after donation. Because of this, employers will have to put more emphasis on random "on the spot" drug testing in the future to prevent subjects from taking actions to negate the accuracy of the testing.

At-home drug-collection systems also have been approved for use. Rather than testing, this system enables collection of urine and then sending it to a certified drug-testing laboratory for definitive results (50). ChemTrak Inc. (Sunnyvale, CA, U.S.A.) began marketing the Parents Alert Home Drug Test kit. A special panel highly encouraged the FDA to include language with these kits indicating that positive results should be confirmed by more elaborate drug assays (e.g., GC/MS).

THERAPEUTIC DRUG MONITORING

The clinical need and commercial interest for POCT devices for therapeutic drug monitoring are not nearly as significant as what exists for drugs-of-abuse testing. With the exception of theophylline (especially in children), tricyclic antidepressants (TCAs), digoxin, acetaminophen, and salicylates, acute overdoses of therapeutic drugs are rarely a clinical problem. Testing for these drugs is also not an issue for workplace drug testing, sports medicine, physician or nurse health, or the criminal justice system. On the other hand, POCT within physician offices can provide real-time results that can lead to changes in dosages made while the patient is still in the office (51).

Some POC devices have been developed and studies conducted as to their accuracy and use. In 1990, Oles (52) reviewed the available physician office laboratory (POL) testing instruments available for therapeutic drug monitoring (TDM). Of the small POL analyzers, all but the Abbott Vision required serum or plasma, making them impractical for bedside testing. Although the Vision permitted use of heparinized whole blood, it was too large to be transported from patient to patient. Currently, only theophylline and phenytoin are available on the Vision. The first true POCT device was the AccuLevel (Syntex, Palo Alto, CA, U.S.A.), a quantitative enzyme immunochromatography assay. AccuLevel assay was developed and evaluated for theophylline and the anticonvulsant drugs carbamazepine, phenobarbital, and phenytoin (53,54). In an ED study, use of the AccuLevel theophylline assay reduced the ED length of stay and time required to achieve a therapeutic drug concentration in

the acute treatment of asthmatic children (55). Nevertheless, the AccuLevel assays have been discontinued by the manufacturer. An improved POC theophylline test is now available (AcuMeter, Chem Trak Co., Sunnyvale, CA, U.S.A.). This assay correlates well to the Abbott TDx (56) and the older AccuLevel assay and is based on the same principle as the over-the-counter AccuMeter cholesterol POC assay (57).

A TDM assay for digoxin would be useful to detect toxicities in the ED. Digoxin overdoses can be treated with digoxin antibodies (Digibind) (58). Unfortunately, POC assays for digoxin are not available because of the technical difficulties of measuring the low therapeutic concentration expected for this drug (1.5–2.0 ng/mL). Whereas therapeutic monitoring of tricyclic antidepressants is rather common, immunoassays for individual drugs have not been developed because of the difficulty in raising antibodies that can distinguish one TCA from another (59). Thus, testing for these drugs is typically performed by liquid chromatography. The POC assay that is available for TCAs, such as the Biosite (San Diego, CA, U.S.A.) Triage has cutoffs designed to detect overdose situations and is not designed for routine therapeutic drug monitoring.

Further development of POC TDM devices will likely be hindered by the incorporation of the TDM assay onto general chemistry analyzers that have large on-board menu capacities. Most laboratories have the capability of delivering results of TDM assays with the same turnaround time and convenience as general chemistry analytes. Other than those discussed already, there is unlikely to be other therapeutic drugs that have a clinical need for turnaround times faster than 1 hour. On the other hand, there may be some market for POL or at-home testing if compact and rapid assays can be developed.

FACTORS FOR POINT-OF-CARE TESTING VERSUS CENTRAL LABORATORY TESTING

The decision to perform drug testing in a central laboratory versus POCT or some combination of the two is highly complex and dependent on a number of factors. Table 15.9 lists some of these issues and the conditions that favor one approach over the other. Each institution must weigh the various factors in deter-

TABLE 15.9. IMPORTANT FACTORS IN COMPARING POC VERSUS CENTRAL LABORATORY TESTING FOR DRUGS OF ABUSE

Factor	Favors POC	Favors Central Lab
Testing volume	Low (5–10/d)	High (>10/d)
Turnaround time needs	Fast (<1 h)	Slow (>1 h)
Reagent costs	Low if volume low ($5–10 each)	Low if volume high (<$1.00 each)
Instrument costs	None	High but equipment may preexist
Specimen delivery	Not required	May be extensive
Labor	Multitasking staff	Dedicated lab staff
Regulatory issues	Not universally approved	Approved

POC, point of care.

mining the most cost-effective approach for their situation. For low-volume off-site testing, PCC may be the best approach because no instrument cost are involved. If the testing is conducted on-site by persons who already have other responsibilities (e.g., nurses on an ED unit or phlebotomists in a collection station), the labor costs for performing POCT will be distributed to a larger pool of responsibilities. This argument is valid only for low toxicology testing volume because if the volume is high, personnel dedicated to drug testing may be required. In this situation, the labor effort will be higher than for the central laboratory unless these persons have other responsibilities. A high testing level environment favors a central laboratory approach. This is particularly true if the turnaround time needs are such that the testing can be performed on a batch basis (e.g., once daily). The costs of performing calibrations and assaying controls will be distributed over the high testing volume, reducing the costs for an individual result. If the laboratory also conducts routine clinical chemistry tests, the same instrumentation can likely be used for drug testing. The reagent costs for drug testing in a central location will be substantially lower than for POCT. Other costs associated with delivery of samples and reports, however, which are not needed for on-site testing, must be considered. For workplace testing, if the delays in sending and testing specimens in a central laboratory result in lost days on the job for an employee, POCT will be overall more cost-effective. Some hospital laboratories who have low testing volumes have elected to use POCT devices within the central laboratory because of limitations in the availability of equipment. In this way, they can deliver rapid turnaround time results while maintaining control of the testing.

A major cooperative effort is under way to standardize the connection between results produced by POCT with clinical information and data management systems (60). Efforts of the Connectivity Industry Consortium will accelerate implementation of POCT within hospitals and medical centers. Although this consortium may be useful for connecting breath-alcohol meters to medical databases, manufacturers of these devices are not yet represented in the group. For POCT drugs of abuse testing, the consortium will also not have a major impact initially, as all current devices make use of a visual endpoint; thus, there is no electronic transfer of results.

Regulatory issues also will play a role in the decision of POC versus the central laboratory. For clinical toxicology, on-site testing must conform to CLIA 88 regulations, which require documentation of proficiency and quality assurance. Usually, POCT is under the control of the central laboratory administrative staff. Some hospitals have a separate CLIA license from the main laboratory. Federal workplace drug-testing regulations currently do not permit on-site drug testing, but it is likely that this situation will change in the near future. On-site testing using POC devices is already widely used in nonregulated workplace and compliance testing. For alcohol, on-site testing using breath or saliva (as opposed to urine testing) is standard practice for most drug-testing programs. It should be recognized that results of screening assays must be confirmed by a second test. For drugs of abuse, this is usually GC/MS. For alcohol, confirmation testing consists of retesting the individual after some time has elapsed.

CONCLUSIONS AND FUTURE CONSIDERATIONS

The POCT platforms have evolved from single analyte latex agglutination assays to multianalyte dipsticks requiring no addition of reagents. If POCT becomes accepted practice for workplace drug testing, the next generation of toxicology dipsticks is likely to incorporate the latest tests for *in vitro* urine adulterants. Also under consideration might be the need to perform quantitative or semiquantitative analysis for positive results using some handheld reflectance readers. Although quantitative results are not currently produced by laboratory-based immunoassays for drugs of abuse, semiquantitative results can be obtained from the raw data of rate absorbances, fluorescence polarization, or radioactive decay counts to permit some idea as to the degree by which the result is positive. SAMHSA regulations require certified laboratories to provide quantitative GC/MS results on all urine samples screened positive for drugs of abuse. Semiquantitative data from screening assays are routinely used by laboratories to determine whether dilution of the sample is necessary before extraction.

New drug assays for the POC platform must always be a future consideration as the patterns for drug abuse evolve. A POC assay for LSD may be warranted today because of the increasing prevalence of use of this drug by teenagers and young adults (61). Fentanyl and fentanyl analogs such as "China white" have had sporadic epidemics in parts of the United States (62). Methcathinone is a designer amphetamine and has been used in parts of the Midwest (63). Improvements in the analytic sensitivity would be required to measure many of these drugs because the expected urine concentrations are very low (0.5 ng/mL) in some cases and cannot be measured using visual POC detection schemes. Other tags, such as fluorescence and chemiluminescence labels, would have the sensitivity needed, but these approaches have not yet been attempted for quantitative POCT because a strip reader would be necessary. Perhaps the next generation of POCT devices will make use of signals that can be amplified while maintaining the convenience of current POCT platforms.

The issue of onsite workplace drug testing of federal employees is coming closer to reality. The Drug Testing Advisory Board (DTAB) made recommendations to HHS for onsite testing. The current recommendations are that the collector and the person conducting the test must be certified by an HHS-approved certification program, similar in principle to the breath-alcohol technician program. The collection facility must satisfy all the requirements for a collection site. Further, the POCT device must be authorized by the HHS. Recommendations on the regular use of quality-control materials also have been made by the DTAB. Once these regulations become enacted for governmental workers, it is likely that there will be a gradual shift from laboratory-based testing to POCT for all employees.

REFERENCES

1. Hoffman JP, Lairson C, Sanderson A. *An analysis of worker drug use and workplace policies and programs.* U.S. Department of Health and Human Services, Office of Applied Studies, Substance Abuse and Mental Health Services Administration, Rockville, MD, 1997. Avail-

able at: www.samhsa.gov/wkplace/workplac.htm. Accessed November 27, 2001.

2. Department of Health and Human Services. Mandatory guidelines for federal workplace drug testing programs; final guidelines notice. *Federal Register* 1988;53:11969–11989.

3. Postal Service to trial onsite testing of all new employees. *Drug Detection Report* 1998;8:65–66.

4. Procedures for transportation workplace drug and alcohol testing programs. *Federal Register* 1994;59:7340–7378.

5. *Preliminary estimates from the Drug Abuse Warning Network.* Rockville, MD: Substance Abuse and Mental Health Administration, U.S. Dept. of Health and Human Services Advance Report no. 8, 1994.

6. National Household Survey on Drug Abuse. *Population estimates 1994.* Rockville, MD: Substance Abuse and Mental Health Services Administration, U.S. Dept. of Health and Human Services, 1995.

7. Wu AHB, Feng YJ, Pajor A, et al. Detection and interpretation of lysergic acid diethylamide (LSD) results by immunoassay screening of urine in various testing groups. *J Anal Toxicol* 1997;21:181–184.

8. Litovitz TL, Smilkstein M, Felberg L, et al. 1996 Annual report of the American Association of Poison Control Centers Toxic Exposure Surveillance System. *Am J Emerg Med* 1997;15:447–500.

9. Hughes PH, Bradenburg N, Baldwin DC, et al. Prevalence of substance use among U.S. physicians. *JAMA* 1992;267:2333–2339.

10. National Institute on Drug Abuse. *National household survey on drug abuse: population estimates 1990.* Rockville, MD: U.S. Department of Health and Human Services, 1990.

11. McClain DA, Hug CC Jr. Intravenous fentanyl kinetics. *Clin Pharmacol Ther* 1980;28:106–114.

12. Henderson GL. Fentanyl-related deaths: demographics, circumstances, and toxicology of 112 cases. *J Forensic Sci* 1991;36:422–433.

13. National Institute of Justice. *Drug treatment needs among adult arrestees in Baltimore.* Document FS 0000168, 1997.

14. Tunis S, Austin J, Morris M, et al. *Evaluation of drug treatment in local corrections.* National Institute of Justice document FS0000171, 1997.

15. Bureau of Justice Assistance. *Drug testing guidelines and practices for adult probation and parole agencies.* Washington, D.C.: Bureau of Justice Assistance, 1990.

16. Wagner JC. Enhancement of athletic performance with drugs: an overview. *Sports Med* 1991;12:250–265.

17. Hatton CK, Catlin DH. Detection of androgenic anabolic steroids in urine. *Clin Lab Med* 1987;7:655–668.

18. Rudis MI, Keyes C. Toxidromes: an approach to the poisoned patient. In: Aghababian RV, ed. *Emergency medicine: the core curriculum.* Philadelphia: Lippincott–Raven; 1998:992–994.

19. Raymond RC, Warren M, Morris RW, et al. Periodicity of presentations of drugs of abuse and overdose in an emergency department. *Clin Toxicol* 1992;30:467–478.

20. Litovitz TL, Clark LR, Soloway RA. 1993 annual report of the American Association of Poison Control Centers Toxic Exposure Surveillance System. *Am J Emerg Med* 1994;12:546–584.

21. Smood J. Acetaminophen and salicylates. In: Aghababian RV, ed. *Emergency medicine: the core curriculum.* Philadelphia: Lippincott–Raven; 1998:1010–1013,1174–1177.

22. Sporer KA, Khayam-Bashi H. Acetaminophen and salicylate serum levels in patients with suicidal ingestion or altered mental status. *Am J Emerg Med* 1996;14:443–446.

23. Gerson B. Alcohol. *Clin Lab Med* 1990;10:355–374.

24. Miller SM. Saliva: new interest in a nontraditional specimen. *Medical Laboratory Observer* 1993;25:31–35.

25. Christopher TA, Zeccardi JA. Evaluation of the Q.E.D. saliva alcohol test: a new, rapid, accurate device for measuring ethanol in saliva. *Ann Emerg Med* 1992;21:1135–1137.

26. *Uniform vehicle code section and model traffic ordinances.* National Committee on Uniform Traffic Laws and Ordinances, Evanston, IL, 1987: 65–66.

27. Aabakken L, Johansen KS, Rydningen EB, et al. Osmolal and anion gaps in patients admitted to an emergency medical department. *Hum Exp Toxicol* 1994;13:131–134.

28. Jortani SA. Point-of-care testing for alcohol. *Ther Drug Monit-Toxicol* 2000;21:121–126.

29. Simpson G. Accuracy and precision of breath alcohol measurements for subjects in the absorptive state. *Clin Chem* 1987;33:753–756.

30. Wu AHB. Near-patient and point-of-care testing for alcohol and drugs of abuse. *Ther Drug Monit-Toxicol* 1995;16:225–236.

31. Blanke RV, Decker WJ. Analysis of toxic substances. In: Tietz NW, ed. *Textbook of clinical chemistry.* Philadelphia: WB Saunders, 1986: 679–683.

32. O'Connor E, Ostheimer D, Wu AHB. Limitations of forensic urine drug testing by methodology and adulteration. *AACC Ther Drug Monit-Toxicol U* 1993;14:275–296.

33. Kasahara Y, Ashihara Y. Simple devices and their possible application in clinical laboratory downsizing. *Clin Chim Acta* 1997;267:87–102.

34. Wu AHB, Wong SS, Johnson KG, et al. Evaluation of the Triage system for emergency testing of phencylidine, amphetamines, opiates, and tetrahydrocannabinol in serum. *J Anal Toxicol* 1993;17:241–245.

35. Koch TR, Raglin RL, Scheree K, et al. Improved screening for benzodiazepine metabolites in urine using the Triage Panel for drugs of abuse. *J Anal Toxicol* 1994;18:168–172.

36. Wennig R, Moeller MR, Haguenoer JM, et al. Development and evaluation of immunochromatographic rapid tests for screening of cannabinoids, cocaine, and opiates in urine. *J Anal Toxicol* 1998;22:148–155.

37. Crouch DJ, Cheever ML, Andrenyak DM, et al. A comparison of ONTRAK TESTCUP, abuscreen ONTRAK, abuscreen ONLINE, and GC/MS urinalysis test results. *J Forens Sci* 1998;43:35–40.

38. HHS evaluation finds on-site device performance encouraging. *Drug Detection Report* 1999;9:17–18.

39. Wu AHB. Integrity of urine specimens submitted for toxicologic analysis: adulteration, mechanisms of action, and laboratory detection. *Forens Sci Rev* 1998;10:47–65.

40. George S, Braithwaite RA. The effect of glutaraldehyde adulteration of urine specimens on Syva EMIT II drugs-of-abuse assays. *J Anal Toxicol* 1996;20:195–196.

41. El Sohly MA, Feng S, Kopycki WJ, et al. A procedure to overcome interferences caused by the adulterant "Klear" in the GC-MS analysis of 11-nor-^{9}-THC-9-COOH. *J Anal Toxicol* 1997;21:240–242.

42. Wu AHB, Bristol B, Sexton K, et al. Adulteration of urine by "Urine Luck." *Clin Chem* 1999;45:1051-1057.

43. Cody JT. Adulteration of urine specimens. In: Liu RH, Goldberger A, eds. *Handbook for workplace drug testing.* Washington, D.C.: AACC Press, 1995:181–208.

44. Cone EJ, Yousenfejad D, Darwin WD, et al. Testing human hair for drugs of abuse. II. Identification of unique cocaine metabolites in hair of drug abusers and evaluation of decontamination procedures. *J Anal Toxicol* 1991;15:250–255.

45. Goldberger BA, Caplan YH, Maguire T, et al . Testing human hair for drugs of abuse. III. Identification of heroin and 6-acetylmorphine as indicators of heroin use. *J Anal Toxicol* 1991;15:226–231.

46. Huestis MA, Cone EJ, Wong CJ, et al. Monitoring opiate use in substance abuse treatment patients with sweat and urine drug testing. *J Anal Toxicol* 2000;24:509–521.

47. Package insert. Oral Screen Morphine. Avitar Technologies, Inc., Canton, MA, 1998.

48. O'Neal CL, Crouch DJ, Rollins DE, et al. The effects of collection methods on oral fluid codeine concentrations. *J Anal Toxicol* 2000; 24:536–542.

49. FDA clears home-based drug screening test kit. *Drug Detection Report* 1998;8:169.

50. Confirmation process urged for on-site home drug tests. *Drug Detection Report* 1997;7:3.

51. Larkin JG, Herrick AL, McGuire GM, et al. Antiepileptic drug monitoring at the epilepsy clinic: a prospective evaluation. *Epilepsia* 1991; 32:89–95.

52. Oles KS. Therapeutic drug monitoring analysis systems for the physician office laboratory: a review of the literature. *Ann Pharmacother* 1990;24:1070–1077.

53. Nguyen QC, Sly RM, Boeckx RL, et al. Determination of theophylline concentrations by AccuLevel. *Ann Allergy* 1988;60:521–522.

54. Nielsen IM, Gram L, Dam M. Comparison of AccuLevel and TD: evaluation of on-site monitoring of antiepileptic drugs. *Epilepsia* 1992; 33:558–563.

55. Shier JM, Sly RM, Boeckx RL, et al. Impact of Acculevel on treatment of acute asthma. *Ann Allergy* 1988;60:523–526.

56. Asmus MJ, Milavetz G, Teresi ME, et al. Evaluation of a noninstrumental disposable method for quantifying serum theophylline concentrations. *Pharmacotherapy* 1998;18:30–34.

57. Volles DF, McKenney JM, Miller WG, et al. Analytic and clinical performance of two compact cholesterol testing devices. *Pharmacotherapy* 1998;18:184–192.

58. Schakenbach L, Arft P. Digoxin toxicity treated with Digibind. *Crit Care Nurse* 1989;9:16–22.

59. Nebinger P, Koel M. Specificity data of the tricyclic antidepressants assay by fluorescent polarization immunoassay. *J Anal Toxicol* 1990;14:219–221.

60. Point-of-Care Connectivity Industry Consortium. Available at: http://www.poccic.org. Accessed November 27, 2001.

61. Gold MS, Schuchard K. LSD use among US high school students. *JAMA* 1994;271:403–404.

62. Martin M, Hecker J, Clark R, et al. China White epidemic: an eastern United States emergency department experience. *Ann Emerg Med* 1991;20:158–164.

63. Goldstone M. "Cat": methcathinone-a new drug of abuse. *JAMA* 1993;269:2508.

16

POINT-OF-CARE TESTING FOR BODY FLUIDS

FREDERICK L. KIECHLE

Rudimentary point-of-care testing (POCT) was described as early as 1883 in London, England (1). The semiquantitative or quantitative nature of the data obtained from such analyses is consistent with physiologic parameters obtained at the bedside, such as temperature, respiratory rate, or blood pressure. Whereas errors in measurement of the latter have been attributed to technique, equipment, or random variability (2–4), adequate training of medical professionals in following established guidelines resulted in improved performance (2). These findings emphasize the need for teamwork (3) and knowledge of established guidelines (5–7) to improve the quality of testing at the bedside. Some procedures at the bedside, however, require evaluation of color, odor, consistency, or a semiqualitative reagent strip reaction (8). The location of a nasogastric tube, for example, can be evaluated by observing the color and pH of the aspirated contents (8). Therefore, not all bedside testing results in a numeric endpoint.

Rules and regulations related to POCT continue to evolve. In general, federal law described by the Centers for Medicare and Medicaid Services (CMS) Administration in the Clinical Laboratory Improvement Amendments of 1988 (CLIA 88) provides the framework for most POCT standards and guidelines (3,5). These federal regulations classify laboratory procedures based on their test complexity using well-defined criteria: waived, moderately complex, highly complex, and provider-performed microscopy.

Traditionally, microscopy of labile specimens was performed by the patient's physician at or near the POC. Because specimen lability could compromise test accuracy, a unique regulatory approach for this testing was defined in the *Federal Register* of April 25, 1995. The procedures included in this category, provider-performed microscopy, are listed in Table 16.1. If a physician, a dentist, a midlevel practitioner, or a physician assistant (under the supervision of a physician or in independent practice authorized by the state) personally performs these tests on patients of his or her medical practice (including a group practice of which the physician is a member), the laboratory may receive a certificate for provider-performed microscopy procedures. Under this certificate, the laboratory is also permitted to conduct waived tests.

BODY FLUIDS

Provider-performed microscopy defines several body fluids used for POCT. Table 16.2 lists these examples as well as other fluids that may be used for analysis in the central laboratory or at the bedside.

Many hospital laboratories have elected to use POCT to cope with the changing laboratory economic environment introduced by capitated reimbursement (9). In the future, large automated core laboratories will provide the most routine testing (3,10). The remaining rapid-turnaround procedures will be divided between the immediate-response laboratory and POCT programs (3,10). Bedside diagnostic testing of body fluids has a variety of applications in the emergency department as well as throughout the hospital (11). Examples of these applications will be described subsequently in this chapter.

TABLE 16.1. PROVIDER-PERFORMED MICROSCOPY PROCEDURES

Wet mounts, including preparation of vaginal, cervical, or skin specimens
All potassium hydroxide (KOH) preparations
Pinworm examinations
Fern test
Postcoital direct, qualitative examination
Vaginal or cervical mucus
Nasal smears for granulocytes
Fecal leukocyte examinations
Qualitative semen analysis (limited to the presence or absence of sperm and detection of motility)

TABLE 16.2. POTENTIAL BODY FLUIDS FOR ANALYSIS IN THE CENTRAL LABORATORY OR AT THE BEDSIDE

Amniotic fluid	Pericardial fluid
Breast milk	Peritoneal fluid
Cerebrospinal fluid	Pleural fluid
Feces	Saliva
Follicular fluid	Seminal fluid
Gastric contents	Synovial fluid
Nasal secretion	Urine

Urine

Urinalysis

Nonautomated urinalysis by dipstick or reagent tablets is classified as waived tests by CLIA '88 (3,7). Although there are limitations in the evaluation of kidney function by observation of urine and reagent dipstick analysis only (12), manual or computerized algorithms have been established for using the dipstick as a biochemical screen prior to microscopic or urine culture (13,14). Four dipstick results (protein, nitrite, leukocyte esterase, and hemoglobin) should constitute the minimum number to be evaluated in a biochemical screen (13). If any one reaction is positive, appropriate additional studies, such as microscopy or urine culture, should be performed. A biochemical screen that excludes leukocyte esterase will yield a higher false-negative rate than a screen that includes it (13). It is important to evaluate any potential urinary biochemical screen for point-of-care use to ensure that no clinically significant positive finding is hidden within the group of false-negative results. A review of the medical record is usually the only way to assess this issue (15).

Initial Evaluation

The ideal urine specimen is acidic and concentrated. Therefore, the pH and specific gravity are useful initially to evaluate the specimen. Two indicator dyes, methyl red and bromthymol blue, are usually used to measure pH. The kidney is capable of producing urine with a pH range of 4.6 to 8.0 (average, 6.0). Table 16.3 reviews some clinical conditions associated with persistently acid or alkaline urine pH. Normally, there is considerable variation in the pH of a random urine specimen attributable to diurnal variation, diet, or the presence of disease. Urinary casts, red cells, and white cells lyse in alkaline urine. Therefore, it is recommended that biochemical and microscopic urinalysis be performed within 2 hours after collection. A College of American Pathologists Q-probe study found, however, that 11.2% of nonrefrigerated urine specimens from hospitalized patients exceeded this 2-hour standard before analysis (16). Refrigeration of urine specimens for 24 hours leads to instability in protein, leukocyte, and erythrocyte detection by urine dipstick (17). The implementation of point-of-care dipstick analysis may improve the quality of the biochemical results in this situation.

The specific gravity of urine normally varies from 1.010 to 1.025. One reagent strip method uses a polyacid, whose acidity varies with the urine's ionic concentration, and the pH indicator bromthymol blue to detect the color change used to estimate specific gravity. A high specific gravity indicates increased urine concentration and is observed in dehydration or in the presence of radio-opaque dyes or dextran in the urine. Dilute urine has a low specific gravity and may be caused by excessive intake of fluids or diabetes insipidus.

Early evaluation of appearance may aid in the interpretation of the biochemical screening results. Fresh urine is usually clear and may become cloudy or turbid at room temperature, which usually indicates the presence of urate or alkaline phosphate crystals. Cloudiness in a fresh specimen may be caused by the presence of white cells, bacteria, fat, blood, crystalloid deposits, or free fat globules. Normal urine color varies from light straw to reddish yellow caused by three primary pigments: urochrome, urobilin, and uroerythrin. Drugs, food, and metabolic disorders may cause unusual coloration, however, such that the pigmentation absorbs in the reagent strip pad and interferes with interpretation of the color reaction. Drugs also can modify the biochemical reaction in the reagent dipstick.

Leukocyte Esterase

Both intact and lysed white cells in urine may be detected by leukocyte esterase reaction of a dipstick (18). Reaction methods differ in the substrate selected; for example, indoxyl carbonic acid ester is enzymatically converted to indoxyl, which is oxidized by atmospheric oxygen to indigo, a blue compound. Several diazonium salts may be used to convert indigo to a colored end product for detection on the dipstick within 2 minutes. False-positive and false-negative reactions have been reported (18). For example, *Trichomonas* organisms may cause a false-positive reaction, and ascorbic acid inhibits the oxidation of indoxyl and leads to a false-negative reaction. Both phenazopyridine and nitrofurantoin introduce pigment in the urine, which interferes with the test's interpretation. The combination of clinical signs and symptoms and leukocyte esterase–positive urine had a 94% sensitivity and 89% specificity in detecting sexually transmitted disease in adolescent males (19).

Nitrite

In urinary tract infections, increased urinary nitrite has been attributed to the conversion of nitrate to nitrite by nitrate reductase, which is found in approximately 80% of uropathogenic bacteria. On the strip, nitrite reacts with a diazonium compound first, followed by reaction with a color indicator that results in a uniform pink spot if it is positive. A negative nitrite reaction does not rule out a urinary tract infection for several reasons (20). First, 20% of uropathogens fail to reduce nitrate to nitrite. Second, because retention of urine in the bladder is required for the reduction reaction to take place if frequent voiding occurs, inadequate incubation time in the bladder may lead to a nitrite concentration too low for dipstick detection. Third, the patient may consume a diet low in nitrates (21). Substances in the urine, such as ascorbic acid (≥ 25 mg/dL) or nitrofurantoin, also can generate a false-negative reaction. Combinations of leukocyte esterase plus nitrite have been evaluated as a screening test for urinary tract infections but with limited success.

TABLE 16.3. CONDITIONS ASSOCIATED WITH URINE pH EXTREMES

Persistently Acid	Persistently Alkaline
Metabolic acidosis	Metabolic alkalosis
Respiratory acidosis	Respiratory alkalosis
Fever	Urea-splitting bacterial urinary tract infection
Phenylketonuria	Hyperaldosteronism
Alkaptonuria	Cushing's syndrome
Methanol intoxication	Renal tubular acidosis
Potassium depletion	Fanconi syndrome

Nitrite and nitrate are also degradation products of nitric oxide, and their rate of excretion in the urine is directly related to renal function (21,22). Nitric oxide or the endothelium-derived relaxing factor is generated from L-arginine by the action of nitric oxide synthase, an enzyme encoded by three different genes (22). It is a gaseous free radical and a highly regulated mediator with diverse biological effects on vasomotor tone, neurotransmission, and host defense. The cellular elements in infected urine contain an increased amount of one of the isoforms of nitric oxide synthase compared with uninfected controls. This enzyme represents an endogenous source of nitrite production in the urine specimen, a conclusion that is supported by the finding that urinary nitrite production was increased if infected urine specimens were incubated with added L-arginine for 4 hours (23). Under appropriate physiologic conditions, nitric oxide—and thus its degradation products, nitrite and nitrate—can be produced nonenzymatically (24). Therefore, inhibition of nitric oxide synthase activity, elevated in septic shock (25), will not completely stop nitric oxide production because the nonenzymatic synthetic pathways would not be altered. In acidic urine, some nitrite is converted to nitric oxide. A variety of disease states will lead to increased or decreased total nitric oxide production and, therefore, to alterations in nitrite excretion in the urine (21). Consequently, urinary nitrite is not only an indicator of a urinary tract infection, but it is also a monitor of total-body nitric oxide production.

Blood, Hemoglobin, and Myoglobin

The peroxidase-like activity of heme from free hemoglobin, lysed red cells, or myoglobin liberates oxygen from organic peroxide located in the reagent strip. Tetramethylbenzidine, an indicator chromogen, is then oxidized, resulting in a color change (green–blue) after 1 minute if heme is present. Falsely low or false-negative results may occur in the presence of ascorbic acid, high nitrite concentration, formalin, or high specific gravity, which may retard red cell lysis. False-positive reactions have been reported in the presence of bleach or microbial peroxidases in patients with bacteriuria (26). Some patients with a history of hematuria for 10 years never develop any clinical disease but have benign familial hematuria, which may be related to a thinner than normal glomerular basement membrane (27). Blood may be present as a result of glomerulonephritis, infection, renal stones, or drugs such as sulfonamides. Of the patients with hematuria, 1% will have bladder cancer.

Rhabdomyolysis, or dissolution of muscle, can occur in a variety of clinical settings, including crush injuries, seizure disorders, prolonged muscle compression, infections, phosphate depletion, staphylococcal toxins, venoms, and drugs (28). Acute renal failure occurs in 4% to 33% of patients after rhabdomyolysis secondary to the combination of renal vasoconstriction, nephrotoxicity, and tubular obstruction by myoglobin plugs and urates (28). The differentiation of myoglobin from hemoglobin in the urine of a patient with skeletal muscle injury is important. At least four rapid, simple, and sensitive methods are available to differentiate myoglobinuria from hemoglobinuria (29). Blondheim and colleagues (30) described the precipitation of hemoglobin tetramers or dimers in urine in an 80% saturated solution of ammonium sulfate. If myoglobin is present, the supernatant remains heme positive after centrifugation (30). It is possible that these two proteins may be bound to other proteins, altering their precipitation characteristics in 80% ammonium sulfate. Although the original description of the method does not address the detection limit for myoglobin in urine, it has been estimated to be 50 g per liter (31). If spectrophotometry is available, the A600/A580 ratio can be calculated. If the ratio is greater than 0.85, myoglobin is present, whereas a ratio lower than 0.80 shows hemoglobin if the benzidine test indicates the presence of heme protein. There is a greater than tenfold discrepancy in the reported detection limit for this absorption ratio method (31). The differential ultrafiltration method is based on myoglobin with a molecular weight of 17,200 Da passing through the filter, whereas hemoglobin (molecular weight of 64,456 Da) will not. The latex agglutination test (Rapi-Tek, Behringwerke, Marburg, Germany) is a semiquantitative assay for the rapid detection of myoglobinuria (29). The reagent consists of a suspension of latex particles coated with antibody to human myoglobin. It is recommended that the urine specimen be assayed for 5 minutes with undiluted and diluted (1:6) urine. The dilution will prevent the postzone phenomenon caused by excess antigen. In an evaluation of trauma patients for myoglobinuria, no false-negative results were seen (29). This assay has been standardized always to be negative when urine myoglobin is less than 4.48 nmol per liter. This assay has also been adapted to serum samples (32). With its limitations, the ammonium sulfate precipitation remains the most common method to differentiate myoglobinuria from hemoglobinuria (30).

Ketone Bodies

Urinary ketone bodies include acetone, acetoacetic acid, and β-hydroxybutyrate. The first two compounds will react with nitroprusside on a reagent strip for urine. Total ketone body concentration increases during fasting, after exercise, in late pregnancy, in early neonatal life, in metabolic disorders such as diabetes, and in some hypoglycemic conditions of childhood where there is a defect in carbohydrate, amino acid, or organic acid metabolism, such as pyruvate decarboxylase deficiency. The reversible reaction of acetoacetate to β-hydroxybutyrate is catalyzed by β-hydroxybutyrate dehydrogenase, which is regulated by the ratio of nicotinamide adenine dinucleotide (NADH) and its oxidized form (NAD^+). This ratio is determined partially by tissue oxygenation. During hypoxia, NADH will increase, and β-hydroxybutyrate, not detected by nitroprusside, will be the predominant ketone body present. If the patient is in diabetic ketoacidosis, a false-negative nitroprusside reaction may be obtained. The addition of 30% hydrogen peroxide to urine specimens at a ratio of 1:10 for peroxide to specimen has been investigated as a method of converting β-hydroxybutyrate to a nitroprusside-positive compound (33). The concentration of β-hydroxybutyrate must be 50 mmol per liter or greater for this method to yield a positive nitroprusside reaction in urine on a dipstick. Blood β-hydroxybutyrate is in the range of 4.2 to 11.0 mmol per liter during diabetic ketoacidosis. False-positive ketone body results may be obtained on a dipstick because nitroprusside also reacts with drugs containing free sulfhydryl groups, such as dimercaprol, D-penicillamine, cysteine, N-acetyl cysteine, mesna, and captopril. An adequate method is needed for rapid urinary β-hydroxybutyrate determination. Several bedside techniques for whole-blood β-hydroxybutyrate have been reported (34).

Glucose

The presence of glucosuria is dependent on three factors: the concentration of glucose in the blood, the glomerular filtration rate, and the degree of tubular reabsorption. When the renal threshold is exceeded (>180–200 mg/dL blood glucose), the excess glucose will not be reabsorbed into the blood but will be eliminated in the urine. Some individuals have a low renal threshold for glucose and will have glucosuria when blood glucose is in the reference range. Glucosuria usually indicates diabetes mellitus. The first urine reagent strip test, Clinistix (Miles, Inc., Elkart, IN, U.S.A.) became available in 1956. Self-monitoring of the adequacy of insulin control by diabetic patients is accomplished primarily by fingerstick blood glucose measurement. For patients who cannot or will not perform self-monitoring of blood glucose, urine glucose represents an alternative (35). A variety of reagent strips are available to monitor adequately glucosuria in diabetic patients. Other clinical conditions associated with glucosuria include pregnancy, post gastric surgery, deranged tubular function (Fanconi syndrome, Wilson disease), and endocrinopathies associated with hyperglycemia, such as Cushing syndrome, thyrotoxicosis, and pheochromocytoma.

The reagent strip for urine glucose is detected by two sequential reactions:

$$Glucose + O_2 + H_2O \xrightarrow[oxidase]{peroxide} gluconic\ acid + H_2O_2$$

$$H_2O_2 + reduced\ chromogen \xrightarrow{peroxidase} oxidized\ chromogen + H_2O$$

Glucose oxidase requires oxygen and is specific for β-D-glucose. The peroxidase is less specific, and various substances, such as uric acid, ascorbic acid, bilirubin, and glutathione, may inhibit the reaction by competing with the chromogen for H_2O_2. Drug interferences with this reaction may be secondary to pigment distorting the color interpretation on the dipstick reaction pad, activation or inhibition of the enzymes within the reaction pad, or combinations of these factors. Urine dipsticks exposed to room air in open vials may generate erroneous results after 7 days of exposure (36). Negative glucose specimens became positive within 7 days of exposure of dipsticks to air.

The following test can be used to screen for galactosemia (galactose-1-phosphate uridyl transferase deficiency) in infants with galactosuria, because the latter would not be detected by the glucose oxidase/peroxidase reagent strip. A reducing substance has the ability to reduce cupric ions (Cu^{2+}) to cuprous ions (Cu^+) in the presence of heat and alkali. Benedict reagent is placed in a tablet. After the addition of urine to the tablet, blue alkaline cupric sulfate reagent is reduced to a red cuprous oxide precipitate. Heat is generated in the test tube during this reaction; therefore, the tube should be picked up by its top. Reducing substances include fructose, pentose, galactose, lactose, maltose, creatinine, uric acid, ascorbic acid, and homogentisic acid. Drugs may interfere with this reaction.

Protein

Normal urinary protein concentration varies from 2 to 8 mg per deciliter, with an upper limit of 150 mg of protein excreted per day. In children, however, this excretion rate varies with age, body surface area, and within individuals. More than 200 protein subunits can be visualized after staining high-resolution two-dimensional electrophoresis of human urinary proteins (37). Normal urinary proteins originate from plasma proteins (60%) or the kidney and the urogenital tract (40%). The glomerular basement membrane presents a charge-selective and size-selective barrier that prevents plasma proteins with a molecular weight greater than 70,000 Da from crossing into Bowman's capsule (38). Most of the filtered proteins are reabsorbed at the proximal tubule. For example, some albumin (molecular weight, 67,000 Da) is normally filtered through the glomerulus and taken up by the renal tubules. Proteinuria (>150 mg protein excreted daily) may be secondary to glomerular damage or decreased reabsorption by the renal tubules (37,38). Three proteins are derived from the kidney: Tamm-Horsfall mucoprotein (40% of total urinary protein), urokinase, and secretory immunoglobulin A (IgA). Tamm-Horsfall mucoprotein is very large and may polymerize into very large aggregates found in the matrix of urinary casts.

Proteinuria may be graded based on the excretion of protein per day: large (>3–4 g daily), moderate (1–3 or 4 g daily), and minimal (<1 g daily). In most diseases associated with significant proteinuria, the major component excreted is albumin. Immunoglobulins and kappa and lambda light chains are excreted in multiple myeloma, systemic amyloidosis, or Waldenström macroglobulinemia. The urine dipstick is impregnated with tetrabromophenol blue and citrate buffer. Protein, primarily albumin, binds to the dye, and a color change occurs based on the phenomenon of protein error of indicators. At a fixed pH, the indicator will have one color in the presence of protein and another in its absence. The citrate buffer maintains the pH at approximately 3.0, at which tetrabromophenol has a yellow color when no protein is present. It changes to yellow–green, green, and blue with increasing amounts of protein. This method may be used to screen for increased albumin excretion in a single voided sample or in serial urine specimens over a 24-hour period to estimate significant proteinuria (>300 mg of protein in 24 hours) in pregnancy (39). To confirm the presence of albumin or determine whether proteins other than albumin are present in urine, protein precipitation by sulfosalicylic acid or trichloroacetic acid may be performed. This reaction will precipitate albumin, glycoproteins, immunoglobulins, light chains (Bence-Jones proteins), and hemoglobin. The identity of monoclonal immunoglobulin and light-chain expression must be confirmed by protein electrophoresis and immunofixation. A variety of drugs or their metabolites and radiocontrast material may cause a urinary precipitate in the presence of sulfosalicylic acid, suggesting the presence of protein in the absence of a positive urine dipstick (ruling out albumin) or positive findings in other total protein assays.

Microalbuminuria

Microalbuminuria is defined as albumin excretion in the urine of 30 to 300 mg in 24 hours (40). It represents reversible glomerular damage and is the earliest stage of diabetic nephropathy. It is likely to progress to clinical albuminuria (≥300 mg in 24 hours) and decreasing filtration rate over years (40). At first, microalbuminuria is present only after exercise (41). Transient elevations in urinary albumin excretion may occur during short-term hyperglycemia, exercise, urinary tract infections, marked hypertension, heart failure, and acute febrile illness. Therapeutic interventions used to prevent progression of early diabetic nephropathy include aggressive treatment of hyperglycemia, antihypertensive therapy, and low-protein diet. This small amount of albumin in the urine cannot be detected by routine reagent strips for urinary protein, which use the protein error-of-indicators method. The American Diabetes Association recommends that screening for microalbuminuria be performed by one of three methods: (1) measurement of the ratio of albumin to creatinine in random spot urine; (2) in a 24-hour specimen along with creatinine clearance; (3) in a timed collection. At least four potential POCT methods are available for screening for microalbuminuria (40–45).

A low-cost nigrosin screening method (2 cents per test) detects total urinary proteins, including Bence-Jones proteins, and urinary albumin between 20 and 200 mg per liter by using the protein-binding dye nigrosin (42). Urine is first dried in spots on cellulose acetate strips before color development by nigrosin solution. Positive results should be evaluated further by a central laboratory method for urinary albumin and creatinine. The Micral-Test II (Roche, Indianapolis, IN) is a gold-labeled antibody, visually read dipstick method designed for semiquantitation of urinary microalbumin concentration (43,44). The gold-labeled antibody and urinary albumin form a complex that turns the detection pad red. A color comparison chart gives albumin values of negative, 20, 50, and 100 mg per liter. The sensitivity of this method varies from 63% to 96.7%, with the variation possibly related to differences in urine volume (43,44). Efforts to correct for this volume fluctuation using specific gravity determined by refractometry, however, improved the sensitivity from 63% to only 69% (44). The newer Micral-Test II strip may perform better than the original and retains its reaction color on the test pad for at least 60 minutes (43). This newer method has a positive interference with oxytetracycline and a negative interference when the temperature is below 10°C. The Clinitek Microalbumin method detects urinary albumin with the high-affinity dye bis(3′,3″-diiodo-4′,4″-dihydroxy-5′,5″-dinitrophenyl)-3,4,5,6-tetrabromosulfonephthalein and creatinine on a second pad. The results may be read visually using a color comparison chart (albumin 10, 30, 80, 150 mg/L; creatinine 300, 1,000, 2,000, 3,000 mg/L) or Clinitek 50 or Clinitek 100 Urine Chemistry Analyzer (Bayer Diagnostics, Tarrytown, NY, U.S.A.). Falsely increased albumin readings occur in the presence of more than 25 mg hemoglobin per liter, alkaline pH greater than 8.0, and in the presence of Tamm-Horsfall mucoprotein. Although creatinine values have not correlated well with quantitative methods, the albumin-to-creatinine ratios calculated from the dipstick compared favorably with the fully quantitative determinations. The DCA 2000 can determine quantitative albumin and creatinine in an undiluted specimen in 7 minutes (45). Because this method provides quantitative results, further evaluation will be required to determine whether these values compare well with more lengthy quantitative methods.

Screening semiquantitative methods for albuminuria should be followed up with quantitative measurements of the albumin-to-creatinine ratio in several first-voided morning urine specimens. Microalbuminuria is associated with coronary heart disease, major cardiovascular risk factors, hypertension, carotid artery stiffness, and elevated serum concentrations of Lp(a) lipoprotein.

Tumor Markers for Urinary Bladder Cancer

Traditionally, a combination of urinary cytology and cytoscopy has been used to detect transitional cell carcinoma of the urinary bladder (46,47). The U.S. Food and Drug Administration (FDA) cleared three noninvasive bladder tumor-marker tests for use only as an adjunct to cytoscopy: bladder tumor antigen (BTA) (Bard Diagnostic Sciences, Inc., Redmond, WA, U.S.A.); nuclear mitotic apparatus protein (NMP22) test (Matritech, Inc., Newton, MA, U.S.A.); and Mentor Accu-Dx assay (PerImmune, Inc., Rockville, MD, U.S.A.) (46). Two of these assays, BTA stat and Accu-Dx, may be used at the point-of-care. The BTA stat is a rapid, qualitative immunochromatographic method that uses monoclonal antibodies to detect complement factor H-related proteins (46,47). These antigens have a similar structure and function as human complement H and prevent cell lysis caused by normal immune surveillance. The assay uses five drops of fresh or frozen (−20°C) urine and requires 5 minutes for a red line (positive result) to develop. The sensitivity of Bard stat, NMP22, and cytology were 52%, 48%, and 17%, respectively, for grade 1 transitional cell carcinoma. These low-grade tumors do not release as many cells in urine, making it difficult for cytology to detect them. False-positive Bard stat results may occur in the presence of urinary tract inflammation, calculi, foreign bodies, ileal conduits/continent diversion, and other genitourinary cancers. The first Bard BTA assay was a latex agglutination assay that quantitatively detected basement membrane-associated proteins in urine (46,47). The amount of these basement membrane protein complexes correlates with tumor stage and grade. This assay required three to four drops of fresh urine added to special test tubes, where a color change occurred within 3 minutes. This assay is being replaced by the BTA stat and BTA Trak assays (46). Careful evaluation of the literature may be required to determine which of the three Bard assays is being evaluated.

The Accu-Dx recurrent bladder cancer test is a rapid, one-step, gold-dye particle, lateral-flow immunoassay for the qualitative detection of fibrinogen and fibrin/fibrinogen degradation products in urine, which are associated with bladder malignancy. Johnston and associates reported comparative results for Accu-Dx (81% sensitive, 75% specific), original BTA (28% sensitive, 87% specific), and urinary cytology (35% sensitive, 90% specific) (48). NMP22 is measured by an enzyme-linked immunoassay using a microplate strip-well format. A comparison of the BTA stat and NMP22 found the lowest sensitivity in the detection of grade 3 transitional cell carcinomas: BTA stat 63%, NMP22 50%. Further investigation is required to determine the financial impact of these two POCTs for bladder tumor on the management of patients with transitional cell carcinoma of the urinary bladder.

In the future, additional bedside assays for bladder tumor markers may be developed. Tumor-associated hyaluronic acid is elevated in all grades of transitional cell carcinoma, whereas tumor-associated hyaluronidase is elevated in grade 2 and 3 cancers (49). Genetic alterations occur in bladder cancer and may be adaptable to POCT using molecular pathologic techniques (46).

Screening for Drugs of Abuse

Quantification of drugs of abuse in urine is performed in the central laboratory by immunoassay or gas chromatography mass spectrometry (GC/MS) (50). Disposable devices are available for determining whether a specific threshold or cutoff concentration of drug is present in urine (Table 16.4) (11,50,51). Most of these devices generate a positive result for drug concentrations at or near the cutoff levels recommended by the U.S. National Institute of Drug Abuse and Substance Abuse and Mental Health Administration (52,53). These values are higher for opiates and amphetamines compared with European Union values (54). All positive results must be confirmed by an alternative method, such as GC/MS. Several immunoassay techniques are used in these commercially available point-of-care devices, including competitive binding microparticle capture immunoassay (Triage; Profile-II), homogeneous microparticle capture immunochemistry (Ontrak Testcup; Verdict), solid-phase competitive enzyme immunoassay (EZ-screen, ID block) and latex-agglutination-inhibition immunoassay (Abuscreen Ontrak) (11,50,51). These devices can be used in emergency departments or by probation officers as a qualitative screen. Care should be exercised, however, in the selection and interpretation of results from these on-site devices, as with values received from the central laboratory. For example, five of these on-site assays have antibodies to phencyclidine that cross-react with dextromethorphan, an antitussive found in many over-the-counter cold medications, such as Nyquil. Adulterants placed in urine specimens have been reported to alter quantitative GC/MS and immunoassays. A variety of these adulterants have been found to have little effect on on-site testing results, with the exception of THC-Free. Other factors that may modify results include temperature and length of specimen storage and the stability of the color formed after the test is performed. The presence of drugs or other toxic agents can be detected qualitatively by classic chemical reactions or spot tests (11). Interfering substances may generate a false-positive result, but this can be ruled out only by a quantitative confirmatory assay. Acetaminophen will generate a blue color in acidified urine after the addition of ammonium hydroxide, copper sulfate, and o-cresol. Trinder's reagent produces a purple color in the presence of salicylic acid, and phenothiazines produce a wide range of color after the addition of ferric, perchloric, and nitric reagent (11). The addition of dichromate to sulfuric, perchloric, and nitric acid creates Forrest's reagent, which will oxidize the tricyclic antidepressants (imipramine, desipramine, and trimipramine) to colored compounds. A Wood's light may be used to detect the fluorescein dye found in some varieties of antifreeze (55).

Pregnancy Tests

The qualitative detection of human chorionic gonadotrophin (hCG) in urine provides a positive reaction above a test-defined cutoff limit. For urine assays, this threshold limit can vary from 2 to 50 U per liter (56,57). This urinary assay for hCG is used clinically for the routine diagnosis of pregnancy, confirmation or exclusion of pregnancy, or detection of ectopic pregnancy (11,56,57). During normal pregnancy, the serum and urine hCG will double every 1.3 to 3.5 days (11,57). Serum hCG is approximately 50,000 U per liter at 7 weeks and peaks at 100,000 U per liter by the end of the first trimester. In fetal loss or ectopic pregnancies, the rate of hCG increase is reduced compared with a normal pregnancy (11,56,57). Therefore, qualitative assays of urinary hCG are useful in confirming pregnancy at approximately 10 days after fertilization and in monitoring the course of pregnancy.

Human chorionic gonadotropin is a noncovalent heterodimer composed of two subunits: α-subunit (92 amino acids) and β-subunit (145 amino acids). It is a glycoprotein, and 30% to 35% of its mass is carbohydrate. The α-subunit is iden-

TABLE 16.4. DEVICES FOR ON-SITE DRUGS OF ABUSE SCREENING IN URINE

Name	Manufacturer and Location
EZ-Screen	Editek, Inc. (Medtox Diagnostics, Burlington, NC)
Profile II	
Verdict	
Ontrak Testcup	Roche Diagnostics Systems (Branchburg, NJ)
Abuscreen Ontrak	
Triage	Biosite Diagnostics (San Diego, CA)
Bionite A/Q One Step Immunochemical Test	Bionite (San Francisco, CA)
EZ-Drug Screen	Biomerica (Newport Beach, CA)
Frontline	Boehringer Mannheim (Mannheim, Germany)
Rapid Drug Screen	Abbott Diagnostics (Abbott Park, IL)
Quick Screen Panel	Bio-Medical Products Corp. (Morris Plains, NJ)
First Check	Worldwide Medical Corp (Irvine, CA)
ID Block	International Diagnostic System Corp. (St Joseph, MI)
Target	V-Tech, Inc. (Pomona, CA)

tical to that found in lutropin, follitropin, and thyrotropin and is primarily responsible for inducing the signal transduction pathway following binding to the hCG receptor on the cell surface. The unique β-subunit structure confers binding specificity. The three-dimensional structure of hCG has been determined and is useful in determining potential monoclonal antibody binding sites for immunoassay development.

In urine and other biological fluids, hCG exists in a variety of forms other than the intact heterodimer (56,57). Free-α and β-subunits and the degradation product (β-core fragment) have been detected. The heterodimer may be modified by nicks in the β-subunit at positions 44 to 45 and/or 47 to 48. These nicks generate a molecule with less biological activity and reduced binding to some specific monoclonal antibodies. During normal pregnancy, the fraction of nicked hCG in urine is approximately threefold greater than intact hCG and the fraction of nicked hCG increases and then decreases during pregnancy. Therefore, prior to selection of a qualitative urinary hCG assay, the specificity of the monoclonal antibodies to hCG variant forms should be evaluated.

A variety of urinary qualitative hCG kits are available (11,56, 58). Most assays have very low cross-reactivity with lutropin, follitropin, and thyrotropin. In general, several drops of urine are placed in a sample well. The enzyme-linked immunosorbent assay uses two monoclonal antibodies. The first is an antihuman chorionic gonadotropin α-subunit monoclonal antibody predried on a porous membrane through which the urine travels by capillary action. The second antibody is specific for hCG β-subunit and may be dye-labeled or attached to an enzyme such as alkaline phosphatase (56,57). If hCG is present, a complex with the second antibody is formed. After washing, the addition of color developer completes the reaction. False-negative results as high as 50% have been reported when volunteers performed qualitative urinary hCG assays at home (58). Primary problems included difficulty in interpretation and in following instructions. Rigorous primary evaluation is required prior to release of a home test kit for urinary hCG. Some drugs may interfere with the assay, and extremes in specific gravity may interfere with test results (11). A modification in the Icon II HCG (Hybritech, San Diego, CA, U.S.A.) procedure retains the manufacturer's sensitivity of 20 U per liter for diluted urine (57). This modification replaced the five drops of urine (normal urine sample) with 20 drops (specific gravity <1.015) or 40 drops (specific gravity <1.005). The Icon II HCG detects intact and nicked hCG and not free α- and β-subunits or β-core fragments. Simple modifications to this assay have lowered the detection limit to 0.6 U per liter. This modified assay was used successfully in rural Bangladesh to detect fetal loss in early pregnancy. Therefore, commercially available qualitative urinary hCG assays may have the lower limit of detection decreased by modification of the manufacturer's protocol for on-site applications.

Miscellaneous Applications

Some inborn errors of metabolism may be screened for initially by using dipsticks or rapid biochemical separations or reactions (59–61). The sulfite dipstick (Sulfitstix Merckoquant, Merck, Darmstadt, Germany), designed for testing grape juice and wine, has been used for rapid semiquantitative detection of elevated urinary sulfite in patients with molybdenum cofactor deficiency. The enzyme activity of sulfite oxidase, aldehyde oxidase, and xanthine dehydrogenase require the molybdenum cofactor. A fresh urine specimen is needed to prevent the oxidation of sulfite to sulfate. False-positive and false-negative results have been reported. The increased excretion of glycosaminoglycans in the urine of patients with mucopolysaccharidosis may be evaluated initially with a quantitative assay (60). Cetyl pyridinium chloride in citrate buffer, pH 4.8, precipitates glycosaminoglycans in a random urine specimen; chondroitin sulfate standards and urine creatinine determination complete the steps required for a quantitative screen. Acute porphyria, including porphobilinogen synthase deficiency, acute intermittent porphyria, hereditary coproporphyria, and variegate porphyria present with abdominal pain and neuropsychiatric manifestations. In this clinical situation, porphobilinogen in a fresh urine specimen should be analyzed. The simple qualitative Watson-Schwartz test has many false-positive and false-negative results and is considered unreliable for detecting increased urinary porphobilinogen concentration (61). A commercial kit (Trace PBG Kit, Alpha Laboratories Ltd, Eastleigh, Hampshire, UK) requires pretreatment of urine with an anion-exchange resin to remove inferring substances prior to color development by Ehrlich's reagent (4-methylaminobenzaldehide in acid solution). This method performed very well at 25 to 50 µmol per liter porphobilinogen concentrations and with pigmented urine specimens. Screening methods for total urinary porphyrins are more time-consuming using column chromatography or spectrophotometry (62).

The rapid detection of parasitic disease in the field is important in developing nations. For example, a rapid card test has been developed for the detection of lymphatic filariasis in blood (63). Identification of ova of *Schistosoma haematobium* in urine is the most direct diagnosis of disease (64). Reagent dipstick screening for the presence of hematuria, proteinuria, and leukouria, or a semiquantitative reagent strip index has been used with limited success to detect urinary schistosomiasis or measure treatment effectiveness. The detection of soluble egg antigen in *S. haematobium* infections was developed as a specific monoclonal antibody-based dipstick. An enzyme-linked immunosorbent assay for soluble egg antigen correlated better with urinary egg counts than dipstick-detected hematuria.

Lutropin or luteinizing hormone is a glycoprotein composed of a unique β-subunit (114 amino acids) and an α-subunit (92 amino acids). Serum or urinary lutropin have been used to detect lutropin surge prior to ovulation, prior to ovulation initiation by hCG during ovarian hyperstimulation, and in planning for endometrial biopsies (65–67). Because lutropin secretion during the menstrual cycle is diurnal and pulsatile, and lutropin secretion is pulsatile, two or more urine determinations per day are recommended. On occasion, a laboratory-based assay rather than a point-of-care lutropin assay may be required to detect the lutropin surge secondary to cross-reactants or other interferences.

Gastric Fluid

The placement of a nasogastric tube is usually confirmed by radiographic demonstration of its location in the stomach (8).

Because the tube may be placed inadvertently in the lung or duodenum, evaluation of aspirated contents for color and pH may aid in evaluating the tube's location (8). Litmus paper with a range of 0 to 14 should be used for the pH determination. Gastric contents usually have a pH in the range of 0 to 4 (8) or greater than 5.0 if efforts are made to reduce the risk of stress ulcer syndrome (68). Intestinal tube placement usually results in a pH of 6.0, and tracheobronchial secretions have a pH of 6.0 or greater, including the presence of mucus.

Pulmonary aspiration in patients receiving nutrients through an enterally placed feeding tube puts the patient at risk for pneumonia. Symptoms of respiratory distress, tachypnea, cyanosis, or tachycardia in tube-fed patients suggest pulmonary aspiration. Two bedside tests are available to help evaluate this problem (8,69,70). In the first method, tracheobronchial secretions are caught in a transparent suction trap to determine whether aspiration of tube-fed formula has occurred. The addition of several drops of a dye (methylene blue or blue food coloring) into the enteral formula should discolor the trapped sputum blue. This method has an inferior sensitivity to the measurement of glucose by the urine dipstick glucose oxidase method in a blood-free sputum sample. This application of the urine glucose oxidase dipstick assay represents another illustration of its use in a manner in which the product was not originally designed (8,69). Therefore, potential matrix effects and other interferences should be evaluated carefully before using this method. If an enteral formula with high glucose concentration is used, a value of 20 mg per deciliter or more usually is obtained in the sputum if aspiration has occurred. Bouillata and colleagues reported that the glucose oxidase dipstick was greater than 20 mg per deciliter after 1:100 dilution only in the enteral feeding product with the highest glucose concentration (440 mg/dL) (69). Additional investigation is required to refine a sensitive and specific POCT method for identifying pulmonary aspiration in these patients.

The guaiac-based method used for detection of blood in feces is unsuitable for acidic gastric samples. Layne and colleagues demonstrated that two different guaiac slide tests for feces failed to turn positive after the addition of 4,000 μL per deciliter of blood to gastric fluid (70). Reactivity was improved if the gastric fluid was buffered by the addition of 0.1 N NaOH. Gastroccult (Smith Kline Diagnostics, Inc., Palo Alto, CA, U.S.A.) uses buffered guaiac designed for blood detection in gastric aspirates and vomitus and has good sensitivity for blood at low pH (68).

Feces

Fecal Leukocytes

The color and consistency of stool are important in initial point-of-care evaluation. Silver stools are associated with carcinoma involving the ampulla of Vater (71). Loose, watery stools observed in patients with diarrhea may be evaluated by bacterial culture, investigation for ova and parasites, and fecal leukocytes. The fecal leukocyte investigation is categorized as provider-performed microscopy (Table 16.1). A fleck of stool or mucus is placed on a glass slide and stained with Wright's or Löffler meth-

ylene blue (72). After placing a coverslip over the mixture, a rough quantitative count of mononuclear and polymorphonuclear cells is distinguished among 200 total cells. The presence of fecal leukocytes indicates the presence of an inflammatory condition caused by either a specific organism (*Salmonella, Shigella,* invasive *Escherichia coli, Yersinia,* or *Entamoeba histolytica*) or nonspecific etiology (ulcerative colitis or antibiotic-associated colitis) (72).

Fecal Occult Blood

Colorectal cancer is the second leading cause of cancer death in the United States, and it affects both men and women (73). It is currently recommended that average-risk patients without a family history of colon cancer should have annual fecal occult blood testing beginning at age 50 years of age (73). Positive results should be followed up with colonoscopy or barium enema plus flexible sigmoidoscopy. Screening with flexible sigmoidoscopy should be done every 5 years and colonoscopy should be done if a 1-cm polyp is found. Several methods are available for fecal occult blood detection in stool specimens: qualitative, guaiac-based (Hemoccult II, Hemoccult SENSA, SmithKline Diagnostics, Palo Alto, CA, U.S.A.; or Coloscreen-VPI, Helena Laboratories, Beaumont, TX, U.S.A.); quantitative (porphyrin fluorescence, HemoQuant, SmithKline Bioscience Laboratories, Palo Alto, CA, U.S.A.); and antibody to intact hemoglobin or globulin (HemeSelect, SmithKline Diagnostics; OC-Hemodia, Eiken Chemical Co., Ltd, Tokyo, Japan) (73–75).

Qualitative assays are rapid estimates of fecal blood loss and can be interpreted by the individual performing the test. Therefore, they are categorized by CLIA '88 as waived tests and are widely used in hospital POCT programs and for screening. Black, tarry stools or melena are suggestive of gastrointestinal bleeding. Small losses of blood, however, may be visually undetectable but positive after fecal occult blood testing. Guaiac is the most widely used chemical reagent. It contains a phenolic compound that is oxidized to a colored quinone in the presence of hydrogen peroxide and the peroxidase-like activity of heme. Heme-derived porphyrin, a heme degradation product, does not react with guaiac-based assays. Therefore, degraded hemoglobin from the upper gastrointestinal tract does not react, and many investigators report the test to be much less sensitive for detection of this problem. Rockey and colleagues, however, reported more upper gastrointestinal lesions than colonic lesions in patients with a positive guaiac-based test and endoscopic follow-up to identify the lesion (76). Therefore, an improved colon-specific cancer screening procedure may be needed.

Today, however, during screening for colorectal cancer, it should be remembered that not all carcinomas or polyps bleed; blood is not uniformly distributed in stool, and the quantity of bleeding varies with the anatomic location. False-positive guaiac reaction may occur after exposure to iodine-containing antiseptic or after consumption of a diet containing high concentrations of hemoglobin or peroxidase (74). Three days before a guaiac-based test, the patient should avoid eating red meat and high-peroxidase foods such as cauliflower, turnip, broccoli, parsnip, radish, horseradish, cucumber, green beans, mushrooms, melon, zucchini, artichoke, and others (73,75). Plant peroxidases are found in raw fruits and vegetables. The Hemoccult developer contains ethanol, which will denature this peroxidase and reduce its interference with the test. Nonhydrated Hemoccult and Hemoccult Sensa were not affected by peroxidase-rich plant foods if the test cards were stored at room temperature for at least 48 hours before developer was added (75). This delay allows reduction of the fecal water content and concentration of fecal peroxidase, which will be denatured by the added ethanol in the developer. The delay did not, however, resolve the dietary interference with rehydrated Hemoccult, and, therefore, dietary restriction of plant peroxidase for 72 hours prior to testing would still be required for this method. The rehydrated Hemoccult assay has improved sensitivity but decreased specificity compared with the Hemoccult Sensa or nonhydrated Hemoccult. The nonhydrated Hemoccult II test is the most cost-effective fecal occult blood screening test compared with HemeSelect and Hemoccult Sensa. The Coloscreen-VPI contains an inhibitor to vegetable peroxidase; however, published data are limited. False-negative reactions occur after excessive fecal drying on the slide or in the presence of large doses of reducing substance such as vitamin C.

Quantitative assays must be sent to a commercial laboratory for testing. In the HemoQuant assay, iron is removed from the heme of hemoglobin, and the fluorescence of all derived porphyrins (normal, 0.11–2.0 mg/g feces on meat-free diet) is measured. The heme in meat is a positive interference for this assay, whereas fish, domestic fowl, and high-peroxidase fruits and vegetables contain little heme and do not interfere. HemeSelect is an immunologic test using antibodies that bind to intact hemoglobin or globin, not to heme, heme-derived porphyrin, or breakdown products of globin. OC-Hemodia uses a human hemoglobin antibody and latex agglutination as endpoints for a positive reaction.

Breast Milk

In general, the yield of breast milk corresponds to the needs of the infant, amounting to about 850 mL per day for a body mass of 5 to 6 kg. Breast milk contains a variety of nutrients, vitamins, and hormones required for the infant's nutrition. It also may contain a variety of drugs of abuse (amphetamine, delta-9-tetrahydrocannabinol, methadone, alcohol), stimulants (caffeine, nicotine), and therapeutic agents (hydroxyurea, theophylline). No on-site testing applications for drugs in breast milk are currently available. At the point-of-care, odor and color may be evaluated. Certain foods, especially garlic, when ingested by the mother may impart an odor to breast milk for about 1 to 2 hours after ingestion (77). Mature breast milk is blue–white, whereas colostrum is yellow to yellow–orange. The color of breast milk can be altered by dietary pigments, medications, or herbal folk remedies. Red and yellow dyes in soda, fruit drinks, or gelatin may result in pink–orange milk. Green milk is associated with the ingestion of Gatorade (green variety), kelp, and other seaweed products. The antibiotic minocycline hydrochloride has been reported to create black milk. Breast milk discoloration usually disappears after the dietary intake stops.

Amniotic Fluid

Volume

The fluid-filled amniotic cavity surrounds the fetus throughout intrauterine life. Human amniotic fluid volume and composition vary during gestation. The volume steadily increases until 30 to 34 weeks and then decreases throughout the remainder of pregnancy (78). Amniotic fluid volume is maintained by fetal fluid production (urine and pulmonary fluid) and amniotic fluid removal (fetal swallowing and gastrointestinal reabsorption) (78). Maternal oral hydration will increase the amniotic fluid volume in women with decreased amniotic fluid levels. Excessive amniotic fluid volume, or *polyhydramnios*, may be caused by congenital problems associated with reduced or no fetal swallowing or increased fetal urine output. *Oligohydramnios*, or reduced amniotic fluid volume, is associated with fetal urinary tract obstruction or malformation (bilateral renal agenesis). The incidence of fetal distress and low Apgar scores was increased in patients with oligohydramnios compared with normal pregnant controls. Amniotic fluid volume can be determined by two ultrasonographic methods (i.e., amniotic fluid index and two-diameter amniotic fluid pocket) or by a dye-dilution technique that involves installation of aminohippurate into the amniotic cavity. At 16 to 18 weeks of gestation, only 5% of total protein in amniotic fluid may be from the fetus or decidua; the remainder is from maternal serum.

Visual Examination

Amniotic fluid can be obtained by transabdominal amniocentesis between weeks 15 and 18 of pregnancy or as early as week 12 to 14 for genetic prenatal diagnosis (78). The procedure can be performed from 20 to 28 weeks' gestation to evaluate Rh-sensitized pregnancies or from 34 to 42 weeks to evaluate fetal lung maturity or suspected chorioamnionitis. Lo and colleagues evaluated maternal plasma samples and found that 80% contained fetal DNA and 17% had fetal cells in the maternal circulation (79). Fetal leukocytes and trophoblasts also have been recovered from maternal blood. These sources of DNA may reduce the need for amniocentesis or chorionic villus biopsies to obtain specimens for genetic prenatal diagnosis in the future.

If blood is detected in the amniotic fluid, the source of the blood (fetal vs. maternal) must be determined. Fetal hemorrhage may be associated with abdominal trauma and suspected placental injury or Rh incompatibility between the fetus and mother (78). Several laboratory procedures are available to determine the presence of fetal blood cells (78,80). During the Kleihauer-Betke staining method, acid elutes adult hemoglobin from maternal red cells, creating "ghosts," but it does not affect fetal hemoglobin in fetal red cells. Complications in technique, staining intensity, and interpretation make this a tedious procedure. A flow cytometric method using a murine monoclonal antibody directed against fetal hemoglobin has been used to determine the degree of fetomaternal hemorrhage (80). The coefficient of variation for the Kleihauer-Betke method was approximately 50%, compared with approximately 5% for the flow cytometric method. There is a need for a rapid point-of-care semiquantitative method to detect the presence of fetal red cells in amniotic fluid.

Green-stained amniotic fluid indicates the presence of meconium. The etiology of meconium stained amniotic fluid is unclear; however, it primarily represents secretions of the fetal intestinal glands, which may increase during fetal hypoxia and acidosis (78). On gross examination, the amount of meconium has been classified as thin (light), moderate, or thick (heavy or pea soup). A method similar to hematocrit has been reported for assessing the amount of meconium ("meconium-crit") (81). The frequency of meconium-stained amniotic fluid ranges from 5.6% to 24.6%, and about 25% of these infants will have a decreased 1-minute Apgar score. *Meconium aspiration syndrome* is defined as respiratory distress in an infant whose birth was associated with meconium-stained amniotic fluid. The incidence of this syndrome varies from 1.7% to 35.8% in these infants. Meconium in amniotic fluid is associated with vasoconstriction, which may lead to fetal brain dysfunction.

Fetal Lung Maturity

All infants at birth, regardless of gestational age, have surface-active compounds in their lungs. If the ability to synthesize these compounds in the lung is inadequate, the infant will have respiratory distress syndrome, and respiratory failure may develop unless prompt and adequate therapy is instituted (82). The economic impact is greatest for infants with the lowest birth weight compared with higher birth weight (82). For example, hospitalization per uncomplicated surviving infant with respiratory distress syndrome is $101,817 for infants who weigh 500 to 1,000 g compared with $27,224 for infants who weight greater than 1,500 g. The pathophysiology is a progressive atelectasis, with progressive consolidation of the lung, pulmonary edema, dilated bronchioles, and, eventually the appearance of hyaline-stained membranes representing detritus (necrotic alveolar duct epithelium, serum proteins, red blood cells, and fibrin).

In type II pneumocytes in the developing fetal lung, phosphatidylcholine (lecithin) begins to be secreted into amniotic fluid at about 24 to 26 weeks' gestation. The process proceeds slowly. Even at 30 to 32 weeks' gestation, the concentration of phosphatidylcholine is relatively low, equal to, or less than sphingomyelin. The phosphatidylinositol concentration also is low at this time. Phosphatidylglycerol is absent. At about 32 to 33 weeks, phosphatidylcholine and sphingomyelin concentrations are about equal. Subsequently, the phosphatidylcholine concentration rises, and, paralleling this, the concentration of phosphatidylinositol, with an abrupt rise in both at 35 weeks. This event is rapidly followed by a decrease in phosphatidylinositol and then the appearance of phosphatidylglycerol from about 36 weeks. The phosphatidylcholine concentration increases steadily until term, whereas sphingomyelin concentrations level off at 32 weeks and begin to decrease thereafter (78).

Biochemical maturity of the fetal lung occurs over a 2- to 3-week period, with a sudden jump in the lecithin/sphingomyelin ratio to 2.0 or more, a concomitant decrease in phosphatidylinositol, and a gradual increase in phosphatidylglycerol. The measurement of lung maturity should indicate that the infant is not going to develop respiratory distress syndrome. This description of biochemical maturity of the fetal lung is based on data originally presented in 1979 using a two-dimensional thin-layer chromatographic method. The data were collected at a time when antenatal intervention to improve fetal lung maturity was uncommon. Today, a variety of laboratory methods are available to evaluate fetal lung maturity (Table 16.5) (83–86). Many of these methods are not readily adaptable to an on-site application because of the need for equipment (cell counter, lamellar body number; fluorescence spectrophotometer, fluorescence polarization) or the requirement for 4 hours or longer to complete numerous procedural steps (one- or two-dimensional thin-layer chromatography, enzymic assays). The simplest rapid evaluation for fetal lung maturity requires a test tube and newsprint (83). Pulmonary maturity is associated with amniotic fluid, which is so turbid that newsprint cannot be read through a test tube in which it is placed. Lamellar bodies, composed of symmetric layers of phospholipids, proteins, and sebaceous and epithelial debris, cause this turbidity (83,86). The light scattering associated with this turbid solution may be quantitated using a spectrophotometer and reading the absorbance at 650 nm. False-positive results may be caused by interfering chromogens, such as meconium, hemoglobin, methemoglobin, and methemalbumin. The shake test or the discontinued commercial product (Lumadex Foam Stability Index; FSI, Beckman Diagnostics, Brea, CA, U.S.A.) evaluate the stability of foam or bubbles formed at the liquid surface of a shaken mixture of ethanol and amniotic fluid. The commercial product's procedure involved the addition of 0.5 mL amniotic fluid to tubes with 95% ethanol so that the final volume fraction of ethanol/amniotic fluid varied from 0.44 to 0.50. False-positive results for the shake test can occur in the presence of blood and meconium. Other potential interfering substances include vaginal secretions, obstetric creams, silicone oils in Vacutainer tubes, and mineral oils used to lubricate plastic syringes.

TABLE 16.5. METHODS FOR EVALUATING FETAL LUNG MATURITY IN AMNIOTIC FLUID

Method	Analyte	Point-of-Care Testing
Turbidity	Total phospholipids	Yes
Foam stability	Total phospholipids	Yes
Absorbance at 650 nm	Total phospholipids	Maybe
Immunologic techniques	Specific phospholipid	Maybe
Thin layer chromatography	Individual phospholipids	No
Enzymic assays	Individual phospholipids	No
Fluorescence polarization	Total phospholipids	No
Lamellar body number	Total phospholipids	No
Near-infrared spectroscopy	Lecithin/sphingomyelin ratio	No

A semiquantitative latex agglutination assay using an antibody specific for phosphatidylglycerol is also available (Amniostat-FLM, Irvine Scientific, Irvine, CA, U.S.A.) (78,84–86). The original kit had a threshold for positivity or a cutoff level set at 2 μg of phosphatidylglycerol per milliliter (0.65 μmol/L) (84). It had poor sensitivity, recording a positive result at ≥25 μmol per liter or more phosphatidylglycerol (84). A modified version of this slide agglutination assay was positive at 6 μmol per liter phosphatidylglycerol, with a sensitivity of 85.3%, a specificity of 83.3%, prediction of fetal lung maturity of 96.7%, and prediction of fetal lung immaturity of 50.0% (85). Blood, meconium, and vaginal secretions do not contain phosphatidylglycerol and therefore do not interfere with this assay. A vaginal pool specimen from a patient with premature rupture of membranes or amniocentesis specimen will provide reliable results. Certain bacteria, however, can synthesize phosphatidylglycerol, which will cause false-positives (78).

A recent practice parameter for the assessment of fetal lung maturity recommends using fluorescence polarization or lamellar body number as the first assay (86). If the result is mature, no further evaluation is required. If the result is immature, the assay not performed initially may be used, and a third assay (immunologic detection of phosphatidylglycerol) may be required to determine fetal lung maturity. Qualitative assays for fetal lung maturity at the bedside (foam stability, turbidity, absorbance at 650 nm) function as screening procedures, which require confirmation by a semiquantitative or quantitative method.

Preterm Labor

Preterm labor may present clinically with spontaneous premature labor, premature rupture of the fetal membranes, or delivery of the premature infant to benefit the mother or infant. Preterm birth occurs in approximately 11% of all pregnancies. Premature rupture of the membranes before the onset of labor is defined as premature rupture of fetal membranes or preterm premature rupture of the membranes if the event occurs before 37 weeks' gestation. If not treated, most women with preterm premature rupture of the membrane will have spontaneous labor and deliver within a week. The risk of preterm delivery can be assessed in symptomatic and asymptomatic women using an enzyme-linked immunosorbent assay (approximately 2 hours) or a rapid, single-use, dry-chemistry test (20 minutes) for fetal fibronectin (Adeza Biomedical Corp, Sunnyvale, CA, U.S.A.) (87). Fetal fibronectin is an isoform of fibronectin found at the uteroplacental junction and in the extracellular matrix of fetal membranes. In the second and third trimesters, the presence of fetal fibronectin in cervicovaginal secretions may indicate extracellular matrix degradation at the interface of the chorionic and decidual layers and impending preterm labor. For the rapid test, a swab of cervicovaginal secretions are reacted for 20 minutes in a membrane device and analyzed in a reader (Adeza TLi System). Values greater than 50 ng per milliliter were considered positive. The rapid test compares well with the longer enzyme immunosorbent assay. Both assays for fetal fibronectin should not be used in the presence of cervical dilation greater than 3 cm, premature rupture of the fetal membranes, cervical cerclage, and placenta previa. Additional evaluation is required to determine the applicability of the rapid fetal fibronectin test for POCT.

Following premature rupture of the fetal membranes, the detection of amniotic fluid may be required. The protein and glucose pads on a urine dipstick can be used to distinguish rapidly amniotic fluid from maternal urine (78). Amniotic fluid will give a positive reaction for both analytes, whereas urine will be negative unless there is maternal diabetes mellitus. Protein and pH also can be evaluated with a urine dipstick. Amniotic fluid is neutral or alkaline, whereas urine is usually acidic. The evaluation of amniotic fluid pH and amniotic fluid crystallization (ferning) has been used to detect amniotic fluid after premature rupture of the fetal membranes (11). Litmus paper, bromthymol blue, and Nitrazine paper (phenaphthazine, Bristol Meyers Squibb, Princeton, NJ, U.S.A.) have been used for pH determination. Nitrazine paper is still used and has a narrow pH range for color change from 6.4 to 6.8. Alkaline amniotic fluid will generate a blue color with sensitivity and specificity greater than 95%. False-positive results may occur in the presence of blood, soaps, or infection. The microscopic detection of amniotic fluid crystallization or the fern test is classified as provider-performed microscopy (Table 16.1). Amniotic fluid after 20 weeks' gestation will crystallize on drying. Estrogen promotes this phenomenon, whereas progesterone inhibits it. Slide arborization occurs in other tissues such as serum, cerebrospinal fluid, and saliva (11,88). The fern test has a similar sensitivity for detecting amniotic fluid in vaginal secretions but is more specific than Nitrazine paper (89). Blood at a dilution of less than 1:1 and meconium do not interfere with the fern test.

Saliva

The salivary glands located in the oral cavity and adjacent areas generate saliva. The appearance varies, depending on the source of production, from a thin liquid (parotid saliva) to thick, tenacious, and ropy mucus (oral mucus). Saliva may be collected following stimulation or no stimulation (resting). A variety of collection techniques have been published. The daily output of saliva is approximately 500 to 1,500 mL, and its chemical composition is influenced by time of collection, age, sex, hormonal status, and oral contraceptive use. Saliva flow may be reduced (*xerostomia*) or increased (*sialorrhea*) in specific pathologic conditions. A variety of analytes can be measured in saliva, and their salivary concentration compares well with that in blood. Analytes measured in saliva include drugs of abuse, steroid hormones, salivary antibodies, infectious agents, and slide arborization. At least two salivary alcohol methods (ON-SITE, Roche Diagnostics, Branchburg, NY, U.S.A.; QED, STC Diagnostics, Bethlehem, PA, U.S.A.) may be used at the point-of-care. Oral mucosal transudate has been used to measure human immunodeficiency virus type 1 (HIV-1) antibody and confirmatory Western blot. The use of a microscopic slide fern test using saliva to determine ovulation in fertile women was found to be unreliable (88). Additional on-site assays using saliva are needed.

Cerebrospinal Fluid

Cerebrospinal fluid (CSF) (70%) is formed from plasma by the filtering and secretory activity of the choroid plexus located in the ventricles. The remaining 30% is formed by nonchoroid sources, such as brain cells, ependyma, and capillary epithelial cells. Domenico Cotugno (1736–1822) was the first to provide a complete description of CSF, including the continuity of the cerebral and spinal fluids. The fluid produced by the choroid plexus moves by bulk flow through the ventricular system of the brain and the subarachnoid space to the arachnoid villi, where most of the reabsorption takes place. Reabsorption also occurs via the cervical lymphatic system.

Cerebrospinal Fluid Pressure

In 1891, Henrich Quinke (1842–1922) perfected the lumbar puncture technique and performed cell counts and total protein measurement and identified bacteria. In one algorithm, a normal open pressure, cell count, and total protein indicate that no further tests are required except in possible childhood meningitis, multiple sclerosis, and immunosuppressed patients (90). Opening CSF pressure may be determined at the bedside with a 2-mm diameter manometer and is usually 60 to 170 mm H_2O. A normal variation of 5 to 10 mm H_2O occurs during the respiratory cycle. Larger increases are seen with nose blowing or breath holding, whereas fluid pressure is decreased during sniffing. Mass lesions in the brain and many other disorders are associated with an increased CSF pressure. A lumbar puncture procedure during the first week of life had a significantly lower yield of diagnostic material compared with procedures performed on patients after 1 week of age. An *in vitro* investigation of various spinal needles demonstrated less CSF leakage with pencil-point needles or the 26-gauge Atraucan needle (B. Braun AG, Melsungen, Germany). Further work is needed to determine whether the use of these spinal needles is associated with fewer postspinal headaches. Local anesthetic solution may be used to enlarge the epidural space in preparation for the insertion of an indwelling catheter. During this procedure, a small volume of fluid may be aspirated. The aspirated material may be anesthetic solution or cerebrospinal fluid. In two studies, four on-site tests (temperature, urine dipstick glucose, urine dipstick pH, and thiopentone-induced turbidity) were evaluated to distinguish bupivacaine (0.25%) or saline from cerebrospinal fluid (91). In both studies, the glucose and pH were the most sensitive (83%–97%), whereas temperature and the thiopentone test were unreliable with a sensitivity of 25% to 84%.

Visual Examination

Normal CSF is clear and colorless like water. Bright red blood in the specimen may be the result of recent intracerebral or subarachnoid hemorrhage or damage to blood vessels during a procedure (traumatic tap) (92,93). A traumatic tap may be distinguished from a subarachnoid hemorrhage by a decrease in cell number from the first tube of cerebrospinal fluid collected compared with the last tube. In subarachnoid hemorrhage, the color intensity and cell count should be similar in the first and last tubes. Also, blood from a traumatic tap may clot and, after centrifugation, the supernatant will be clear and colorless. Subsequent color changes occur as blood and hemoglobin break down: oxyhemoglobin (pink to pink–orange), bilirubin (yellow) or (rarely) methemoglobin (yellow) (93). *Xanthochromia*, or yellow discoloration, also may be seen with CSF in the presence of

total protein greater than 100 mg per deciliter, merthiolate contamination, melanin (meningeal melanosarcoma), or carotene. In the presence of a normal radiographic computerized tomography study of the head and clinical headache, some researchers recommend performing a spectrophotometric scan from 400 to 600 nm to rule out the presence of visually undetectable bilirubin/methemoglobin in subarachnoid hemorrhage (93). Red cells and their components (especially hemoglobin) are cytotoxic to cerebral endothelial cells. Turbid CSF may result from high protein concentration, increased red cells, increased white cells, or numerous microorganisms.

Cerebrospinal Fluid Leakage

Following head trauma, skull-base tumor operations, or rupture of a cerebrospinal fluid fistula, clear fluid may drain from the ear (*otorrhea*) or nose (*rhinorrhea*). The differential diagnosis of CSF from other body fluid does not include qualitative (urine dipstick) or quantitative glucose determination. In the laboratory, electrophoresis with immunofixation for transferrin is the method of choice (94). CSF has two isoforms of transferrin, whereas serum, nasal secretions, saliva, tears, perilymph, endolymph, and other body fluids have only isoform. CSF leakage also can be detected by laborious radiographic isotopic techniques or computed tomographic cisternography. A rapid on-site method is needed for distinguishing cerebrospinal fluid from other body fluids in the emergency center in patients with head trauma and possible fractured skull.

Serous Fluids

Fluids that accumulate in the pleural, pericardial, or peritoneal cavities are called *serous effusions* and are divided into *transudates* or *exudates* (95). Transudates are not caused by direct disease involvement of the mesothelial surface but are produced by imbalances in hydrostatic or oncotic pressures. They are characterized by low protein, low lactate dehydrogenase, low specific gravity, and relatively few cells. Exudates suggest a much wider range of diagnoses and indicate the presence of disease involving the lining of the cavity, such as infection, infarction, or malignancy.

Pleural Fluid

Pleural fluid (3–5 mL) is present to lubricate the pleural surfaces during respiration. After strenuous exercise or normal labor, there may be an increase in pleural fluid volume. Pleural fluid forms on the surface of the parietal pleura at a rate of 100 mL per hour. Lymph vessels remove most of the protein and red cells (20 mL pleural fluid hourly) and capillaries in the visceral pleura absorb most of the fluid (300 mL pleural fluid hourly).

Light and colleagues published the criteria for distinguishing a pleural exudate from a transudate (95).

An exudate must meet one of the following three criteria: (1) pleural fluid protein divided by serum protein is greater than 0.5; (2) pleural fluid lactate dehydrogenase divided by serum lactate dehydrogenase is greater than 0.6; (3) pleural fluid lactate dehydrogenase is greater than 200 IU or more than two-thirds the upper limit of normal for serum lactate dehydrogenase (96). Transudates meet none of these three criteria. Other clues include visual appearance. An exudate will be cloudy to turbid, purulent, or bloody, whereas a transudate is clear or pale yellow. Chylothorax has a milky white or yellow bloody effusion. Some investigators extended Light's original criteria of an exudate to include pleural fluid cholesterol greater than 55 mg per deciliter and pleural fluid cholesterol divided by serum cholesterol greater than 0.3. Costa and colleagues reported a sensitivity of 99% and a specificity of 98% using only two criteria for an exudate: pleural fluid cholesterol greater than 45 mg per deciliter and pleural fluid lactate dehydrogenase greater than 200 IU per liter (97). Many biochemical investigations may be undertaken using a pleural fluid specimen, but once the presence of a transudate has been established, there is little benefit to proceeding with additional laboratory studies (96). Table 16.6 lists some clinical conditions associated with pleural exudates and transudates (95).

Pleural fluid is obtained by thoracentesis, usually performed with the patient in the upright position (98). If the patient has been supine and the thoracentesis is performed immediately after the patient sits up, pleural fluid pH, protein lactate dehydrogenase, and red cell count will be significantly lower than if the patient remains upright for at least 30 minutes before the procedure.

Pleural fluid pH measurements have received increased attention recently. Although the pH values do not indicate a specific disease, they narrow the differential diagnosis (99). Normal pleural fluid is 7.6. A pleural pH less than 7.30 is associated with six different disease processes: empyema, malignancy, collagen vascular disease, tuberculosis, esophageal rupture, and hemothorax. A patient with bacterial pneumonia and associated parapneumonic effusion may need tube thoracostomy if the pleural fluid pH is below 7.0 and pleural fluid glucose is below 40 mg per deciliter. A pleural fluid pH less than 7.3 in a patient with a malignant effusion is a poor prognostic indicator. The use of a paper pH indicator strip or a pH meter is not as reliable as a pH determined by a blood gas machine using pleural fluid collected in a heparinized syringe without air bubbles (99). Non-heparinized syringes may be adequate if the analysis is per-

formed within 30 minutes of collection. The blood gas machine was not designed to analyze body fluids, and care must be taken in evaluating the specimen for clumps or clots before injecting the specimen into the machine. Thick, purulent pleural fluid specimens do not need to be analyzed. On-site biochemical evaluation for pleural, pericardial, and peritoneal fluid is currently unavailable. Physical examination and visual examination of the pleural fluid may be performed at the point of care.

Pericardial Fluid

Pericardial fluid is primarily a plasma ultrafiltrate consisting of 15 to 35 mL. Pericardial fluid can be collected by pericardiocentesis or by surgical pericardiotomy. Evaluation of this fluid should begin with differentiation of exudate vs. transudate using four criteria for an exudate: pericardial fluid total protein, greater than 3.0 g per deciliter; pericardial fluid total protein divided by serum protein, greater than 0.5; pericardial fluid lactate dehydrogenase divided by serum lactate dehydrogenase, greater than 0.6; pericardial fluid lactate dehydrogenase less than 300 U per deciliter (100). Bacterial culture and cytology are the only two tests that may add specificity to the differential diagnosis.

Peritoneal Fluid

Free fluid in the abdominal cavity is ascitic fluid or peritoneal fluid. Fluid aspiration by paracentesis or peritoneal lavage may be used to collect this fluid for laboratory evaluation. This fluid also can be visualized by ultrasound or computed tomography. The pathophysiologic etiology of ascitic fluid includes elevated hydrostatic pressure, decreased osmotic pressure, fluid production exceeding resorptive capacity, and urinary bladder rupture. A single calculation (ascitic fluid bilirubin divided by serum bilirubin >0.6) defines an exudate with a sensitivity of 72% and a specificity of 86%. Combination of these criteria with others did not improve the sensitivity or specificity (100). Nephrogenic ascites associated with end-stage renal disease usually has an ascitic fluid total protein greater than 25 g per liter (101). Ascitic fluid creatinine divided by serum creatinine greater than 1.0 is diagnostic of intraperitoneal urinary leak. Transudates are clear and colorless. Cirrhotic ascites is clear and pale yellow, whereas in abdominal trauma, it is bloody and chylous. Pseudochylous ascites is milky.

Seminal Fluid

Seminal fluid, or semen, consists of products from various male reproductive organs: seminal vesicles (60% by volume); prostate (20%); epididymis, vas deferens, bulbourethral glands and urethral glands (10%–15%) (102). Spermatozoa are maintained in seminal fluid. Semen analysis is performed for a variety of reasons that dictate the complexity of the analysis required including infertile couple evaluation, detecting sexual assault, vasectomy effectiveness, and suitability for use in artificial insemination procedures.

Semen should be collected by masturbation after a minimum of 48 hours, but not longer than 7 days, of sexual abstinence. The viscous yellow–gray semen forms a coagulum in which the

TABLE 16.6. SOME CAUSES OF PLEURAL TRANSUDATES AND EXUDATES

Transudates	Exudates
Congestive heart failure	Parapneumonic effusion
Cirrhosis with ascites	Pulmonary infarction
Nephrotic syndrome	Malignancy (direct pleural
Hypoalbuminemia	involvement; late
Peritoneal dialysis	mediastinal involvement)
Acute atelectasis	Viral fungal, parasitic diseases
Superior vena cava obstruction	Tuberculosis
Subclavian catheter misplacement	Connective tissue disease
Early mediastinal malignancy	Gastrointestinal disease
	Uremic pleurisy
	Chronic atelectasis
	Chylothorax
	Drug reaction (nitrofurantoin,
	methylsergide)

sperm are trapped. Liquefaction begins within 10 to 20 minutes and is complete within 1 hour (102). Laboratory evaluation should be performed within 1.5 to 2 hours after collection. Post-vasectomy patients should provide several semen specimens to ensure that no viable or nonviable sperm are present. Qualitative semen analysis (limited to the presence or absence of sperm and detection of motility) is classified as provider-performed microscopy (Table 16.1). A wet-mount preparation on a glass slide with a coverslip is adequate. In the emergency center, a saline wet mount of a swab of a specimen obtained from a sexual assault victim may be used for a point-of-care search for motile or nonmotile sperm under a microscope.

Semen analysis for evaluation of the infertile couple and adequacy for artificial insemination procedures requires additional procedures, including viscosity, volume, pH, sperm concentration or count, sperm mobility, sperm morphology, and viability studies (102). Reproductive laboratories that perform assisted reproductive technology are accredited on a voluntary basis by the Reproductive Laboratory Accreditation Program, started in 1992 as a joint venture of the College of American Pathologists and the American Society for Reproductive Medicine. Approximately 36% of these laboratories have been accredited.

Synovial Fluid

Synovial fluid is an ultrafiltrate of plasma that provides nutrients for the articular cartilage. The total protein and immunoglobulin concentration is lower than that of plasma. A high-molecular-weight mucopolysaccharide, hyaluronate or hyaluronic acid, creates the high viscosity of synovial fluid. Type B cells in the synovial lining are abundant in endoplasmic reticulum and produce hyaluronic acid and lamellar bodies composed of proteolipids and phospholipids for joint lubrication. Synovial fluid is collected by sterile needle aspiration from the affected joint; this procedure is called *arthrocentesis*. Treatment of synovial fluid with hyaluronidase will degrade hyaluronic acid and reduce the viscosity of the fluid, facilitating cytocentrifuge preparations and biochemical analysis.

Arthritides are classified into five major groups: noninflammatory, inflammatory, infectious, crystal-induced, and hemorrhagic (104). Normal synovial fluid is clear, viscous, and colorless or pale yellow. Bright-red color suggests a hemorrhagic process. Turbid, opalescent fluid is observed in crystal-induced arthritides, such as gout (monosodium urate crystals) and pseudogout (calcium pyrophosphate dihydrate crystals). In acute attacks of gout, the synovial fluid may appear chalky and milky white and is referred to as *urate milk*. Turbidity is associated with noninflammatory and inflammatory arthritides. The measurement of synovial fluid hyaluronic acid concentration or viscosity may be used to distinguish these two groups of joint disease. Although total white blood cell count and the number of polymorphonuclear leukocytes are higher in synovial fluid from inflammatory joint diseases, there is an overlap with non-inflammatory joint diseases. Clayburne and colleagues reported that finding none to two white blood cells per high-power field in ten different fields on a wet-drop preparation of synovial fluid will predict fewer than 1,000 white cells per millimeter of white cells counted by hemocytometer (3,105). This screen provides a

rapid on-site method for placing the joint disease in the inflammatory or noninflammatory category.

The stability of formed elements in synovial fluid specimens was studied by Kerolus et al., who examined specimens at different times following collection and storage at room temperature (22°C) and at refrigerator temperature (4°C) (106). They found that the white blood cell count decreased in 3 to 6 hours. Calcium pyrophosphate dihydrate crystals dissolved significantly within 24 hours, and monosodium urate crystals were detectable for 8 weeks but became smaller and less numerous. As the storage time increased, new artifactual crystals developed in the form of star-shaped arrays, plate-like structures, and positive birefringent Maltese crosses. Synovial fluid should be evaluated within 1 hour of collection.

Microscopic evaluation of crystals in synovial fluid may be performed initially with an ordinary light microscope, but definitive identification of the crystals requires a polarizing microscope. The correct classification of gout and pseudogout is greatly improved if synovial fluid microscopy is included in the patient's evaluation. Monosodium urate and calcium pyrophosphate dihydrate crystals can be distinguished by the sign of their birefringence. Monosodium urate crystals are negatively birefringent, which in practice means that the slow wave along the longitudinal axis of the crystal subtracts from the slow wave of the color compensatory filter. When the background is adjusted to magenta, the crystals appear reddish. The crystals are usually needle-like but may be spherules or "beach ball like." They may be intracytoplasmic or extracytoplasmic. Corticosteroid preparations such as betamethasone acetate therapeutically injected in the joint space to reduce inflammation may appear morphologically identical to monosodium urate. The crystals of calcium pyrophosphate dihydrate deposition disease (chondrocalcinosis or pseudogout) are positively birefringent, and when oriented longitudinally with respect to the slow wave of the compensation filter, appear blue to green. These crystals may be needle-like but are more frequently rhomboidal or shaped like irregular parallelograms. Although these crystals are characteristic of pseudogout, they are not pathognomonic and may be seen in other joint diseases, such as septic arthritis and osteoarthritis. It is essential that a control monosodium urate slide be kept near the microscope and reviewed daily to ensure that no alteration in alignment has occurred.

Quality assurance programs to evaluate synovial fluid crystal identification have used a variety of preparations for shipping to other hospital laboratories, including cytocentrifuge slides, sealing synovial fluid on a slide inside a resin ring with a coverslip, or sending fresh synovial fluid in a sealed capillary or in a plastic tube. There is an overall need to improve the accuracy of crystal identification. The crystals, however, especially calcium pyrophosphate dihydrate, are unstable in liquid synovial fluid used as quality control checks. Alternative crystal stabilization methods for liquid challenges or new dried preparations should be investigated to improve laboratory performance in synovial fluid crystal identification.

Clinical suspicion of joint sepsis should prompt immediate synovial fluid aspiration. Gram stain and culture are required for the definitive diagnosis of bacteria in synovial fluid; however, routine culture of all synovial fluid specimens is not recommended.

CONCLUSIONS

Because body fluids are collected at or near the bedside, their evaluation on-site is convenient and time saving. For some body fluids (urine), or some common diseases (diabetes mellitus), there are numerous POCT applications. For many body fluids, however, laboratory testing has not been adapted to the bedside. In this case, visual examination at the bedside may provide an initial assessment of the patient's clinical condition. In the future, new point-of-care assays will be developed for a variety of body fluids, especially saliva, urine, and amniotic fluid, and for therapeutic drug monitoring, identification of tumor markers, autoantibody detection, and assays for fetal lung maturity, preterm labor, and other conditions. This enlargement in the POCT repertoire would be facilitated by parallel development of data management systems for POCT (3). This next frontier will provide connectivity or transfer of results from the point-of-care site to the laboratory or hospital information system. Without a data management solution, the results generated by POCT programs will remain recorded in a variety of unorthodox methods, with subsequent missing results and potential therapeutic misadventures. Additional POCT tests for body fluids will improve therapeutic turnaround time, clinical decision-making, and patient outcome.

ACKNOWLEDGMENT

Thanks are extended to Pat Schmidt for her skill in typing this manuscript.

REFERENCES

1. Anonymous. The tests for albumen and sugar in the urine. [Editorial]. *Lancet* 1883;i:956.
2. Shuler CL, Allison N, Holcomb S, et al. Accuracy of an automated blood pressure device in stable inpatients. Optimum vs routine use. *Arch Intern Med* 1998;158:714–721.
3. Kiechle FL. *Point-of-care testing*. Rainey P, ed. Washington, D.C.: American Association for Clinical Chemistry, Inc., 1998:1–98.
4. Miller KA, Miller NA. Joining forces to improve point-of-care testing. *Nurs Manage* 1998;28:34–37.
5. Kost GJ. Guidelines for point-of-care testing: improving patient outcomes. Pathology patterns. *Am J Clin Pathol* 1995;104(Suppl 1):S111–S127.
6. Cembrowski GS, Kiechle FL. Point-of-care testing: critical analysis and practical application. *Adv Pathol Lab Med* 1994;7:3–26.
7. Kiechle FL, Ingram-Main R. Quality improvement and point-of-care testing. *J Clin Ligand Assay* 1995;18:14–20.
8. Methany NA, Clouse RE. Bedside methods for detecting aspiration in tube-fed patients. *Chest* 1997;111:724–731.
9. Jahn M. The managed care era strikes in the lab. *Medical Laboratory Observer* 1995;27:38–43.
10. Boyd JC, Felder RA, Savory J. Robotics and the changing face of the clinical laboratory. *Clin Chem* 1996;42:1901–1910.
11. Peredy TR, Powers RD. Bedside diagnostic testing of body fluids. *Am J Emerg Med* 1997;15:400–407.
12. Cohen EP, Lemann J. The role of the laboratory in evaluation of kidney function. *Clin Chem* 1991;3:785–796.
13. Kiechle FL, Idlibi O. Biochemical screening in urinalysis. *Am J Clin Pathol* 1987;87:423–424.
14. Davis GM. Autoverification of macroscopic urinalysis. *Lab Med* 1999;30:56–60.
15. Kiechle FL, Karcher RE, Epstein E. Routine microscopic examination of the urine sediment revisited. *Arch Pathol Lab Med* 1984;108:855–856.
16. Howanitz PJ, Saladino AJ, Dale JC. Timeliness of urinalysis: a College of American Pathologists Q-Probe study of 346 small hospitals. *Arch Pathol Lab Med* 1997;121:667–672.
17. Froom P, Bieganiec B, Ehrenrich Z, et al. Stability of common analytes in urine refrigerated for 24 h before automated analysis by test strips. *Clin Chem* 2000;46:1384–1389.
18. Gillenwater JY. Detection of urinary leukocytes by Chemstrip-L. *J Urol* 1981;125:383–384.
19. Sadof MD, Woods ER, Emans SJ. Dipstick leukocyte esterase activity in first-catch urine specimens: a useful screening test for detecting sexually transmitted disease in the adolescent male. *JAMA* 1987;258:1932–1934.
20. Walters CS. Why can a urine specimen have a negative nitrite result on a dipstick reagent test yield a positive urine culture? *Lab Med* 1999;30:22–23.
21. Ellis G, Adatia I, Yazdanpanah M, et al. Nitrite and nitrate analyses: a clinical biochemistry perspective. *Clin Biochem* 1998;31:195–220.
22. Kiechle FL, Malinski T. Indirect detection of nitric oxide effects: a review. *Ann Clin Lab Sci* 1996;26:501–511.
23. Smith SD, Wheeler MA, Weiss RM. Nitric oxide synthase: an endogenous source of elevated nitrite in infected urine. *Kidney Int* 1994;45:586–591.
24. Nagase S, Takemura K, Meda A, et al. A novel nonenzymatic pathway for the generation of nitric oxide by the reaction of hydrogen peroxide and D- or L-arginine. *Biochem Biophys Res Commun* 1997;233:150–153.
25. Annane D, Sanquer S, Sébille V, et al. Compartmentalised inducible nitric-oxide synthase activity in septic shock. *Lancet* 2000;355:1143–1148.
26. Lam MH. False 'hematuria' due to bacteriuria. *Arch Pathol Lab Med* 1995;119:717–721.
27. Yoshikawa N, Matsuyama S, Iijima K, et al. Benign familial hematuria. *Arch Pathol Lab Med* 1988;112:794–797.
28. Beetham R. Biochemical investigation of suspected rhabdomyolysis. *Ann Clin Biochem* 2000;37:581–587.
29. Anderson PT, Jorgenson PJ, Nielson LK, et al. Semiquantitative measurement of myoglobunuria in trauma patients with a latex-agglutination test (Rapi-Tex). *Scand J Clin Lab Invest* 1992;52:847–851.
30. Blondheim SH, Margoliash E, Shafrir E. A simple test for myohemoglobinuria (myoglobinuria). *JAMA* 1958;167:453–454.
31. Agosti SJ, Foulis PR, Vandor S. Rapid differentiation of hemoglobinuria from myoglobinuria. [Abstract]. *Am J Clin Pathol* 1989;91:356.
32. Andersen PT, Jorgensen PJ, Toft E, et al. Rapid estimation of serum myoglobin concentration during rhabdomyolysis with a latex-agglutination test (Rapi-Tex). *Acta Chir Scand* 1990;156:515–519.
33. Oster JR, Rietberg B, Taylor AL, et al. Can β-hydroxybutyrate be detected at the bedside by *in vitro* oxidation with hydrogen peroxide. *Diabetes Care* 1984;7:80–82.
34. Wiggam MI, O'Kane MJ, Harper R, et al. Treatment of diabetic ketoacidosis using normalization of blood 3-hydroxybutyrate concentration as the endpoint of emergency management. *Diabetes Care* 1997;20:1347–1352.
35. American Diabetes Association. Tests of glycemia in diabetes. *Diabetes Care* 1999;22(Suppl 1):S77–S81.
36. Cohen HT, Spiegel DM. Air exposed urine dipsticks give false-positive results for glucose and false-negative results for blood. *Am J Clin Pathol* 1991;96:398–400.
37. Edwards JJ, Tollaksen SL, Andersen NG. Proteins of human urine. III. Identification and two-dimensional electrophoretic map positions of some major urinary proteins. *Clin Chem* 1982;28:941–948.
38. Orth SR, Ritz E. The nephrotic syndrome. *N Engl J Med* 1998;338:1202–1211.
39. Jazayeri A, Chez RA, Porter KB, et al. Urine protein dipstick measurements. A screen for a standard, 24-hour urine collection. *J Reprod Med* 1998;43:687–690.

40. American Diabetes Association. Diabetic nephropathy. *Diabetes Care* 1999;22(Suppl 1):S66–S69.

41. Hidaka S, Kaneko O, Shirai M, et al. Do obesity and non-insulin dependent diabetes mellitus aggravate exercise-induced microproteinuria? *Clin Chim Acta* 1998;275:115–126.

42. Kutter D, Kremer A, Bousser F, et al. A simple and inexpensive screening test for low protein levels in urine. *Clin Chim Acta* 1997;258:231–239.

43. Mogensen CE, Viberti GC, Peheim E, et al. Multicenter evaluation of the Micral-Test II test strip, an immunologic rapid test for the detection of microalbuminuria. *Diabetes Care* 1997;20:1642–1646.

44. Moore RR, Hirata-Dulas CA, Kasiske BL. Use of urine specific gravity to improve screening for albuminuria. *Kidney Int* 1997;52:240–243.

45. Poulsen PL, Mogensen CE. Clinical evaluation of a test for immediate and quantitative determination of urinary albumin-to-creatinine ratio. *Diabetes Care* 1998;21:97–98.

46. Burchardt M, Burchardt T, Shabsigh A, et al. Current concepts in biomarker technology for bladder cancers. *Clin Chem* 2000;46:595–605.

47. Hruszkewycz AM. *New urine tests for bladder cancer detection*. American Society of Clinical Pathologists Teleconference no. 2840, 1998, audiotape.

48. Johnston B, Morales A, Emerson L, et al. Rapid detection of bladder cancer: a comparative study of point of care tests. *J Urol* 1997;158:2098–2101.

49. Lokeshwar VB, Öbek C, Soloway MS, et al. Tumor-associated hyaluronic acid: a new sensitive and specific urine marker for bladder cancer. *Cancer Res* 1997;57:773–777.

50. Simpson D, Braithwaite RA, Jarvie DR, et al. Screening for drugs of abuse (II): cannabinoids, lysergic acid diethylamide, buprenorphine, methadone, barbiturates, benzodiazepines, and other drugs. *Ann Clin Biochem* 1997;34:460–510.

51. Crouch DJ, Frank JF, Farell LJ, et al. A multiple-site laboratory evaluation of three on-site urinalysis drug-testing devices. *J Anal Toxicol* 1998;22:493–502.

52. National Institute of Drug Abuse. Mandatory guidelines for federal workplace drug testing program. *Federal Register* 1988;53:11970–11989.

53. Substance Abuse and Mental Health Administration. Mandatory guidelines for federal workplace drug testing program. *Federal Register* 1997;62:51118–51119.

54. de la Torre R, Segura J, de Zeeuw R, et al. Recommendations for the reliable detection of illicit drugs in urine in the European Union, with special attention to the workplace. *Ann Clin Biochem* 1997;34:339–344.

55. Osterloh JD. Utility and reliability of emergency toxicology. *Emerg Med Clin N Am* 1990;8:693–723.

56. Sturgeon CM, McAllister EJ. Analysis of hCG: clinical applications and assay requirements. *Ann Clin Biochem* 1998;35:460–491.

57. Udoji WC, Victory DF, Cartwright PS, et al. Diagnostic problems with variant forms of human chorionic gonadotrophin. *Lab Med* 1998;29:243–246.

58. Daviaud J, Fournet D, Ballongue C, et al. Reliability and feasibility of pregnancy home-use tests: laboratory validation and diagnostic evaluation of 638 volunteers. *Clin Chem* 1993;39:53–59.

59. Koch H. Dipsticks and convulsions. *Lancet* 1998;352:1824.

60. Stone JE. Urine analysis in the diagnosis of mucopolysaccharide disorders. *Ann Clin Biochem* 1998;35:207–225.

61. Kiechle FL. The porphyrias. In: Bick RL, Bennet JM, Brynes RK, et al., editors. *Hematology: clinical and laboratory practice*. St. Louis: Mosby, 1993:553–573.

62. Zuijderhoudt FMJ, de Bok JD. Comparison of the Bio-Rad prophyrin column test with a simple spectrophotometric test for total urine porphyrin concentration. *Ann Clin Biochem* 1998;35:418–421.

63. Friedman DO, de Almeida A, Miranda J, et al. Field test of a rapid card test for *Wuchereria bancrofti*. *Lancet* 1997;350:1681.

64. Gundersen SG, Kjetland EF, Poggensee G, et al. Urine reagent strips for diagnosis of schistosomiasis haematobium in women of fertile age. *Acta Trop* 1996;62:281–287.

65. Kesner JS, Knecht EA, Krieg EF Jr, et al. Detecting pre-ovulatory luteinizing hormone surges in urine. *Hum Reprod* 1998;13:15–21.

66. Kiechle FL, Quattrociocchi-Longe TM, Brinton DA. Quality improvement in the laboratory assessment of *in vitro* fertilization. *Arch Pathol Lab Med* 1992;116:410–417.

67. Martinez AB, Voorhorst FJ, Schoemaker J. Reliability of urinary LH tests for planning endometrial biopsies. *Eur J Obstet Gyn Reprod Biol* 1992;43:137–142.

68. Eisenberg P, Muhs SMJ. GI study in the ICU bedside testing of gastric contents. *Nurs Manage* 1996;27:48J–48M.

69. Bouillata JI, Kim YC, Dean S. Glucose oxidase test for *in vitro* detection of enteral feeding products. *Am J Hosp Pharm* 1994;51:2424–2426.

70. Layne EA, Mellow MH, Lipman TO. Insensitivity of guaiac slide tests for detection of blood in gastric juice. *Ann Intern Med* 1981;94:774–776.

71. Ong YYT, Pintauro WM. Silver stools. *JAMA* 1979;242:2433.

72. Harrie JC, Dupont HL, Hornick RB. Fecal leukocytes in diarrhea illness. *Ann Intern Med* 1972;76:697–703.

73. Jednak MA, Nostrant TT. Screening for colorectal cancer. *Primary Care* 1998;25:293–308.

74. UKCCR. *Faecal occult blood testing: report of United Kingdom Coordinating Committee on Cancer Research Working Party*. London: UKCCR, Africa House, 1989.

75. Sinatra MC, St John JB, Young GP. Interference of plant peroxidases with guaiac-based fecal occult blood tests is avoidable. *Clin Chem* 1999;45:123–126.

76. Rockey DC, Koch J, Cello JP, et al. Relative frequency of upper gastrointestinal and colonic lesions in patients with positive fecal occult blood tests. *N Engl J Med* 1998;339:153–159.

77. Lawrence RA. *Breastfeeding: a guide for the medical profession*. St. Louis: Mosby, 1994:305–306.

78. Kjeldsberg CR, Knight JA. Amniotic fluid. In: Kjeldsberg CR, Knight JA, eds. *Body fluids: laboratory examination of amniotic, cerebrospinal, seminal, serous and synovial fluids*. Chicago: American Society of Clinical Pathologists, 1993:1–63.

79. Lo YMD, Corbetta N, Chamberlain PF, et al. Presence of fetal DNA in maternal plasma and serum. *Lancet* 1997;350:485–487.

80. Davis H, Olsen S, Bigelow NC, et al. Detection of fetal red cells in fetomaternal hemorrhage using a fetal hemoglobin monoclonal antibody by flow cytometry. *Transfusion* 1998;38:749–756.

81. Weitzner JS, Strassner HT, Rowlens RG, et al. Objective assessment of meconium content of amniotic fluid. *Obstet Gynecol* 1990;76:1143–1144.

82. Neil N, Sullivan SD, Lessler DS. The economics of treatment for infants with respiratory distress syndrome. *Med Decis Making* 1998;18:44–51.

83. Strong TH Jr, Hayes AS, Sawyer AT, et al. Amniotic fluid turbidity: a useful adjunct for assessing fetal pulmonary maturity status. *Int J Gynecol Obstet* 1992;38:97–100.

84. Coapman-Hankin RA, Kiechle FL, Epstein E, et al. Three methods compared for determining phosphatidylglycerol in amniotic fluid. *Clin Chem* 1985;31:1374–1176.

85. Eisenbrey AB, Epstein E, Zak B, et al. Phosphatidylglycerol in amniotic fluid. Comparison of an "ultrasensitive" immunologic assay with TLC and enzymatic assay. *Am J Clin Pathol* 1989;91:293–297.

86. Dubin SB. Assessment of fetal lung maturity practice parameter. *Am J Clin Pathol* 1998;110:723–732.

87. Lockwood CJ, Senyei AE, Dische MR, et al. Fetal fibronectin in cervical and vaginal secretions as a predictor of preterm delivery. *N Engl J Med* 1991;325:669–674.

88. Braat DDM, Smeenk JMJ, Manger AP, et al. Saliva test as ovulation predictor. *Lancet* 1998;352:1283–1284.

89. Smith RW, Callagen DA. Amniotic fluid crystallization test for ruptured membranes. *Obstet Gynecol* 1962;20:155–660.

90. Hayward RA, Shapiro MF, Oye RK. Laboratory testing on cerebrospinal fluid: a reappraisal. *Lancet* 1987;i:1–4.

91. Walker DS, Brock-Utne JG. A comparison of simple tests to distinguish cerebrospinal fluid from saline. *Can J Anaesth* 1997;44:494–497.

92. Kjeldsberg CR, Knight JA. Cerebrospinal fluid. In: Kjeldsberg CR, Knight JA, eds. *Body fluids: laboratory examination of amniotic, cere-*

brospinal, seminal, serous and synovial fluids. Chicago: American Society of Clinical Pathologists, 1993:65–71.

93. Beetham R, Fabie-Wilson MN, Park D. What is the role of CSF spectrophotometry in the diagnosis of subarachnoid hemorrhage? *Ann Clin Biochem* 1998;35:1–4.

94. Rouch E, Rogers BB, Buffone GJ. Transferrin analysis by immunofixation as an aid in the diagnosis of cerebrospinal fluid otorrhea. *Arch Pathol Lab Med* 1987;111:756–757.

95. Light RW, Macgregor MI, Luchsinger PC, et al. Pleural effusions: the diagnostic separation of transudates and exudates. *Ann Intern Med* 1972;77:507–513.

96. Peterman TA, Speicher CE. Evaluating pleural effusions: a two-stage laboratory approach. *JAMA* 1984;252:1051–1053.

97. Costa M, Quiroga T, Cruz E. Measurement of pleural fluid cholesterol and lactate dehydrogenase: a simple and accurate set of indicators for separating exudates from transudates. *Chest* 1995;103:1210–1213.

98. Brandstetter RD, Velazquez V, Viejo C, et al. Postural changes in pleural fluid constituents. *Chest* 1994;105:1458–1461.

99. Cheng D-S, Rodriquez M, Rogers J, et al. Comparison of pleural fluid pH values obtained using blood gas machine, pH meter, and pH indicator strip. *Chest* 1998;114:1368–1372.

100. Meyers DG, Meyers RE, Prendergast TW. The usefulness of diagnostic tests on pericardial fluid. *Chest* 1997;111:1213–1221.

101. Mauk PM, Schwartz JT, Lowe JF, et al. Diagnosis and course of nephrogenic ascites. *Arch Intern Med* 1998;148:1577–1579.

102. Sinton E. Seminal fluid. In: Kjeldsberg CR, Knight JA, eds. *Body fluids: laboratory examination of amniotic, cerebrospinal, seminal, serous and synovial fluids.* Chicago: American Society of Clinical Pathologists, 1993:255–264.

103. Pool TB. Practices contributing to quality performance in the embryo laboratory and the status of laboratory regulation in the US. *Hum Reprod* 1997;12:2591–2593.

104. Rippey JH. Synovial fluid analysis. *Lab Med* 1979;10:140–145.

105. Clayburne G, Baker DG, Schumacher HR Jr. Estimated synovial fluid leukocyte numbers on wet drop preparations as a potential substitute for actual leukocyte counts. *J Rheumatol* 1992;19:60–62.

106. Kerolus G, Clayburne G, Schumacher HR Jr. Is it mandatory to examine synovial fluids promptly after arthrocentesis? *Arthritis Rheum* 1989;32:271–278.

17

IN VITRO, *EX VIVO*, AND *IN VIVO* MONITORING OF THE NEONATE AND PREMATURE INFANT

JOHN W. BERKENBOSCH
RYAN E. GRUEBER
JOSEPH D. TOBIAS

GOALS OF POINT-OF-CARE TESTING IN THE NEONATE

From the earliest days, the goals of medicine have been, and must continue to be, delivery of the highest quality patient-centered care. Whereas the development of technology for biochemical analysis has added much to the practice of medicine, these advances have not necessarily enhanced the patient-directed aspect of care. Until recently, most biochemical analyses were performed in centralized laboratories, often far removed from the bedside. Samples required multiple processing steps and often were run in batches. Although efficient from the laboratory standpoint, such steps may result in unacceptably lengthy turnaround times. This is of particular concern in the critical care environment, where the need for immediate action mandates rapid delivery of laboratory results. Therefore, the concept of point-of-care testing (POCT), testing performed at or near the bedside, has become increasingly popular and exciting. Although the technologies used in various aspects of bedside testing have been in use for as long as 30 years, the development of whole-blood analysis has facilitated the recent acceleration of POCT utilization. These advances are vital to practice in critical care areas, such as the emergency department, intensive care unit (ICU), and operating suite, where patient care and survival depend on the availability of relevant information. This chapter reviews applications of POCT that are of particular importance, or that mandate particular caution, in infant and neonatal critical care (Table 17.1).

BIOCHEMICAL ANALYSES

The Benefits of Whole-blood Analysis

The development of whole-blood analysis has been instrumental in enabling the transfer of biochemical analysis from centralized laboratories to the bedside. The principles and advantages of whole-blood analysis have been extensively reviewed (1–3) and can be summarized in three areas. First, the reduction in processing steps, such as sample transport, centrifugation, and data entry into central computers, has facilitated a reduction in turnaround time

from 30 to 60 minutes in most centralized "statim" laboratories to minutes with bedside or near-patient whole-blood analysis technology (4). Second, whole-blood testing allows reporting of more physiologically relevant results (e.g., ionized versus total calcium concentrations) (5) and avoids some of the pitfalls of plasma-based testing that can result in potentially disastrous treatment decisions (e.g., *Pseudohyponatremia*) (6). Third, whole blood analysis can reduce the volume required for performing analyses.

Conservation of Blood Volume

Third and of particular benefit to the neonate, whole-blood analysis allows testing to be performed on much smaller quantities of blood (4). With an average blood volume of 80 to 100 mL per kilogram of body weight (7), this reduction is important, especially in the very preterm or growth-retarded infant, in whom total blood volumes may be as low as 40 to 50 mL. Indeed, blood loss associated with laboratory testing is the primary causative factor of anemia and the need for transfusions during the preterm infant's first few weeks of life (8). This is compounded by a relatively reduced ability of neonates to maintain their circulating red blood cell mass. Both term and especially preterm infants are relatively deficient in erythropoietin, with circulating levels at birth less than 25% of those found in anemic adults (7). Subsequently, Ohls and colleagues measured erythropoietin levels in 11 preterm infants with progressive anemia secondary to phlebotomy losses. In contrast to older children and adults, in whom erythropoietin levels rise in response to blood loss, erythropoietin levels in these infants did not increase, suggesting an impaired ability to compensate for red cell losses (9). Furthermore, the life span of red blood cells in neonates is only 60 to 90 days, roughly one-half to two-thirds that of an adult red blood cell (7). Therefore, anemia in the neonatal ICU, both for iatrogenic and physiologic reasons, is an ongoing concern. Multiple randomized trials have shown that erythropoietin effectively stimulates erythropoiesis and can decrease transfusion requirements in these patients (10,11), and this will continue to be an important component of neonatal care. Along with this, however, is a growing recognition that decreasing unnecessary blood losses is vital (12). Therefore, strategies designed to minimize

TABLE 17.1. INDICATIONS FOR POINT-OF-CARE TESTING IN NEONATES AND INFANTS

General	More rapid and relevant answers
	Test interpretation within a patient context
	Remove risks associated with patient movement, i.e., endotracheal extubation
Biochemical analysis	Decreased phlebotomy losses and transfusion requirements
Glucose	Screening for and prevention of neonatal hypoglycemia
	Gestational diabetes, improved neonatal outcomes
Calcium	Neonatal seizures, rapid detection of hypocalcemia
	Avoidance of hypocalcemia during cardiopulmonary bypass
Lactate	Perinatal assessment, scalp lactate
	Evaluating therapy for shock states and need for ECMO
Coagulation	Assessing coagulation during CPB, ECMO
Cerebral function	Outcome prediction following asphyxial injury
EEG	Evaluation/diagnosis of neonatal brain death
	Adequacy of sedation during mechanical ventilation, (BIS)
Cerebral perfusion	Evaluation/diagnosis of neonatal brain death
Mechanical ventilation	Continuous versus intermittent monitoring, proactive versus reactive management
Noninvasive	All are continuous
	Decreased need for ABG analysis and phlebotomy
	Documentation of ETT placement (end-tidal CO_2)
In-line ABG analysis	Decreased need for ABG analysis and phlebotomy
	Can do more frequent analyses than with *in vitro* ABGs
Fiberoptic technology	Continuous monitoring
	Decreased need for ABG analysis and phlebotomy
	May be used intravenously if arterial access unavailable

ECMO, extracorporeal membrane oxyenation; CPB, cardiopulmonary bypass; EEG, electroencephalography; ABG, arterial blood gas; ETT, endotracheal tube; BIS, bispectral index.

blood loss in this high-risk population, both by decreasing the amount of blood required to perform analyses as well as decreasing the number of analyses performed, should be welcomed.

Analytes of Specific Interest in the Neonate

The spectrum of analytes which now can be assessed by whole-blood analysis has become quite extensive, and many of these will be discussed at length in other areas of this text. The complex metabolic adaptions that occur in the perinatal and neonatal period, however, magnify the importance of certain analytes; the focus of this section is limited to those analytes.

Glucose

Neonates are uniquely susceptible to developing hypoglycemia. During development, 80% of fetal nutrition is carbohydrate. Whereas glucose is obtained solely by transplacental transfer, insulin production is fetal. At birth, with clamping of the umbilical cord, glucose supply ceases and blood glucose levels drop dramatically in the first 60 to 90 minutes of life. These levels recover spontaneously, but levels of 40 to 50 mg per deciliter (2.2–2.8 mmol/L) remain the norm during the first few days of life (13). Although the fetal liver contains all of the enzymes required for glycogen synthesis and storage, most glycogen deposition does not occur until late gestation and may be additionally impaired in the setting of placental insufficiency. This leaves the newborn relatively glycogen deficient and, particularly in the premature and growth retarded infant, glycogen stores at

birth are rapidly depleted in the absence of exogenous glucose. The increased basal metabolic rate present in newborns further contributes to this depletion (14). Hypoglycemia is also an important component of many metabolic disorders that present in the neonate. Therefore, rapid and accurate monitoring of glucose levels is particularly important in this population.

Some controversy remains, but most studies define neonatal hypoglycemia as a glucose level below 35 to 40 mg per deciliter (1.9–2.2 mmol/L). The incidence of early (within 24 hours) hypoglycemia by these definitions is reported to be 35% to 73% (13,15,16). Although these levels typically are well tolerated, symptomatic hypoglycemia may occur. Symptoms may be mild or subtle (e.g., lethargy, jitteriness, hypothermia) or more life threatening (e.g., apnea/bradycardia, cyanosis and hypoxemia, seizures) (14). Whereas these symptoms are very nonspecific, the risks of neurologic and neurodevelopmental sequelae are well known (17), making rapid diagnosis and treatment of these infants essential. Additionally, there is growing evidence that neurodevelopmental outcome may be affected in neonates with asymptomatic hypoglycemia. Pildes and colleagues prospectively compared 39 term infants with asymptomatic hypoglycemia (<30 mg/dL, 1.7 mmol/L) with 41 euglycemic controls (18). Hypoglycemic infants were found to have smaller head circumferences and intelligence quotient (IQ) scores were lower by 5 to 7 points. Lucas and colleagues retrospectively reviewed the effects of hypoglycemia in 661 premature infants (19). When glucose levels were less than 47 mg per deciliter (2.6 mmol/L) on at least 5 days, the relative risk for significant neurodevelopmental impairment at 18 months of age was 3.5. Whereas some of these impairments appeared to resolve with time, other deficiencies persisted. Subsequently, Duvanel and co-workers prospectively studied the effects of hypoglycemia (<47 mg/dL, 2.6 mmol/L) in 85 low-birth-weight babies (15). Intravenous glucose was provided for glucose values lower than 36 mg per deciliter (2 mmol/L), regardless of symptoms. By this definition, 73% of babies developed hypoglycemia. Despite rapid treatment, these investigators also found that repeated (five or more) episodes of hypoglycemia were associated with decreased head circumference at 18 months of age and decreased psychomotor scores at 5 years of age. Moderate, recurrent hypoglycemia was more ominous than single episodes of severe hypoglycemia. These data suggest that aggressive assessment for and treatment of moderate, asymptomatic hypoglycemia would be prudent.

Because of the widespread need for outpatient glucose monitoring, portable, POC glucose monitors have become widely available. First-generation monitors used semiquantitative reagent strips and were inconsistent in detecting hypoglycemia. Present-day analyzers utilize photometric or electrochemical biosensor technology to produce quantitative results rapidly (20). Because of the presence of relatively glucose-deficient red blood cells, whole-blood glucose levels are on average 10% to 15% lower than plasma levels (14). This may be particularly important in the neonate because hematocrit levels at birth are especially high. Four reflectance photometry-based glucometers have been evaluated in neonates: HemoCue and HemoCue-B (Mallinkrodt), Ames Glucometer 3 (Bayer), and One Touch II glucometer (Lifescan). All require only a single drop of blood, and results are available in 1 to 4 minutes. The first-generation HemoCue consistently overestimated plasma glucose levels by as much as 2.5 mmol per liter (45 mg/dL) (21,22). Consistent with the reported low range of 40 mg per deciliter (2.2 mmol/L) for this device, these differences were greatest at the lowest glucose levels, and these investigators concluded that this device could not be used safely in neonates. Deshpande and colleagues evaluated the HemoCue B in 113 samples and found that, although this device also overestimated plasma glucose, the difference was less than with the HemoCue device (23). In contrast, Schlebusch and colleagues found excellent correlation between the HemoCue-B and plasma glucose levels (r = 0.965) and concluded that this device could be safely and appropriately used in neonates (24). Because only a small number of the samples in this study were less than 40 mg per deciliter (2.2 mmol/L), the range in which accurate glucose measurement is most important, some caution must be used in interpreting this conclusion. Kirkham and Watkins evaluated the accuracy of the Ames Glucometer 3 in 50 paired whole-blood and plasma samples from 30 neonates (25). They found that the Ames device consistently overestimated plasma glucose values by 0.7 ± 1.1 mmol per liter (12.6 ± 19.8mg/dL) and concluded that it may be of limited use in the neonate (25). These results are somewhat surprising because whole-blood glucose values should be lower than plasma values. In contrast, in 327 paired samples, the One Touch II glucometer consistently underestimated plasma glucose levels by 10% (26). The magnitude of this difference did not vary with glucose concentration, leading to the conclusion that this device is acceptably reliable for the detection of neonatal hypoglycemia. Schlebusch and colleagues also reported a consistent underestimation of plasma glucose with the One Touch II, but the greater magnitude

of this underestimation (8.5 mg/dL) was such that they concluded the device was not appropriate for routine clinical use. The sample size of this study was small (n = 52), however, suggesting that this conclusion may be somewhat premature.

Fewer data exist regarding the neonatal use of electrochemical biosensor-based glucometers. In 50 cord blood samples, the YSI glucometer (Yellow Springs Instruments) compared well with plasma values, with a mean difference of 3 mg per deciliter (0.17 mmol/L) over a wide range (2–94 mg/dL, 0.1–5.2 mmol/L) of values (27). Innanen and colleagues analyzed 188 heel-stick samples with the Ames Glucometer Elite (Bayer) and found only a 5% coefficient of variation from plasma values (28). Finally, Demers and Smith evaluated the Precision-G glucometer (MediSense) in 74 heel-stick samples (29). The Precision-G underestimated plasma glucose by an average of 5.6 mg per deciliter (0.31 mmol/L). In 14 samples that were less than 40 mg per deciliter (2.2 mmol/L), this difference was even smaller. Despite some variation, these studies suggest that (POC) glucose testing is more accurately performed with electrochemical biosensor-based glucometers and that these devices remain accurate in the hypoglycemic range. Data do not yet exist to determine whether more rapid diagnosis and treatment of hypoglycemia using these devices will positively impact neurodevelopmental outcome.

In contrast, antenatal POC glucometry during diabetic pregnancy appears to have had a positive impact on perinatal outcome. Whereas neonatal hypoglycemia is a well-known risk of gestational diabetes, these infants are also at increased risk for congenital abnormalities, cardiomyopathy, renal vein thrombosis, respiratory distress syndrome, birth trauma secondary to macrosomia, and fetal demise (14). The development of these problems is believed to correlate with glycemic control during pregnancy, suggesting a potential beneficial role for home glucose monitoring in pregnant diabetic mothers. Goldberg and colleagues (30) randomized 116 diabetic mothers to either conventional gestational diabetes management (diabetic diet and weekly postprandial glucose checks) or a rigorous home glucose monitoring regimen, which included the use of insulin for fasting glucose levels greater than 95 mg per deciliter (5.3 mmol/L) or postprandial levels greater than 120 mg/dL (6.7 mmol/L). This management was associated with a significant decrease in average birth weight and the incidence of macrosomia and large-for-gestational-age infants. Similarly, Wechter and colleagues (31) managed 153 gestational diabetic patients with an intensive home glucose monitoring/insulin therapy regimen and found that the incidence of macrosomia and average birth weight were identical to those in a reference population of nondiabetic women. Although not specifically addressed, the decrease in macrosomia in these studies suggests that perinatal morbidity should also be decreased. Therefore, Langer and colleagues (32) prospectively evaluated neonatal outcomes in 2,461 gestational diabetics assigned to either intensive quantitative (7 times/day) or semiquantitative (4 times/day) home glucose testing. Both groups received insulin therapy as needed. Birth weight was lower in infants born to mothers on the intensive regimen and similar to birth weights in nondiabetic pregnancies. Labor complications were reduced; fewer deliveries were by caesarean section; and neonatal mortality, morbidity, and metabolic complications were reduced.

Ionized Calcium

Traditionally, central hospital laboratories report total serum calcium, often in conjunction with other analyte panels. Particularly in the critical care environment, measurement of whole-blood ionized calcium (Ca^{2+}) is more clinically relevant. Calcium is physiologically active only in its ionized state (5) and plays a vital role in many important physiologic processes. Of particular importance in the critical care setting are its roles in myocardial action potential generation and excitation–contraction coupling, vascular smooth-muscle tone, release of acetylcholine at the neuromuscular junction, and neuronal function/homeostasis within the central nervous system (CNS). Blood-borne calcium exists in three forms: ionized (50%), protein bound (40%–45%), and in complex with anions such as lactate, bicarbonate, and citrate (5%–10%) (14). Alterations in these percentages, protein levels, or anion concentrations make interpretation of total calcium levels misleading. Whereas numerous algorithms have been developed to predict Ca^{2+} from total calcium levels, none has been consistently useful clinically (33). This is especially true in the critically ill child. Vascular endothelial dysfunction, capillary leak, and liver or renal dysfunction decrease both serum protein and total calcium levels but variably affect Ca^{2+}. Alternatively, citrate from massive transfusions or bicarbonate for correction of acidosis may alter Ca^{2+} levels without significantly altering total calcium. Therefore, interpretation of serum calcium levels in the critically ill is difficult at best.

The transition to extrauterine life is associated with marked changes in calcium metabolism. Although the fetus contains the enzymes required for calcium regulation, the major source of fetal calcium is active transport across the placenta. In fact, neonates have higher total calcium levels than their mothers. Ionized calcium levels fall over the next 24 to 48 hours (34,35), reach adult values after 48 to 72 hours (34), and are not significantly different between preterm and full-term infants. The mechanism for this is believed to be both decreased calcium intake and absorption as well as increased serum calcitonin levels in the immediate newborn period (14). The normal range for Ca^{2+} in both premature and full-term infants is 1.05 to 1.40 mmol/l (34, 36), and values below 1.0 mmol per liter should be considered hypocalcemic (36).

Ionized calcium is measured in whole blood with an ion-selective electrode (1). Care must be taken because changes in pH alter calcium binding to protein, causing Ca^{2+} levels to increase as pH decreases (37). This may be significant in the critically ill patient, in whom pH levels may be widely variable. Decreased pH resulting from use of a tourniquet during venipuncture, particularly if the draw is difficult, also will cause an artificially elevated Ca^{2+} result. Although the technology for measurement of Ca^{2+} has been available since the early 1980s, the need to monitor for and treat transfusion-induced ionized hypocalcemia during liver and cardiac transplantation represented a major step in the rapid dissemination of whole blood electrolyte and subsequent POCT (38). Since then, whole-blood calcium testing has become vital to the practice of critical care. Rapid, relevant results facilitate informed clinical decisions, and there is a growing realization that ionized hypocalcemia has prognostic implications.

In the neonate, hypocalcemia is a far greater clinical problem than hypercalcemia, with symptoms beginning to emerge when Ca^{2+} levels drop below 1.0 mmol per liter (39). Hypocalcemia most significantly affects the CNS and cardiovascular system (CVS). Jitteriness is an early sign but is nonspecific in neonates and does not correlate well with calcium level. Hypocalcemia is a well-known cause of seizures and accounts for 12% to 34% of neonatal seizures (40,41). The reported seizure thresholds are based on total serum calcium measurement, however, and new studies to determine this threshold for ionized hypocalcemia are indicated. Hypocalcemic seizures are relatively rare, and the critical care practitioner more commonly encounters the adverse effects of hypocalcemia on myocardial function. Ca^{2+} plays vital roles in automaticity, pacemaker function, and excitation–contraction coupling. Levels below 0.7 mmol per liter are associated with hypotension, whereas levels below 0.6 can lead to dysrhythmias and cardiac arrest (1). Venkataramen and colleagues measured the effects of both serum and ionized calcium on myocardial function in 15 preterm neonates (42). In the eight neonates whose serum Ca levels were below 6 mg per deciliter (1.5 mmol/L), a single bolus of 18 mg per kilogram of elemental calcium had no effect on heart rate (HR), blood pressure (BP), or echographic assessment. The mean Ca^{2+} concentration in these infants, however, was 3.8 mg per deciliter (0.95 mmol/L), a level unlikely to cause myocardial impairment. In contrast, Bifano and colleagues assessed the effects of 200 mg per kilogram of Ca gluconate in ten critically ill neonates with persistent pulmonary hypertension and ionized hypocalcemia (<3 mg/dL, 0.75 mmol/L) (43). Postinfusion Ca^{2+} levels increased to 3.7 to 6.1 mg per deciliter (0.93–1.53 mmol/L) and, whereas HR and BP were unchanged, left ventricular function as measured by echocardiogram was improved. Meliones amd associates observed that hypotension frequently developed during institution of extracorporeal membrane oxygenation (ECMO) and measured serial Ca^{2+} levels in 19 patients (16 neonates) immediately after initiation of ECMO (44). In the first 5 minutes, Ca^{2+} levels had decreased from 3.8 mg per deciliter (0.94 mmol/L) to 2.8 mg/dl (0.7 mmol/L). Spontaneous return to baseline occurred by 30 minutes. These changes correlated temporally with the onset and subsequent resolution of hypotension. Increasing the Ca^{2+} level in the ECMO priming solution from 1.7 mg per deciliter (0.42 mmol/L) to 4.1 mg per deciliter (1.02 mmol/L) prevented this hypocalcemia and was associated with improved, rather than decreased, blood pressure on ECMO institution (45). Finally, whereas data specific to the neonate do not exist, Ca^{2+} levels in critically ill children have been shown to correlate with outcome. Sanchez and colleagues measured serum and ionized calcium levels in 15 critically ill children (46). Ca^{2+} levels were lower compared with noncritically ill controls. In the 14 survivors, Ca^{2+} levels rose progressively but declined in the single nonsurvivor. Cardenas-Rivero and colleagues prospectively measured total and ionized calcium concentrations in 145 critically ill children (47). Of 71 patients with low total serum calcium, only 26 (37%) had ionized hypocalcemia. In seven patients with normal serum calcium, three had ionized hypocalcemia. Patients with ionized hypocalcemia were sicker and had higher injury severity scores; these patients also had increased use of neuromuscular blockers, glucocorticoids, diuretics, antacids, vasopressors, and transfusions. Although neither sensitive nor specific, the mortality rate was higher in the hypocalcemic group (31% versus 2.5%). Finally, Broner and colleagues (48) compared total and ionized calcium levels in 98 critically ill children. The incidence of ionized hypocalcemia was 12.9%, and the mortality rate in this group was significantly higher (55%) than in patients with normocalcemia or hypercalcemia. As predicted, no correlation existed between total and ionized calcium levels (47,48), thus underscoring the importance of measuring Ca^{2+} in this population.

Lactate

Metabolic acidosis is a relatively common finding in critically ill patients and, when associated with an elevated anion gap, is frequently due to lactate accumulation. In the neonate one must additionally consider inborn errors of metabolism, although the most common causes of lactic acidosis are circulatory failure (i.e., cardiac failure, hypovolemia, sepsis) or deficiencies in oxygen transport (e.g., anemia, severe hypoxemia) (49). In either case, oxygen delivery is inadequate to meet oxygen consumption. Although the traditional belief has been that lactate production during cellular hypoxia represents a shift from aerobic to anaerobic metabolism, there is growing evidence that direct insults to both mitochondria and the pyruvate dehydrogenase complex during shock states also contribute (50). Because lactate undergoes hepatic metabolism, the concurrent development of liver failure during shock states may further contribute to lactic acidemia. Mixed venous oxygen desaturation is one of the earliest findings in shock, but there is some consensus that lactic acidosis better indicates the severity of shock (1).

In the early 1990s, development of an amperometric, enzymatic, substrate-specific electrode biosensor enabled measurement of lactate levels on small quantities of whole blood. This biosensor has since been incorporated in a handheld portable device. The Accusport portable lactate analyzer (Boehringer Mannheim) measures whole blood or serum lactate on a single drop of blood. Results are available in 60 to 90 seconds with an accuracy range of 0.8 to 22 mmol per liter. Two separate studies evaluated this device in 86 critically ill patients, and both found excellent correlation with slower central laboratory measurements (51,52), confirming simple, rapid, and accurate availability of bedside lactate analysis. This Accusport is also relatively inexpensive ($230 U.S.) and, at a cost of $1.80 per test strip, appears quite cost-effective compared with central laboratory costs of $2.50 and charges of $11.80 per lactate sample (51).

In the perinatal environment, access to the fetus is limited, and most monitoring is indirect. Scalp pH measurement is commonly performed when fetal HR recordings are abnormal. This approach is suboptimal, however, because differentiation between respiratory and metabolic causes of acidosis cannot be made. Scalp lactate measurement may be a more useful tool for the assessment of fetal well-being. Smith and colleagues measured simultaneous scalp pH and lactate levels in 215 fetuses and found that abnormalities in both correlated well with ominous fetal HR patterns and low Apgar scores (53). Subsequently, Westgren and associates randomized 341 fetuses to either scalp whole-blood lactate or scalp pH measurements when scalp blood sampling was believed to be indicated (54). Scalp lactate measurements were more successfully obtained than pH measurements, primarily

because of the need for a much smaller quantity of blood (5 versus 35 µL). Although these studies did not assess the effect of testing on obstetric decisions and outcome, concerns exist that more invasive fetal monitoring may lead to inappropriate obstetric interventions (53). Therefore, further studies are required to determine whether these measurements lead to improved obstetric and perinatal decision making.

Conversely, the correlation between neonatal lactic acidosis and outcome has been well documented. Lactate levels are increased in infants who show evidence of birth asphyxia, and the degree of elevation correlates with outcome. da Silva and colleagues measured lactate levels 30 minutes after birth in 115 neonates with clinical signs and symptoms of hypoxic–ischemic encephalopathy (HIE) (55). At 3 days of life, HIE was mild or absent when lactate levels were below 5 mmol per liter, whereas 80% of infants with lactate levels greater than 14 mmol per liter had persistent moderate or severe encephalopathy. Without further follow-up, the significance of these early elevations for long-term neurologic outcome remains to be determined. Of greater clinical importance may be the pattern of lactate progression. Beca and Scopes measured lactate levels every 4 hours in 21 neonates with respiratory distress syndrome (56). Initial lactate levels were higher in nonsurvivors than in survivors. Lactate levels progressively increased in all eight nonsurvivors; a decline was universally associated with survival, leading these investigators to conclude that, to be useful prognostically, serial lactate measurements are required. Deshpande and Ward-Platt prospectively compared serial lactate levels with pH and base deficit in 75 ventilated neonates (57). Both peak lactate level and persistence of lactic acidemia correlated positively with outcome. Whereas the mortality rate was 11% in patients without lactic acidosis, it increased to 57% if lactate levels reached a level greater than 5 mmol per liter. Lactate levels fell by 44% in survivors, compared with only 7% in nonsurvivors. Base deficit did not correlate with lactate level, suggesting that, contrary to common belief, it may be a poor predictor of tissue perfusion. Charpie and colleagues further quantified this with serial lactate measurements in 46 infants following cardiac surgery (58). An increase in lactate concentration of more than 0.75 mmol per hour predicted a poor outcome (death or need for ECMO), normalization by 24 hours strongly predicted survival. In addition to mortality correlations, lactate levels appear to be useful in predicting morbidity. Cheung and Finer evaluated the effect of lactate on mortality and neurodevelopmental outcome in 29 neonates requiring ECMO for hypoxemic respiratory failure (59). Admission and peak lactate levels were higher in nonsurvivors and, contrary to survivors, failed to decrease during the first 12 hours of ECMO. Neurodevelopmental assessment 10 to 30 months after decannulation in 17 survivors revealed that a peak lactate level greater than 15 mmol per liter predicted neurologic impairment (60). Neurologic outcome was normal when admission and peak lactate levels remained below 15 mmol per liter. Furthermore, Duke and colleagues found that lactate levels greater than 4.5 mmol per liter at admission to the pediatric ICU or greater than 4 mmol per liter at 4 and 8 hours after admission predicted significant adverse events in 12 of 96 infants following cardiac surgery (61). Similarly, Deshpande and Ward Platt (57) documented an increase in lactate level just prior to significant clinical deterioration in 6 of 44 critically ill neonates, implying a predictive role for serial lactate levels in at-risk infants.

Finally, lactate levels also have been used to guide therapeutic decisions. An increase of more than 0.75 mmol per hour in cardiac surgical patients (58) or to greater than 5 mmol per liter in infants with hypoxemic respiratory failure (59) has been used to predict the need for ECMO. Failure of lactate levels to decrease has been used to direct decisions regarding hematocrit, ECMO flows, or a change from venovenous to venoarterial ECMO (59). Israeli and colleagues found that lactate levels were greater than 1.8 mmol per liter in 46% of 37 infants transfused for asymptomatic anemia of prematurity (hematocrit <0.3) and concluded that lactate measurement prior to transfusion in these infants may be used to avoid possibly unnecessary transfusions (62).

Assessment of Coagulation

Rapid assessment of coagulation in the adult has numerous applications, both diagnostic and therapeutic. Thrombolytic therapy may decrease mortality and morbidity rates in coronary artery, pulmonary vascular, and cerebrovascular disease. The complications of these therapies can be disastrous, however, mandating tight control of anticoagulation. The utility of POC assessment of hemostasis in these patients is well recognized (63). Conversely, these disorders are exceedingly rare in infants and children and, outside of the use of cardiopulmonary bypass (CPB) and ECMO, POC evaluation of hemostasis is uncommon. During CPB or ECMO, the thrombogenic nature of the bypass circuit mandates high levels of anticoagulation, with the attendant risks of hemorrhagic complications. In neonates, intraventricular hemorrhage during ECMO is of particular concern. Heparin requirements are also widely variable in neonates and infants (64,65), preventing accurate prediction of "standard" doses of heparin. Therefore, rapid and accurate assessment of coagulation status in these situations is essential. The most commonly used measure of anticoagulation during neonatal ECMO and CPB is the activated clotting time (ACT), specifically defined as the time required for a clot to form in the presence of a coagulation stimulant, either celite or kaolin (66). Blood is placed within a tube containing the stimulant and a small magnet; it is vigorously mixed and then placed in a heated block, which continuously rotates the tube. When clot forms, the magnet becomes trapped against the side of the tube, the magnetic field is interrupted, and the timer stops (67). In the absence of anticoagulation, ACTs range from 81 to 133 seconds. During ECMO, ACTs greater than 400 seconds may be required during cannulation (67), whereas maintenance ACTs of 160 to 220 seconds appear adequate to prevent clot formation (68,69). Of interest, in 7 of 50 infants who developed an intracranial hemorrhage while on ECMO, increasing difficulties in controlling the ACT developed in the time just preceding the event, implying that coagulation status may be a predictor of intracranial catastrophe (70). Given the importance of intracranial hemorrhage to neurodevelopmental outcome after ECMO, POC coagulation assessment is useful in guiding therapeutic decisions in these patients.

Other Analytes

Although the preceding discussion certainly does not encompass the range of analytes that may be assessed in the neonate, an exhaustive discussion of all these analytes is beyond the scope of this chapter. Additionally, many of the remaining analytes of importance will be discussed elsewhere in this text and, although brief mention of some of these analytes is included here, the reader is referred to these chapters for more detailed description.

Sodium

The newborn kidney is characterized by a decreased capacity for sodium regulation secondary to immaturity of renal tubular cells, incomplete glomerular development, decreased expression, and less efficient hormonal regulation, of salt-transporting proteins (71). Consequently, with increasing prematurity, salt and water homeostasis is impaired, and up to 40% of infants less than 30 weeks' gestation are reported to develop hyponatremia (serum sodium <130 mmol/L) (72). Prevention of this and progression to severe hyponatremia, with the attendant risk of seizures, mandate strict management of sodium and water intake in these infants, including frequent assessments of electrolyte levels. Whole-blood sodium levels are measured using an ion-selective electrode, which is often coupled to other such electrodes so that comprehensive electrolyte panels can be simultaneously performed. The i-STAT (i-STAT Corporation, Princeton, NJ, U.S.A.) is a portable blood analyzer that can perform a variety of electrolyte or hematologic assessments on 0.06 mL of whole blood and results are available in less than 2 minutes. Murthy and colleagues compared 77 paired sodium measurements performed with the i-STAT and Ciba Corning 288 analyzer and reported excellent correlation between the two methods (slope = 0.989, r = 0.954) (73). Similarly, Alex and colleagues compared the i-STAT with centralized laboratory plasma analysis in 88 samples from 42 infants (74). Samples were obtained from indwelling umbilical artery catheters. Correlation between the i-STAT and plasma sodium values was good (r = 0.86) with a bias of less than 1 mmol per liter and a precision of 5 mmol per liter. In contrast, the same group evaluated the i-STAT using blood samples obtained via heel stick and reported a poor correlation between the i-STAT and plasma analysis (75), implying that sample site can significantly alter the usefulness of this device. Further study into this apparent discrepancy would be helpful because the acquisition or maintenance of indwelling arterial access in neonates is not always feasible.

Potassium

Whereas more than 98% of the body's potassium is contained within the intracellular milieu, much clinical effort is spent in maintaining extracellular potassium levels within a very tight physiologic range. Potassium levels are regulated primarily by the kidney. Compared with the older child or adult, most potassium secretion in the neonate occurs distal to the loop of Henle (76). In addition, this secretion is dependent on distal delivery of sodium; so, during hyponatremic states, the neonate's ability to secrete potassium may be impaired. This, combined with relative immaturity of the distal secretory mechanisms (77) and decreased activity of the Na^+,K^+-adenosine triphosphatase (ATPase) (78), decreases the ability of the neonatal kidney to excrete a potassium load. Disorders of potassium homeostasis contribute to morbidity and mortality rates, primarily through the arrhythmogenic effects of hyperkalemia. In the older child or adult, significant hyperkalemia (serum K^+ > 6.5–7 mmol/L) generally occurs in the setting of oliguria or anuria; so, in the critical care environment, the possibility of hyperkalemia usually can be anticipated. In contrast, hyperkalemia is common in the premature infant, with an incidence of 30% to 52% and frequently occurs in the absence of oliguria (79,80). Acidemia, also relatively common in critically ill neonates, is associated with the development of this disorder (80). The contribution to morbidity is significant. Leslie and colleagues reported serum K+ levels greater than 7 mmol per liter in 10 of 26 premature infants (79). Five of these infants developed cardiac arrhythmias, which were lethal in four, leading these investigators to recommend early and frequent potassium analysis in these infants. Underscoring the ability of the neonate to handle potassium loads, Hall and colleagues reported lethal hyperkalemia in a 2-week-old neonate following transfusion of a 32-day-old unit of packed red blood cells that had measured potassium levels of approximately 60 mmol per liter (81). Bedside analysis of whole-blood potassium levels has been evaluated with the portable i-STAT analyzer and appears to be reliable. Murthy and associates reported a slope of 0.96 with an *r* value of 0.989 when comparing whole blood with serum potassium levels in 76 samples taken from critically ill infants and children (73). Similarly, Alex and colleagues reported an *r* value of 0.97 when comparing paired analysis of whole blood and serum potassium levels from 42 critically ill neonates (74). The clinician must be wary that, as has long been recognized, the presence of red blood cell hemolysis can significantly alter reported potassium measurements (82). This alteration occurs most commonly when difficulties are encountered in sample collection, particularly with sampling by heel stick, as is commonly performed in neonates. Whereas the presence of hemolysis is often reported with results obtained from centralized laboratory analysis, this does not occur with the use of the i-STAT and mandates additional care in the interpretation of potassium values obtained with this device.

POINT-OF-CARE ASSESSMENT OF CEREBRAL FUNCTION AND PERFUSION

The ability to predict neurologic outcome accurately after severe brain injury remains a significant source of frustration in neonatal and pediatric critical care. Parents often request such predictions and are frequently disappointed by the lack of conviction in the reply. Useful prognostic information is vital when families need to make decisions regarding the duration and aggressiveness of their child's therapy, especially because discontinuation of therapy increasingly is viewed as acceptable when neurologically meaningful survival appears unlikely. Although imaging studies such as computed tomography (CT) or magnetic resonance imaging (MRI) scans can provide information regarding the degree of CNS structural injury or infarct, this information does not necessarily correlate with long-term functional outcome. Additionally, many infants in whom this information is sought are too unstable to be removed from the ICU to undergo these investigations. Similarly, neonatal and pediatric brain death declaration has been an area of much controversy. Recent recommendations from various sources, including the American Academy of Pediatrics, have recommended the use of ancillary tests in making this diagnosis in children (83–85). Accurate diagnosis of brain death is vitally important in these patients. Continuation of aggressive and costly therapy in the child with no hope of survival represents a difficult ethical dilemma for the critical care practitioner, and a declaration of brain death removes some of this dilemma. Additionally, because brain death inevitably is followed by cardiovascular arrest, this has implications for organ donation. Especially in neonates and infants, in whom the need for organs far outweighs the supply, a timely, accurate declaration of brain death optimizes the likelihood of successful organ harvest and transplantation. Conversely, from most parents' standpoint, declaration of death in the presence of cardiac activity is counterintuitive. Being presented with objective evidence of absent brain function may make this transition easier, at least cognitively, and may give families the reassurance that a decision to discontinue support was not premature. POCT has long been available for assessment of both cerebral function and perfusion and may be helpful in making these predictions and diagnoses.

Cerebral Function: Electroencephalography

Developed more than 100 years ago, the concept of electroencephalographic (EEG) monitoring refers to the measurement of electric activity at specific locations on the scalp and ears and, by analysis of the amplitudes and patterns of activity, making conclusions about the state of brain activity. This technology is crucial to evaluation of the critically ill child with neurologic disease. Although full-function, portable EEG monitors have been in clinical use for some time, newer, simpler monitors are also available and allow high-quality EEG recordings to be performed easily at the bedside. In the older child and adult, EEG monitoring is used predominantly for seizure evaluation or during pharmacologic therapy for increased intracranial pressure (ICP). In the neonate, however, the pattern of background EEG activity also has become useful in predicting neurologic outcome after perinatal asphyxial insult. In such infants, moderate to severe background disturbances, with the exception of modified burst suppression, have been associated with poor neurologic outcome, and isoelectric or very-low-voltage recordings are predictive of death (86,87). Conversely, outcome appears to be good if the EEG is normal or shows only mild disturbances. Of concern, however, is the fact that standard EEG analysis in infants requires considerable technical skill to obtain and interpret, limiting the speed of analysis in many hospitals. With optimism that newer therapies, instituted early, may improve the outcome of neonatal HIE, these delays may be significant, particularly because these therapies may have significant side effects and should, therefore, be offered only to infants at greatest long-term risk (88).

The amplitude-integrated EEG (aEEG) records a single-channel EEG from biparietal electrodes, correlates well with standard EEG monitoring, and can be placed and interpreted easily by the bedside practitioner (89). Hellstrom-Westas and colleagues recorded aEEGs within 6 hours of birth in 47 neonates with signs of intrapartum distress (88). Follow-up at a median of 2.75 years revealed that, of the 26 infants with a normal aEEG, 25 were neurologically normal, whereas all seven infants with either flat or extremely low-voltage aEEGs died or were severely handicapped. Similarly, Toet and associates recorded an EEG at 3 and 6 hours of life in 73 asphyxiated infants and evaluated neurologic outcome 1 to 6 years later (90). In infants in whom the aEEG pattern improved, outcome was normal, whereas deterioration predicted death or severe handicap. A persistently flat or extremely low-voltage pattern predicted universally poor outcome. Although a burst-suppression pattern tended to predict a poor outcome, the predictive power was not adequate to be clinically useful (88,90).

There is consensus that, under most circumstances, the diagnosis of brain death in adults can be reliably made by clinical examination; however, rapid neurodevelopment during late gestation and early infancy makes this application more suspect in young children (91). Therefore, in 1987, a Task Force of the American Academy of Pediatrics recommended that, in children less than 1 year of age, the diagnosis of brain death also includes documentation of electrocerebral silence (ECS) on EEG (83). Although controversial, subsequent recommendations have continued to include this suggestion (84,85), albeit with certain provisos. The criteria for determination of ECS on EEG are specific. Voltages must be lower than 10 μV during maximal signal amplification, body temperature must be greater than 36°C, and CNS depressants must have levels documented below the toxic range (92). Despite this, controversy remains. Although it is well documented that ECS is incompatible with a good neurologic outcome (86,88,90), it does not appear to predict death with the same certainty because there are reports of survival in neonates with ECS on EEG (93,94). The EEG of the very preterm infant is characterized by discontinuous, low-voltage activity and, in the presence of nonlethal CNS insult, may appear silent, leading to an inappropriate prediction of severe, permanent neurologic insult. Conversely, EEG activity persists in up to 20% of children meeting the clinical criteria for brain death (84). To encourage the rational use of EEG during determination of infant brain death, Ashwal made the following suggestions (84). When two clinical examinations, 24 hours apart, are consistent with brain death, an isoelectric EEG in the absence of other confounders (sedatives, hypothermia) is confirmatory of brain death, and a repeat EEG or additional ancillary tests are not necessary. Furthermore, although phenobarbital levels below 40 to 60 μg per milliliter generally do not suppress EEG activity, this threshold may be as low as 25 to 35 μg per milliliter in the sick neonate; therefore, increased caution must be used in these patients.

Finally, EEG technology may be a useful adjunct for monitoring sedation in the ICU. Mechanically ventilated infants frequently require sedation with or without analgesia to facilitate ventilator synchrony and to prevent the inadvertent removal of endotracheal tubes or intravascular catheters. Whereas alterations in physical examination and physiologic parameters are usually adequate for assessing sedation, concurrent use of neuromuscular blockade makes this assessment difficult. Physical reactions are lost, and commonly used physiologic parameters may be misleading. To minimize the risk of consciousness and suffering during neuromuscular blockade, the tendency appears to be to oversedate, and concern exists that this may be associated with an increased incidence of drug withdrawal (95). A modified EEG produced by the BIS monitor may be helpful in this scenario. EEG waveforms are recorded from three electrodes placed on the scalp and are internally processed to provide a "sedation score" between 0 (isoelectric)

and 100 (awake). First developed for use in the operating room, studies suggest that a BIS score less than 60 is associated with amnesia (96). Few data exist, however, regarding lengthier use of this monitor in the critical care setting. As part of an ongoing prospective evaluation of the BIS monitor during mechanical ventilation in critically ill children, we recently reported the effects of opioid and benzodiazepine tolerance on the BIS monitor in a 10-year-old child being treated for septic shock (97). As the doses of fentanyl and midazolam required to maintain the same level of sedation and BIS score increased over a 5-day period, BIS scores correlated well with clinical sedation scores and patient agitation. We have now completed an evaluation of the BIS monitor in 24 intubated pediatric patients. The BIS value correlated well with clinical sedation score as assessed by the modified Ramsay sedation score and was effective in differentiating clinically adequate from inadequate levels of sedation (97a). Further study to evaluate the usefulness of the BIS during neuromuscular blockade would be valuable.

Cerebral Perfusion

In addition to EEG, ancillary testing for the confirmation of brain death may include assessment of cerebral perfusion. In fact, this modality may be superior to EEG in this setting. Whereas ECS or EEG does not absolutely predict brain death, especially in infants, sustained absence of cerebral blood flow correlates absolutely with the development of brain death (98). Additionally, flow studies are not altered by the presence of CNS-depressing drugs or hypothermia. The gold standard for assessment of cerebral perfusion is direct four-vessel cerebral angiography; however, issues regarding vascular access and the need to remove patients from the critical care environment often make this procedure impractical in neonates and premature infants. Accurate bedside assessment of cerebral perfusion represents an important addition to the evaluation of these patients.

Transcranial Doppler

Transcranial Doppler (TCD) is based on the fact that arterial flow is pulsatile and that absence of pulsation within the cerebral vasculature indicates absence of flow. This technique is particularly useful in the neonate, where an open anterior fontanelle allows easy visualization of intracerebral vessels. In adults and older children, anterograde and retrograde flow in the internal carotid or middle cerebral arteries is assessed via transtemporal windows. Because of the low-resistance nature of the cerebral circulation, both systolic and diastolic flow velocities are normally obtained (99). Ducrocq and colleagues performed TCD evaluation of 130 patients meeting clinical criteria for brain death (100). In 129 of these patients, cerebral circulatory arrest was diagnosed by the presence of an oscillating to and fro, systolic spike, or zero-flow pattern. In the 64 patients who also underwent cerebral angiography, concordance was perfect. The one patient in whom flow was retained had undergone an extensive skull flap performed because of massive cerebral edema. No differences in interpretation were necessary in the 13 children included in this series. Similarly, Hadani and colleagues performed TCD on 137 patients with severe neurologic injury (101). Of these, 84 met clinical criteria for brain death and, in 81 TCD was consistent with absent cerebral circulation. One patient had retained flow, whereas adequate examination could not be performed in two patients. In the 53 patients who were not clinically brain dead, TCD patterns were variable but never consistent with bilateral circulatory arrest, confirming both the sensitivity (96.5%) and specificity (100%) of this modality. Both studies included children, but uniquely neonatal or pediatric data are scarce. McMenamin and Volpe noted a consistent pattern of anterior cerebral artery flow in six neonates with clinical, and in some EEGs, evidence of brain death (99). First, diastolic flow ceased and then became retrograde. This was followed by attenuation, and finally cessation, of anterograde systolic flow. This progression correlated closely with elevations in ICP, leading these researchers to conclude that loss of cerebral blood flow in brain death is due to progressive cerebral edema and increased cerebrovascular resistance. These patterns differed somewhat from those found in the predominantly adult studies. The significance of this is unclear and may represent important differences in intracranial dynamics that accompany an open fontanelle or simply technical differences between the studies. Because of the ease of performance of TCD and the apparent accuracy of the results, it is important that further neonatal studies be performed.

Radionuclide Angiography

The development of portable, bedside gamma counters enabled the use of radionuclide angiography (RA) as a safe alternative to direct angiography in the assessment of cerebral perfusion. The procedure is simply and rapidly performed via intravenous injection of technitium-99m-labelled substrates (albumin, glucoheptonate, pertechnetate). Serial dynamic images are obtained with a gamma counter placed over the head and neck region for 30 to 60 seconds, followed by static images 10 to 20 minutes later to evaluate the sagittal sinus. Absence of radioactivity above the base of the skull confirms absent cerebral perfusion (102–104). Schwartz and colleagues compared RA with direct angiography in nine children meeting clinical criteria for brain death (103). In all nine cases, both modalities revealed absent cerebral circulation. Holzman and colleagues then used RA in the evaluation of 18 comatose children, 11 of whom ultimately were diagnosed as brain dead (104). In eight of these patients, RA demonstrated no flow; in two, only faint activity in the sagittal sinus was noted on delayed static images. One patient with a normal study was diagnosed as brain dead. Studies were normal in the seven patients who never fulfilled brain death criteria. Of note, in four cases of absent flow, mean arterial pressure exceeded ICP by a mean of 55 torr, suggesting that factors other than, or in addition to, ICP elevations are important in the development of cerebral circulatory arrest. Whereas these studies suggest that RA may be helpful in establishing the diagnosis of brain death in older children, neonatal data are limited and somewhat less optimistic. In a retrospective analysis of 18 term and preterm infants diagnosed with brain death, Ashwal and Schneider reported intact RA-assessed cerebral perfusion in 6 (105). This suggests that RA may be less sensitive in this age group, reemphasizing the possible changes in intracranial dynamics that accompany an open fontanelle. They did find, however, that the predictive value was increased with simultaneous use of EEG and RA. Despite the lack of prospective data, demonstration of absent flow

by RA still may play a useful role in the diagnosis of neonatal brain death. As with TCD technology, further study in this area is both indicated and important.

POINT-OF-CARE MONITORING DURING MECHANICAL VENTILATION

Respiratory insufficiency, with or without the need for mechanical ventilation, is one of the most common reasons for admission to the neonatal or pediatric ICU. Routine assessment of these patients includes accurate monitoring of oxygenation and ventilation. Traditionally, these are performed by intermittent sampling and analysis of arterial blood using a glass electrode to measure pH, a Stow-Severinghaus electrode to measure PCO_2, and a Clark electrode to measure PO_2. Care must be taken during sampling because air bubbles artificially decrease PCO_2, and move PO_2 toward that of room air. Delays in analysis, particularly when the sample is maintained at room temperature, allow cellular metabolism to continue, which artificially decreases PO_2 and increases PCO_2 (106). Intermittent arterial blood gas (ABG) analysis has other limitations as well. Arterial vascular access may be difficult to obtain or maintain for a long time; when this access is not available, repetitive sampling can be difficult and painful. When patient status is rapidly changing or persistently unstable, frequent acquisition of ABG analysis becomes costly and contributes to the development of iatrogenic anemia and the need for blood transfusions. Intermittent monitoring may be suboptimal in certain clinical situations where avoidance of toxicities (i.e., hyperoxia and retinopathy of prematurity) or complications (i.e., hypercarbia and pulmonary hypertension, pH, and intraventricular hemorrhage) mandates tight control of oxygenation and ventilation. Utilization of the now numerous methods of continuous respiratory monitoring available may therefore offer many advantages.

Ex Vivo Assessment
Noninvasive Methods

Noninvasive methods exist for accurate estimation of both the oxygenation and ventilation status of critically ill neonates and children. Pulse-oximetry technology is used to estimate oxyhemoglobin saturation while end-tidal capnometry provides an estimate of arterial CO_2 levels. Transcutaneous monitoring offers the potential for simultaneous estimation of both oxygenation and ventilation. The advantages and limitations of each technology are summarized in Table 17.2.

Pulse Oximetry
Microprocessor advances facilitated a rapid dissemination of pulse-oximeter technology in the 1980s, and pulse oximetry is now a widely used and accepted means of continuously monitoring oxygenation. It is based on the Beer-Lambert law, which states that the concentration of an unknown solute may be determined by its pattern of light absorption. A light-emitting, photosensitive diode is applied to an area of the body that is narrow enough for light to traverse. Wavelengths of 660 nm (red) and 940 nm (infrared) are specifically analyzed because the

TABLE 17.2. COMPARISON OF NONINVASIVE VENTILATORY MONITORING TECHNOLOGIES

	Pulse Oximetry	Transcutaneous O$_2$ and CO$_2$ Monitoring	End-tidal Capnometry
Advantages	Inexpensive	Inexpensive	Inexpensive
	Can use in both intubated and nonintubated patients	Can use in both intubated and nonintubated patients	Can use in both intubated and nonintubated patients
	Continuous assessment	Simultaneous P$_{O_2}$ and P$_{CO_2}$	Rapid response
	Easily obtained	P$_{O_2}$ accurate in neonates	Most reliable in healthy patients
	Physiologically relevant	May detect hyperoxia better	Verification of ETT position
		Accurate over wide range of CO$_2$	
Disadvantages	Unreliable when perfusion poor	P$_{O_2}$ not reliable outside neonates	Less accurate when pulmonary
	Unreliable at low SaO$_2$ values	Slow response time	function abnormal
	Dyshemoglobinemia detection	Thermal injury, especially in	Increased dead space
	Less sensitive to oxygen toxicity	preterm infants	Added weight on ETT
Limitations	Movement artifact	Poor perfusion states	Moderate to severe lung disease
	Cyanotic congenital heart disease	Insensitive to inadvertent	Preterm infants (dead space, weight)
	Poor perfusion states	endotracheal extubation	
		Sensitivity to thermal injury	

ETT, endotracheal tube; P$_{O_2}$, partial pressure of oxygen; P$_{CO_2}$, partial pressure of carbon dioxide.

absorption patterns of oxyhemoglobin and deoxyhemoglobin differ greatly at these lengths. Elimination of interference by nonarterial sources (i.e., tissues, venous flow) is accomplished by analysis of only AC (pulsatile) currents and, from comparison of the absorption characteristics at both baseline and peak amplitude, an arterial oxyhemoglobin saturation (SaO$_2$) is calculated (107). Present pulse-oximetry technology incorporates an automatic internal calibration process that is activated when the machine is turned on and at periodic intervals during use. This is also activated when the sensor is changed; each sensor contains its own encoded calibration resistor indicating the specific wavelengths at which it operates.

The use of pulse oximetry has been evaluated extensively within the neonatal population. It is reliable, inexpensive, correlates very well with co-oximetry measurements of arterial saturation (108,109), and has become a standard of care in many ICU's. Limitations, however, do exist. Most importantly, patient movement may be interpreted as an arterial pulsation, resulting in a spurious reading. Although the oximeter alarm usually indicates a device failure, such artifact may constitute up to 20% of the recording time in the nonsedated infant (108). Newer pulse oximeters appear to be less sensitive to these artifacts, and the entirely new algorithm for processing light absorption and noise interpretation recently developed by Masimo is particularly exciting. Although data are preliminary, this Signal Extraction Technology (Masimo SET) appears to be much more sensitive to detection of true desaturation events and more successfully decreases false alarms due to motion artifact (110).

Second, the accuracy of pulse oximeters diminishes greatly below SaO$_2$ values of 75% to 80% (111). This is of concern in the neonate with cyanotic congenital heart disease where SaO$_2$ values of 60% to 70% are common. In infants with single-ventricle physiology, accurate assessment of SaO$_2$ in the immediate perioperative and postoperative periods is vital because SaO$_2$ values are commonly used to assess and manipulate the balance between systemic and pulmonary blood flow. The decreased amplitude of arterial pulsation during situations of poor perfu-

sion, such as severe shock or the use of vasoconstrictors, may further decrease pulse oximeter reliability. Although the data are again preliminary, there is optimism that the Masimo SET oximeter may be more reliable at both lower SaO$_2$ values and during low-perfusion states (112). Of unique importance in the neonate is probe placement position. Intermittent right-to-left shunting across the ductus arteriosus, particularly in the critically preterm infant with pulmonary hypertension, may falsely indicate arterial desaturation if the probe is placed postductally, and care must be taken to ensure preductal monitoring in these patients. Pulse oximetry is also unreliable in the setting of dyshemoglobinemias. The absorption pattern of carboxyhemoglobin is such that it is interpreted by the oximeter as oxyhemoglobin, resulting in an overestimation of SaO$_2$. The implications of this can be disastrous, and the use of pulse oximetry cannot be recommended in patients at risk for carboxyhemoglobinemia. Similarly, the absorption spectrum of methemoglobin is roughly equal at both pulse oximetry wavelengths. This tends to spuriously bring the pulse oximeter reading toward 85% with increasing concentrations of methemoglobin (107). Finally, whereas prevention of hypoxemia is the usual concern, hyperoxia also has significant toxicity in the neonate and is associated with the development of both retinopathy of prematurity and bronchopulmonary dysplasia. At values greater than 95%, small changes in SaO$_2$ may be associated with large changes in PaO$_2$. Although most researchers believe SaO$_2$ is a more physiologic measure of oxygen content, others believe that PaO$_2$, rather than SaO$_2$, is a better indicator of oxygen toxicity. Few data exist to support this, but some have therefore voiced concern that pulse oximetry may be inadequately sensitive to limit these morbidities (111). Others, however, have suggested that with appropriate, monitor-specific alarm limits, pulse oximetry is accurate and reliable for the detection of hyperoxia (113). Therefore, although pulse oximetry is easily, inexpensively, and accurately used in most clinical scenarios, the practitioner is encouraged to use sound judgment and apply this technology in conjunction with the unique needs of each patient.

Transcutaneous Monitoring

Transcutaneous monitoring offers the advantages of assessing both oxygenation and ventilation and can be used effectively in both intubated and nonintubated patients. At ambient temperatures, O_2 and CO_2 levels at the skin surface are essentially zero because of the lack of metabolic activity in the surface skin layers and the relative impermeability of the stratum corneum skin layer to gas diffusion. Heating of the skin surface to 42° to 43°C disrupts the stratum corneum, enhancing the diffusion of capillary gases to the skin surface and effectively removing the capillary to skin surface gradients for O_2 and CO_2. A Clark-type platinum cathode and pH glass-type electrode housed within the transcutaneous probe measure PO_2 and PCO_2, respectively (114).

O_2 diffuses through the skin less effectively than CO_2, which can make transcutaneous O_2 monitoring a challenge. The thin skin of neonates, particularly preterm infants, decreases this problem, however, and transcutaneous O_2 measurements are reported to be quite reliable in this age group. Palmisano and colleagues reported that, below PaO_2 levels of 80 mm Hg, the ratio of transcutaneous O_2/PaO_2 was 1.05; at PaO_2 greater than 80 mm Hg, this ratio dropped to 0.88 and was associated with a marked increase in variability (115). Conversely, the respective transcutaneous O_2/PaO_2 ratios were 0.93 and 0.74 in patients greater than 4 weeks of age. Because PaO_2 levels greater than 80 mm Hg are usually quite undesirable in the neonate, they concluded that transcutaneous O_2 monitoring would be clinically relevant in this population, whereas its utility was more limited in the older child and adult. In fact, despite the widespread dissemination of pulse oximetry, transcutaneous O_2 remains widely used in neonatal critical care, and some researchers still believe it is more sensitive to the detection of hyperoxia and, therefore, superior to pulse oximetry in this population (111).

Conversely, transcutaneous CO_2 monitoring appears to be more widely applicable and constitutes a more diversely useful application of this technology. Most studies suggested that transcutaneous CO_2 correlates well with $PaCO_2$ in neonates (115, 116), although others describe a consistent overestimation of $PaCO_2$ (117). This may be related to the use of higher electrode temperatures because an increase in skin surface temperature of 1°C increases local CO_2 production by 4.5%. We have studied transcutaneous CO_2 monitoring extensively and have shown an accurate estimation of arterial CO_2 in both infants and toddlers (118) as well as older children (119) over a wide range of arterial CO_2 values. The mean differences between transcutaneous and arterial CO_2 values in these studies were 2.3 and 2.6 mm Hg, respectively. This difference was consistent over the range of $PaCO_2$ values and is well within clinical relevance. We also recently completed an evaluation of transcutaneous CO_2 monitoring during high-frequency oscillatory ventilation, a therapy not amenable to the use of end-tidal CO_2 monitoring. The mean $PaCO_2$ to transcutaneous CO_2 difference was 2.8 ± 1.9 mm Hg, similar to our findings during conventional ventilation (119a). We now routinely use transcutaneous CO_2 monitoring in both intubated and nonintubated patients in our pediatric ICU. We believe this has facilitated more proactive, rather than reactive, patient management decisions and has, additionally, decreased our use of blood gas analysis. Our usual practice is to perform a single daily ABG, primarily to confirm continued correlation with the transcutaneous monitor and we may not even do this if

the monitor consistently correlates well. Although we have not formally studied it, this practice should help decrease the incidence of iatrogenic anemia and also may help limit the rising costs of ICU care.

Numerous issues, however, affect the usefulness of transcutaneous monitoring. Similar to pulse oximetry, the accuracy of transcutaneous monitoring is limited in states of decreased perfusion. Hypotension and hypoperfusion decrease local oxygen delivery, and transcutaneous O_2 underestimates PaO_2(120). Similarly, we reported that high doses of vasoconstricting drugs increased the transcutaneous to arterial CO_2 difference in children after cardiac surgery (121). Increased skin thickness and edema, factors that may develop during critical illness, further limit the success of transcutaneous monitoring. Transcutaneous electrodes must be recalibrated every 3 to 4 hours. Although this takes about 5 minutes, an additional 15 minutes is required for the electrode to equilibrate once it is repositioned, leaving the patient effectively unmonitored 15% to 20% of the time. At standard electrode temperatures of 43° to 44°C, the electrode must also be repositioned every 3 to 4 hours to avoid significant thermal injury (118). For convenience, this is usually done in conjunction with electrode recalibration. Technical issues such as improper electrode calibration or placement, entrapment of air bubbles under the electrode, or membrane damage further diminish accuracy. Whereas these issues make transcutaneous monitoring somewhat more cumbersome, they are not overly difficult to overcome with careful training of respiratory therapy staff, and transcutaneous monitoring should continue to be a valuable tool in the care of critically ill infants and children.

End-tidal Capnometry

Capnometry refers to the measurement of CO_2 during the respiratory cycle and subsequent estimation of arterial CO_2 content from the end-tidal CO_2 (ET CO_2) concentration. This has become the standard for monitoring the adequacy of ventilation and to confirm the intratracheal placement of the endotracheal tube during anesthesia (122), and some have suggested a similar role in the critical care setting (123). Normally, CO_2 is absent in inspired air, and the capnometer reads zero. The capnogram remains flat during the clearance of anatomic dead space in early exhalation. A sharp rise signals the exhalation of CO_2-rich alveolar gas, and the remainder of exhalation is characterized by a plateau on the capnogram. Failure to reach this plateau before the sharp fall in CO_2 that signals a new inspiration indicates failure to achieve alveolar ventilation completely, which is usually indicative of significant airflow obstruction. A capnometer is either in-line, where exhaled air flows directly past the CO_2 detector, or side stream, where air is continuously aspirated from the ventilator circuit to a detector located downstream within the capnometer box. Both detectors most commonly measure CO_2 by infrared spectroscopy. Whereas in-line and side-stream detectors appear equally accurate, side-stream devices tend to be preferred in neonatal applications because they are lighter and add less dead space than most in-line devices (124). They have the disadvantages, however, of being more easily occluded by secretions and a slower response to CO_2 changes (125).

Portable, nonelectric, capnometers are also available for qualitative assessment of CO_2. They contain a disk coated with hygroscopic material. This material produces H^+ ions on contact with CO_2, causing the disk to change color from purple to yellow. These devices are used primarily to differentiate endotracheal (yellow) from esophageal (purple) intubation and, therefore, may be of particular value in the transport environment when capnography may not be as easily available and clinical assessment of ventilation may be limited.

The accuracy of ET CO_2 estimation of arterial CO_2 in infants and children with normal lung function has been well documented during both mechanical (126) and spontaneous ventilation (127,128). In the critical care environment, however, capnometry is somewhat limited because accurate ET CO_2 monitoring is dependent on a high degree of ventilation–perfusion matching. The presence of alveolar infiltrates or atelectasis, common in critically ill children, increases alveolar dead space. This tends to dilute CO_2 from areas of healthy lung with normal ventilation–perfusion ratios, resulting in an underestimation of $PaCO_2$ (129). The presence of significant obstructive lung disease additionally limits ET CO_2 monitoring because marked prolongation of the exhalation phase may prevent failure to achieve, and thereby truly document, actual alveolar ventilation. This has been confirmed in both neonatal and pediatric studies. Rozycki and colleagues evaluated ET CO_2 monitoring in 45 mechanically ventilated neonates and found that ET CO_2 underestimated $PaCO_2$ by a mean of 6.9 mm Hg with a 95% confidence interval of 12.9 mm Hg (130). Similarly, we compared the accuracy of ET and transcutaneous CO_2 monitoring in 25 infants and toddlers with respiratory failure (118). ET CO_2 to $PaCO_2$ comparison revealed a bias of −6.7 and a precision of 5.0 mm Hg; transcutaneous CO_2 to $PaCO_2$ comparison revealed a bias of only −0.7 and a precision of 2.4 mm Hg. A subsequent study in older children revealed similar findings (119), with transcutaneous CO_2 monitoring proving to be more accurate and well within the limits of clinical usefulness in both age groups. Of note, we found that removal of patients with significant parenchymal lung disease or status asthmaticus from the analysis significantly improved the accuracy of ET CO_2 monitoring, suggesting that, despite significant limitations, this technology still may have useful applications in neonatal and pediatric critical care (119). Additionally, ET CO_2 monitoring may be of unique assistance during cardiopulmonary resuscitation efforts. In the absence of pulmonary blood flow, CO_2 exchange ceases and ET CO_2 levels decrease to zero. Whereas ET CO_2 levels increase slightly with the initiation of cardiopulmonary resuscitation, a sharp rise in ET CO_2 occurs with restoration of spontaneous circulation and may be the first indicator of reperfusion (131). This has led some researchers to suggest a promising role for ET CO_2 monitoring as an objective measure of the effectiveness of resuscitative efforts during cardiopulmonary arrest (125).

Applications during Neonatal and Pediatric Transport

The demonstration by Usher of improved neonatal outcomes through the use of dedicated neonatal ICUs (132) was a key step in the evolution of our present-day system of regionalized neonatal critical care. This consequently necessitated the development of comprehensive neonatal transport systems, and thousands of critically ill infants are now transported yearly. The noise and turbulence present in both air and ground transport vehicles, however, make accurate clinical assessment during transport challenging (133), and the transport team relies heav-

ily on patient monitors, particularly for the assessment of pulmonary status. With the possible exception of the Masimo SET technology (110), pulse oximeters may function poorly during transport. Transcutaneous monitors, however, are both reliable in the neonate and are less sensitive to the effects of motion and turbulence and may offer a distinct advantage in assessing oxygenation during transport. Additionally, we previously documented the usefulness of transcutaneous CO_2 monitoring for guiding adjustments to ventilatory support during transport (134). Conversely, in the tiny preterm infant, the difference between endotracheal intubation and extubation is measured in millimeters, and accidental extubation is a real concern. In this setting, transcutaneous monitors are of little clinical usefulness because they react relatively slowly to changes in $PaCO_2$. On the other hand, the immediate response and graphic representation of CO_2 patterns make capnography ideally suited to rapid detection of endotracheal tube problems, particularly extubation (135). In fact, the transport section of the American Academy of Pediatrics considers the ET capnometer as standard equipment during pediatric and neonatal transport (136). Although the less bulky colorimetric capnograph may also be helpful, its greater dead space may limit its usefulness, at least for continuous monitoring, in the tiny neonate or preterm infant. Finally, recent advances in technology have enabled the transport of infants on high-frequency ventilation, inhaled nitric oxide, and ECMO. Although these advances are exciting, they also place increased demands on the quality of intratransport monitoring and will necessitate continued improvements in these technologies.

Invasive Methods

Ex Vivo, Whole-blood Gas Analysis

An additional advance on the use of near-patient blood-gas analysis has been the development of in-line whole-blood gas analyzers, two of which were evaluated in the clinical environment. The CDI 2000 (CDI-3M Healthcare) was developed in the late 1980s. It uses fluorescent optode technology to measure independently pH, Po_2, and Pco_2. The optodes are housed within a sensor cassette, which is placed in series with the arterial catheter tubing system. A single-sensor calibration is required prior to insertion. This process takes roughly 30 minutes and can be performed easily with a calibration cuvette containing two gases of known concentration that is packaged with the sensor (137). The VIA V-ABG bedside monitoring system (VIA Medical) was designed for in-line placement with an indwelling arterial catheter and has since been modified (VIA LVM Blood Gas and Chemistry Monitoring System) for use with umbilical arterial catheters. This system uses ion-sensitive electrodes to measure pH and Pco_2, and an amperometric Clark electrode to measure Po_2. This device has the added advantage of also measuring sodium and potassium (ion-sensitive electrode) and hematocrit (electric conductance) (138). With this device, calibration fluid continuously flows through the sensor, and calibration occurs automatically every 30 minutes (139). With both devices, intermittent blood-gas analysis is performed by stopping the flow of arterial-line fluid into the patient and allowing arterial blood to flow retrograde into the sensor cassette. The analysis takes less than 2 minutes and, on completion, the sample blood is returned to the patient by flushing the cassette with the arterial-line solution. Therefore, direct blood-gas measurement is performed without resultant blood loss. This design could be of particular benefit to the neonate in whom, as previously mentioned, iatrogenic anemia is a significant clinical problem. These devices also may avoid some of the problems associated with the use of *in vivo* fiberoptic technology (see later). Fluorescent dyes are stable over time, and problems with drift are less likely (140). Because nothing is inserted directly into the arterial catheter itself, there should be minimal problems with catheter thrombosis and dampening of the arterial waveform. The need for a larger-bore cannula is also removed, which should facilitate easier application to smaller children. By decreasing the frequency with which the system is accessed for *in vitro* blood analyses, these systems may decrease the risk of arterial-line infection. These advantages are offset by the fact that analysis is still intermittent and therefore not continuous. Although analyses can be performed as often as every 3 to 6 minutes, automatic cycling is not yet possible, making this near approximation of continuous monitoring highly impractical.

Applications of this technology are still limited and have occurred mostly in adults. Shapiro and colleagues evaluated the CDI 2000 in 117 critically ill patients (141). The device was used for 1 to 4 days and functioned well with no significant effect on the arterial waveform tracing, no sensor failures, and no evidence of thrombus formation within the device. A total of 1,341 simultaneous in-line and conventional ABGs were compared. This comparison revealed a bias and precision of 0.004 and 0.027 for pH, 2.2 and 8.7 torr for PO_2, and 0.8 and 2.4 torr for PCO_2, leading these researchers to conclude that this system could replace the use of blood-gas analyzers in critically ill patients with indwelling arterial access. Subsequently, Mahutte and colleagues compared the CDI 2000 with conventional *in vitro* ABG analysis in 683 samples from 50 critically ill adults and reported similar results (142). Despite these promising results, further evaluation of this device has not been reported, and its present clinical status appears unclear. Initial experience with the VIA V-ABG device in 19 healthy volunteers was positive, with a reported bias and precision of 0.01 and 0.04 for pH, 0.4 and 4.8 for PCO_2, and 1 and 17 for PO_2 (138). A single study has evaluated the VIA LVM system in 16 neonates (139). In-line results were compared with conventional ABG analysis in 229 paired samples. No sensor failures occurred during in-line use. Analysis of the effluent from the sensor revealed an average of 24 μL of blood loss per sample tested, compared with 250 μL required for conventional analysis (excluding discard). No evidence of significant hemolysis within the device was detected. These investigators also found excellent concordance with conventional ABG analysis, with a bias and precision of 0.003 and 0.024 for pH, 0.39 and 7.3 for PO_2, and 0.35 and 2.84 for PCO_2, differences that are well within the range of clinical acceptability. These researchers concluded that routine use of this technology in neonatal critical care holds promise and may be important in reducing the need for transfusions in this setting but recognized the need for further study.

In Vivo Assessment

Fiberoptic Technology

Continuous measurement of pH using an *in vivo* device was described originally in 1927 (143). In the 1960s and 1970s,

ongoing refinement of the technology resulted in the availability of single-parameter sensors capable of measuring *in vivo* pH, PCO_2, or PO_2. The initial technology was fraught with several problems, however, most importantly thrombus formation, vessel occlusion, and excessive drift of the values, thereby limiting their clinical utility. The Paratrend 7 (Agilent Technologies) has refined this technology into a single filament containing a Clark electrochemical sensor to measure PO_2, optical sensors to measure PCO_2 and pH, and a thermocoupler to determine temperature, enabling temperature correction of blood gas values. These components are held together in a heparin-coated, microporous, polyethylene filament that has an outside diameter of less than 0.5 mm, thereby allowing placement through a 20-gauge cannula. Prior to placement, three precision gas mixtures are used to calibrate PO_2, PCO_2, and pH. This process requires 20 to 30 minutes. The manufacturer's operating handbook reports the following specifications for the measured variables: (a) range—PO_2 20 to 500 mm Hg, PCO_2 10 to 80 mm Hg, pH 6.80 to 7.80, temperature 10° to 42°C; (b) accuracy—PO_2 ± 5% with a PO_2 less than 120 mm Hg and ±10% with a PO_2 greater than or equal to 120 mm Hg, PCO_2 ±3 mm Hg, pH ± 0.03, temperature ± 0.2°C; and (c) drift—PO_2 less than 1% per hour; PCO_2 less than 1% per hour, pH less than 0.005 per hour. Following calibration, the device is inserted through the cannula so that the distal end of the filament floats freely in blood. A recent modification of the original design (the Neotrend) is longer than the original version, thereby allowing placement through an umbilical artery catheter for use in the neonatal population.

The initial applications of the Paratrend system included adults in both the critical care and the perioperative settings (144,145). Subsequent clinical experience and trials demonstrated the efficacy of this device in the neonatal, infant, and pediatric populations. Weiss and colleagues evaluated the Paratrend in 24 patients aged 1 to 21 years who were receiving mechanical ventilation for respiratory failure (146). The device was placed through a 20-gauge cannula in either the radial or femoral artery and was used for a mean of 101 hours and a maximum of 238 hours in one patient. A total of 414 ABGs were obtained. The bias and precision were 0.005 and 0.030 for pH, −1.8 and 6.3 mm Hg for PCO_2, and 1.2 and 24 mm Hg for PO_2. Technical problems on insertion occurred in five patients and included clot formation around the sensor in three and failure of the sensor in two patients as a result of either sensor malfunction or kinking during the insertion process. These researchers concluded that the sensor provided an accurate and clinically useful tool in the pediatric patient. Hatherill and associates evaluated the Paratrend sensor in ten infants following cardiac surgical procedures, including Norwood stage I, Glenn shunt arterial switch, and tetralogy of Fallot repair (147). Ten simultaneous ABG and Paratrend values were obtained from each patient. These investigators reported a bias and precision of 0.02 and 0.06 for pH, −0.44 and 0.74 kPa for PCO_2, and 0.04 and 0.87 kPa for PO_2, confirming the accuracy and utility of this monitor in pediatric patients.

One disadvantage of this system, however, is the requirement for a 20-gauge arterial cannula. In the younger patient, this may necessitate femoral artery cannulation, whereas peripheral arterial access tends to be the more common and preferred practice in pediatric ICU patients. Additionally, our clinical experience suggests that when the Paratrend 7 sensor is inserted through a 20-gauge arterial catheter, the waveform is slightly dampened, making BP measurements somewhat inaccurate. In an attempt to overcome such problems, we evaluated the use of the Paratrend 7 sensor inserted into the venous system through a peripheral intravenous site (148). This study included 23 children aged 2 months to 18 years who required mechanical ventilation for respiratory failure. The catheter was inserted through an 18- to 22-gauge catheter into an antecubital ($n = 13$), forearm ($n = 6$), or saphenous ($n = 4$) vein. The duration of sensor use ranged from 3 to 12 days. Three catheters required replacement because of breakage caused by excessive patient movement. Accurate reading occasionally necessitated withdrawal, saline flushing, and reinsertion of the sensor. In two patients treated with hypothermia for control of ICP, significant deviation of the sensor values from the ABG values was corrected by wrapping the extremity in blankets to return its temperature to core body temperature. The bias and precision for arterial values and those obtained from the venous Paratrend 7 sensor were 0.03 and 0.03 for pH and −2.1 and 2.7 mm Hg for PCO_2. During venous insertion, the monitor may be calibrated and corrected for arterial–venous differences. We have found, however, that when there is a decrease in cardiac output, the arterial–venous gradient for PCO_2 may widen substantially (149). Therefore, although venous use of the Paratrend may be of clinical utility, values must be interpreted with caution and in the context of the patient's hemodynamic status. Additionally, venous placement eliminates the possibility of measuring PaO_2, although this may be of little consequence because arterial oxygenation is most commonly estimated noninvasively with pulse oximetry. As a follow-up to the preceding study, Tobias investigated the use of the longer Neotrend sensor inserted through a pulmonary artery or central venous catheter in three infants (149). In two of these infants, the sensor was inserted through a 4-French catheter, surgically placed into the pulmonary artery during repair of congenital heart disease and through the distal port of a 5-French, 8-cm, triple-lumen catheter in one infant treated for sepsis. This application has the advantage of eliminating the need for peripheral intravenous access, sometimes difficult in critically ill infants. The sensor initially was calibrated against an arterial value to compensate for the normal venous to arterial gradient. In 14 sample sets, the differences between Neotrend and arterial values were 0.02 ± 0.009 for pH and 2.4 ± 0.8 mm Hg for PCO_2. Of note, there was a significant discrepancy between the sensor values for oxygen saturation and the mixed venous oxygen saturation values measured by co-oximetry ($9\% \pm 5\%$). The Paratrend sensor calculates oxygen saturation from the measured PO_2 using the normal hemoglobin saturation nomograph. The normal variability of PO_2 measurement is $\pm 5\%$ at PO_2 values lower than 120 mm Hg. This minor variation is of no clinical significance on the arterial side. On the venous side, however, where PO_2 is 60 mm Hg or lower, small discrepancies can alter PO_2 by 2 to 3 mm Hg and oxygen saturation by 3% to 5% because of the steep slope of the oxyhemoglobin dissociation curve. Because mixed venous oxygen saturation is used as an indicator of cardiovascular function and cardiac output in various pathologic processes, this difference may be clinically significant and may limit the value of the Paratrend for this application.

Finally, although most studies to date focused on the use of the Paratrend/Neotrend for measuring PO_2 and PCO_2 during respiratory failure and mechanical ventilation, other clinical sce-

narios exist (e.g., diabetic ketoacidosis or lactic acidosis from shock or metabolic defects) during which the measurement of pH is of primary interest (150,151). Whereas only individual case reports exist, the correlation found between measured values for pH and those reported by the monitor provided a clinically useful estimate of this physiologic variable.

CONCLUSIONS

Advances in both biochemical and other diagnostic technology continue to revolutionize the practice of medicine. The traditional milieu of centralized biochemical and radiologic facilities, however, frequently separates the test from both the subject and his or her health care providers, which can both delay and depersonalize health care provision. Clearly, the development of POCT capabilities has helped to remedy some of these concerns. Rapid test results are now the norm instead of the exception, enabling management decisions to be made on the basis of relevant rather than outdated data. Particularly in the critical care environment, this is both necessary and invaluable. As testing and approval of therapeutic advances for children tend to occur frustratingly slowly; it is encouraging that pediatric and neonatal applications of POCT do not appear to have met with the same delays. Biochemical analyzers have, where clinically relevant, been well evaluated, and newer, more invasive technologies such as *in vivo* blood gas analyzers have been adapted relatively rapidly for neonatal and pediatric applications. The data show without a doubt that applications of POCT are possible, accurate, and relevant in this population. Of particular value to the neonate will be evaluation of in-line analyzers to assess electrolytes and blood gases in an effort to decrease phlebotomy-related anemia. The use of fluorescent dyes in these analyzers raises the interesting, if maybe overoptimistic, possibility of expanding transcutaneous technology to the assessment of hematologic and electrolyte variables, further decreasing the need for phlebotomy. In addition, expansions within the transport environment, particularly the transport of patients receiving ECMO support or other highly invasive technologies, will mandate increased evaluation of available portable biochemical analyzers. We live in a time, however, when technologic advances must be evaluated against two additional, and sometimes conflicting, yardsticks: the ability to improve patient care and outcome and the ability to do so in a more cost-effective manner. Whereas there are many reasons to believe that these yardsticks can be surpassed, convincing data remain to be gathered and must become the next focus of study if the necessary advancement of pediatric patient-focused care is to continue.

REFERENCES

1. Kost GJ. Point-of-care testing in intensive care. In: Tobin MJ, ed. *Principles and practice of intensive care monitoring.* New York: McGraw-Hill, 1997:1267–1296.
2. Kost GJ, Wiese DA, Bowen TP. New whole blood methods and instruments: glucose measurement and test menus for critical care. *J Int Fed Clin Chem* 1991;3:160–172.
3. Collison ME, Meyerhoff ME. Chemical sensors for bedside monitoring of critically ill patients. *Biochim Clin* 1990;14:1288–1296.
4. Salem M, Chernow B, Burke R, et al. Bedside diagnostic testing: its

accuracy, rapidity, and utility in blood conservation. *JAMA* 1991;266: 382–389.

5. McLean FC, Hastings AB. A biological method for the estimation of calcium ion concentration. *J Biol Chem* 1934;107:337–350.

6. Forrest ARW, Shenkin. Dangerous pseudohyponatremia. *Lancet* 1980; 2:1256.

7. Ohls RK. Developmental erythropoiesis. In: Polin RA, Fox WW, eds. *Fetal and neonatal physiology*. 2nd ed. Philadelphia: WB Saunders, 1998:1762–1786.

8. Ramasethu J, Luban NLC. Red blood cell transfusions in the newborn. *Semin Neonatol* 1999;4:5–16.

9. Ohls RK, Harcum J, Davila G, et al. Serum erythropoietin levels fail to increase after significant phlebotomy losses in preterm infants. *J Perinatol* 1997;17:465–467.

10. Maier RF, Obladen M, Scigalla P, et al. The effect of epoetin beta (recombinant human erythropoietin) on the need for transfusions in very low birth weight infants. *N Engl J Med* 1994;330:1173–1178.

11. Ohls RK, Harcum J, Schibler KR, et al. The effect of erythropoietin on the transfusion requirements of preterm infants weighing 750 grams or less: a randomized, double-blind, placebo-controlled study. *J Pediatr* 1997;131:661–665.

12. Wilson JR, Gaedeke MK. Blood conservation in neonatal and pediatric populations. *AACN Clin Issues* 1996;7:229–237.

13. Cole MD, Peevy K. Hypoglycemia in normal neonates appropriate for gestational age. *J Perinatol* 1994;14:118–120.

14. Kalhan SC, Saker F. Metabolic and endocrine disorders. In: Fanaroff AA, Martin RJ eds. *Neonatal-perinatal medicine: diseases of the fetus and infant*, 6th ed. St. Louis: Mosby, 1997:1439–1563.

15. Duvanel CB, Fawer C-L, Cotting J, et al. Long-term effects of neonatal hypoglycemia on brain growth and psychomotor development in small-for-gestational-age preterm infants. *J Pediatr* 1999;134:492–498.

16. Zanardo V, Cagdas S, Golin R, et al. Risk factors for hypoglycemia in premature infants. *Fetal Diagn Ther* 1999;14:63–67.

17. Halamek LP, Stevenson DK. Neonatal hypoglycemia, Part II: pathophysiology and therapy. *Clin Pediatr* 1998;37:11–16.

18. Pildes RS, Cornblath M, Warren I, et al. A prospective, controlled study of neonatal hypoglycemia. *Pediatrics* 1974;54:5–15.

19. Lucas A, Morley R. Cole TJ. Adverse neurodevelopmental outcome of moderate neonatal hypoglycaemia. *BMJ* 1988;297:1304–1308.

20. Chmielewski SA. Advances and strategies for glucose monitoring. *Am J Clin Pathol* 1995;104(Suppl 1):S59–S71.

21. Ellis M, Manandhar DS, Manandhar N, et al. Comparison of two cotside methods for the detection of hypoglycaemia among neonates in Nepal. *Arch Dis Child* 1996;75:F122–F125.

22. Leonard M, Chessall M, Manning D. The use of a HemoCue blood glucose analyser in a neonatal unit. *Ann Clin Biochem* 1997;34:287–290.

23. Deshpande SA, Matthews JNS, Ward Platt MP. Measuring blood glucose in neonatal units: how does Hemocue compare? *Arch Dis Child* 1996;75:F202–F208.

24. Schlebusch H, Niesen M, Sorger M, et al. Blood glucose determinations in newborns: four instruments compared. *Pediatr Pathol Lab Med* 1998;18:41–48.

25. Kirkham P, Watkins A. Comparison of two reflectance photometers in the assessment of neonatal hypoglycaemia. *Arch Dis Child* 1995;73: F170–F173.

26. Altimier LB, Roberts W. One Touch II hospital system for neonates: correlation with serum glucose values. *Neonatal Network* 1996;15:15–19.

27. Conrad PD, Sparks JW, Osberg I, et al. Clinical application of a new glucose analyzer in the neonatal intensive care unit: comparison with other methods. *J Pediatr* 1989;114:281–287.

28. Innanen VT, DeLand ME, deCampos FM, et al. Point-of-care glucose testing in the neonatal intensive care unit is facilitated by the use of the Ames Glucometer Elite electrochemical glucose meter. *J Pediatr* 1995;130:151–155.

29. Demers LM, Smith B. Application of the MediSense Precision-G blood glucose testing system in a neonatal intensive care unit. *Clin Chem* 1999;45:1578–1579.

30. Goldberg JD, Franklin B, Lasser D. et al. Gestational diabetes: impact of home glucose monitoring on neonatal birth weight. *Am J Obstet Gynecol* 1986;154:546–550.

31. Wechter DJ, Kaufmann RC, Amankwah KS, et al. Prevention of neona-tal macrosomia in gestational diabetes by the use of intensive dietary therapy and home glucose monitoring. *Am J Perinatol* 1991;8:131–134.

32. Langer O, Rodriguez DA, Xenakis EMJ, et al. Intensified versus conventional management of gestational diabetes. *Am J Obstet Gynecol* 1994;170:1036–1047.

33. Ladenson JH, Lewis JW, Boyd JC. Failure of total calcium corrected for protein, albumin, and pH to correctly assess free calcium status. *J Clin Endocrinol Metab* 1978;46:986–993.

34. Wandrup J, Kroner J, Pryds O, et al. Age-related reference values for ionized calcium in the first week of life in premature and full-term infants. *Scand J Clin Lab Invest* 1988;48:255–260.

35. Lougheed JL, Mimouni F, Tsang RC. Serum ionized calcium concentrations in normal neonates. *Am J Dis Child* 1988;142:516–518.

36. Mimouni F, Tsang RC. Neonatal hypocalcemia: to treat or not to treat (a review). *J Am Coll Nutr* 1994;13:408–415.

37. Brauman J, Delvigne CH, Deconnick I, et al. Factors affecting the determination of ionized calcium in blood. *Scand J Clin Lab Invest* 1983;43(Suppl165): 27–31.

38. Kost GJ, Jammel MA, Ward RE, et al. Monitoring of ionized calcium during human hepatic transplantation: critical values and their relevance to cardiac and hemodynamic function. *Am J Clin Pathol* 1986; 86:61–70.

39. Toffaletti J. Physiology and regulation: ionized calcium, magnesium and lactate measurements in critical care settings. *Am J Clin Pathol* 1995;104(Suppl 1):S88–S94.

40. Eriksson M, Zetterstrom R. Neonatal convulsions. Incidence and causes in the Stockholm area. *Acta Paediatr Scand* 1979;68:807–811.

41. Keen JH. Significance of hypocalcaemia in neonatal convulsions. *Arch Dis Child* 1969;44:356–361.

42. Venkataramen PS, Wilson DA, Sheldon RE, et al. Effect of hypocalcemia on cardiac function in very-low-birth-weight preterm neonates: studies of blood ionized calcium, echocardiography, and cardiac effect of intravenous calcium therapy. *Pediatrics* 1985;76:543–550.

43. Bifano E, Kavey RE, Pergolizzi J, et al. The cardiopulmonary effects of calcium infusion in infants with persistent pulmonary hypertension of the newborn. *Pediatr Res* 1989;25:262–265.

44. Meliones JN, Moler FW, Custer JR, et al. Hemodynamic instability after the initiation of extracorporeal membrane oxygenation: role of ionized calcium. *Crit Care Med* 1991;19:1247–1251.

45. Meliones JN, Moler FW, Custer JR, et al. Normalization of priming solution ionized calcium concentration improves hemodynamic instability of neonates receiving venovenous ECMO. *ASAOI J* 1995;41: 884–888.

46. Sanchez GJ, Venkataramen PS, Pryor RW, et al. Hypercalcitonemia and hypocalcemia in acutely ill children: studies in serum calcium, blood ionized calcium, and calcium-regulating hormones. *J Pediatr* 1989;114:952–956.

47. Cardenas-Rivero N, Chernow B, Stolko MA, et al. Hypocalcemia in critically ill children. *J Pediatr* 1989;114:946–951.

48. Broner CW, Stidham GL, Westenkirchner DF, et al. Hypermagnesemia and hypocalcemia as predictors of high mortality in critically ill pediatric patients. *Crit Care Med* 1990;18:921–928.

49. Vincent J-L. Lactate levels in critically ill patients. *Acta Anesthesiol Scand* 1995;39:261–266.

50. Hotchkiss RS, Karl IE. Reevaluation of the role of cellular hypoxia and bioenergetic failure in sepsis. *JAMA* 1992;18:1503–1510.

51. Brinkert W, Rommes JH, Bakker J. Lactate measurement in critically ill patients with a hand-held analyser. *Intensive Care Med* 1999;25: 966–969.

52. Slomovitz BM, Lavery RF, Tortella BJ, et al. Validation of a hand-held lactate device in determination of blood lactate in critically injured patients. *Crit Care Med* 1998;26:1523-1528.

53. Smith NC, Soutter WP, Sharp F, et al. Fetal scalp blood lactate as an indicator of intrapartum hypoxia. *Br J Obstet Gynaecol* 1983;90: 821–831.

54. Westgren N, Kruger K, Ek S, et al. Lactate compared with pH analysis at fetal scalp blood sampling: a prospective randomised study. *Br J Obstet Gynaecol* 1998;105:29–33.

55. da Silva S, Hennebert N, Denis R, et al. Clinical value of a single postnatal lactate measurement after intrapartum asphyxia. *Acta Pediatr* 2000;89:320–323.

56. Beca JP, Scopes JW. Serial determination of blood lactate in respiratory distress syndrome. *Arch Dis Child* 1972;47:550–557.

57. Deshpande SA, Ward-Platt MP. Association between blood lactate and acid-base status and mortality in ventilated babies. *Arch Dis Child* 1997;76:F15–F20.

58. Charpie JR, Dekeon MK, Goldberg CS, et al. Serial blood lactate measurements predict early outcome after neonatal repair or palliation for complex congenital heart disease. *J Thorac Cardiovasc Surg* 2000;120:73–80.

59. Cheung P-Y, Finer NN. Plasma lactate concentration as a predictor of death in neonates with severe hypoxemia requiring extracorporeal membrane oxygenation. *J Pediatr* 1994;125:763–768.

60. Cheung P-Y, Robertson CMT, Finer NN. Plasma lactate as a predictor of early childhood neurodevelopmental outcome of neonates with severe hypoxaemia requiring extracorporeal membrane oxygenation. *Arch Dis Child* 1996;74:F47–F50.

61. Duke T, Butt W, South M, et al. Early markers of major adverse events in children after cardiac operations. *J Thorac Cardiovasc Surg* 1997;114:1042–1052.

62. Izraeli S, Ben-Sira L, Harrell D, et al. Lactic acid as a predictor for erythrocyte transfusion in healthy preterm infants with anemia of prematurity. *J Pediatr* 1993;1222:629–631.

63. Oberhardt BJ. Thrombosis and hemostasis testing at the point of care. *Am J Clin Pathol* 1995;104(Suppl 1):S72–S78.

64. Nuss R, Hays T, Manco-Johnson M. Efficacy and safety of heparin anticoagulation for neonatal renal vein thrombosis. *Am J Pediatr Hem Oncol* 1994;16:127–132.

65. D'Errico C, Shayevitz JR, Martindale SJ. Age-related differences in heparin sensitivity and heparin-protamine interactions in cardiac surgery patients. *J Cardiothorac Vasc Anesth* 1996;10:451–457.

66. Graves DF, Chernin JM, Kurusz M, Zwischenberger JB. Anticoagulation practices during neonatal extracorporeal membrane oxygenation: survey results. *Perfusion* 1996;11:461–466.

67. Malviya S. Monitoring and management of anticoagulation in children requiring extracorporeal circulation. *Semin Hemost Thromb* 1997;23:563–567.

68. Urlesberger B, Zobel G, Zenz W, et al. Activation of the clotting system during extracorporeal membrane oxygenation in term newborn infants. *J Pediatr* 1996;129:264–268.

69. Howell GC, Hatley RM, Davis JB, et al. Successful gastrorrhaphy on ECMO. *J Pediatr Surg* 1988;23:1161–1162.

70. Hirthler MA, Blackwell E, Abbe D, et al. Coagulation parameter instability as an early predictor of intracranial hemorrhage during extracorporeal membrane oxygenation. *J Pediatr Surg* 1992;27:40–43.

71. Haycock GB, Aperia A. Salt and the newborn kidney. *Pediatr Nephrol* 1991;5:65–70.

72. Al-Dahhan J, Haycock GB, Chantler C, et al. Sodium homeostasis in term and preterm neonates. I: Renal aspects. *Arch Dis Child* 1983;58:335–342.

73. Murthy JN, Hicks JM, Soldin SJ. Evaluation of i-STAT portable clinical analyzer in a neonatal and pediatric intensive care unit. *Clin Biochem* 1997;30:385–389.

74. Alex CP, Manto JC, Garland JS. Clinical utility of a bedside blood analyzer for measuring blood chemistry values in neonates. *J Perinatol* 1998;18:45–48.

75. Garland JS, Manto J. Clinical accuracy of a bedside laboratory analyzer (BLA) for rapid determination of blood hematocrit and chemistries. *Pediatr Res* 1995;37:206A(abst).

76. Lelievre-Pegorier M, Merlet-Benichou C, Roinel N, et al. Developmental pattern of water and electrolyte transport in rat superficial nephrons. *Am J Physiol* 1983;245:F15–F21.

77. Engle WD. Potassium transport in early development. In: Polin RA, Fox WW, eds. *Fetal and neonatal physiology,* 2nd ed. Philadelphia: WB Saunders, 1998:1612–1615.

78. Stefano JL, Norman ME, Morales MC, et al. Decreased erythrocyte Na+,K+-ATPase activity associated with cellular potassium loss in extremely low birth weight infants with nonoliguric hyperkalemia. *J Pediatr* 1993;122:276–284.

79. Leslie GI, Carman G, Arnold JD. Early neonatal hyperkalemia in the extremely premature newborn infant. *J Paediatr Child Health* 1990;26:58–61.

80. Shaffer SG, Kilbride HW, Hayen LK, et al. Hyperkalemia in very low birth weight infants. *J Pediatr* 1992;121:275–279.

81. Hall TL, Barnes A, Miller JR, et al. Neonatal mortality following transfusion of red cells with high plasma potassium levels. *Transfusion* 1993;33:606–609.

82. Yucel D, Dalva K. Effect of *in vitro* hemolysis on 25 common biochemical tests. *Clin Chem* 1992;38:575–577.

83. Task Force on Brain Death in Children. Guidelines for the determination of brain death in children. *Pediatrics* 1987;80:298–300.

84. Ashwal S. Brain death in the newborn. *Clin Perinatol* 1989;16:501–518.

85. Canadian Neurocritical Care Group. Guidelines for the diagnosis of brain death. *Can J Neurol Sci* 1999;26:64–66.

86. Van Lieshout HBM, Jacobs JWFM, Rottveel JJ, et al. The prognostic value of the EEG in asphyxiated newborns. *Acta Neurol Scand* 1995;91:203–207.

87. Sinclair DB, Campbell M, Byrne P, et al. EEG and long-term outcome of term infants with neonatal hypoxic-ischemic encephalopathy. *Clin Neurophysiol* 1999;110:655–659.

88. Hellstrom-Westas L, Rosen I, Svenningsen NW. Predictive value of early continuous amplitude integrated EEG recordings on outcome after severe birth asphyxia in full term infants. *Arch Dis Child* 1995;72:F34–F38.

89. Hellstrom-Westas L. Comparison between tape-recorded and amplitude-integrated EEG in sick neonates. *Acta Paediatr* 1993;81:812–818.

90. Toet MC, Hellstrom-Westas L, Groenendaal F, et al. Amplitude integrated EEG 3 and 6 hours after birth in full term neonates with hypoxic-ischaemic encephalopathy. *Arch Dis Child* 1999;81:F19–F23.

91. Volpe JJ. Commentary: brain death determination in the newborn. *Pediatrics* 1987;80:293–297.

92. American Electroencephalographic Society. Guidelines in EEG 1-7 (revised 1985). *J Clin Neurophysiol* 1986;3:131–168.

93. Green JB, Lauber A. Return of EEG activity after electrocerebral silence: two case reports. *J Neurol Neurosurg Psychiatry* 1972;35:103–107.

94. Pezzani C, Radvanyi-Bouvet MF, Relier J-P, et al. Neonatal electroencephalography during the first twenty-four hours of life in full-term newborn infants. *Neuropediatrics* 1986;17:11–18.

95. Cammarano WB, Pittet JF, Weitz S, et al. Acute withdrawal syndrome related to the administration of analgesic and sedative medications in adult intensive care unit patients. *Crit Care Med* 1998;26:676–684.

96. Vernon JM, Lang E, Sebel PS, et al. Prediction of movement using bispectral electroencephalographic analysis during propofol/alfentanil or isoflurane/alfentanil anesthesia. *Anesth Analg* 1995;80:780–785.

97. Tobias JD, Berkenbosch JW. Tolerance during sedation in a pediatric ICU patient: effects on the BIS monitor. *J Clin Anesth* 2001;13:122–124.

97a. Berkenbosch JW, Fichter CR, Tobias JD. Correlation of the BIS monitor with clinical sedation scores during mechanical ventilation in the pediatric intesive care unit. *Anesth Analg* (in press).

98. Ashwal S, Schneider S, Thompson J. Xenon computed tomography cerebral flow in the determination of brain death in children. *Ann Neurol* 1989;25:539–546.

99. McMenamin JB, Volpe JJ. Doppler ultrasonography in the determination of neonatal brain death. *Ann Neurol* 1983;14:302–307.

100. Ducrocq X, Braun M, Debouverie M, et al. Brain death and transcranial doppler: experience in 130 cases of brain dead patients. *J Neurol Sci* 1998;160:41–46.

101. Hadani M, Bruk B, Ram Z, et al. Application of transcranial doppler ultrasonography for the diagnosis of brain death. *Intensive Care Med* 1999;25:822–828.

102. Goodman J, Heck L. Confirmation of brain death at bedside by isotope angiography. *JAMA* 1977;238:966–968.

103. Schwartz JA, Baxter J, Brill DR. Diagnosis of brain death in children by radionuclide cerebral imaging. *Pediatrics* 1984;73:14–18.

104. Holzman BH, Curless RG, Sfakianakis GN, et al. Radionuclide cerebral perfusion scintigraphy in determination of brain death in children. *Neurology* 1983;33:1027–1031.

105. Ashwal S, Schneider S. Brain death in the newborn. *Pediatrics* 1989;84:429–437.

106. Zimmerman JL, Dellinger RP. Blood gas monitoring. *Crit Care Clin* 1996;12:865–874.

107. Meliones JN, Wilson BG, Cheifetz IM. Respiratory monitoring. In: Rogers MC, ed. *Textbook of pediatric intensive care.* Baltimore: Williams & Wilkins, 1996:331–363.

108. Barrington KJ, Finer NN, Ryan CA. Evaluation of pulse oximetry as a continuous monitoring technique in the neonatal intensive care unit. *Crit Care Med* 1988;16:1147–1153.

109. Hay WW, Brockway JM, Eyzaguirre M. Neonatal pulse oximetry: accuracy and reliability. *Pediatrics* 1989;83:717–722.

110. Malviya S, Reynolds PI, Voepel-Lewis T, et al. False alarms and sensitivity of conventional pulse oximetry versus the Masimo SET™ technology in the pediatric postanesthetic care unit. *Anesth Analg* 2000; 90:1336–1340.

111. Moyle JTB. Uses and abuses of pulse oximetry. *Arch Dis Child* 1996; 74:77–80.

112. Barker SJ, Novak S, Morgan S. The performance of three pulse oximeters during low perfusion in volunteers. *Anesthesiology* 1997; 87:A409.

113. Bucher HU, Fanconi S, Baeckert P, et al. Hyperoxia in newborn infants: detection by pulse oximetry. *Pediatrics* 1989;84:226–230.

114. Jubran A, Tobin MJ. Monitoring gas exchange during mechanical ventilation. In: Tobin MJ, ed. *Principles and practice of mechanical ventilation.* New York: McGraw-Hill, 1994:991–943.

115. Palmisano BW, Severinghaus JW. Transcutaneous PCO_2 and PO_2: a multicenter study of accuracy. *J Clin Monit Comput* 1990;6:189–195.

116. McEvedy BAB, McLeod ME, Mulera M, et al. End-tidal, transcutaneous, and arterial PCO_2 measurements in critically ill neonates: a comparative study. *Anesthesiology* 1988;69:112–116.

117. Bhat R, Kim WD, Shukla A, et al. Simultaneous tissue pH and transcutaneous carbon dioxide monitoring in critically ill neonates. *Crit Care Med* 1981;9:744–749.

118. Tobias JD, Meyer DJ. Noninvasive monitoring of carbon dioxide during respiratory failure in toddlers and infants: end-tidal versus transcutaneous carbon dioxide. *Anesth Analg* 1997;85:55–58.

119. Berkenbosch JW, Lam J, Burd RS, et al. Noninvasive monitoring of carbon dioxide during mechanical ventilation in older children: end-tidal versus transcutaneous techniques. *Anesth Analg* 2001;92:1427–1431.

119a Berkenbosch JW, Tobias JD. Transcutaneous carbon dioxide monitoring during high frequency oscillatory ventilation in infants and children. *Crit Care Med* (2002).

120. Versmold HT, Linderkamp O, Holzmann M, et al. Transcutaneous monitoring of PO_2 in newborn infants: where are the limits? Influence of blood pressure, blood volume, blood flow, viscosity, and acid base state. *Birth Defects* 1979;15:285–294.

121. Tobias JD, Wilson WR, Meyer DJ. Transcutaneous monitoring of carbon dioxide tension after cardiothoracic surgery in infants and children. *Anesth Analg* 1999;88:531–534.

122. Duncan PG, Cohen MM. Pulse oximetry and capnography in anesthetic practice: an epidemiological appraisal. *Can J Anaesth* 1991;38: 619–625.

123. Recommendations for services and personnel for delivery of care in a critical care setting. *Crit Care Med* 1988;16:809–811.

124. Badgwell JM, Heavner JE. End-tidal carbon dioxide pressure in neonates and infants measured by aspiration and flow-through capnography. *J Clin Monit Comput* 1991;7:285–288.

125. Hess DR. Capnometry. In: Tobin MJ, ed. *Principles and practice of intensive care monitoring.* New York: McGraw-Hill, 1997:377–400.

126. Lindahl SG, Yates AP, Hatch DJ. Relationship between invasive and noninvasive measurements of gas exchange in anesthetized infants and children. *Anesthesiology* 1987;66:168—175.

127. Tobias JD, Flanagan JF, Wheeler TJ, et al. Noninvasive monitoring of end-tidal CO_2 via nasal cannula in spontaneously breathing children during the perioperative period. *Crit Care Med* 1994;22:1805–1808.

128. Flanagan JF, Garrett JS, McDuffee A, et al. Noninvasive monitoring of end-tidal carbon dioxide tension via nasal cannulas in spontaneously breathing children with profound hypocarbia. *Crit Care Med* 1995;23:1140–1142.

129. Yamanaka MK, Sue DY. Comparison of arterial-end-tidal PCO_2 dif-

130. Rozycki HJ, Sysyn GD, Marshall MK, et al. Mainstream end-tidal carbon dioxide monitoring in the neonatal intensive care unit. *Pediatrics* 1998;101:648–653.

131. Steedman DJ, Robertson CE. Measurement of end-tidal carbon dioxide concentration during cardiopulmonary resuscitation. *Arch Emerg Med* 1990;7:129–134.

132. Usher RH. The role of the neonatologist. *Pediatr Clin North Am* 1970;19:199–202.

133. Brown LH, Gough JE, Bryan-Berg DM, et al. Assessment of breath sounds during ambulance transport. *Ann Emerg Med* 1997;29: 228–231.

134. O'Connor TA, Grueber R. Transcutaneous measurement of carbon dioxide tension during long-distance transport of neonates receiving mechanical ventilation. *J Perinatol* 1998;18:189–192.

135. Bhende MS, Karr VA, Wiltsie DC, et al. Evaluation of a portable infrared end-tidal carbon dioxide monitor during pediatric interhospital transport. *Pediatrics* 1995;95:875–878.

136. Task Force on Interhospital Transport. *Guidelines for air and ground transport of neonatal and pediatric patients.* American Academy of Pediatrics, 1999:110.

137. Mahutte CK, Sassoon CSH, Muro JR, et al. Progress in the development of a fluorescent intravascular blood gas system in man. *J Clin Monit Comput* 1990;6:147–157.

138. Bailey PL, McJames SW, Chaff ML, et al. Evaluation in volunteers of the VIA V-ABG automated bedside blood gas, chemistry, and hematocrit monitor. *J Clin Monit Comput* 1998;14:339–346.

139. Widness JA, Kulhavey JC, Johnson KJ, et al. Clinical performance of an in-line point-of-care monitor in neonates. *Pediatrics* 2000;106:497–504.

140. Shapiro BA. Clinical and economic performance criteria for intraarterial and extraarterial blood gas monitors, with comparison with *in vitro* testing. *Am J Clin Pathol* 1995;104(Suppl 1):S100–S106.

141. Shapiro BA, Mahutte KC, Cane RD, et al. Clinical performance of a blood gas monitor: a prospective, multicenter trial. *Crit Care Med* 1993;21:487–494.

142. Mahutte CK, Sasse SA, Chen PA, et al. Performance of a patient dedicated, on-demand blood gas monitor in medical ICU patients. *Am J Respir Crit Care Med* 1994;150:865–869.

143. Buytendijk F. The use of the antinomy electrode in the determination of pH *in vivo. Arch Neerland Physiol* 1927;12:319.

144. Pappert D, Rossaint R, Lewandowski K, et al. Preliminary evaluation of a new continuous intra-arterial blood gas monitoring system. *Acta Anaesthesiol Scand* 1995;39(Suppl):67–70.

145. Zollinger A, Spahn DR, Singer T, et al. Accuracy and clinical performance of a continuous intra-arterial blood-gas monitoring system during thoracoscopic surgery. *Br J Anaesth* 1997;79:47–52.

146. Weiss IK, Fink S, Harrison R, et al. Clinical use of continuous arterial blood gas monitoring in the pediatric intensive care unit. *Pediatrics* 1999;103:440–445.

147. Hatherill M, Tibby SM, Durward A, et al. Continuous intra-arterial blood-gas monitoring in infants and children with cyanotic heart disease. *Br J Anaesth* 1997;79:665–667.

148. Tobias JD, Connors D, Strauser L, et al. Continuous pH and PCO_2 monitoring during respiratory failure in children with the Paratrend 7 sensor inserted into the peripheral venous system. *J Pediatr* 2000; 136:623–627.

149. Tobias JD. Continuous pH and PCO_2 monitoring using the Paratrend inserted through a pulmonary artery or central venous catheter. *J Intensive Care Med* 2001;16:151–154.

150. Tobias JD. pH monitoring during diabetic ketoacidosis using the Paratrend 7 continuous blood gas monitoring system. *Pediatr Emerg Care* 1998;14:259–260.

151. Easley RB, Johnson TR, Tobias JD. Continuous pH monitoring using the Paratrend 7 inserted into a peripheral vein during severe metabolic acidosis in a patient with shock and congenital lactic acidosis. *Clin Pediatr* (in press).

18

POINT-OF-CARE TESTING IN THE CHILDREN'S HOSPITAL

THEODORE J. PYSHER
PHILLIP R. BACH
DAVID H. PEDERSEN

POINT-OF-CARE TESTING IN PEDIATRICS

The most important roles for point-of-care testing (POCT) in pediatrics are monitoring critically ill patients and streamlining the patient care process. Rapid acquisition of laboratory results is essential in pediatrics because the patient often cannot provide a reliable clinical history, physical findings may significantly underrepresent the severity of disease, and the patient's condition can change rapidly. In less acute settings, the availability of diagnostic results while the patient and family are still present can greatly facilitate counseling, improve compliance with treatment, and obviate the need for a return visit that would be inconvenient to the patient's family and the health care provider. The small sample required for most POCT is especially appropriate for infants and small children, and the portability of analyzers allows testing to be performed in a variety of inpatient and outpatient settings that have not had access to immediate laboratory testing in the past.

The ideal system for the pediatric patient would provide accurate measurement of key analytes noninvasively or with little or no consumption of blood. Indwelling or so-called patient-attached monitors have been shown to reduce blood loss in critically ill neonates by 90% compared with analysis of similar blood gas and electrolyte tests by *in vitro* micromethods (1). Controversy surrounds the frequency of invasive analysis that is required for optimal patient care (2), however, and as that frequency decreases, the costs and risks of indwelling monitors become prohibitive. Analyses of the costs of other forms of near-patient testing have generally shown them to be more expensive than centralized testing unless one factors in the savings from improved patient care processes (3), but these savings are difficult to convert to actual cost reductions. Further complicating the analysis are the different perceptions clinicians and laboratorians have regarding what constitutes an adequate turnaround time for laboratory results (4). Near-patient testing is almost always well received by clinicians, but efforts to demonstrate a real improvement in the overall patient care process have had mixed results (5,6). The goal of the laboratory service should be to create "patient proximity," either by testing at the point of care (POC) or through optimization of the process of transporting the specimen to the laboratory, performing the analysis, and reporting the results back to the point of care (7). The challenges to achieving this goal are likely to be similar in any institution serving the health care needs of children, and we describe herein how we have dealt with these in our institution.

OVERVIEW OF POINT-OF-CARE TESTING AT PRIMARY CHILDREN'S MEDICAL CENTER

Primary Children's Medical Center (PCMC) developed an approach to POCT that included oversight of approved testing by the clinical laboratory and review of requests for near-patient testing by a committee composed of directors of medical, nursing and laboratory services, and hospital administration and information systems. This committee considered the clinical arguments of the requesting service, the availability of centralized testing, and the relative costs of providing the testing in different venues. In some cases, a request would be approved as submitted. In others, it would be approved with a recommendation that testing be limited to certain categories of patients or that it be performed by different personnel than requested (e.g., phlebotomists or respiratory therapists rather than nurses because the former groups were smaller in number or had more background in laboratory testing). In still other cases, the request would be denied, but the clinical laboratory would be directed to work with the requesting service to improve the situation that led to the request for near-patient testing. The committee was convened in response to a large number of requests for near-patient testing. After these requests were reviewed, there have been few additional requests, and it has been possible for the laboratory director to deal with these by going through the preceding process with the director of the clinical services requesting the testing.

The laboratory director was given the responsibility of implementing approved POCT in accordance with applicable regulations. The laboratory has the primary responsibility for the writing of standard operating procedures (SOPs), the training and competency testing of the personnel who would perform near-patient testing, the maintenance of instruments, and the review of results. Testing personnel perform all quality control and external proficiency tests. Each SOP specifies that results must be communicated immediately to a health care provider responsible for the patient, and, as an added precaution, a printout of the results of blood gas and electrolyte determinations must be given to that provider. The responsibility for documentation of results in the patient's medical record is shared by laboratory and testing personnel. The fundamental tenet is that there is one standard for laboratory testing throughout the hospital and that this standard must include both the quality of testing and the capture of data in the patient's medical and financial records. Initially, near-patient testing was performed under the Clinical Laboratory Improvement Act (CLIA) license of the laboratory director, but in some instances it has been necessary or desirable for a clinical service to obtain its own licensure. These circumstances are discussed in greater detail in the following sections.

Facilities

Children's hospitals and related facilities are usually regional centers for comprehensive pediatric care, and they often serve as the base for a university department of pediatrics or a group of pediatric medical and surgical subspecialists. Local medical history and politics, financial considerations, and the proximity of other facilities providing maternal and child health care determine the actual inpatient and ambulatory services offered by each pediatric medical center. These clinical services, in turn, dictate the laboratory services needed in each facility. The plan to address the need for laboratory services, including near-patient testing, will be influenced by the organization of laboratory services, the quality of laboratory and hospital information systems, the availability of a pneumatic tube system within the institution, and the opportunities for consolidation or sharing of laboratory services in the region. These factors are also important when comparing models for laboratory services, including POCT, between institutions. We, therefore, provide the following description of PCMC.

A tertiary-level pediatric hospital located in Salt Lake City, Utah, PCMC serves the largest geographic area of any children's hospital in the United States, including all of Utah and parts of Idaho, Montana, Nevada, and Wyoming. The hospital is owned by Intermountain Health Care (IHC), a not-for-profit corporation with more than 60 facilities in Utah, Idaho, and Wyoming. PCMC is located on the campus of the University of Utah adjacent to the state-owned University Hospital and 2 miles from the central facility of Associated Regional and University Pathologists (ARUP) Laboratories, a national reference laboratory that is operated by the university's Department of Pathology. PCMC is the principal teaching facility for the university's Department of Pediatrics, and all hospital-based clinicians and surgeons are members of the university faculty.

In the year 2000, PCMC admitted 9,849 patients, performed 10,359 operations, had more than 120,000 outpatient visits, transported 1,363 critically ill patients by air, and saw 33,043 patients in the emergency department. The hospital has 232 inpatient beds, including a 35-bed neonatal and a 26-bed

pediatric intensive care unit (ICU), eight operating rooms, and active endoscopy and cardiac catheterization suites. Outpatient services include all pediatric medical and surgical specialties, outpatient surgery, and diagnostic testing. Many of the subspeciality groups also conduct outreach clinics at several urban and rural sites in Utah and Idaho, some of which are several hundred miles from the hospital.

The building, which was built in 1990, is a single structure encompassing 520,000 square feet (48,000 m²) on four floors. A pneumatic tube system (TransLogic Corporation, Denver, CO, U.S.A.) links nursing units, the laboratory, the pharmacy, outpatient clinics, and supply areas within the hospital; and there is a station in the blood bank of the adjacent University Hospital. About 65% of the 1,000 to 1,500 daily transactions on this system involve the laboratory. Although the system handles one tube at a time, wait times (the delay from when a tube is placed on the system until it begins moving) average 5 to 10 seconds except at peak hours (10:00–18:00), when the wait averages about 30 seconds but seldom exceeds 2 minutes (Fig. 18.1). Tubes are transported in the order in which they are loaded into sending stations, but a tube can be designated as critical and taken ahead of others. To avoid abuse of this feature, it has been limited to delivery of emergency blood products. Transit times are 20 to 40 seconds within the building and 75 to 145 seconds to the University Hospital blood-bank station. Because of the speed of the tube system, the standard phlebotomy practice for essentially all patients is to draw specimens from a patient at the bedside or in the outpatient clinic, immediately tube those specimens to the laboratory and then go to the next patient.

In the year 2000, the laboratory performed 567,153 billable tests (414,908 on inpatients, 152,245 on outpatients). Laboratory orders are received from and results are reported to the hospital information system (HIS, HELP Patient Care System, 3M Health Information Systems, Murray, UT, U.S.A.), which is interfaced to the laboratory information system (LIS, Flexilab, Sunquest Informations Systems, Tucson, AZ, U.S.A.). Labora-

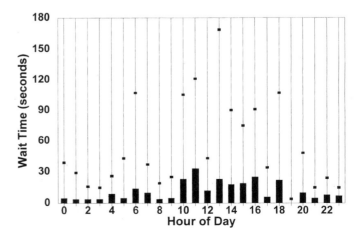

FIGURE 18.1. Tube system wait time by hour of the day. The average time (bars) from when a tube is placed on the system until it begins moving is 5 to 10 seconds except at peak hours (10:00–18:00) when the wait averages about 30 seconds but seldom exceeds 2 minutes (points represent maximum times).

tory instrumentation currently includes Vitros 950 and 250 chemistry analyzers (Ortho-Clinical Diagnostics, Rochester, NY, U.S.A.); AxSYM, TDx, and IMx immunochemistry analyzers (Abbott Diagnostics, Abbott Park, IL, U.S.A.); MaxM automated hematology analyzers and ACL100 and ACL3000 coagulation analyzers (Beckman Coulter Corporation, Brea, CA, U.S.A.); ABL520 and 725 blood-gas analyzers (Radiometer America, Westlake, OH, U.S.A.); and a variety of smaller instruments. Major instruments are interfaced to the LIS and results are displayed on HIS terminals at each nursing station or at each bedside in the ICU within seconds of verification in the LIS. The rapid transport of specimens to the laboratory via the pneumatic tube system, use of whole-blood analyzers or heparinized plasma for most chemistry testing (which avoids waiting for the specimen to clot), and immediate reporting of results to the HIS have resulted in short (5–30 minutes) turnaround times for critical tests sent to the central laboratory, eliminating the need for near-patient testing in many circumstances.

Quality Assurance

A supervisor-level medical technologist is in charge of POCT. This supervisor is responsible for writing a procedure for each approved test, for developing a training program and competency checklist (Fig. 18.2) for personnel, for creating a log for the documentation of results of quality control and patient tests (Fig. 18.3), and for obtaining computer codes to allow reporting of results directly to the LIS and HIS. Testing is performed by as small a group of individuals as possible to minimize the time and expense of training and documentation, and, whenever possible, we prefer to use personnel with some experience in laboratory testing, such as clinical laboratory assistants and respiratory therapists (Table 18.1). More recently, we adopted the model of training a small cadre of support staff in high-intensity areas to perform phlebotomy and POCT. Review of results by the POC supervisor includes verification of the qualifications of testing personnel. Newer instruments include a variety of options to ensure that controls have been performed and that an operator is qualified before patient testing is done.

The results of all POCT are entered into the LIS in the same manner as testing performed in the laboratory. This process is facilitated by instruments that can be interfaced electronically. For example, results of tests performed on the i-STAT® analyzer (Abbott Diagnostics, Abbott Park, IL, U.S.A.) are stored in the analyzer until they can be uploaded to the Central Data Station, a personal computer that is interfaced to the LIS. Quality control and patient results are reviewed daily on this computer by a laboratory supervisor. For methods that cannot be interfaced, test results are recorded on the data-capture form by testing personnel and entered into the LIS no later than the next working day by laboratory personnel. Review of patient and quality control results is accomplished at that time. Billing for all testing is captured from the LIS.

Many POC methods use traditional liquid controls, whereas others use a combination of electronic and traditional controls. In either case, daily controls are run by testing personnel. When the manufacturer recommends daily electronic controls and less frequent liquid-based controls, for example,

to verify the integrity of a new lot of reagents, testing personnel also run the liquid controls. Samples from external proficiency testing programs are reconstituted or otherwise prepared by the laboratory POCT supervisor and circulated to testing personnel for performance. Correlation between POC and central laboratory methods using patient samples is determined daily for blood gas and electrolyte tests and at least twice yearly for other tests.

POINT-OF-CARE TESTING ON PEDIATRIC INPATIENT UNITS

Blood Gas and Electrolyte Determinations in the Neonatal Intensive Care Unit

The PCMC neonatal intensive care unit (NICU) is populated exclusively by infants transported from other facilities. Rapid turnaround times for laboratory tests are especially important in this setting because these tiny patients are in critical condition on arrival and can deteriorate rapidly at any time without apparent warning. For many years, we operated a satellite laboratory adjacent to the NICU that was staffed 24 hours a day by a medical technologist. The technologist performed an average of two blood gases per hour and a small number of serum glucose determinations and occult blood tests each shift. The satellite laboratory was a major expense, but the medical need was real.

Our first attempt at cost reduction was to train selected respiratory therapists to operate the blood-gas analyzer during evenings, nights, and weekends and to staff the laboratory with a technologist only during the eight busiest hours of the day. The technologist did instrument maintenance and performed testing during those hours. This approach worked well, but pressures for cost reduction continued to increase, and a team was formed with representatives from the laboratory, NICU, respiratory therapy, and clinical engineering (which maintains the tube system). The team proposed a plan in which the bulk of blood gases from NICU would be sent to the main laboratory via the tube system, and an i-STAT analyzer would reside permanently in the NICU area to provide faster turnaround time when needed. Selected respiratory therapists and NICU phlebotomists would be trained to use the analyzer. The NICU clinical staff insisted that results continue to appear on bedside terminals in a tabular format. Therefore, an interface was installed in the NICU so that results from the i-STAT could be uploaded immediately to the LIS. Concerned that overuse of the i-STAT analyzer would nullify the savings gained by closing the satellite laboratory, the team defined criteria for determining when a blood gas should be run on the i-STAT. Any blood-gas specimens not meeting one of these criteria would be sent to the main laboratory. The criteria were new admission, unstable patient (as determined by the neonatologist), and unavailability of the tube system.

A 6-month pilot study was carried out to determine whether this approach could meet the clinical need while achieving the desired cost reduction. Acceptance criteria included tube system reliability, central laboratory blood gas turnaround time, performance of the i-STAT system, and timely display of results on the bedside terminals. During the 6 months of the pilot study, 4,679

PRIMARY CHILDREN'S MEDICAL CENTER DIVISION OF LABORATORIES

Competency testing is performed annually for each employee.
Competency testing is performed twice during the first year of service.

Training and Competency Testing for i-STAT Handheld Blood Gas Analyzer														
Name	First		First		First		First		First		First			
	Last		Last		Last		Last		Last		Last			
Tech ID	1235		323		328		339		1626		342			
Date	12-98		12-98		12-98		11-98		11-98		12-98			
Read procedure	Yes	No	Yes	No	Yes	No	Yes	No	Yes	No	Yes	No	Yes	No
Intended use	Yes	No	Yes	No	Yes	No	Yes	No	Yes	No	Yes	No	Yes	No
Sample handling	Yes	No	Yes	No	Yes	No	Yes	No	Yes	No	Yes	No	Yes	No
Gloves required	Yes	No	Yes	No	Yes	No	Yes	No	Yes	No	Yes	No	Yes	No
Expiration dating	Yes	No	Yes	No	Yes	No	Yes	No	Yes	No	Yes	No	Yes	No
Warming cartridge	Yes	No	Yes	No	Yes	No	Yes	No	Yes	No	Yes	No	Yes	No
Filling cartridge	Yes	No	Yes	No	Yes	No	Yes	No	Yes	No	Yes	No	Yes	No
Operator ID	Yes	No	Yes	No	Yes	No	Yes	No	Yes	No	Yes	No	Yes	No
Patient ID (account number)	Yes	No	Yes	No	Yes	No	Yes	No	Yes	No	Yes	No	Yes	No
Entering other data	Yes	No	Yes	No	Yes	No	Yes	No	Yes	No	Yes	No	Yes	No
Reading results	Yes	No	Yes	No	Yes	No	Yes	No	Yes	No	Yes	No	Yes	No
Transmitting results	Yes	No	Yes	No	Yes	No	Yes	No	Yes	No	Yes	No	Yes	No
Printing results	Yes	No	Yes	No	Yes	No	Yes	No	Yes	No	Yes	No	Yes	No
Calculated results	Yes	No	Yes	No	Yes	No	Yes	No	Yes	No	Yes	No	Yes	No
Questionable results	Yes	No	Yes	No	Yes	No	Yes	No	Yes	No	Yes	No	Yes	No
Error messages	Yes	No	Yes	No	Yes	No	Yes	No	Yes	No	Yes	No	Yes	No
Simulator (built in)	Yes	No	Yes	No	Yes	No	Yes	No	Yes	No	Yes	No	Yes	No
Reagent storage	Yes	No	Yes	No	Yes	No	Yes	No	Yes	No	Yes	No	Yes	No
Data storage	Yes	No	Yes	No	Yes	No	Yes	No	Yes	No	Yes	No	Yes	No
All results to care giver	Yes	No	Yes	No	Yes	No	Yes	No	Yes	No	Yes	No	Yes	No
Date of next training														

Trainer: John Doe

Reviewed by _____   Date: _____

FIGURE 18.2. Training checklist for i-STAT. A training program for each point-of-care test is developed from the procedure manual, and the checklist must be completed by personnel before they can perform patient testing.

H. Pylori **QUALITY CONTROL AND RESULTS**
(Return to lab each day of use.)

Date_____

Control Lot No. _____   Receive Date _____   Refrigerated Exp. Date _____

Date at Room Temp. _____   Room Temp. Exp. Date _____

NAME	ACCOUNT #	START TIME	END TIME	TECH	RESULT	POS Control	NEG Control
1.							
2.							
3.							
4.							
5.							
6.							
7.							
8.							
9.							
10.							

RESULTS REVIEWED BY_____   DATE_____   TIME_____

ENTERED IN SUNQUEST BY_____   DATE_____   TIME_____

SUNQUEST CODE   **UREAS**   Give results to Dave

FIGURE 18.3. Data capture form for *Helicobacter pylori* testing. For methods that cannot be interfaced, daily quality control and test results are recorded on the data capture form by testing personnel and subsequently entered manually into the laboratory information service. Review of patient and quality control results is accomplished at that time.

TABLE 18.1. PERSONNEL PERFORMING POCT

Analyzer	Used By	Educational Background
i-STAT	MT	B.S. degree
	Nurse	B.S. degree or nursing degree
	CLA	High school
	RT	50% Associate degree, 50% B.S. degree
Hemochron	Nurse	B.S. degree or nursing degree
	CLA	High school
AVOX	Nurse	B.S. degree or nursing degree
DCA 2000	CLA	High school
H. Pylori	Nurse	B.S. degree or nursing degree
UA	Nurse	B.S. degree or nursing degree
	CLA	High school
Thrombelastograph	MT	B.S. degree

POCT, point-of-care testing; MT, Medical Technologist; CLA, Certified Laboratory Assistant.

blood-gas analyses were performed for patients in the NICU. Only 102 (2.2%) of these were performed on the i-STAT analyzer. The pneumatic tube system was down, on average, less than 5 minutes per day. The median time for a specimen to reach the central laboratory via the pneumatic tube system was 3 minutes, and the median time for analysis and on-line reporting was 4 minutes, compared with a median time for analysis on the i-STAT of 2 minutes (Fig. 18.4a). In general, central laboratory turnaround times of greater than 10 minutes (Fig. 18.4b) were due to the simultaneous receipt of samples from two or more patients, a problem that, by definition, never complicated testing with the point-of-care analyzer. The central laboratory turnaround time was considered acceptable for most specimens, and there were no incidents of compromised patient care. An annualized cost saving of $20,000 (not including labor) was realized, largely by moving the blood-gas analyzer from the satellite to the main laboratory and retiring an older instrument (8). The pilot configuration was made permanent after approval by NICU staff.

The process, which led to replacing a satellite laboratory with a pneumatic tube system and a point-of-care analyzer, illustrates that there is no single solution to every need for faster turnaround

times. When available, a pneumatic tube system can save a great deal of time by providing rapid transportation of specimens to a central laboratory (3). Without such a system, a satellite laboratory may be the least expensive option. Even with reliable pneumatic tube and computer systems in place, however, a few patients may require a turnaround time that can only be met by POCT.

Bedside Glucose Determinations for Patients Receiving Insulin Infusions

Dedicated glucose meters are not used in PCMC. This decision was made more than a decade ago because a critical issue with glucose levels in pediatrics is hypoglycemia, and the glucose meters at that time lacked adequate accuracy and precision in the hypoglycemic range (9); and results from these instruments could not be uploaded to the LIS. Although the performance of glucose meters has improved since then (10,11), we still do not use them in PCMC because of concerns about connectivity to the LIS, control of the quality process, and comparability of results with those obtained on larger laboratory instruments (12). With the pneumatic tube, whole-blood analyzers, and integrated information systems, the laboratory is able to provide 15- to 30-minute turnaround times on stat requests for glucose determinations. When faster turnaround is needed, typically for patients receiving continuous insulin infusions, the i-STAT analyzer is used. To avoid the effort and expense of training and certifying the competency of more than 1,000 medical and nursing staff who might care for one of these patients, the analyzers are operated by laboratory phlebotomists. Bedside glucose determinations are also done when newly diagnosed patients are learning to use their glucose meters because nurse educators report that having patients compare meter results with laboratory-quality results in real time is a very effective teaching tool.

Bedside Determination of Occult Bleeding

At one time, the laboratory supplied testing cards and developing reagent to nursing units as needed. With the advent of CLIA '88, it became necessary to control this test in the same manner

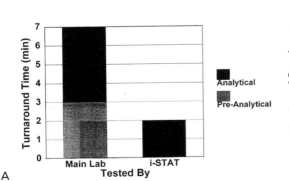

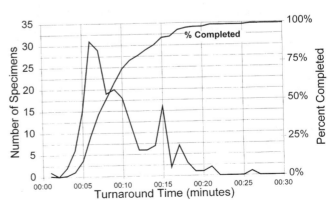

FIGURE 18.4. A: Comparison of turnaround time for blood-gas analysis from patients in the neonatal intensive care unit (NICU) sent to the hospital's main clinical laboratory via a pneumatic tube system or performed at the point-of-care with an i-STAT analyzer. **B**: Distribution of total turnaround time for blood-gas analysis performed in the main laboratory for patients in the NICU.

as tests done in the laboratory. The laboratory's first effort at this was to continue to distribute the cards and reagents to nursing units and to develop procedures for training and documentation. Follow-up investigation revealed poor compliance with these procedures and with our attempt to limit testing to small groups of nurses on each unit. An unexpected finding that emerged in discussions with the nursing units was that although it was most convenient to inoculate the cards with specimens at the bedside, results were typically not developed or recorded for 1 to 2 hours. Therefore, POCT was discontinued and inoculated cards were tubed to the laboratory, where the card is developed and the results are entered into the LIS within 30 minutes of collection. The need for turnaround time is met, compliance with regulatory requirements is maintained in the same manner as for other laboratory tests, and cost is greatly reduced, both because it is not necessary to train and periodically test dozens of nurses and also because the developing reagent is kept in the laboratory.

Bedside Determination of the pH of Gastrointestinal Secretions

Measurement of the pH of fluid withdrawn from a nasogastric tube is a convenient way to ascertain whether the tip of the tube is in the stomach (acid pH) or small intestine (alkaline pH). It is difficult to transfer this specimen to a tube for transport to the laboratory, and because the clinician is at the bedside positioning the tube, it is impractical to wait several minutes for the results. Therefore, the laboratory validated the performance of pH paper with a range of 4 to 8, wrote a procedure, and trained a small group of technicians in the pediatric ICU to perform point-of-care pH testing. Note that because testing personnel must be able to discriminate colors to correctly interpret pH testing, color discrimination testing must be included in the initial and subsequent competency testing. Controls consist of buffered pH calibrators in small dropper bottles, and unlabeled bottles of calibrators are periodically circulated to testing personnel as proficiency testing material. Results of quality control and patient testing are recorded on log sheets that also have the names of trained personnel, and these logs are reviewed and results transcribed to the LIS by laboratory personnel.

POINT-OF-CARE TESTING FOR PEDIATRIC SURGERY, CARDIAC CATHETERIZATION, AND EXTRACORPOREAL MEMBRANE OXYGENATION

Blood Gas and Electrolyte Determinations in Operating Rooms

Numerous blood gas determinations are performed during surgery for congenital heart disease, and specimens from several sites may be collected in a short time frame when the patient is being removed from bypass or to determine the degree of shunting. It was not feasible to place tube stations in each operating room; so to meet the need for rapid turnaround of these blood-gas results, the laboratory placed a blood-gas analyzer on a cart in the operating suite and trained a small group of anes-

thesia technicians to operate it. Once a day, a technologist from the laboratory went into the operating suite to perform maintenance procedures. As discussed already for the NICU, maintaining this instrument for a few specimens per day was very expensive, and it became increasingly difficult to free a technologist from the laboratory to do the daily maintenance. The solution again was the i-STAT analyzer. Anesthesia technicians trained to operate this analyzer obtained one from the laboratory as needed. They run blood gases during surgery, provide a printed result to the anesthesiologist, and enter results into the HIS, from which they are displayed on a large monitor for the surgical team. At the end of the day, the analyzer is returned to the laboratory, where results are uploaded to the LIS and reviewed by a laboratory supervisor. This approach has allowed us to maintain the turnaround time for critical blood gases during surgery while reducing the cost per test from $40 to $5 (considering the expense of maintaining the underused blood-gas instrument.)

Blood Gas and Oximetry Determinations during Cardiac Catheterization

A situation similar to that described in the preceding section exists in the cardiac catheterization suites that are located one floor below the clinical laboratory and are also without a pneumatic tube station. To determine blood gases and hemoglobin oxygen saturation of blood taken from various locations by catheter, the catheterization technicians use an i-STAT analyzer and an oximeter (A-VOX, Radiometer America, Fair Oaks Ranch, TX, U.S.A.), both of which are maintained by the laboratory.

Activated Clotting Time in Operating Rooms and during Cardiac Catheterization, Hemodialysis, and Extracorporeal Membrane Oxygenation

Activated clotting time (ACT) is a test used to monitor patients who have been anticoagulated with heparin, and it can be performed only at the point of care because the blood sample must be added to the reagent tube immediately after collection. The tube must be observed almost continuously. The most common applications of this test in pediatrics are during cardiovascular surgery and extracorporeal membrane oxygenation (ECMO) therapy. ECMO utilizes perfusion devices similar to those used in cardiac surgery, but they are connected to peripheral vessels for several days to allow the lungs of patients with potentially reversible acute respiratory failure to recover without the trauma of mechanical ventilation. ACT testing is requested infrequently for patients undergoing cardiac catheterization or hemodialysis. The test is performed at PCMC using a Hemachron analyzer (International Technidyne Corporation, Edison, NJ, U.S.A.) by the small group of operating room personnel trained to use the i-STAT analyzers and the catheterization laboratory personnel trained to perform blood gas tests and oximetry. We have evaluated newer instruments that require less sample and have a wider linear range but have had difficulty correlating results on specimens obtained while the patient is on bypass. This may be due, in part, to interference by substances in banked blood because in infants and small children, it is necessary to prime the bypass devices with blood rather than saline. A saline prime would result in significant hemodilution because of the infant's small blood volume relative to the size of the chamber in the perfusion device, but use of a blood prime results in a greater proportion of the blood in the circuit being banked blood.

Thromboelastography during Liver Transplantation

The thromboelastograph provides a continuous measure of the process of clot formation, and characteristic abnormal curves are seen in a variety of coagulopathies. Essentially the only application of this test in pediatrics is during liver transplantation. A specimen of whole blood is placed in a cup on the instrument, a probe is lowered into the specimen, and the force required to move the probe in the specimen as it clots is plotted against time, sometimes up to 90 minutes. The plot is a visual representation of clot formation and lysis. The Thromboelastograph 3000S (Heamoscope Corporation, Skokie, IL, U.S.A.) is classified as a moderately complex test if the specimen is native whole blood and highly complex if the specimen is modified whole blood or plasma (13). At PCMC, the clinical laboratory is responsible for operating and maintaining the instrument, which remains in the laboratory between uses. Two medical technologists are trained in its operation and share on-call duties. When needed, the instrument is moved to the operating room, where it is calibrated and brought into control by the on-call technologist, who then runs the patient samples. The curve is interpreted by the anesthesiologist as it is being generated.

POINT-OF-CARE TESTING IN PEDIATRIC EMERGENCY AND OUTPATIENT SETTINGS

Blood Gas, Electrolytes, Glucose, Ionized Calcium, and Hemoglobin in Support Of Air Transport

Intermountain Health Care's air transport system, LifeFlight, uses helicopters and fixed-wing aircraft to fly critically ill patients from outlying areas to major hospitals, including PCMC. Before transporting a critically ill neonate, the transport team often requests a blood-gas determination at the referring hospital. In rural facilities, this could entail a delay and added expense as an off-duty medical technologist was called in. Once in the air, the transport team had to rely on clinical findings and a pulse oximeter to monitor the patient. With an i-STAT analyzer, the transport team can measure blood gases, electrolytes, glucose, ionized calcium, and hemoglobin anytime during the transport process. This clinical need was well established before technology was available to meet it, and POCT was the only feasible solution. Financially, the cost of the testing is much less than the cost of delaying a transport, and the results from the analyzer can be downloaded to the LIS when the patient arrives at PCMC. Because the air transport teams fly to several hospitals, the service is administered at a corporate rather than at a hospital level and has obtained its own CLIA license.

Blood Gas, Electrolytes, Glucose, Ionized Calcium, and Hemoglobin in the Emergency Department

The PCMC emergency department (ED) sees more than 30,000 patients annually, and PCMC is the only pediatric trauma facility in the intermountain west. Because of the pneumatic tube and integrated information systems, most laboratory tests in support of ED patients can be performed in the hospital's central laboratory. A phlebotomist armed with an i-STAT analyzer is included in the team, which is paged whenever a patient with major trauma or in cardiopulmonary arrest is *en route* to the emergency department. In addition to delivering emergency blood products and assisting with the collection of blood samples and labeling of tubes, the phlebotomist can perform critical determinations of blood gases, electrolytes, glucose, ionized calcium, and hemoglobin as needed. As noted in the introduction, studies of the effect of POTC on the length of a patient's stay in the ED have shown either no effect (5) or significant reduction (6). Both these studies were conducted in EDs that serve adults, and in the latter study most of the reduction occurred in patients who were not admitted to the hospital. Kendall and colleagues found that the faster turnaround time of POCT in the ED reduced the time to decision-making, even if it did not shorten the length of stay (14). Aximos and colleagues studied the impact of POCT on the ED management of trauma and concluded that determinations of hemoglobin, glucose, blood gas, and lactate measurements might influence management but that determinations of electrolytes and blood urea nitrogen did not (15). Thus, the impact of the POCT in the ED will depend on the rapidity with which results can be obtained from the central laboratory and the acuity of patients seen in the emergency department.

Glycosylated Hemoglobin in Diabetes Clinics

The PCMC diabetes clinic sees about 1,200 patients annually at PCMC and another 1,200 in off-site clinics around the region. Hemoglobin A1c is a key indicator of long-term glucose control, and providing results at the beginning of the clinic visit allows clinic personnel to identify patients who will need additional education or more intensive intervention during the visit. This has proved to be even more important at outlying clinics, where specimens previously had to be transported back to PCMC for analysis by the laboratory, incurring an additional delay of several days. Now a clinic employee is trained by the laboratory to collect specimens and measure hemoglobin A1c in the clinic using a DCA2000+ (Bayer Diagnostics, Tarrytown, NY, U.S.A.). In this context, POCT brings a standard of care to patients in rural areas that is similar to that in the clinic in the hospital. Testing is more expensive than it would be if performed in batch mode on an automated analyzer, but the advantages of the point-of-care approach include the ability to tailor the patient's visit based on the results of the test, and the time saved by clinic personnel in pulling files and contacting patients when results were returned after the clinic visit. Because the clinic operates at several different sites, it has obtained its own CLIA license.

Macroscopic Urinalysis in the Nephrology Clinic

In the PCMC laboratory, macroscopic urinalysis is performed by certified laboratory analysts (CLA) using an automated instrument (Clinitek 200+, Bayer, Elkhart, IN, U.S.A.). Microscopic urinalysis is performed by medical technologists based on the results of the macroscopic findings or on a specific order from a physician. In the hospital's pediatric nephrology clinic, a clinic nurse performs the macroscopic urinalysis and prepares microscopic slides for examination by a nephrologist. Because only a single nurse needs to be trained and tested, and because that nurse has sufficient marginal time to perform the testing and daily quality control, there is a slight financial advantage and considerable advantage to the care process to perform testing in this manner.

Blood Counts in the Hematology–Oncology Clinic

The PCMC hematology–oncology clinic sees about 7,000 patients annually. To improve patient processing, the clinic director requested a satellite laboratory equipped with an automated cell counter and staffed by a medical technologist. Workflow and financial analyses indicated that this would cost in excess of $100,000 annually. Moreover, the full-time medical technologist assigned to the satellite laboratory would experience considerable variation in workload, and the necessary reduction in staff in the central laboratory would make it difficult for technologists in the central laboratory to assist during peak periods. Because the clinic area is closed after hours, an instrument placed there would not be available to back up the central laboratory's analyzer. POCT was not implemented in this instance, but the request for it precipitated creation of a process improvement team. Galloway and colleagues reported that operation of a backup analyzer in a hematology clinic by nurse specialists could consistently achieve the goal of a 30-minute turnaround time, whereas utilization of a pneumatic tube system and electronic transfer of results could not (16). Our team found that the greatest delays in complete blood count turnaround time occurred before receipt of the specimen in the laboratory. The median within-laboratory turnaround time (from receipt of specimen to verification of results) was 8 minutes. Streamlining the process of patient registration, collection of the specimen soon after arrival, and expeditious delivery of the specimen to the laboratory would ensure that most results would be available before the oncologist saw the patient. Without such changes, however, turnaround times would not be expected to improve even if a satellite laboratory was created.

Rapid Diagnosis of Group A Streptococcal Pharyngitis

Very few laboratory tests are required in a general pediatrics practice, and even fewer tests need to be performed at the point of care (17). Perhaps the most important exception, however, is a rapid test for the diagnosis of group A streptococcal pharyngitis. A prompt diagnosis allows the practitioner to initiate appropriate therapy and provide immediate counseling. Although it is highly specific, the rapid tests are still less sensitive than culture, and current recommendations call for the confirmation of negative results with a blood agar culture. Rather than attempt to train and document the performance of a large number of ED and outpatient clinic staff to perform this test, we trained personnel on the day shift in the microbiology laboratory and the evening and night shift personnel in the central laboratory. Throat culture swabs are tubed to the main laboratory, and a rapid test is performed on receipt. Results are called to the physician and entered into the LIS. A culture is set up if the rapid test is negative.

Tests for *Helicobacter pylori* Infection

Helicobacter pylori is an important cause of gastritis in children, and early diagnosis and treatment can relieve symptoms and may prevent the more serious complications seen in adults. The diagnosis can be made by culturing the organism, observing it in gastric biopsy specimens, or by detecting it via immediate analysis of a gastric biopsy specimen for evidence of urea splitting or antigens unique to the organism (18). Specimens must be placed in the test kits soon after collection in the endoscopy suite. Therefore, the clinical laboratory, in conjunction with the test kit manufacturer, trained eight endoscopy nurses, one of whom is always present at a procedure, to perform and interpret the rapid test. Each test kit (Pyloritek, C. R. Bard, Inc., Billerica, MA, U.S.A.) contains positive and negative control samples that are developed along with the patient sample; in the absence of an external proficiency testing program, the laboratory provides a surrogate proficiency test consisting of five cubes of agar, some of which contain urease.

Other Point-of-Care Tests in Ambulatory Pediatrics

The advantages of POCT described in the preceding sections can be applied to a number of specialized situations in pediatrics. Pediatric and adult patients on long-term therapy with a growing number of drugs require frequent monitoring, and, as noted in preceding discussions, receiving the laboratory results at the time of the office visit allows for timely adjustment of therapy. POCT for anemia, hematuria and proteinuria, lead poisoning, and screening for genetic diseases or predispositions in the context of a well-child visit can allow timely and efficient counseling and therapy. As rapid tests become available for infectious agents, these, too, may be appropriate for near-patient testing if the quality, sensitivity, and specificity of the result are such that an immediate management decision can be made. In all the preceding scenarios, the same end can be achieved if the patient has the laboratory test performed before the office visit; or the clinician or associate communicates with the family when all testing is completed. There is clearly a tradeoff between convenience and cost. The numbers of patients in the practice with a specific testing need, the availability of alternate testing sites, and the balance between cost and reimbursement will favor POCT in some circumstances and referral to central laboratories in others.

CONCLUSIONS

Although fully aware that some of our solutions are unique to our circumstances, we think our experience allows the following generalizations about POCT in pediatrics. They are strikingly similar to those that came from a conference on POCT convened by the College of American Pathologists (19).

- Point-of-care testing can improve the *process* of pediatric patient care in both inpatient and outpatient settings and may have its greatest impact beyond the walls of the hospital: during the transport of infants and children to the regional center and in the off-site subspeciality ambulatory clinic.

- In evaluating the need for POCT, the focus should remain on the *process* of patient care. The question should not be what testing can be done but what testing *should* be done at the point of care to improve patient care.

- Administrative direction of point-of-care services by the laboratory serves both to assure a single standard of laboratory testing in the hospital and to expand the possibilities for POCT to moderate and even high-complexity testing.

- Testing should be limited to as small a group of testing personnel as possible to maintain proficiency and minimize the cost and time for implementing and maintaining the test.

- Tests and reagents should be selected on the basis of the comparability of results to similar tests performed in the central laboratory, ease of performance by nonlaboratory personnel, incorporation of quality control features, and connectivity to the LIS.

- The results of quality control and patient tests should be captured in the LIS, and results of near-patient testing should be made a part of patients' medical records in the same way as tests performed in the central laboratory.

REFERENCES

1. Widness JA, Kulhavy JC, Johnson KJ, et al. Clinical performance of an in-line point-of-care monitor in neonates. *Pediatrics* 2000;106:497–504.
2. Shapiro BA, Peruzzi WT. Blood gas analysis. In: Civetta JM, Taylor RW, Kirby RR, eds. *Critical care*, 3rd ed. Philadelphia: Lippincott–Raven Publishers, 1997:921–939.
3. Steindel SJ, Howanitz PJ. Changes in emergency department turnaround time performance from 1990 to 1993. *Arch Pathol Lab Med* 1997;121:1031–1041.
4. Bailey TM, Topham TM, Wantz S, et al. Laboratory process improvement through point-of-care testing. *Journal of Quality Improvement* 1997;23:362–380.
5. Parvin CA, Lo SF, Deuser SM, et al. Impact of point-of-care testing on patients' length of stay in a large emergency department. *Clin Chem* 1996;42:711–717.
6. Murray RP, Leroux M, Sabga E, et al. Effect of point of care testing on length of stay in an adult emergency department. *J Emerg Med* 1999;17:811–814.
7. Kost GJ. Point-of care testing in intensive care. In: Tobin MJ, ed. *Principles and practice of intensive care monitoring*. New York: McGraw-Hill, 1998:1267–1297.
8. Ballard J, Salyer J, Pedersen D, et al. Implementing a point-of-care blood gas-testing system in a NICU. *Respir Care* 1998;43:859 (abst).
9. Maser RE, Butler MA, DeCherney GS. Use of arterial blood with bedside glucose reflectance meters in an intensive care unit: are they accurate? *Crit Care Med* 1994;22:595–599.
10. Kost GJ, Vu HT, Lee JH, et al. Multicenter study of oxygen-insensitive handheld glucose point-of-care testing in critical care/hospital/ambulatory patients in the United States and Canada. *Crit Care Med* 1998;26:581–590.
11. Weitgasser R, Gappmayer B, Pichler M. Newer portable glucose meters—analytical improvement compared with previous generation devices? *Clin Chem* 1999;45:1821–1825.
12. Aller R. Bedside glucose testing systems. *CAP Today* 2001;15:26–34.
13. *Federal Register*. Point-of-care testing in the children's hospital. July 8, 1996 (Volume 61, Number 131), pp. 35736–35762.
14. Kendall J, Reeves B, Clancy M. Point-of-care testing: randomised controlled trial of clinical outcome. *BMJ* 1998;316:1052–1057.
15. Aximos AW, Gibbs MA, Marx JA, et al. Value of point-of-care blood testing in emergent trauma management. *J Trauma* 2000;48:1101–1108.
16. Galloway MJ, Woods RS, Nicholson SC, et al. An audit of waiting times in a haematology clinic before and after the introduction of point-of-care testing. *Clin Lab Haematol* 1999;21:201–205.
17. Pysher TJ, Daly JA. The pediatric office laboratory: a look at recent trends. *Pediatr Clin North Am* 1989;36:1–22.
18. Bourke B, Jones N, Sherman P. *Helicobacter pylori* infection and peptic ulcer disease in children. *Pediatr Infect Dis J* 1996;15:1–13.
19. Handorf CR. College of American Pathologists Conference XXVIII on alternate site testing: introduction. *Arch Pathol Lab Med* 1995;119:867–871.

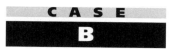

CASE
B

POCT FOR VASCULAR DISORDERS AND ANTICOAGULATION THERAPY IN EUROPE

ROSANNA ABBATE
DOMENICO PRISCO
DANIELA POLI
ALESSANDRA LOMBARDI
ANDREA A. CONTI

This study represents a review of data from the literature and from personal communications about the use of point-of-care testing (POCT) in Europe for diagnosis of cardiovascular disorders and monitoring of antithrombotic therapy. In the last ten years, we have seen a significant increase in the accessibility of services dedicated to acute coronary syndromes and in the use of thrombolytic treatment. Care units where reperfusion procedures such as percutaneous transluminal coronary angioplasty and stent application can be performed have become more widely available, underscoring the clinical relevance of obtaining rapid laboratory test results. In addition to their importance in clinical evaluations, biochemical analyses provide the diagnostic criteria necessary to decide the actual need for hospitalization and the most appropriate therapeutic approach.

CARDIAC INJURY MARKERS

In recent years, immunoassays have become available for determining blood levels of troponins I and T (1), which have high diagnostic value because they usually are not detectable in patients without myocardial injury. Although the sensitivity of cardiac troponin I is similar to myocardial muscle creatine kinase isoenzyme (CK-MB) in detecting acute myocardial infarction, it has a higher specificity for myocardial tissue, shows a greater proportional increase, and remains elevated for a longer period. In patients with mild myocardial infarction, troponin I levels are of particular value in patients with borderline CK-MB values and, coupled with echocardiography, provide a powerful tool in establishing a diagnosis. Troponin T also has proved to be a better marker than CK-MB for risk stratification of patients with acute myocardial ischemia (2,3). In patients with unstable angina, troponin I appeared to be an independent risk factor in predicting mortality, and the prognostic value of this protein was greater in patients who presented more than 6 hours after the onset of symptoms (4). Moreover, myocardial infarction was more frequent in unstable angina patients with high troponin T levels, which had a significantly higher prognostic accuracy than both symptoms and electrocardiographic results (5). The new rapid bedside assays for the detection of troponins have been particularly useful in the emergency department setting, where evaluation of chest pain must be as quick and precise as possible (6–8). Several studies confirm that one positive test identifies high-risk patients who require hospitalization, and two negative tests (together with negative standard diagnostic tests) rule out the necessity for hospitalization in patients who can be discharged safely (9,10).

MONITORING THERAPEUTIC EFFICACY

Troponin levels also may be useful for noninvasive prediction of reperfusion of the infarcted area (11). Some evidence indicates that troponin measurements during the first 48 hours after onset of myocardial symptoms can contribute to the early success of thrombolytic therapy (12). Troponin T has been shown to be capable of predicting the benefit of the glycoprotein IIb-IIIa inhibitor abciximab in subjects with unstable angina (13). Although these results are preliminary, the measurement of a humoral index to guide therapeutic decision making holds promise. In Sweden, a troponin T substudy performed in 15 hospitals to evaluate the efficacy of low-molecular-weight heparin in unstable angina has validated the usefulness of biochemical markers for prognostic evaluation in unstable coronary artery disease (14). Lindahl and colleagues suggest that low-risk patients are identifiable by troponin T concentrations, thereby avoiding intensive treatment and longer observation (12). In Great Britain, circulating troponin T levels were found to be useful for selecting unstable angina patients to be revascularized because revascularization of patients with more than 0.2 μg per liter troponin T resulted in an eightfold difference in mortality rates (15). The significance of a surrogate marker for active thrombus formation makes the use of a rapid assay of cardiac-specific proteins particularly interesting in light of new therapeutic perspectives accompanied by increasing costs.

DIAGNOSIS OF VENOUS THROMBOEMBOLISM

Since the introduction of D-dimer assays to measure fibrin degradation products, many clinical studies have shown that D-dimer measurements are useful for diagnosing deep venous thrombosis and pulmonary embolism, provided that reliable methods such as enzyme-linked immunosorbent assay (ELISA) are used (16). The latest rapid methods also have been shown to be reliable as thrombosis-excluding tests. One such method, performed at the bedside on whole blood, is SimpliRed (Agen, Brisbane, Australia), which uses bispecific antibodies directed toward both a D-dimer epitope and a red cell surface epitope, thus making possible the detection of D-dimer in whole blood within a few minutes after blood sampling (17). The combined approach of pretest probability, determined by clinical model and noninvasive tests such as ultrasound, with D-dimer tests may improve the diagnosis of venous thromboembolism.

ANTICOAGULANT MONITORING

Antithrombotic treatment of cardiovascular inpatients requires appropriate monitoring. The greatest challenge in daily practice is heparin therapy because information is needed quickly, whereas for oral anticoagulants prothrombin time (PT), performed in central laboratories, is usually appropriate. Heparin therapy must be closely monitored to modify dosages and to determine whether there is no longer a bleeding risk after cardiac surgery. Although the laboratory activated partial thromboplastin time (APTT) procedure has the highest diagnostic accuracy and should be considered the primary method for monitoring heparin therapy (18), a significant disadvantage is the overly long turnaround time. POCT devices can significantly reduce the time between blood sampling and a decision regarding heparin titration adjustments (19). Activated clotting time (ACT) was the first POCT device used for coagulation evaluation and is the most common hemostasis test used in Europe to monitor heparin anticoagulation, both in cardiac surgery and during percutaneous revascularization. Other bedside devices are used also to perform common coagulation tests rapidly, such as APTT and PT on whole blood. In France, a comparison of the performances of APTT Biotrack (Ciba Corning, Mountain View, CA, U.S.A.) and ACT with central laboratory APTT in monitoring heparin therapy showed that the best concordance with the latter was obtained with the APTT Biotrack (20). Both APTT systems are limited in their application, however, because of a high sensitivity to heparin.

CONCLUSIONS

The POCT devices offer a potential benefit for critical care and oral anticoagulant management, but their use has not yet been standardized in Europe. We sent a questionnaire to cardiology and thrombosis centers throughout Europe to determine the degree of use of POCT devices. Although the results have not been sufficiently informative, we note that POCT devices are not used routinely except in Germany, where guidelines for POCT procedures were published in 1998 by the German Association for Clinical Chemistry and the German Association for Laboratory Medicine. The availability of POCT offers the possibility of improving diagnostic efficiency of cardiovascular disorders and management of anticoagulant therapy. This opportunity is underused in Europe today. A critical issue is the underuse of oral anticoagulants; in Great Britain, about 40% of the patients with atrial fibrillation eligible for anticoagulation did not receive antithrombotic therapy (21). The possibility of monitoring anticoagulation by decentralized systems could possibly prevent 3,000 to 5,000 strokes per year in Great Britain alone as calculated by a projection of the results based on the Stroke Preven-

tion in Atrial Fibrillation study (22). We recommend that European guidelines be established for implementing POCT programs and that health agencies at the national, regional, and local levels be identified for regulating these programs.

REFERENCES

1. Coudrey L. The troponins. *Arch Intern Med* 1998;158:1173–1180.
2. Ohman EM, Armstrong PW, Christenson RH, et al. Cardiac troponin T levels for risk stratification in acute myocardial ischemia. *N Engl J Med* 1996;335:1333–1341.
3. Roberts R, Fromm RE. Management of acute coronary syndromes based on risk stratification by biochemical markers. An idea whose time has come. *Circulation* 1998;98:1831–1833.
4. Antman EM, Tanasijevic MJ, Thompson B, et al. Cardiac-specific troponin I levels to predict the risk of mortality in patients with acute coronary syndromes. *N Engl J Med* 1996;335:1342–1349.
5. Rebuzzi AG, Quaranta G, Liuzzo G, et al. Incremental prognostic value of serum levels of troponin T and C-reactive protein on admission in patients with unstable angina pectoris. *Am J Cardiol* 1998;82:715–719.
6. Heeschen C, Goldmann BU, Moeller RH, et al. Analytical performance and clinical application of a new rapid bedside assay for the detection of serum cardiac troponin I. *Clin Chem* 1998;44:1925–1930.
7. Luscher MS, Ravkilde J, Thygesen K. Clinical application of two novel rapid bedside tests for the detection of troponin T and creatine kinase-MB mass/myoglobin in whole blood in acute myocardial infarction. *Cardiology* 1998;89:222–228.
8. Baum H, Braun S, Gerhardt W. Multicenter evaluation of a second-generation assay for cardiac troponin T. *Clin Chem* 1997;43:1877–1884.
9. Hamm CW, Goldmann BU, Heeschen C, et al. Emergency room triage of patients with acute chest pain by means of rapid testing for cardiac troponin T or troponin I. *N Engl J Med* 1997;337:1648–1653.
10. Meinertz T, Hamm CW. Rapid testing for cardiac troponins in patients with acute chest pain in the emergency room. *Eur Heart J* 1998;19:973–974.
11. Remppis A, Scheffold T, Karrer O, et al. Assessment of reperfusion of the infarct zone after acute myocardial infarction by serial cardiac troponin T measurements in serum. *Br Heart J* 1994;71:242–248.
12. Lindahl B, Venge P, Wallentin L (for the FRISC Study Group). Relation between troponin T and the risk of subsequent cardiac events in unstable coronary artery disease. *Circulation* 1996;93:1651–1657.
13. Hamm CW, Heeschen C, Goldmann B, et al. Troponin T predicts the benefit of abciximab in patients with unstable angina in the CAPTURE study. *Eur Heart J* 1998;19(Suppl):117(abst).
14. Fragmin during Instability in Coronary Artery Disease (FRISC) Study Group. Low-molecular-weight heparin during instability in coronary artery disease. *Lancet* 1996;347:561–568.
15. Collinson PO. Troponin T or Troponin I or CK-MB (or none?). *Eur Heart J* 1998;19(Suppl N):N16–N24.
16. Bounameaux H, DeMoerloose P, Perrier A, et al. Plasma measurement of D-dimer as diagnostic aid in suspected venous thromboembolism: an overview. *Thromb Haemost* 1994;71:71–76.
17. John MA, Elms MJ, O'Reilly EJ, et al. The SimpliRED D-dimer test: a novel assay for the detection of crosslinked fibrin degradation products in whole blood. *Thromb Res* 1990;68:273–281.
18. Solomon HM, Mullins RE, Lyden P, et al. The diagnostic accuracy of bedside and laboratory coagulation: procedures used to monitor the anticoagulation status of patients treated with heparin. *Am J Clin Pathol* 1998;109:371–378.
19. Becker RC, Cyr J, Corrao JM, et al. Bedside coagulation monitoring in heparin-treated patients with active thromboembolic disease: a coronary care unit experience. *Am Heart J* 1994;128:719–723.
20. Hezard N, Metz D, Potron G, et al. Monitoring the effect of heparin bolus during percutaneous angioplasty (PTCA): assessment of three bedside coagulation monitors. *Thromb Haemost* 1998;80:865–866.
21. Sudlow M, Thomson R, Thwaites B, et al. Prevalence of atrial fibrillation and eligibility for anticoagulants in the community. *Lancet* 1998;352:1167–1171.
22. The Stroke Prevention in Atrial Fibrillation Investigators. Adjusted-dose warfarin versus low-intensity fixed dose warfarin plus aspirin for high-risk patients with atrial fibrillation: Stroke Prevention in Atrial Fibrillation III randomised clinical trial. *Lancet* 1996;348:633–638.

ADVANCEMENT OF POCT IN SWEDEN

LASSE LARSSON
EVA FREMNER

The health care system in Sweden is changing, as in many other parts of the world. In our county of Östergötland, we have seen a strong political effort to strengthen primary health care (PHC), increase home-based health care, and create a new role for hospitals as technical centers to support home- and PHC-based care. These changes have gone hand in hand with the technologic advances to perform all common clinical chemistry, hematology, and even former esoteric tests (e.g., HbA$_{1c}$) in a point-of-care testing (POCT) setup. The miniaturization of instruments, development of ready and prepacked reagents, and immune technology have opened the doors for the relatively new and evolving possibility of POCT in PHC settings. These new possibilities for improving both patient and physician convenience have created a national interest in testing the POCT concept, initiating the development of an advanced system for near-patient testing.

In Sweden, the organization of health care is rather uniform, although financial arrangements for laboratory services may vary. In some parts, physicians are given the funding for laboratory services and can buy whatever testing they choose, whereas in other parts the central hospital laboratories are given a budget to serve the practitioners, who can order any test without having to consider its cost. The fact that general practitioners (GPs) in Östergötland are in the former category has probably been the single most important factor responsible for the change from centralized to decentralized laboratory services. This sort of economic power, together with a close cooperation between GPs and clinical chemists interested in exploring the possibilities of POCT, has hastened the development of extensive decentralized services in this county.

There are approximately 900 primary health care centers (PHCCs) with laboratories in Sweden and considerable variation with respect to the existing analytic panel. In most decentralized laboratories of this kind, only waived tests are performed (hemoglobin, glucose, sedimentation rate, and urinary strips). In 24 decentralized laboratories in the county of Östergötland, more than 90% of tests needed by physicians are performed by a medical technologist with a bachelor of science degree, fully competent to handle all aspects of the analytic work, from sampling to reporting of results. Within our four county hospitals, about 80% of the critical care analytes also are performed in each intensive care unit (ICU). Table C.1 lists the analytic tests available in these setups. The tests are ordered selectively as needed and are performed in each PHCC, either in a near-patient laboratory or at the point of care. They also are offered in intensive care sites by means of stationary or mobile instruments used within the healthcare system.

Only about 40% of all the PHCCs in Sweden have professionally trained laboratory staff. Although the Swedish health care authorities do not require medical technologists, it is expected that anyone performing analytic work should have proper and accurate training for the task, with documented knowledge in preanalytic and analytic problems as well as quality assurance. Quality assurance is of extreme importance, particularly in ICUs, where the most critically ill patients are (1). In view of this, the Swedish accreditation bureau (Swedac) recently issued rules for accreditation, not only for primary health care but also for decentralized laboratories run by non-laboratorians within hospitals. Health care authorities also have declared that POCT is accepted anywhere but that every decentralized laboratory site should be quality controlled and accredited.

After several years of preparation, ten of our PHCC laboratories were the first such laboratories in Europe to be accredited by Swedac in 1995 and to perform according to an established quality assurance system (2). Because conventional quality assurance is not easily adopted for an advanced POCT system (3), the quality assurance procedures were developed further, and another 14 PHCC laboratories were accredited in early 2000, along with the first decentralized ICU laboratory in Europe, in the department of neonatology at the University of Linkoping. We now have an organization in which all procedures are documented, mistakes are registered, and information noted on action taken to prevent a repeat of mistakes (4).

The cost-effectiveness of POCT has been debated in Sweden as everywhere else. Few studies have made cost comparisons, but some report considerably higher costs in a decentralized setting (5–7). To clarify further the analytic costs of decentralized testing, we performed a cost study for eight basic laboratory procedures in two kinds of laboratory settings: a midsize hospital (300 beds) and PHCC laboratories in the same geographic area. In both settings, medical technologists performed all testing, and the same system was used for quality control and instrument calibration. The distribution of direct costs was similar in both settings; personnel costs were 55% and 52% of total costs for the PHCC and hospital laboratories, respectively,

TABLE C.1. ANALYTIC PROGRAM AT THE MJOLBY PHCC LABORATORY[a]

Hematology	Hb EVF, MCV, MCHC, red cell distribution width, platelet distribution width, leukocyte particle concentration, TPC, lymphocytes, monocytes, granulocytes, ferritin
Coagulation	Prothrombin complex, TPC, clotting time (Ivy0, D-dimer)
Infection	Sedimentation rate, C-reactive protein, mononucleosis quicktest (Monospot), streptococcus quicktest (Strep-A)
Electrolytes	Sodium, potassium, calcium, albumin
Renal function	Creatinine, microalbumin, ADH-test
Heart	Myoglobin, troponin-T, CK, CK-MB[b]
Liver	α-GT (glutamyltransferase), LDH, bilirubin, ALP, ALT, AST
Pancreas	Total amylase
Thyroid	TSH, FT_4
Lipids	Cholesterol, triglycerides (TC), HDL cholesterol, LDL cholesterol
Diabetes	Glucose, hemoglobin A1c, microalbumin, creatinine
Prostate	PSA
Pregnancy	hCG
Oral tolerance tests	Glycose tolerance test according to WHO, lactose tolerance test
Intensive care	pH, PCO_2, PO_2, SO_4 oxygen saturation, standard bicarbonate, base excess, sodium, potassium, chloride, Ca^{2+}, urea, glucose, lactate, Hb, EVF

PHCC, primary health care centers; Hb, hemoglobin; EVF, erythrocyte volume fraction; MCV, mean corpuscular volume; MCHC, mean corpuscular hemoglobin concentration; TPC, thrombocyte particle concentration; CK, creatine kinase; CK-MB, myocardial muscle creatine kinase isoenzyme; ADH, antidiuretic hormone; LDH, lactate dehydrogenase; ALP, alkaline phosphatase; ALT, alanine aminotransferase; AST, aspartate aminotransferase; TSH, thyroid-stimulating hormone; FT_4, free thyroxine; HDL, high-density lipoprotein; LDL, low-density lipoprotein; PSA, prostate-specific antigen; hCG, human chorionic gonadotropin; WHO, World Health Organization; PCO_2, partial pressure of carbon dioxide; PO_2, partial pressure of oxygen.
[a]Serves nine general practitioners. Program is based on the most common disease conditions encountered in the actual PHCC area and covers >90% of all tests needed by the physicians in any outpatient clinic in Sweden. Also includes analyses performed at any intensive care unit at the University Hospital of Linkoping.
[b]Myoglobin and troponin T are always the first analyses performed in connection with myocardial infarction (MI). CK is not used often in point-of-care testing in connection with MI but more in questions related to different diffuse muscle problems.

and variable costs were 27% and 25%, respectively. The amount of time used by personnel for direct productive work was the same for both laboratory settings. After allocating working time to each of the studied procedures, the total direct cost per procedure was calculated. Three analyses (glucose, urine screening, and sedimentation rate) were found to have about the same costs, two (sampling, HDL-cholesterol) were more expensive in the hospital laboratory, and three (blood status, potassium, alanine aminotransferase) were more costly in the PHCC laboratories. Our study indicated that the results were very dependent on the allocation of personnel and fixed costs, that clinical chemistry analytical costs are complex and difficult to calculate, and that comparisons between different laboratory setups must be made carefully (8). Thus, the assumption (9) that POCT should be considerably more expensive could not be verified in our study. Furthermore, the reduction in total administrative time for general practitioners could be considerable. Physicians in Östergötland believe that only those with experience with advanced POCT can fully appreciate the value of the service.

REFERENCES

1. Larsson L, Sandhagen B, Kallner A. Quality assurance in blood gas analysis: a medical risk zone. *Lakartidningen* 1999;96:2368–2373.
2. Fremner E, Kalerud B, Mengel A-C, et al. Quality control in decentralized primary health care laboratories. *Clin Chem* 1997;43:S143.
3. Phillips DL. Quality systems for unit-use testing devices. *Clin Chem* 1997;43:893–896.
4. Fremner E, Larsson L. Organization of point-of-care testing (POCT): an administrative challenge. *Clin Chem* 2000;46:A7–A8.
5. Jacobs E. Analysis of economic models used in point-of-care testing. In: D'Orazio P, ed. *Preparing for critical care analyses in the 21st century, 16th International Symposium*, Waikoloa, Hawaii, 1996:126.
6. Tsai WW, Nash DB, Seamonds B, Weir GJ. Point of care versus central laboratory testing: an economic analysis in an academic medical center. *Clin Ther* 1994;16:898–910.
7. Winkelmann JW, et al. The fiscal consequences of central versus distributed testing of glucose. *Clin Chem* 1994;40:1628–30.
8. Larsson L, Fremner E, Mengel A-C, et al. Decentralized versus central laboratory testing: a cost comparison. In: *Proceedings of the Confluence of Critical Care Analysis and Near Patient Testing, 17th International Symposium*, Nice, France, June 4–7, 1998.
9. Scott MG. Faster is better: it's rarely that simple! *Clin Chem* 2000;46: 441–442.

POINT-OF-CARE PARATHYROID HORMONE TESTING

LORI J. SOKOLL
PATRICIA I. DONOVAN
ROBERT UDELSMAN

When thinking about point-of-care testing (POCT), it is unlikely that parathyroid hormone (PTH), a test used in the diagnosis of calcium and parathyroid disorders and analyzed using immunoassays, comes to mind. The definition of POCT includes any test or diagnostic procedure performed at or near the site of patient care, regardless of the method or device characteristics. Thus, PTH, now performed in the operating and angiography suites, can be included in the rapidly growing list of point-of-care tests (1,2).

Although the surgical treatment for hyperparathyroidism has a success rate greater than 95%, persistent or recurrent hypercalcemia may result from residual hyperfunctioning parathyroid tissue from an unrecognized or inaccessible adenoma, insufficient excision of hyperplastic tissue, or difficulty in distinguishing adenomatous and hyperplastic tissue. Because repeat surgeries have higher complication and lower success rates, numerous approaches have been proposed to ensure parathyroidectomy success. In 1988, the intraoperative use of PTH was investigated following the development of an immunoradiometric assay (IRMA) for the intact PTH molecule and a subsequent modified version of the assay reducing the assay incubation time from 22 hours to 15 minutes (3). PTH was proposed as a monitor of parathyroid surgery because (a) PTH production is limited to the parathyroid glands, (b) the intact molecule has a half-life of less than 5 minutes, and (c) PTH secretion is suppressed in normal parathyroid glands after hyperfunctioning tissue has been removed. Therefore, circulating PTH concentrations should decline rapidly after all hypersecreting parathyroid tissue has been removed (4). In the typical paradigm, PTH concentrations are measured at baseline, prior to exploration, and then at 5 to 10 minutes following tumor excision; a 50% decline in values should be observed if all hypersecreting tissue has been removed (5,6).

The first rapid PTH assays used a radioactive label, and therefore it was not until chemiluminescent labels were introduced that the ability to perform the assay in the operating room was realized (6). The first commercialized assay was a modified version of the Nichols Institute Diagnostics intact PTH immunochemiluminometric assay (ICMA). Use of vibratory shaking and increased temperature to 45°C altered assay kinetics to allow a decrease in incubation time from 22 hours to 7 minutes. The entire assay can be performed in EDTA plasma in approximately 15 minutes, including pipetting, centrifuging, incubation, washing, and reaction/reading steps. Instrumentation required for the assay, consisting of a microcentrifuge, heater-shaker apparatus, bead washer, and single-well luminometer, fits on a cart that can be transported in or near the operating suite. The standard curve, required with each assay, is stored in the luminometer and can be performed in the laboratory prior to patient testing.

A second rapid PTH assay was introduced subsequently by Diagnostic Products Corporation on the IMMULITE analyzer. The *Turbo* intact PTH assay is a modified version of the chemiluminescent sandwich IMMULITE intact PTH assay. The assay has two incubation times totaling 10 minutes and an overall assay time, including specimen preparation, of approximately 15 minutes. The IMMULITE is a totally automated instrument with a calibration stability of 2 weeks. Although the instrument and controlling personal computer (PC) theoretically could be transported to the operating room, the size of the analyzer makes it more suitable for a satellite or a central laboratory location in conjunction with specimen transport by pneumatic tube or messenger (7).

Since the commercialization of the rapid intact PTH assay in 1997, use of the assay has increased and found acceptance primarily at large medical centers that specialize in endocrine surgery (8). In a series of 200 consecutive patients, we found that the assay was a useful guide for the surgeon in cases of primary or secondary/tertiary hyperparathyroidism, initial or reoperative cases, as well as uniglandular and multiglandular disease (1). Using a benchmark of a 50% decline in PTH concentrations following resection, the rapid assay predicted surgical success in 97% of cases overall, although a subset of patients (9%) demonstrated a delayed decrease in PTH, which may be related to factors affecting PTH clearance or specimen integrity. This study also illustrated that the rapid assay is not intended to replace the experience of the surgeon. For example, postexcision values in several patients were close but not greater than or equal to the 50% guideline, and the judgment of the surgeon that these patients were cured proved correct.

One of the significant outcomes of the introduction of the rapid PTH assay has been the evolution of surgery for primary hyperparathyroidism from an approach using a bilateral neck exploration under general anesthesia, with associated hospital admission and significant surgical incisions, to a minimally invasive approach (9). Of patients with primary hyperparathyroidism, 85 to 90% have a single parathyroid adenoma and thus, using preoperative sestamibi-SPECT (single-photon emission computed tomography), the operation can be performed in a directed manner using local or regional anesthesia and a small incision. Use of the rapid PTH assay confirms the adequacy of resection, and patients are discharged within 1 to 3 hours of surgery (10). In our institution, adoption of this technique has radically changed the logistics of the surgeries, with operations now performed in our same-day surgery facility in our outpatient center, as opposed to the hospital's general operating facilities, allowing four to five surgeries per day to be performed by a dedicated parathyroid team.

The following case illustrates the role of the rapid PTH assay in the minimally invasive parathyroid exploration approach. A 52-year-old white woman was referred to an endocrinologist for evaluation of recurrent nephrolithiasis dating back 10 years. The patient had a history of hypercalciuria, and previous bone-density studies revealed osteopenia of the spine and hip. Laboratory studies had the following results: total serum calcium, 11.0 mg per deciliter (8.4–10.5 mg/dL); ionized calcium, 1.40 mmol per liter (1.13–1.32 mmol/L); intact PTH, 128 pg per milliliter (10–65 pg/mL); and serum phosphate, 2.3 mg per deciliter (2.5–4.9 mg/dL). A diagnosis of primary hyperparathyroidism was made, and the patient was referred to an endocrine surgeon for parathyroidectomy. Preoperative sestamibi-SPECT imaging revealed a single parathyroid adenoma in the inferior right neck posteriorly near the level of the sternal notch. Using the minimally invasive approach, a 1,150-mg parathyroid gland was removed. As shown in Figure D.1, the baseline intact PTH concentration was 90 pg per milliliter, and 5 minutes following resection, the PTH concentration dropped to 28 pg per milliliter. The patient was discharged the same day, and laboratory tests performed 1 month following the procedure indicated that the patient had been cured of her disease (total serum calcium, 9.2 mg/dL; ionized calcium, 1.22 mmol/L; intact PTH, 35 pg/mL).

A second case illustrates the role of the rapid PTH assay in assisting the surgeon in identifying occult multiglandular disease in patients with primary hyperparathyroidism. A 54-year-old white woman with a history of increasing serum calcium concentrations over a 1-year period was diagnosed with osteoporosis by DEXA scan, kidney stones, and gastrointestinal ulcers. Her most recent intact PTH level was 85 pg per milliliter. No definite parathyroid adenoma was identified with sestamibi-SPECT imaging, although slightly increased activity was observed in the region of the left inferior thyroid gland. The first baseline PTH obtained during surgery was 43 pg per milliliter; however, a subsequent baseline specimen was 71 pg per milliliter. A most likely explanation for the discrepancy was dilution of the first specimen with intravenous fluids. The left lower parathyroid gland was resected first, but PTH concentrations remained elevated at 51 pg per milliliter 6 minutes postexcision. Although the right lower gland was subsequently removed, PTH concentrations at 7 minutes postresection remained at 54 pg per milliliter. The surgeon thus determined that the patient had multiglandular disease. A formal bilateral exploration was performed, an enlarged right upper gland was removed, and a subtotal resection performed on an enlarged left upper gland. Five minutes post-subtotal parathyroidectomy, the patient's PTH concentration was less than 11 pg per milliliter. After the operation, the patient exhibited symptoms of hypocalcemia, but her follow-up calcium values were within the reference range (total serum calcium, 9.8 mg/dL; ionized calcium, 1.18 mmol/L).

These cases illustrate that the rapid PTH assay has many advantages for both the patient and surgeon. Improvements in patient care include minimizing the need for remedial surgeries, allowing a minimally invasive surgical approach, and allowing the surgery to be performed on an outpatient basis. The rapid assay aids the surgeon in identifying multiglandular disease and reducing the extent of neck exploration as well as confirming the success of the surgical procedure. In addition, financial benefits can be realized through decreased frozen sections, decreased operating room time and associated fees, and elimination of overnight hospital stays. Although we have shown that avoiding both general anesthesia and overnight hospital stays results in cost savings of greater than 50% compared with conventional surgical approaches (10), the rapid assay performed on-site requires a dedicated technologist as well as purchase of reagents priced significantly higher than standard PTH assay reagents. Cost to the laboratory for labor and reagents can be reduced by performing the rapid assay in the central laboratory; however, turnaround times and the ability to interact with the surgical team to ensure specimen integrity may be compromised (11).

These case studies indicate that introduction of PTH testing at the point of care has been highly successful, providing improved outcomes for the patient, increased assurance for surgical success, potential increased savings for the hospital, and increased patient care and visibility for the laboratory. It is expected that future developments in instrumentation will help to alleviate some of the financial implications of providing this service for the laboratory while also paving the way for the introduction of additional hormone assays as real-time monitors for surgical and localization procedures.

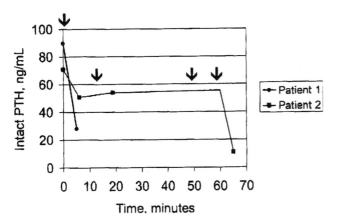

FIGURE D.1. Rapid intact parathyroid hormone results in two patients undergoing surgery for primary hyperparathyroidism. Arrows indicate time of parathyroid gland resection.

REFERENCES

1. Sokoll LJ, Drew H, Udelsman R. Intraoperative parathyroid hormone analysis: a study of 200 cases. *Clin Chem* 2000;46:1262–1268.
2. Udelsman R, Osterman F, Sokoll LJ, et al. Rapid parathyroid hormone measurement during venous localization. *Clin Chim Acta* 2000;295:193–198.

3. Nussbaum SR, Thompson AR, Hutcheson KA, et al. Intraoperative measurement of parathyroid hormone in the surgical management of hyperparathyroidism. *Surgery* 1988;104:1121–1127.

4. Brasier AR, Wang CA, Nussbaum SR. Recovery of parathyroid hormone secretion after parathyroid adenomectomy. *J Clin Endocrinol Metab* 1988;66:495–500.

5. Irvin GL III, Dembrow VD, Prudhomme DL. Operative monitoring of parathyroid gland hyperfunction. *Am J Surg* 1991;162:299–302.

6. Irvin GL III, Deserio GT III. A new, practical intraoperative parathyroid hormone assay. *Am J Surg* 1994;168:466–468.

7. Wenk RE, Efron G, Madamba L. Central laboratory analyses of intact PTH using intraoperative samples. *Lab Med* 2000;31:158–161.

8. Garner SC, Light GS Jr. Initial experience with intraoperative PTH determinations in the surgical management of 130 cases of primary hyperparathyroidism. *Surgery* 1999;126:1132–1138.

9. Irvin GL III, Sfakianakis G, Yeung L, et al. Ambulatory parathyroidectomy for primary hyperparathyroidism. *Arch Surg* 1996;131: 1074–1078.

10. Udelsman R, Donovan PI, Sokoll LJ. One hundred consecutive minimally invasive parathyroid explorations. *Ann Surg* 2000;232: 331–339.

11. Wians FH Jr, Balko JA, Hsu RM, et al. Intraoperative vs central laboratory PTH testing during parathyroidectomy surgery. *Lab Med* 2000; 31:616–621.

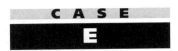
POCT PROGRAM AT THE TEXAS CHILDREN'S HOSPITAL

CHING-NAN OU
LAURA A. TOWNSEND-COLLYMORE

Texas Children's Hospital in Houston is a 715-licensed bed, nonprofit pediatric specialty hospital and is the largest children's hospital in the United States. Within its spectrum of more than 40 pediatric specialties, the pathology department provides all laboratory services and oversees the point-of-care testing (POCT) program throughout the hospital and outreach clinics. Our POCT program encompasses 41 inpatient nursing units and outpatient clinics, such as the neonatal and pediatric intensive care units, the premature nurseries, diabetes clinic, emergency center, dialysis unit, and operating room. There are also two areas performing near-patient testing in satellite laboratories within the hospital to enable optimum service to patients with critical needs. In the past 2 years, the hospital's POCT program expanded into the community to support testing performed in five suburban health center clinics. These suburban laboratories are not managed by the hospital's pathology department staff but typically are assisted with expertise and initial training to facilitate their compliance with regulatory requirements. Texas Children's also has assumed oversight of near-patient testing in 44 physicians' office laboratories within a 25-mile radius; these constitute the Texas Children's Pediatric Associates (TCPA). Laboratory pro-

cedures and instrumentation available to perform POCT are shown in Table E.1.

Our POCT program is managed collaboratively by a multidisciplinary team that includes pathology, nursing, and medical staff. Nursing personnel perform virtually all testing within the hospital, with the exception of KOH preps and microscopy (performed by physicians) and the activated clotting times test (performed by our nurses and by perfusionists staffed by an outside agency). Nurse managers review quality control records weekly, nurse educators participate in training, and directors of nursing review periodic reports prepared by the pathology department regarding the significant findings of our review of quality control documentation and proficiency survey testing results.

Although POCT is indicated in virtually every area of the hospital, the following areas have the most critical needs:

DIALYSIS UNIT

Activated clotting times must be monitored closely during dialysis procedures to prevent loss of extracorporeal blood volume

TABLE E.1. POINT-OF-CARE TESTING INSTRUMENTS AND TESTS AVAILABLE AT TEXAS CHILDREN'S HOSPITAL (TCH) AND THE TEXAS CHILDREN'S PEDIATRIC ASSOCIATES (TCPA) OFFICE PRACTICE SITES

Instruments	One Touch II Hospital Glucose Analyzer		
	HEMOCHRON whole blood coagulation system		
	Oxycom 3000 oxygen saturation machine		
	Gem Premier blood gas and elecrolyte analyzer		
	Radiometer ABL735 Analyzer		
	Bayer DCA 2000 Analyzer for hemoglobin A1c measurements		
	HemoCue for whole blood hemoglobin		
	iSTAT blood gas analyzer		
Tests performed at TCH	Urine dipstick	Hemoccult	Gastroccult
	Group A strep screen	Pregnancy test	Glucose
	Activated clotting time	KOH prep	Blood gas/electrolytes
	Hemoglobin A1c	Urine pH	Urine microscopic
	Hemoglobin	Co-oxymetry	
Tests performed at TCPA clinics	Urine dipstick	Microhematocrit	Hemoccult
	Stool pH	Pregnancy	Glucose
	KOH	Skin tests for scabies	CBC

resulting from clotting difficulties from inadequate heparinization of the extracorporeal circuit (1).

OPERATING ROOM

Activated clotting times are measured during surgery to monitor the patient's status during cardiopulmonary bypasses when heparin therapy is used. Blood gases also are measured to provide urgently needed information about the acid-base status of patients during cardiovascular surgery. Measurement of blood glucose is also indicated to prevent hypoglycemia or hyperglycemia in patients who are receiving citrated blood or who are losing blood volume. The measurement of hemoglobins during surgery is currently being implemented.

NEONATAL INTENSIVE CARE

Activated clotting times are used to monitor the system during extracorporeal membrane oxygenation (ECMO) of premature infants. This testing provides rapid feedback regarding clotting status of an infant whose blood is circulating through the ECMO machine. Additionally, urine glucose levels of infants who are receiving total parenteral nutrition or insulin are monitored to follow-up with blood glucose testing if needed. Immediate information is required to guard against hyperglycemia.

EMERGENCY DEPARTMENT

The test menu includes urine dipsticks, hemoccult, gastroccult, strep screen, pregnancy, glucose, and urine pH. When there is an urgent need for electrolyte results, the whole-blood electrolytes, including sodium, potassium, chloride, carbon dioxide, and ionized calcium, can be obtained by sending the specimen, via a pneumatic tube system, to a satellite laboratory that provides blood gases and whole blood electrolytes with a 15-minute turnaround time.

DIABETES CLINIC

Point-of-care testing includes glucose Chemstrips, One-Touch Glucose monitor, urine dipsticks, and hemoglobin A1c testing, which enables patients to receive timely counseling during the visit by the physician and dietitian.

PEDIATRIC INTENSIVE CARE

Activated clotting time (ACT) is needed almost immediately for optimization of heparin treatment of these typically unstable, acutely ill patients. ACTs are performed usually every 30 min in an acute care situation (1). Other tests performed include urine dipsticks, hemoccult, gastroccult, glucose, and urine pH. Blood gases and whole-blood electrolytes, including blood glucose and lactic acid, are provided by a nearby satellite laboratory with a 15-minute turnaround time.

OUTPATIENT CLINICS

In our outpatient clinics, POCT includes urine dipsticks, hemoccult, strep screens, glucose, and urine pH.

NEONATAL TRANSPORT

We transport sick neonates to our neonatal intensive care unit from hospitals located within an 85-mile radius. Glucose testing is frequently required during the transport and enables timely adjustments to prevent potential harm from hypoglycemia or hyperglycemia.

SPECIAL REQUIREMENTS FOR PREMATURE, NEWBORN, AND PEDIATRIC PATIENTS

Our patient population consists of premature infants, newborns, children at different developmental stages, and young adults. To accommodate such a heterogeneous population, the selection of methods and instrumentation becomes quite a challenge for laboratorians. Although much of modern instrumentations use small sample volumes, specimen size remains of prime concern, especially when dealing with premature infants who weigh less than 1,000 g in total body weight. Because the hematocrit in a newborn infant can be 60% or more, the yield of serum or plasma often is expected to be less than that of the same volume of blood collected from an older child or adult. In addition, the high hematocrit also could affect the accuracy of analyte measurement when whole blood is used. We selected the One-Touch II hospital blood glucose meter because it enables glucose measurements to be performed in either the neonatal or non-neonatal mode. The neonatal mode expands the hematocrit range from 25% to 60% up to 25% to 76% because neonatal blood usually has a high hematocrit (2,3). In addition, the neonatal mode subtracts 5 mg from the glucose reading and thus ensures against the dangers of hypoglycemia by erring on the safe side (4). After completing correlation studies with various handheld glucose analyzers, we concluded that the One-Touch was the most suitable for our needs.

The requirements of pediatric patients also have driven special modifications to some test methodologies. For example, we implemented the testing of pH and glucose of watery stools using Nitrazine pH paper and the glucose Chemstrips, although the Chemstrip manufacturer did not support its use for testing stool samples. Correlation studies indicated that our modified procedure provided sufficient information to be useful for medical decisions regarding treatment of patients with severe diarrhea from various causes.

RECOMMENDATIONS

Based on our experience at Texas Children's Hospital, we offer the following recommendations: (a) streamline quality control forms to facilitate compliance with documentation; (b) educate physicians and nurses regarding the importance of regulatory requirements; and (c) be innovative in implementing protocols that are different from those required by regulators, especially nongovernment regulators, provided they do not adversely impact patient care. Regulatory inspectors generally will accept your rationale if it is properly documented.

REFERENCES

1. Lancaster L, ed. *Core curriculum for nephrology nursing*. Pitman, NJ: American Nephrology Nurses' Association, 1992.
2. Soldin SJ, Rifai N, Hicks JMB, eds. *Biochemical basis of pediatric disease*, 2nd ed. Washington, DC: AACC Press, 1995:4–5.
3. Lifescan. One Touch II hospital blood glucose monitoring system. In: *Manual and inservice guide for hospitals and clinics*. Milpitas, CA: Johnson & Johnson, 1996.
4. Lifescan. One Touch II Hospital System in NEO and NOTNEO test modes: a comparison with the Accu-Check III and Chemstrip bG reagent strips *(abstract). Clinical study report*. Milpitas, CA: Johnson & Johnson, 1995.

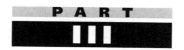

POINT-OF-CARE TESTING IN THE HEALTH SYSTEM, COMMUNITY, AND FIELD

19

POINT-OF-CARE TESTING IN PRIMARY CARE NETWORKS AND MANAGED CARE

JAY B. JONES

POINT-OF-CARE TESTING IN REGIONAL NETWORKS

Design, Menu, and Response Time

With increasing focus on access to large multientity primary care networks delivering services to health maintenance organizations (HMOs), clinical laboratory functions have been distributed to an increasing number of locations (1–3). Incorporation of hospitals into integrated delivery systems (IDSs) with merged outpatient populations and facilities have enlarged and accelerated this distribution phenomenon (4,5). In many cases and in particular the case of the Geisinger Health System (GHS), *managed care* describes the enterprise of HMO insurance of IDS benefit (6,7). As the congealing of such large IDS networks continues, the laboratory industry will face challenges to maintain unified distributed laboratory operations within increasing numbers of primary care sites and diverse health care facilities (8–10). Point-of-care testing (POCT) surely will have a place in the dynamics of managed care but will be subject to prevailing economic and technologic realities (11,12).

A description of the evolution of such a distributed laboratory, the Geisinger Medical Laboratories (GML), is presented herein. This description shares the experience of maintaining a unified operation during 15 years of expansion, merger, and diversification (1,8). Aspects of POCT are stressed, and it is important to recognize how this testing fits into the whole of the integrated delivery system (13). It was noted time after time during evolution of the subject health care system that a "balanced" solution to implementing laboratory support at primary care practice sites was most practical. Decentralization and centralization of laboratory testing did not compete but rather complemented each other in decision-making.

In a successful IDS, freestanding facilities do not exist but are part of a system. Solutions must be created that react to the emerging "big picture," and these solutions almost always are multifaceted and balanced (14,15).

Little has been written directly about the evolution of such distributed laboratories because models are relatively new and in the midst of constant change. Consultants are looking increasingly to this type of distributed laboratory operation as a successful model (5) just as technology enables POCT at locations geographically farther from the traditional clinical laboratory

(16,17). Just as total laboratory automation (TLA) is enabling formation of "core laboratories," POCT is enabling decentralization of testing (18). Hence opposite trends are impacting decisions as to how to configure distributed laboratories in the enlarging IDS, or, as aptly put, "The winds of change are blowing in two directions, leading to a vortex in the middle." Again, solutions for properly distributing laboratory support in large provider networks require balance, and this balance may be between opposite extremes.

Point-of-care testing in the evolving GHS continues to find valuable niches (19–21) in the midst of dynamic change. In fact, POCT has provided "off-the-shelf" rapid solutions to problems in several instances. As a relatively mature distributed laboratory, it is helpful to judge the basis of stable POCT in the GHS from a historical as well as a contemporary perspective.

Design of an Integrated Point-of-Care Testing Model in a Regional Integrated Delivery System Network

The current GHS, an IDS in central Pennsylvania consisting of two hospitals and 70 owned community practice sites, exemplifies the evolution of a distributed laboratory network. The GHS community practice network of 2001 has evolved into a distributed laboratory where both physician office laboratories (POLs) and hospitals perform standardized POCT.

In 1984, a plan was established to evolve a Geisinger Regional Laboratory (GRL) at the Geisinger Clinic, then a 190-physician group practice in rural central Pennsylvania, restructured into a diversified primary care network providing services to its own HMO (i.e., Geisinger Health Plan). This foresighted plan enabled the laboratory to establish operations at physician practice sites as they were built *de novo* or acquired by physician joining. The luxury of time was afforded by this proactive plan as laboratory infrastructure was integrated into an expanding network during the course of 15 years. The foundation for the GRL-distributed laboratory evolved as 65 network sites, and a community hospital, Geisinger Wyoming Valley Medical Center, entered the Geisinger organization. This infrastructure was created around owned facilities employing salaried Geisinger physicians and support staff. By 1995, the Geisinger Health Plan (GHP) serviced 200,000 members in 22 counties of central Pennsylvania, and expansion shifted toward contracting with or impaneling physicians and other providers to service GHP patients. Table 19.1 shows the timeline of network expansion. The design and plan of the laboratory in integrating its services, especially POCT services, into this diversified network are detailed in the following sections.

In July 1997, the Geisinger Clinic merged with the Hershey Medical Center to become the PennState Geisinger Healthcare System (PSGHS). The Division of Laboratory Medicine remained an autonomous, albeit integrated, operating division of the PSGHS. Renamed the PennState Geisinger Medical Laboratories (PSGML), the distributed laboratory organized itself as shown in Figure 19.1. The decentralized network of laboratories that had evolved as the GRL is shown as an enlarged entity renamed PennState Geisinger Health Group Laboratories, or HGL, and remained an operational unit separate from but integrated with the three hospitals. The basic technical and information system infrastructure remained essentially the same as the PSGML merged. A single pathologist chairman of the PSGML was appointed in July 1997, and standardization efforts between the two parts of the system (i.e., the old Geisinger and Hershey organizations) began.

Although the merger between POCT operations and PSGML operations in general were largely successful, the parent organizations decided to demerge in July 2000. Despite this demerger of PSGML operations, it remains important to describe the dynamics and infrastructure of a successfully consolidated PSGML. Note, however, that the HGL nomenclature has returned to the preexisting GRL nomenclature as part of the GHS. For purposes of describing the overall infrastructure of this distributed laboratory model that evolved to July 2000, the terms HGL and GRL can be used interchangeably.

Point-of-care testing services, including those at HGL sites and the three hospitals, and distributed laboratory informational systems had continued to evolve much as they had since 1984. A "design team" of persons involved with decentralized laboratory testing rapidly merged the POCT activities of the PennState and Geisinger portions of the system that differed only minimally to begin with. POCT at the three medical centers (both inpatient and outpatient) was regulated largely by a single Clinical Laboratories Improvement Act (CLIA) license at each hospital. This hospital testing in turn was standardized with POCT at each of the 83 CLIA-licensed practice sites in the HGL.

The HGL evolution was somewhat "organic" and adaptive as necessities of the market and changing physician practice patterns were manifested. Standardized POCT systems have been found to be highly adaptable when tests need to be centralized,

TABLE 19.1. EVOLUTION OF THE PENN STATE GEISINGER HEALTH GROUP LABORATORY NETWORK

1984: Geisinger Regional Laboratory (GRL) Task Force convened. Commercial lab joint venture proposal declined. Health Maintenance Organization (HMO), the Geisinger Health Plan, established.

1985: GRL Project Team supports first physician office laboratory (POL). Standardization begins with simple point-of-care tests with formation of Laboratory Technical Advisory Committee (LTAC). POL network begun as primary practice sites purchased or built.

1986: Eight POLs and two hospitals standardize point-of-care tests. POL educational program begun with support of Pennsylvania Bureau of Laboratories.

1987: Fourteen POLs and two hospitals linked by courier system. 24-hour referral laboratory testing begun. Medical technologist assigned GRL quality oversight and support duties.

1988: Five "Clusters" of POLs established with medical technologist oversight. Regulatory issues including CLIA '88 prioritized as GRL gains greater recognition.

1990: Common laboratory information system (LIS) installed for two (2) hospitals and 28 GRL network sites. Standardized methods, quality assurance, leadership structure, financial relationships established in LIS.

1992: First point-of-care testing electronic interface to LIS established. Fifty site GRL and point-of-care tests in two medical centers fully standardized with group purchasing generating $250K in incremental discounts.

1993: Two hospitals and GRL formally consolidate testing to a 24-hour core laboratory operation. System-wide client services department established. Single pathologist director of unified Geisinger Medical Laboratories.

1995: Wide-area network (WAN) installed to integrate information systems at 65 GRL sites. Consolidated testing reduces point-of-care tests by 20%–30%. Formal for-profit outreach program begun.

1997: Merger of Geisinger System with Hershey Medical Center to form PennState Geisinger Health System (PSGHS). Addition of eight POL "Clusters." Retrieval of tests from HMO patients, home visiting nurses, and skilled nursing facilities increases activities of five GRL "Cluster" supervisors. HMO at 250,000 members, 1.8 million outpatient visits per year.

1998: Eighty-three POL GRL and three hospital point-of-care testing activities reorganized as PennState Geisinger Health Group Labs (HGL). Common LIS expanded on WAN. Tests referred from HGL sites approach 1 million.

2000: PSGHS demerges to original Geisinger and Hershey organizations. Reconstituted GRL reduced to 70 POLs and two hospitals. EpicCare with Sunquest LIS results interface established at most GRL sites.

CLIA '88, Clinical Laboratories Improvement Act of 1988.

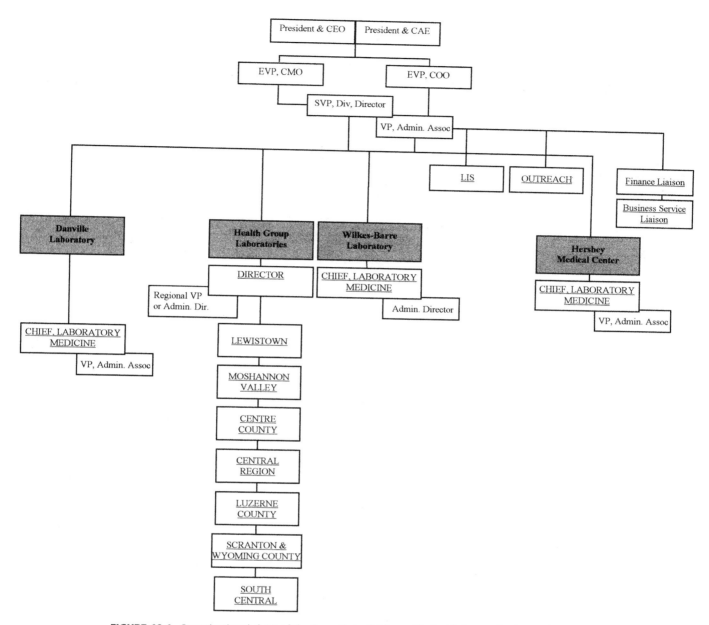

FIGURE 19.1. Organizational chart of the Penn State Geisinger Medical Laboratories (PSGML), including the Health Group Laboratories (HGL) in 1998.

decentralized, or rapidly deployed at selected POLs. Conditions constantly change in an IDS, and portions of the POCT configuration likewise must change. Change involves not just finding new solutions to laboratory testing problems but more problematically removing old entrenched infrastructure. The basic model of the current Geisinger-distributed laboratory, however, has remained essentially constant during the last 15 years. Fifteen years of "change management" teaches one to take change in stride—mergers, demergers, and possibly even remergers.

The core HGL system consisted of 83 practice sites with the topology shown in Figure 19.2. Decisions to centralize or decentralize laboratory testing in the HGL network had largely achieved a steady state of equilibrium between niche POCT

applications and a preponderance of specimens transported into hospital referral laboratories. The growth of this referral testing in the Geisinger portion of the PSGHL (mostly at Geisinger Medical Center in Danville, PA) is shown in Figure 19.3. Growth of this referral testing exceeded one million outpatient tests by the year 2000.

Similar growth (i.e., >30% per year) of referral testing from HGL network sites was experienced at the Hershey Medical Center and Geisinger Wyoming Valley Medical Center sites of the PSGML. A distributed laboratory presence at expanding numbers of HGL network sites was instrumental in facilitating this phenomenal growth of referred testing. Maintaining quality POCT in an IDS is only a part of the advantage of evolving a

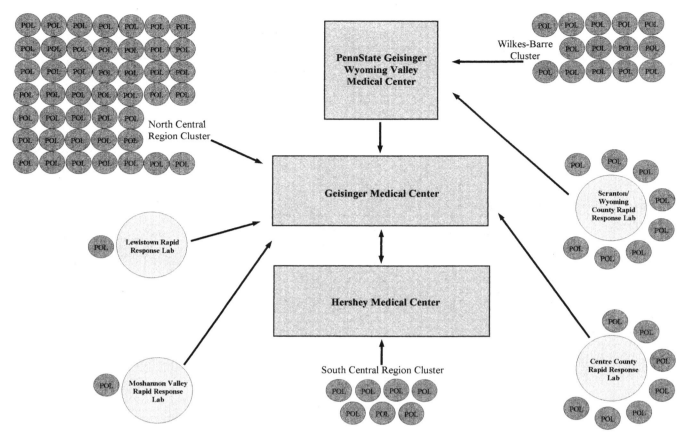

FIGURE 19.2. Topology of "clusters" of Health Group Laboratory (HGL) sites in the Penn State Geisinger Medical Laboratory System (PSGML). *Small circles*, physician office laboratories (POL); *large circles*, rapid-response decentralized group practice laboratories; *boxes*, medical centers. Each *incoming arrow* to medical center indicates an HGL cluster; *arrows* between medical centers indicate test referral patterns. PSGML demerger in 2000 removed the Hershey Medical Center from the associated cluster. The Geisinger Medical Laboratory (GML) with associated Geisinger Regional Laboratory (GRL) was reestablished.

distributed laboratory because many aspects of client services operate hand in glove with on-site testing. POCT volumes are still a small fraction of the total PSGML test volume, but applications of POCT are increasing.

The important principle of "niche testing" has been maintained during the evolution of the GRL. POCT was implemented in niches of clinical need where "real-time" laboratory testing results were clinically and financially necessary. The mainstream of operational efficiency and economy of scale remains in transporting specimens to 24-hour hospital laboratories operating increasingly like traditional commercial laboratories. Again, opposite trends coexist in practical balance as more diverse POCT and consolidated total laboratory automation increase in prevalence. As POCT technology becomes more reliable (e.g., accurate, precise, convenient) and integrated (e.g., electronically connected to the LIS), it will increasingly become part of the infrastructure of the specimen collection process. As the efficiency of concurrently obtaining a specimen and a test result improves, POCT niche applications will become more mainstream. The strategy of our GRL organization is to adapt to

POCT when to do so is judged economically and technically practical. Our standardized and "organic" approach to managing GRL operations will help facilitate the placement of POCT in the mainstream when process improvement dictates.

Point-of-Care Testing Menu in a Regional Integrated Delivery System Network

In the distributed laboratory, there are often different levels or "tiers" of laboratory testing that lend themselves to practice sites of different size or physician specialty. These levels of laboratory testing lend themselves to different models of laboratory operations with associated POCT. The three predominant models that have evolved in the GRL with associated POCT are listed in Table 19.2. The simpler level one or level two models have at times been rapidly deployed in as little as 1 week when physician practices have joined the GHS. Having predefined models with lists of approved methods in the distributed laboratory has removed confusion and given clear direction to physicians when their practices join the GHS. This prepackaged laboratory

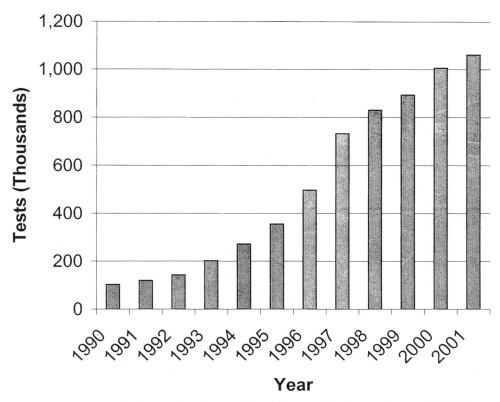

FIGURE 19.3. Increase in the number of tests referred from Health Group Laboratory (HGL) sites to central laboratories, 1990 to 2001.

TABLE 19.2. PREDOMINANT MODELS FOR CLIA PHYSICIAN OFFICE LABORATORY SITES IN THE GEISINGER REGIONAL LABORATORY

"Level one" or "waived" model
 Quantitative glucose (HemoCue)
 Hemoglobin (HemoCue)
 Urinalysis by dipstick
 Rapid strep
 Pregnancy test
 Provider-performed microscopy (PPM)
"Level two" model
 Tests in level one plus:
  BUN (I-stat)
  Electrolytes (I-stat)
  Cell counts (WBC, RBC, H/H, plt)
  Prothrombin time
"Level three" or "cluster" lab site
 Tests in levels one and two plus:
  ALT
  AST
  ALP
  Calcium
  Total protein
  Albumin
  Total bilirubin
  Creatinine
  CBC with partial diff
  Blood gases

CLIA, Clinical Laboratories Improvement Act; BUN, blood urea nitrogen; WBC, white blood cells; RBC, red blood cells; H/H, hemoglobin and hematocrit; plt, platelets; ALT, alanine aminotransferase; AST, aspartate aminotransferase; ALP, alkaline phosphate.

model approach resembles a franchise and has been referred to affectionately as "McLab."

The predominant model in our 83-site distributed laboratory network fell under the category of level one. Several of these sites do only minimal testing, mostly urinalysis by dipstick, occult blood, and pregnancy testing. Of the 68 sites that fell under this model, approximately 20 perform quantitative glucose or hemoglobin measurements with the HemoCue device (22,23). Test menus are established within a given model but are used selectively as clinical need justifies. A test being "approved" for use within a given model of laboratory does not automatically justify the expense of implementing it. A careful explanation is given to clinician users of the infrastructure (24–26) required for implementation of a POCT (e.g., data logging, proficiency testing, quality control, preventative maintenance). Because testing personnel are predominantly nursing personnel, and nursing time in busy outpatient clinics is already at a premium, the demand for expanded POCT has been very conservative. Tests that are implemented at a site are formally added to the site CLIA license and fully supported by HGL technical staff. The commonly held fear that if POCT devices are made available they will be overused did not materialize in the HGL network. In fact, during 1997 through 1999, the number of tests performed in the HGL as POCT declined by about 20% because twice-a-day courier pickup increased centralized referral. Again, the PSGML had achieved balance between POCT and centralized referral.

Response Time for Point-of-Care Testing in a Regional Integrated Delivery System Network

With the distribution of POCT to practice sites, access to medically necessary tests on an emergent or clinically convenient basis has been largely available for 15 years. The availability of a selective menu of tests has served almost all the emergent needs of our practice sites. Alternatives to performing POCT at our practice sites include the following: (a) primarily, referral to one of the hospital laboratories or (b) secondarily, referral to local non-GHS community hospital laboratories. The former is enabled by twice-daily routine pickup by a GHS courier or an emergency-dispatched PSGML laboratory courier. The latter usually involves referring the patient to a local emergency department or laboratory for specimen collection. Some local community hospitals are contracted with our GHP and offer discounted laboratory services. Hence, collaboration with local providers is another factor that impacts the necessity of placing POCT in community practice sites of an IDS.

The referral of patients or specimens outside the GML for laboratory services (commonly termed *leakage*) is discouraged except for emergent or priority patient convenience purposes. It has been found that charges for referral of such testing, even at discounted pricing, are much greater than GML costs. A single referral of a pediatric patient for electrolyte testing to diagnose dehydration, for example, may result in out-of-system "leakage" of several hundred dollars (e.g., emergency department fees, intravenous rehydration therapy, and professional charges). The use of I-Stat electrolyte testing (27–29) at selected level two and level three sites has been judged cost-effective compared with such out-of-system charges. This "charge avoidance" philosophy has entered into decision-making for deploying some "level two" POCT. We have not restricted ourselves to the narrow cost comparison of POCT versus centralized tests on solely a reagent cost basis, but rather we factor in issues of access and charge avoidance.

Medical necessity is a term we also have taken seriously from a regulatory standpoint when deciding where to deploy POCT. We established Medicare panels (i.e., hepatic function, electrolyte, basic metabolic, comprehensive metabolic panels) at the medical centers and, where technically practicable, at community practice sites. At the larger level three or "cluster" laboratory sites, these panels are tested at a point of care with four Roche Cobas MIRAS, which offers the capability of the basic metabolic [glucose, blood urea nitrogen (BUN), creatinine, Na, K, Cl, CO_2] and comprehensive metabolic (renal plus, aspartate aminotransferase, alkaline phosphate, Ca, total bilirubin, albumin, total protein) panels. In general, we avoid splitting panels, testing some components as POCT and testing the remaining tests at a hospital laboratory. This splitting practice creates some problems from a billing standpoint because the potential exists for double billing redundantly tested components. At GRL sites, which test discrete panel components such as glucose, the remainder of the panel components are individually ordered if medically necessary. Access to POCT in an IDS must include these integrated billing considerations. Capturing correct billing information, including International Classification of Diseases (ICD)-9 code and medical necessity documentation, at the point of service is another cost burden to performing POCT at multiple locations.

In summary, response-time necessity has not been a primary driving factor for decentralizing POCT in the GHS. Some POCT is conveniently provided while the patient waits. In more emergent situations, outpatients can be referred to local community hospitals, or specimens can be transported to a GHS hospital for statim testing. The largest measures of practicality for decentralizing POCT stem from "charge avoidance" and system integration issues.

Integrating Point-of-Care Testing across the Continuum of Care

In a seamless IDS, a continuum of care exists at ever increasing numbers of locations that require standardization not only of the laboratory testing method but also of patient preparation, specimen collection, and information processing (30,31). Standardized protocol is integral to the entire testing process and is complied with predominantly at the point of care. Point-of-care locations across this continuum include patient homes, skilled nursing facilities, schools, community service organizations, workplaces, physician offices, group practice clinics, phlebotomy stations, as well as larger established laboratories in hospitals.

This access to testing locations across the continuum of care has been an impetus to enlarge our focus from testing locations within owned GHS facilities, staffed by salaried GHS personnel (i.e., in Fig. 19.4 locations within the triple line) to "outside-of-system" testing locations. As diagrammed in Figure 19.4, concentric circles grow out of traditional core laboratory testing at the three hospitals. The three domains of laboratory growth are (a) owned GRL laboratories with diversified services, including respiratory therapy (RT) and home nursing; (b) support of GHP patient laboratory testing be it in "impaneled" physician offices (i.e., contracted physicians caring for GHP HMO patients), skilled nursing facilities, or contracted hospitals; and (c) for-profit "outreach" testing, including a variety of marketable services. The basic service-delivery system that supports the GHS-owned facilities has become enlarged and refined to launch into the competitive regional marketplace. The time required to develop a service-oriented outreach culture and organization is shortened as the distributed laboratory grows with its own primary care network. The full description of this transition process from a hospital-based service to a full-fledged outreach service (i.e., akin to a three-shift commercial laboratory operation) is beyond the scope of this chapter. Suffice to say that as a distributed laboratory extends itself across the continuum of care [e.g., with couriers and dial-up personal computer (PC) systems] within its own health care system, opportunities abound to launch into the commercial sector.

In the GML, the term *point of care*, and to some degree *point-of-care testing*, has expanded to include all laboratory activities at all continua of care locations. The early establishment of POCT at primary care network sites provided valuable exposure to laboratorians to master an understanding of information needs in the continuum of care. It was learned early on that actual generation of a result from a POCT device, although important, is

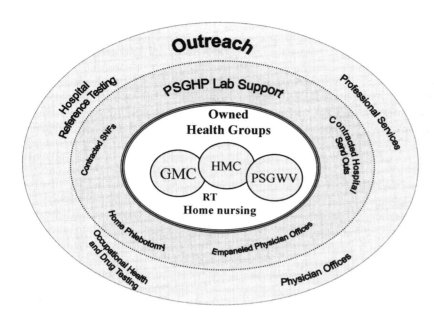

FIGURE 19.4. Outgrowth of laboratory outreach from an integrated primary care network.

a relatively minor component responsible for the overall program success of the GRL. Because the product of POCT activity is *information*, the importance of integrating information into the IDS to meet clinical and informational needs has overshadowed the actual "pushing of buttons" on the POCT device. At all locations in the continuum of care—from home-visiting nurse glucose testing to central laboratorian glycosylated hemoglobin (HbA1c) testing—the quality of information integration has become as important as the testing itself (30,32,33).

Point-of-care testing data must be seamlessly integrated into an IDS and its large continuum of care in such a way to produce test results that are interchangeable with central laboratory tests. The same rules that govern central laboratory testing must be applied at all locations where results are derived (34). CLIA regulations, Medicare rules, and clinical pathways all must be integrated into the laboratory testing system in a standardized manner across the continuum of care. This information integration has been a daunting task at times in the GHS, but where electronic archiving of test results currently exists, standardization has largely been achieved.

Because a single unified Division of Laboratory Medicine has established laboratory infrastructure across the continuum of care as it has evolved over the last 10 years in the GHS, a relatively seamless system now exists. Laboratorians who helped establish this infrastructure in POCT in the last 10 to 15 years are now experienced in expanded operational systems and have taken on an expanded role in PSGHS "system analysis." The role of "system analyst" includes assignment to committees and design teams that install new information systems (e.g., billing and ambulatory care physician practice systems), refine operational efficiency in reception and related ancillary areas (e.g., outpatient coagulation testing by pharmacy program), and launch outreach activities in the local community.

It is of utmost importance that the laboratorian practicing at the point of care recognizes this expanded role across the continuum of care. Total responsibility for POCT in a given specialty (e.g., coagulation testing in hematology, glucose testing in chemistry) in an IDS cannot be partitioned into a specialty laboratory *per se* but must be organized into the flow of *information*. Laboratorians must avoid the rigid thinking that POCT must emulate the factory setting of a hospital laboratory to produce the same quality results. Assuring quality of preanalytic and postanalytic information and being part of the flow of *information* at point of care contributes immensely to the success of the overall laboratory. The term *distributed laboratory* aptly describes the new laboratory structure in the GRL as POCT and associated information processing continues to migrate into the continuum of care.

Some examples of POCT-based activities, which should be planned in a distributed laboratory across the continuum of care, are listed in Table 19.3. Distributed HGL laboratory operations exist at various levels of maturity for all these activities.

TABLE 19.3. ACTIVITIES ASSOCIATED WITH POINT-OF-CARE TESTING IN AN INTEGRATED DELIVERY SYSTEM

Supporting community based point-of-care testing (e.g., diabetes screening)
Receiving and processing specimens from home health nurses at point-of-care testing locations
Dispatching phlebotomy services to home health and SNFs
Dispatching testing services to home health and SNFs (e.g., blood gas testing)
Ensuring proper supply utilization by nursing (e.g., designing supply order forms)
Ensuring proper supply distribution (e.g., dispensing home tests)
Directing patients to "next step" (e.g., go to pharmacy anticoagulation clinic after PT result)
Performing QC checks on patient home glucose meters
Assuring adherence of point-of-care testing and specimen processing to clinical pathways
Providing real-time results communication for real-time treatment (e.g., P_{O_2} with F_{IO_2} for home oxygen prescription)

SNF, skilled nursing facilities; PT, prothrombin time; QC, quality control; P_{O_2}, partial pressure of oxygen; F_{IO_2}, fraction of inspired oxygen.

A specific example of how a system POCT standard was applied to a continuum of care testing need was the use of the HemoCue whole-blood glucose testing device for employer-sponsored "health fairs." Nurses from the GHP continuous health improvement program (CHIP) asked the laboratory for help in certifying its testing program with the State of Pennsylvania, which requires a temporary site license for the testing event. The POCT coordinator at Geisinger Medical Center in Danville provided CHIP nurses with HemoCue devices; these devices had data managers kept in a modular tray for rapid deployment. The laboratory provided a batch sheet for resulting individual glucose results (for local use) and archived downloaded electronic results (for laboratory use). The laboratory helped CHIP register each testing event with the state for a $25.00 fee and charged the CHIP program $1.00 per electronically logged test to cover the cost of consumables. The laboratory trained a select number of CHIP nurses and maintained competency and quality control records. This entire program was put in place in 2 weeks and, within 6 months the number of screening glucose tests performed has climbed to approximately 1,000 per month (average of 10 events per month with 100 tests per event). This type of rapidly deployed yet well-monitored POCT program in the continuum of care exemplifies the current demand for services in a growing IDS and for service excellence that the GML has learned to deliver.

All these examples involve understanding broader-based systems than POCT alone. The most important new understanding that laboratorians will need to achieve resides in the preanalytic and postanalytic aspects of the testing process. Laboratorians who migrate to POCT locations must be empowered to make decisions affecting laboratory testing that reside in these parts of the testing process. A subsequent section describes dynamics that unfolded in the PSGHS as empowerment was gained for technologists working at POCT locations.

Standardizing Point-of-Care Testing via Group Purchasing Organizations

One of the first things to do in unifying laboratory testing within an IDS, especially after a merger, is to standardize technical methods, including those performed at point of care. There are numerous positive gains with minimal risk when achieving technical standardization. To overcome inertia of user resistance to change, it is useful to develop a standardization strategy that includes combined purchasing through a group purchasing organization (GPO) (35,36). A rapid group decision by affected laboratorians and POCT users is facilitated by (a) perceived supply savings projected by combined volume discounts, (b) a more select number of GPO vendors to choose from, (c) greater efficiency of supply requisitioning, and (d) assured compliance with the selected vendor products. It is important that senior leadership in the IDS and the laboratory create a mandate and deadline for vendor selection under guidelines of the designated GPO. The dynamics of such a group decision process frequently are cited as a stumbling block. Selecting vendors from a GPO need not produce disharmony if approached from a positive and practical mindset.

Leadership from the laboratory standardization group as well as encouragement from senior leadership should produce a "we are all in this together" camaraderie (37). Well-designed facilitator training programs are available to bring together the decision process, but most laboratories have natural leaders who, if empowered by senior leadership, should be able to accomplish consensus in vendor selection. It is important that a clear understanding exists with senior leadership of the IDS that the laboratory must make vendor selections and maintain tight, unfettered relationships with these suppliers.

Often, hospital systems are merged and a rapid standardization process is started for major laboratory systems, such as chemistry analyzers, hematology analyzers, and laboratory information systems. Many of these efforts do not succeed because parties with major vested interests draw "turf lines" and protect themselves from change. If given the luxury of time (e.g., a year), it is much more productive to start with POCT methods standardization, which is viewed as more benign by affected hospital laboratorians who rally together to improve the perceived quality of POCT. For example, standardizing a qualitative pregnancy test from a dual source GPO vendor agreement should get a standardization team working together constructively and a selection achieved with comparative ease. Once the selection is made, the standardization group can support the decision and immediately help in implementing the change.

It is imperative that laboratorians be involved in implementing the milieu of details that are involved in a change as "simple" as standardizing qualitative pregnancy testing. It is also important to recognize that ultimately the laboratory will be responsible for supporting standardized POCT and that the IDS will need to incorporate the specified technology into clinical pathways for years to come. Vendors should not expect to work solely with material management or purchasing departments to leverage distribution of their product. The distribution of product requires a substantial effort from the laboratory (e.g., setting up laboratory supply requisitions that track expenses to the proper laboratory cost center).

Once a POCT product is chosen as a standard, a great deal of infrastructure must be built around it. Ongoing user training, supply distribution, CLIA regulatory compliance, and information system input are a few of the laboratory infrastructural details that must be supported. For this reason, it is important to make long-term (3–5 years) vendor selections around which infrastructure will stabilize. Short-term decisions with changes every few years to save a few pennies per test or gain small increments of performance improvement are not wise in an IDS.

The real work of integrating POCT into an IDS is just that—integrating the delivery of POCT services to a broad range of customers. Once decisions are made in standardizing a POCT method, it takes at least a year to finalize the details of integration. With yearly turnover of a few hundred POCT users typical in a large IDS, retraining should settle on a stable ongoing method. IDSs do have economy of scale and "clout" with GPOs but also suffer unwieldiness from this large scale on the implementation side. Making changes in POCT in an IDS can seem like steering a supertanker in that implementing a small change in direction requires much time and effort to bring closure. In the preceding example of qualitative pregnancy testing, the PSGML had used the same testing device for the last 10 years without losing appreciable savings or performance.

Standardizing POCT products also must take into account a host of IDS considerations. Does the product integrate into larger clinical laboratory testing systems (e.g., qualitative urine microalbumin dipstick and quantitative urine albumin/creatinine ratio)? Does the GPO designated vendor have a strategy of developing a range of products to support disease management? Will the product eventually be used in home testing, and will it be distributed by HMO and local pharmacies (e.g., HMO-supplied glucose meters for home use versus those used in clinics and at the bedside)? Will the product be available from the vendor and GPO in 5 years (e.g., will the vendor and GPO form a strategic or corporate partnership)?

In the PSGHS a "premier corporate partner" relationship was established with the Premier GPO. Under this relationship, financial incentives were offered PSGHS not only for compliance within our own organization but also for the financial success of Premier. The PSGHS had in essence become a business partner of this GPO. Such a strong alliance stiffens resolve to comply with selected vendors. This may seem at first glance to take authority from the laboratory in making vendor selections, but in actuality it strengthened the combined laboratory position. In every instance of vendor selection, POCT, and otherwise, one of the vendors we had standardized to was offered as a choice under the Premier GPO. By choosing larger "mainstream" vendors over the last 10 years, we have positioned ourselves to move rather painlessly into the GPO era. Table 19.4 lists the POCT vendors we purchased technology from during the last 5 to 10 years (our a priori standards), the vendors we selected under the Premier partnership, and the vendors designated by Premier in sole source to trisource agreements.

Standardization decisions were made at a very opportune time because they have enabled a very aggressive time frame for

installation of a Sunquest laboratory information system ("Mulhos" configuration on a wide area network, or WAN) at HMC. The advantages of implementing standardized methods with common LIS test codes will be expanded on in a later section. Suffice it to say that achieving method standardization (starting with simple POCT) generates momentum to achieve a unified distributed laboratory, so necessary for supporting a seamless IDS. In fact, the PSGML was regarded in the PSGHS as a positive example and driving force for integrating clinic operations and information systems.

Parameters for Centralized Versus Decentralized Laboratory Testing Decisions

One parameter used in deciding whether a test method is deployed decentrally is its frequency of emergent use. As already mentioned, there are options of dispatching a courier or using a local hospital resource to meet most emergent testing needs of our 83 practice sites. If the frequency of emergent need reaches the level of several times per month and the out-of-system charges clearly exceed the cost of bringing the test method to a given practice site, it is targeted for implementation. Blanket decisions are not made that all or most practice sites qualify for emergent POCT. Because practice sites differ in their location, patient population, and provider practice style, they are treated individually. Providers at individual practice sites have not insisted on "me too" implementation of technology seen at sister practice sites. One may be somewhat assured that negative assumptions of "if you give it to one, they will all want it" rarely materialize.

Site-by-site and test-by-test assessments are made by cluster supervisors, site medical directors, and HGL leadership based on actual site utilization to determine which tests should be supported. Although the 83 sites generally fell into the aforementioned "levels" or models of laboratories, not every test was implemented within a given model. Instead, standardized test methods were "taken off the shelf" to meet site needs. Some level one sites opted for rapid strep testing, whereas others opted for referring a swab for probe testing to the central laboratory. In general, in the PSGML, we preferred to refer as many tests to centralized hospital laboratories operating around the clock as possible with POCT used selectively.

Another parameter used in deciding the location of testing is "clinical efficiency" at the point of care (38). If a patient's care can be modified because of an immediately available laboratory test, it may be done at point of care. Most clinical services have not matured to the point of being able to incorporate immediately available laboratory testing data into real-time decision-making; therefore, only selective applications of POCT have been made to enhance clinical efficiency in our outpatient setting.

Two clinical applications that have benefited from POCT in terms of clinical efficiency are outpatient pulmonology and coagulation clinics (39,40). An I-Stat device supports the former and Dade MLA-750s supports the latter. These two test methods are standardized across the entire GHS. Both methods use reagent or cartridges from a system-wide sequestered lot number. Both methods use quality control materials (with identical

TABLE 19.4. EFFECT OF GROUP PURCHASING ORGANIZATION ON LAB PRODUCTS USED IN THE PSGHS

Product Category	Before Premier	After Premier	Premier Source(s)
Glucose meter	Lifescan	Lifescan	Lifescan BMD
Pregnancy test	Abbott	Abbott	Abbott Quidel
Strep test	Abbott	Abbott	Abbott Quidel
Urinalysis	Bayer BMD	Bayer	Bayer
Blood gas, POCT	I-Stat	I-Stat	I-Stat
Blood gas	Chiron Radiometer	Chiron	Chiron IL
Chemistry	Roche Ortho	Roche	Roche Ortho Dade
Coagulation	Dade Pacific HS	Dade	Dade Ortho
Hematology	Sysmex Coulter	Sysmex	Sysmex Coulter

PSGHS, Penn State Geisinger Health System; POCT, point-of-care testing.

lot numbers and data reduction services) as the entire system. As patients are seen and tested at different GRL and hospital sites, their laboratory results are available with a single standard of interpretability and quality. Clinical efficiency is also enhanced by the transportability of test results between sites without the need for retesting.

Initial outcome studies (40) from three decentralized coagulation clinics in the PSGHS showed system savings in terms of avoided complications from inadequate anticoagulation. These coagulation clinics demonstrated clinical efficiency by enabling the alteration of a patient's anticoagulation therapy dose based on a prothrombin time (PT) during a single short visit to a convenient accessible location. In a cohort of PSGHS patients with atrial fibrillation, those tightly monitored for PT ($n = 66$) by a pharmacy-managed anticoagulation clinic versus those patients managed by the normal means ($n = 228$), the difference in complication outcome was established. The cost per member per month (pm/pm) of the tightly monitored group was substantially less at $1.80 pm/pm than the normally monitored group at $27.27 pm/pm. Over the 12 months of this study, 39 cerebral vascular accidents (CVA) were found from claims data for the normally monitored group ($n = 228$) versus one for the tightly monitored group ($n = 66$). A focused coagulation clinic performing rapid or point-of-care PT with immediate clinical intervention was also a great patient satisfier. The ongoing usefulness of this outcome data will be enhanced as information systems package it into clinical pathways via the clinical repository.

Although clinical efficiency has yet to become a major driving force for extensive POCT, we are positioned to expand current methodologies and operating systems rapidly as clinical services become better accommodated to such real-time laboratory support. Although this chapter focuses mainly on the outpatient aspect of POCT, the GHS has also selectively integrated POCT in hospital inpatient niches for several years using clinical efficiency as a major deciding parameter.

STANDARDIZATION OF COMPUTERIZATION AND INFORMATICS IN AN INTEGRATED HEALTH CARE DELIVERY SYSTEM

As IDSs expand and merge, extremely complex information systems aggregate. These aggregated information systems are increasingly complex because most frequently "best of breed" departmental systems become intermixed at merger. In essence, the IDS has the challenge of integrating customized information systems, producing customization to accommodate customization.

With the accelerated pace of mergers and inflated expectations of information system functionality, a major crisis looms in these expanding IDSs. One may whimsically state that perhaps the "year 2000 bug" is a blessing in disguise. IDSs continue to carry forward patchwork information systems. Certainly, this state of nonstandardized information system linkage in the current IDS landscape will require major dollar investments to maintain and upgrade for years to come (41).

Fortunately, POCT is a relatively new health care activity that may opportune information systems that avoid the pitfalls and problems of the past. Given proper planning, POCT information

flow may be integrated more easily and appropriately into health care informatics at large (42). Standardization efforts for creating POCT data managers (also commonly referred to as data concentrators or POCT workstations) have recently begun. Standardization development organizations (SDOs), such as the American Society for Testing and Materials (ASTM), the National Committee for Clinical Laboratory Standards (NCCLS), the Institute of Electrical and Electronics Engineers (IEEE), Health Level 7 (HL7), and the International Standards Organization (ISO), have pioneered standards for acquiring data from POCT devices for import into the computerized patient record (49).

Recently, the Connectivity Industrial Consortium (CIC) produced specifications using many of these preexisting standards. These CIC specifications promise enabling of a PC data manager/workstation(s) for interfacing multivendor POCT devices to LISs and computerized patient records. CIC specifications are targeted for adoption by instrument and information systems vendors as well as users in 2001. Ongoing refinement and maintenance of these CIC specifications will likely be the responsibility of at least two of these SDOs, namely HL7 and NCCLS.

Because POCT results must be integrated into the medical and business records of an IDS, and access to this information resides largely at the point of care, there is abundant information that needs to flow through this standardized data manager to the LIS. The diversity and amount of information that crosses the interface between the testing device and its data manager are much greater than that which typically flows through an instrument interface to an LIS. Hence the approach taken to develop POCT device interfaces is not limited to the classic approach of developing an instrument interface.

The PC revolution is also enhancing functionality for capturing and sharing information from multiple information systems across WANs using Internet connectivity. With this increased capability, common conventions and standards are acutely needed to make the integration of POCT data managers practical.

A straightforward example of a need for improved conventions and standards in the PSGHS involves the use of location identifiers or codes. Where is the patient when he or she is tested? Where was the patient transferred to (i.e., does the admission/transfer/discharge, A/D/T, information system update the location identifier)? Where should the laboratory test results be sent? Traditionally, in most health care systems, location is a geographic place. As IDSs such as the PSGHS diffuse across multiple locations, entities, and collaborative services, however, the term *location* becomes more confused. Because POCT requires location of the patient to be input to information system(s) to archive a test result, consideration must be given to location when integrating across the continuum of care.

In the PSGHS, location code was not universally standardized within multiple information systems. In fact, there is lack of agreement as to what location code should actually signify. Should location code designate the physical location of the patient (e.g., bed, room, and ward)? Should it designate the clinical service (e.g., dialysis, nephrology, outpatient)? Should it designate a physician's or group of physicians' activity (e.g., three dermatologists practicing outreach at several network locations)? Despite several efforts, there is not a location code in the GHS either at the alpha-numeric field length level or at the "What does location code signify?" level. Despite this lack of standardization, disparate information systems do share this information element in the GHS—but at a price. Multiple conversion tables are maintained to convert location codes from one information system to another(s) as interfaces pass this key demographic.

Because the lack of standard identifiers such as location code will likely be problematic for IDS informatics for years to come, POCT data managers will have to maintain the flexibility to connect to multiple disparate systems. It is unlikely that POCT data manager standardization efforts will attempt to force standardization of location codes. Rather, field length and message content specifications will need to be spelled out to adapt to multiple host systems. The task of standardizing location codes will likely remain the task of the individual IDS or the medical informatics community at large. Foresighted IDSs will have to discipline themselves to standardize such straightforward data elements to remain integrated across the continuum of care as integration becomes more important for "cradle to grave" health coverage.

Using Laboratory Information System Test Method Codes to Drive Standardization

Once standardized test methods are placed at point of care and a multientity IDS is using the same LIS, it becomes compelling and logical to establish common LIS test codes. Standardization of methods enables all the advantages of reporting results from various locations with the same clinical interpretability (43,44). A longitudinal laboratory test record as patients intermingle their visits at different primary care and hospital sites is a growing necessity for IDSs.

In essence, method standardization enables database standardization which enables outcome studies. A major goal of an IDS with associated HMO is to ensure risk using laboratory parameters based on outcome studies to quantitate risk. Standardizing laboratory test results in a clinical database, or repository, moves an IDS toward effective monitoring of population risk and appropriate treatment for desired outcome (see later section on the importance of the IDS clinical repository).

All these advantages to the IDS encourage a strong standardization effort at the LIS test method and test code levels. It has been the experience of PSGML POCT laboratories that once a method is established in the LIS with its associated test code, it is almost invariably used "off the shelf." As a given POCT method proliferates through different sites in the IDS, LIS test codes are rarely modified if enough foresight was exercised in establishing them with broad application. Once properly established, the time and effort to maintain standardized LIS method and test codes become minimal. This type of standardization proliferation is exemplified by how I-Stat to LIS interfaces evolved at multiple point-of-care testing locations in our IDS.

In January 1992, the first "autoscripting" (i.e., terminal emulation) interface was established (1) from the I-Stat central data station (CDS) to our Community Health Computing (CHC) LIS for the 6+ cartridge (Glucose, BUN, Na, K, Cl, CO_2, hematocrit). Test codes were established and tables built in the LIS that were separate from but standardized to the same whole-blood tests performed on Nova Stat 5 whole-blood instruments. These

tests were identified with an extension pneumonic of ISTAT (e.g., GLU-ISTAT). In this way, even though the whole-blood studies performed from a pneumatically tubed syringe specimen or an I-Stat test done at point of care were printed sequentially in the same cumulative summary in the patient's chart, they were easily discernible. Comparability testing on patient specimens was performed at regular intervals to confirm that the pairs of test results did not show clinically significant difference. Hematocrit did show enough difference so that protocols were written to establish the central lab as the primary method (in this case hematocrit from a Coulter counter) that was to be used for clinically significant treatment decisions such as neonate transfusion. Again, having the results interspersed but discernable suited clinical needs in the inpatient hospital setting.

When I-Stat cartridges became available for additional tests such as blood gases and ionized calcium, we took much the same tack. Besides LIS test code parameters, we also standardized associated patient clinical parameters (e.g., temperature, O_2 delivery, FiO_2, specimen source, pulse oximetry). All these test code and clinical parameters were synchronized between the LIS and the I-Stat central data station.

Once established in the LIS, I-Stat test results settled into stable information flow in clinic operations. Maintenance of the integrated data was minimal. All test codes and clinical parameters were ported from CHC to our new Sunquest LIS when it went live under version 5.2 software in April 1997. Except for the aforementioned mnemonic identifiers, blood-gas results are reported from POCT sites and central stat laboratory sites transparently to the clinician in the same location in the chart.

Because laboratory billing is accomplished via a Sunquest interface, standardized Current Procedural Terminology (CPT) codes, charges, and billing numbers were also built for the billing system. Critical limits (reported visually by the handheld device at point of care), reference ranges, and patient identification requirements (by medical record number) were all standardized to central stat laboratory parameters. These same parameters initially built for broad application are now shared across three medical centers and five community practice sites using I-Stat. The initial battery of test codes built in the 1992 CHC LIS were expanded and continue to provide an easily maintained template for future expansion.

A particular I-Stat device placed at a community practice site to support outpatient pulmonology is configured with blood-gas LIS parameters identical to those used in hospital POCT (1,28). There were, however, implementation issues when this technology was decentralized to the practice site 90 miles from the main hospital in Danville.

The I-Stat arterial blood gas (ABG) cartridge is filled and tested in the phlebotomy or physician office areas of this practice site, depending on whether the laboratory or the physician obtains the specimen. ABG results are reported locally from the I-Stat device and archived after input into the Sunquest LIS, usually on a daily basis. For this specialty testing, Medicare regulations state that the physician needs to be in proximity to the phlebotomy area and must medically direct the obtaining of specimens. Phlebotomists needed to be trained under the direction of the pulmonologist physician. By reporting blood gas (with FiO_2) as a POCT, treatment may be modified and oxygen prescribed in a single visit. Out-of-system costs and patient inconvenience are avoided if the patient does not need to be referred to a local hospital for an ABG. Implementation of data integrated into the LIS was a major factor in encouraging physicians to perform these tests at point of care in the HGL rather than sending patients to a nearby hospital. All these implementation issues were addressed by a growing team of forward-looking laboratorians with an on-site "cluster" supervisor taking the lead in actual installation.

A similar approach was taken in standardizing quantitative glucose testing at point of care by the HemoCue device. Although a Sunquest LIS interface has been prototyped (20), glucose results currently remain manually input to the LIS from paper slips. The result in the chart utilizes a "GLU-HEMO-CUE" nomenclature and is used in locations where more accurate and precise measurements, especially at less than 50 mg per deciliter, are required (e.g., surgical preoperative area, neonatology, intensive care) than is afforded by the ubiquitous glucose meter. HemoCue glucose testing devices are currently used at approximately 30 primary care network sites and billed with the CPT code for quantitative glucose. One Touch Lifescan Glucose meters are used at most of these primary care sites largely for diabetic patient education for home testing.

Glucose meter results are currently interfaced to the SunQuest LIS at all three PSGML inpatient hospitals. An electronic data interface (EDI) is installed at the three hospitals. As of January 1999, two hospital sites were using modem connections between PC data managers and "Sure Step Pro" upload cradles and one was using Ethernet. Ethernet connectivity for all three hospitals is planned within the next few years.

Stratifying Informatics in a Multientity Integrated Delivery System

There is a quiet and sometimes not so quiet movement occurring in medical informatics, especially in IDSs. Classic departmental information systems (e.g., laboratory, radiology, pharmacy) are being criticized for lack of functionality and user friendliness as PC-based specialty systems, either as stand-alone workstations or as server-based PC networks, are demonstrating enhanced functionality and ease of use. Medical informatics, especially in IDSs, may be well on the road of evolving to point of care just as laboratory testing is evolving to point of care.

Personal computer–based specialty systems do create a challenge for integration into an evolving IDS. Although diabetes, coagulation, or cardiology PC-based specialty systems may provide enhanced functionality at the local level compared with large departmental systems, they are currently hard to integrate and maintain. The same may also be said for PC-based POCT testing data managers from a host of different POCT device vendors (e.g., glucose, ABG, PT, chemistry, urinalysis). As network technology improves, more flexible server application software evolves, and IDSs discipline themselves to standardized operations, integration problems eventually will be overcome and integrated networks will almost assuredly become predominant. In the near term as the PC informatics revolution gathers momentum, there will remain significant and at times overwhelming challenges to implementation and integration of POCT and specialty systems.

A major challenge to implementing these user-friendly local PC-based systems involves adapting them to the front end of the health care operation. These systems are designed to capture patient information as the patient presents and may evolve into the order entry console for multiple departmental information systems at strata deeper in the integrated delivery system. A prime example of this supplanting of the order entry process is occurring in the GHS with the installation of a PC-based ambulatory care and practice management system, EpicCare. EpicCare will be the outer strata of information entry and retrieval whose screen will face most PSGHS outpatient users.

The EpicCare System, consisting of approximately 1,200 PC workstations, is being installed at 70 practice sites in the GHS and eventually most outpatient clinics in the two hospitals. It is designed to be the primary physician interface for placing departmental outpatient orders (i.e., laboratory, radiology, pharmacy) for the entire IDS. The specifics of implementing POCT with this EpicCare System are described in detail later. Suffice it to say that a new paradigm is being approached in laboratory informatics that will change the way laboratorians receive and process information from the point of care.

The laboratory that understands fundamental medical informatics at the point of care will be a key operative in implementing the new strata of WAN-based information systems. Laboratorians who ignore the impact of decentralized PC-based information systems risk losing control of their product: *information.*

Unifying Patient Demographic Information in an Integrated Delivery System

Some of the most difficult aspects of implementing a POCT program at multiple sites in an IDS involve obtaining patient demographics that meet the requirements for LIS ordering and resulting. At owned GRL practice sites, which are not part of a medical center, the use of a common medical record number (MRN) is mandatory in our system. When a new practice site joins the GHS, one of the first changes made is converting patients and their records to a GHS MRN. Old patient MRNs might not change initially at a few excepted sites, but usually even they are replaced within 2 years. As new patients are enrolled at a newly joined site and as old patients are seem during return visits, the standardized MRN is used.

Location codes, provider numbers, insurance-carrier information, and ICD-9 codes all are important information elements requiring input for a valid laboratory order and result. In an IDS like GHS spread across 28 counties with thousands of providers, obtaining this information in a consistent manner requires a major ongoing effort. As mentioned, this type of information management has supplanted technologic management in terms of time consumed by the laboratory in operating its POCT program. Cluster supervisors, client service technologists, and other GRL personnel spend a great deal of time attending to preanalytic and postanalytical information quality as CLIA-mandated technical quality requires less ongoing attention. Our 15 years of experience in decentralizing POCT across 28 (or 35) counties and 70 (or 83) CLIA licenses in the GHS (or PSGHS) has taught us that laboratorians make expert information concentrators and processors. The challenge continues to transplant this expertise to increasing numbers of users. Training a few nurses in proper order entry in an intensive care area of a hospital is much easier than training a few hundred country doctors entering orders in busy primary care examining rooms.

Another problem encountered in POCT is the lack of real time patient identification and MRN assignment. In our trauma unit, "John or Jane Doe" patients are admitted and tested by POCT prior to assignment of a permanent MRN. In these cases, a temporary MRN is assigned and placed as a bar-coded wristband and a case number assigned (e.g., M14 for fourteenth male trauma case of day). I-Stat results such as ABG and electrolytes, commonly performed for these patients, are tagged with the temporary identification numbers and then merged with the permanent MRN prior to or after verification to the LIS. Significant patient misidentification has not occurred since the inception of this trauma POCT system in 1992.

Real-time verification of I-Stat test results to the LIS does not occur, largely because of the lack of real-time patient registration and associated "encounter number." In the outpatient areas of our IDS, where patients present as part of a clinical appointment, patient identification is not problematic as new patients are registered and old patients are updated in the admission/discharge/transfer (A/D/T) system.

A major time consumer in POCT at diverse locations in the IDS is assigning a proper diagnosis code (i.e., ICD-9 code), especially when it is not initially provided with the physician order. Medical technologist cluster supervisors and other testing personnel who receive specimens for POCT must obtain this information at the front end of our operation. POCT personnel are best positioned to reestablish the testing request in the mind of the provider to obtain ICD-9 codes. They also diplomatically issue a gentle reminder to fill out complete requisitions the next time. We have found that this practice is more productive and ultimately more efficient than obtaining the ICD-9 codes at the back end of the operation (i.e., in the billing office). In most HGL locations, compliance in supplying ICD-9 codes and complying with "medical necessity" requirements is good or improving. Medical necessity compliance as per a documented PSGML Medicare Fraud and Abuse Compliance Plan is established at all GRL sites in the GHS.

Importance of Decision Support Systems and a Clinical Repository

Decision support systems (DSS) are increasingly used in managed care organizations to track financial performance of various health care activities. These information systems generate financial data that will assist in making business decisions, especially when benchmarks become available to compare peer organizations. One may view the future of DSS analysis in the same light as laboratory proficiency testing. As these systems mature, the basic question of "how are we doing financially, compared to our peers" may be addressed with peer comparison benchmarks. DSS analysis is currently very popular in IDSs and managed care organizations because of shrinking reimbursement, increasing cost, and increasing price sensitivity in the laboratory outreach market. By and large, DSS analysis focusses on financial

rather than clinical outcomes, although theoretically some overlap may occur in the future. Clinical outcome studies for the foreseeable future will likely be performed on clinical repository systems separate from DSSs. The DSSs were Transition Systems Incorporated (TSI) for the old Geisinger portion of the PSGHS and Trend Star for the old Hershey Medical Center portion of the PSGHS, respectively.

It is generally recognized that POCT is more expensive than central laboratory tests on a supply and laboratory labor basis; however, the clinical value or efficiency of POCT frequently justifies this cost difference. One must draw this distinction when interpreting DSS information because the true institutional cost savings are often missed in DSS analysis. These missed cost savings, oftentimes referred to as *intangibles*, are not intangible at all but represent major cost savings that may be gained by increased clinical efficiency. A major component of cost that is saved by POCT is the labor of information processing and assimilation. This component is also not assessed in current DSSs.

Point-of-care testing will need to be justified with methods that currently are lacking in DSSs. In fact, DSS analysis may inhibit the growth of POCT unless hidden costs of performing lab testing are factored into cost analysis. One project informally performed in the HGL that demonstrates such hidden costs is assessment of the labor cost of the entire testing process: preanalytic, analytic, and postanalytic. Initial assessment confirms that most of the labor costs are in the preanalytic step of the process. Estimates stated elsewhere confirm our own perceptions, that 50% to 75% of labor costs exist in procuring, processing, and delivering a specimen to the laboratory from the point of care. In one example, obtaining a specimen for electrolyte analysis where order entry and specimen processing were performed at a GRL site, only 5% of attended or "hands-on" time (i.e. labor) was associated with actually performing batch testing in the central laboratory (Table 19.5). Ninety percent of attended time for generating the test results was spent at the point of care.

Clearly, we must focus on efficiency at the front end of the testing process (i.e., near or at the point-of-care) to find labor savings in the future. As we streamline the pre-analytical laboratory testing process, we may very well find that the analytic process folds into it. A handheld device may accomplish paperless order entry, testing without specimen processing, and initial results reporting during the patient encounter. If properly integrated into front-end information flow, the clinical efficiency of POCT may result in substantial labor savings. Time studies will need to be extensively and more formally done to present usable data to DSSs to quantitate such savings. Fiscally conservative IDSs are slow to move to POCT because of a lack of documented preanalytic labor savings. Most financial decisions are made with classic DSS data "counting widgets" that lag behind practical reality.

A paramount goal of an IDS is to concentrate data in a clinical repository for clinical outcome studies. The potential value to an IDS is enormous in establishing clinical pathways based on validated outcome. These outcome data may also be used from a financial standpoint much as an insurance actuarial would do. It may not be an understatement that the ultimate success of an IDS, and its most valuable asset will reside in its clinical repository.

TABLE 19.5. REPRESENTATIVE ATTENDED TIMES TO COMPLETE LABORATORY TESTING CYCLE

Step	Attended Time, s	Step Time, s (%)
Preanalytic		
1. Check in patient and generate "face sheet" containing insurance, provider, testing information	90	
2. Phlebotomy reception, converting "face sheet" into LIS order	60	
3. Phlebotomy procedure, verify LIS order, label tubes, rack tubes	480	
4. Centrifuge specimens, label aliquot tubes	20	
5. Aliquot specimens, prepare for transport, place in transport bag	15	665 *(90%)*
Analytic		
1. Unpack specimen(s), place in rack	15	
2. Place specimen rack on instrument, verify results	15	
3. Discard specimen(s)	10	40 *(5%)*
Postanalytic		
1. Start result printing, clarify "copy to" reports	10	
2. Sort, review, route hard copy reports	25	35 *(5%)*
Total *(100%)*	**740**	**740**

LIS, laboratory information system.

Point-of-care tests with associated patient demographics and clinical information must also reside in the clinical repository (44). As testing and the ability to capture test results migrate out into the continuum of care in an IDS, clinical treatment will require POCT. Clinical pathways will be established utilizing remote tests performed in clinics, doctor's offices, skilled nursing facilities, and the home. Results in the clinical repository will be used not only for retrospective studies but also contribute data to assist real-time decision support.

In the GHS, one clinical repository is envisioned as a back-end repository, whereas more real-time interactive systems assist real-time decision-making. In outpatient areas of the GHS, the EpicCare System described in detail later will be the primary tool in doctor's examining rooms to aid in clinical decision-making and will serve as the clinical repository. A mirrored clinical repository in a separate Cerner Millenium clinical information system was abandoned as the PSGHS demerged (Fig. 19.5).

Eventually, all laboratory results will reside in the EpicCare clinical repository; therefore, the aforementioned method and LIS method code standardization will be an important construct for the relational database of the repository.

COMMUNICATION SYSTEMS AND REMOTE ACCESS

Emergence of Ambulatory Care and Practice Management Information Systems

Primary care practice sites in an IDS are ever increasingly installing networked PC-based practice management systems. These PC-based practice management systems (e.g., EpicCare, Oceana) offer the practicing primary care physician a very user-friendly efficiency tool to document patient visits and treatment. In-baskets, out-baskets, and desktops are graphical user interface (GUI, or "gooey") presentations that doctors can relate to and master rapidly. The simplification of the graphic user interface has facilitated the growth of these types of systems.

The enormous amounts of information that must be input via GUI by clinicians present a major challenge to proper integration of these systems into IDSs. Important patient information including ICD-9 codes must accompany laboratory orders placed by physicians. Detailed input by keyboard and mouse replacing a scribbled note on a patient's chart to be "taken off" by clerical and nursing personnel constitute major cultural changes for physicians. "Information overload" in creating detailed lab orders, including those tested at point of care, it is hoped will be ameliorated for physicians by simplified GUI in increasingly busy clinical practice.

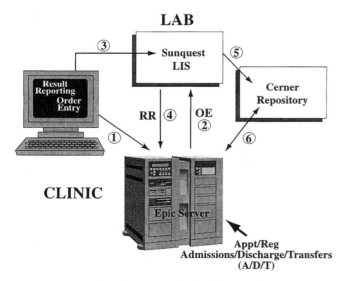

FIGURE 19.5. Design of integrated physician practice management (EpicCare) and laboratory information system (Sunquest LIS) computers in the PennState Geisinger Health System. Test order entry (OE) from EpicCare to Sunquest LIS, steps 1 and 2; test result reporting (RR), steps 3 and 4; test result archiving, steps 5 and 6.

Admission, discharge, and transfer information must also be a part of the ordering transaction. The EpicCare system that the GHS is installing has a portion of the A/D/T system embedded in application software (i.e., Cadence). The integration of front-end order entry activity (i.e., Cadence) is mission critical for the enlarging GML because accurate information is paramount to producing a valid laboratory test order and bill. Because multiple systems are responsible for departmental orders and departmental bills, implementation of the Cadence portion of the EpicCare System has been an ongoing difficult process.

The EpicCare system has been rolling out to the PSGHS in several phases beginning in 1996. The initial phase for implementation of EpicCare in the GHS involved hardware installation - 1200 PC's in examining rooms at all practice sites with connectivity to a WAN. This installation project was popularized with the term *microwave*. Older PC-based systems were replaced with the new PC terminals during the microwave project. Cable was pulled, connections to communication closets made, and terminals placed in all examining rooms at 83 primary care practice sites and several hospital outpatient areas. The placement of "intelligent" PC terminals also initiated a familiarization project for Windows-based applications for those physicians and medical professionals who were not familiar with its GUI at the time. The mere presence of microwaved PCs accelerated the training and adaptation process that was clearly intended to evolve into a paperless electronic medical record. Early installation of hardware helped to gauge and then overcome some natural resistance by some physicians who preferred practicing "the way we always have."

Of course, POCT was one of the things that physicians had always done and recorded manually in the patient's chart. Therefore, at hand was and continues to be the necessity to integrate POCT orders and results. Before this could be accomplished the integration of front-end information input (i.e., Cadence) remains to be fully implemented. Valid orders for laboratory tests, including those done at the point of care, require much initial input and hence integration between the LIS and the ambulatory care systems (Table 19.6). These information items in many cases also need to be standardized because straightforward information like patient location is shared by multiple information systems.

Although the EpicCare system is a very efficient tool for physicians to document clinical intervention, there are drawbacks to how laboratory information, including POCT, is

TABLE 19.6. DATA ELEMENTS REQUIRED FOR ELECTRONIC POINT-OF-CARE TEST ORDERING

Medical record number
Name
Date of birth
Sex
Location
Provider number
Provider Service
Collection time/date
Episode ("encounter" or "billing") number
ICD-9 number(s)

ICD, International Classification of Diseases.

archived. This Massachusetts General Hospital Utility Multiprogramming System (MUMPS)-based system is not a table-driven system in terms of archived laboratory results. Laboratory results are not stored with tabular database elements such as reference ranges, stratified by age and sex, critical limits, test and method codes, or specimen numbers. Rather, information elements in the EpicCare database are sorted by textual descriptors, or "smart text." EpicCare textual description of laboratory tests is very important to differentiate, for example, glucose test results from serum, urine, or cerebrospinal fluid (CSF) specimens. The "smart text" feature of EpicCare would find intermingled serial results for "glucose" unless additional descriptors (e.g., "serum," "urine," "CSF") were present. A cursory review of the number of tables built for different glucose test codes is found in in our Sunquest LIS number 16.

It is of utmost importance that POCT results enter the EpicCare database from a structured table-based Sunquest LIS. Because of the importance of this concept, the laboratory at the GHS has been closely involved in developing the order entry and result-reporting interface between EpicCare and Sunquest (Fig. 19.5). Because EpicCare will evolve to the predominant inquiry device for laboratory information in our primary care network, it is imperative that data pass through the LIS and be validated prior to archiving in EpicCare.

The diagram in Figure 19.5 shows the means for order entry (OE), steps 1 and 2, result reporting (RR), steps 3 and 4, from PC terminals at GRL network clinic sites. The initial order, step 1, is placed from office or examining room by the physician into the Epic Server and as it collates with appointment and registration (A/D/T) information, it completes a valid order that then is passed, step 2, to the Sunquest LIS. These appointment and registration data are supplied during the patient encounter within the EpicCare system by the aforementioned Cadence module and contain vital information listed in Table 19.6. An order is thus placed on a real-time basis to Sunquest, step 2 OE, which "creates a hole" awaiting a point-of-care laboratory test result, step 3.

In the meantime, POCT at the HGL site proceeds with specimens collected in the designated clinic area based on EpicCare worksheets. When results are manually or electronically entered into the laboratory PC terminal, a Sunquest terminal device shared among several applications, they match tests preordered as described previously. The results are verified, step 3, in the Sunquest LIS under the structure of the all-important standardized PSGML table-driven database.

Results that "fill the hole" of the SQ test request, step 3, are in turn reported back, step 4 RR, to the EpicCare server and hence made available to the physician's office or examining room terminal. Results verified in the Sunquest LIS thus could be released to the Cerner clinical repository, step 5, in a form that would meet requirements for outcome-based research. Also released to the Cerner repository, step 6, could be accessory information from EpicCare (e.g., medications, treatments, diagnoses, and a wide variety of clinical information) that would form the basis of extensive cross-related outcome-based research. As already mentioned, this mirrored clinical repository approach was abandoned during the PSGHS demerger, but it illustrates how IDS enterprises might function in the future.

As in other IDSs, such as Kaiser North West in Clackamas County, Washington, EpicCare will serve as the primary outpatient tool with a GUI terminal view to funnel information conveniently from and to the user. Clinical pathways will be developed for presentation particularly to outpatient areas by the EpicCare system using its own clinical repository.

Of great concern to GRL/HGL personnel for POCT of the future is that the laboratory would not "own the data," especially quality assurance data, from such testing if it went directly into the nonstructured database of EpicCare. All the efforts of standardizing and producing quality POCT would be for naught if test data were reported in nonstandard formats (e.g., different reference ranges, test pneumonics, result units). The specter loomed of "gospel in, garbage out" for POCT. It is of the utmost importance that laboratories consider this aspect of POCT for the future.

The EpicCare system is constantly being customized, in many cases to the site application level, as it rolls out into the GHS primary care network. Physicians who have a primary role and stake in the use and implementation of this tool are involved in this customization. It is a time of "retooling" in the GHS to meet the challenges of efficient ambulatory care practice management in the future. An investment of 20 million dollars during the course of the initial 5 years of EpicCare rollout has been made, a high financial and operational priority in the PSGHS.

Acceptance by physicians and other health care professionals of the EpicCare rollout has been mixed and at times difficult. The "retooling" of clinic operations around electronic input and inquiry has been difficult for some practitioners who have used paper systems for decades. Most clinicians who have participated in the EpicCare rollout are enthusiastic about its potential for simplifying clinic operations and creating greater time efficiency. Physicians, in general, have felt empowered by the prospect of "a physician practice system" being tailored to their clinical needs given such a high priority for implementation. Many see the EpicCare system as revolutionizing the way they practice medicine.

Much remains to be done, not just in implementing EpicCare application software but also in converting the old paper medical record to an electronic format. Physicians and other health professionals will be responsible for abstracting data from a given medical record as that patient is now followed in EpicCare. Individual practice styles should be maintained to a large degree because of the flexibility of EpicCare to be customized by practice site and provider. The early practice sites to be implemented on EpicCare in the PSGHS will tend to be a template for later site implementations. This will help to standardize clinical practice to some degree (e.g., medication lists, nomenclature, and clinical pathway development). EpicCare being the primary inquiry system for an anticipated 600 providers in primary care practice will increase the value of the GML by associating clinical laboratory results with those from other departmental systems (i.e., pharmacy, radiology, HMO, cardiology, diabetes disease management) on a real-time basis. Properly constructed, this PC network will be almost as important as point-of-care laboratory testing itself in presenting a quality laboratory product: *information*.

"Autoscripting" Versus Electronic Data Integration for Interfacing Point-of-Care Testing Data Managers

Electronic data integration (EDI) of POCT results into information systems required to deliver data to providers on a real-time basis is only in its infancy. Currently, the most common configuration for delivering this information to where and when a provider needs it involves batch uploading of information from a POCT device to a PC data manager and from this location batch uploading to the LIS. This two-step process typically involves a single vendor's POCT device and a matched data manager but infrequently archives results to the LIS on a real-time basis. Also, different communication devices and protocols are used for transmission of necessary data elements from the different PC data managers to the LIS. As multiple POCT devices with data managers are integrated into a host of information systems, the laboratory is left with the specter of having multiple PC and LIS interfaces to maintain.

Because these POCT products are only in their infancy, one may hope a more standardized approach eventually can be taken to POCT data management. Conceptually, many vendors have begun designing universal POCT data managers whereby a single PC will manage a number of testing devices. The diversity of needs for POCT data management is expanding into areas where clear specifications do not exist.

Means need to be developed to define the needs and develop specifications for increasing diversity and complexity of the POCT data management. The aforementioned CIC specification is a major unifying step in this direction. Because this is an expanding field in terms of POCT applications, it is likely there will be stages of development to meet user needs. One may view current POCT data management as in its infancy and existing in the first of three stages of development.

Stage 1 has existed for approximately 8 years. Early POCT data management systems became commercially available *circa* 1992. The I-Stat (Princeton, NJ, U.S.A.) Central Data Station was initially interfaced to the LIS via terminal emulation from an MS-DOS–based PC manager in 1992. One may view this initial POCT data integrated system as launching the era of POCT data management. The Geisinger System was involved in the initial prototyping of this system, using Cross-Talk Mark IV terminal emulation or "autoscripting" software between an I-Stat central data station running under MS-DOS and the Community Health Computing (CHC) LIS. This system in 1992 was considered a breakthrough in that valid test orders on registered patients were uploaded to the LIS through the "autoscripting" process, and results in the LIS were reported and billed "in the mainstream" of information flow. In essence, a paperless OE and RR system was implemented for POCT in 1992 as patient and operator identification was input, a testing cartridge was inserted, and a result read from a liquid crystal display. "Flash" reports could be generated from a local thermal strip printer, and results were batch processed to the central data station and LIS.

This basic design has become much more prevalent as various vendors develop PC-based data managers for their particular devices. Bidirectional interfaces between the device and the data manager are now the norm and part of a vendor's integrated system. Various autoscripting algorithms are used to upload data from the data manager to the LIS. "Autoscripting" has become the nearly universal means of creating the data link to the LIS.

Autoscripting can provide only uploaded information to the LIS that exists in the data manager. The basic elements for a valid order typically exist (e.g., patient identification, time and date of test, test code, operator identification, some comment fields). This stage 1 data manager to LIS interface functions well for a freestanding POCT device; however, there are increasing marketplace pressures for consolidated POCT workstations. For this reason, one can foresee the need for a stage 2 level of development of integrated POCT data management.

A stage 2 level of development may include a single PC workstation receiving data from diverse POCT testing devices. A single graphic user interface for viewing data from diverse POCT devices and applications will be needed to gate data into the LIS. A single workstation may exist to verify test results into the LIS for coagulation testing, bedside glucose testing, electrolyte and arterial blood-gas testing, therapeutic drug testing, urinalysis, and many other soon-to-be-developed applications. For a universal POCT data manager/workstation to be developed, vendors will have to adopt some standardized specifications for using a common database. Database tools exist for creating a data repository from multiple diverse devices. These databases should be nonproprietary to accommodate expanding complexity and diversity of POCT devices. Many relational database PC-based products may be selected for use in these applications. One also can envision that in stage 2 the POCT data repository database may exist either in a PC workstation separate from the LIS or as a module within the LIS. For this reason, LIS vendors must work closely with POCT device/data manager vendors to develop truly integrated products for the medical and laboratory community.

At this stage of development, one must also consider whether there are advantages to developing a more rapid and interactive LIS interface than may be achieved with "autoscripting." Ideally, POCT devices should provide data to the LIS on a real-time basis. Typical stage 1 data managers, although they offer this option, often cannot provide such data flow practically. Necessary patient registration demographics must accompany a valid test order, and autoscripting from the data manager often does not have this necessary data element. If the point-of-care data manager does not have an "encounter" or "billing" number to match with the LIS, the LIS typically cannot receive a valid order and result from the data manager. Data elements from multiple health care information systems, including A/D/T and billing systems, which can assign real-time encounter or billing numbers, will need to be shared with the POCT device or its data manager.

More direct EDI interfaces are becoming favored for linkage of data managers to LISs because they integrate these order demographics in the LIS. The aforementioned SureStep Pro bedside glucose meter system is an example of such an EDI. This configuration, in use in the PSGHS since June 1999, allows for A/D/T/ information collected at near real time by the LIS to be added to the electronic order within the LIS. It has been our observation that the 0.2 seconds it typically takes to order and file a glucose meter result in the LIS is 500 times faster than a comparable autoscripting process. The CIS specifications also designate the EDI as the preferred interface.

For this reason, more enterprise-wide integrated solutions for POCT data integration will need to evolve in stage 3. In stage 3, highly interactive WAN exchange of POCT and patient demographic data must occur. As conceptualized in Figure 19.6, multiple bidirectional interfaces from POCT devices, the POCT workstation (and database). This workstation will function with the laboratory information system and overlapping computerized patient as interfaced or integral hardware.

If one can envision a POCT device with user interface polling for pertinent clinical information from the computerized patient record to guide the next step of the testing process (47), one can envision the need for WAN interactivity. For example, should not an operator of a coagulation POCT device on entering patient identification be presented with the previous anticoagulant therapy dose information immediately prior to performing a coagulation test? This pharmaceutical information would not exist in the LIS or the POCT database necessarily, but it might need to be retrieved in real time from the computerized patient record/pharmacy record. In stage 3, some pertinent data for POCT may reside in the database or database segment (if integral to LIS or computerized patient record) of the POCT workstation as well as in the computerized patient record. This workstation would thence become a temporary repository of clinical and demographic information for a particular patient undergoing POCT.

One should not over-forecast that the POCT device will become a general inquiry terminal but rather remain a gateway to pertinent clinical information for POCT. The POCT data repository in stage 3 (see "Database") would remain a data management tool for the clinical laboratory legally to maintain the scientific and clinical record of POCT events from multiple devices. POCT devices would evolve as primarily testing instruments with intelligent, highly interactive user interfaces for obtaining real-time information likely through wireless WAN communication.

The expertise for managing POCT in all three stages of workstation/database/repository evolution resides with the clinical laboratory. One must envision the core competency in the clinical laboratory as moving ever increasingly into areas of information management. The clinical laboratory must remain responsible for the archiving of POCT data into an LIS into whatever form it may evolve. Hence, working at integrating

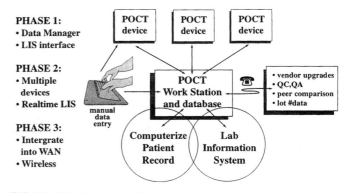

FIGURE 19.6. Evolution of a point-of-care testing workstation integral to a computerized patient record.

diverse clinical systems into a focus of POCT data management will remain a challenge to clinical laboratorians. Information will be shared increasingly between different departments of a clinical enterprise (especially in an IDS), but the legal responsibility for archiving clinical laboratory test data will remain that of the clinical laboratory. For this reason, clinical laboratorians must aggressively participate in the evolution of information systems in the IDS and "carve out" a niche of well-structured POCT data management of valid clinical laboratory data.

Also shown in Figure 19.6 is a projected need for a real time interface to the vendor of the POCT device via modem or Internet connection. It is common even under stage 1 for workstation/data manager software to be remotely updated by modem by the vendor. This telecommunication link may expand into areas that the user and vendor are jointly responsible for, such as peer comparison quality control, lot number tracking, and calibration verification. Therefore, vendors must partner with clinical laboratory enterprises in developing such flexible user applications. It is likely that security issues will need to be resolved as vendors are granted remote access to increasingly data rich POCT workstations, workstation databases, and other WAN data repositories. At

Geisinger, remote diagnostics by vendors are allowed only if the session is terminal monitored by laboratory personnel. This restriction is in place since once on the GHS WAN, a remote terminal could have access to sensitive patient data.

In summary, there is a growing need for more diverse sophisticated data management of POCT (49). Partnerships between users and vendors applying flexible customized applications must be maintained in this growing enterprise. Resources and responsibilities for developing and paying for the maintenance of highly integrated POCT applications on open architecture TCP/IP WANS, computerized patient records, LIS, and POCT data managers will require an increasingly close relationship between health care providers and vendors. POCT devices will be viewed increasingly as simply the operator front end of a highly complex information-processing system.

Wide Area Network Use in Expanding an Integrated Delivery System

Point-of-care testing in an IDS requires support from a very interactive communication system. Management of increasing

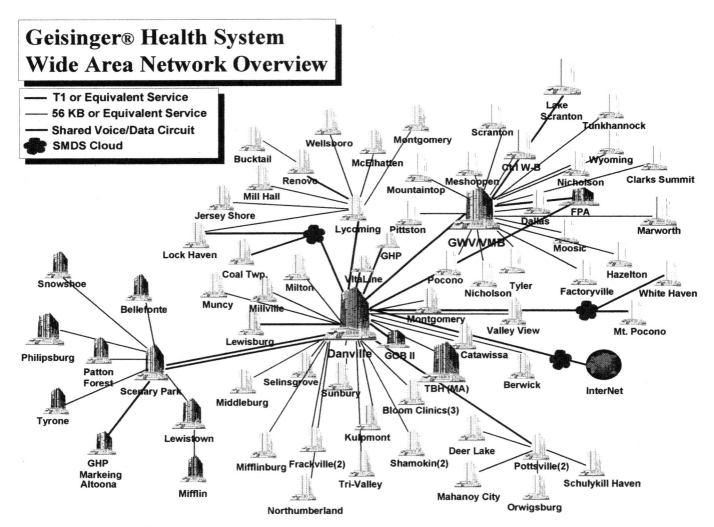

FIGURE 19.7. Configuration of the wide area network (WAN) used in the Geisinger System.

numbers of POCT devices as well as increasing numbers of operators requires attention by laboratory professionals through a highly communicative process. In the PSGHS, cluster supervisors have one-on-one interaction with users at hundreds of testing locations. A handful of laboratorians cannot physically attend to the daily supervision of the thousands of POCT device users who have appeared in the last decade.

As shown in Figure 19.7, the WAN contains links of fiberoptic T1 and T3 lines between multiple remote locations and central "hubs" within the old Geisinger enterprise. This WAN was expanded to include the Hershey component of the merged PSGHS prior to the demerger. Standardizing network connectivity hardware and support, removing firewalls, consolidating departmental local area networks, and upgrading fiberoptic lines to accomplish a seamless functional PSGHS WAN was accomplished in little over a year. Standardized network hardware was agreed on so that e-mail, audiovisual data, and voice could be communicated seamlessly. Asynchronous telecommunication has been replaced steadily with Ethernet connectivity. Network node hardware, cabling, and file servers are some of the items that were standardized. The PSGHS has been very progressive in terms of wiring the system for this interconnectivity as witnessed by recent awards (45). This fiberoptic "backbone," which was initially installed in 1995, has enabled the evolution of a progressively integrated LIS and was and continues to be a vital link between all PSGHS operational systems. If it were not for this link, all the standardization of testing methodologies, including those of POCT, would not have evolved into an integrated cohesive laboratory system.

Electronic communication through e-mail has become an indispensable tool. A single e-mail system, Groupwise, operating on a WAN, has become more useful than the telephone for serving most communication needs in the GRL/HGL. Cluster supervisors are able to communicate with key contact personnel in the user community by posting to e-mail message groups. A record of important technical and or regulatory information being sent and received by e-mail is maintained as an audit trail in this communicative process.

Audiovisual educational programs sponsored or conducted by the GRL/HGL have been broadcast live or by video recording across the WAN for several years. Videotape or live simulcast (46) to three remote nodes across the WAN has become an indispensable educational tool as education of operators has become an ever increasingly challenging task in the managing of POCT across 28 counties. Legal requirements for competency testing often can be achieved with such educational programs. Increasingly in our IDS we must think of operator training in terms of batch control as the number of POCTs enlarges into the thousands. Efficient electronic and telecommunication means are the only feasible tools to document contact with the thousands of operators who perform POCT.

An *intra*net "infoweb" was developed by PSGHS, and it permits communication of policy and procedure for POCT. The WAN, with at least 1,200 connected PCs in the PSGHS, allows access to this intranet information. The GHS is in the process of consolidating all method manuals onto the infoweb in a common format. The high degree of standardization that has evolved in the GML has allowed for common method manuals.

It is envisioned that practical daily information, such as forms to obtain supplies with a designated product number, will be posted on the infoweb in the future. As opposed to mere "advertisement" on the infoweb, it is our goal to use this as a practical interactive tool for disseminating information to thousands of POCT operators. It has been repeatedly observed during the last 15 years of supporting POCT in the Geisinger primary care network that the better supported the technical standard is, the more it is complied with, and less policing is required.

As POCT expands into the continuum of care, the PSGHS intranet and, if security issues are resolved, the *Inter*net, may be used as an information source for other health care providers. Preliminary discussions have been started for the use of the PSGHS Internet for disseminating patient information (e.g., patient preparation for elective procedures). Time efficiency of disseminating information in a very large enterprise is a focus of our future planning. The practical application of Internet and intranet technology to health care, especially in the clinical laboratory, is at hand.

QUALITY MANAGEMENT AND PROFESSIONAL OVERSIGHT

A primary motivation for laboratorians to become involved in managing networks of POCT laboratories is quality. In the old GRL system, much of the quality oversight we did was established prior to the inception of CLIA '88. A rational approach was started in 1984 to standardize not only testing methods but also the quality control of testing. Beginning with testing methods such as urine pregnancy, urine dipstick, and glucose testing, standardized quality control material was chosen as well as standardized procedures for documenting quality control for these procedures. Initial training of operators in POLs and hospital POCT areas to perform correct quality control on a daily basis involved explanation and education of the "why" of the procedure. The training process was enhanced by educating operators that what they were doing was part of a uniform standardized system across dozens of peer sites in the Geisinger System. Having a standardized approach to quality control material and procedures helped to gain user acceptance of the quality control program.

Prior to the introduction of CLIA '88 regulations, the laboratory used State of Pennsylvania regulations to establish the notion that doing quality control was not just a good idea but was required for regulatory compliance. User acceptance of the quality control program, although tenuous at the start in 1985, gained support gradually over the course of a few years. By 1988, the Geisinger Regional Laboratory had, in essence, implemented all quality control requirements mandated by CLIA '88.

Instrumental in the implementation of the quality control program were medical technologists who functioned as a "cluster" supervisor in a sizable network laboratory, a supervisor of several smaller POLs, or both. Overseeing quality improvement at the beginning stages of laboratory regionalization was initially a frustrating, although rewarding, activity for these medical technologists.

At the beginning stages of laboratory regionalization, as the GRL grew, much quality control simply was not performed.

During the years 1988 through 1995, approximately 40 practice sites joined the Geisinger System and largely had to be taught basic quality control principles. These regional laboratory sites (each site joining was licensed as a separate CLIA certificate) were assigned to a cluster supervisor, who was responsible for quality oversight, training and management. As these practice sites were converted to standardized methods and documentation procedures, the cluster supervisor was responsible for implementation details. Implementation details included not just the implementation of standardized methods but also the completion of the CLIA certificate application with noted testing, supervisory, and medical director personnel. Proficiency testing continues to be enrolled with the College of American Pathologists (CAP) under the Excel program.

Proficiency testing was and is the primary tool for assessment of quality in the regional network. The outcome of this proficiency testing is shared not just with a designated site medical director (commonly the physician leader of the practice site) but also the regional laboratory, or GRL, director. The GRL director has a role in reviewing proficiency testing consultant copies and assuring that failed events are being addressed.

There were 83 CLIA licenses and 7 clusters in the HGL network, four of which were complex enough to require a board certified clinical laboratorian. With the demerger of the Hershey cluster, this number dropped to 70 CLIA licenses and 6 clusters. Three doctoral-level directors continue to fulfill CLIA and State of Pennsylvania requirements for licensure at these moderate- to high-complexity GRL sites as well as smaller physician office laboratories within the associated cluster. Overall quality oversight is hence a shared responsibility between the GRL director, the doctoral director within a cluster, the cluster supervisor, and the site medical director. Expertise is shared between these responsible laboratorians to address any particular quality problem. Because all laboratorians have functioned for several years within the distributed GRL structure and a true team philosophy has been ingrained, "turf" issues are virtually nonexistent.

All site-specific proficiency testing data is retained at the CLIA-registered site. The designated site medical director, although initiated by the cluster supervisor and shared with the doctoral and GRL director, must sign responses to the State of Pennsylvania or the CAP.

Site medical directors of the 70-site regional GRL network are involved with technical assessment to varying degrees. The site medical director must be involved in the resolution of proficiency testing failures for his or her specific CLIA-licensed site and sign off on documented course of action. The cluster supervisor and doctoral directors largely accomplish resolution of the technical details in responding to a proficiency testing failure.

To date, over the course of the last 14 years of proficiency testing in POLs of the Geisinger System, the only systematic ongoing problem with quality has been observed with provider-performed microscopy (PPM). Occasional proficiency testing failures with other testing methods are sporadic and typically have been resolved easily. Proficiency testing problems with PPM have been more difficult to improve, although a plan of remediation has been implemented. This plan for remediation includes identifying the provider who input the faulty PPM data and contacting that person with suggested means of improve-

ment. Resources made available for PPM remediation include a CD-ROM tutorial, proficiency testing 2 × 2 slides, atlases, and wall charts for urinalysis identification, didactic lectures by pathologists or regional laboratory personnel, and other teaching sessions. To date, the most successful and provider-accepted means of education has been the CD-ROM tutorial "UA Tutor." Fortunately, many of the PCs installed on the WAN are configured with CD-ROM drives. It is interesting to see how the GHS has grown into efficient use of PC hardware at the point of care that initially was thought to be luxuriantly over-configured.

Besides the aforementioned operational oversight of quality in the regional laboratory network, systematic group oversight was established in 1985. A Laboratory Technical Advisory Committee (LTAC) was charged with establishing quality expectations for the regional laboratory system and establishing standardized testing methods. These quality expectations in the Regional Laboratory System often exceed the minimum regulatory requirements for documentation and performance. Frequency of quality control, subscribing to proficiency testing, and performance of technical methods were prescribed by LTAC and designed to create system standards for quality.

For example, LTAC established glucose testing in whole blood by the HemoCue device as the desirable method for quantitative glucose testing (including use of the designated CPT code for billing) at regional sites based on a coefficient of variation (%CV) precision of 4% or less. Although arguably more convenient, reflectance meter testing of glucose for diagnostic purposes has not been adopted because of less desirable accuracy and precision compared with spectrophotometric methods.

Likewise, the decision was made by LTAC to maintain a standardized PT-measuring method using the aforementioned MLA750 instruments with a standardized reagent system at GRL sites. A single sequestered lot number of reagent and quality control material is distributed to network laboratory sites to document comparative quality performance of these methods. Because of this process, standardization results can be reported to the LIS with common test codes. Because there is such a high degree of standardization and strict quality oversight, physicians are ensured of site neutrality in the quality of their test results. As performance, cost, and data integration of handheld coagulation devices improve, it is likely that they will be recommended for use by LTAC in the future.

A sequestered lot number of chemistry quality control material is also used in the hospital laboratories and GRL sites performing POCT. For example, identical quality control material is currently used on main laboratory automated chemistry analyzers (Roche Modular, 917, 717), Roche Cobas MIRAs at larger HGL sites, and I-Stat handheld devices at hospital and outpatient POCT sites. Troubleshooting by comparing peer lot means and coefficients of variation have been performed at multiple sites. Although it is possible to do so, the GRL has not systematically adopted ongoing peer comparison of quality control statistics site by site. It is planned in the future to adopt a more system-wide comparison review of quality control when all laboratory quality control data are input to the Sunquest LIS. Again, quality control statistics are not the ongoing outcome statistic for judging quality in our system; rather, quality of testing is judged primarily by proficiency testing.

Use of "Clusters" in Supporting Large Primary Care Networks

As large multisite networks of primary care providers with their associated POCT expand, it is important to manage testing activities in a manageable scale (48). Organizing groups of primary care practice sites into clusters allows for such management of operational scale. One technologist acting as a cluster supervisor can manage up to 35 individual CLIA certificates, depending on the size and complexity of the practice sites. It is important in establishing such groups of laboratories into clusters to keep several characteristics in mind.

Geographic location is but one of many characteristics that must be recognized in establishing a cluster. Types of specialty practice at outpatient sites, cross-coverage of physician practitioners at multiple sites, management structure of clinical operations, political affiliations of sites with hospitals, and transportation logistics to a system hospital are important considerations in designing a cluster. It must be remembered that more than logistics are involved in successfully managing such a cluster operation.

The cluster supervisor must interact on a daily basis with both operational personnel doing POCT in the laboratory as well as clinical operational managers to maintain a unified operation. Once laboratory standardization settles into routine operation, the operation largely takes care of itself. Most of the time and energy of the cluster supervisor becomes directed toward solving other operational problems. Experience in the GRL shows 90% of the time of the cluster supervisor is focused on problems with information systems, safety, human resources, billing, logistics of laboratory outreach, clinical process improvement, and performing system duties in general—not POCT itself. Cluster supervisors are viewed as the "fingertips of the HGL system." Problems and suggestions are encountered by cluster supervisors long before they surface as complaints to the central laboratory. Having cluster supervisors in the field interacting with customers of the laboratory is invaluable in formulating proactive solutions to problems. Because different geographic and regional parts of the GHS have different problems, politics, and priorities, the designated cluster supervisor can advise the laboratory of specific site issues.

Besides being the reconnaissance or "fingertips of the laboratory," the cluster supervisor also functions as the "face of the laboratory." Site personnel recognize these friendly faces as the people who solve problems for them. Cluster supervisors in turn have become quite loyal in advocating for their customers. Functioning outside the central laboratory and in clinic operations has proved an extremely rewarding career for seven GML medical technologists who have taken this track during the last several years of GRL operation.

Financial Management of Point-of-Care Testing in Primary Care Networks

Financial management in an IDS, including that of POCT in primary care networks, is much more structured and systematic than in health care systems that exist as part of a loose alliance.

Programmatic financial management, not just of purchasing (e.g., the aforementioned GPO alignment) but also the distribution of revenue collected from the billing process, is part of the accepted culture in the GHS and most IDSs.

A much greater economy of scale for purchasing supplies and services is achievable in large "seamless" IDSs. To achieve economy of scale and integration, a large view must be taken of laboratory testing across all entities of the IDS. This large view encourages the aforementioned group purchasing and standardization efforts and builds much stronger infrastructure to ensure compliance of agreed on POCT methods. Stringent financial management of the budgeting process, the purchasing process, and the supply distribution process all help to control costs as well as monitor compliance with agreed on technical standards. System agreements replace individual "deals" made with supply vendors. For these reasons, IDSs have a great advantage for delivery of POCT and indeed all laboratory testing at a much lower cost per test than "voluntary" alliances of regional testing facilities.

To manage financially all the various entities that perform POCT in large multisite IDSs, a global strategy of neutralizing financial incentives for testing is paramount. In the GHS, CLIA licenses are owned by a single laboratory organization. As such, all revenue as well as expenses are rolled into the financial management structure of the single laboratory division.

At each of the two Geisinger medical centers, a single site CLIA license covers all POCT locations within their campus addresses. Outpatient clinics, specialty practices, as well as inpatient POCT are the responsibility of the designated hospital laboratory. A single cost and revenue center for "ancillary testing" has been operating for 8 years within the Geisinger Medical Center in Danville (as of 2001). Expense from operations is assigned to this single cost center. Costs for operational personnel performing POCT (e.g., nursing, respiratory therapists) are not included in these expenses. Supplies and other consumables are included in the expense category of this "ancillary testing" cost center. Laboratory administration of POCT within this ancillary testing cost center, with the exception of the salary for the medical technologist supervisor, is not included as an expense. Hence, only costs most directly attributable to performing POCT are tracked. On the revenue side, all collected revenue flows back to "ancillary testing," and any surplus of revenue over expenses helps to offset operational costs in the hospital. This surplus revenue is not allocated to the laboratory, alleviating the perception that the laboratory is charging for testing done by hospital operational personnel.

At 70 decentralized CLIA-licensed sites in the GHS, a laboratory cost center is established for each site. Larger GRL sites are staffed and operated by medical technologists and staff paid by the laboratory division. Smaller GRL sites without stationed laboratory personnel receive a yearly offset of salary expense to cover time spent on laboratory services, including POCT. This salary offset (predominantly for nursing time) is credited by an interdepartmental charge transfer. All supplies costs are assigned to the GML for all practice sites because they perform their own supply requisitioning.

The aforementioned cluster supervisors of the primary care network are assigned to and report through the GRL. Directly attributable salary and operational expenses managed by the medical technologist cluster supervisor are carried within the GRL and tracked within its individual cluster. Likewise, other laboratory assigned personnel (phlebotomists, laboratory assistants, and medical technicians/technologists) are assigned as an expense to one of the six clusters within the GRL. On the revenue side, tests that are billed as POCT generate revenue tracked by both the individual CLIA-licensed site performing the test and the cluster to which the specific site belongs. Cluster supervisors are responsible for yearly formulation of budgets and monthly tracking of expenses. All expenses and revenues accrued by an individual CLIA-licensed site in the primary care network are rolled up (a) into the designated cluster, (b) to the GRL operating division, and (c) to the entire GML.

Individual practice sites within the primary care network do not book expenses or revenue to their internal clinic operations. There is no incentive for practitioners at a given practice site to produce revenue by doing POCT. Likewise, there is no penalty in cost for performing POCT. Because of this revenue and cost neutrality, decisions tend to be made according to clinical need, not financial pressures. If a test can be performed with greater cost-efficiency and can produce required clinical service centrally, it will be referred to one of three hospital laboratories (i.e., by courier). On the other hand, if clinical necessity dictates formation of a POCT, an appropriate standardized and information system-integrated method is brought to a practice site.

Over the last several years, the GRL/HGL has established infrastructure to meet the operational, technical, and medical needs for POCT at the satellite practice sites. A state of equilibrium has been reached in terms of operational efficiency and financial cost-effectiveness. Because of the integrated nature of our at-large practice network, an increasing amount of time at GRL sites has been devoted to information processing rather than POCT. Medical technologists who serve as cluster supervisors at larger GRL network sites have become quite astute at judging whether a test is needed at point of care or would be more cost-effectively performed at a central site. The need to justify one's function as a medical technologist has changed from that of performing more tests at the bench to one of getting information to clinicians quickly, accurately, and cost-effectively. Medical technologists have become very business oriented in delivering services to local customers in their cluster.

It is the intention of the GRL to deliver laboratory testing services to GHS salaried physicians at a capitated rate that reflects overall laboratory costs rather than traditional laboratory charges. Almost invariably, this capitated cost will be a small fraction of a traditional laboratory charge. This capitated cost charge transfer mechanism almost assuredly will beat the price of any local competitor in the GHS region, including local providers and commercial laboratories. For this reason, integrated delivery systems performing efficient, standardized, inexpensive, data integrated, and quality laboratory testing services will likely dominate regional markets.

Roles of Director, Manager, Technologist in Operating Point-of-Care Testing in an Integrated Delivery System

In an IDS, leadership is also integrated. A common term used for the last decade in IDS is *seamless*. *Team* is another popular term in current management structures of an IDS. The need to attain true integration of laboratory leadership, or a seamless team, is even more necessary in large primary-care practice-site networks performing POCT.

The diversity of practice specialties, local customer needs, and information processing requirements dictates a very fluid and responsive management structure. Unlike the "factory setting" of the traditional hospital laboratory, the IDS distributed laboratory requires leadership and expertise in a large number of areas. The role of doctoral-level directors in quality oversight already has been described.

No one person or professional group can be expected to have the depth of expertise to lead all the activities required by such an enterprise. Leaders in technical areas, operational areas, and financial areas must coordinate their activities to meet the goals of the IDS. The politics of "turf" and "control" are a hindrance to the evolution of a truly integrated primary care network. For this reason, the titles of director, administrator, manager, and technologist, although they still exist in the GML, have blurred and become less important.

The traditional role of director has changed. Although a principal party in evolving a primary care network and integrated POCT program in an IDS, the director must take an increased coordinating and delegating role. Although the core competency of an IDS laboratory activity is still technical, the day-to-day challenges are not. Day-to-day challenges include regulatory compliance (e.g., "medical necessity"), client services, logistical support, strategizing business opportunities, supporting clinical programs in disease management, understanding information system linkages, and keeping costs under control to name a few. Most of these daily challenges were not taught as a core curriculum in a medical or scientific training program that prepared M.D. or Ph.D. directors for their clinical lab responsibilities. Skills to direct a laboratory were likely achieved by on-the-job training and learned from other professionals in the health care enterprise. To expand the necessary skills to direct an evolutionary IDS laboratory, one must team with administrators, managers, technologists, and other professionals in the health care system. The laboratory director should feel increasingly comfortable as a "Jack or Jane of all trades" but should not feel uncomfortable being the master of none.

Although the pathologist director maintains the role of oversight of the distributed IDS laboratory, new areas for POCT in the continuum of care must be mastered as they arrive in the health care setting. Any number of health care professionals (e.g., home health nurses, chief financial officers, material managers, clinicians, HMO marketers, and nursing home administrative directors) bring these new areas, often in the form of an immediate problem, to the laboratory. To be an effective director, one must have open channels of communication and interpersonal skills to learn evolving needs for POCT support.

As roles blur and overlap, administrators of laboratories are put into an expanded role and must team effectively with laboratory directors. In the GHS, a common partnership is seen between directors of clinical services and a chief administrator. To partner effectively, traditional roles of laboratory director and administrative director must not be held onto tenaciously but rather blended synergistically into a team approach. It has been the experience of the PSGHS that a greater capacity for meeting ever-enlarging challenges is created with these effective partnerships. It must be stated, however, that a single pathologist chairman of the unified laboratory division has been a cornerstone of its success.

Traditionally, administrative directors are more entrepreneurial and tied to business success than are most technical and medical directors. Because most daily challenges, as noted already, involve business aspects of the evolving IDS laboratory, the administrative director plays a key role in meeting current and future challenges.

The traditional laboratory manager faces new challenges of the ever-expanding laboratory operation. Most of the "nuts and bolts" of implementing daily operations across multiple clinical services fall to the laboratory manager. A key role for the laboratory manager is in creating realistic expectations for evolving POCT laboratory services for medical and administrative directors. The effort of the laboratory manager has become focused increasingly on accomplishing change while maintaining stability of operations. New POCT information system integration, especially with billing and financial computer systems, is a major challenge to laboratory managers.

Point-of-care testing evolution in an IDS requires much of the skill of an experienced laboratory manager in maintaining integration of testing across all shifts of the laboratory. Laboratory managers often need to negotiate coverage of POCT in the hospital setting across a 21-shift-per-week operation. Laboratory managers being very close to operational staffs of medical technologists are front-line leaders maintaining a continuous operation.

In the evolving GML, an increasing amount of the traditional work of the laboratory manager has been delegated to the supervisory level of the laboratory, a cadre now termed *team leaders*. Personnel management, budgeting, acquisition of instrumentation, and supply requisition are less part of a laboratory manager's daily activity now than in the past. In the GRL, cluster supervisors have been regarded as being at the same level as "team leaders" in the medical centers.

The technologist has an increasingly important role in ensuring good laboratory practice at point of care. The important role of technologists as cluster supervisors in the primary care network already has been described. Medical technologist supervisors of ancillary testing in the medical centers likewise face a very challenging position. The technologist, in performing front-line duties shoulder to shoulder with testing personnel (i.e., nurses, respiratory therapists, and other operational personnel), is regarded as a key resource for troubleshooting technologic procedures, including information management.

All these professional categories need to cross-fertilize in terms of expertise, information, and operational experience. POCT management is a physically, emotionally, and intellectually challenging endeavor. Effective teams of medical, scientific, administrative, management, and technologist groups can make work easier and more rewarding in an increasingly demanding IDS. Fluid communication and teamwork achieve mutual empowerment. A director is most effective when well informed by front-line personnel bringing back daily "reconnaissance" from evolving operational systems. POCT supervisory personnel empower laboratory directors just as laboratory directors empower supervisory personnel, all to the benefit of the laboratory profession. It is through this empowerment that the necessary expertise will be applied to solve the immense information system problems facing the health care industry in the immediate future. Successful distributed laboratories will create successful IDSs as they continue to be recognized as the experts of not just POCT but the information systems that integrate POCT.

CONCLUSIONS

To understand the role of POCT in an IDS, one must take a broad view. This broad view, or "big picture," is presented in the conservative implementation of POCT in the GHS in niche applications across an expanding continuum of care. The implementation pathway taken by a cadre of laboratorians during 15 years has produced a fundamental and profound change in their understanding of clinical need and clinic operations in a physician's office laboratory network.

This enhanced understanding of basic clinic operations at the point of care in the now 70-site GRL network has enabled the laboratory to integrate effectively WAN-based laboratory information systems into a dynamically expanding IDS. Just as information processing has become "distributed," laboratory operations have likewise become "distributed." This case study of an IDS distributed laboratory shows some organizational principles that helped to integrate diversified POCT and core laboratory operations.

The actual performance of POCT was not as critical to success as was the understanding of clinic operations at the point of care by the laboratorian. Pathologists, laboratory directors, administrators, managers, and technologists must develop and use this understanding to empower mutually their role in evolving functional laboratory information systems. The laboratory's product—*information*—must be integrated into ever-diversifying information systems that will require a multidisciplinary approach to guarantee its integrity. Registration systems, DSS, billing systems, clinical repositories, ambulatory care practice systems, and other departmental systems will all require involvement from a broad base of savvy laboratorians. The successful integration of POCT data into diversified PC and file server based information systems on WANs remains an ongoing challenge to the GHS clinical laboratory.

Point-of-care testing will likely grow as its clinical efficiency is demonstrated. Access to important medical information (e.g., patient clinical status, billing information, provider diagnosis) is integral to the specimen collection process. The preanalytic, analytic, and postanalytic portions of the laboratory testing process in many cases may merge during specimen collection and may produce an optimal and more clinically efficient encounter. The patient and health care provider, "customers" of the laboratory, may benefit greatly from such a merged encounter. The GHS laboratory is strategically positioned in integrating information systems at the point of service to enable this clinical efficiency.

The laboratory will need to help develop improved DSS measurement tools to show cost savings to the overall organization for such POCT. Shrinking reimbursement, increased costs, and overall complexity of doing business in the era of managed care initially may inhibit the growth of appropriate POCT unless the laboratory cost justifies its use. The challenge continues in demonstrating cost savings as the laboratory intuitively prepares for point-of-service clinical efficiency.

Information system technology is growing at an astounding pace, and it offers a tremendous opportunity for the laboratory to increase its value to an IDS. PC hardware used by the laboratory, from the point-of-care data manager to terminals on a WAN, has many accessory applications. The GHS laboratory is beginning to harvest the opportunities provided by WAN connectivity with several information-sharing tools. The laboratory community has a great opportunity in mastering these tools to distribute not only test results but also laboratory information.

Graphic user interface PC systems on WANs will be used increasingly for information retrieval from clinical repositories and real-time clinical and financial decision-making. It is imperative that the laboratory understand the dynamics and content that will be used in this decision-making process. Real-time distribution of laboratory information across the continuum of care will increasingly be used in clinical decision-making and will be the driving force for POCT.

In conclusion, a core requirement for IDS laboratories emerges: The laboratory must own its laboratory data. An LIS as a "source of truth" data repository ensures quality laboratory data for clinical decision-making and input to a clinical repository. There is a growing risk of POCT data escaping rigorous validation by such an established LIS data repository. It may well be the challenge of the new millennium for laboratorians to validate all archived testing data, including that generated at expanding points of care, in a clinical repository with solid clinical interpretability.

REFERENCES

1. Jones JB. *Creation and maintenance of a distributed laboratory network: proceedings of Medical Automation Research Center (MARC) Workshop.* Charlottesville, VA: MARC, 1997.
2. Bickford GR. Decentralized testing in the 1990s: a survey of United States hospitals. *Clinical Laboratory Management Review* 1994;8: 327–338.
3. Kost G. Point-of-care testing: current and future directions. *LabAutomation* 1998;131.
4. Steiner JW, et al. Networks and integrated lab systems: models and strategies. *Strategic Directions* 1996;Sept/Oct:3–6.
5. Michel RL, et al. Laboratory consolidation within a non-profit integrated healthcare system. *CLMA* 1995; 51–73.
6. Anders G, Winslow R. HMOs' woes reflect conflicting demands of American public. *Wall Street Journal* 1997 Dec 22.
7. Davidoff F, ed. Medicine and commerce. I. Is managed care a "monstrous hybrid"? *Ann Intern Med* 1998;128:496–499.
8. Jones JB. Regional laboratory integration via laboratory information system (LIS) integration. *Proceedings of Sixth International LIMS Conference*, Pittsburgh, PA. June 1992.
9. Michel R, et al. Building laboratory alliances: what successful networks have in common. *Strategic Directions* 1998;June:3–6.
10. Jones JB, et al. Point-of-care testing in an era of laboratory consolidation. *In Vivo* 1996;May.
11. Michel RL. Why clinical laboratory consolidation will fragment the industry. *The Dark Report* 1998;April:1–6.
12. Warner K, Luce B. *Cost-benefit and cost-effectiveness analysis in health care: principles, practice and potential.* Ann Arbor, MI: Health Administration Press, 1982:1–100.
13. Lebo R, Faett J, Jones JB. Integration of laboratory point of care PC workstations into a regional lab network. *Proceedings of Towards an Electronic Patient Record (TEPR 1997).* Nashville, TN, April 1997.
14. Dark RL. Consolidation: threat or opportunity? *The Dark Report* 1998;5:1.
15. Diller W, Erickson D. To consolidate or network: for laboratories, that's the question. *In vivo* 1996;14, 30–37.
16. Jones JB, Shulski A, Sharretts S. A systems approach to multisite decentralized chemistry testing utilizing Kodak DT-60 analyzers. *Clin Chem* 1990;36:1076.
17. Kost GJ. Point-of-care testing: patient focusing for the future. In: Howanitz PJ, McBride JH, eds. *Professional practice in clinical chemistry: a review.* Washington, DC: American Association for Clinical Chemistry Press, 1994:443–454.
18. Felder R. Clinical laboratory automation in the next century: from process control to point-of-care. *Clinical LabAutomation* 1998;51.
19. Bailey TM, Topham TM, Wantz S, et al. Laboratory process improvement through point-of-care testing. *Journal on Quality Improvement* 1997;23:7.
20. Volz D. Managing "value" on the front line. *Integrated Healthcare Report* 1998;Sept:13–15.
21. Saltz J, Rottman J, Kroll M. An electronic clinical repository: how labs can add value to lab data. *Clinical Laboratory News* 1998;Oct: 16–17.
22. Lebo R, Jones JB. Operational experience with the HemoCue glucose spectrophotometer in a neonatal unit. *Clin Chem* 1997;43:S122.
23. Chen PP, Short TG, Leung DHY, et al. A clinical evaluation of the Hemocue haemoglobinometer using capillary, venous, and arterial samples. *Anaesth Intens Care* 1992;20:497–503.
24. Ehrmeyer SS, Laessig RH. Regulatory requirements (CLIA '88, JCAHO, CAP) for decentralized testing. *Am J Clin Pathol* 1995;104 (Suppl 1):S40–S49.
25. Ehrmeyer SH, Laessig RH. POCT regulations and inspections. In: *New approaches to point of-care testing.* Washington, DC: American Association for Clinical Chemistry; Audioconference Series, February 25, 1997.
26. College of American Pathologists. *Point-of-care testing inspection checklist.* Northfield, IL: CAP Commission on Laboratory Accreditation, section 30, 1997.
27. Jacobs E, Vadasdi E. Sarkozi L, et al. Analytical evaluation of the i-STAT portable clinical analyzer and use by nonlaboratory health-care professionals. *Clin Chem* 1993;39:1069–1074.
28. Jones JB, Danielson L, Shulski A, et al. Integration of the i-stat testing device into laboratory operational and information systems. Presented at: American Association for Clinical Chemistry Meeting. New York. *Clin Chem* 1993;39:1224.
29. Tortella BJ, Lavery RF, Doran JV, et al. Precision, accuracy, and managed care implications of a hand-held whole blood analyzer in the prehospital setting. *Am J Clin Pathol* 1996;106:124–127.
30. Kost GJ. Point-of-care testing: the hybrid laboratory (Knowledge Optimization). In: Kost GJ, ed. *Handbook of clinical automation, robotics, and optimization.* New York: John Wiley and Sons, 1996: 757–838.
31. Integrating point-of care testing with continuity of care: effects on outcome. *Proceedings of the National Academy of Clinical Biochemistry* Sept. 1997:19–20.
32. Scott FI. Integrating point-of-care testing with continuity of care: more on the use of outcomes for the assessment of value. *Am Clin Lab* 1998, 4–5.
33. Auerbach PS. Impact of point-of-care testing on healthcare delivery. *Clin Chem* 1996;42:2052–2053.
34. Hurst J, Nickel K, Hilborne LH. Are physicians' office laboratory results of comparable quality to those produced in other laboratory settings? *JAMA* 1998;279:468–471.
35. Cassak D. AmeriNet and Hospital Consolidation's endgame. *In Vivo: the Business and Medicine Report* 1997;15, 53–63.

36. Diller W. Premier and Quest Bet on the ultimate deal. *In Vivo: the Business and Medicine Report* 1998;16, 5–10.

37. Kasper JF, Mulley AG, Wennberg JE. Developing shared decision-making programs to improve quality of health care. *Qual Rev Bull* 1992;18:183–190.

38. Cassak D. Physician practice management: the doctor is in. *In Vivo* 1996;14, 36–47.

39. Oberhardt BJ. Thrombosis and hemostasis testing at the point of care. *Am J Clin Pathol* 1995;104:S72–S78.

40. Hanus PM, Evans-Shields J, Macri T, et al. Cost-benefit analysis of pharmacist-managed anticoagulation clinic for patients with atrial fibrillation. *Proceedings meeting on Neurology Outcomes Research: Current Science and Future Directions.* Montreal, Oct 1998.

41. Blick K. How IT can be your lab's best friend. *Health Management* 1998;Sept. 12–14.

42. Nichols J. Data management for point-of-care testing. *LabAutomation* 1998;133.

43. Hagland M. IT and point-of-care. *Health Management Technology* 1998;Oct., pg. 10.

44. Kost GJ. Guidelines for point-of-care testing: improving patient outcomes. *Am J Clin Pathol* 1995;104:S111–S127.

45. Golob R. Best networked: Geisinger gets the gold. *Healthcare Informatics* 1996;21:32–35.

46. Rasmussen T. Keeping pace: video communications in a managed care environment. *Managed Care Quarterly* 1998;6:36–42.

47. Fitzmaurice DA, Hobbs FD, Murray ET, et al. Oral anticoagulation management in primary care with the use of computerized decision support and near patient testing: a randomized, controlled trial. *Arch Intern Med* 2000;160:2343–2348.

48. Crook MA. Near patient testing and pathology in the new millenium. *J Clin Pathol* 2000;53:27–30.

49. Point-of-care connectivity specification. POCT1-A. National Committee for Clinical Laboratory Standards (NCCLS). Approved Guidelines 2002.

20

POINT-OF-CARE TESTING IN THE VETERANS AFFAIRS SYSTEM

DANIEL M. BAER
WALDEMAR A. SCHMIDT

This chapter describes the point-of-care testing (POCT) program at one Veterans Affairs Hospital Medical Center and discusses the Veterans Affairs (VA) corporate program for POCT.

REGULATORY REQUIREMENTS

Medical facilities operated by the Department of Veterans Affairs are subject to multiple layers of regulation and accreditation. All VA medical centers (hospitals) are inspected and accredited by Joint Commission on Accreditation of Healthcare Organizations (JCAHO), and laboratories, including POCT, within hospitals and clinics are inspected and accredited by JCAHO or the College of American Pathologists (CAP). All facilities, including clinics, hospitals, and domiciliaries are subjected to numerous specific VA regulations (1,2). Each of these regulatory bodies has numerous and often idiosyncratic and, at times, conflicting requirements for POCT.

PORTLAND VETERANS AFFAIRS MEDICAL CENTER PLAN

History

At the Portland Veterans Affairs Medical Center (PVAMC), an organized plan for capillary blood glucose testing began in 1982 with discussions between the chiefs of Nursing and Pathology & Laboratory Medicine (P&LMS) Services. This led to formation of a Nursing Service and P&LMS working group. Soon, other members of the medical center staff were added, including a diabetes nurse–educator, an endocrinologist, a pharmacist, and supply service representative. This committee began developing plans for standardization of testing procedures, quality control, supplies, and equipment. By 1991, the working group achieved formal status within the medical center as the Ancillary Testing Committee, having produced policies and procedures that were endorsed by the medical staff.

Policy

The point-of-care policy developed by the Ancillary Testing Committee addresses the topics shown in Table 20.1 (PVAMC Policy on Point-of-Care Testing).

Approval of New Tests

The policy requires any new test, as well as tests not specifically authorized when the policy was implemented, to be evaluated by the Ancillary Testing Committee prior to implementation. "Privileges" to perform the specific POCT are granted by the Medical Staff Council. This means that even though a specific test may be authorized within the medical center, if a new site wishes to perform the test, it must seek specific authorization.

Process for Approval of New Tests and Sites

All new tests, as well as tests not currently authorized for a specific test site, are approved by the Ancillary Testing Committee prior to implementation. Criteria for approval include demonstration of medical necessity for rapid testing, willingness and ability of the staff at the testing site to perform high-quality testing, and demonstrated compliance with all accreditation and regulatory requirements.

In their request for approval, applicants for test authorization specify the following:

- The medical, administrative, and fiscal rationale for performing the test at the point of care;
- The ancillary test site director
- The specific test methods, reagents, and equipment to be used
- A quality management and quality control plan
- The names and numbers of persons who will perform testing. If personnel from another service (such as the nursing service) will perform testing, the concurrence of the other service chief is required.
- The plan for personnel training, certification of competency, and authorization to perform testing
- An estimate of numbers of tests to be performed per month
- The indications for performing the test at the point of care
- The policies and procedures related to testing

Before testing can be started at an approved testing site, a complete policy and procedure manual must be available at the testing site, and all personnel who will do testing must be trained, certified competent, and authorized to perform the testing by the ancillary test site director.

TABLE 20.1. PORTLAND VA MEDICAL CENTER POLICY ON POINT-OF-CARE TESTING

Definitions
The committee meeting time
Committee members
Approved ancillary testing sites and tests
Approval of new tests
Authorization to perform tests
Designation of ancillary testing site directors
Training of individuals performing testing
Demonstration of adequate level of competency and its documentation
Quality management documentation
Definition of compliance with accreditation and regulatory standards
Procedure for dealing with significant compliance problems
Ensuring proper patient and sample identity
Policies regarding specific tests
    Confirmatory testing
    Procedure for performing capillary blood glucose testing
    Authorized glucose testing methods
    Quality control for capillary testing

Authorization of Personnel to Perform Tests

The Clinical Laboratories Improvement Act (CLIA), as well as the VA and JCAHO, require all persons, including nonlaboratory personnel, who perform testing to be trained, certified competent, and authorized to do the testing. This requirement applies to staff working at the VA Medical Center, but not employed by the VA, as well as VA employees. It is clear from all the rules that this requirement applies to house staff and attending physicians as well as nonphysician personnel. Although it is a manageable task to apply these rules to employees, there are problems in documentation of training, competency, and authorization for physicians, especially house staff.

There are certain specific exceptions for providers who perform specific tests. These tests, which are defined to fall within the scope of practice and training of physicians, physician assistants, and nurses, require no additional training or certification beyond their basic medical or nursing education. House staff at PVAMC are exempt in their context as *supervised trainees* whose "privileges" are managed by other means. PVAMC faced the problem of some common tests performed by medical and nursing staff by adopting the following policies:

- All house staff and staff physicians are deemed qualified, competent, and authorized to perform the following tests: stool occult blood, gastric occult blood, spun hematocrit, capillary blood glucose, and urine dipstick chemistry.
- All registered nurses are deemed trained, competent, and authorized to perform the following tests, without additional training or authorization: stool occult blood, gastric occult blood, urine dipstick chemistry.
- No additional documentation of authorization, competency, or training is required for these staff to perform the preceding tests. Basic medical and nursing education and experience are adequate for these commonly performed tests without risk to patients.

Assignment of Responsibility for Ancillary Testing

The Chief of Pathology and Laboratory Medicine is responsible for the oversight of quality management of all ancillary testing. The chief of each service area (i.e., the urology clinic) is usually the ancillary test site director, although that task may be designated to another qualified individual. We agree with Nichols and Poe (3) that success depends on recognizing the multidisciplinary nature of ancillary testing.

Responsibility of Ancillary Testing Site Directors

The ancillary test site director is responsible for proper conduct of testing and its quality management. The ancillary test site director, or the designee, is responsible for ensuring that all applicable VA and accrediting agency requirements, rules, and regulations are met.

Training of Staff Performing Testing

The ancillary test site director, or designee, is responsible for ensuring that all persons performing tests at that site have received adequate training, the training has been documented, and their competency is verified and documented.

Committee Functions

The functions of the Ancillary Testing Committee are as follows:

- Develop general policies for ancillary testing
- Approve ancillary testing sites and tests
- Deal with problems of compliance

At the beginning of the ancillary testing program, the committee met on a monthly basis to develop policies and procedures. As the program matured, meetings have been much less frequent and have dealt mostly with discussion and approval of new tests or testing sites.

Role of the Quality Management Staff

A member of the quality management service staff is designated to assist the chief of P&LMS in ensuring all ancillary testing programs meet all regulations and licensing requirements. This person acts as liaison between the ancillary testing program and quality management service and serves as the expert information resource on regulatory requirements and inspections by various agencies. We agree with Bennett and colleagues (4) that having an ongoing survey readiness program is central to ensuring passing inspections.

Role of the Laboratory

At PVAMC, the chief of P&LMS does not serve as the laboratory director for POCT sites. The P&LMS staff members serve as technical consultants as defined in CLIA regulations. The laboratory staff also manages the distribution and return of proficiency testing materials, performs compliance inspections of the ancillary testing sites to ensure that quality control and other functions are properly documented, and manages accreditation and inspection matters. In the case of capillary blood glucose, laboratory personnel also oversee application of the RALS-GJ (Medical Automation Systems, Charlottesville, VA, U.S.A.) data collection system.

Role of the Ancillary Test Site Director

The directors of testing sites have the ultimate authority over the conduct of testing in their areas. Because these persons are usually the supervisors of the testing staff, it is reasonable for them to be the ancillary test site directors; therefore, they are responsible for testing. Although the chief of P&LMS in some medical centers is directly responsible for testing in point-of-care locations, it has proven efficacious to us that the person with supervisory and disciplinary authority over the testing staff be the person responsible for their POCT activities. Hence, when there is a compliance problem, it is the site director's responsibility to take corrective actions. The site director is also ultimately responsible for the training, authorization of personnel to perform testing, and documentation of all aspects of the testing. When there are compliance problems, it is expected that communications will be directed to the site director, who is expected to correct the problem.

DETAILS OF THE PORTLAND PROGRAM
Ancillary Testing Committee Membership and Roles

At PVAMC, the Ancillary Testing Committee is composed of the chief of P&LMS (who serves as the chairman), the designated P&LMS ancillary testing coordinator; all the ancillary testing site directors, the chief of the Acquisition & Materiel Management Service (i.e., supply), the chief of biomedical engineering, and the designated quality management specialist. One reason for including all the ancillary testing site directors is that this committee has an educational role as well. The chief of Acquisition & Materiel Management is a member because of that service's important function of monitoring purchases of laboratory supplies and equipment by unauthorized sites. Biomedical engineering is a part of the committee because this department has responsibility for maintenance of all laboratory equipment.

Scope of Testing

Although POCT began at the PVAMC with capillary blood glucose testing, the list of tests quickly expanded. Current POCT tests and their locations are shown in Table 20.2.

Compliance Oversight

The P&LMS and quality management service staffs share responsibilities for compliance oversight. VA regulations assign to the P&LMS chief the responsibility for quality management of the POCT program. Assisting the P&LMS chief are the assigned quality management staff liaison and the designated P&LMS ancillary testing coordinator. These persons perform regular periodic compliance inspections and review quality control and proficiency testing data.

When lapses of compliance occur, the P&LMS chief confers with the ancillary testing site director. Usually, a resolution is found when the site director understands the regulatory and accreditation requirements. If the problem is not resolved and requirements are not met, the chief of P&LMs has the power to end testing at the POCT site, although that is usually done through the chief medical executive (i.e., the chief of the medical staff).

The most frequent lapses of compliance at the PVAMC are listed in Table 20.3. We found that virtually all sites are cooperative once the background, needs, rules, and regulations are explained. There tends to be "entropic decay" of record keeping at all sites, however, some worse than others. Therefore, we review POCT sites for compliance on a quarterly schedule.

Training

Responsibility for training of testing personnel resides with the ancillary testing site director. In most cases, especially when new procedures or equipment are first installed, the vendor provides training and will certify the initial competence of the staff. With personnel turnover, adequate training and certification of personnel are more problematic. Some manufacturers provide training manuals and videotapes for training new testing personnel. These training materials may even contain quizzes for use in certifying the initial competency of newly trained testing personnel. If vendor-prepared training materials or a representative of the vendor cannot be available to provide training, we have a knowledgeable P&LMS staff member train the new employees. In our opinion, initial training by testing site personnel who are not specifically trained laboratory personnel is hazardous and should be avoided.

Competency Assessment

After initial training, competency assurance, and authorization to perform testing, regulatory and accreditation agencies require that each person who performs testing be periodically assessed for competency to perform tests. At PVAMC, the ancillary testing site director is responsible for competency assessment and certification. Often the laboratory can assist in this task.

Methods we have used for competency assessment include examination and documentation of successful quality control testing and successful performance on periodic proficiency surveys (5). In some POCT applications, such as capillary blood glucose testing, the vendor may provide written testing materials for competency assessment. Whereas observation of testing technique by an individual can be used, this has often proven time consuming and difficult to coordinate.

Quality Control Issues

Staff resistance to quality control testing is predictable and has occurred at each new testing site. Uniformly, it has been necessary to educate and explain to new POCT personnel how the regulatory requirements apply and how compliance with rules and regulations is achieved.

TABLE 20.2. ANCILLARY TESTING LIST OF SITES, TESTS AND INDICATIONS

Emergency care unit
  Stool occult blood test
  Gastric occult blood test
  Spun hematocrit
  Urine dipstick chemistry
  Urine microscopic exam
  KOH skin and vaginal preparation
  Vaginal wet mount
  Sputum Gram stain
  Capillary blood glucose
  Indications: Rapid assessment of patient's condition as a guide to immediate therapy
Operating room (anesthesia)
  Blood gas: GEM (Instrumentation Laboratory, Lexington, MA)
  Electrolytes: GEM (Instrumentation Laboratory, Lexington, MA)
  Hematocrit: GEM (Instrumentation Laboratory, Lexington, MA)
  Oximetry
  Capillary blood glucose
  Indications: Rapid assessment of patient's ventilatory status as a guide to regulation of anesthesia.
    Rapid assessment of blood glucose as a guide to use of insulin or glucose solutions in diabetic
    patients undergoing surgery or recovering from anesthesia
Operating room (perfusion)
  Activated clotting time
  Indications: Control of heparinization and its reversal during procedure
  Blood gases with electrolytes and hematocrit
  Indications: Monitoring of perfusion and ventilation
Cardiac catheterization lab
  Oximetry
  Indications: Rapid assessment of blood oxygenation as a guide to the placement of the catheter
  Activated clotting time
  Indications: Control of heparinization and its reversal during procedure
Dialysis
  Activated clotting time
  Indications: Control of heparinization and its reversal during procedure
  Capillary blood glucose
  Indications: Rapid assessment of blood glucose as a guide to use of insulin in diabetic patients
Endoscopy
  Helicobacter: CLO spot test for urease activity (Ballard Medical Products, Draper, UT)
  Gastric pH
  Indications: Rapid diagnosis of *Helicobacter*-induced ulceration
Entire hospital, including extended care sites (Nursing Service function)
  Capillary blood glucose
  Indications: Rapid assessment of blood glucose as a guide to use of insulin and oral hypoglycemic
    agents in diabetic patients and initiation of rapid treatment of hypoglycemia
  Stool occult blood
  Gastric occult blood test
  Indications: Rapid detection of the presence of GI bleeding
Home-based health care
  Prothrombin time (CoaguChek [Roche Diagnostics, Indianapolis, IN])
  Indications: Rapid determination of prothrombin time to advise patient and regulate therapy while
    at the patient's home
  Capillary blood glucose
  Indications: Rapid assessment of blood glucose as a guide to use of insulin and oral hypoglycemic
    agents in diabetic patients, and initiation of rapid treatment of hypoglycemia
Urology (clinic)
  (Cystoscopy)
  Urine dipstick chemistry
  Urine microscopic exam
  Indications: Rapid screening for the presence of infection or glycosuria prior to a procedure
General medical clinic
  Urine dipstick chemistry
  Urine microscopic exam
  Indications: Rapid screening for the presence of infection or glycosuria prior to a procedure
  Joint fluid microscopy (rheumatology clinic)
  Indications: Diagnostic procedure
Medical intensive care unit
  Activated clotting time
  Indications: Monitoring of coagulation at time of coronary stent removal

(continued)

TABLE 20.2. *(continued)*

Emergency care unit
  KOH preparation
  Spun hematocrit
  Gastric occult blood and pH
  Fecal occult blood
  Urine dipstick chemistry
Imaging service
  Schilling test
  ^{51}Cr RBC volume with hematocrit
  Indications: Diagnostic procedures
  Activated clotting time
  Indications: Control of heparinization and its reversal during procedure
Surgical service
  Urine dipstick chemistry
  Urine microscopic exam
  Indications: Rapid screening for the presence of infection or glycosuria prior to a procedure
  Gastric pH
  KOH preparation
  Indications: Diagnostic procedures
Primary care (includes 2 remote clinic sites)
  Vaginal wet mounts
  KOH preparations
  Fecal occult blood
  Urine dipstick chemistry
  Indications: Diagnostic procedures
Behavioral medicine
  Breath alcohol
  Indications: Monitoring of alcohol use in patients returning from leave

GI, gastrointestinal; RBC, red blood cells.

TABLE 20.3. MOST COMMON PROBLEMS ENCOUNTERED IN POINT-OF-CARE PROGRAM MANAGEMENT

Regulation and accreditation
  Site director (SD) or coordinator (ATC) lacks understanding of, or is reluctant to conform with, the
    VA directives dealing with point-of-care testing
  SD or ATC lacks understanding of, or is reluctant to conform with, standards and requirements from
    CAP and JCAHO
  SD or ATC and/or those performing testing do not understand difference between training and
    authorization to perform testing
Quality management
  Failure to perform quality control testing on each day of testing
  Failure to perform proficiency testing in timely manner
  SD or ATC or those performing tests do not understand difference between QC and proficiency
    testing
  Failure to investigate out of control QC or unacceptable proficiency testing result
  Use of expired reagents
  Failure to date reagents at time of placing them in use
  Performance of QC on one instrument and patient testing on a different instrument on the same
    day
Documentation
  Failure to document any of the above
  SD or ATC or those performing tests reluctant to maintain records
  Failure to enter data into patient record
  Lack of review of QC or proficiency testing results by the SD
  Failure to authorize new testing person before testing of patients

ATC, Ancillary Testing Coordinator; VA, Veterans Affairs; CAP, College of American Pathologists; JCAHO, Joint
Commission on Accreditation of Healthcare Organizations; QC, quality control.

When the capillary blood glucose testing program was first implemented, we were convinced that all POCT personnel should perform quality control testing each day the individual performed patient testing. We thought quality control testing had educational value and that its performance improved testing technique. We also believed that traditional quality control techniques were relatively ineffective for POCT, where errors tend to be random rather than systematic (6). In a compromise with the nursing staff, we initially planned that only one level (elevated) would be tested. This policy, however, was in conflict with the regulatory and accreditation requirements and was changed to a system in which two levels of control materials (high and low) were tested daily by only one operator at each testing site.

Capillary blood prothrombin time, on the other hand, presents a different kind of quality control problem. With this test, the most critical technical point is skin puncture and rapid transfer of the drop of blood to the test cartridge. Unfortunately, there is no adequate quality control material that tests this critical element. For this reason, we require that a venipuncture and conventional prothrombin time test be compared with the capillary blood method every tenth time the test is performed.

Proficiency Testing Issues

Proficiency testing (PT) must be performed by the personnel who actually perform the tests. At PVAMC, the proficiency testing program is managed by the laboratory. Following receipt of the survey material in the laboratory, the relevant POCT sites are informed and the specimens are obtained by POCT site personnel. All proficiency testing specimens are tracked by P&LMS to ensure timely return of data to the proficiency testing agency. In most cases, we find it necessary to follow up actively the reporting of these proficiency testing surveys because testing site personnel either do not understand or fail to remember the seriousness of failure to report promptly the results of the survey. Prior to returning the results to the agency conducting the proficiency testing, we obtain a copy of the answer sheet for our records.

When proficiency testing results and scores are returned from the testing agency, the P&LMS staff reviews the results. If the results are within the acceptable range, the results are returned to the ancillary testing site director. If the results are out of acceptable range, the laboratory staff prepares a "Proficiency Test Error Response Form," which is sent along with the test results to the site director. Laboratory staff monitors the return of the "Proficiency Test Error Response Form" and maintains records of such events.

Except for capillary blood glucose testing, proficiency tests are performed at all testing sites in the medical center. Because capillary blood glucose testing occurs in numerous locations, we have chosen to participate in the CAP Capillary Blood Glucose Program, which provides 20 samples of survey material. These are tested at different sites on a rotating basis. The persons who do the patient testing at a site also do the sample proficiency testing, on a rotating basis. In this manner, each site and each person doing the testing participate in the PT program while at the same time minimizing PT costs. The designated P&LMS ancillary testing coordinator collects and analyzes these PT data and prepares a report showing the proficiency testing results for capillary blood glucose ancillary testing throughout the medical center.

Ensuring Proper Patient and Sample Identity

Good medical practice requires that procedures be in place to verify sample identity and integrity. In the laboratory, this principle leads to procedures for labeling specimens that are relatively standardized between laboratories. We have encountered problems during point-of-care testing site accreditation inspections because standard laboratory techniques for specimen identification are not always appropriate for point-of-care testing. As a result, we use the following policy and procedure for point-of-care testing specimen identification.

In situations where samples from more than one patient can be misidentified prior to definitive analysis, the sample container must be identified with the patient's name and another unique identifier. In situations where the test is performed at the bedside or other site, where there is only one patient, where the sample is taken directly from the patient to the analyzer, and where there is no possibility of misidentification, such detailed labeling is unnecessary and might delay analysis.

Specific requirements include the following: Specimens removed from patients for analysis must have a label on the primary container. At a minimum, the label must show the full name and last four digits of the social security number. An exception can be made to the labeling requirement if all of the following conditions are met:

1. The sample to be analyzed is taken directly from the patient to the analyzer.
2. The patient and analyzer are in the same or adjacent rooms.
3. The analyst has personally obtained the sample or was given the sample in the presence of the patient.
4. No samples from other patients are being analyzed at the same time.
5. Test results are given directly to the care provider *and* are documented in the patient's chart or a log bearing the patient's identification.

Confirmatory Testing

It is generally recognized that confirmatory testing of capillary blood glucose tests should be performed in the laboratory for values greater than 350 mg per deciliter or lower than 50 mg per deciliter. Therapeutic intervention based on initial capillary blood glucose test results outside this range is usually withheld until the results are confirmed by the designated confirmatory test method. Although this method is practical in the hospital setting, we have found this approach impractical in the nursing home or clinic located at a distance from a laboratory. As a result, we *require* confirmatory testing of abnormal capillary blood glucose only in the hospital. Of course, providers may obtain confirmatory testing at any time they deem it necessary.

Although no other *policies* requiring confirmatory testing exist, it is good practice to confirm unexpected test results in the laboratory. We have no data indicating the extent to which this is done.

Site Director Review of Documentation

Regulations direct the ancillary site testing director to review and sign off on quality control, maintenance, and proficiency testing on a monthly basis. We find it difficult to obtain uniform compliance with this requirement. Consequently, in our periodic compliance inspections, we constantly must look for documentation of these events.

Cost

Cost analysis of POCT is a complex issue (7). The direct costs of reagents, other consumable supplies, and labor to perform tests can be tabulated on the basis of numbers of tests performed. When cost analyses are reported in the literature, these costs usually are provided. We show ancillary testing costs for PVAMC in Table 20.4 (direct POCT costs) and Table 20.5

TABLE 20.4. DIRECT POINT-OF-CARE PROGRAM COSTS

Item	Time (h/yr)	Cost ($/yr)
Operating room		
Blood gases		
GEM packs		13,200
Labor for patient tests	200	5,320
Service contract		2,500
Capillary blood glucose		
Reagent strips		33,000
Labor for patient tests	6,333	168,458
Prothrombin time		
Reagent cassettes		11,658
Labor for patient tests	362	9,642
Total		243,777

TABLE 20.5. INDIRECT POINT-OF-CARE TESTING COSTS

Activity	Personnel Involved or Notes	Time (h/yr/person)	Cost ($/yr)
Accreditation			
Annual fee for 10 sites, plus 26 CBG locations			250
Preparation for inspection	ATC Site personnel	½ h per site	266
Quarterly compliance inspections		26	1383
Annual compliance inspection	ATC QM staff Chief P&LMS Site personnel SD	13	3,300
Proficiency testing			
Program fees			2793
Compliance and review of data	ATC	CBG: 48 Others: 96	3,830
Reagents			CBG: 195 Others: 50
Testing labor	Site personnel	CBG: 20 Others: 20	665 665
Quality control			
QC control solutions	CBG: 8/site × 26 sites		CBG Inpatient 768 Outpatient 1,007 GEM 1,020 Prothrombin 1,162
Reagents for QC	CBG: 2 strips daily × 26 sites		CBG Inpatient 9,500 Outpatient unknown GEM no cost Prothrombin 11,658
Labor for QC	Site personnel (RN)	CBG 791 Prothrombin 362	21,014 9,642
Compliance inspections	ATC	288	7,661
Instrument maintenance	ATC	52	1,383
Meetings	ATC QM staff Chief P&LMS MLO	60	10,212
Total			Labor 60,021 Fees 3,043 Reagents 25,360
Total		1,662	88,424

CBG, capillary blood glucose; ATC, Ancillary Testing Coordinator; QC, quality control; QM, quality management; P&LMS, Pathology and Laboratory Medicine; SD, site director; RN, registered nurse; MLO, medical laboratory observer.

(indirect POCT costs). Reports of cost analyses frequently do not report these indirect costs. Our cost data for capillary blood glucose testing also indicate costs for strips and quality control solutions dispensed by the pharmacy to some, but not all, of our outpatients. These strip costs for home testing are more than three times the costs for inpatients.

Point-of-care testing cost savings are almost never reported. These are associated with a shortened hospital length of stay for an episode of care and include costs for the following:

- Hospital facilities
- Physician services
- Technical and professional services
- Drugs and intravenous catheters
- Avoidance of collateral diseases and complications related to hospitalization.

We have not attempted to estimate the cost savings of the episode of care because there is no good method to do so. The few studies that have considered cost avoidance associated with POCT suggest that the cost savings far exceed the direct and indirect costs of the testing (7).

Patient Self-Testing

The policy of the VA addresses patient self-testing as well as ancillary testing performed by employees. Outpatients who are going to perform ancillary testing must receive training in the use of the testing devices. Further, the devices used require periodic checking by trained personnel, usually the caregiver. In the case of capillary blood glucose ancillary testing, diabetes nurse–educators are charged with the patient training and device testing roles. At PVAMC, the diabetes care group makes the choice of capillary blood glucose testing systems. As a result, ancillary testing capillary blood glucose results involving PVAMC patients come from the same instrument and methodology, no matter who is doing the testing.

Self-testing by inpatients, with the use of test results in therapy, is not allowed in the VA. Inpatients can, however, use their test systems as part of educational and quality control activities.

GENERALIZATION TO THE ENTIRE VETERANS AFFAIRS

Nature of Central Control

At present, the VA does not exert strong central control on the day-to-day practice of medicine. General policies are developed at the central level, but the details of their implementation are left to the field organization. As a result, there is no uniform pattern of POCT management in the VA. We expect that attempts to standardize systems, control testing indications, or manage costs of POCT will take place at the local or network level rather than from the VA Headquarters in Washington.

Network Organization

Recently, a new organizational structure was introduced in the VA. Medical facilities were grouped into regional "networks." Each network contains a group of hospitals and other medical facilities in a relatively large geographic area. Patterns of medical practice vary considerably from one network to another. In some networks, including ours, each medical facility operates relatively independently. In others, there is pronounced standardization.

Standardization of POCT has received little attention in the networks. A few have standardized test systems for capillary blood glucose testing. There are now attempts to standardize quality control materials and to use a single lot number within at least one network. We found no examples of a centralized quality assurance system for POCT within any network. There is also no nationally mandated management plan for POCT. We are aware of no VA-wide attempts to reduce the cost of POCT. One means of doing this could be the development of a set of indications for capillary blood glucose testing for hospitalized patients.

Electronic Data Capture

The VA policy establishing POCT requires that all POCT laboratory data be integrated into the patient's computerized medical record. Until very recently, the only way to do this is was to enter laboratory results manually, either at the time of testing or later. As a result, most POCT data were recorded on flow charts or progress notes in the patient record but did not become part of the patient's computerized laboratory database.

All VA medical centers use a hospital and laboratory information system developed by the VA, known as *VistA*. Interfaces for the more popular hospital capillary blood glucose systems have been written for the VistA LIS system. Entry of all testing data used in the medical care of veteran patients is required by VA policy to be entered into the VistA LIS laboratory data file. There is, however, no VA policy on how this is to be done or a requirement to use any specific software or system to accomplish the data entry. Our medical center uses Medical Automation System's RALS-G point-of-care data management system. The potential of electronic data capture, tracking, and computerized patient management for POCT is being realized at some medical centers in the VA.

CONCLUSIONS

Point-of-care testing within the VA medical care system is much like POCT in private sector hospitals. Although the VA is the country's largest medical care provider, no standard organization of POCT has taken place, and only general guidelines for the implementation of POCT exist.

The following are the major policies relating to POCT:

- Point-of-care testing activities will be inspected and accredited by JCAHO or CAP.
- The chief of pathology and laboratory service is responsible for and has authority over all point-of-care testing activities within each medical center.

Our system works. Sites that need POCT capability have it available. Sites that do not really need the capability usually opt out because of the regulatory requirements. Medical and nursing staff compliance is possible, but it requires close personal interaction and monitoring, which is difficult for P&LMS staff. We in the laboratory know what quality management procedures are needed, and it is a part of our lives; it is difficult for the ancillary testing sites because their personnel are not oriented toward or trained in this aspect of medical care.

With close personal supervision and monitoring, it is possible to acquire CAP and JCAHO accreditation, but the reader should be forewarned that there is considerably more emphasis and attention to detail in this area than there has been before.

REFERENCES

1. VA Manual M2, Part VI, Chapter 10, Ancillary testing. Department of Veterans Affairs, 1993.
2. VA Handbook 1106.1, Chapter 7, Ancillary testing. Department of Veterans Affairs, February 12, 1998.
3. Nichols JH, Poe SS. Quality assurance, practical management, and outcomes of point-of-care testing: laboratory perspectives, part I. *Clin Lab Manage Rev* 1999;13:341–350.
4. Bennett J, Cervantes C, Pacheco S. Point-of-care testing: inspection preparedness. *Perfusion* 2000;15:137–142.
5. Baer DM. An operational approach to competency assessment. *Medical Laboratory Observer* 1997;29:55–57.
6. Baer DM, Belsey RE. Limitations of quality control in physicians offices and other decentralized testing situations: the challenge to develop new methods of test validation. *Clin Chem* 1993;39:9–12.
7. Baer DM. Point-of-care testing versus central lab costs. *Medical Laboratory Observer* 1998;30(Suppl 9):46–56.

21

POINT-OF-CARE TESTING IN THE COMMUNITY HEALTH SYSTEM

RHONDA M. PIKELNY

ORGANIZATION OF THE GROUP HEALTH SYSTEM

Group Health Cooperative (GHC) is a not-for-profit, consumer-governed health care organization that provides health care to more than 590,000 enrollees in central, northern, and eastern Washington and northern Idaho. In the Puget Sound area, it encompasses two hospitals, 24 clinics, a long-term care facility, a hospice program, and a large distribution center. Laboratory services are provided through an integrated system of laboratories located in each of the clinics and hospitals and a centralized reference laboratory.

DISTRIBUTION OF TESTING SITES

Point-of-care testing (POCT) in the GHC system is performed at the bedside in both hospitals, in the long-term health facility, and in some nonlaboratory clinical sites. Tests performed by POCT sites include whole-blood glucose, urine dipstick, stool occult blood, gastroccult, and rapid strep testing. Blood gases are drawn and performed by respiratory therapists and in the laboratory. Whole-blood prothrombin times are performed by doctors of pharmacy at selected clinical sites, and provider-performed microscopic procedures are performed by providers at various hospital and clinical sites.

The number of sites and large physical area covered by the program present special problems in the design and implementation of a point-of-care program. This chapter describes how the GHC point-of-care program was established to meet these special needs.

GROUP HEALTH COOPERATIVE POINT-OF-CARE TESTING PROGRAM MISSION

The mission of the POCT program of the GHC is to ensure that accurate, timely, and reliable patient test results performed outside a clinical laboratory comply with regulations and are effective for patient outcomes.

POINT-OF-CARE TESTING COMMITTEE

Working with the Staff Credentialing Committee, the laboratory quality assurance/education coordinator organized the Group Health Cooperative Point-of-Care Committee (POCC), which is the foundation of the GHC point-of-care program. The members of this committee were carefully selected and consist of managers who have an understanding of the operations needed to design and the authority to implement a point-of-care program. The members of the POCC include the medical director of Laboratory Services, the coordinator of Laboratory Services Quality Assurance/Point-of-Care, two hospital-system laboratory supervisors, two hospital laboratory point-of-care coordinators, the nurse managers/clinical nurse specialists from five hospital units, the coordinator of Ambulatory Care/Hospice/Specialty Clinics Staff Development, the coordinator of Long-Term Care Unit Quality Assurance, and an occasional special guest manager or coordinator.

The POCC meets every month. The laboratory members and the chair of the committee meet the week prior to the POCC meeting, if necessary, to develop the agenda and to discuss laboratory responsibilities.

QUALITY MANAGEMENT

The Policy

The POCC agreed that the program would accomplish its mission by the development of protocols and procedures, which define methods, equipment, training, competency evaluation, limits and uses of the results. Whole-blood glucose POCT results are used for screening and to monitor treatment but must not be used for diagnostic purposes. Other specific tests may be used for diagnosis, such as arterial blood gas and positive rapid strep screening. Point-of-care results are intended to supplement, rather than substitute for, clinical laboratory testing. The point-of-care testing program is crucial to providing quality patient care, achieving good outcomes, and ensuring compliance with the Washington State Medical Test Site Law (MTS), the Joint Commission on Accreditation of Healthcare Organizations (JCAHO) standards, the Occupational Safety and Health Administration (OSHA)/(WISHA) regulations.

Responsibilities

Point-of-Care Committee

All members of the POCC serve as contacts for POCT in the GHC and are expected to communicate the mission, policies, expectations, and procedures related to POCT to their peers who are not part of the committee. The POCC develops the policies and procedures that define the methods, equipment, limits, training, and uses of the results. The committee oversees the planning and implementation of the program. It also identifies, reviews, and evaluates new POCT and equipment. The POCC monitors and ensures compliance with the POCT program with the aid of the quality assurance reports. Individual responsibilities for members of the POCC were identified as described in the following sections.

Medical Director

The laboratory medical director, a clinical pathologist, is responsible for the oversight and approval of all policies, procedures, and equipment related to testing performed outside the laboratory by nonlaboratory personnel. He or she reviews and approves appropriate use of POCT methods, oversees all POCC activity, and is the liaison to the medical staff regarding POCT issues and uses.

Office of Laboratory Quality Assurance and Education

The coordinator of Quality Assurance for Laboratory Services (LQA) is the coordinator of the POCT program and chair of the POCC. The LQA department maintains the point-of-care database for the system, collates downloaded information, prepares quality assurance monitor reports for the hospital laboratories, coordinates linearity studies, collates proficiency results, evaluates performance, instigates any necessary corrective action, and prepares quality assurance reports on the proficiency programs. The coordinator of Quality Assurance/Education serves as the contact for manufacturers and coordinates the evaluation and selection of methods and equipment used in the program.

The LQA office provides continuing education, as needed, on POCT. The LQA office prepares, distributes, and grades provider-performed microscopic procedures (PPMP) test validation results to medical staff performing postvasectomy semen checks for sperm, urine microscopy, nasal smears for eosinophils, pinworm preps, fern tests, and vaginal wet preps.

Group Health Quality Services Department

The GHC Quality Services Department provides staff support to the POCC. The staff-supports member plans the agenda for the monthly meeting with the chair of the committee. He or she records and distributes minutes of the meetings and identifies continuing agenda items.

In addition, the chair supports the POCT annual and weekly training programs, providing oversight of schedules and departmental key contacts. He or she coordinates POCT registration, provides POCT training packets to campuses, and ensures that the training packets are updated and readily available. The quality services representative coordinates the development of the POCC annual work plan and ensures that the work plan is implemented in coordination with the chair and the POCC. He or she assures that the program evaluations and documentation are in place.

Since disciplines have various formats for procedures and policies, the quality services representative has the responsibility of coordinating the content and format of these between the various disciplines and assures annual review by the POCC. The quality services representative also provides consultation and information on changes back to the GHC quality service managers and collates budget information for POCC activities.

Hospital Laboratory Staff

The laboratory staff members write, organize, maintain, and update procedures, manuals, logs, checklists, and training material as needed. They review monthly compliance reports and mail recommendations to the hospital testing units, as needed. They are responsible for oversight of the supply and maintenance of instruments, performance of linearity studies, and distribution of proficiency testing to the units with follow-up of the results. The staff also assists in the planning and training of annual certification classes and training weekly certification classes and maintains recertification records. Hospital laboratory managers report to the Hospital Quality Committee.

The hospital staff goes to the testing units where they download data from the glucose monitor system. At this time they survey the testing sites for compliance to the program and adjust instruments, as needed.

In the laboratories the technologists print the data downloaded at the testing sites, troubleshoot blood glucose monitoring instrument problems, review and enter all point-of-care results into the laboratory computer system, and maintain the glucose monitor database at the hospital site. They also perform controls on the urine test strip vials and label the vials prior to distribution to floors.

Nursing Managers, Clinical Nurse Specialists, or Designees

Nursing managers, clinical nurse specialists, or their designees review quality assurance reports and take appropriate action when necessary. They ensure compliance with the POCT program by identifying and reporting any testing performed in their areas of responsibility to the POCC. They ensure that staff is trained and adhere to the POCT program, including participation in proficiency testing. They also maintain department certification records and participate in standards review and development.

Nonlaboratory Testing Personnel

All POCT personnel must attend the GHC POCT training program and keep their certification current. They must know and follow current testing procedures and comply with regulations. All testing personnel must use a current GHC user identification number and perform testing according to the program including proficiency testing, control documentation, equipment maintenance, and the dating of control and strip vials.

Gathering Information

The POCC developed and distributed a "Limits and Uses of Point of Care Testing Form" (Fig. 21.1) with which they obtained the following information: Who is performing POCT? Why must this test be performed as POCT? How is the POCT performed and recorded at present? Who is responsible for training of personnel at this point?

Whole-blood Glucose Testing Program

Instrument Selection

The coordinator of quality assurance/education of Laboratory Services was asked to select the monitor to be used in the POCT program. Several criteria had to be met. The monitor must meet the laboratory equipment standards as set by the technical director of Laboratory Services. It must easily pass the bloodborne

pathogen standard and must be able to be used easily by non-technical personnel. The testing system must have adequate memory to facilitate the needs in all testing sites. The manufacturer must have adequate staff and support to meet the decentralized glucose-monitoring program in all regions to include training and monitor maintenance. It must include a computerized system for use in the hospitals and long-term care facility. Finally, the system must be cost-effective. A glucose monitor system that met the above criteria was recommended by the coordinator of assurance/education and approved by Laboratory Services and the POCC.

Training

Each hospital and long-term care facility unit has a POCC approved "Limits and Uses of Blood Glucose Monitoring Form" (Fig. 21.1). This form indicates: the patient population for which the whole blood glucose is to be used, the name of the standard in which it is described, and limitations that may apply.

All testing personnel in the two hospital systems and the long-term care facility were trained according to the program developed by the POCC. This training also was given to nurses employed by temporary nursing service agencies. Each employee

Group Health Cooperative
Limits and Uses of Blood Glucose Monitoring
Bedside Blood Glucose monitoring indications can be modified and customized at any time by an M.D. order.

Name of Department/Unit_____   **Campus**: Eastside __ Central _____ KCC _____

Patient Population	Applies to this unit	Name of Standard		Limitation apply?	
				Yes	No
Adult Diabetic Patients		▪ Blood Glucose Management's Protocol		✓	
Ketoacidosis		▪ Insulin Drip Protocol ▪ Management Of Adult Or Pediatric Patient Of Insulin Drip ▪ Care Plan For Patient With Diabetes		✓	
TPN		▪ TPN Protocol		✓	
Unexpected coma/shock		▪ Blood Glucose Management Protocol		✓	
Patients with AIDS receiving IV Pentamidine		▪ Nursing Management Of Patient Receiving IV Pentamidine		✓	
Patients receiving Enteral Feedings		▪ Enternal Feeding Protocol ▪ Nursing Management Of The Adult And Pediatric Patient Receiving Enternal Feeding		✓	
Pediatric Diabetic Patients		▪ Pediatric Standard Of Care ▪ Type I Diabetes Soc ▪ Insulin Drip Protocol ▪ Nursing Management Of The Adult Or Pediatric Patient On Insulin Drip		✓	
Neonate		▪ Nursing Management Of Neonate At Risk Of Hypo/Hyperglycemia		✓	
Insulin Dependant Diabetic Or Insulin Dependent Gestational Diabetic in Labor		▪ IV Insulin With Infusion Protocol ▪ Nursing Management Of Pregnant Patient On Insulin ▪ Drip		✓	
Diet Controlled Diabetic in Labor				✓	
Gestational Diabetic on Tocolytic Therapy				✓	

Director Point of Care Testing _____ Date: _____ NM/CNS/Signature: _____ Date: _____

FIGURE 21.1. Limits and uses of blood glucose monitoring. This form is filled out by each department or unit for each point-of-care analyte, defining why the test must be performed at point of care.

receives a packet prior to the training program. The packet includes a copy of the GHC policy on POCT, the appropriate test procedures to be read, and a written examination to be taken prior to the training session. The test is to be taken prior to the training session. The trainer reviews any incorrect responses with the employee. A score of 100% is necessary before the employee moves to a competency demonstration table, where the employee must perform accurate, competent testing. The training program covers JCAHO standards, GHC POCT policies, user identification, patient identification, instrument operation and troubleshooting, quality control/pro-

ficiency testing performance and documentation, comment codes, result reporting, fingerstick techniques, and bloodborne pathogen regulations. The training program takes approximately one and a half hours per session, during which the trainer completes a POCT training checklist (Fig. 21.2). At completion of satisfactory training, the employee receives a "Point-of-Care Certification Card" (Fig. 21.3). No employee is permitted to perform POCT in the system without being certified in the GHC POCT program. Staff trained on monitors outside the GHC system must retrain in the GHC training program. New employees, staff, and agency personnel who were unable to

GROUP HEALTH COOPERATIVE
POCT Training Checklist

Name: _____   User ID: _____   SS#_____

Mgr/Supvr's Name: _____   Dept Code: _____   Job Class #:_____

Unit: _____   Date: _____

Circle your location: CH   Eastside   KCC

Color Blind Testing: ☐ Neg   ☐ Pos

Check each activity as it is demonstrated or described.

Plan		Accucheck Adv. WB Glucose	Urine dipstick (chemistries)	Clinitest Reducing Sub.	Refractometer Specif. Gravity	Occult Blood	Gastroccult
Policy							
Procedure							
Competency							
User identification							
Patient identification							
Infection control							
Proficiency testing							
Equipment							
BGM test strips, GTS, Blood drawing equipment							
Chemstrip test strips							
Clinitest tablets, tube, H_2O							
Refractometer							
Hemoccult Sensa Cards, developer							
Gastrocult Cards, developer							
Procedures / Skills							
Aware of appropriate specimen collection, test reagents, test reagent storage, control handling/storage, and PPE.							
Checks expiration date(s).							
Demonstrates proper technique when inoculating strip, preparing sample.							
Observes accurate timing per requirement of specific test.							
Properly disposes of test equipment/sample.							
Correctly performs/interprets test & controls per specific test requirements.							
Maintains accurate and complete QC logs /paper work where appropriate.							
Completes Laboratory Test Worksheet with all required information.							
Verifies that 3-digit code numbers match.							
Inserts test strip correctly.							
Obtains blood sample and applies to test strip correctly.							
Reads and enters results, uses comment codes as needed.							
Knows/follows trouble-shooting steps, when instrument/controls do not perform correctly.							
Demonstrate good finger-stick technique.							
Signature of Verifier:							

Circle one for each.

Demo Results: Pass or Needs Review   **Exam Results:** Pass or Needs Review

FIGURE 21.2. Point-of-care training checklist. This form is completed and signed by the trainer at the time of point-of-care training.

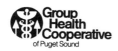

Point of Care Testing

Certification Document

Kelsey Creek

Eastside Laboratory	425-883-5141
Central Laboratory	206-326-3366
Tacoma Specialty Lab	253-596-3337

↑

Front of Certification Card

Point of Care Testing

Has completed GHC approved training for those categories checked below.

User ID #_____   **Exp. Date**

Whole Blood Glucose   Date   Trainer

QC (high & low)
Patient Testing
Fingerstick

Hemoccult   Gastroccult

Urine Dipstick

Reducing Substances (Clinitest)

Other

This card constitutes verification of skills.

↑

Reverse of Certification Card

FIGURE 21.3. Point-of-Care certification card: Each employee who has completed a point-of-care training session receives a point-of-care certification card valid for 1 year.

attend the initial training must attend a POCT training session held weekly in a hospital laboratory. Laboratory staff conducts these training sessions at specific times. Attendees must register ahead for the training.

Recertification

Recertification is held on an annual basis. Each employee receives a training packet prior to the recertification session. The packet includes a copy of the test procedures and a written examination with a Scantron answer sheet covering all POCT. The employee answers only questions relating to the tests for which he/she is to be certified. The trainer reviews any incorrect answers with the employee. A score of 100% is required before the employee moves to a competency demonstration table, where he or she must perform accurate, competent testing. If the employee has the test completed on arrival and can demonstrate competency, the recertification process takes approximately 25 minutes. On satisfactory completion, the employee receives a current GHC "Point-of-Care Certification Card" (Fig. 21.3).

Other Point-of-Care Testing in the Program

After successful implementation of the whole-blood glucose point-of-care program, the POCC addressed the testing of

visual urine dipstick, gastroccults, stool occult blood, and rapid strep screen. The director of Laboratory Services reviewed the "Limits and Uses of Point-of-Care Testing Form" (see Fig. 21.1) for each test and each area where it was being performed. Staff performing visual urine dipsticks, stool occult bloods, gastroccults, or rapid strep screens were contacted, and the need for POCT was discussed. Personnel performing these procedures were identified. The training, certification, and annual recertification of these tests were added to the whole-blood glucose monitoring program using the same format. The written examination was expanded to cover all POCT included in the training program. The employees answer only questions that pertain to the tests in which they need to be certified. The program has been renamed the GHC point-of-care certification program. Additionally, a test for color-blindness is given to each employee performing visual urine dipstick, stool occult blood, gastroccults, and rapid strep screens. Those found to be color-blind may not perform these tests because of the necessity to observe specific color changes that may occur and are asked to sign a form (Fig. 21.4) stating that they understand these limitations. The current GHC point-of-care certification (see Fig. 21.3) indicates the tests for which each employee is certified.

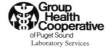
Laboratory Services

To:_____
      Employee

_____
      Position/Department

POSITIVE COLOR BLIND TEST
Job Performance Limitations

Statement of Understanding

I understand that I have a type of color abnormality or deficiency, as identified in screening. I also understand that I will not perform patient laboratory or Point of Care tests that require visual interpretation of color. I may continue to perform those tests that are interpreted by electronic or non-color dependant means as long as I am employed at Group Health Cooperative.

_____   _____
Employee Signature   Manager/Supervisor Signature

_____
Date

FIGURE 21.4. Positive color-blindness test statement of understanding: Each trainee who is found to be color-blind must sign this form stating he or she understands that he or she cannot perform laboratory tests that require visual identification of color. The form is placed in the personnel file of the color-blind employee.

Quality Control

Whole-blood Glucose

A 1-year supply of a sequestered lot of strips and controls are purchased. Acceptable ranges are validated by the quality assurance coordinator and are entered into the glucose monitor's computer system by the laboratory staff. Two levels of controls, high and low, are performed on each monitor each day of testing. Patient testing cannot be performed unless both control results are within acceptable range. Control and patient data are downloaded into a laboratory computer system monthly by laboratory staff.

Urine Dipstick

All vials of dipsticks are delivered to the laboratory, where a positive control is performed and recorded, and the vial is labeled with "QC-OK," the date, and the initial of the tech performing the control. The nursing staff obtains the controlled vials from the laboratory and takes them to the specified department for urine testing. Laboratory staff checks for vials that have been left open or that are expired when they download the glucose data. If such problems are found, they are discarded, the unit staff is informed, and a note is left apprising the staff that the vial was found unacceptable and discarded.

Occult Blood

The performance control monitor is read on the card by the testing person and recorded on the "Lab Test Worksheet" (Fig. 21.5).

Rapid Strep Screen

External positive and negative controls are performed every time a new kit is opened. These results and the internal control are recorded on a "Rapid Strep Screen QC Log" (Fig. 21.6).

Lab Test Worksheet

Specimen Type: (circle one) Urine Stool (reducing substance only) Chemstrip 10/Clinitest Tablets (circle one) Lot # _____ Exp. Date: _____	
	Patient Results:
Spec. Gravity (chemstrip or refract)	
pH	
Leucocytes	
Nitrite	
Protein	
Glucose	
Ketones	
Urobilinogen	
Bilirubin	
Blood	
Hgb.	
Red. Subst.	
*Colo	
*Appearance/ transparency	

Test performed by:_____
(Lab test user ID)

```
Addressograph /ARPA Label
_____

Date          Time          _____

Name:         _____

Medical History #          _____

Requesting MD (Name & #)          _____

Diagnosis Code
```

Hemoccult or Gastroccult (circle one)

Card Lot #_____   Exp Date. _____
Developer Lot #_____   Exp. Date: _____

Controls: Positive (blue)   OK   If control not OK:
                                    Circle   1) use another card

              Negative (clear)   OK   2) Open new reagent vial and repeat
                                    Circle

Do not report patient results until control is OK!

pH results (gastroccult only)_____

Patient Result (circle one)   Positive   Negative

Place top copy in patient's chart. Remove copy when hospital report is issued to chart. Send second copy to lab.

FIGURE 21.5. Laboratory test worksheet: Hospital units performing point-of-care testing document results on this form. One sheet is kept in the chart temporarily, and the other is sent to the laboratory where it is resulted into the laboratory computer system.

LOCATION:											
KIT NAME: Rapid Strep A											
Kit Lot Number:								Exp. Date:			
External Positive Cont. Lot#:								Exp. Date:			
External Negative Cont. Lot#:								Exp. Date:			

Test	Date	PATIENT NAME	Patient Results	Internal RED control line seen ✔	TECH INIT.	Test	Date	PATIENT NAME	PATIENT RESULTS	Internal RED control line seen ✔	TECH INIT.
1		Positive External Control				15					
2		Negative External Control				16					
3						17					
4						18					
5						19					
6						20					
7						21					
8						22					
9						23					
10						24					
11						24					
12						25					
13						26					
14						Perform External Controls on each new QC Sheet! REVIEWED BY: Date:					

FIGURE 21.6. Rapid strep screen log sheet: Rapid strep controls and patient results are documented on this log sheet.

Patient Results

Glucose results are placed in the patient's chart directly by the testing personnel. The testing personnel fill out a two-part "Lab Test Worksheet" (see Fig. 21.5) for urine dipstick, stool occult blood, and gastroccult and rapid strep screen results. The top copy is sent to the laboratory, where the results are entered into the laboratory information system and a permanent laboratory report is generated. The bottom is sent to the chart as a temporary report.

Whole-blood Coagulation Clinics

Group Health Cooperative has three anticoagulation clinics using whole-blood prothrombin time instruments. These are located in GHC clinics and are run by doctors of pharmacy with prescriptive authority to manage warfarin therapy. Changes to dosage are made according to international normalized ratio (INR) results and a preapproved algorithm. The pharmacists consult directly with the attending physician when a visit is required for the management of any medical complication of therapy or other conditions noted during the visit. Results and all routine care are documented in a computerized information system. The "Anticoagulation Clinic Progress Note" is printed for the outpatient medical record if there is a change in dose, a significant change in the patient's clinical condition, or other pertinent information to the managing physician. Monthly Anticoagulation Clinic meetings are attended by the testing pharmacists, the medical director of Laboratory Services, the hematology/coagulation manager for Laboratory Services, and the quality assurance/education coordinator for Laboratory Services.

The preceding laboratory representatives and the testing pharmacists developed the testing program. Electronic controls are performed each day of testing. Liquid controls are performed on each shipment of cartridges and on new lot numbers. Laboratory personnel enter testing results into the laboratory computer system. All new testing employees are evaluated for competency prior to independent patient testing, according to the laboratory competency policy. All clinics participate in a Washington State Medical Test Site/Clinical Laboratory Improvement Act of 1988 (CLIA '88) approved proficiency program. The LQA office and the director of laboratory services review all proficiency testing results. Quality assurance reports that include diagnosis distribution, patient population, percentage of INRs in and out of therapeutic range, percentage of INRs less than 1.5 or greater than 4.0 on stabilized or established patients, and reportable events are submitted to the GHC Quality Improvement Council. Copies are kept in the LQA office. A member of this group also attends the Heart Care Pathway Committee. This program has developed excellent coordination between the pharmacists and laboratory administration. The Washington State Pharmacy Board licenses these clinics.

New Point-of-Care Testing

Two other nonlaboratory sites performing testing are respiratory therapy performing blood gases and nuclear medicine performing the Schilling test. Laboratory administration evaluates all requests for new POCT, according to GHC laboratory method/equipment validation procedure. Once laboratory administration and the POCC approve the test and method, the POCC implements the program using the format described.

PERFORMANCE MONITORING

An essential part of the POCT program is preparation of the reports that are generated and issued to the appropriate persons. In addition to training reports that are sent to the managers of the appropriate units, the following reports are issued:

1. Quarterly managers report: Quarterly, each manager receives a list of all testing personnel (users) for every department for which they are responsible. The list includes the department code, the users' names, the users' unique identification codes, and the tests for which each user has been trained and certified.
2. Monthly managers/laboratory update report (Fig. 21.7): Each month, every manager and hospital laboratory point-of-care coordinator receives a report listing testing personnel who have been trained during the month by department, name, and user identification number and the tests for which they were certified.
3. Monthly manager-performance analysis report (Fig. 21.8): During the download of the glucose monitors, laboratory staff inspects each area for compliance to the program. Monthly, each manager receives a report from the hospital laboratory regarding the performance by department listing any deficiencies observed or obtained during the download process.

Cost Analysis

Group Health Cooperative is a not-for-profit managed care organization, and it is important that the point-of-care program is cost-effective. The cost of strip, reagent, and control use; training and management of the program; and time in meetings are tracked.

Proficiency and Test Validation Programs

Whole-blood Glucose, Urine Dipstick, and Rapid Strep Screen

Group Health Cooperative subscribes to a Washington State Medical Test Site/CLIA-'88-approved proficiency program for whole-blood glucose, rapid strep screen testing, and visual urine dipstick. The proficiency samples are delivered to the hospital laboratories, and a laboratory staff member takes the proficiency samples to each unit performing these tests. Results are recorded on a GHC "Proficiency Result Form" and are returned to the laboratory for submission to the proficiency program for grading. Graded results from the proficiency company are sent to the LQA office, where results are evaluated. Managers of each testing unit receive a report on the performance of all testing personnel on their units. Corrective actions are arranged with the manager and include retraining in the laboratory, as necessary.

Certification 12/2/00-12/31/00

DEPT NAME	DEPTCD	UserID	LastName	FirstName	ClassName	Date Cert.
AGENCY	*Department Code.*	*ID #*	*Name*		Color Blind Test-Negative	
					BGM-New	
					Hemoccult-New	
CEN URGENT CARE	*Department Code.*	*ID #*	*Name*		Hemoccult-New	
					BGM-New	
					Urine Testing-New	
		ID #	*Name*		BGM-Recertification	
		ID #	*Name*		BGM-Recertification	
CEN HSP-NSG-FAM BEG	*Department Code.*	*ID #*	*Name*		Color Blind Test-Negative	
					Urine Testing-New	
					BGM-Recertification	
CEN HSP-NSG-FLOAT POOL	*Department Code.*	*ID #*	*Name*		BGM-New	
					Clinitest-New	
					Color Blind Test-Negative	
					Gastroccult-New	
					Hemoccult-New	
					Urine Testing-New	
CEN HSP-NSG-SPEC NRSRY	*Department Code.*	*ID #*	*Name*		Hemoccult-New	
					BGM-Recertification	
					Clinitest-New	
					Urine Testing-New	
					Gastroccult-New	
					Color Blind Test-Negative	
					Clinitest-Recertification	
					BGM-Recertification	
					Hemoccult-Recertification	
					Urine Testing-Recertification	
ES HSP-NSG-PEDS	*Department Code.*	*ID #*	*Name*		Hemoccult-New	
					Urine Testing-New	
					Color Blind Test-Negative	
					BGM-New	
					Clinitest-New	
ES HSP-NSG-PEDS	*Department Code.*	*ID #*	*Name*		BGM-New	

FIGURE 21.7. Point-of-care certification report: Laboratory managers receive this report monthly.

PARAMETER MEASURED (EXAMPLE ONLY)	1/1-1/31 2000	2/1-2/28 2000	3/1/-3/31 2000	4/1-4/30 2000	5/1-5/31 2000	6/1-6/30 2000	7/1-7/31 2000	8/1-8/31 2000	9/1-9/30 2000	10/1-10/31 2000	11/1-11/30 2000	12/1-21/31 2000	1/1-1/31 2001
Operator ID present and authorized	90%	98%	90%	94%	91%	99%	97%	100%	98%	99%	100%	96%	100%
Patient Medical History Number Present	98%	98%	99%	96%	88%	99%	100%	98%	100%	100%	99%	100%	100%
Comment code inappropriate or missing for patient	2	5	4	48	65	10	1	13	0	7	10	5	0
Lab confirmation requested on out of range patients	0	1	4	4	2	2	38	2	3	5	2	4	1
Control comment code inappropriate or missing	7	2	4	10	1	5	5	0	2	9	4	1	0
All strip vials have lid on tightly when not in use	Yes	Yes	Yes	5-Yes 1-No	Yes	Yes	Yes	Yes	Yes	4-Yes 1-No	Yes	Yes	Yes
All strip vials within expiration date	Yes	Yes	Yes	Yes	Yes	Yes	Yes	Yes	Yes	4-Yes 1-No	Yes	Yes	Yes
All control vials within expiration date (Non-dated or expired vials discarded)	3 of 5	5 of 5	Yes	Yes	5-Yes 3-No	4-Yes 1-No	Yes	Yes	4-Yes 1-No	Yes	Yes	4-Yes 1-No	Yes
All control vials dated when opened	4 of 5	2 of 5	Yes	5-Yes 1-No	5-Yes 3-No	Yes	Yes	Yes	4-Yes 2-No	4-Yes 1-No	2-Yes 3-No	4-Yes 1-No	3-Yes 3-No
GTS & monitor clean	Yes	Yes	Yes	Yes	6-Yes 2-No	4-Yes 1-No	Yes	Yes	Yes	Yes	Yes	4-Yes 3-No	Yes
Total # of patients run	214	134	250	235	293	277	231	210	270	182	268	241	215
Total # of QC run	267	211	215	223	235	268	195	174	184	140	182	158	222
Total tests run	481	345	465	458	528	545	426	384	454	322	450	399	450

FIGURE 21.8. Monthly unit report forms: Reports prepared by the quality assurance of the Laboratory Services office and submitted to unit managers as indicators of performance.

Stool Occult Blood Test Validation

The laboratory staff prepares a mixture of bananas or peanut butter and blood that has tested negative for human immunodeficiency virus (HIV) and hepatitis to simulate a stool sample. When the laboratory staff delivers the proficiency samples for glucose or urine dipstick in a hospital setting, they also take the fake stool mixture for stool occult blood testing by the unit testing personnel. Results are recorded on the proficiency result form.

Twice per year in all nonhospital sites where stool occult blood testing is performed, an unknown occult blood sample is sent to the testing personnel on an individual basis for testing. The sample is prepared and distributed by the (LQA) department using the fake stool sample described above. The "Lab Test Worksheet" (see Fig. 21.5), which includes performance control monitor results, lot numbers, and expiration dates of the cards and developer, is returned to the LQA office and evaluated. An acceptable or unacceptable score is returned to the testing personnel. Another set of unknowns is sent to those with unacceptable results. If this sample is also unacceptable, the LQA office arranges retraining of the staff member.

Provider-Performed Microscopic Procedures

Twice a year, the LQA Department prepares a "PPMP Test Validation Unknown Sheet" with photographs to be identified. A sheet is sent to each individual employee, including physicians and laboratory staff, who perform urine microscopic examination, wet preps, fern tests, nasal smears for eosinophils, pinworm preps, fern tests, sperm morphology, and post vas sperm checks. Results are returned to the LQA department, where they are evaluated and documented into the database. Graded results are returned to the individual staff member. If there are errors, continuing education material appropriate to the errors and to the correct answers are sent to the testing individual. If an employee has an error in three or more of four sets, he or she is notified of an unsatisfactory performance, and notification is also sent to his/her manager or chief of staff.

COMPETENCY EVALUATION

Competency evaluation is part of the POCT recertification program. Annual recertification with demonstration of specimen collection by all testing personnel allows one-on-one evaluation and retraining with a trainer, if necessary. Managers also consider the performance of proficiency samples and controls when evaluating the competency of testing personnel.

CONCLUSIONS

Point-of-care testing is a fundamental part of the GHC patient care program. The foundation of the GHC POCT program is the POCC. All POCT proposed must be submitted to the POCC for approval. Without the input of members of the committee and the authority they possess to design, implement, monitor, and redesign the program, it would not be successful. The program is ongoing and is in constant development. It is a tremendous amount of work to design, implement, and monitor this program; however, it is the consensus of the committee that the program is a good example of how disciplines can work together for better patient care. Each member of the committee now has more knowledge of and respect for the work performed by each other. This promotes closer working relationships and benefits patient care.

SUGGESTED READINGS

Belsey R, Baer D. Protocols for bedside testing. *Medical Laboratory Observer* 1988; 63–72.

Point-of-care testing. *Medical Laboratory Observer* 1992;24(Special Suppl): 1–41.

Ingram-Main R, Kiechle FL. Implementing a successful bedside glucose program. *Medical Laboratory Observer* 1993;25:25–28.

Kiechle FL, Ingram-Main R. Bedside testing: beyond glucose. *Medical Laboratory Observer* 1993;25:65–68.

Point-of-care testing. *Medical Laboratory Observer* 1993;25(Suppl):2–47.

Measuring the cost savings of point-of-care testing. *Medical Laboratory Observer* 1996;27(Suppl 9):2–18.

College of American Pathologists (CAP). *Standards on decentralized lab testing.* Approved, Joint Commission Accreditation. Northfield, IL: Commission on Laboratory Accreditation, 1988:2.

Roby PV, Kenny MA, Garza D. The laboratory outside the laboratory: our role in point-of-care testing. *Clin Lab Sci* 1993;6:222–230.

Hendricks C. POL dipstick testing. *Advance* 1997;9:12:6–7.

Kost GJ. Point-of-care testing in intensive care and planning and implementing point-of-care testing systems. In: Tobin MJ, ed. *Principles and practice of intensive care monitoring.* New York: McGraw-Hill, 1998: 1267–1297,1297–1328.

Price CP, Hicks JM. *Point-of-care testing,* USA. AACC Press, 1999.

22

PATIENT SELF-TESTING AND PATIENT SELF-MANAGEMENT OF ORAL ANTICOAGULATION WITH POINT-OF-CARE TESTING

JACK E. ANSELL

PROBLEMS WITH THE CURRENT MANAGEMENT OF ORAL ANTICOAGULATION

For over 50 years, oral anticoagulation with warfarin sodium has proven to be an effective and useful therapy for patients at risk for thromboembolism (1). Unfortunately, many physicians are reluctant to treat patients with an anticoagulant due to its high risk/benefit profile (2,3). Many factors contribute to this high risk/benefit ratio. Oral anticoagulants have a narrow therapeutic index, and response varies with individuals and time (4); they therefore require fastidious monitoring. Problems with laboratory monitoring include the lack of a standardized thromboplastin resulting in a prothrombin time (PT) that is not standardized from one laboratory to another even with the use of the international normalized ratio (INR) for results reporting (5). The logistics of communications from the laboratory to the physician to the patient are often time consuming and may be flawed. Prescribing doctors must be aware of the risk factors associated with adverse events, willing to educate patients, and able to take the time required to manage patients properly. These and other deterrents have led to the widespread underuse of a drug that, when used and managed more effectively, could spare many patients the adverse events associated with thromboembolic disease or its treatment, and reduce healthcare costs enormously.

Over the last decade, developments have occurred that do effectively lower the risk/benefit profile. Standardization of the PT using the INR has been one important advance (6). Data from the College of American Pathologists' Comprehensive Coagulation Survey shows that 97.3% of participants in the United States were utilizing the INR in 1997 compared to only 21.1% in 1991 (7). Another development is the growing reliance on anticoagulation clinics to manage therapy (8). The focused and coordinated care these clinics provide facilitates the monitoring process for the physician and maximizes the potential for therapeutic effectiveness (9). Studies of the effectiveness of these anticoagulation clinics indicate that patients actually spend more time in the desired therapeutic range and have a 50% to 75% reduction in adverse events compared to those patients monitored by their physicians (8–10).

The third advancement in anticoagulation management is the advent of new point-of-care (POC) PT monitoring technologies that allow for capillary whole-blood testing, and are small, lightweight, portable, and ultimately designed for home use (8). The following discussion reviews the development of capillary whole-blood PT monitoring focusing on the technology, the accuracy and precision of instrumentation, and innovative strategies to improve the efficacy and safety of oral anticoagulation.

INSTRUMENTATION

Technical Aspects of Instrument Operation

There are currently four different portable PT monitors approved for POC diagnostic testing that have the potential for patient self-testing at home; three of these are currently approved for home use in the United States (Table 22.1). Each of these monitors measures the time to clotting, induced by thromboplastin, which is then converted to a plasma PT equivalent by a microprocessor and expressed as a PT or INR (11). Other POC PT instruments are available, but are intended for professional use in the office or hospital, are not adaptable for home use, and are not discussed in this chapter.

The first group of monitors includes the original Protime Monitor 1000® (Biotrack) and its subsequent versions, the Coumatrak® (DuPont), the Ciba Corning 512 Coagulation Monitor® (Ciba Corning Diagnostics), the CoaguChek Plus®, and the CoaguChek Pro/DM® (Roche Diagnostics). These instruments are derived from a common prototype developed by Biotrack, and have been marketed under different names and licensing rights. Earlier models were intended for home use, but later models have added capabilities and are intended for professional use only. Each monitor functions according to the same methodology. A microsample of fresh whole blood (approximately 25 μl) is drawn by capillary action into a reagent chamber within a cuvette inserted in the instrument, where it mixes with dry rabbit-brain thromboplastin (international sensitivity index [ISI] approximately 2.0) to initiate coagulation.

TABLE 22.1. CAPILLARY WHOLE-BLOOD (POINT-OF-CARE) PROTHROMBIN TIME INSTRUMENTS

Instrument	Clot Detection Methodology	Home Use Approval
Protime Monitor 1000 Coumatrak[a] Ciba Corning 512 Coagulation Monitor[a] CoaguChek Plus[a]	Clot initiation: thromboplastin Clot detection: cessation of blood flow through capillary channel	—
CoaguChek Thrombolytic Assessment System	Clot initiation: thromboplastin Clot detection: cessation of movement of iron particles	Yes
ProTIME Monitor	Clot initiation: thromboplastin Clot detection: cessation of blood flow through capillary channel	Yes
AvoSure	Clot initiation: thromboplastin Clot detection: thrombin generation detected by fluorescent thrombin probe	Yes

[a]All instruments are based on original Biotrack model (Protime Monitor 1000) and licensed under different names and now marketed as CoaguChek Pro or Pro/DM (more recent models with added capabilities).

Clot formation is detected by a photodetector sensing the cessation of blood flow as clotting proceeds. The optical signal is converted into an electrical signal and subsequently converted to a quantitative result shown on a liquid crystal display as the PT, PT ratio, or INR. The time from application of blood to cessation of flow is mathematically converted to a plasma-equivalent PT based on a formula derived from comparative instrument and laboratory results in preclinical studies.

A second type of PT monitor is the CoaguChek® (Roche Diagnostics). The test cartridge contains paramagnetic iron oxide particles coated with dry reagent thromboplastin (ISI approximately 2.6). A microsample of fresh whole blood (approximately 25 µl) is applied to the test strip and drawn into the reagent chamber by capillary action, where it reconstitutes the test reagents. An oscillating magnetic field in the analyzer initiates a particle wave motion that is read optically. Particle movement slows until coagulation stops the particles completely. The time from application of the blood sample to cessation of particle movement represents the time to clotting, which is measured by a microprocessor and displayed on the screen as the PT or INR, with the correlation formula having been derived in preclinical studies.

A third type of POC capillary whole-blood PT instrumentation is the ProTime Monitor® (International Technidyne). The PT determination is based on capillary whole-blood mixing with dry thromboplastin (recombinant human thromboplastin; Ortho Recomboplastin, ISI = 1.0) in a capillary channel, but this instrument differs from the previously described instruments in that it performs a PT in triplicate (three capillary channels) as well as internal level 1 and level 2 controls in two additional capillary channels (the previously described monitors both require external liquid controls). The two control channels contain normal and abnormal control material. These channels run concurrently with the PT test and identify sample collection error as well as reagent error. The PT test is run in triplicate (50

µl of capillary whole blood required) and the median value is used in calculating the plasma equivalent PT result or the INR. The end point is determined by an optical detection system (infrared LED light source and detector) and the instrument contains computer capabilities to record and compute data.

The fourth type of instrument, known as the AvoSure® PT test system (Avocet), uses a different technology for clot detection. The reagent test strips contain an ultrathin, sponge-like, asymmetric polysulfone membrane. When whole blood from a fingerstick is applied to the membrane (plasma can also be used), the red blood cells are separated from the plasma. The membrane contains thromboplastin (ISI approximately 1.5), which when hydrated by the blood sample, activates coagulation. As thrombin is generated, it comes in contact with a Rhodamine-110-based fluorescent thrombin substrate. The reaction liberates free rhodamine, an intense fluorophore, and fluorescence is monitored. The time from the initial application of the sample, detected by a resistance drop between two electrodes, to the onset of fluorescence is proportional to the PT. Preclinical studies established the mathematical correlation relationship.

Additional monitors are in preclinical testing. Two such instruments that are near FDA approval at this time include one from HemoSense, where clot detection is based on electrical impedance, and one from LifeScan.

VALIDATION OF MONITORS

The Biotrack prototype model was initially validated in 1987 by Lucas et al. (12). Using 858 samples from 732 subjects (controls and warfarin- and heparin-treated patients), the investigators found correlation coefficients of 0.96 between reference plasma PTs and capillary whole-blood PTs. Results were similar for capillary and venous whole blood measured on the instrument. Within-day precision using two different levels of controls revealed coefficients of variation of 4.9% (Level 1 control) and 2.9% (Level 2 control). Replicate capillary whole-blood PTs from two different fingersticks and two different instruments revealed a correlation coefficient of 0.99. Lastly, hematocrits from 23% to 54% did not compromise the accuracy of the instrument. Overall, the investigators found the monitor comparable to standard laboratory methods. Other studies have confirmed the accuracy of this model compared to reference laboratory methods with correlation coefficients of 0.95 and 0.91 (13,14).

Other investigators have published more qualified support of this instrument's accuracy. A study of the Ciba Corning 512 Coagulation Monitor® by Jennings et al. (15) examined 104 patients on warfarin and 20 healthy subjects with the capillary PT and compared it to two standard laboratory methods. They found the best INR correlation with the Manchester Reagent, which had a lower thromboplastin ISI, and the worst with the capillary thrombotest INR. They suggested that the relatively high ISI of the capillary instrument's thromboplastin (approximately 2.0) and an inability to determine a local geometric mean normal PT resulted in poor comparability with some thromboplastins, especially the thrombotest. McCurdy and White (16), rather than using the correlation coefficient (which measures adherence to a regression line that does not necessarily conform to X = Y), characterized the performance of the portable monitor by focusing on the differences between the monitor and reference laboratory measurements (ISIs approximately 2.4 to 2.6) in standardized units. In 143 paired specimens, they noted that the capillary method yielded the most accurate results in an INR range of 2.0 to 3.0. As the INR increased, the discrepancy between methods increased; the capillary PT was up to 0.5 units lower for INRs of 3.0 to 4.5. The best correlation was found when the INR was approximately 3.0. They also assessed precision of two repeated measurements in 54 patients and found a within-patient standard deviation of 0.23 INR units for the capillary whole-blood PT and 0.19 INR units for paired clinical laboratory measurements. Their conclusions are consistent with those of Tripodi et al. (17), who, using the 512 Coagulation Monitor, recalibrated the ISI of the instrument's thromboplastin against the secondary international reference preparation for rabbit thromboplastin to assess the precision of the INR specifically. The ISI calculated in the study was systematically higher (ISI = 2.715) than that reported by the manufacturer (ISI = 2.036). They found that the between-assay reproducibility of the monitors was acceptable when results were expressed as PT (coefficient of variation [CV] = 9.7%), but became unacceptable when results were expressed as INR (CV = 18.8%). Like McCurdy and White (16), Tripodi et al. (17) found that the monitor underestimated the result as the INR increased (INR >4.0). This error did not occur if they calculated the INR using their recalibrated ISI. The investigators concluded that the monitor might be suitable for oral anticoagulation monitoring if the manufacturers used a more sensitive thromboplastin in the cartridges.

Oberhardt et al. (18) initially described the technology of the second class of PT monitor (CoaguChek®) and its ability to measure PTs from capillary whole blood, citrated and nonanticoagulated venous whole blood, and citrated plasma. They reported a correlation coefficient of 0.96 in 271 samples of citrated plasma tested on the instrument versus standard laboratory methodology. They found no effect of hematocrit (from 0%, i.e., plasma, to 57%), or of platelet concentration, on their results. Rose et al. (19) further tested this instrument in a clinical setting. Within-day precision for normal and abnormal control plasmas in 20 tests each yielded CVs of 3.7% and 3.6%, respectively. A correlation coefficient of 0.86 was obtained from 50 outpatients (using capillary whole blood) compared to reference plasma PTs.

Fabbrini et al. (20) compared this technology to standard laboratory methods using an MLA 1000 instrument with two different thromboplastins (ISI = 2.46 and 1.01) for two groups of anticoagulated patients (*n* = 100 and 96, respectively). Using citrated blood, reasonable precision was demonstrated (CV = 6% and 4%) with excellent correlation coefficients of 0.92 and 0.91 compared to reference plasma PTs. Van den Besselaar et al. (21), in a multicenter study, found similar correlations in 359 paired results between the CoaguChek® and two reference assays (Hepato Quick, *r* = 0.888 and Thromborel™ S, *r* = 0.895).

Kapiotis et al. (22) compared CoaguChek® performance with that of the Thrombotest® on a KC-1 instrument. In 76 patients on oral anticoagulants investigators found a coefficient of correlation of 0.91 when INRs were compared from each instrument on capillary samples from the same fingerstick. On three samples each from 30 anticoagulated patients tested on three CoaguChek instruments they found coefficients of correlation between 0.98 and 0.99 (instrument 1 versus 2 and 1 versus 3). Finally, a correlation of 0.98 was measured when two lots of test strips were tested on the same instrument from capillary samples from 30 anticoagulated patients.

Lastly, Tripodi et al. (23) evaluated the calibration of the ISI in this system based on an international reference preparation. The calibrated ISIs for both whole blood and plasma determined by the investigators were extremely close to those adopted by the manufacturer, although slight differences in INRs were detected in anticoagulated patients because the manufacturer's mean normal PT was slightly lower than that determined in the study (INRs ~0.3 to 0.5 INR units lower using study calibration compared to manufacturer calibration at an INR of ~3.0). Although the CVs of the slopes of the regression lines comparing the system with an international reference were excellent (CV of 2.2 for both whole blood and plasma on the instrument compared with the international reference), the instrument reported significantly higher INRs (3.20 and 3.41 in whole blood and plasma versus 2.92 for plasma in the reference system) using the manufacturer's calibration. The differences were due to a lower mean normal PT adopted by the manufacturer.

A study by Kaatz et al. (24) evaluated both classes of monitors (CoaguChek® and Coumatrak®) as well as four clinical laboratories against the criterion standard established by the World Health Organization. The criterion standard INR was determined using an international reference thromboplastin and the manual tilt-tube technique. Determinations of INR from four laboratories (using four different thromboplastins and three different instruments) were compared to INR determinations of both monitors. Kaatz et al. (24) found that laboratories 1 and 2, which used a more sensitive thromboplastin (ISI = 1.99 and 2.0), showed close agreement with the criterion standard, whereas laboratories 3 and 4, which used an insensitive thromboplastin (ISI = 2.84 and 2.98), showed poor agreement. The two monitors fell between these two extremes. As in the study by McCurdy and White (16), the Coumatrak® underestimated the INR at values above 3.5, whereas the CoaguChek® simply showed more scatter at INR values above 2.75. INR determinations of the Coumatrak® monitor and the CoaguChek were only slightly less accurate than those of the best clinical laboratories. *The Medical Letter*'s review of the CoaguChek® and Coumatrak® in March 1995 (25) cited several studies discussed above and presents the two instruments as viable PT monitoring options.

The third instrument class or ProTime Monitor® was evaluated in a multiinstitutional trial (26), where simultaneous capillary whole-blood and venous samples from 201 warfarin-treated patients and 52 controls were compared with standard laboratory methodology at each institution as well as with a reference laboratory. The study also analyzed the ability and accuracy of patients to perform their own measurements compared to the healthcare provider. The ProTime® INR significantly correlated to the reference lab for both the healthcare provider (venous sample, r = 0.93) and the patient (capillary sample, r = 0.93). PT results for fingersticks performed by both the patient and the healthcare provider were also equivalent and correlated highly (r = 0.91).

In a separate report in children, Andrew et al. (27), reported on the instrument's accuracy and precision in 76 warfarin-treated children and 9 healthy controls. Venous and capillary whole blood tested on the instrument yielded a correlation of r = 0.89. Both results, compared to venous blood tested in a reference laboratory (ISI = 1.0), revealed correlation coefficients of 0.90 and 0.92, respectively.

The technology of the AvoSure® monitor was originally described by Zweig et al. (28) and its accuracy and precision only recently reported (29). Within-day precision was assessed by measuring 30 repeat tests each from citrated whole-blood and citrated plasma on the instrument resulting in CVs of 4.8% and 5.5%. Level 1 and level 2 controls were run daily for between-day precision producing CVs of 11.2% (n = 72) and 7.1% (n = 72) respectively. Accuracy was evaluated with capillary whole blood and citrated venous blood tested on the monitor compared to citrated plasma in the reference laboratory using an MLA Electra 800 with Innovin (ISI ~1.0). In samples from 160 patients from three medical centers, a correlation of 0.97 was noted for both capillary blood and citrated venous blood (n = 153 and 157, respectively).

CLINICAL STUDIES

Patient Self-Testing

Given the simplicity and portability of these capillary whole-blood PT monitors, it was not long before studies were conducted to determine the suitability of patient self-testing and home monitoring with an eye toward improving clinical outcomes (safety and efficacy) and patient satisfaction. There are several possible reasons why patient self-testing and patient self-management might result in better therapeutic control or outcomes. Testing at home allows not only for an increased frequency of testing, but also an improved timeliness of testing, providing the ability to test when it is needed. The use of the same instrument can provide a degree of consistency not always obtained by patients who might otherwise be tested in different laboratories from time to time. Patient self-testing might allow better management of patients who need to stop taking anticoagulants for invasive procedures. Finally, patient self-management may have a subtle impact on patient empowerment, compliance, and satisfaction that may be important elements in achieving better outcomes. To date, only a few studies summarized below (Table 22.2), have been conducted solely to address the potential of patient self-testing or self-monitoring. Additional investigations assessing the potential for patients to adjust their own dose incorporate the concept of self-testing and are discussed subsequently.

Self-testing has been evaluated primarily with regard to achieving a certain frequency of therapeutic effectiveness as measured by the PT or INR. A study by Belsey et al. (30) showed that the capillary PT instrument could be used by individuals with little laboratory experience and was subject to few operational problems. Trained technologists and nontechnically trained staff achieved comparable results with the portable monitor. White et al. (31), in a prospective randomized study, reported on a model of care where patients were given portable PT monitors at the time of hospital discharge, instructed in their use, and asked to perform their own PT test at home. Patients then reported their results to a physician who adjusted the warfarin dose. These self-monitoring patients (n = 23), compared to a control group (n = 23) who visited an anticoagulation clinic for monitoring, spent a greater percentage of the time within the therapeutic range (87% versus 68%; p<0.001) during the follow-up period.

Anderson et al. (32), in a cohort study, confirmed the feasibility and accuracy of patient self-testing at home in a group of 40 individuals who monitored their own therapy over a period of 6 to 24 months. Patients monitored their own PT every 2 weeks and periodically had a venous sample drawn within 4 hours of self-testing for a reference plasma PT. Based on either a narrow- or expanded-target therapeutic range, they observed a mean level of agreement per patient with reference plasma PTs of 83% by narrow criteria and 96% by expanded criteria. Ninety-seven percent of the patients preferred home testing to standard management.

In a larger randomized study, Byeth et al. (33) reported on 325 newly treated elderly patients, 163 of whom were managed by a single investigator based on INR results from patient self-testing at home compared to 162 managed by their private physicians based on venous sampling. Over a 6-month period, the investigators recorded a rate of major hemorrhage of 12% in the latter group versus 5.7% in the self-testing group. This finding was based on an intention-to-treat analysis. For those actually performing self-testing, there was only a 1.2% incidence of major hemorrhage.

TABLE 22.2. SUMMARY OF STUDIES ASSESSING TIME IN THERAPEUTIC RANGE OR ADVERSE EVENTS USING PATIENT SELF-TESTING OR PATIENT SELF-MANAGEMENT

Study	Study Design	Study Groups	# of Patients	Time in Major Range (% or days)	Hemorrhage (% pt-yr)	Thromboembolism (% pt-yr)	Indications
White 1989 (31)	RCT	PST	23	93	0	0	Mixed
		ACC	23	75	0	0	Mixed
Anderson 1993 (32)	Inception Cohort	PST	40	2.3	0	0	Mixed
Byeth 2000 (33)	RCT	PST	162	56	5.7	9	Mixed
		UC	163	33	12	13	Mixed
Ansell 1995 (37)	Obs	PSM	20	89	0	0	Mixed
	Matched controlled	ACC	20	68	0	0	Mixed
Bernardo 1996 (38)	Obs	PSM	216	83	NA	NA	Heart valves
Horstkotte 1996 (39)	RCT	PSM	75	92	4.5[a]	0.9	Heart valves
		UC	75	59	10.9[a]	3.6	Heart valves
Hasenkam 1997 (40)	Obs	PSM	20	77	NA	NA	Heart valves
	Matched controlled	UC	20	53	NA	NA	Heart valves
Sawicki 1999 (41)	RCT	PSM	90	57 / 53[b]	2.2	2.2	Mixed
		UC	89	34 / 43[b]	2.2	4.5	Mixed
Watzke 2000 (42)	Prospective	PSM	49	86	4[c]	0	Mixed
	Controlled	ACC	53	80	0	0	Mixed
Cromheecke 2000 (43)	Randomized	PSM	50	55	0	0	Mixed
	Controlled cross-over	ACC	50	49	0	16	Mixed

[a]Major and minor bleeding.
[b]Time in range at 3 months and 6 months.
[c]Percent of episodes in 49 patients.
RCT, randomized controlled trial; Obs, observational; PST, patient self-testing; PSM, patient self-management;
ACC, anticoagulation clinic; UC, usual care; Mixed, mixed indications.

Patient Self-Management

Patient self-management is the logical endpoint for the clinical use of these POC instruments and a small handful of studies have demonstrated the potential for this model of care. Over 25 years ago, Erdman et al. (34) published the first study of the potential role patients could play in facilitating the management of anticoagulants by adjusting their own dose. Two hundred patients with prosthetic heart valves managed their own therapy based on a personalized guidance table indicating the correct dose for that patient given a particular PT result. PTs were performed in the usual manner with a venous sample in a central laboratory. Investigators found that of patients managed before the introduction of this study, 71% were satisfactorily anticoagulated at any given time, while 98% of patients participating in the study were satisfactorily anticoagulated.

Schachner et al. (35) continued and updated the study of Erdman et al. (34). Comparison of 59 patients in the self-managed group and 60 in the physician-managed group demonstrated that patients in the self-managed group were more likely to have a therapeutic PT (0.53 PTs per patient out of range versus 2.9 PTs per patient out of range). Self-managed patients also experienced fewer embolic episodes (1.1% per patient-year versus 4.7% per patient-year; $p<0.0005$) and fewer bleeding episodes (5.7% per patient-year versus 7.5% per patient-year; $p<0.05$) than physician-managed patients.

Ansell et al. (36,37), in a case-controlled retrospective study, recently analyzed the results of patient self-management with the Biotrack® instrument in a cohort of 20 patients ranging in age from 3 to 87 years with diverse indications for anticoagula-

tion over a span of 7 years. These patients (or their caretakers) performed their own PT test at home and adjusted their own warfarin dose based on physician guidelines. Results were compared to an age-, sex-, and diagnosis-matched control group managed by an anticoagulation clinic. Self-managed patients were found to be in therapeutic range for 88.6% of the PT determinations versus 68% for the controls ($p<0.001$). There were also fewer dose changes for study patients (10.7%) than for controls (28.2%; $p<0.001$), while complications rates did not differ between the groups. Patient satisfaction was extremely high with this mode of therapy based on a patient survey of attitudes.

Bernardo (38) has published similar experience from her work in Germany where patient self-management is widespread. In 216 self-monitored and self-managed patients between 1986 and 1992, 83.1% of the PT results were within the target therapeutic range, and no serious adverse events occurred. In a randomly selected subgroup of 92 self-managed patients compared to a retrospective comparison of 317 patients managed by traditional means (118 patient-years versus 374 patient-years), investigators found fewer hemorrhagic events (3.38% versus 4.38%) and fewer embolic events.

Horstkotte et al. (39) published in abstract form the outcome from a randomized prospective study of 150 patients with prosthetic heart valves who managed their own therapy ($n = 75$) compared to a control group ($n = 75$) who were managed by their private physicians. The self-managed patients tested themselves approximately every 4 days and achieved a 92% degree of satisfactory anticoagulation as determined by the INR. The physician-managed patients were tested approximately every 19 days and only 59% of INRs were in therapeutic range. These individuals experienced an 11% incidence of any type of bleeding and a 3.6% rate of thromboembolism ($p<0.001$ between the two groups). Hasenkam et al. (40) confirmed the effectiveness of self-management in 20 patients with prosthetic valves, reporting that these patients were in the therapeutic range 77% of the time compared to 53% of the time for 20 retrospectively matched control patients.

Most recently, Sawicki et al. (41) reported on patients randomized between self-management ($n = 90$) and management by their personal physicians ($n = 89$). As an outcome measure, they compared the distribution of INRs from the midpoint of each patient's therapeutic range at 3 months and 6 months (cross-section of the files method) compared to baseline. Patients in the self-managed group were significantly closer to their target INR and had a greater percentage of values within therapeutic range at 3 months (57% versus 34% within range), while the differences were not significant at 6 months, although the study design may have accounted for the improvement in the control group at 6 months. Based on a survey of patient preferences, general treatment satisfaction and daily hassle scores improved in the self-management group and remained unchanged in the routine care group. Watzke et al. (42) also compared weekly INR patient self-management in 49 patients with management by an anticoagulation clinic in 53 patients. The self-management group was within therapeutic range a greater percentage of time and had a significantly smaller mean deviation from the target INR. Lastly, Cromheecke et al. (43) conducted a randomized cross-over study with 50 patients managed by an anticoagulation clinic or by self-management. Although the differences did not achieve statistical significance, there was a trend toward greater time in therapeutic range in the self-management group (55% versus 49%).

None of these patient self-management studies were adequately designed to answer the important questions of what might account for better therapeutic control and whether such management is better than the gold standard of anticoagulation clinic management. The major variables not adequately controlled include the levels of patient education, the subtle impact on compliance, the frequency of monitoring, and the consistency of reagent and instrumentation. Further studies are needed to define the importance of these parameters.

PATIENT SELECTION AND EDUCATION FOR PATIENT SELF-TESTING

Patient education in the use of capillary whole-blood monitors should begin with the identification of good candidates who are able or willing to perform the test and keep the necessary records to ensure safe and accurate monitoring. The important consideration in the identification of a good candidate is incentive. Incentives differ among patients and often depend on their individual circumstances. Less-frequent clinic visits, particularly for patients who have difficulty reaching the clinic, might be sufficient incentive to learn the information. Patients who have an aversion to phlebotomy or who have poor venous access might appreciate the ease in obtaining results from a fingerstick. Some

patients will be grateful for the opportunity to learn about their conditions and to take an active role in their treatments. Patients at increased risk for hemorrhage, or individuals whose PT seems to fluctuate widely for a variety of reasons, might welcome the opportunity for more frequent (and less invasive) monitoring. For some patients, the recommendation of self-testing by a trusted physician will suffice. Other important considerations in the identification of good candidates are adequate motor skills to perform the test; sufficient mentation and memory; sufficient reading and writing capabilities; and adequate eyesight, with or without glasses, to see the screen. For some patients who lack these abilities, at-home caregivers might be willing to take the responsibility for monitoring.

Patients must also be educated about anticoagulation so that they understand what they are being asked to do and why, and they must be trained in the use of the monitor. Ensuring that patients have the skills and information required for correct use of the PT monitor involves a different yet complementary approach than that required for teaching about anticoagulation. The challenge for the healthcare provider is to convey the necessary information to the patient and train the patient in the use of the monitor without conveying excessive or superfluous information. Trainers should simplify the process as much as possible and provide backup written instructions. Instructions for performing the actual test should be written in short, clear sentences or phrases, and the test print should be large and clear.

When instructing patients in the actual use of the instrument, the trainer must remember that the majority of patients may not be able to program a VCR or coffee machine and perhaps are uncomfortable with computers. Consequently, they might be intimidated by the apparent complexity of the monitoring device and accompanying materials. The transition from clinic to home testing can be facilitated if patients have been monitored in a clinic that uses the capillary whole-blood monitor.

Once patients have performed the test, they must record their results. Large, clearly marked spaces should be provided for writing the results. Often, a printed calendar to use both as a testing schedule and a place for recording results is helpful. The trainer must discuss the following points with each patient and verify that the patient understands the instructions before leaving the clinic: the days the patient will perform the test; where the patient writes down the results, preferably in an easily accessible place for the patient to refer again (e.g., on the calendar); time of day when it is most convenient for the patient to perform the test; what the patient must do to plan the test at that time and how the trainer can help with the plan; where in the house it will be most convenient to perform the test; and how the patient pictures the process running smoothly in the home and how the trainer can help in clarifying the picture.

Follow-up visits should be scheduled and recorded on the calendar. More than one visit might be necessary to train a patient in all aspects of home testing. Patients should know whom to call when they have problems and should have that individual's telephone number. Ideally, this would be the same person to call for a medical problem, such as bruising, or to make appointments.

Finally, the trainer must give patients the opportunity to express concerns and ask questions. Many patients look forward to interacting with a healthcare provider, especially one whom they know, and they should be assured that the trainer will be available for them. It is also important for the trainer to reinforce the incentive identified by each patient and the trainer at the beginning of the session.

CONCLUSIONS

Although POC PT testing has been available for professionals for over 12 years, the potential for patient self-testing and patient self-management is only now being realized. This technology offers the possibility of an increased frequency of testing that is unlikely to be achievable with standard care, a consistency of instrumentation and reagents that may reduce the variability of results, and a model of care that truly invests patients in their own management leading to greater satisfaction and compliance. Large randomized studies are just beginning to emerge to document these outcomes and to examine the cost effectiveness of this approach to the management of oral anticoagulation.

REFERENCES

1. Ansell J. Oral anticoagulant therapy: fifty years later. *Arch Intern Med* 1993;153:586–596.
2. Kutner M, Nixon G, Silverstone F. Physicians' attitudes toward oral anticoagulants and antiplatelet agents for stroke prevention in elderly patients with atrial fibrillation. *Arch Intern Med* 1991;151:1950–1953.
3. McCrory DC, Matchar DB, Samsa G, et al. Physician attitudes about anticoagulation for nonvalvular atrial fibrillation in the elderly. *Arch Intern Med* 1995;155:277–281.
4. Cannegieter SC, Rosendaal FR, Wintzen AR, et al. Optimal oral anticoagulant therapy in patients with mechanical heart valves. *N Engl J Med* 1995;33:11–17.
5. Fairweather RB, Ansell J, van den Besselaar AMHP, et al. College of American Pathologists Conference XXXI on Laboratory Monitoring of Anticoagulant Therapy. Laboratory monitoring of oral anticoagulant therapy. *Arch Pathol Lab Med* 1998;122:768–781.
6. Kirkwood TBL. Calibration of reference thromboplastins and standardization of the prothrombin time ratio. *Thromb Haemost* 1983;49:238–244.
7. College of American Pathologists. *Coagulation survey set 1997.* Doc. CG2-C. Northfield, IL: College of American Pathologists, 1997.
8. Ansell JE, Hughes R. Evolving models of warfarin management: anticoagulation clinics, patient self-monitoring and patient self-management. *Am Heart J* 1996;132:1095–1100.
9. Ansell JE, Buttaro ML, Voltis-Thomas O, et al. Consensus guidelines for coordinated outpatient oral anticoagulation therapy management. *Ann Pharmacother* 1997;31:604–615.
10. Hirsh J, Dalen JE, Anderson D, et al. Oral anticoagulants: mechanism of action, clinical effectiveness, and optimal therapeutic range. *Chest* 1998;114:445S–469S.
11. Leaning KE, Ansell JE. Advances in the monitoring of oral anticoagulation: point-of-care testing, patient self-monitoring, and patient self-management. *J Thrombo Thrombolysis* 1996;3:377–383.
12. Lucas FV, Duncan A, Jay R, et al. A novel whole blood capillary technique for measuring prothrombin time. *Am J Clin Pathol* 1987;88:442–446.
13. Yano Y, Kambayashi J, Murata K, et al. Bedside monitoring of warfarin therapy by a whole blood capillary coagulation monitor. *Thromb Res* 1992;66:583–590.
14. Weibert RT, Adler DS. Evaluation of a capillary whole blood prothrombin time measurement system. *Clin Pharm* 1989;8:864–867.
15. Jennings I, Luddington RJ, Baglin T. Evaluation of the Ciba Corning Biotrack 512 coagulation monitor for the control of oral anticoagulation. *J Clin Pathol* 1991;44:950–953.
16. McCurdy SA, White RH. Accuracy and precision of a portable anticoagulation monitor in a clinical setting. *Arch Intern Med* 1992:152:589–592.
17. Tripodi A, Arbini AA, Chantarangkul V, et al. Are capillary whole blood coagulation monitors suitable for the control of oral anticoagulant treatment by the international normalized ratio? *Thrombo Haemost* 1993;70:921–924.
18. Oberhardt BJ, Dermott SC, Taylor M, et al. Dry reagent technology for rapid, convenient measurements of blood coagulation and fibrinolysis. *Clin Chem* 1991;37:520–526.
19. Rose VL, Dermott SC, Murray BF, et al. Decentralized testing for prothrombin time and activated partial thromboplastin time using a dry chemistry portable analyzer. *Arch Pathol Lab Med* 1993;117:611–617.
20. Fabbrini N, Messmore H, Balbale S, et al. Pilot study to determine use of a TAS analyzer in an anticoagulation clinic setting. *Blood* 1995;86 [Suppl 1]:869a(abst).
21. van den Besselaar AMHP, Breddin K, Lutze G, et al. Multicenter evaluation of a new capillary blood prothrombin time monitoring system. *Blood Coag Fibrinolysis* 1995;6:726–732.
22. Kapiotis S, Puehenberger P, Speiser W. Evaluation of the new method CoaguChek for the determination of prothrombin time from capillary blood: comparison with Thrombotest on KC-1. *Thromb Res* 1995;77:563–567.
23. Tripodi A, Chantarangkul V, Clerici M, et al. Determination of the international sensitivity index of a new near-patient testing device to monitor oral anticoagulant therapy. *Thromb Haemost* 1997;78:855–858.
24. Kaatz AA, White RH, Hill J, et al. Accuracy of laboratory and portable monitor International Normalized Ratio determinations. *Arch Intern Med* 1995;155:1861–1867.
25. The Medical Letter. Portable prothrombin time monitors. *The Medical Letter* 1995;37:24–25.
26. Ansell J, Becker D, Andrew M, et al. Accurate and precise prothrombin time measurement in a multicenter anticoagulation trial employing patient self-testing. *Blood* 1995;86[Suppl 1]:864a(abst).
27. Andrew M, Marzinotto V, Adams M, et al. Monitoring of oral anticoagulant therapy in pediatric patients using a new microsample PT device. *Blood* 1995;86[Suppl 1]:863a(abst).
28. Zweig SE, Meyer BG, Sharma S, et al. Membrane-based, dry-reagent prothrombin time tests. *Biomed Instrumentation Technol* 1996;30:245–256.
29. Ansell JE, Zweig S, Meyer B, et al. Performance of the Avocet$_{PT}$ prothrombin time system. *Blood* 1998;92[Suppl 1]:112b(abst).
30. Belsey RE, Fischer PM, Baer DM. An evaluation of a whole blood prothrombin analyzer designed for use by individuals without formal laboratory training. *J Fam Pract* 1991;33:266–271.
31. White RH, McCurdy SA, von Marensdorff H, et al. Home prothrombin time monitoring after initiation of warfarin therapy. *Ann Intern Med* 1989;111:730–737.
32. Anderson D, Harrison L, Hirsh J. Evaluation of a portable prothrombin time monitor for home use by patients who require long-term oral anticoagulant therapy. *Arch Intern Med* 1993;153:1441–1447.
33. Byeth RJ, Quinn L, Landefeld CS. A multicomponent intervention to prevent major bleeding complications in older patients receiving warfarin: a randomized controlled trial. *Ann Intern Med* 2000;133:687–695.
34. Erdman S, Vidne B, Levy MJ. A self-control method for long-term anticoagulation therapy. *J Cardiovasc Surg* 1974;15:454–457.
35. Schachner A, Deviri E, Shabat S. Patient-regulated anticoagulation. In: Butchart EG, Bodnar E, eds. *Thrombosis, embolism, and bleeding.* London: ICR Publishers, 1992:318–324.
36. Ansell J, Holden A, Knapic N. Patient self-management of oral anticoagulation guided by capillary (fingerstick) whole blood prothrombin times. *Arch Intern Med* 1989;149:2509–2511.
37. Ansell J, Patel N, Ostrovsky D, et al. Long-term patient self-management of oral anticoagulation. *Arch Intern Med* 1995;155:2185–2189.

38. Bernardo A. Experience with patient self-management of oral anticoagulation. *J Thromb Thrombolysis* 1996;2:321–325.
39. Horstkotte D, Piper C, Wiemer M, et al. Improvement of prognosis by home prothrombin estimation in patients with life-long anticoagulant therapy. *Eur Heart J* 1996;17[Suppl]:230.
40. Hasenkam JM, Kimose II, Knudsen L, et al. Self-management of oral anticoagulant therapy after heart valve replacement. *Eur J Cardiothorac Surg* 1997;11:935–942.
41. Sawicki PT. A structured teaching and self-management program for patients receiving oral anticoagulation: a randomized controlled trial. *JAMA* 1999;281:145–150.
42. Watzke HH, Forberg E, Svolba G, et al. A prospective controlled trial comparing weekly self-testing and self-dosing with the standard management of patients on stable oral anticoagulation. *Thromb Haemost* 2000;83:661–665.
43. Cromheecke ME, Levi M, Colly LP, et al. Oral anticoagulation self-management and management by a specialist anticoagulation clinic: a randomized cross-over comparison. *Lancet* 2000;356:97–102.

23

HOME-BASED POINT-OF-CARE TESTING

SHEILA G. DUNN
MICHAEL R. VISNICH

Consumers can now perform tests ranging from simple urine dip-strip tests to relatively sophisticated instrument-based pro-thrombin time (PT) assays in the privacy of their own homes. In most instances, consumers report test results to their healthcare provider, but in some cases, notably diabetes, patients actually self-manage their condition. In either case, home-based tests can provide clinicians with valuable information, reduce complications and costs associated with chronic disease state management, and improve patient outcomes.

Home-based testing is perhaps the least understood and most frequently maligned segment of point-of-care testing. This is primarily attributable to the fact that home-based testing is virtually unregulated and the most difficult for laboratory professionals to control. Other valid concerns involve the quality, reliability, and liability surrounding self-testing.

The objective of this chapter is to augment current information, albeit scarce, about home-based testing. Hopefully, interested readers will take appropriate steps to gain experience with patient self-testing programs and substantiate the clinical and economic benefits of home-based testing presented in this chapter.

First, the dramatic growth of patient self-testing, its indications, and its many forms are discussed. Patient self-testing and self-management are highlighted with particular emphasis on glucose and PT testing and their accuracy compared to traditional laboratory methods. Key components of a home-based testing program are discussed including needs and cost analyses, a patient training program, and a results-reporting system. Communications and informatics are discussed toward the end of the chapter. These are the key ingredients that will facilitate the expansion and acceptance of home-based testing into mainstream medicine. Finally, the future of home-based testing is forecasted.

THE HOME-TESTING REVOLUTION

Proponents of the home-testing movement proclaim it as the way of the future, a paradigm shift that will reduce unnecessary testing, provide timely measurement of test values, and reduce mistakes. Opponents from the laboratory industry are mostly concerned with accuracy or turf issues, whereas most concerned parties are proceeding with caution. Is home testing simply another blip on the radar screen or can it truly change for the better the way we practice medicine? As for any market segment in its infancy, there are no simple answers.

HOME TESTING: A GROWING SEGMENT OF THE LABORATORY MARKET

Gone are the days when a thermometer was the only medical diagnostic device in the home. Consumers are increasingly turning to technologically sophisticated healthcare products that can be used privately and conveniently in their homes. In the last 15 years, there has been an explosion of home diagnostic tests on the market allowing consumers to test for pregnancy, blood pressure, glucose, cholesterol, cancer, and HIV. Table 23-1 lists the types of laboratory tests available today for home use.

The concept of patients, their families, or a caretaker performing certain diagnostic tests in the home is not new. The simple act of taking one's temperature is a type of diagnostic test. Currently, most home testing consists of blood glucose monitoring, which is performed by about 8.5 million Americans.

The use of home-testing devices will continue to increase because of rising consumer expectations, managed care and Medicare payment limitations, and the fact that patients are taking more responsibility for their health. Television advertising by pharmaceutical companies has presented consumers with information about improving their health through medications, and consumers have mounted a tremendous response to these ads. Patients are empowered to ask their physician to prescribe a medication or to go to the pharmacy and buy ones that are available over the counter. The future will certainly bring more "direct-to-consumer" advertising for home-testing products.

In the pipeline are heart attack monitors, ulcer and gastritis tests, and sexually transmitted disease tests, among others. As technology continues to advance, more sophisticated testing will be developed for home use.

According to a 1998 strategic market engineering study by Frost & Sullivan, *U.S. Home Diagnostics and Monitoring Device Markets*, the most significant areas for growth in the home diagnostics market will be in the home blood-glucose monitoring and drugs-of-abuse device markets. This study

TABLE 23.1. HOME TESTS[a]

Analyte/Test	Device/Specimen	Indication/Comments
Alcohol	Breath	Two-minute test determines capacity to drive. Detects to 0.08% alcohol.
Body fat	Bioimpedance monitor	Test determines percent body fat.
Blood, occult	Kit/stool	Widely used in both professional and consumer market. Expected to grow to $43 million in 2002.
Blood pressure monitoring	Instrument with digital display	Screening for hypertension. Eliminates white-coat hypertension. Mature professional and consumer market predicted to grow by 5% annually to $244 million in 2002.
Cholesterol	Card type test kits/whole blood	Screens for hypercholesterolemia. Available over the counter. Expected revenues of $127 million by 2002.
Drugs of abuse: cocaine, marijuana, opiates, amphetamines, and phencyclidine (PCP), methamphetamine.	Kit/urine	Test performed at home in 10 minutes. Requires referral for confirmation of positive results.
Ear infection	Tympanometer	Product for OTC use comes with picture training manual.
Fructosamine	Instrument/whole blood	Used to evaluate diabetes control over 2–3 weeks.
Glucose	Dip strip/urine	Intended to screen for diabetes.
Glucose	Instrument/whole blood	8.5 million diabetics regularly monitor glucose levels.
Glycosylated hemoglobin	Instrument/whole blood	Used to evaluate diabetes control over the last month.
Heart rate, pulse, oxygen use	Instrument	Measures fitness indicators (heart rate, oxygen use, caloric expenditure, and duration of exercise) for cardiac patients.
Human chorionic gonadotropin (hCG)	Kit/urine	Introduced in 1977, home pregnancy tests account for 23% of the home diagnostics market.
Human immunodeficiency virus (HIV)	Blood	Screens for HIV infection. Collection kits only in USA but patient self-screening is performed in numerous other countries.
Ketones	Dip strip/urine	Used by diabetics and, for some, to monitor ketones during weight-loss programs.
Leutinizing hormone (LH)	Kit/urine	Predicts ovulation.
Lung function	Peak flow meter	Performed at home by asthmatics.
Lung function	Spirometer	Usually performed/supervised by home health personnel due to the expense of the instrument.
Protein	Dip strip/urine	Useful for diabetics and renal patients.
Prothrombin time (PT)	Instrument/whole blood	Used by patients taking anticoagulant therapy.
Temperature	Glass bulb, electronic and tympanic thermometry	Detects fever. The first home-based test.
Urinary tract infections (leukocyte esterase and nitrite)	Dip strip/urine	Detects the main causes of urinary tract infections, including *Escherichia coli*.
Urine chemistry tests	Dip strip/urine	Detects bilirubin, glucose, ketones, pH, protein, and urobilinogen.

[a]Self-tests that consist mainly of patient education materials, such as vision-screening charts and skin-growth monitoring systems are not included in this table.

deals strictly with the over-the-counter (OTC) portion of the home-testing market but does not take into account the emerging prescription-only segment. This other segment encompasses some diabetes products as well as products that test the effectiveness of anticoagulation therapy. More prescription-only tests will surely follow.

In 1998, the total U.S. home diagnostics and monitoring device market, which includes those available to consumers OTC in retail outlets, was valued at approximately $1.9 billion. It is expected to double to $4 billion in the next 4 years.

Many factors are fueling the explosive growth of home testing. The way Americans view and receive health care has changed dramatically in the last several years. Consumers today are becoming aware of the need to participate in the management of their own health and to stay fit. Moreover, consumers are barraged with a variety of healthcare information not formerly available to the general public. Those with access to the Internet can find information about diagnosing and treating a variety of illnesses. Dubbed "cyberchondriacs,"

these informed Americans may treat their healthcare concerns without ever seeing a doctor.

The second major reason for the growth of home testing is technological advances in diagnostic test kits and instruments. The rapid pace of technology developments allows faster, easier, more accurate, and less expensive products to diagnose and monitor a variety of conditions.

Third, patients are being released from acute care settings much sooner than in previous years, due to the demands of third-party payers. These patients tend to need the services of home healthcare providers and close monitoring of their conditions via various types of testing. Some of this testing is performed in the home by a healthcare professional, whereas some becomes the responsibility of the patient or concerned family members.

Finally, a large aging population, the "baby boomers," has become more involved in managing their own health than in any previous generation. Medicare reimbursement limitations may prohibit physicians from performing the tests in their office, so an empowered senior citizen may opt to test at home.

Indications for Home Testing

Home testing is particularly suited to a variety of situations:

- Patients who must take warfarin (Coumadin) or heparin therapy and need to have appropriate drug levels established, or are in one of the following categories: high risk; newly anti-coagulated with unstable drug levels; and those who are taking warfarin for a limited amount of time, such as a few weeks of prophylaxis following hospital discharge for orthopedic surgery.
- Patients starting or stopping a drug that interferes with anti-coagulation therapy.
- Patients with a high-risk condition that requires frequent monitoring.
- Patients with poor venous access. Point-of-care testing that uses whole-blood fingerstick, urine, or saliva samples is more comfortable for these patients.
- Patients who do not have easy access to laboratory services and require frequent testing. Many seniors relocate to warmer climates in the winter months or travel extensively and find home testing quite convenient for their mobile lifestyle.
- Patients who meet one or more of the above requirements and are capable of performing a test themselves and can afford the cost to purchase and perform these tests.

Factors that Motivate Patients to Perform Testing

One important motivator for potential home testers to proceed is the perceived medical urgency of the test. Patients who believe that self-testing will eliminate negative consequences of unreliable test results are motivated to self-test based on medical urgency. A good example is the insulin-dependent diabetic who has experienced the negative impact of unstable, out-of-control glucose levels, or a patient taking warfarin who does not get his or her prescribed PT test and experiences a complication that requires hospitalization. In these examples, patients were motivated to self-test out of fear of poor health outcomes.

Not all patients with the ability to test and the access to self-testing choose to perform it. Only those who are motivated by one or more of the following factors will purchase and perform tests. Some of the most common factors are the patients' desire to:

- Avoid frequent venipuncture
- Avoid traveling long distances to a laboratory
- Gain better control of their condition
- Avoid costly complications
- Travel and still monitor health
- Get more accurate results (mistrust of the referral laboratory)
- Escape frequent laboratory visits
- Participate in their own care
- Take less time off work
- Maintain privacy (e.g., tests for sexually transmitted diseases, ovulation, and pregnancy)
- Show concern for a family member (e.g., a parent who performs a home test on her child)
- Save money (although self-testing is not yet embraced by all third-party payers, except in the case of diabetes)

- Avoid assistance such as an ambulance, specialized transport, or the time and resources of a family member to get to a laboratory or clinic for a test (when patients are homebound)

Most self-testers learn about tests available to them, such as PT test equipment, via word of mouth, websites, and chat rooms. They often bring the information to their physician and, in many cases, insist that their physician write them a prescription to purchase the test. These patients often change doctors or healthcare facilities if their requests are denied.

A surprising number of patients are willing to pay their expenses out of pocket when unable to obtain insurance coverage. Even Medicare-eligible patients often opt to pay themselves, since Medicare does not currently cover PT self-testing. These active consumers of health care are many in number and are not limited to "baby boomers." Their fervent desire to be more involved in their own health care is one of the most important predictors of successful self-testing.

Benefits of Home Testing

Home tests offer quick—often immediate—results that allow faster treatment or adjustment of therapy. Tests approved for the consumer market are easy to administer, usually with a simple fingerstick device that patients quickly master. Home testing, performed properly, can enhance patient care in the following nine ways:

1. Patient mobility is important for patients who do not wish to accept the constraints imposed by a disease state requiring ongoing, regular monitoring. Self-testing releases them to move about, travel, and work without interruption. Productivity, quality of life, and continuity of care can all be well served via self-testing.
2. Patient comfort, especially for those with poor venous access. Fingerstick technology is very attractive to those who require frequent blood collection.
3. Convenience for both patient and provider, especially for those patients who need frequent monitoring or who live in rural areas and for whom travel to a referral laboratory is burdensome.
4. Increased compliance and flexibility to perform tests. Patients who self-test usually manage their conditions better and perform tests whenever a problem is suspected or otherwise needed.
5. Faster results for some home-based tests (e.g., glucose or PT) contribute to more stable drug dosages. Delays in turn-around time occur mainly in the preanalytic phase (1) (from the time tests are ordered until the laboratory receives the test), which is negated by patient self-testing.
6. Home testers generally test more frequently than those who must travel to a remote laboratory. More frequent testing results in closer monitoring of high-risk patients, especially those discharged from the hospital "quicker and sicker."
7. Removing specimen transport issues.
8. Consistency of testing results when the same person uses the same instrument rather than a test result derived from different instruments or different laboratories.

9. Home testing can have a subtle impact on patient empowerment, compliance, and satisfaction that may be important elements in achieving better outcomes (2).

Due to these factors, a greater therapeutic efficacy is often achieved when patients perform tests at home. One example of better outcomes derived from home-based testing is in the case of anticoagulation monitoring (3). The objective of monitoring anticoagulant therapy is to detect a change in steady state, which requires more than one data point. For the greatest reliability, many data points are desirable. Unfortunately, long-term routine testing using referral laboratories at a frequency of more than once per month is impractical for most patients. Instruments that allow patients to determine their own levels of anticoagulant can provide results within 2 to 3 minutes.

Diversity of Home Testing

Tests designed for use by consumers range from simple urine dip strips to black box instruments for fructosamine and PT. Some of these tests are not "laboratory" tests in the traditional sense. Rather, they are "physiological" diagnostic tests, such as peak flow meters, spirometers, and ambulatory blood pressure monitors. Table 23-1 contains a list of currently available home tests.

Figure 23.1 depicts the many configurations of self-testing or home testing. These range from patient self-management where patients not only perform tests in their homes, but also adjust therapy on their own, to self-referral, specimen collection, and

home health testing. Because some of these test modalities may not be considered home testing, per se, this chapter will focus on three areas of patient self-testing: (a) those tests provided in the home by home health personnel, (b) patient self-testing, and (c) patient self-management.

Patient self-referral involves a patient selecting the desired laboratory tests and then contracting with a laboratory or pharmacy that provides these tests. The tests most commonly ordered by patients on a self-referral basis are HIV, drugs of abuse, and lipids, followed by such tests as prostate-specific antigen, complete blood count, thyroid-stimulating hormone, and wellness chemistries (4). Many states place restrictions on patient direct-access testing; New York forbids it, but 21 states and the District of Columbia have no restrictions on this type of testing (5). When patients self-refer, they not only order their own tests, but they may not share test results with their personal physician.

Another form of patient self-testing, patient specimen collection, is not self-testing per se, because it involves purchasing a kit to collect a specimen and mailing the specimen to a laboratory for analysis. Two examples of this form of testing are one for HIV screening (6) and one for estriol, a saliva-based test to identify females at risk for spontaneous preterm labor and delivery (7). Other mail-in tests are also available for prostate-specific antigen, hepatitis C, female hormone levels, mineral status, and osteoporosis. As with patient self-referral, patients often do not share test results with their physician. Regardless of whether these two types of tests—patient self-referral and patient speci-

Consumer Participation/Independence from Physician	Type of Testing
High	**Patient Self Management** Patient performs test and can adjust therapy independent of physician
Moderate	**Patient Self Testing** Patient performs test and relays results to physician. Physician must follow up on test results by adjusting therapy, scheduling an appointment, etc.
Moderate	**Patient Specimen Collection** Patient collects urine, saliva, blood, etc. and mails to testing facility. Consultation is available via telephone. Laboratory does not share results with physician.
Moderate	**Patient Self Referral** Patient has tests performed in pharmacy or retail lab without a physician's orders. Results are not shared with physician.
Low	**Home Health Testing** Patient has tests performed at home by home health personnel. Results become part of the patient chart and are acted on immediately.

FIGURE 23.1. Types of home-based testing.

TABLE 23.2. CLIA-WAIVED TESTS NOT CURRENTLY APPROVED FOR PATIENT SELF-TESTING

Test	Rationale for Exclusion from PST
Erythrocyte sedimentation rate	Not clinically appropriate for home use
Hemoglobin instrument	Not yet offered by manufacturers for home use
Microhematocrit test	Requires centrifugation
Helicobacter pylori kit	Not yet offered by manufacturers for home use
Streptococcus pyogenes (Group A strep) kit	Not yet offered by manufacturers for home use
Influenza virus test kit	Not yet offered by manufacturers for home use
Gastric occult blood card test	Not clinically appropriate for home testing
Glycosylated hemoglobin (A1c) instrument	Not yet offered by manufacturers for home use
Mononucleosis test kit	Not yet offered by manufacturers for home use
Nicotine urine test	Not yet offered by manufacturers for home use
Vaginal pH test	Not yet offered by manufacturers for home use

PST, patient self-testing.

men collection—are considered "self-tests," they do place the responsibility for ordering the test, collecting the specimen, and interpreting the test result squarely on the shoulders of the patient.

Patient specimen collection tests for HIV are controversial mostly because of the way that results are reported. To retrieve test results, patients telephone the manufacturer, identify themselves via a randomly assigned number to maintain anonymity, and are informed as to their HIV status. Those with positive results are encouraged to speak directly with trained personnel for result interpretation and counseling.

Laboratory tests that are approved by the Food and Drug Administration (FDA) for patient self-testing are usually (but not automatically) waived under the Clinical Laboratory Improvement Amendments of 1988 (CLIA '88). Not every CLIA-waived test is approved for home use. Examples of CLIA-waived tests that are not currently approved for patient self-testing are in Table 23.2.

HOME TESTING PROVIDED BY HOME HEALTHCARE PERSONNEL

Approximately 14% of the gross domestic product in the United States is spent on health care, and of that, 3% is attributed to home healthcare services. In 2015, the number of people who will need long-term home care will grow to about 4 million, a 2.3-million increase from the approximately 1.7 million people who require it now. The home healthcare market is growing rapidly. In 1997, there were 306 million home-care visits and the demand for home-care services is growing by about 12% per year (8).

Most people who receive home health care are Medicare or Medicaid beneficiaries. Medicare has traditionally been the largest payer source, accounting for about 60% of home healthcare revenues.

Home healthcare workers are mostly nurses, but other healthcare professionals, technicians, and home health aides also make patient visits.

The number of disease states that can be successfully treated in the home has expanded to more than 1,000 (8). The major indications for home care are:

- Cardiovascular disease
- Diabetes and endocrine disorders
- Respiratory disease
- Stroke
- Alzheimer's disease
- AIDS
- Psychiatric disorders
- Cancer
- Renal failure
- Nutrition
- Arthritis and other musculoskeletal disorders
- Wound therapy
- Injury and poisoning
- Nervous system disorders

Information presented at the 1998 meeting of the American Association for Clinical Chemistry suggests that home testing *by medical professionals* is a major growth area for the clinical laboratory testing industry. At this time, however, most home testing through home healthcare agencies—with the exception of glucose monitoring by diabetics, peak flow meters, pulse oximeters, and coagulation monitors—simply involves collecting a patient's blood sample. These samples are transported to commercial or hospital laboratories, or to the patient's physician who has an office-based laboratory.

The most common tests ordered in this fashion are:

- Prothrombin times
- Complete blood counts
- Erythrocyte sedimentation rates
- Blood chemistry panels
- Serum drug levels including peaks and troughs for antibiotic therapy
- Bacteriology cultures and antibiotic susceptibility tests

There are myriad flaws with this method of testing, including poor turnaround time. Transporting specimens to the laboratory creates logistical problems for home healthcare nurses, who spend unproductive time on these duties. More obvious specimen transport issues exist as well, such as specimen temperature, transport time, vibrations, and the inability to separate serum from cells before reaching the referral laboratory.

Regulation of Lab Testing Performed by Home Healthcare Workers

Currently, all tests intended for patient self-testing are waived under the CLIA. Waived tests have no personnel educational or experiential requirements or quality standards, except that the manufacturer's instructions must be followed. When performed by home health personnel, the CLIA-waived requirements exist. Testing by patients in the home, however, is not regulated by the CLIA.

Many home health agencies must meet Joint Commission of Accreditation of Healthcare Organizations (JCAHO) standards. The JCAHO has requirements for personnel competency as well as calibration, maintenance, and quality control efforts for tests performed by home healthcare personnel (9,10).

PATIENT SELF-TESTING

To gain access to tests that can be performed at home, a patient may or may not need a prescription from a physician. Examples of direct access tests, that is, those that do not require a prescription, are glucose meters and accessories, urine dip strips, fecal occult blood tests, cholesterol tests, and most of the other tests or instruments found in pharmacies. The only home test that requires a prescription to purchase, at this time, is an instrument for PT. In any case, for patients to receive insurance coverage, the home-test device must have been prescribed.

Glucose Monitors

Blood glucose monitors, introduced in 1980, are the most frequently used self-testing products. With more than 600,000 new cases of diabetes diagnosed each year in the United States, home testing for diabetes is predicted to grow to $1.4 billion in 2002 (8). Blood glucose instruments and the related supplies—strips, lancets, and platforms—are expected to grow the most rapidly of any other self-test devices. This is due, in part, to recent Medicare coverage for both type 1 and type 2 diabetes mellitus. Effective in mid-1998, Medicare began to reimburse certain providers for training patients to use their glucose monitors (Table 23.3) and also began covering related supplies.

The majority of patients who perform glucose monitoring at home have chronic conditions such as diabetes, hypertension, or asthma, and check their blood glucose levels frequently to ensure that they are taking medications properly.

The American Diabetes Association (ADA) recommends blood glucose testing at home for people with diabetes who are pregnant, take oral hypoglycemics or insulin, have difficulty controlling their blood glucose levels, have extremely low blood glucose levels or ketoacidosis, or experience low blood glucose levels without warning (11).

Prothrombin Time Monitors

Properly selected and trained patients cannot only obtain results equivalent to professionals, but improved access to testing allows for increased testing frequency and results in improvements in the safety and efficacy of Coumadin therapy (12). In a study that included elementary and high school children, 85% of patients rated the ProTime instrument (International Technidyne) easy to use at home. Less than 1% had difficulty operating the instrument.

PATIENT SELF-MANAGEMENT

Patient self-management is a term for patients who have been instructed to perform tests at home and then manage their own therapy within certain parameters based on their own test results. This model of care places more responsibility in the hands of patients for therapeutic decision-making and is expected to gain in popularity. The most common test involving patient self-management is whole-blood glucose testing for monitoring blood sugar levels.

In the treatment of diabetes mellitus and hypertension, self-management combined with structured educational programs has resulted in major improvements of patient compliance, medical outcomes, and quality of life (13). By achieving glycemic control, the ADA expects the following benefits:

■ Prolong life by approximately 5 years
■ Delay onset of complications by about 15 years
■ Delay blindness by about 8 years
■ Delay by 6 years end-stage renal disease and lower extremity amputation

TABLE 23.3. GLUCOSE SELF-TESTING MEDICARE COVERAGE LIMITATIONS

Description	Coverage Limitations
Diabetes training	Individual session, each 60 minutes
Diabetes training	Group session, per person, each 60 minutes
Glucose self test device	For all diabetic beneficiaries
Test strips, box 50	Up to 100/month for insulin-treated diabetics[a]
Lancets, box 100	Up to 50/2 months for noninsulin-treated diabetics[b]
Spring device for fingerstick	One/6 months
Battery, replacement	No limits
Control solutions	No limits

[a]Medicare will pay for more than 100 test strips and lancets/month if physician documents beneficiary's medical need.
[b]Medicare will pay for more than 50 test strips and lancets every 2 months for the noninsulin-treated beneficiary if one of the following indicators is present: management of medical condition by adjusting therapy and/or oral agents, or detection of hypoglycemia when symptoms are present.

Oral anticoagulation management is slowly evolving into a model of patient self-management, where patients not only perform the test, but also adjust their therapy based on the results of that test. This new model of care has great potential, even though more studies are needed (14).

The idea of patient self-management is well accepted in some European countries. In 1997, there were more than 18,000 patients in Germany performing both self-testing of PTs and self-adjustment of medication dosage. One longitudinal study (12) with more than 200 patient-years of follow-up, testing on average every 4 days, found the anticoagulant to be in the therapeutic range 92% of the time with patient home testing, compared to 60% in a well-managed, standard anticoagulation clinic.

In retrospective and prospective studies, Ansell et al. (15,16) and Tripoldi et al. (17) reported that patient self management of oral anticoagulation based on self-measurement of PT is feasible and safe, and that it results in control at least as good as specialized anticoagulation clinics.

A recent German study (18) indicates that patients' self-adjustment of oral anticoagulation therapy improves control and results in improved quality of life. Patients in the self-management group were significantly closer to their target international normalized ratio (INR), had a greater percentage of values within therapeutic range, and reported greater satisfaction with this management approach when compared to patients in the traditional care group.

ACCURACY OF HOME-BASED TESTING

Home-based test devices, in themselves, compare favorably to reference methods. Reliability decreases with untrained patients or patients who either do not have the capacity or are not motivated to test.

Cholesterol

Home-based, whole-blood cholesterol tests were shown to produce acceptable results for 486 volunteers of varying age, occupation, and educational backgrounds (19). Participants received only written instructions provided in the kit and access to a toll-free telephone number for additional help. A short instructional video was available to consumers on request. Fingerstick cholesterol values obtained by these volunteers correlated well with the reference method and were within the biases of the National Cholesterol Education Program (NCEP) cutoffs.

Glucose Monitors

The most common home-based instrument is the glucose monitor, used to enable diabetics to keep close control of their blood sugar. Several studies verify that many patients are capable of attaining therapeutically reliable results after extensive training.

Most existing glucose monitors are based on the glucose oxidase method and are quite reliable (20) for patient use. A newer method employs the glucose dehydrogenase method and has also been found to meet the acceptable criteria for glucose levels used for therapeutic management (21,22).

The accuracy of home instruments depends not only on their analytical performance but also the proficiency of the operator and the quality of the test strips. With certain conditions, such as very low blood sugar, home glucose meters become less accurate. Once within the range of 100 mg/dL to 300 mg/dL, the accuracy of home meters increases. Meters that use whole blood generally provide a reading that is somewhat lower (approximately 12%) than one from plasma done in a laboratory. Several meters have the capability to calibrate whole-blood samples to plasma to account for the 12% difference between blood and plasma (7).

Pregnancy Test Kits

Five studies evaluating 16 home pregnancy test kits found ranges of sensitivity of 52% to 100% (23). In studies where volunteers tested urine samples, sensitivity was 91%, but was less in studies where subjects were actual patients (75%). The authors of this literature search concluded that the diagnostic efficacy of home pregnancy test kits is greatly affected by the characteristics of the users, and expressed concern about their diagnostic efficacy when used by actual patients. The authors suggested that manufacturers of these kits publish results of trials on actual patients (23).

Ovulation Test Kits

Although by most accounts, home ovulation tests are reliable for family planning purposes, one study found them to be counterproductive in fertility clinics when used for artificial insemination. In this study, home ovulation testing actually reduced the chance of pregnancy, especially for women with high baseline concentrations of leutinizing hormone (LH). Moreover, both patients and clinic staff reported increased frustration with home testing (24).

Sensory Tool for Diabetes

One study of a self-administered sensory tool to identify individuals at risk for diabetes-related foot problems found discrepant test results in 18 of 145 cases, which were directly related to the age of the patient (25). The authors concluded that self-administered sensory tests are valuable for involving the patient in preventive care, but that the tests should not replace routine foot evaluation by a provider.

Tuberculosis Skin Tests

Another study that assessed patients' ability to accurately interpret their tuberculosis skin test found discrepant results in 17 of 27 cases (26). The authors attributed this, in part, to the patients' lack of education, foreign birth, and denial of illness. They recommended that an experienced professional check these test results.

Whole-blood Prothrombin Time and International Normalized Ratio Instruments

Instruments for home-based PT testing are easy and accurate and provide a PT-INR from a few drops of blood. The majority of current studies indicate that these tests provide adequate clinical efficacy, provided patients are motivated and trained (27–30). Using several different PT instruments, studies show home-test PT-INR results comparable to results from standard plasma PT determinations (31–35).

In a university-affiliated coagulation clinic study, anticoagulation testing performed by the fingerstick method was less variable than routine laboratory methods. Moreover, routine laboratory results indicated anticoagulant dosage changes erroneously more often than did the fingerstick method (36).

Patients who switch testing from one laboratory to another are more likely to have strokes and heart attacks. Whatever the reason for patients switching laboratories, the odds of a stroke following a switch have been reported to be 1.57 times higher than for patients who stayed with the same laboratory (37). For myocardial infarctions, the odds were 1.32 times greater. This may indicate that physicians are more likely to make errors in adjusting medications when they are dealing with an unfamiliar laboratory.

ADMINISTRATION OF HOME-BASED TESTING PROGRAM

Patient selection is a key consideration both for determining patient eligibility and selecting an appropriate test method. For instance, not all patients on Coumadin are candidates for monitoring themselves using a PT instrument. Patient reliability, competence, and initiative help to determine which type of monitoring is best.

Patients who self-test must be depended upon to carry out all instructions regarding:

- Performing the test
- Self-monitoring of diet and lifestyle changes
- Bleeding indicators
- Appropriate communication with the clinician

A patient self-testing program administered by an ambulatory care facility such as a physician practice or an anticoagulation clinic should contain, at minimum, a needs analysis, cost analysis, instrument selection criteria, training program, and results-reporting system (Fig. 23.2).

Needs Analysis

Prior to developing a self-testing program, perform a needs analysis (38). Consider the following questions for each potential program:

Needs Analysis

Cost Analysis

Make Go/No Go Decision

           Abort Project

Select Instrument(s)

Design and Implement Training Program

Design a Results Reporting System, or, if Patient is to Self-Manage, Indicate When Interaction With Caregiver is Required.

FIGURE 23.2. Components of a home testing program.

- Justification: Why is the program needed? What are the advantages/disadvantages of providing this program? What are the clinical applications?
- Logistics: What types of patients will be accepted into the program? Who will coordinate the program (documentation, instrument maintenance, and training)? How many instruments are required? Where and how will results be recorded?
- Technical issues: What quality control/quality assurance programs are needed? (internal/external controls and ongoing proficiency checks)? At what frequency should patients test? When/how should results be transmitted to the caregiver? For patients who will manage their disease at home, at what point should the physician be consulted?

Cost Analysis

Perform an assessment of both direct and indirect costs. Cost savings associated with providing the program may also be assessed, including improved timeliness of assessment and intervention. Compare the total cost of the program with the cost associated with current test methods.

The direct costs associated with home-based testing include: instruments, reagents, supplies, waste associated with repeat testing (assume 5% repeat rate), personnel, training, and program coordination. Indirect costs include medical interventions, computer resources, and telephone or pagers.

Some insurance plans, such as Medicare, reimburse for the cost of glucose monitors and supplies as well as diabetes patient education under certain conditions (Table 23.4) when

TABLE 23.4. CRITERIA FOR SELECTING AND EVALUATING INSTRUMENTS FOR HOME-TESTING PROGRAMS

Manufacturer support
Device warranty and repair policies
Training program for staff/patients (interactive, video, CD-ROM, virtual, Internet)
Instructions for meeting CLIA/JCAHO requirements
Instrument characteristics
Therapeutic turnaround time
Number and efficiency of preanalytical, analytical, and postanalytical steps
Flexibility, modularity, expandability, and upgrade capability
Networking or interfacing capability
Information system, data storage, and archiving capability
Small sample volume
Automated calibration
Interrupt capability
Short analysis cycle
Compact, reliable, durable, lightweight, mobile, and power efficient with battery operation
Reagent stability, shelf life, and lot size
Instrument performance
Accuracy, precision, bias, resolution, reproducibility, stability, and response time
Linearity in both high and low extremes of measurement
Consistency and relationship to tests performed in the parent laboratory
Artifact elimination, error detection, interference warning, and specimen flagging

CLIA, Clinical Laboratory Improvement Amendments; JCAHO, Joint Commission on Accreditation of Healthcare Organizations.

prescribed by a physician. It is also now possible for physicians or other qualified providers to attain Medicare reimbursement for training their patients about use of these instruments. The ADA's National Standards for Diabetes Self-Management Education Programs spell out the requisite components of a quality self-management education program. These standards are listed in Table 23.5. Providers must meet these ADA standards to attain reimbursement from Medicare for training.

Many insurance companies follow Medicare's lead on coverage issues. Managed care organizations may or may not cover these services; physicians must examine their individual contractual agreements.

Instrument Selection

Consider the following criteria when evaluating instruments for home-based testing (38,39). Table 23.4 depicts the most common criteria for selecting and evaluating instruments for a home-based testing program.

Manufacturer Support

Obtain references concerning the instrument's reliability and quality of support. Find out where the most qualified distributor is located and the approximate lead time once orders are placed. Be sure the manufacturer or distributor has a toll-free (24 hours a day, 7 days a week) technical assistance department. Will the manufacturer supply a replacement instrument while repairs are being performed? Determine whether the manufacturer will supply a training program for the medical facility's staff. Examine patient educational materials for quality and content. The manufacturer should provide an instruction/operator's manual and cue cards outlining critical steps. Finally, the instrument's specifications and limitations should be clearly indicated.

Instrument Characteristics

The testing procedure should be acceptable to both the patient and the operator. Determine the complexity of the testing procedure; complex procedures are not well suited for use with patients. Speed, ease, simplicity, and user-friendly operation are essential. Assess the functional turnaround time capability, including patient preparation, sample collection, test performance, and result documentation.

Low sample-volume requirements are preferable because this generally means that the collection procedure will be less invasive and less painful for the patient. This is also important for patients who require frequent blood glucose sampling and may have poor peripheral circulation.

Instruments designed for home testing should have built-in calibration and fast, simple maintenance. Ideally, reagents and supplies will be compact and easy to store, not require refrigeration, and have a long shelf life. Error messages should be easy to interpret by operators.

Patients who are visually impaired require a meter with large numbers and letters or one that is compatible with a voice synthesizer. Those who, because of diabetic neuropathy or callused fingers, may not have sufficient blood flow to their fingers may need a meter that does not require a large drop of blood (7). The size of the instrument, amount of test supplies, and storage should afford easy handling and access for most operators. The instrument must be rugged enough to survive home use, including all kinds of conditions and accidents, as well as travel. Supplies should be environmentally friendly, and ease of waste disposal should be considered. The instrument should include a "low battery" indicator that can be tested routinely. Possible sources of error should be identified on the cue cards, and they should be minimized whenever possible.

Instrument Reliability

Assess the accuracy of the instrument and strive for results within 10% of laboratory values, or define acceptable limitations for imprecision at each specific medical decision limit. A number of interferences, such as lipemia, hemolysis, hyperbilirubinemia, and abnormal hematocrit, may interfere with the test and must be evaluated.

Design and Implement Training Program

Training and education programs should be designed to match test complexity, system types, intended use (self-testing versus self-management), and professional disciplines. Hence, training programs will differ from facility to facility. Apart from training patients to use the testing device, there are several other variables that can affect test reliability. Some of these factors are listed below.

Preanalytical variables:

- Specimens are collected properly
- Patient performs test at the right time
- Patient has undergone the proper preparations (e.g., fasting)

Postanalytical factors:

- Clerical errors (transposing numbers, writing the wrong result, placing the result in the wrong place, and sending the wrong caregiver the result)
- Results not appropriately acted upon
- Wrong patient information (e.g., age, gender) used to calculate reference ranges

Employee and patient training program should include:

- Patient preparation
- Sample handling
- Test performance
- Preventive maintenance, troubleshooting, and calibration
- Reagent storage and stability
- Knowledge of pertinent preanalytic and postanalytic variables
- Test result evaluation, including proper follow-up procedures
- Performance and evaluation of quality control results
- Result reporting and steps to take if results indicate further action
- Therapy adjustment

The ADA states that education is the cornerstone of treatment for all people with diabetes. An example of a training pro-

TABLE 23.5. NATIONAL STANDARDS FOR DIABETES SELF-MANAGEMENT EDUCATION PROGRAMS

1. The sponsoring organization shall have a written policy that affirms education as an integral component of diabetes care.
2. The sponsoring organization shall identify and provide the educational resources required to achieve its educational objectives in terms of its target population. These resources include adequate space, personnel, budget, and instructional materials.
3. The organizational relationships, lines of authority, staffing, job descriptions, and operational policies shall be clearly defined and documented.
4. The service area shall be assessed in order to define the target population and determine appropriate allocation of personnel and resources to serve the educational needs of the target population.
5. A standing advisory committee consisting of a physician, a nurse educator, a dietitian, an individual with behavioral science expertise, a consumer, and a community representative, at a minimum, shall be established to oversee the program.
6. The advisory committee shall participate in the annual planning process, including the determination of target audience, program objectives, participant access mechanisms, instructional methods, resource requirements (including space, personnel, budget, and materials), participant follow-up mechanisms, and program evaluation.
7. Professional program staff shall have sufficient time and resources for lesson planning, instruction, documentation, evaluation, and follow-up.
8. Community resources shall be assessed periodically.
9. A coordinator shall be designated who is responsible for program planning, implementation, and evaluation.
10. Healthcare professionals with recent didactic and experiential preparation in diabetes clinical and educational issues shall serve as the program instructors.
11. Professional program staff shall obtain education about diabetes, educational principles, and behavioral change strategies on a continuing basis.
12. Based on the needs of the target population, the program shall be capable of offering instruction in the following content areas:
    Diabetes overview
    Stress and psychosocial adjustment
    Family involvement and social support
    Nutrition
    Exercise and activity
    Medications
    Monitoring and use of results
    Relationships among nutrition, exercise, medication, and blood glucose levels
    Prevention, detection, and treatment of acute complications
    Prevention, detection, and treatment of chronic complications
    Foot, skin, and dental care
    Behavior change strategies, goal setting, risk factor reduction, and problem solving
    Benefits, risks, and management options for improving glucose control
    Preconception care, pregnancy, and gestational diabetes
    Use of healthcare systems and community resources
13. The program shall use instructional methods and materials that are appropriate for the target population and the participants being served.
14. A system shall be in place to inform the target population and potential referral sources of the availability and benefits of the program.
15. The program shall be conveniently and regularly available.
16. The program shall be responsive to requests for information and referrals from consumers and healthcare agencies.
17. An individualized assessment shall be developed and updated in collaboration with each participant.
18. An individualized education plan, based on the assessment, shall be developed in collaboration with each participant.
19. The participants' educational experience, including assessment, intervention, evaluation, and follow-up, shall be documented in a permanent medical or education record. There shall be documentation of collaboration and coordination among program staff and other providers.
20. The program shall offer appropriate and timely educational interventions based on periodic reassessments of health status, knowledge, skills, attitudes, goals, and self-care behaviors.
21. The advisory committee shall review program performance annually, including all components of the annual program plan and curriculum, and use the information in subsequent planning and program modification.
22. The advisory committee shall annually review and evaluate predetermined outcomes for program participants.

gram for diabetes self-management is presented in Table 23.5 (40). Providers who wish to be reimbursed by Medicare for diabetes training and education must develop a program equivalent to these standards.

The Loma Linda Veterans Administration (VA) clinics initiated patient self-testing for PT in 1996 after satisfactory evaluations of devices and ensuring equivalence of patient and professional monitoring results. Loma Linda's training session consisted of two 3-hour sessions in which patients became familiar with the theory and operation of the device. The Loma Linda program included several levels of safeguards such as comparisons of patient results with professionals, quality control testing, electronic calibration, and optional proficiency testing.

In addition to initial employee and patient training, periodic competence evaluations are recommended. Any one (or a combination of) the following may be used:

- Blind samples
- Testing a sample in the presence of another trained observer
- Checklists to ensure conformance with the proper procedures

Devise Results-Reporting System

Determine the method for documenting test results. Is the instrument capable of interfacing with the laboratory/patient care information system? If not, determine how patients are to record results. If patients are to keep logs, determine what information needs to be included (date, time, test result, etc.).

A home-based testing program must stipulate under what circumstances patients are to contact their physician and exactly how the physician is to be notified.

COMMUNICATIONS/INFORMATICS ISSUES

Logistical problems arise when patients must telephone their caregivers to coordinate management of their home-test results. Traditional telephone triage of patient test results takes a total time commitment of about 15 minutes per patient to contact the patient, discuss the results, and perform charting. This allows for only 30 results to be handled per day per full-time staff member. This is not cost effective for most physician practices.

The evolution of home testing will accelerate as methods to communicate between healthcare professionals and patients improve to keep pace with developing testing technologies. Currently, several venues are under development for data transmission of home-test results.

Telemedicine is one such venue, which allows medical information to be exchanged from one site to another via electronic communications both for patient education and education of healthcare providers. Telemedicine began in the 1960s when the space program monitored the health of astronauts as they traveled through space. Today, telemedicine continues to evolve and is used to communicate test data via fax, telephone, computer, or the Internet. Applications today include the transmission of radiology and imaging data, laboratory results, and physician training programs over great distances. These applications are particularly appealing in rural and underserved areas.

Significant progress toward secure patient/physician information transfer has been made in the last year. New Internet sites are being established to facilitate information management and patient education. These efforts are well under way but it is too early to determine their long-term viability. Still, the logic of Internet-based information sharing makes sense from several standpoints. It costs less on the patient's part to obtain information without leaving home. It is also more efficient for physicians or staff members to issue instructions to large numbers of patients in a relatively short time. Examples of these uses might be reminders to self-test, adjust medication, or simply to deliver "custom" patient education material. All of this is available today, but choices are limited and most are not part of a complete system.

Internet information for diabetics, by far the largest population of self-testers, has attracted the most investment to date. The online diabetes management programs currently offered are seeking to contract with insurance carriers and health management organizations that recognize the savings which can be realized when patients are more involved and better managed by their physician.

Still, many questions remain. Who pays for the physician's time when remote, Internet/e-mail management of self-testing occurs? Is an electronic or "virtual" visit the same as an office visit? How should this be documented? These and other practical questions must be answered before online or telemedicine truly becomes part of the fabric of our healthcare system.

Most home-testing instruments manufactured today include provisions for automated data transmission. Data storage is a common built-in feature of most instruments but most designs rely upon external programs to receive and manipulate data. Some tests are performed without the use of an instrument, such as diagnostic test kits and, in these cases, the consumer must communicate results directly to his or her physician. This is usually accomplished via telephone and is an inefficient, error-prone, and costly process (41).

E-mail may prove to be a better medium for patient-doctor communication than the telephone. Unlike voice mail, e-mail can be checked quickly and answered as time allows and priority dictates. For certain patients, e-mail provides a number of advantages (42–44). Asynchronous communications makes sending and responding to messages much more convenient for both the doctor and the patient, and phone tag is eliminated. Another important advantage of e-mail is that it is self-documenting. The language used in an e-mail message can be more carefully chosen than that in a telephone conversation and responses can be reused for patients with identical circumstances. E-mail may also be used to display logic trees, flow diagrams, and a variety of graphics. As a result, there may be less confusion and less need for follow-up questions.

A final issue with e-mail is security of test results transmitted in this fashion. Browser encryption standards are expected to eliminate this problem soon, but other types of security issues also warrant consideration. For example, some patients may share computer and e-mail accounts. Many companies maintain the right to read employee e-mail. A physician's laptop computer may be stolen, containing patient correspondence and test results.

Reporting test results and medical conditions over an unsecured Internet connection raises concerns about protecting patient confidentiality and about physicians' legal liability related to electronic patient interaction. In 1998, the American Medical Informatics Association (AMIA) released guidelines for the clinical use of e-mail, addressing both effective patient-physician communication and medicolegal prudence (45).

The AMIA guidelines recommend that physicians ask patients how they want to communicate with the practice and document in the chart which form of communication patients prefer for different purposes. The guidelines also recommend that physicians consider obtaining formal informed consent for the use of e-mail, a view seconded by a healthcare attorney recently in the *Journal of the American Medical Association* (46).

Home testing that requires close professional supervision is greatly enhanced with automated data communication with caregivers. The security of knowing that results are "true" is an important element of successful self-testing, especially when trust is an issue. More development is needed in the area of automated data transmission. Various individuals and organizations are working on or have developed improved methods of information exchange between the healthcare professional and the patient (47–49). These efforts are designed to help improve outcomes and reduce expenses, and many include a home-testing component.

The Veterans Administration Hospital in Tampa, Florida, is a good example of a pilot project, slated to begin soon, which will use diagnostic equipment and computer, video cameras and telephony, to communicate test results, coach patients, and monitor patients' condition. The equipment will first be installed in clinics that are remote from the hospital, and then to people in their homes who are patients of those remote clinics. An entity large enough to deploy the necessary equipment and support infrastructure might save considerable expense while still providing above-average care.

Another project recently undertaken equipped chronically ill patients with a physiologic vital-signs monitor and modem that allowed for transmission of weight, blood pressure, heart rate, oxygen saturation, glucose, and PT/INR results. This approach produced promising results from a clinical and economic perspective. When results are not within clinical guidelines, the patient is counseled and directed to adjust or change medication by phone. Unfortunately, the start-up cost puts access to this type of program out of reach of most individuals and smaller medical entities, but this could change as the technology gains widespread use.

The Loma Linda VA clinics have instituted a system effective in integrating home testing with the central clinic (50). The patient at home calls in the INR to a computer with interactive voice response. These calls take approximately 2 minutes during which the patient can confirm the dosage, the next appointment, and if needed, request a call from a staff member. Staff members enter the INR results via the telephone touch pad directly into the computer that automatically prints off a label. From the label printer, a nurse can review a number of patient test results without the need to make phone calls to individual patients. To master the system, patients receive brief verbal instructions lasting less than 5 minutes and a single-page instruction sheet. The majority of patients were reliable and accurate in their data entry; an error rate of 3.6% occurred between the test values telephoned to the clinic versus the actual results stored in the PT instrument's memory. Loma Linda continues to refine its techniques in patient selection, patient education, and collection of data for patient self-testing.

CONCLUSIONS AND FUTURE TRENDS

Home-based testing is a growing alternative to traditional laboratory testing for a variety of reasons. Educated, empowered consumers coupled with an ever-expanding array of technology are fueling this growth. Continued development of secure, reliable information-sharing mechanisms are key to widespread, standardized use of patient self-testing for a variety of medical conditions.

Anticipating growth in the home-testing market, manufacturers are devoting significant resources to develop noninvasive tests. The fact that patients dislike needles is well known, yet the extent to which it compromises care and undermines public health has not been determined. It is recognized that diabetics do not monitor their blood glucose level or take their insulin as often as they should because of this distaste for needle sticks. Now it appears that a virtually needle-less future may be plausible (51,52).

Several companies are working to develop noninvasive systems (53). Tests for which technology is currently available to be performed noninvasively include bilirubin, hemoglobin, glucose, WBC, hematocrit, and tests for *H. pylori*. At this time, only certain noninvasive glucose devices are available for home use.

Efforts to find less-invasive glucose tests were bolstered by recent findings that the glucose level in interstitial fluid just below the skin is proportional to blood glucose concentrations. Devices in development use "minimally invasive" processes to extract small amounts of interstitial fluid to be analyzed instead of blood.

One manufacturer has developed a noninvasive device (GlucoWatch, Cygnus, Redwood City, CA) that monitors blood glucose levels and sounds an alarm when an intervention is needed. The $300 GlucoWatch is strapped to the wrist and beeps when insulin levels need to be adjusted. It is calibrated by a fingerstick glucose determination and uses reverse iontophoresis to monitor glucose levels continuously. By applying a small electrical current to the skin under the device, the monitor beeps whenever the wearer's glucose falls below a predetermined cutoff, prompting him/her to perform a fingerstick glucose.

One study (54) found a close agreement between Glucowatch and blood glucose measurements using repeated fingerstick blood samples. The automatic, frequent, and noninvasive measurements obtained with this device provided more information about glucose levels than the current standard of care.

One manufacturer, Abbott Laboratories, is currently developing noninvasive devices for glucose monitoring. Rather than applying an electric current to the skin, SpectRx uses a patch to make microscopic perforations in the outer layer of the skin, then uses suction to pull interstitial fluid into the patch. Fingersticks may be replaced completely with this device, which resembles a pager in size, since the patch may be worn for 3 days, most likely tethered to an adhesive patch affixed to a patient's abdomen. It does not irritate the skin or require a traditional fingerstick for initial calibration (55). The product will likely be available in 2002.

Another continuous glucose monitoring system (MiniMed, MiniMed Corporation) was recently approved for home use with a doctor's prescription. It consists of a small, pager-like device that is connected to a tiny, glucose oxidase-based subcutaneous sensor. The system provides continuous Holter-type monitoring of glucose levels diabetes (56).

If indicated by the blood glucose level, patients could then administer insulin through a noninvasive drug delivery system, such as a skin patch or a painless microneedle (e.g., PowderJect or SpectRx). This handheld device blasts drugs in powder form through the skin at high speed.

The future of self-testing could also include a laser beam that creates a tiny port from which fluid is extracted. Still other research focuses on electromagnetic radiation to measure blood glucose in such areas as the eye, which is a painless process.

Laser technology can now be applied to phlebotomy. The Lasette (Cell Robotics International, Albuquerque, NM) is a laser skin perforator cleared by the FDA for use in the home. Devices that perforate the skin with a finely focused laser beam may substitute for lancets to obtain minute quantities of blood. Producing near-painless capillary access, laser devices direct a pulse of light energy onto the skin vaporizing it to 1 to 2 mm into the capillary bed, yielding blood in quantities sufficient for most POCT. Instead of the sharp pain associated with traditional lancets, patients feel a sensation similar to mild heat or pressure. Wounds generated by this technology heal faster than those produced by lancets; however, laser skin perforation devices are not recommended in areas where oxygen is in use.

On January 19, 2000, the FDA cleared a virtually pain-free blood glucose test, FreeStyle, developed by TheraSense (Alameda, CA). The device provides a blood glucose value using a fraction of the blood sample currently required by other products on the market. The device allows diabetics to obtain a blood sample from places other than fingertips, such as the thigh or forearm.

Efforts are under way to develop assays using noninvasive techniques including infrared and nearinfrared measurements coupled with signature analysis and photo-acoustic means (57). An analyzer that utilizes noninvasive laser technology (Futrex 900 NIR transmittance blood chemistry analyzer) has been developed, but requires further evaluation before clinical use. The advantage of this system is its speed, portability, lack of consumables, dry chemistry, noninvasiveness, and virtual absence of moving parts. This method is purported to provide a more pleasant, less-invasive method of drawing blood. It is likely that the first application for this type of technology will be where there is a requirement for multiple assays and where sample size is a limitation (55).

A saliva analyzer is under development (LifePoint, Rancho Cucamanga, CA) to measure the concentration of as many as ten chemical analytes using less than a drop of saliva. The system will be useful in screening, diagnosis, and therapeutic drug monitoring in ambulances, the workplace, the home, and law enforcement facilities. The first application will be tests for alcohol and drugs of abuse.

Skin cholesterol is an effective means of monitoring individual patients' response to cholesterol-lowering medications. Using the skin cholesterol test every 3 months is suggested to measure a treatment's effectiveness (58).

Cholesterol 1,2,3 (International Medical Innovations, Mississauga, Ontario, Canada) is a noninvasive test that measures cholesterol in the skin rather than in the blood. The test takes 3 minutes and is administered by placing two drops of liquid on an applicator pad in the palm of the hand. A digitonin-peroxidase conjugate is added to a well in the pad with a dropper bottle. After a 1-minute incubation, the hand is rinsed briefly with tap water and blotted dry. Peroxide substrate solution is added to the well and incubated for 2 minutes. A color change in the second drop shows the patient's level of skin cholesterol. A negative control well in the pad remains colorless in a valid assay.

Oral mucosal transudate (OMT), a serum-derived fluid that enters saliva from the gingival crevice and across oral mucosal surfaces, can be preferentially concentrated by a novel collecting system to yield detectable levels of immunoglobulins (i.e., IgG and IgM antibodies) against various bacterial and viral diseases (59). Assays based on reliable and accurate OMT-based tests may aid in the diagnosis of viral hepatitis, measles, mumps, and rubella. Future applications also include monitoring levels of hormones and therapeutic drugs such as theophylline (59).

Expect to see in the near future technology that integrates training capabilities within analyzers designed for home use, even small handheld devices. The further shrinking of electronics and optics both at the detector stage and data processing stage will enable even a greater degree of portability than presently available.

Future home-test devices must be fully integrated into the medical information system. As communication links become smaller and less expensive, direct infrared links between instruments and referral laboratories or physician practices will further enhance the development of controlled independence (50).

The overriding factor impeding rapid deployment of automated data transmission in the home setting is cost. If prices decline on a scale of typical computer technology, this limiting factor should be eliminated over time. It is also likely that further integration of technologies, such as personal organizers, data recorders, telecommunications hardware, and so on, will have an increasing presence in home-testing applications.

Liability concerns may slow the growth of home testing, especially therapeutic drug monitoring and other tests associated with ongoing disease state management. There are no easy answers to the liability issue. Ultimately, a patient who has the capacity should be responsible for compliance with a plan laid out by her or his physician. As in conventional treatment plans, some patients will comply and some will not. The challenge for the future is to lay out and follow uniform guidelines for medical personnel as well as home testers. Formal patient self-testing/patient self-management policies, written orders, and instructions and notes, in addition to prescriptions, are important. Advances in electronic communication may eliminate some, but not all, liability concerns.

One unresolved issue is whether to allow patients access to tests that, if positive, have grave consequences. Currently, the technology exists to allow tests for HIV to be performed and read by the consumer with acceptable accuracy, but how to handle a positive HIV test is currently unresolved. The question of trust becomes a valid consideration in this case. Emotional reactions to the news of a positive test result could range from an appropriate one—seeking professional advice and care—to simply ignoring the results altogether or the acting-out behavior of a few individuals who have made the headlines via a determination to infect as many others as possible. What about parents who discover, via a home test, that their child is using cocaine? The answer to both situations, so far, has been telemedicine in the form of remote phone counseling.

Until more automated data transference is developed and priced to reach the masses, the patient must be relied upon to initiate communication with her or his healthcare provider. Should control be removed from the patient and given to a third party? Third-party involvement makes sense in situations requiring immediate intervention or consultation, but ultimately the rapidly growing population of consumer-patients will demand participation and reasonable control.

One promising technology with potential applications to home testing is the adaptation of computer chips for both testing and patient medication capabilities. Currently, research is under way to develop an implantable microchip that provides time-release medication or performs diagnostic tests at the patient's bedside and delivers immediate results. Extending this idea to home testing, one could reasonably anticipate development of similar microchips to perform tests and report results to both the patient and a physician at a remote terminal. The physician would program a dosage adjustment based on the test result. Further, the most common dosage adjustments could be preprogrammed onto the microchip.

The direction this new technology is taking indicates that there may become a time when the current barriers to information management—compliance, security, and liability—become moot.

Despite obstacles to overcome, the future of home testing is bright. In the next decade POCT networks will extend from the home to the most sophisticated acute care settings (57). Resembling modern electrical utility grids, workload will be distributed to the most efficient laboratory site, that is, that which optimizes therapeutic turnaround time and economic effectiveness. Throughout the network, clinical and managerial information will be accessible at all points in a manner that maintains patient confidentiality and data security.

Current home-test programs in use show significant benefits in terms of outcomes and costs. Motivated and trained patients can and do produce results on par, if not superior to other methods.

The forces of change are moving toward patient home-based testing. The appropriate response to this force is careful study, innovative approaches, and continued education for patients/consumers who, in growing numbers, are demanding greater participation in their own care. Home-based testing is a valuable tool in the hands of a motivated, trained patient in partnership with an enlightened, progressive clinician. Ulti-

mately, patient demand will fuel the growth of home testing, which will comprise products that are easy to use and that directly communicate with clinicians when needed. Once these objectives are attained, consumers can actively participate in their own health care.

REFERENCES

1. Scott FI. Integrating point-of-care testing with continuity of care, part 3. *Am Clin Lab* 1998;6:4–5.
2. Ansell JE. Empowering patients to monitor and manage oral anticoagulation therapy. *JAMA* 1999;281:182–183.
3. Becker RC. *Anticoagulant management and the growing role of patient self-testing.* Paper presented at American Society of Hematology meeting, New Orleans, LA, November 11, 1996.
4. Paxton A. "Retail revolution" on horizon for laboratories? *CAP Today* 1998;12:5–15.
5. Schulze M. Direct access testing: a state-by-state analysis. *Lab Med* 1999;30:371–373.
6. Goetsch R, Minor JR, Piscitelli SC. Home collection and non-blood-based methods of testing for the human immunodeficiency virus. *Am J Health Syst Pharm* 1997;54:2232–2235.
7. LoBuono C. Taking advantage of home testing and monitoring. *Patient Care* 2000;3:144–159.
8. Home testing market gets favorable prognosis. Genesis Report special report. October–November 1998.
9. Carlson DA. Point of care testing: regulation and accreditation. *Clin Lab Sci* 1996;5:298–302.
10. Belanger AC. Point-of-care testing: the JCAHO perspective. *Med Lab Obs* 1994;6:46–49.
11. American Diabetes Association. *Diabetes self-testing.* Available at: http://www.diabetes.org/ada/c30j.asp. Accessed on January 12, 2001.
12. Scott FI. Integrating point-of-care testing with continuity of care. Part 4: Case studies in anticoagulant therapy, cardiac marker, and blood gases. *Am Clin Lab* 1998;8:4–6.
13. Muhlhauser I, Berger M. Diabetes education and insulin therapy: when will they ever learn? *J Intern Med* 1993;233:321–326.
14. Ansell JE. Empowering patients to monitor and manage oral anticoagulation therapy. *JAMA* 1999;281:182–183.
15. Ansell JE, Patel N, Ostrovsky D, et al. Long-term patients' self-management of oral anticoagulation. *Arch Intern Med* 1995;155:2185–2189.
16. Ansell JE, Holden A, Knapic N. Patients' self-management of oral anticoagulation guided by capillary (fingerstick) whole blood prothrombin times. *Arch Intern Med* 1989;149:2509–2511.
17. Tripoldi A, Chantarangkul V, Clerici M, et al. Determination of the International Sensitivity Index of a new near-patient testing device to monitor oral anticoagulant therapy—overview of the assessment of conformity to the calibration model. *Thromb Haemost* 1997;78:855–858.
18. Sawicki PT. A structured teaching and self-management program for patients receiving oral anticoagulation: a randomized controlled trial. *JAMA* 1999;281:145–150.
19. McNamara JR, Warnick GR, Leary ET, et al. Multicenter evaluation of a patient-administered test for blood cholesterol measurement. *Prev Med* 1996;25:583–592.
20. Bennett BD. Blood glucose determination: point of care testing. *South Med J* 1997;90:678–680.
21. Kost GJ, Vu HT, Lee JH, et al. Multicenter study of oxygen-insensitive handheld glucose point-of-care testing in critical care/hospital/ambulatory patients in the United States and Canada. *Crit Care Med* 1998;26:581–590.
22. Kabadi UM, Kabadi M, O'Connell KM. Acceptability of capillary blood glucose testing with Companion 2 after intensive individual patient training. *Diabet Res Clin Pract* 1994;26:25–32.
23. Bastian LA, Nanda K, Hasselblad V, et al. Diagnostic efficiency of

home pregnancy test kits: a meta-analysis. *Arch Fam Med* 1998;7:
465–469.

24. Anderson RA, Eccles SM, Irvine DS. Home ovulation testing in a
donor insemination service. *Hum Reprod* 1996;11:1674–1677.

25. Birke JA, Rolfsen RJ. Evaluation of a self-administered sensory testing
tool to identify patients at risk of diabetes-related foot problems. *Diabet Care* 1998;21:23–25.

26. Colp C, Goldfarb A, Wei I, et al. Patient's self-interpretation of tuberculin skin tests. *Chest* 1996;110:1275–1277.

27. Landefeld CS, Anderson PA, Cavanaugh LT, et al. The bleeding severity index: validation and comparison to other methods for classifying
bleeding complications of medical therapy. *J Clin Hem* 1989;42:
711–718.

28. White RH, McCurdy SA, Woodruff DE, et al. Home prothrombin
time monitoring after initiation of warfarin therapy. *Arch Intern Med*
1989;111:730–737.

29. Anderson D, Harrison L, Hirsch J. Evaluation of a portable prothrombin time monitor for home use by patients who require longterm oral anticoagulation therapy. *Arch Intern Med* 1993;153:
1441–1444.

30. Massicotte P, Marzinotto V, Adams M, et al. Home monitoring of warfarin therapy in children with a whole blood prothrombin time monitor. *J Pediatr* 1995;127:389–394.

31. Lucas LV, Duncan A, Jay R, et al. A novel whole blood capillary technique for measuring prothrombin time. *Am J Clin Pathol* 1987;88:
442–446.

32. McCurdy SA, White RH. Accuracy and precision of a portable anticoagulation monitor in a clinical setting. *Arch Intern Med* 1991;152:
589–592.

33. Cachia PG, McGregor E, Adlakha S, et al. Accuracy and precision of
the TAS analyzer for near-patient INR testing by non-pathology staff
in the community. *J Clin Pathol* 1998;51:68–72.

34. Becker R, Andrew M, Ansell J, et al. *Multicenter trial of accurate home
self-testing in oral anticoagulant patients with a novel whole blood system.*
Paper presented at American College of Cardiology annual meetings,
March 16–19, 1997, Anaheim, California.

35. Ansell J, Becker D, Andrew M, et al. Accurate and precise prothrombin time measurement in a multicenter anticoagulation trial employing
patient self-testing. *Blood* 1995;86[Suppl 1]:864a(abst).

36. Bussey H, Chiquett E, Bianco T, et al. A statistical and clinical evaluation of fingerstick and routine laboratory prothrombin time measurements. *Pharmacotherapy* 1997;17:861–866.

37. Mennemeyer ST, Winkelman JW. Searching for inaccuracy in clinical
laboratory testing using Medicare data: evidence for prothrombin time.
JAMA 1993;269:1030–1033.

38. Collier CP, Houlden RL, Rhymer SL. How to develop an effective
decentralized laboratory program. *Clin Lab Mgmt Rev* 1998;12:
418–423.

39. Kost GJ. Planning and implementing point-of-care testing systems. In:

40. Tobin MJ, ed. *Principles and practice of intensive care monitoring.* New
York: McGraw-Hill, 1997:1297–1299.

40. American Diabetes Association. National standards for diabetes selfmanagement education programs and American Diabetes Association
review criteria. *Diabet Care* 1998;21[Suppl 1]:2–3.

41. Buckner F. Telemedicine: the state of the art and current issues. *J Med
Pract Mgmt* 1998;14:145–149.

42. Hoffman J. The risks of patient encounters by telephone. *J Med Pract
Mgmt* 1998;14:160.

43. Stevens L. Virtually there. *Am Med News* 1998;41:24–27.

44. Baldwin G. Doctor benefits from e-mail efficiency with patients. *Am
Med News* 1998;41:29–30.

45. Kane B, Sands DZ, Task Force on Guidelines for the Use of ClinicPatient Electronic Mail. Guidelines for the clinical use of electronic
mail with patients. *J Am Med Informatics Assoc* 1998;5:104–111.

46. Spielberg AR. On call and online: sociohistorical, legal and ethical
implications of e-mail for the patient-physician relationship. *JAMA*
1998;280:1353–1359.

47. Bergeron BP, Bailin MT. The technological underpinnings of a modern clinical practice. *J Med Pract Mgmt* 1998;7:150–153.

48. Cublio NA, Carevic K, Mowrey KA, et al. *Application of telemedicine to
pharmacy practice: the concept of telepharmacy.* Abstract presented at the
1998 American Society of Health-System Pharmacists mid-year clinical meeting, Las Vegas, NV, December 6–10, 1998.

49. Bondmass M. *Home care by telephone: integration of technology to
improve outcomes.* Abstract presented at American Society of HealthSystem Pharmacists mid-year clinical meeting, Las Vegas, NV, December 6–10, 1998.

50. Elevitch FR. Multimedia communications networks: patient care
through interactive point-of-care testing. *Clin Lab Med* 1994;14:
559–567.

51. Maclin E, Mahoney WC. Point-of-care testing technology. *J Clin Ligand Assay* 1995;18:21–33.

52. Wiebe C. Ouchless medicine. *Am Med News* 1998;39:29–30.

53. Kahn J. Emerging technologies target point-of-care settings. *Clin Chem
News* 1993;19:1.

54. Tamada JA, Garg S, Jovanovid L, et al. Noninvasive glucose monitoring. *JAMA* 1999;282:1839–1844.

55. Uehling M. Under the skin: sorting through the hype and hope for
noninvasive POC devices. *CAP Today* 2000;7:56–68.

56. Titus K. Future of self-test market not in the bag. *CAP Today* 1999;13:
80–81.

57. Stevens JF, Vadgama P. Infrared analysis in clinical chemistry: its use in
the laboratory and in non-invasive near patient testing. *Ann Clin
Biochem* 1997;34:215–221.

58. Sunheimer RR. En route to non-invasive cholesterol testing. *AdvanceLab* November 2000;74–77.

59. George JR, Fitchen JH. Future applications of oral fluid specimen
technology. *Am J Med* 1997;102:21–25.

24

ADVANCES IN THE PHYSICIAN OFFICE LABORATORY

JOHN T. BENJAMIN
C. ROBERT BAISDEN

THE OFFICE LABORATORY AND CLIA '88 LEGISLATION

Introduction

The office laboratory has undergone significant changes over the past ten years. This chapter reviews the history of those changes and some of the forces that have brought about those changes. Test complexity and personnel requirements will be explained. We also discuss the physical setup of a laboratory, laboratory safety, nine steps needed to follow in order to establish a laboratory, and tests to consider performing in an office laboratory. The overall goal of this chapter is to provide the reader with a historical background in the office laboratory, and also to provide practical information of how to start up and maintain an office laboratory.

In 1988, Congress passed the Clinical Laboratory Improvement Amendments of 1988 (CLIA '88), replacing the then-current Medicare/Medicaid and CLIA '67 standards with a single set of requirements that applied to all laboratory testing of human specimens (1). CLIA '88 set the standards for laboratory personnel, quality control (QC), and quality assurance (QA) based on test complexity and risk factors. For the first time, laboratory tests had been divided according to the level of complexity in performing the procedures. The three categories of complexity are waived tests, tests of moderate complexity, and tests of high complexity. In 1993, the provider-performed microscopy (PPM) category was added as a subgroup under the moderately complex category. The secretary of the Department of Health and Human Services (DHHS) published the final rules implementing the Clinical Laboratory Improvement Amendments of 1988 on February 28, 1992.

For laboratories performing moderate and/or high complexity tests, there were now requirements for proficiency testing, written QC procedures, a comprehensive QA program, and personnel standards. The personnel standards included the qualifications for laboratory director, technical consultant, clinical consultant, and testing personnel. In addition, the CLIA '88 regulations required that user fees finance the program. The regulated laboratories were required to pay all costs involved in issuing certificates, conducting special studies mandated by CLIA '88, developing and conducting surveyor training and the cost of a biennial on-site inspection. The fees are based on laboratory test volume and the number of test specialties. The test volume for purposes of determining fee amounts excludes tests performed for QC and proficiency testing.

Test Complexity

Waived Tests

CLIA '88 provided that the secretary of the DHHS may determine that simple tests which have an insignificant risk of an erroneous result be classified as waived. Waived tests may include tests approved by the Food and Drug Administration (FDA) for home use, tests employing methods that are so simple and accurate as to be unlikely to render erroneous results, and tests determined by the secretary to pose no reasonable risk of patient harm if performed incorrectly.

The original list of waived tests included dipstick or tablet reagent urinalysis, ovulation tests (visual color test for human lutenizing hormone), urine pregnancy test (vision color comparison test), erythrocyte sedimentation rate (nonautomated), hemoglobin copper sulfate, fecal occult blood, spun microhematocrit, and blood glucose by glucose monitoring devices cleared by the FDA specifically for home use. In 2000, the number of waived analytes had increased from eight to 26 (Table 24.1).

All office laboratories and laboratories not associated with a hospital must obtain a certificate of waiver before performing any of the waived tests. The application for certificate of waiver is made to the DHHS on a form prescribed by DHHS. The form must be signed by the laboratory owner or an authorized representative of the laboratory who attests that the laboratory will be operated in accordance with requirements established by the secretary as defined by CLIA '88. The application includes a description of the characteristics of the laboratory operation and the test procedures performed by the laboratory including the names and total number of test procedures and examinations performed annually. Excluded are tests the laboratory may run for QC, QA, or proficiency testing procedures. The methodologies for each laboratory procedure or examination performed must be stated. The educational background, training, and experience of the personnel directing and supervising the laboratory as well as those performing laboratory examinations and test procedures must be specifically stated.

TABLE 24.1. WAIVED TESTS (JANUARY, 2002)

Category	Name of Analyte
Bacteriology/virology	Helicobacter pylori
	Group A streptococcus
	Influenza A and B
Endocrinology	HCG urine
	Ovulation test (visual color comparison)
	Urine hCG (visual color comparison)
	N-telopeptides (for osteoporosis)
	FSH and LH
	Estrone-3 glucuronide
	Semen (for male fertility screen)
General chemistry	Amines
	Lactic acid
	Cholesterol
	Fecal occult blood
	Fructosamine
	Gastric occult Blood
	Glucose (glucose monitoring)
	Hemoglobin A_1C
	Microalbumin
	Triglycerides
	HDL cholesterol
	Ketones (blood and urine)
	Lyme disease antibodies
	Bladder tumor associated antigen
	Vaginal pH
	Alanine aminotransferase (ALT)
General immunology	H. pylori antibodies
	Infectious mononucleosis
Hematology	Sedimentation rate
	Hematocrit
	Hemoglobin
	Prothrombin time (PT)
Toxicology	Nicotine
	Ethanol (saliva alcohol)
	Cocaine
	Metabolites
	Cannabinoids
	Opiates
	PCP
	Amphetamines/methamphetamines
Urinalysis	Urine catalase
	Urine dipstick
	Urine qualitative dipstick (automated)

hCG, human chroionic gonadotropin; HDL, high-density lipoprotein.

The laboratory agrees to provide access to the DHHS or its representative in order to determine compliance with the requirements for waived testing. The laboratory must also agree to permit announced and unannounced inspections by the DHHS. In addition, the laboratory must permit access to the premises for the DHHS when there is a requirement to evaluate complaints from the public, or when it should determine whether the laboratory is performing tests not listed as waived tests.

A certificate of waiver is issued for no more than 2 years. The current address for forwarding remittance is HCFA Laboratory Program, P.O. Box 849036, Dallas, TX 75284-9036.

TABLE 24.2. PROVIDER-PERFORMED MICROSCOPY TESTS

Wet mounts, including preparations of vaginal, cervical or skin specimens.
All potassium hydroxide preparations
Pinworm examinations
Fern test
Post-coital direct exams, qualitative examinations of vaginal or cervical mucous
Urinalysis: microscopic only
Urinalysis: by dipstick or tablet reagent for bilirubin, glucose, hemoglobin, ketones, leukocytes, nitrite, pH, protein, specific gravity, urobilinogen, nonautomated with microscopy
Urinalysis: by dipstick or tablet reagent for bilirubin, glucose, hemoglobin, ketones, leukocytes, nitrite, pH, protein, specific gravity, urobilinogen, automated (waived) with microscopy
Fecal leukocyte examination
Semen analysis; presence and/or motility of sperm excluding Huhner
Nasal smear for eosinophils and granulocytes
Wet mount-prostate secretions

Provider-Performed Microscopy

A provider-performed microscopy (PPM) certificate may be issued to a laboratory in which a physician, mid-level practitioner, or dentist performs no test other than PPM procedures, and, if desired, specific waived tests listed on the certificate of waiver. A midlevel practitioner is defined as a nurse midwife, nurse practitioner, or physician assistant licensed by the state within which the individual practices.

A provider-performed microscopy procedure is defined as an examination that must be personally performed by one of the following practitioners: a physician during the patient's visit on a specimen obtained from his or her patient, or from a patient of a group medical practice of which the physician is a member or an employee. A midlevel practitioner, under the supervision of the physician or an independent practice authorized by the state, may examine during the patient's visit a specimen obtained from his or her own patient or from a patient of a clinic, group medical practice, or other healthcare provider of which the midlevel practitioner is a member or an employee. During the patient's visit a dentist may examine a specimen obtained from his or her patient or from a patient of a group dental practice of which the dentist is a member or an employee. The ten PPM tests are listed in Table 24.2. Even though PPM tests do not require inspection, a PPM procedure is categorized as moderately complex. The primary instrument for performing a PPM test is the microscope, limited to bright field or phase contrast microscopy. A laboratory performing PPM procedures must obtain a certificate for PPM procedures.

Moderate Complexity Tests

Physicians may choose to perform several moderately complex tests in their offices in order to expedite diagnoses and treatments for their patients. Moderate complexity tests include certain bacteriology, microbacteriology, mycology, parasitology, limited virology, immunology, routine chemistry, urinalysis, hematology, and limited immunohematology tests. Other tests such as semen analysis, occult blood on body fluids, crystal

TABLE 24.3. EXAMPLES OF MODERATELY COMPLEX TESTS

Complete blood count
Differential
Reticulocyte count
Throat culture
Automated chemistries
Blood gases
Urine culture: identification of positive or negative only
Limited gram stain
Some rapid streptococcal antigen tests
Rapid-slide infectious mononucleosis tests done on serum or plasma
Rapid *H. pylori* antibody tests done on serum or plasma
Influenza A tests; Influenza A and B test
Lead level tests
DNA probe tests for gardnerella, candida, and trichimonas
Immunology tests for T4, T3 uptake, quantitative hCG

analysis on joint fluid, and viscosity are moderately complex tests. Some moderately complex tests that are frequently used in the office laboratory are listed in Table 24.3.

Laboratories performing tests of moderate complexity must use an instrument, kit, or test system cleared by the FDA through premarket notification or approval, and the laboratory must follow the manufacturer's instructions for the instrument of test system operation and test performance. In addition, the laboratory must have a procedure manual describing the processes for testing and reporting patient results. Laboratories also must perform and document calibration procedures or check calibration at least once every 6 months; perform and document a control procedure using at least two levels of control materials each day of testing; perform and document applicable specialty and subspecialty control procedures; perform and document that remedial action has been taken when problems or errors are identified; and maintain records of all QC activities for 2 years. QC records for immunohematology and blood and blood products must be maintained for 5 years after completion of the tests.

Personnel Requirements

While there are no personnel requirements for a laboratory certified to perform waived tests, laboratories performing tests of moderate complexity must meet requirements for positions of laboratory director, technical consultant, clinical consultant, and testing personnel.

The laboratory director may be a pathologist, licensed MD or DO, and have 1 year of experience directing/supervising non-waived tests or have at least 20 CME credit hours in laboratory practice commensurate with director responsibilities or laboratory training during residency equivalent to the above, or certification in hematology or hematology/oncology. The director may be a PhD with a degree in science plus laboratory-related board certification or 1 year of full-time experience supervising nonwaived testing. The director may have a master's degree in science with 1 year of laboratory training or experience, and 1 year of supervisory experience. A person with a master's degree in science may serve as a laboratory director of a moderately complex laboratory if he or she has 2 years of laboratory training or experience and 2 years of supervisory experience.

A technical consultant is responsible for the technical and scientific oversight of the laboratory. The laboratory director may qualify as the technical consultant with the above listed requirements. The clinical consultant can provide information about the appropriateness of the laboratory testing done, and about how diagnosis and treatment of patients is affected by utilization of the office laboratory. The clinical consultant must be an MD, DO, or PhD who qualifies as a laboratory director.

Testing personnel must have at least a high school graduate or equivalent degree with documented training appropriate for the testing performed in the laboratory. Knowledge about specimen collection, proper instrument use, and assessment of validity of patient test results is required.

The laboratory performing moderately complex tests must pay a current registration fee for a certificate of accreditation or certificate of compliance, and a volume-related fee. Laboratories performing moderate or high complexity tests must submit to unannounced inspections that are conducted at least on a biennial basis unless the laboratory is located in a state whose licensure program is approved by the Center for Medicare and Medicaid Services (CMS). The laboratory may be accredited by a Center for Medicare and Medicaid Services-approved, private, nonprofit accrediting agency such as the College of American Pathologists' Laboratory Accreditation Program or a similar program provided by the Joint Commission on Accreditation of Healthcare Organizations. Laboratories performing only waived tests and/or PPM are not routinely inspected. The HCFA reserves the right to conduct inspections to investigate complaints or to ensure that only waived tests are being performed in such a laboratory. Failure to permit an inspection of the laboratory results in immediate suspension of Medicare or Medicaid payments and in the initiation of action to revoke the laboratory certificate.

FACTORS RECENTLY AFFECTING THE OFFICE LABORATORY

The Changing Effects of CLIA '88 on the Office Laboratory

The initial passage of CLIA '88 sent shock waves through the private physician community. The original language of the legislation was quite punitive, and resulted in many physicians either limiting their test menus (number of tests performed in the office laboratory), or even closing their laboratories. For example, in a survey of 1,030 practices in 1995, 72% of pediatricians, 69% of family practitioners, and 14% of internal medicine groups had either modified their test menus or eliminated their office laboratories (2). Respondents to the survey gave as their reasons the expense, onerous paperwork, and punitive approach of the CLIA '88, as well as the effects of managed care.

Over recent years, however, the original punitive approach of CLIA '88 has been replaced by a more educational approach. Laboratories are still inspected carefully for QA, but severe sanctions have been infrequent. Instead of levying monetary fines or forcing laboratories to close—as recommended in the original legislation—inspectors now give corrective advice to laboratory personnel. For example, the original legislation indicated that if a specific office laboratory failed two out of three proficiency tests, that laboratory could no longer test for that analyte. Now, when errors are made in the office laboratory, the personnel are asked to present a written plan that demonstrates the changes they have made to improve their results. During the time period of this corrective action, the laboratory continues to run the analyte, and, if improved proficiency testing is demonstrated, nothing further needs to be done. In the past several years, this focus on education has encouraged many physicians—who had earlier closed their office laboratories in reaction to CLIA '88—to reopen their laboratories and reexpand their test menus. Information compiled by the American Association of Family Physicians between 1992 and 1997 (3) shows that the percentage of family practitioners doing office laboratory tests dropped from 93% in 1992 to 88% in 1993 to 79% in 1994, but rose to 82% in 1995 and to 92% in 1996 and 1997. Since CLIA '88 inspections emphasized QA, office laboratory testing became more nearly accurate, and the results more reproducible. A number of publications have confirmed that laboratory testing has improved in recent years (4). Despite the concern expressed by physicians when CLIA '88 was first passed, this legislation has ultimately improved office laboratory testing, and therefore, has resulted in a major advance for the office laboratory.

The Effects of Managed Care on the Office Laboratory

A second major influence on the office laboratory in recent years has been the effect of managed care organizations on the office laboratory. In the early 1990s, few of these administrative groups were supportive of doctors doing tests in their office laboratories. Their reasoning was that if a test could be performed at a lower cost in a reference laboratory, it made little sense to allow fee-for-service in-house testing. However, in recent years, the relationship between managed care companies and physician office laboratories has undergone a significant change. Many managed care companies now understand that office laboratories allow physicians to make earlier diagnoses and start treatment earlier, thus preventing more serious illnesses and even hospital admissions. In other words, instead of looking at office laboratories as cost centers, many managed care companies now see office laboratories as cost savers. In 1996, a group of 14 managed care companies allowed an average of six tests per office laboratory to be done on a fee-for-service basis; in 1998, that figure had increased to 14 tests allowed (5). Not all managed care companies have changed their approach to office testing, and some physicians are unaware that they can negotiate with them on this issue. However, the greater tendency for managed care companies to support the use of office laboratories has helped open the way for physicians to expand or to reopen their laboratories.

The Effects of Technology on the Office Laboratory

In addition to changes in CLIA '88 regulations and a new awareness among managed care companies, a third significant factor promoting the office laboratory has been the technological explosion in laboratory equipment. Manufacturers recognized that physicians would prefer waived testing to moderately complex testing with its requirement of increased paperwork and resultant costs of inspection. Over the past few years, the efforts of manufacturers have been highly successful. When CLIA '88 was first enforced in 1992, only eight tests were waived. By 2000, the number had risen to 26 (Table 24.1). Technology, in the form of new office instruments, has been responsible for this increase. In addition, the federal government expedited its procedures for the approval of new waived laboratory equipment by utilizing personnel from the laboratory branch of the Centers for Disease Control and Prevention.

Not only is the new laboratory technology highly accurate and easy to use, it also is less expensive than earlier instruments. For example, an instrument testing for cholesterol and HDL costs $1,800, and a fingerstick hemoglobin test can be done on a $600 instrument. The cost of moderately complex equipment has also recently become more affordable. Some complete-blood-count instruments, formerly available only in the $20,000 to $25,000 range, can now be purchased for between $7,000 and $12,000. Also, a moderately complex lead-testing instrument, formerly available only as a $10,000 to $15,000 tabletop model, can now be purchased as a handheld instrument for about $1,800.

It is not surprising, given these technological developments, that the number of waived office laboratories increased. In 1997, the total number of waived office laboratories was 29,749; by 1999, that number had increased to 37,730. In that 2-year time period, the percentage of waived office laboratories rose from 34% to 41% of all office laboratories, while moderately complex laboratories decreased from 34% to 20% of the total (6).

Additional changes in CLIA regulations that may occur in the near future are expected to further strengthen the office laboratory. In late 1999, a major overhaul of CLIA '88 regulations was expected, including changes in QC that would ease the administrative procedure for classifying tests as waived and facilitate inspection procedures for the moderately complex laboratory. In February 1999, Bill Archer (R-TX) reintroduced a bill in Congress recommending the exemption of all office laboratory testing from CLIA '88 requirements. A similar bill failed in 1995 (7).

Effect of Development of the Provider Performed Microscopy Category on the Office Laboratory

A fourth major influence on the promotion of the office laboratory was the creation, in 1993, of the PPM category. As described above, while PPM laboratories must comply with the same personnel standards as moderately complex laboratories, these ten tests do not require inspection. In 1999, combined with the 26 waived tests, the total number of tests that can be done in the office laboratory without an inspection now numbers 36—quite a different figure from the eight tests originally waived in 1992. Between 1997 and 1999, the number of PPM laboratories has risen from 22,861 to 28,446, representing an increase from 26% to 31% of the total number of office laboratories in that time period. In 1999, 72% of all office laboratories were waived and PPM laboratories—a remarkable combined increase of 16% in the previous 2-year time period (8).

With this background, we now discuss the nine steps that can be followed to begin an office laboratory and provide a summary of some of the more frequently used tests in the office laboratory. Clinical scenarios are presented that illustrate the advantages of doing these tests in the office laboratory.

ESTABLISHING AN OFFICE LABORATORY

Physical Setup of an Office Laboratory

Office laboratories vary considerably in size and location within the office. Whatever the space restrictions might be, most laboratories can be divided into three distinct areas: a receiving area, a testing area, and an administrative area. The administrative area is the only truly clean area; all other areas of the laboratory are considered dirty areas (9,10).

If space allows, it is desirable for each laboratory to have at least two sinks, two refrigerators, and plentiful storage cabinets and drawers, and all should provide adequate ventilation. Office laboratories should follow Occupational Safety and Health Administration (OSHA) safety regulations, which include the availability of eyewash, a fire extinguisher, and material safety data sheets. Records and reports should document the disposition of waste and chemicals and the immunization and continuing medical education credits of the personnel doing the laboratory work.

It has been estimated that there should be 114 to 220 square feet of space for each person performing technical procedures in the laboratory. On the average, 140 square feet per technician are adequate for performing most procedures in an office laboratory that is used for a variety of tests. It is obvious that if only hematocrits or dipstick urinalyses are being performed, this figure is somewhat generous. However, the variety and the complexity of procedures tend to increase with the growth of a physician's practice. For this reason, future expansion must be kept in mind when first locating the laboratory in the office complex. If the physician intends to take on an associate or

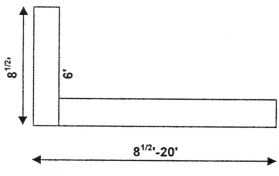

FIGURE 24.2. The "L-shaped" laboratory.

develop a group practice, plans must be made for laboratory expansion, because the number as well as the variety and complexity of the procedures performed will increase geometrically.

Since a significant percentage of the patients visiting the office will require a laboratory procedure, we urge that the physician locate the laboratory, especially the specimen procurement area, in a place that is convenient both to the office personnel and the patients. The laboratory should be centralized so as to increase the efficiency of the technician.

The simplest small laboratory has a *straight bench,* which should be at least 5 feet to 6 feet long and 30″ in depth (Fig. 24.1). The bench should be 28″ to 30″ in height above the floor. There should be a leg space, usually 24″ to 26″ wide and 24″ to 26″ in height, which permits the technician to sit comfortably at the bench while using a microscope or writing. A suitable chair with good back support that the technician can roll comfortably under the bench should be provided.

For the somewhat larger laboratory, an *L-shaped configuration* is very efficient since it will fit into a corner (Fig. 24.2). One portion of the L may be used as a sit-down area while the other portion may be raised to 36″, which is a convenient height for a benchtop in a stand-up work area. This counter should be 30″ in depth and a minimum of 5 feet to 6 feet in length. One should consider the advisability of having leg space available under this elevated bench. Sitting down while working at an elevated bench requires a bar-stool type of seat, which has a higher center of gravity and is somewhat of a safety hazard. There are high stools available that have five casters instead of the more tiltable four casters in the base.

A *C-shaped laboratory* (Fig. 24.3) is very efficient and especially convenient for one technologist who is performing several

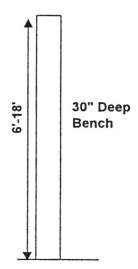

FIGURE 24.1. The "bench" laboratory.

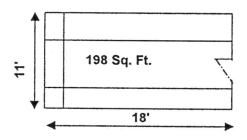

FIGURE 24.3. The "C-shaped" laboratory.

different procedures. Each side of the C should allow at least 6 feet of bench space, which would result in a total space requirement of 93.5 square feet. This is obviously significantly less than the 140 square feet that was noted as adequate earlier; however, it provides the minimal functional space requirement for a laboratory offering procedures from more than two of the major categories. It is most important that the space be sufficient. For example, a centrifuge should not be placed beside the microscope because this will result in vibrations that prohibit the simultaneous use of the microscope. Again, it is important not to place the chemistry or microbiology incubator next to the refrigerator for obvious reasons of heat transfer.

As the laboratory grows, more space will be needed for refrigeration. The leg space under a stand-up bench may be used for an under-the-counter refrigerator; however, these are generally much more expensive than a small- to moderate-size household freezer/refrigerator combination, which can be purchased at a local discount store. A word of caution: space should be allowed for a larger refrigerator during initial planning of the laboratory, but plans must not be made to store food, drugs, and other consumables in the same refrigerator in which specimens are stored. The possibility of contaminating an employee's lunch with a specimen containing hepatitis virus is just too great. Likewise, the possibility of a busy nurse picking up an ampule of reagents and inadvertently injecting the contents into a patient should be seriously considered.

If the workload in the office requires two technicians to be present in the laboratory at the same time, the planner will most likely want to consider a larger C-shaped module of 11 feet × 18 feet, which requires 198 square feet of space. Such an arrangement permits a 6-foot bench on the backside of the C and two 15.5-foot sections of bench space on the top and bottom portion of the C. If three to four technicians are required to perform the tests on a daily basis, the planner will want to consider combining two of the C-shaped modules into an E-shaped laboratory (Fig. 24.4). A minimum of 396 square feet

will be required for this laboratory configuration. This again yields less than the amount of space considered adequate per technician (140 square feet, or 560 square feet for four technicians). However, additional space will be needed to provide for such things as a large refrigerator, file cabinets for permanent records, and storage space for large shipments of reagents and supplies, which will allow the purchasing of supplies at volume discounts.

Laboratory Safety

The following laboratory safety rules (10) should be posted in each laboratory work area. Every laboratory technical worker in addition to nurses and office personnel who visit the laboratory should review a list of laboratory safety rules and acknowledge having read such rules by means of signature or initials. The following list is strongly recommended:

1. Smoking is prohibited in the laboratory.
2. Food and drink are prohibited in the laboratory.
3. Cosmetics may not be applied while in the laboratory.
4. Safety glasses or facial shields must be worn when handling caustic or toxic materials. Eye protection devices must be worn when handling blood or other specimens that may contain infectious agents.
5. Gowns, aprons, or laboratory coats are required when working in the laboratory area. Shoes should cover the entire foot. Canvas shoes are not recommended.
6. Hair should be secured back and off the shoulders in such a manner as to prevent it from contact with contaminated materials and to prevent shedding organisms in the working area. Hair and long beards must be kept out of moving equipment such as centrifuges.
7. Hands should be washed after removing gloves, before leaving the laboratory, before and after contact with each patient, and before eating and smoking.
8. An eyewash should be readily available where ever acids, caustics, corrosives, and other hazardous chemicals are used. The eyewash should be tested each week to ensure proper functioning and to flush stagnant water.
9. Mouth pipetting is prohibited.
10. Gloves should be worn at all times while obtaining a specimen from a patient. Gloves should be worn while handling patient specimens and performing procedures.
11. Discard broken or chipped glassware.
12. Centrifuges may not be operated unless the covers are closed. Specimen tubes are to remain capped while being centrifuged. The centrifuge must be properly balanced prior to operation. Centrifuges should be routinely cleaned with a 1:10 dilution of sodium hypochlorite or other appropriate disinfectant.

Nine Steps of Establishing an Office Laboratory

After a room is chosen and prepared and safety procedures identified and listed, there are nine specific steps that, if followed, will help ensure the development of a smoothly functioning lab-

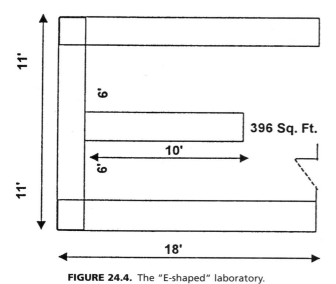

FIGURE 24.4. The "E-shaped" laboratory.

TABLE 24.4. NINE STEPS TO STARTING AN OFFICE LABORATORY

Steps	Comments
1. Decide on the complexity of the laboratory.	Consider waived, moderately complex, PPM, or highly complex.
2. Decide which instruments to obtain and how to pay for them.	See worksheet in Table 24.5. Consider buying or leasing.
3. Decide which personnel are going to be responsible for doing the testing.	Medical technologist versus high school graduate: consider pros and cons.
4. Choose the accrediting agency: Centers for Medicare & Medicaid Services or COLA.	Call other offices in the area and check with them.
5. Choose a proficiency testing agency.	Most physicians sign up with agency in their academy's home office.
6. Fill out Centers for Medicare & Medicaid Services form 116.	Must be completed even if accredited by COLA.
7. Prepare for inspection.	Moderate or high complexity only.
8. Keep up with the changes after inspection.	Newsletters and meetings should be considered.
9. Do a financial analysis (Table 24.5).	Will laboratory pay for itself?

COLA, Commission on Office Laboratory Accreditation.

oratory (11). Some of these steps, such as choosing a proficiency testing agency, and preparing for inspection, would not be necessary if developing a waived or PPM laboratory. These nine steps are summarized in Table 24.4.

The first step in establishing an office laboratory is to decide whether the laboratory will be characterized as waived, moderately complex, PPM, or highly complex. Few office laboratories are in the highly complex category, and, therefore, are not discussed here. In general, most physicians will opt for the waived or PPM, unless they want to do a complete blood count (CBC), cultures or blood chemistry, which require moderately complex laboratories. If only one of the many tests performed in an office laboratory is moderately complex, then that laboratory would be classified as moderately complex.

Once the decision has been made about the desired test menu, the second step in establishing an office laboratory is to decide what instruments to use and how to pay for them. The physician needs to make a judgment about the number of tests envisioned in the office laboratory, what the cost of each test will be (cost of reagents, controls, proficiency testing, personnel time, and other overhead), and what the most likely source and amount of reimbursement for that test might be. Ideally, most instruments should pay for themselves after 12 to 18 months of use. Comparison of the costs of leasing should be done before considering buying an instrument. Prior to any purchase of laboratory equipment, physicians must make sure that their managed care companies will allow them to perform the tests in the office laboratory, and should also call other physicians who have used the instrument to make sure that the technology is easy to use and reliable. The worksheet in Table 24.5 can be utilized to make the financial calculations.

In a recent development, manufacturers of instruments now partner much more closely with office laboratory personnel than in the past. Manufacturers provide in-depth analyses of the cost feasibility of buying new instruments, provide in-office training for using their instruments, demonstrate the paperwork necessary under CLIA '88 regulations, and also allow testing the equipment in the office prior to purchase. Package inserts provided by the manufacturer have been written so that they can become part of the procedure manual. In other words, these

TABLE 24.5. FINANCIAL CHECKLIST: COST VERSUS REIMBURSEMENT

Reminder #1: Most instruments should pay for themselves in 12 to 18 months.
#2: Always check with managed care company before obtaining instrument!

Expenses of all instruments/month	
Monthly cost of buying or leasing instruments/month	_____
Maintenance cost of instrument/month: 10% × purchase price/year/12	_____
CLIA costs to be considered for inspection per month	_____
Proficiency testing costs per month	_____
Personnel costs per month: include all benefits	_____
Space costs: will vary with rent and size of instrument	_____
All reagent, control, calibration costs per month	_____
Structural costs needed in laboratory if any, per month	_____
Total cost per month for laboratory	_____
Income calculation	
Reimbursement per test[a]	
Number of tests anticipate doing per month	_____
Drawing fee per venipuncture per month	_____
Reimbursement/month: # tests × reimbursement + drawing fee per month	_____
Total profit (or loss): reimbursement minus cost per month	_____

[a]Need to calculate managed care reimbursement, Medicaid or Medicare reimbursement, private insurance reimbursement, and decide what percentages of each apply to your practice.

companies help minimize the effects of CLIA '88 on the office laboratory for physicians.

The third step in creating an office laboratory is to decide which personnel will be responsible for doing the testing, the controls, and all the paperwork. The minimum requirement to do testing in a moderately complex office laboratory is a high school degree, and many physicians train their laboratory personnel on the job. On the other hand, other groups choose to hire medical technologists. This decision is often based on weighing the advantages of having a knowledgeable person in the laboratory against the costs of hiring a technologist. Larger groups of doctors (three to five) usually can afford the salary and fringe benefits of a medical technologist more easily than smaller groups.

Another decision is whether the physician or the person working in the laboratory should become the laboratory director. Medical technologists with 2 years of training/experience plus 2 years of supervisory experience are qualified to serve as laboratory directors of moderately complex laboratories. Physicians who had not directed a laboratory prior to February 28, 1992, must obtain 20 hours of CME in lab practice to qualify to direct a moderate complexity lab. Most private offices now have one designated person in charge of the entire lab even if many people do the testing.

After deciding on the test menu, the instruments that are to be used, and the personnel involved in running the laboratory, the fourth step in establishing an office laboratory is to choose the accrediting agent—either the CMS, a governmental agency, or the Commission on Office Laboratory Accreditation (COLA), a private physician-directed organization. A confusing point is that, even if an office chooses COLA to inspect its laboratory, it still must register with CMS (see sixth step below). The costs of the two agencies are similar, but the choice of agency can often depend on the approach of the individual inspector to the office laboratory. Recent data have shown that of the 35,000 moderately or highly complex office laboratories that require inspection, CMS has about three times more registrants than COLA.

The fifth step in establishing an office laboratory is to choose a proficiency testing agency. Proficiency testing—the testing and reporting of unknown samples provided through a central agency—helps assure the accuracy of the testing done in office laboratories. Other than the pinworm test, proficiency testing is not necessary for the waived and PPM laboratories. Only the moderately and highly complex labs require proficiency testing. In most proficiency testing programs, unknown specimens are sent to the participating office laboratory three to six times a year. Ten to 14 days are usually allowed for reporting test results to the proficiency testing provider. Summary reports indicating whether a laboratory has passed or failed are provided to each laboratory. If proficiency testing is failed, a plan of corrective action must be devised, implemented immediately, and reported to the provider. The most important reason to do proficiency testing is that it proves that a laboratory can get reproducible test results. By obtaining such reliable results, the patient is much better served. Office laboratories have improved greatly in recent years in their proficiency testing, meaning that patients are getting more reliable test results.

There are now over 20 approved proficiency testing agencies for office laboratories. The American Academy of Pediatrics, the American Academy of Family Medicine, and the American Society of Internal Medicine each has its own proficiency testing organization. The physician chooses the agency. Comparative costs for most of the organizations are similar.

The sixth step in establishing an office laboratory is to fill out CMS form 116, which requests demographic information about the laboratory, the name of the laboratory director, the level of certificate requested (waived, PPM, or regular), the lab's hours of operation, and whether the lab is accredited by a non-CMS accrediting agency. If you have a shared lab, only one certificate for that lab need be obtained.

The seventh step in creating an office laboratory is to prepare for inspection. Quality assurance and QC are emphasized in laboratory inspections. Documentation of all activities in the laboratory must be carefully done. The results of all tests performed must be documented, including controls run, instrument calibrations, proficiency testing, and correction of errors. In addition, all laboratory results for the past 2 years must be kept in an orderly fashion, and a complete procedure manual detailing all testing procedures must be available for the inspector. Personnel information, including demonstration of hepatitis B vaccination or declination form, OSHA bloodborne-pathogen training records, diplomas and other educational certificates, continuing education records, job descriptions, and competency assessment evaluation forms must also be documented and available.

Paper-based self-surveys are now available from the CMS (Alternate Quality Assessment Survey) and the Committee on Office Laboratory Accreditation (Performance Based Survey). These surveys are alternatives for those laboratories who had few or no deficiencies on their initial on-site survey, no proficiency testing failures since their last survey, and can substitute for the on-site survey in an every other 2-year cycle.

Consultants are available to help physicians prepare for laboratory inspections. There are a number of very qualified consultants, but physicians find those with office laboratory experience more helpful than those with only hospital laboratory experience.

Very few office laboratories have been sanctioned or closed down as a result of failed inspections. When laboratories have been forced to close, it has almost always been the result of a total disregard for quality laboratory testing methods and a refusal to implement changes that were recommended by the accrediting agency.

The eighth step in establishing and maintaining an office laboratory is to keep up with the changes that occur after inspection. Reinspections, whether by paper or on site, will occur every 2 years, and it is the duty of the physician to keep up with the changes in the office laboratory that might have occurred during that interval. Consultants can share these changes by calling the COLA toll-free number (1-800-298-8044), or by attending meetings on the subject of office laboratories. In addition, newsletters such as the *Washington G-2 Reports* (1-800-LAB-REGS) are helpful in keeping physicians current about legislative changes.

The ninth step in establishing an office laboratory is to take all the information gathered in the first eight steps and do a financial analysis, which should help determine whether the laboratory will be a cost center or a profit center. Some physicians will continue to have an office laboratory even if it represents a cost center; most will not start a laboratory. Some physicians think that an office laboratory is so important to their practice of medicine that they absorb some cost in running the laboratory. Others will be more interested in running a laboratory only if it is a profit center.

All costs need to be summarized and subtracted from the income anticipated, so that a profit margin can be calculated. Costs and income are most easily calculated per month. A worksheet, provided in Table 24.5, can be utilized when starting a laboratory, or when considering adding a new test to the office laboratory menu. The following items need to be considered when determining the *costs* of running an office laboratory:

- Cost of equipment. A decision must be made whether to buy or lease the instrument (calculation: cost per month for each instrument).
- Maintenance cost of each instrument per month. Maintenance agreements typically cost 10% of the purchase price per year. If a yearly maintenance agreement is to be obtained, that cost will need to be divided by 12 to get the monthly cost.
- CLIA or inspection costs depending on the agency. These costs will vary with the size of the laboratory, and the number and the specialties of the tests performed. Registration costs are based on the volume of tests performed—the higher the volume, the greater the costs. Each laboratory should calculate a monthly figure for CLIA and inspection costs.
- Proficiency testing costs per month for moderately and highly complex tests. After a proficiency testing agency is chosen, monthly costs can be easily obtained.
- Cost of personnel. More than just the monthly salary must be included in this calculation. The true cost of an employee includes the total economic package: health insurance, pension plan, vacation coverage, sick leave, continuing education fees, and so on (calculation: monthly amount for entire cost of employee).
- Size and space of the room used for the laboratory. An estimated amount of rent can be calculated for the monthly use of this room (calculations: square footage × $/square foot per month).
- Cost of reagents and controls. This figure will depend on the number of tests to be performed in the laboratory and must be determined for all instruments in the laboratory (calculation: monthly cost of all reagents and controls).
- Structural costs needed in laboratory if any. When obtaining instruments for a laboratory, some manufacturers will bear the burden of extra cabinets, shelving, and so on that might be needed to accommodate their instrument. If not, this figure needs to be included.
- Write-offs. In any calculation of expenses, the number of write-offs must be considered. Some managed care companies will not allow physicians to be reimbursed for certain tests done in their laboratories. These expenses need to be considered. For instance, if Company X is the managed care company for 20% of the patients, and the company does not allow a CBC to be reimbursed when performed in the office

laboratory, 20% of anticipated income needs to be considered a cost item. Also, if Medicare reimburses less than the charged amount, that figure needs to be determined as well (calculation: monthly expense of write-offs).

The *income* from an office laboratory should then be determined. Of course, the income will depend on the size of the physician group—the larger the number of doctors, the more tests will be ordered, and the more likely profit can be achieved. A general rule of thumb is that the smallest group for which an office laboratory is profitable is three physicians. The following items should be included in the calculations of income:

- Reimbursement per test and number of procedures anticipated for each instrument. Reimbursement figures are readily obtainable through the appropriate insurance companies, but the number of procedures may be more difficult to predict. If, for instance, the decision has been made to buy a CBC instrument, the number of CBCs performed over the previous month should be determined. That number should then be multiplied by the number of dollars charged for each test and a monthly figure determined. In fact, most groups find that once they have an instrument in their office laboratory, they order more tests than in the past. However, conservative estimates should be employed (calculation: number of tests/month × $/test). This calculation must be done for each test considered for the office laboratory.
- Drawing fee. Medicare will reimburse $3 for each venipuncture. Multiply the number of venipunctures anticipated by $3 to obtain a monthly income figure.
- Calculate profit or loss anticipated from the laboratory. Subtract monthly income from monthly expenses. That figure represents the profit or loss per month.

TESTS TO CONSIDER PERFORMING IN THE OFFICE LABORATORY

Introduction

This section focuses on some of the most frequently used office laboratory tests, typical clinical scenarios demonstrating the importance of having those tests available in the office laboratory, and discussion of some of the most frequently used types of instruments. Waived, PPM, and moderately complex tests are discussed. Many of the tests that are now waived had formerly been available only as moderately complex tests, while some tests are still available in both the moderately complex and the waived categories.

The discussion of examples of specific laboratory equipment is not intended to be all-inclusive and should not be interpreted as endorsements of specific instruments. Further, the cost/reimbursement information presented here is based on current information, is subject to change, and reflects only the cost of the test—not the costs of personnel and laboratory space. These figures should be used only as guidelines.

When choosing a suitable procedure for detecting or excluding a disease in a patient, the physician should select one that is acceptable to the patient and readily available. The procedure should allow the sorting of sick from well patients with a low incidence of false-negative results (i.e., normal results in persons having the disease). In most practices, the acceptable level of false-positive results (abnormal results in persons who are well) is set higher than that for false-negative results. This is because false-positive results can usually be discovered during subsequent evaluations, but false-negative results may have more serious consequences in terms of misdiagnoses and a lost opportunity for therapy.

The suitability of the test can be evaluated by means of its sensitivity and its specificity. *Sensitivity* allows the physician to evaluate the use of a test detecting a disease in a patient or a population that is being tested.

Specificity defines the ability of a test to rule out a disease in a particular patient or population. The specificity of a test may also be described as the percentage or frequency of a true-negative (or normal) test result among all patients without the particular disease in question. A patient with a positive test result may not have a disease.

The *predictive value* of a positive test is a statement of the probability, expressed as a percentage, that a patient with a positive test result does have the disease for which she or he is being tested. The predictive value is obtained by dividing the number of true-positives multiplied by 100 by the sum of the true-positives and the false-positives. The predictive value of a negative result, also expressed as a percentage, indicates the probability that a patient with a negative result is in fact free of the disease for which the test is being performed.

The *efficiency* of a diagnostic test is expressed as a percentage that gives the probability that a patient's test result, be it positive or negative, correctly corresponds with the disease state for which he is being evaluated.

Prevalence, or the frequency with which a disease occurs in a given population, is of the utmost importance in evaluating the usefulness of a test result in detecting the presence or absence of disease. Prevalence is the number of persons having the disease in a population at a given time. For example, if three or four abnormally high calcium results were obtained for different patients from the laboratory in 1 day, the physician should be highly suspicious of the existence of a technical or clerical problem in the laboratory, since the prevalence of parathyroid abnormalities is approximately 1 in 1,000 patients. If a patient gives a history in the office of aches, pains, fever, and chills during the flu season, a physician might correctly suspect that the patient has the flu. However, if the patient were in the hospital and receiving a blood transfusion, the physician would be more nearly correct in suspecting a transfusion reaction or septicemia.

Specific Tests to Consider Performing in the Office Laboratory

Streptococcal Antigen Testing (12–18)

Clinical scenario. A 5-year-old child comes to a pediatrician's office with a sore throat and fever. Physical findings are nonspecific other than a red throat. A throat swab is obtained and the diagnosis of streptococcal pharyngitis is made after results of the 5-minute rapid strep test are available; a prescription for antibiotics is given to the child's parent before he/she leaves the office.

The advent of rapid streptococcal testing in the office has simplified the approach for physicians taking care of patients presenting with sore throats. Prior to the availability of rapid streptococcal antigen testing, physicians had to make clinical judgments, and either start antibiotics that might not be needed, or delay treatment until throat culture results were available 24 to 48 hours later. The rapid streptococcus antigen test allows physicians to prescribe only when necessary, thus avoiding the overuse of unnecessary antibiotics—an important issue in this day of resistant organisms.

Most rapid streptococcal antigen tests can be performed in 5 minutes, are inexpensive to run, and have sensitivities in the 90% to 95% range. It is recommended that all negative rapid streptococcal antigen tests be followed up by an overnight throat culture—a moderately complex test. Many physicians send out throat cultures to hospital or reference laboratories in order to avoid making their laboratories moderately complex.

In January 1999, there were nine different brand names of waived testing for Group A beta hemolytic streptococcus. Even though this list is long, there are actually only three different methodologies used in all nine of these rapid tests. The reason for this confusion is that after a company develops a test, it names it one thing, and then sells the marketing rights to other companies who rename the same test, and then market it under different names. For instance, Smith-Kline bought the marketing rights to Binax NOW and renamed that test ICON Fx. Also, the marketing rights to Wyntek OSOM have been bought by seven different companies; that one test has now been renamed the Biostar Acceava, the Abbott Signify Strep A test, the Surestep Strep A Test from Applied Biotech, Remel RIM A.R.C. Strep A test, Meridian Diagnostics ImmunoCard STAT Strep A, Jant Pharmacal AccuStrip Strep A, Mainline Technology Strep A Dots Test, and the Link 2 Strep A Rapid test. The third different type of rapid strep test is named the Quidel One-Step.

Included in the list of moderately complex rapid streptococcal antigen tests are ICON from Smith-Kline, the Biostar OIA Max, the Abbott Strep Plus, and the BD Directogen. Like the waived tests, moderately complex tests are simple to perform and give results in about 5 minutes. Sensitivity and specificity results have varied, but are similar for these tests, and comparable to the moderately complex tests. All tests are less sensitive with lower colony counts. Cost/reimbursement figures show that profit per test ranges can vary significantly. There are minimal differences in reimbursement between the waived and moderately complex tests (19). For this reason, most physicians are now opting to utilize waived testing for rapid streptococcal antigen testing.

Helicobacter Pylori Testing (20–27)

Clinical scenario. A 22-year-old man comes to the office complaining of an upset stomach and pain of several months' duration. Another doctor had performed an upper gastrointestinal series, which was normal. A 5-minute rapid *H. pylori* test on two drops of blood is done, the result is positive, and treatment for this infection is begun.

Unfortunately, there is no general agreement on what action should be taken with a positive rapid *H. pylori* test. Some physicians use this test as a screening method and refer patients to specialists for confirmation of the *H. pylori* infection; other physicians treat on the basis of a positive test. In children particularly there is little baseline information about the incidence of false-positive *H. pylori* screening tests. Each physician will need to decide whether rapid testing for *H. pylori* is clinically a useful office laboratory test.

There are three major waived *Helicobacter pylori* rapid tests that can be performed in the office laboratory: Quidel Quick-Vue One Step H. Pylori Test; FlexSure HP Test; and the Abbott FlexPack HP Test. The only difference between these waived tests and the moderately complex tests is that the waived tests are performed on whole blood, and the moderately complex tests are done on serum or plasma. Otherwise, the waived and moderately complex test kits are identical, are performed in the same way, take 5 minutes to run, and have the same sensitivity and specificity (93% and 89%, respectively). Cost/reimbursement information is similar for the two categories of tests (19).

Infectious Mononucleosis Testing

Clinical scenario. An 18-year-old college student is due to return to school the next day. She comes into your office late in the afternoon complaining of nonspecific fatigue and a mild sore throat. Physical examination shows a red throat with an exudate. A rapid mononucleosis test is performed; 5 minutes later the positive test result allows the physician to share the diagnosis with the patient and give the proper anticipatory guidance.

The diagnosis of infectious mononucleosis is often difficult. Symptoms, as in the above case, are frequently vague and nonspecific, and they occur most often in busy teenagers who do not want to admit the intensity of their symptoms. In this condition, anticipatory guidance can be critical in the prevention of long-term sequelae. Having a test available in the office laboratory allows a rapid diagnosis that can be shared immediately with the patient. As of July 2000, there were nine waived rapid tests available: Genzyme Contrast Mono, Color Q, Biostar Acceava Mono Test, LifeSign UniStep Mono, Princeton Bio-Meditech BioSign Mono WB, Quidel CARDS O.S. Mono, Seradyn Color Q Mono, and Wampole Mono-Plus WB. Examples of moderately complex rapid infectious mononucleosis tests include Wampole Mono-Plus Serum Test, Seradyn Color Slide Mono II test, and Card QS Mono/Quidel test. Like the rapid tests for *H. pylori*, the waived tests use whole blood, and the moderately complex tests use serum. Otherwise, the kits are identical, the cost/reimbursement comparisons are the same (19), and take only 5 minutes to get results. As in the rapid streptococcal tests and the *H. pylori* tests, most physicians will prefer using the waived type of infectious mononucleosis test kits.

Complete Blood Count Testing (28–33)

Clinical scenario. A 9-month-old child comes to the office with a 105-degree temperature. His physical examination is normal; no site of infection can be identified. A CBC is drawn and, 10 minutes later, the white count returns at 38,000 with a differential of 92% polymorphonuclear leukocytes. A presumptive

diagnosis of pneumococcal bacteremia is made, a blood culture drawn, and antibiotics are given. The child is seen the next day feeling well and afebrile.

The CBC is a frequently performed moderately complex test in office laboratories. Most CBC instruments now test for total white count, red blood cell count, hemoglobin, hematocrit, red cell indices, red cell distribution width, and platelet count, and provide either a three-part or a five-part differential. The information that can be obtained in an office laboratory from a CBC can be a major help in diagnosing patients' illnesses.

The QBC instrument by Becton Dickinson is the least expensive and the most frequently used instrument in the office laboratory. It gives a three-part differential (percentage of granulocytes, lymphocytes, and monocytes), and can do up to 30 tests an hour on fingerstick samples. The QBC is most often utilized in smaller office laboratories.

The Coulter counter is another popular CBC instrument for the office laboratory. There are different models available including MD 16, MD II, ACT 8, ACT 10, and ACT differential. A relatively recent addition—the Spirit by Biochem Immunosystems—is less expensive to run than either the QBC or Coulter. A number of other CBC instruments are available, such as the Sysmex and the Abbott Cell-Dyn and Baker.

If physicians are going to use a CBC in their office laboratories, they should try the instrument out for several weeks before actually purchasing it. It is hoped that in the near future, the platelet count and the white count will be categorized as waived tests.

Cholesterol Testing in the Office Laboratory

Clinical scenario. A 45-year-old man comes into the office with concerns about his cholesterol level. He has avoided having his cholesterol checked, because he did not want to change his lifestyle. He states that his father and his brother both have cholesterol levels over 300 mg%. He is finally ready to have it checked, and wants an immediate answer. After a 5-minute test, he is told that his cholesterol is normal (180 mg%) and that he does not need to worry.

Screening for cholesterol has been done for years in doctors' offices (34). Now the public is aware that this testing is readily available to them and that doctors should be able to do this in their office laboratories. Some patients even request information about the levels of their low-density lipoprotein fraction of cholesterol. Cholesterol testing can now be done in such nonphysician settings as Wal-Marts and pharmacies, as well as in office laboratories.

In 1999, there were three waived techniques for testing for cholesterol in physicians' office laboratories. The first method of testing is the disposable kit CholesTrak. Formerly named the Accumeter, this is the same test that was named "Advanced Care." It requires only two drops of blood to run; results are available in 15 minutes. Reimbursement is only slightly higher than the cost per test, but this technology may be considered for those physicians with a small demand for cholesterol tests.

The second waived instrument that tests cholesterol is the Accu-Chek cholesterol instrument, which also only needs a few drops of blood to run; results are available in 3 minutes.

A third waived instrument that is being used in office laboratories, as well as in pharmacies and Wal-Marts, is the Cholestech LDX. This analyzer was waived in 1996 and can test for glucose, HDL, and triglycerides as well as total cholesterol. Cartridges are available to test for any or all of these analytes in combination; results are available in 5 minutes. Reimbursement with this analyzer is complicated: when a total cholesterol is run alone, the cost of the test is greater than the reimbursement; when a lipid profile is run (cholesterol, HDL, and triglyceride), the profit can be substantial. Since most physicians screen by checking only total cholesterol, this instrument—like the other waived tests for cholesterol—may not be profitable in the office laboratory.

There are a number of moderately complex tests that are available for testing cholesterol. Examples of these instruments are the Vitros DT series and the Reflotron Plus. (See discussion of chemistry testing in the office laboratory.)

Hemoglobin and Hematocrit Testing (35–38)

Clinical scenario. A 33-year-old woman visits the family medicine doctor's office 2 months after having delivered a baby. Since that time she has been unusually tired and fatigued. On physical examination she looks quite pale, and has an elevated heart rate at rest. A hemoglobin is done in the examining room, which is 7.2 gm%. A presumptive diagnosis of iron deficiency anemia is made, etiologies sought, and supplemental iron is prescribed.

Testing for hemoglobin or hematocrit in the office laboratory is done often. Now that portable instruments are available, screening for hemoglobin can be done in rural offices or malls as well as the standard office laboratory. While the diagnosis of anemia is only the first step in identifying the underlying problem, having an instrument available to diagnose anemia can be critical in caring for patients.

The centrifuging of a capillary tube filled with whole blood determines the hematocrit. There are three major waived tests that can test for hemoglobin. The most popular and the instrument waived first is called the HemoCueB-Hemoglobin Analyzer. This easy-to-use method requires one drop of blood that is put into a disposable microcurette and entered into the instrument, with results available in 45 seconds. In 1997, HemoCue added a data management system that stores up to 1,000 records at a time. Another waived method for testing hemoglobin is the stat-crit test by Wampole Laboratories. This instrument requires only one drop of blood, and measures the hematocrit with calculated hemoglobin.

Hemoglobin A1C Testing

Clinical scenario. A 55-year-old woman comes into the office for routine follow-up of her diabetes mellitus. She has been a known diabetic for many years, but compliance with insulin regimens has been a problem. Even though she states that her blood sugars have been in good control recently, the physician wants to get an objective measure of her control. A capillary sample is obtained, and a hemoglobin A1C test is run with results in 6 minutes. The patient is found to have an elevated hemoglobin A1C that implies poor diabetic control. When presented with this evidence, the patient agrees to see a nutritionist and improve her eating habits.

The hemoglobin A1C measures long-term glycemic control over the previous 90 to 120 days. It is an objective measure of long-term diabetes control; testing for it has become a standard in following diabetic children as well as adults. There are two waived instruments: the Ames 2000 and the Bayer DCA 2000+. The equipment stores up to 16 results in memory at a time. For any physician who follows diabetic patients, the availability of this instrument in the office laboratory can be quite helpful. There have been definite correlations between physicians' use of this instrument and glycemic control (39).

Prothrombin Time Testing (40–43)

Clinical scenario. A 58-year-old man who had suffered a pulmonary embolus was put on medication to prevent clotting. He returns to the office for routine follow-up. A sample of blood is taken and within 5 minutes the results of the prothrombin time are available, and the medication dosage altered.

Anticoagulant therapy is prescribed for a number of reasons: angina, strokes, and myocardial infarctions, as well as congenital defects of clotting such as protein S deficiency, protein C deficiency, and antithrombin III deficiency. The coumarin derivatives act by decreasing the rate of synthesis of the vitamin K-dependent clotting factors II, VII, IX, and X. The proper dosage of oral medications can sometimes be difficult to attain; if the prothrombin time is too prolonged, the possibility of hemorrhage exists; if the prothrombin time is not prolonged, the patient is not protected from recurrent clotting. It is important to monitor this test in patients on coumarin.

There are two waived tests that can be done in the office laboratory: the CoaguChek Plus System and the ProTime Microcoagulation system. Reimbursement requires claiming two CPT codes for the test: CPT 85610QW and CPT99211 (the physician evaluation and management fee, respectively). Without the addition of the latter fee, reimbursement would be about the same as the cost for the test. Even if running this test proves not to be financially beneficial, many physicians still run these tests in the office laboratory because of their ease of use and clinical importance. A number of studies have found that office follow-up with these instruments is as good as hospital follow-up.

Moderately complex tests also exist for office laboratory prothrombin time calculations. These include Coag-A-Mate (800-682-2666), which is an inexpensive instrument that can test prothrombin time, partial thromboplastin time, and thrombin time, and do factor assays. Controls are expensive. Cost/reimbursement information was not available at the time of this writing.

Glucose Testing (44–53)

Clinical scenario. A known diabetic is brought to the office feeling faint and shaky. She states that her diabetes has been under poor control recently, and that she is never quite sure how much insulin she should give herself. This morning, she doubled her insulin. A blood sugar is obtained from a drop of capillary blood; a result of 35 mg% is obtained, and the patient started on intravenous fluids with dextrose. She returns home in 2 hours feeling fine. A repeat blood sugar before leaving the office is 75 mg%.

Whether concerned about hypoglycemia or hyperglycemia, a method for testing glucose in the office setting can be extremely valuable. Particularly if diabetic patients arrive in the office confused and semialert, a rapidly obtained blood sugar will help the physician determine whether the patient has had too much or too little insulin.

There are two waived analyzers on the market that test for blood glucose. HemoCue B—in addition to its hemoglobin instrument—has another instrument that tests for glucose. It also requires a very small drop of capillary blood to run and gets results in 40 to 240 seconds. In addition, the Accuchek, similar to the instrument used to test cholesterol, is available for rapid glucose results in the office setting. Results are available in 12 seconds. Patients monitoring blood sugars at home often use the Accuchek.

In addition to these two waived glucose analyzers, as of March 2000, there are 128 other waived glucose-monitoring devices that are cleared for home use. In addition, glucose can be obtained as part of profiles included in other instruments. For instance, the waived Cholestech LDX instrument can run glucose as part of its profile; in addition, it is available in a number of moderately complex instruments, such as i-STAT (i-STAT, East Windsor, NJ); Vitros DT, DT 60, DTSC, and DTE from Ortho-Clinical Diagnostics; and Reflotron Plus from Roche. While results vary depending on the operator, point-of-care testing has been shown reliable for glucose testing with these instruments.

Chemistry Testing (54–59)

Clinical scenario. A 40-year-old woman comes to the office with a new onset of fatigue. Her physical examination shows a slightly enlarged liver, and screening liver function tests are performed from a fingerstick. Test results are available after 15 minutes. A diagnosis of hepatitis is made based on those results and further testing is then sent to the reference laboratory to identify the cause of the hepatitis.

Usually, only larger office laboratories of family practitioners and internists perform testing for such chemistries as liver function studies, renal function studies, calcium, phosphorus, amylase, bilirubin, and electrolytes. All chemistries are in the moderately complex category. A few examples of the instruments available are discussed.

The i-STAT is a handheld instrument that tests for blood gases (pH, PO_2, PCO_2, HCO_3, and O_2 saturation), electrolytes, glucose, and hematocrit from two drops of blood, and gives results in 90 seconds. It has been widely utilized in emergency rooms, intensive care units, and neonatal transport teams. It can store up to 50 results at a time. For those interested in having these values available in the office laboratory, this instrument should be considered.

The Vitros DT series is an example of a desktop instrument that could be utilized in the office laboratory. It requires about 3 minutes to load a fingerstick sample into the instrument and results are available in 6 minutes or less. It tests for a total of up to 18 tests including a panel of liver function and renal function tests, lipid tests, and electrolytes.

Another example of a desktop instrument that could be considered for the office laboratory is the Reflotron Plus, which tests for a total of 16 analytes including a liver panel, amylase, triglyceride, and HDL.

Urinalysis Testing in the Office Laboratory

Clinical scenario. A 30-year-old woman comes to the office complaining of burning on urination, urinary frequency, and nocturia. She has never had a urinary tract infection before. A dipstick and microscopic urinalysis is performed showing multiple white cells and a few white-cell casts. A urine culture is obtained, the diagnosis of a urinary tract infection made, and the patient begun on antibiotic therapy.

Most office laboratories perform at least a urine dipstick if not a microscopic urinalysis. In March 2000, there were 144 waived urine dipsticks or tablet analytes. Many urine dipsticks can test for glucose, ketones, protein, specific gravity, leukocytes, nitrites, red cells, and urobilinogen. Microscopic examination is done by looking at either the unspun or the spun urine; some technologists use methylene blue to analyze the specimen while others look at the sediment without a stain.

Recently, the CLINITEK 50 automated instrument has been waived. The technique of doing the test is the same as that described above, except that the dipstick is entered into the CLINITEK 50 instrument, which reads the stick and makes a hard copy of the results that can become a part of the permanent record. The microscopic examination of the urine is done as described above. Other CLINITEK instruments, such as the CLINITEK 100, are larger, can do larger volumes, and are mostly used in hospital laboratories. This equipment can also be used to test for hCG and for creatinine/microalbumin.

Another recently waived automated urine test is the Roche/Boehringer Mannheim Chemstrip 101 Urine Analyzer, which became available in late 1999.

Provider-Performed Microscopy Testing

Clinical scenario. A 14-year-old sexually active girl comes to a rural clinic complaining of a vaginal discharge. A physical examination is performed, which is negative except for the discharge. A wet prep is performed that shows an infection with trichimonas; anticipatory guidance is provided and a prescription to treat the infection is given to the patient.

The PPM category is actually classified as a subgroup under the moderately complex category, even though, like the waived category, the tests performed in it do not require inspection. The reason for this is that personnel requirements of the more stringent moderately complex category do apply to PPM testing. The PPM category, begun in 1993, is now comprised of ten tests; laboratories performing these tests also do not require inspection, but they are subject to all the QA standards that exist for moderately complex tests.

The most frequently used tests in the PPM category include the urinalysis with microscopy, the wet prep, and the potassium hydroxide prep. Wet preps are performed by placing one drop of specimen on a glass slide with one drop of saline; under a coverslip, yeast, budding hyphae, trichimonas, and clue cells (diagnostic for bacterial vaginosis) can be identified. A drop of potassium hydroxide is then added to look for yeast infection or to do a "whiff" test—also suggestive of bacterial vaginosis. Much less frequently needed are the pinworm test (a slide test looking for pinworm eggs), fern test, semen analysis, examination of prostate secretions, nasal and rectal smear analyses (nasal smear for eosinophils tests for allergic tendencies), rectal smear for granulocytes, and post-coital direct examinations.

Other Laboratory Tests to Consider

Waived. A number of other waived tests could be performed in the office laboratory. As of December 2000, there were 255 urine pregnancy tests, 33 fecal occult blood tests, 38 ovulation tests by visual color comparison, erythrocyte sedimentation rates, a microalbumin test, a gastric occult blood test; an influenza test (Zstat Flu from ZymeTX); and an ethanol test by saliva analysis (19).

Moderately complex. Many moderately complex tests are available for use in the office laboratory (Table 24.3). Urine cultures and throat cultures are done in many office laboratories. Urine cultures can only be identified as positive or negative; the actual organism can be identified only in highly complex laboratories. While a number of systems of doing urine cultures are available, most physicians culture on EMB (eosin and methylene blue) and McConkey plates. Physicians seeing children may consider obtaining the ESA handheld, lead-level test, which costs about $1,800. This test requires only a few drops of blood and gets results quickly. Other moderately complex tests include the Affirm VPIII (Becton Dickinson), which tests for candida, gardnerella, and trichimonas, and the Immunodiagnostic Testing System (IOS), which tests for thyroid and hCG.

There are a number of relatively recent moderately complex tests for the office laboratory that have been developed. For example, several tests identify Influenza A or B (the recently waived Zstat Flu and the moderately complex Biostar AB FLU OIA) (60). The first test requires up to an hour to be run, although it takes only 2 to 3 minutes of hands-on time. The Biostar test takes 15 minutes. In late 2000, Becton Dickinson released a moderately complex influenza test (Directogen Influenza A + B) that can identify either Influenza A or Influenza B specifically. With the advent of medications that treat only Influenza A (Amantadine) or only Influenza B (Oseltamivir, Relenza), these tests identify the specific type of influenza infecting the patient.

Other recently available tests include a rotavirus test that has 93% sensitivity and 95.8% specificity, a hydrogen breath monitor that measures hydrogen in the breath, and a chromatic, color-sciences noninvasive technique of measuring bilirubin in babies.

CONCLUSIONS AND SUMMARY

Over the last ten years, the office laboratory has experienced the following major advances:

- In the early 1990s, the effects of CLIA '88 and managed care were not positive to the office laboratory: many office laboratories closed, and, in the remaining laboratories, the number of tests performed decreased. However, ultimately the office laboratory benefited from those effects.
- Manufacturers responded to this situation by creating many inexpensive, easy-to-use, rapid, and accurate instruments suitable for benchtop use in office laboratories.
- Many of these instruments ended up being classified as waived or PPM, not moderately complex. As a result of this technological explosion and a mellowing of CLIA '88 and managed care orientations, office laboratories reopened and test menus reexpanded. Instead of the majority of laboratories being classified as moderately complex, now 72% of office laboratories are now either waived or PPM.
- The total number of tests that can be performed in an office laboratory without inspection increased from 8 to 36 (26 waived and 10 PPM). Doctors have found that the need to do less paperwork and undergo costly laboratory inspections is positive. Physicians can now do tests on instruments that are inexpensive, accurate, easy to use, require small samples of blood, and get results in minutes.
- The ultimate long-term effects of CLIA '88 and managed care have been beneficial to the office laboratory.

This chapter summarized the method by which an office laboratory can be started, and suggested a number of specific tests that can be run. The final step in developing a laboratory is to determine its financial feasibility. A worksheet is provided to help physicians calculate whether the laboratory will be a profit or a cost center. Because of the availability of easy-to-use technology, some physicians will decide to run tests in their office laboratory that are not fully cost effective. They and their patients find the earlier diagnoses made possible with the utilization of an office laboratory are beneficial—patients can be diagnosed and treated more quickly, feel better sooner, and can go back to work or school earlier. Physicians find that their patients are well served when their doctors have office laboratories.

It is expected that the major advances made by the office laboratory will continue in the future. Currently, there are many companies doing research on simplifying testing techniques so that their instruments can become waived. In the future, it is expected that the office laboratory will become an even more valuable resource for practicing physicians and their patients.

REFERENCES

1. U.S. Department of Health and Human Services. Public Law 100-578, Clinical Laboratory Improvement Amendments of 1988. *Federal Register* 1988 Oct 31: .
2. Needels K, Strouse R, Hall J. *1995 survey of physicians' office laboratories*. Submitted to American Medical Association. Princeton, NJ: Mathematica Policy Research, Inc., 1995.
3. Mitchell B (Manager, Laboratory Issues, American Academy of Family Physicians). Personal communication, 1997.
4. St John TM, Lipman HB, Krolak JM, et al. Improvement in physician's office laboratory practices, 1989–1994. *Arch Pathol Lab Med* 2000;124:1066–1073.
5. Smith T. Tests allowed in the office laboratory by managed care com-

panies. Presentation at 13th Physician Office Laboratory Annual Symposium, Commission on Office Laboratory Accreditation, September 1998.

6. Weissman DW. *Washington G-2 Reports Newsletter* 1999 Jan:1.
7. Bill to amend section 353 of the Public Health Service Act, Clinical Laboratory Improvement Act of 1988, H.R. 1386 (15 April 1995).
8. Yost J (Director, Center for Laboratories, Health Care Financing Administration). Personal communication, January 1999.
9. Pysher TJ, Daly JA. The pediatric office laboratory: a look at recent trends [Review]. *Pediatr Clin North Am* 1989;36:1–28.
10. Baisden CR. *The office practice laboratory.* Rockville, MD: Aspen Systems, 1985.
11. Benjamin JT, Janzen VK. Eight steps to office lab survival under CLIA regulations. *AAP News* 1997;13:22.
12. Schwartz B, Fries S, Fitzgibbon AM, et al. Pediatricians' diagnostic approach to pharyngitis: impact of CLIA 1988 on office diagnostic tests. *JAMA* 1994;271:234–238.
13. Dagnelie CF, Bartelink ML, Van der Graaf Y, et al. Towards a better diagnostic of throat infections (with group A beta-haemolytic streptococcus) in general practice. *Br J Gen Pract* 1998;48:959–962.
14. Webb KH. Does culture confirmation of high-sensitivity rapid streptococcal tests make sense? A medical decision analysis. *Pediatrics* 1998; 101:E2.
15. Badgett JT, Hesterberg LK. Management of group A streptococcus pharyngitis with a second-generation rapid strep screen: Strep A QIA [Review]. *Microbiol Drug Resistance* 1996;2:371–376.
16. Heiter BJ, Bourbeau PP. Comparison of two rapid streptococcal antigen detection assays with culture for diagnosis of streptococcal pharyngitis. *J Clin Microbiol* 1995;33:1408–1410.
17. Hurst J, Nickel K, Hilborne LH. Are physicians' office laboratory results of comparable quality to those produced in other laboratory settings? [Comment]. *JAMA* 1998;279:468–471.
18. American Academy of Pediatrics. *Red book: report of the Committee on Infectious Diseases*, 24th ed. Elk Grove Village, IL: American Academy of Pediatrics, 1997.
19. Benjamin JT, Bassali RW. Which tests should you perform in your office laboratory? A cost/benefit analysis of some frequently used tests. *Pediatr Ann* 1998;27:505–511.
20. Talley NJ, Lambert JR, Howell S, et al. An evaluation of whole blood testing for Helicobacter pylori in general practice. *Aliment Pharmacol Ther* 1998;12:641–645.
21. Harrison JR, Bevan J, Furth EE, et al. AccuStat whole blood fingerstick test for Helicobacter pylori infection: a reliable screening method. *J Clin Gastroenterol* 1998;27:50–53.
22. Vaira D, Holton J, Menegatti M, et al. Blood tests in the management of Helicobacter pylori infection: Italian Helicobacter Pylori Study Group [Review]. *Gut* 1998;43[Suppl 1]:S39–S46.
23. Oksanen A, Veijola L, Sipponen P, et al. Evaluation of Pyloriset Screen, a rapid whole-blood diagnostic test for Helicobacter pylori infection. *J Clin Microbiol* 1998;36:955–957.
24. Moayyedi P, Carter AM, Catto A, et al. Validation of a rapid whole blood test for diagnosing Helicobacter Pylori infection [Comment]. *BMJ* 1997;314:119.
25. Enroth H, Engstrand L. Rapid detection of Helicobacter pylori infection in serum and whole-blood samples. *APMIS* 1997;105:951–955.
26. Borody TJ, Andrews P, Shortis NP. Evaluation of whole blood antibody kit to detect active Helicobacter Pylori infection. *Am J Gastroenterol* 1996;91:2509–2512.
27. Asante MA, Mendall MA, Finlayson C, et al. Screening dyspeptic patients for Helicobacter Pylori prior to endoscopy: laboratory or near-patient testing? *Eur J Gastroenterol Hepatol* 1998;10(10):843–846.
28. Despotis GJ, Alsoufiev A, Hogue CW Jr, et al. Evaluation of complete blood count results from a new, on-site hemocytometer compared with a laboratory-based hemocytometer. *Crit Care Med* 1996;24:1163–1167.
29. Procop GW, Hartman JS, Sedor F. Laboratory tests in evaluation of acute febrile illness in pediatric emergency room patients. *Am J Clin Pathol* 1997;107:114–121.
30. Vives-Corrons J, Besson I, Jou JM, et al. Evaluation of the Abbott Cell-DYN 3500 hematology analyzer in a university hospital. *Am J Clin Pathol* 1996;105:553–559.

31. Walters MC, Abelson HT. Interpretation of the complete blood count. *Pediatr Clin North Am* 1996;43:599–622.
32. Winkelman JW, Tanasijevic MJ, Wybenga DR, et al. How fast is fast enough for clinical laboratory turnaround time? Measurement of the interval between result entry and inquiries for reports [Comment]. *Am J Clin Pathol* 1997;108:400–405.
33. Silver BE, Patterson JW, Kulick M, et al. Effect of CBC results on ED management of women with lower abdominal pain. *Am J Emerg Med* 1995;13:304–306.
34. Ey JL, Aldous MB, Duncan B, et al. Office laboratory procedures, office economics, patient and parent education, and urinary tract infection [Review]. *Curr Opin Pediatr* 1996;8:639–649.
35. Centers for Disease Control and Prevention. Compliance with the Clinical Laboratory Improvement Amendments of 1988 for hemoglobin screening—California, 1995. *MMWR Morb Mort Wkly Rep* 1996;45:419–422.
36. Conway AM, Hinchliffe RF, Earland J, et al. Measurement of haemoglobin using single drops of skin puncture blood: is precision acceptable? *J Clin Pathol* 1998;51:248–250.
37. Leonard M, Chessall M, Manning D. The use of a Hemocue blood glucose analyzer in a neonatal unit. *Ann Clin Biochem* 1997;34:287–290.
38. McNulty SE, Torjman M, Grodecki W, et al. A comparison of four bedside methods of hemoglobin assessment during cardiac surgery. *Anesth Analg* 1995;81:1197–1202.
39. Deichmann RE, Castello E, Horswell R, et al. Improvements in diabetic care as measured by HbAlc after a physician education project. *Diabet Care* 1999;22:1612–1616.
40. Macik BG. Designing a point-of-care program for coagulation testing [Review]. *Arch Pathol Lab Med* 1995;119:929–938.
41. Solomon HM, Mullins RE, Lyden P, et al. The diagnosis accuracy of bedside and laboratory coagulation: procedures used to monitor the anticoagulation status of patients treated with heparin. *Am J Clin Pathol* 1998;109:371–378.
42. Oberhardt BJ, Mize PD, Prithcard CG. Point-of-care fibrinolytic tests: the other side of blood coagulation. *Clin Chem* 1997;43:1697–1702.
43. Fitzmaurice DA, Hobbs FD, Murray ET, et al. Oral anticoagulation management in primary care with the use of computerized decision support and near-patient testing: a randomized, controlled trial. *Arch Intern Med* 2000;160:2343–2348.
44. Bennett BD. Blood glucose determination: point-of-care testing. *South Med J* 1997;90:678–680.
45. Innanen VT, Barqueira de Campos F. Point-of-care glucose testing: cost savings and ease of use with the Ames Glucometer Elite. *Clin Chem* 1995;41:1537–1538.
46. Innanen VT, DeLand ME, DeCampos FM, et al. Point-of-care glucose testing in the neonatal intensive care unit is facilitated by the use of the Ames Glucometer Elite electrochemical glucose meter. *J Pediatr* 1997;130:151–155.
47. Kost GJ, Vu HT, Lee JH, et al. Multicenter study of oxygen-insensitive handheld glucose point-of-care testing in critical care/hospital/ambulatory patients in the United States and Canada. *Crit Care Med* 1998;26:581–590.
48. Schlebusch H, Niesen M, Sorger M. Blood glucose determinations in newborns: four instruments compared. *Pediatr Pathol Lab Med* 1998; 18:41–48.
49. Elimam A, Horal M, Gerstrom M, et al. Diagnosis of hypoglycaemia: effects of blood sample handling and evaluation of a glucose photometer in the low glucose range. *Acta Paediatr* 1997;86:474–478.
50. Carr SR, Slocum J, Tefft L, et al. Precision of office-based blood glucose meters in screening for gestational diabetes [Comment]. *Am J Obstet Gynecol* 1995;173:1267–1272.
51. Nichols JH, Howard C, Loman K, et al. Laboratory and bedside evaluation of portable glucose meters [Comment]. *Am J Clin Pathol* 1995;103:244–251.
52. Lee-Lewandrowski E, Laposata M, Eschenbach K, et al. Utilization and cost analysis of bedside capillary glucose testing in a large teaching hospital: implications for managing point-of-care testing [Comment]. *Am J Med* 1994;97:222–230.

53. Louie RF, Tang Z, Sutton DV, et al. Point-of-care glucose testing: effects of critical care variables, influence of reference instruments, and a modular glucose meter design. *Arch Pathol Lab Med* 2000;124: 257–266.

54. Meier S, Ehrmeyer S, Laessig R, et al. Performance of the Kodak DT-60 physicians' office analyzer as measured by CLIA-88 proposed evaluation criteria: assessment of demographic and quality assurance factors influencing performance [Comment]. *Arch Pathol Lab Med* 1992;116:524–530.

55. Murthy JN, Hicks JM, Soldin SJ. Evaluation of i-STAT portable clinical analyzer in a neonatal and pediatric intensive care unit. *Clin Biochem* 1997;30:385–389.

56. Adams DA, Buus-Frank M. Point-of-care technology: the i-STAT system for bedside blood analysis. *J Pediatr Nurs* 1995;10:194–198.

57. Mock T, Morrison D, Yatscoff R. Evaluation of the i-STAT system: a portable chemistry analyzer for the measurement of sodium, potassium, chloride, urea, glucose, and hematocrit. *Clin Biochem* 1995;28:187–192.

58. Connelly NR, Magee M, Kiessling B. The use of the i-STAT portable analyzer in patients undergoing cardiopulmonary bypass. *J Clin Monit* 1996;12:311–315.

59. Gault MH, Harding CE. Evaluation of i-STAT portable clinical analyzer in a hemodialysis unit. *Clin Biochem* 1996;29:117–124.

60. Benjamin JT. Diagnosing and treating influenza in children in 1999–2000. *Contemp Pediatr* 2000;17:75–81.

POCT FOR EARTHQUAKES AND DISASTER PREPAREDNESS

TADASHI KAWAI
NORIYUKI TATSUMI

Disasters occur unexpectedly and can be divided into two major categories: natural and artifactual. Natural disasters often occur in a wide area and include earthquakes, floods, and volcano eruptions, while artifactual disasters may occur in localized areas and include regional wars, gas explosions, radiation diffusion, and epidemic disease outbreaks. Local disasters often can be handled following established emergency protocols, but natural and artifactual disasters occurring in a wide area need special attention because life-sustaining lines such as electricity, gas, and water supplies may be partially or completely damaged, transportation systems immobilized, and communication systems limited. In the initial state of most disasters, prevention of secondary disasters, rescue of the injured survivors, and emergency treatment become paramount. Temporary mobile or transportable laboratories become necessary for emergency laboratory testing, which can be performed with field-ready, small, point-of-care testing (POCT) devices (1). Historically, electricity supply systems have required a few days to a month to be restored, depending on the magnitude of the disaster. Because the water supply may be limited, liquid reagent-free analytical (dry-chemistry type) or cassette-based instruments should be available for emergency laboratory testing. Reagent films or small cassettes also are preferable because disposable wastes are minimal (2).

THE HANSHIN-AWAJI GREAT EARTHQUAKE

In the early morning of January 17, 1995, just before the super-express trains were about to start moving, an extraordinarily strong earthquake (7.5 Richter) occurred on the island of Awaji and in the Hanshin district, including the heavily populated southern part of the Hyogo Prefecture (Kobe, Ashiya, Nishinomiya and Amagasaki cities and their neighboring zones) and the northern part of the Osaka Prefecture. Although the earthquake lasted only for about 45 seconds, over 100,000 people were wounded or killed, and over 145,600 houses and portions of the superhighway collapsed instantaneously. All life-sustaining lines were completely destroyed. Gas leaks were ignited by electrical sparks, and fires spread rapidly throughout the damaged areas. The total number of deaths related directly to the earthquake reached 5,372. Hospitals affected by the earthquake were not able to function as medical centers under those conditions, and many temporary clinics were established. Tent-house clinics were set up in the damaged areas and, although they were supplied with electricity, no water lines were available. Under these extraordinary circumstances, certain POCT devices became the most valuable of medical instruments.

Rescue Operations

Every clinic initially received patients with trauma, dehydration, and fever of unknown origin. Two to 3 days later, some patients suffered from muscle crush syndrome with or without renal insufficiency, others showed bacterial diarrhea or pneumonia due to smoke inhalation, and several weeks later aged patients were seen suffering from posttraumatic stress disorders. Standard laboratory analyzers were useless because of the lack of water and reagents. Full sets of laboratory tests could not be performed in tent-house field laboratories. Instead, mobile POCT devices were invaluable in these clinics because they could be used with minimal electricity, no water, fewer technologists, the least operational training practice, and faster turnaround time. The most frequently requested tests were glucose, urinalysis, and complete blood count (Table F.1). Before POCT devices were introduced fully in the tent-house field laboratories, quality assessments were performed by analyzing fresh patient and control samples with five dry-chemistry type instruments for confirming intra- and inter-instrumental reproducibility. The results were compared with those obtained in the central clinical laboratories at Kobe University Hospital, since most of the physicians in the tent-house clinics were from there. Internal quality control measures were applied daily as in the routine clinical laboratory. It was confirmed that all of the POCT devices could give fairly satisfactory results, provided random errors were watched for, as is done in the clinical laboratory (3).

Experience gained from practical application of POCT devices in these temporary field clinics has proven their clinical utility, durability, and reliability. Immediately after the earthquake, most patients needed surgical treatment for traumatic injury and compression, in addition to dehydration. Patients with muscle crush syndrome and subsequent renal insufficiency due to long-term compression of the body under a collapsed

TABLE F.1. POCT DEVICES NECESSARY IN A FIELD TENT-HOUSE CLINIC

Instruments	Specimen	Test Item(s)	TAT
Urine test strips with or without analyzer	Urine	Semiquantitative	2 min
Blood chemistry analyzer	Whole blood, plasma, serum	Blood chemistry	<30 min
Glucose analyzer	Heparinized blood, plasma	Glucose	2 min
Blood-gas analyzer	Whole blood	pH, pCO_2, pO_2	3 min
Hematology analyzer	EDTA blood	Complete blood count	2 min
Coagulometer	Citrated blood	PT, APTT, fbg	10 min
Glass hemocytometer	Whole blood, urine, spinal fluid	WBC, platelet count	10 min
Microscope	Blood smear, urine, gram stain film	Cell morphology, bacterial typing	<30 min
Blood sedimentation rate	Citrated blood	ESR	40 min
ECG			3 min

APTT, activated partial thromboplastin time; ECG, electrocardiogram; EDTA, ethylenediaminetetraacetic acid; ESR, electron spin resonance; fbg, fasting blood glucose; PT, prothrombin time; TAT, turnaround time; WBC, white blood count.

building were brought to the clinic 2 to 5 days later. Patients with muscle crush syndrome showed characteristic elevations in potassium, creatine kinase, and lactate dehydrogenase, and high myoglobulin levels in urine. Diagnosis could be made easily based on medical history and observed elevations in serum potassium and other analytes.

CONCLUSIONS

Based on experience gained in the Hanshin-Awaji earthquake, a number of objectives should be considered in the preparation for disasters. The most important follow:

- POCT devices should be used regularly under normal conditions in hospital laboratories, not only by laboratory personnel, but also by other medical to enable medical personnel to establish a hybrid laboratory system for near-patient testing.
- Trained laboratory technicians, the lack of which was experienced in the earthquake, must be available for emergency medical teams as much as possible.
- A laboratory information system or knowledge-based diagnostic system, using laboratory results obtained by POCT devices, should be prepared in general community or university hospitals to avoid inappropriate use of laboratory data

and misdiagnosis or mistreatment by any future volunteer medical staff in emergency care settings.

- The necessity of POCT is beyond cost considerations in cases of disaster. The need for clinical laboratory testing will not disappear as long as modern medicine continues to progress (4). While the distribution of POCT devices in disaster is easily done, familiarization with their application and use requires advance training. Although cost benefit is important for the clinical laboratory, it is secondary to the advantages of convenience, simplicity, and speed critical in disaster situations.

REFERENCES

1. Kost GJ. Point-of-care testing in intensive care. In: Tobin MJ, ed. *Principles and practice of intensive care monitoring.* New York: McGraw-Hill, 1997:1267–1396.
2. Okuda K. Basic principles of dry chemistry. *Jpn J Clin Pathol* 1997;106: 3–11.
3. Hyogo Association of Medical Technologists. *Record on Hanshin-Awaji earthquake, medical support activity.* Hyogo, Japan: Hyogo Association of Medical Technologists, 1996.
4. Kawai T. Challenging changes in health care. In: Moeller G, Fischer EP, eds. *The long road to molecular medicine.* Munich: Piper, 1997: 183–190.

POCT IN REMOTE AND EXTREME ENVIRONMENTS

RICHARD M. SATAVA
SHAUN B. JONES

The need for point-of-care testing (POCT) may be most critical in remote environments that lack expert medical resources and a full logistics infrastructure. These environments include the military battlefield, scientific and exploratory expeditions, space voyages, disaster sites, and remote isolated populations. Often, the user of the diagnostic information is a nonexpert healthcare provider, such as a battlefield medic, an expeditionary first-aid provider, an emergency or disaster medical technician, or a nurse. Their limited capabilities must be supported by appropriate immediate information, using telemedicine to link these first responders to medical specialists in a central location. Over the past 5 years, the Defense Advanced Research Projects Agency (DARPA) has explored the use of advanced medical technologies to perform point-of-care (POC) medicine at the far-forward battlefield (1). This research was undertaken after an analysis of battlefield casualties over the past 200 years revealed that about 90% of the wounded died on the far-forward battlefield. If the wounded were stabilized and evacuated to rear-echelon hospitals, mortality was diminished (2), since 30% to 40% had injuries from which they could recover. The cause of death among casualties was usually bleeding to death or the inability of the medic to be aware of or locate the wounded soldier.

POINT-OF-CARE SYSTEMS

In order to decrease casualties on the battlefield, a revolutionary program was developed combining information technologies and advanced medical technologies such as miniaturized microelectromechanical systems integrated by means of a battlefield telemedicine network. The result was an integrated system of devices that communicate over a secure telecommunication network. One of the centerpieces is a wearable suite of communication, computing, and monitoring devices called the Personnel Status Monitor (PSM) system (3). The PSM is a sophisticated system of sensors worn on the body and connected to a central processing unit, which conveys the information to the radio transmission components for relay to the medic or central location. The system consists of three components worn by a soldier: (a) a telecommunications system that processes and then transmits information back to the closest medic or commander; (b) a geopositioning satellite system to determine the location of the soldier on the battlefield; and (c) vital signs monitors on various parts of the body to acquire heart rate, temperature, respiration,

motion, and shivering. In July 1966, the system underwent field testing with the military at a jungle training site in Camp Rudder, Florida. Five soldiers wore the system for 5 continuous days during a ranger field-training exercise. Position, heart rate, temperature, and motion were monitored. Vital signs and locations were tracked successfully to within 3 meters the entire time, including crawling through sandy ground or crossing a river neck deep in water. At the end of the exercise, no adverse effects from wearing the sensors were noted, including no rash or abrasions. Complementing the PSM is a "smart T-shirt" (4), an undergarment with vital signs monitors woven into the fabric, which sends the information to the PSM. Our goal was to provide a more user-friendly platform for mounting the sensors and to provide additional information about wounding. The garment is woven in three dimensions and incorporates fiber-optic and piezoelectric fibers into the actual fabric in a grid-like pattern. When the garment is penetrated as in wounding, the location of the entrance and exit wounds are instantly calculated, and the possible organs injured are estimated. In addition, DARPA developed the Life Support for Trauma and Transport (LSTAT), a portable intensive-care unit built into a stretcher, which has all the components of a typical hospital-based, intensive care unit (5). Using modern microelectromechanical systems technologies, the size and weight of the equipment were miniaturized to a point where ventilator, oxygen generator, suction, IV fluid administration, computer, telecommunications system, and sensors could all be built in a 6″-wide platform that sits under a standard North Atlantic Treaty Organization stretcher and provides full monitoring, ventilatory, and cardiorespiratory support to the casualty. In June 1998, the LSTAT was approved by the Food and Drug Administration and soon will be available commercially.

POINT-OF-CARE INSTRUMENT CRITERIA

Extreme environments impose special requirements on POCT. Under most circumstances, the equipment must be carried by the individual, whether it be battlefield, expedition, or hazardous site. Thus, there must be trade-offs among a number of factors, each of which must be optimized. These include but are not limited to the following criteria for POCT devices: (a) lightweight and small in size, since they must be carried or worn and thus will compete with other survival equipment such as weapons and food; (b) require low power, since batteries and fuel cells are extremely heavy, are expended quickly, and usually cannot be recharged in the far-forward field environment; (c) rugged and dependable, since there is no local support, and the devices must be able to work under the most difficult of conditions; (d) simple to use, since the devices cannot take much attention from the user while performing critical diagnostic testing in an extreme environment; and (e) telecommunication enabled, since effectiveness in these isolated environments requires communication.

OTHER ENVIRONMENTS

Virtually no medical data are available in extreme environments, and the immediate requirements would mandate the priority of the data that should be acquired. The military developed devices based on the need to monitor the health and fitness of soldiers and to identify soldiers that have sustained acute trauma. Thus, the data needed are those that reflect wounding, particularly severe bleeding, from projectiles (bullets) or shrapnel. On the other hand, an expedition on Mt. Everest would require slightly different parameters to be measured, because the threat is mainly from hypoxia, hypothermia, and exhaustion. Measurements that have been studied with wearable devices include heart rate, single-lead electrocardiogram, respiratory rate, temperature, motion, hemoglobin, hematocrit, and oxygen saturation. Measurements studied with portable and handheld devices include electrolytes, renal and liver function tests, blood sugar, blood gases, cardiac output, pulmonary function, Doppler flow of various arteries, and 3-D portable teleultrasound.

CONCLUSIONS

POCT is now emerging in even the most remote and challenging environments, including the battlefield and scientific expeditions. In addition to the uses the military has explored for combat casualty care, chronic diseases such as asthma (bronchodilator levels), diabetes (insulin as well as glucose), rheumatoid arthritis (salicylate or steroid levels), and others, all would benefit from POC diagnostics and immediate access to medical information, which not only will enhance the quality of patient care, but also, in combination with prediction and prevention, will reduce the overall cost of health care on the battlefield and other extreme environments.

REFERENCES

1. Satava RM. Virtual reality and telepresence for military medicine. *Comput Biol Med* 1995;25:229–236.
2. Zajtchuck R, Jenkins DP, Bellamy RF. *Textbook of military medicine: part 1, warfare, weaponry and the casualty.* Vol. 5. Washington, DC: Office of the Surgeon General of the Army, 1998:64–72.
3. Satava RM. Surgery 2001: a technologic framework for the future. *Surg Endosc* 1992;7:111–113.
4. Park S, Gopalsamy C, Rajasanickam R, et al. The wearable motherboard: a flexible information infrastructure or sensate liner for medical applications. In: Westwood JD, Hoffman HM, Robb RA, et al., eds. *Medicine meets virtual reality: the convergence of physical and informational technologies; options for a new era in healthcare.* Vol. 62. Amsterdam: IOS Press, 1999:252–258.
5. Satava RM. Virtual reality and telepresence for military medicine. *Ann Acad Med Singapore* 1997;26:118–120.

MILITARY POCT: FIELD CARE AND AEROMEDICAL EVACUATION

JAMES A. KING
SEAN E. BOURKE

Use of point-of-care testing (POCT) in the prehospital environment has been approached with limited success to date. In 1995, for example, Herr et al. (1) and Burritt et al. (2) used a helicopter-based POCT device to guide the administration of blood transfusions prior to emergency department arrival. Asimos et al. (3) showed that in the emergency department management of blunt trauma, POCT devices occasionally reduce morbidity or conserve resources. Prehospital testing of cardiac injury markers (4) offers potential to identify high-risk patients presenting with acute myocardial infarction who could benefit from prehospital definitive treatment. Future use of prehospital POCT could improve patient care in the critically ill (5,6). Because the U.S. Air Force (USAF) deploys throughout the world in austere environments often far from medical care, it needs to minimize the risks inherent in delayed definitive care. In POCT, the USAF recognizes tremendous potential to effect prehospital medical decision making and improve patient outcomes and resource management.

USAF medical teams generally are involved with four types of missions: combat care, disaster relief, humanitarian relief, and primary care for units deployed in the field. Their smallest rapidly deployable medical unit, the 25-person EMEDS Basic (Expeditionary Medical Support/Air Force Transportable Hospital), relies on portable POCT devices to carry out missions. With the help of POCT devices, seriously ill patients are identified, stabilized, and urgently evacuated to distant definitive care by Critical Care Air Transport (CCAT) teams. Elsewhere, POCT devices are used to risk stratify those who do not need evacuation but can instead be returned to duty in the field.

Resuscitative and monitoring equipment employed by the EMEDS Basic and CCAT teams include ventilators, hemodynamic monitors, electrocardiography, defibrillators, handheld ultrasonography, and rapid infusion pumps. The EMEDS Basic can perform up to ten major trauma surgeries or 20 nonoperative resuscitations. Definitive care is not the goal, but rather salvage surgery prior to evacuation. Surgeons will control life-threatening bleeding, externally fix orthopedic injuries, and provide temporary vascular bypass for limb salvage or fasciotomies for burn victims. Nonoperative care includes airway and ventilator management, tube thoracostomy, hemodynamic resuscitation, and treatment for life-threatening medical illnesses (e.g., acute myocardial infarction).

Seriously ill casualties would then be transported to definitive care by a CCAT team composed of a medical doctor (anesthesiologist, intensivist, or emergency medicine physician), critical care nurse, and respiratory therapist. Aircraft employed for aeromedical evacuation include the Lockheed C-130 and Lockheed C-141 and other aircraft. The C-130 can transport up to 92 ambulatory patients, 74 litter patients, or a combination of the two. The C-141 can transport up to 103 litter patients.

The EMEDS Basic and CCAT teams formulate field diagnosis and treatment using several POCT devices. Both use the i-STAT portable blood analyzer using either the cartridge that determines whole-blood pH, P_{CO_2}, P_{O_2}, sodium, potassium, ionized calcium, and hematocrit or a cartridge that determines sodium, potassium, glucose, and hematocrit. As if situated in a hospital-based intensive care unit, such data can be used to evaluate hemodynamic resuscitation, need for transfusion, ventilator management, severity of respiratory failure, electrolyte abnormalities, and re-triage of deteriorating patients.

Currently, the i-STAT is the only portable blood analyzer certified by the USAF Armstrong Labs for use in flight on military aircraft. Field use of this device, however, has several limitations. For example, cartridges need refrigeration at 2°C to 8°C to maintain a shelf life of 6 months. At room temperature, 18°C to 30°C, the cartridges possess a shelf life of 2 weeks. If exposed to heat, as might occur in the desert or other warm climate, cartridges are rendered useless. In a cold climate, cartridges must be brought up to room temperature before a test result can be obtained. Additionally, the software of the i-STAT must be updated every 6 months. When deployed, this becomes problematic, although updates can be performed over the Internet or using another i-STAT device containing the software update.

POC devices also can help risk stratify patients able to return to duty. For example, qualitative tests for cardiac troponin I, CK-MB, and myoglobin assist a physician triaging patients with atypical chest pain. Normal electrocardiogram and cardiac injury markers may allow a patient to return to duty, while abnormalities merit emergent aeromedical transport for treatment of acute myocardial infarction. Similarly, patients presenting with symptoms of deep-vein thrombosis who have normal D-dimer levels may return to duty instead of being evacuated for further care. Diagnosis of acute cystitis and prevention of pyelonephritis is facilitated using urine dipsticks. Vaginal bleeding is risk stratified using qualitative beta-HCG pregnancy tests and hematocrit levels. Screening for altered mental status is accomplished using qualitative urine screening for alcohol and drugs of abuse including PCP, benzodiazepines, amphetamines, THC, opiates, and barbiturates. Further screening capabilities include monospot and fecal occult blood. In sum, POCT facilitates triage, aids resuscitation, and differentiates between those who may return to duty or require aeromedical evacuation.

CONCLUSIONS

USAF medical teams continue to search for ways to improve field-based medical care. One of the areas where they are forging new ground is in field and prehospital POCT. We believe that use of POCT leads to improved patient outcomes and better use of resources as critically sick patients far from definitive care are appropriately treated, stabilized, and evacuated, while those who are capable remain on duty.

Disclaimer

This writing represents the views of the authors and is not to be interpreted as official or as representing the USAF or Department of Defense.

REFERENCES

1. Herr DM, Newton NC, Santrach PJ, et al. Airborne and rescue point-of-care testing. *Am J Clin Pathol* 1995;104:S54–S58.
2. Burritt MF, Santrach PJ, Hankins DG, et al. Evaluation of the I-STAT portable clinical analyzer for use in a helicopter. *Scand J Clin Lab Invest* 1996;56[Suppl 224]:121–128.
3. Asimos AW, Gibbs MA, Marx JA, et al. Value of point-of-care blood testing in emergent trauma management. *J Trauma* 2000;48: 1101–1108.
4. Schuchert A, Hamm C, Scholz J, et al. Prehospital testing for troponin T in patients with suspected acute myocardial infarction. *Am Heart J* 1999;138:45–48.
5. Fukuda A, Ishida H, Kubota M, et al. Usefulness of POCT in critical care medicine. *Jpn J Clin Pathol* 1999;47:1113–1118.
6. Backer HD, Collins S. Use of a handheld, battery-operated chemistry analyzer for evaluation of heat-related symptoms in the backcountry of Grand Canyon National Park: a brief report. *Ann Emerg Med* 1999;33: 418–422.

POCT IN SPACE AND AT HIGH ALTITUDE

SCOTT M. SMITH
DANIEL L. FEEBACK

Space flight and the microgravity environment of space introduce new technical challenges to point-of-care testing (POCT) that are not encountered on Earth. Because instrumentation developed for use in the terrestrial environment usually depends on gravity for proper operation, the performance of any analytical equipment must be validated in a microgravity environment prior to use on a space vehicle (Table I.1). Stringent construction standards related to off-gassing, electromagnetic interference, vibration/g-force endurance, and other parameters must be met by equipment and instruments on space vehicles. Other environmental parameters of spacecraft, such as atmospheric pressure, partial pressures of ambient gases, ambient temperature, vibration, and radiation, may also affect operation of POCT equipment. Instrumentation must be small, lightweight, and have low power requirements for operation, since launch mass, storage space, and power are premium resources on spacecraft. POCT during space flight is intended mainly for assessment of crew health, treatment of potential illnesses that may arise during the mission, or for life sciences research studies, since preexisting medical conditions that require monitoring are ruled out by intensive medical screening of the astronauts.

SHORT-TERM FLIGHT

POCT generally has not been performed on short-duration missions (less than 30 days). Nonetheless, research studies have been conducted to demonstrate the technology for POCT on-orbit while determining changes in routine clinical measurements during flight. One such study involved the use of a glucose meter to check blood glucose levels from fingerstick blood samples. This instrument appeared to work well on three Space Shuttle flights. Another study conducted on the Shuttle involved the use of a portable clinical blood analyzer (1), including pre-, in-, and postflight analyses of both control solutions and subject samples. Fingerstick samples were obtained, and capillary tubes were used for sample handling/transfer. The disposable cartridges used for this experiment allowed measurement of sodium, potassium, ionized calcium, pH, glucose, and hematocrit. In general, the instrument worked well, and there were very few problems.

LONG-TERM FLIGHT

On longer-term missions (30 days to 1 year), there is clearly a greater need for on-orbit medical evaluation and POCT. The Russian space program used in situ testing in early Mir missions, but this was intended more for research than medical testing. Fingerstick blood samples have been analyzed using a Reflotron (Boehringer Mannheim) and a "Biokhim" analyzer (Labotron, Germany) (2–4). A microcapillary centrifuge has also flown on Mir and Shuttle missions to provide real-time fingerstick hematocrit data. The Mir 18 mission included an extensive life sciences research program involving numerous experiments. A portable clinical blood analyzer flew on this first mission to provide ionized calcium and pH data (5). These analyses were performed on venous samples, using Monovette® syringes (Sarstedt, Newton, NC) for sample collection and transfer.

Russian investigators have used a small, handheld lactate analyzer (Accusport, Hoffman-LaRoche, Basel, Switzerland) as part of scientific studies on the Mir. Although its use was largely for research purposes, it is another example of how small, portable, battery-powered devices can provide useful POCT results in environments as remote as space. The International Space Station will house an international team whose individual crew members will remain in space for an average of 3 to 4 months. Unlike Shuttle missions in which all crew members participating in the mission remain together for a fixed duration, International Space Station missions will be characterized by frequent changes in the crew complement. Thus, the International Space Station environment will be less well controlled for protection against introduction of new pathogens with potential worldwide origins, obviating the need for a more robust healthcare monitoring and response system, including diagnostic POCT. Since infectious disease is a major concern, the capability to provide hematologic analyses for diagnosis of infection, inflammatory disease, and anemia during long-duration space flight or planetary exploration is paramount.

The National Aeronautics and Space Administration (NASA) is currently evaluating a commercial off-the-shelf instrument using the Quantitative Buffy Coat analysis method (Becton-Dickinson Primary Care Division, Sparks, MD) for potential space-flight use (6). This system was tested aboard NASA's KC-135 parabolic flight aircraft during level flight, microgravity, and hypergravity conditions. The capillary tubes performed well in all conditions, but the tubes floated out of the analyzer's loading platform during the microgravity phase. In collaboration with the manufacturer, several modifications were made to the system, and a method for mixing blood with the dry chemicals in the tubes under microgravity conditions was

TABLE I.1. DESIGN/PERFORMANCE CRITERIA FOR SPACE FLIGHT HARDWARE

Criteria	Constraints
Function	All processes must work without gravity
Materials	Must be of flight-certified, nontoxic, low/inflammable materials
Environment	Must pass off-gassing, electromagnetic interference, vibration/g-force endurance specifications
	Must function in spacecraft environment (atmospheric pressure, partial pressures of ambient gases, temperature, humidity, radio frequency interference, vibration, and radiation)
Power	Must use the typical low-voltage direct current of the spacecraft or batteries of an approved type
Equipment size	Volume and mass must be minimized
Fluid handling/transfer	Ability to collect/transfer biological samples in microgravity is problematic
Reagents	Conditioned storage (refrigeration) very limited
	Limited shelf-life items are problematic on long missions

developed by modifying a pipettor. On two subsequent KC-135 flights, both the modified analyzer and centrifuge performed exceptionally, yielding reproducible results on two subjects that correlated well with analyses performed on the ground.

FUTURE OF POINT-OF-CARE TESTING IN SPACE

The most critical need for POCT will be during interplanetary missions, as these will require space travelers to spend extended periods (perhaps years) beyond the outer limits of conventional healthcare systems. An interplanetary mission and establishment of a remote planetary base such as on the surface of Mars will be isolated from effective radio communications. Additionally, due to the rotation of Mars, long periods when no communications are available will be encountered. Together, telemedicine and POCT will provide the only means of medical monitoring, diagnosis, and disease intervention. The limitations of communications will further impact the effectiveness of telemedicine. Thus, the most crucial diagnostic tools, therapeutic modalities, and POCT elements should be components

of such missions, and the crew members should be well trained in the use of such tools.

REFERENCES

1. Smith SM, Davis-Street JE, Fontenot TB, et al. Assessment of a portable clinical blood analyzer during space flight. *Clin Chem* 1997;43:1056–1065.
2. Leach Huntoon CS, Grigoriev AI, Natochin YV. Long flights. In: *Fluid and electrolyte regulation in spaceflight.* Vol. 94, Science and Technology Series, A Supplement to Advances in the Astronautical Sciences. San Diego: Univelt, 1998:41–80.
3. Grigoriev AI, Polyakov VV, Noskov VV, et al. Evaluation of the state of health and characteristics of metabolism in cosmonauts on long-term space flight. *Kosmicheskiya Biologiya I Avakosmicheskaya Meditsina* 1991; 26:48–49.
4. Grigoriev AI, Arzamazov GS, Dorokhova BR, et al. Methodological recommendations for using fluid and fluid-salt loading tests to evaluate the functional status of human kidneys. Institute for Biomedical Problems. Moscow, 1979.
5. Smith SM, Wastney ME, Morukov BV, et al. Calcium metabolism before, during, and after a 3-month space flight: kinetic and biochemical changes. *Am J Physiol* 1999;277:R1–R10.
6. Prow SJ, Gunter K, Clarke MSF, et al. Evaluation of a microgravity operated clinical hematology analyzer. *Gravit Space Biol Bull* 1997;11:67.

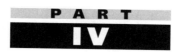

MANAGEMENT, PERFORMANCE, ACCREDITATION, AND EDUCATION

25

ASSESSING POINT-OF-CARE TESTING PROGRAMS

MARCY ANDERSON

An assessment of an institution's point-of-care testing (POCT) program is essential for enhancement and continued growth in this diverse area. Many programs lack several important elements needed to make a comprehensive and beneficial POCT program (1,2). To assess a program, the point-of-care coordinator (POCC) must identify key areas that need help as the first step toward resolving problems and reaching the performance level desired. Gathering information and using resources within the facility will help identify these key areas needing improvement. This chapter provides an understanding of how to assess a POCT program as well as information on outcomes, or what most programs lack or need.

OVERVIEW AND ROLE OF THE POINT-OF-CARE COORDINATOR

It is often difficult to evaluate one's own program objectively. Taking a close look at the policies, procedures, regulatory/accreditation compliance, and costs can be one sided and skewed. The POCC has a number of duties and responsibilities but oftentimes little authority. His or her goal is to help meet the POCT needs of the institution. To reach that goal the POCC must:

- Ensure that all POCT testing sites within the hospital are in compliance with the current regulatory and accreditation standards.
- Write procedures in National Committee on Clinical Laboratory Standards (NCCLS) format for point-of-care (POC) tests and distribute up-to-date procedures to the appropriate hospital testing sites.
- Advise and assist POCT contact persons at each site by helping with test method selection, procedural changes, and in-servicing of old or new testing procedures.
- Ensure that patient testing is consistent by using standardized normal ranges and panic values, and ensure standardization of recording and reporting of patient results.
- Establish a quality control (QC) program and a proficiency testing program for each test method used. Monitor these

results for compliance, precision, accuracy, trending, and shifting.
- Assist with annual training for the POCT personnel to assess competence. Keep records of this training and include aspects of the standard operating procedure, documentation of patient and QC records, handling of critical/erroneous values, maintenance and storage requirements, as well as safety.
- Review patient tests and QC results for technical or clerical errors/problems.
- Review corrective action documentation and make recommendations for improvement among POCT personnel.
- Reside as the chair of the POCT committee that meets when necessary to discuss issues such as new test selection criteria, any deviations from established procedures, performance improvement measurements, and billing/financial decisions (3).

Therefore, it is necessary to involve the institution's POCT committee to help perform this assessment and reach that goal efficiently (4). The objectives, scope, and time line must be discussed and agreed upon before the assessment can begin. The committee must agree to meet on a regular basis to check progress and reevaluate the time line and objectives if necessary. Once many of the logistics have been decided, the committee must determine who will take on the various tasks of assessing the program.

If there is no formal committee in place, an ad hoc committee should be instituted for the purpose of assessing the POCT program. Members of this committee could include but may not be limited to nursing personnel, administration, physicians, respiratory therapy, materials management, finance, billing, information technology, and education.

PREPARING FOR THE ASSESSMENT
Data Gathering Checklists

A series of questions and data-gathering steps are required for the performance of the POC assessment. This requires several hours of time from the POCC and assigned members of the committee (5,6). In addition to gathering this information,

TABLE 25.1. DATA GATHERING CHECKLIST

#	Process	Responsible Individual
1	Develop a comprehensive list of what floors are performing which tests throughout the entire organization.	
2	Check all QC log sheets to determine if all appropriate information is requested and documented, that is, reference ranges, lot numbers, staff initials, dates, times, and corrective action.	
3	Evaluate the POCT policy. Determine what it should address, such as personnel duties and requirements, who is responsible for competencies, ordering and safety information, troubleshooting, and PI processes.	
4	Determine if procedures are in NCCLS format or in acceptable JCAHO format. If not, who can amend and update them?	
5	Observe if cheat sheets are available on patient floors and whether they are acceptable. If not, who can enhance them?	
6	Check for proficiency testing enrollment. This must be found acceptable as per the regulatory/accrediting body.	
7	Determine if the PI plan reflects the needs of the institution.	
8	Investigate the CLIA numbers to make sure they represent the types of testing performed in the facility.	
9	Assess how competencies are handled throughout the institution and whether they can become standardized systemwide.	
10	Evaluate the POCT committee. Is it meeting the needs of the institution with on-target agenda items and numerous cross-discipline members?	
11	Determine if PPMPs occur within your institution and who oversees QC and training.	
12	Investigate to determine if a new test request form is available and whether it places ownership appropriately.	
13	Determine if tests are standardized. If not, is there a good reason for this?	
14	Check to ensure that MSDSs are readily available where necessary.	
15	Choose four representative floors to audit (Table 25.2).	
16	Interview key decision makers: finance and billing—which tests are billed; materials management—cost and volumes of supplies used for all POCT; and IT—data management capabilities	

CLIA, Clinical Laboratory Improvement Amendments; IT, information technology; JCAHO, Joint Commission on Accreditation of Healthcare Organizations; MSDS, material safety data sheet; NCCLS, National Committee for Clinical Laboratory Standards; PI, phase I; POCT, point-of-care testing; PPMP, provider-performed microscopy procedures; QC, quality control.

interviews with key decision makers within the facility must be performed. Table 25.1 lists the data-gathering checklist. Question 9 states: How are competencies handled? Many institutions handle competencies differently on each patient floor. Is there a way to streamline this so that each floor is not reinventing the wheel? Are these competencies kept in an ideal central location? In what format are they? Can there be recommendations made which simplify this tedious process and enable floors to use the same competency for like tests? (3).

Audit Questions

Once much of the data has been collected and the POCC and other members of the assessment committee are familiar with the policy and procedures, the floor audits need to be performed in which several questions are asked of the patient-care staff. A sample of these questions is detailed in Table 25.2. The unit audits give the assessment team information on regulatory/accreditation compliance, whether the staff is following the institution's policy and procedures, and what type of rapport there is between patient-care services and the laboratory (7). Observations on work flow and how the staff feels about performing POCT are also key elements that help assess the program. These findings should be summarized in table format for all members of the team to analyze.

The next step of the assessment process is to interview key decision makers to understand institutional needs concerning

the POCT program (7,8). The interviews include asking questions about what is important to the lab and to the end user or what the future holds for POCT within that facility. Many of the answers to these types of questions are stepping stones to uncovering important information that later becomes a strength, issue, or recommendation.

Once unit audits and interviews are completed, the assessment team can then sift through the various reports and information obtained. Typically, the team discovers additional questions that have not been answered or missing information. Log

TABLE 25.2. AUDIT QUESTIONS SAMPLE

General questions
What tests are performed on this floor?
What is the QC schedule for each?
Are the QC logs complete?
How do you identify patients before testing?
When do you notify the physician?
Who performs POCT?
How are you deemed competent to perform POCT?
Do you get feedback from POC coordinators?
How do you troubleshoot problems with POC tests?
Chart review
Are the results on the chart?
Are there units of measurement? Or reference ranges?
Is a physician order present?

POC, point of care; POCT, point-of-care testing; QC, quality control.

TABLE 25.3. SUMMARY OF POC TESTS

Data management capable?			
Performed in . . .			
Procedure?		NCCLS format?	
Last review QC requirements			
Normal range		Critical range	
Proficiency testing			
Disposable supply cost			
Supply	CPT	Yearly volume	Cost/pkg
Proficiency testing			
Total CPT (disposable)			
Yearly disposable cost			
CPT		Description	
Medicare fee schedule		Billing	

CPT, cost per test; NCCLS, National Committee for Clinical Laboratory Standards; POC, point of care; QC, quality control.

sheets, tracking mechanisms, additional performance improvement/quality assurance, and materials management documents are oftentimes missing and are needed to assess the program thoroughly.

Summary of Point-of-Care Tests

Meeting and seeking answers from the finance and materials management departments can take a lot of time and effort. A continuous flow of information is requested and obtained from these departments until all the necessary data are gathered to complete the program summary sheets for each test (10). See Table 25.3 for a sample summary sheet.

ANALYSIS OF DATA
Detailed List of What Is Needed

Once the policies and procedures, audit results, and interview summaries have been compiled, the analysis of the data must begin immediately. Lists are developed, which contain the information yet to be collected and the information already collected that has been placed into the appropriate category. These categories are strengths, issues, recommendations, and supportive material.

Development of Strengths

The strengths are developed from the observations made during the unit audits, interviews, chart review, procedure and documentation review, and interaction seen in the laboratory as well as on the patient floors. Oftentimes strengths will point to how well the institution follows the regulatory/accreditation guidelines defined by the Clinical Laboratory Improvement Amendments of 1988, Joint Commission on Accreditation of Healthcare Organizations, and the College of American Pathologists (CAP) (8–10). Additional strengths that have often been found through the assessments include the fact that the POCC is very accessible and always a phone call away for any issues or troubleshooting problems that surface. The proficiency testing programs show high acceptance levels for most all of the POC ana-

lytes. A result can be tracked back to a physician order located on the patient chart. Staff members on the patient floors are well aware of the critical ranges, and when to notify physicians of questionable results. The list is most often a comprehensive evaluation of the strong points of the program. This brings recognition to the program, and also emphasizes the hard work and dedication that the POCC and staff members have put into the program. In addition, key decision makers can identify opportunities for the POCT program to expand and grow in the future.

Development of Recommendations

As with the strengths of the POCT program, the recommendations are discerned from the unit audits, interviews, chart review, and procedure and documentation review. Each recommendation is developed through the recognition of an issue or problem in the POCT program. The recommendations document should not only describe (a) the issue and (b) recommendation, but also address (c) the regulatory/accreditation reference, (d) who is responsible to implement this recommendation, (e) the rationale, (f) the investment of time and resources, and (g) the benefit (13). All seven key components should be detailed for every recommendation that is made to the POCT program. Oftentimes recommendations do not take much time or effort to correct. For instance, placing QC ranges on QC log sheets or eliminating a proficiency testing kit are examples of minor recommendations. The recommendations generally fit into the categories of efficiency, regulatory/accreditation, or financial.

Efficiency recommendations are intended to bring to light tasks that take a lot of unnecessary time and effort on the part of the POCC or the staff members performing the tests. Transcribing results onto several different flow sheets on the patient floor, or the nonexistence of a POCT committee would be examples of efficiency recommendations.

Regulatory/accreditation recommendations are recognizable in the document when the regulatory/accreditation reference section is filled out with a CLIA, JCAHO, or CAP reference. JCAHO standards are often cited for staff members not initialing results or the fact that signatures cannot be associated in any way to the result on the flow sheet. Following a manufacturer's procedural recommendations according to the package insert is another issue that is often cited. Reagents and test kits are frequently not being dated when they are opened. One of the most frequently cited standards is the fact that activated clotting time, prothrombin time, and activated partial thromboplastin time controls are not run every 8 hours of patient testing (9,10).

The CAP regulations that are overlooked include proficiency testing samples that are performed consistently by only one staff member. Two levels of QC should be performed daily for most POC quantitative tests. The procedures must be written in NCCLS GP2-A3 format, and each test must have the staff member's initials accompanying each result (10,11).

The financial/cost-savings piece includes the recommendation to hire additional POCT staff if applicable. Eliminating low-volume testing performed on patient floors is another cost-saving recommendation. Standardizing tests performed by several different instruments is certainly another highly used recommendation (12). In addition, ways in which to save on QC and proficiency testing kits are also key recommendations that are given to POCT programs. Finally, opportunities to capture revenue generation for billing POCT are addressed (13,14).

Documents to Support Recommendations

The supporting documents are really considered the backbone for enhancing the facility's POCT program for the future. These documents contain the tools needed to implement the program and include other relevant information requested by the individuals involved in the assessment. The program can improve from any of these templates, references, or resources that have been gathered as supportive documents. This material supports the rationale, investment, and benefit listed in the recommendations document (6). A representation of the different types of documents includes but is not limited to abbreviations and terminology, new test request form, new procedures for every type of POCT instrument and manual test, comparison studies for different types of instruments, material safety data sheets, POCT policies, job descriptions, and data management information.

Revenue Generation Information

A spreadsheet should be prepared that includes several specific financial pieces of information obtained from the billing and finance departments. The spreadsheet contains a number of columns for calculating net potential revenue. It lists the type of test, the CPT code, annual test volume, payer mix for the institution, the Medicare fee schedule, volume adjustments, and what the institution is billing for each POC test (13,14). The more precise and accurate an institution can be about the information provided, the more accurate the potential revenue will be. Other considerations, such as inpatient versus outpatient and core laboratory testing versus POCT on the same patient on the same day, are used in determining what the institution can expect. The fiscal intermediary and carrier are also investigated to determine contractual information that may help obtain revenue generation data (14).

The total annual disposable cost for each test is also used to help determine the actual net potential revenue generation. These figures are subtracted from the potential revenue to get an actual dollar number for the institution.

PRESENTING THE FINDINGS

An executive summary meeting should be scheduled soon after the assessment is performed and all the information has been formatted and collated. All of the same key decision makers should be invited as well as staff members who contributed to the assessment. The assessment team can then present their findings at the meeting. The findings may include basic program information, what types of POCT are performed on the patient-care floors, and a cost-potential revenue spreadsheet. An action plan may then be developed for implementation of all recom-

mendations. The action plan could be divided into phases. Phase 0 is a list of recommendations that can be implemented immediately. Phase I recommendations are to be implemented within the next 12 months. These may require some investigative work, some buy-in from other departments within the facility, or some auditing processes to be put in place. Phase II recommendations require up to 18 months or more to implement, and include complete process or hospital changes. Examples of phase II recommendations are the introduction of bar-coded armbands, researching data management solutions for all POCT, and billing for POCT.

Once the executive summary meeting has addressed the findings and the action plan, the attendees have an opportunity to ask questions, voice concerns, and give feedback to the assessment team. This exchange of information is crucial for continuous enhancement and development of the institution's POCT program.

VALIDATION OF ASSESSMENT AND OUTCOMES

Table 25.4 details the most common recommendations obtained from the performance of seven POCT assessments over a year and a half. Table 25.5 details the top five requirements of POCCs when looking to expand and enhance their POCT program for their institution. The POCT programs assessed are

TABLE 25.4. COMMON RECOMMENDATIONS

#	Recommendation
1	Comply with the correct QC frequency on moderate complexity tests according to accreditation body standards. Perform two levels of QC every 8 hours for coagulation testing.
2	Develop a better tracking mechanism for POCT materials and supplies. Oftentimes this information is scattered and unobtainable in a single central location.
3	Document units of measure, staff initials, and reference ranges on the patient's chart, regardless of the accrediting body.
4	Obtain a data management solution for all POCT.
5	Prepare all procedures in NCCLS format.
6	Involve all appropriate parties in developing a comprehensive competency program for the institution.
7	Educate nurse managers/staff members to realize what testing is being performed on each particular floor (oftentimes a test or two is missed).
8	Create a comprehensive and standard process for requesting new POC tests.
9	Eliminate testing performed infrequently on patient floors.
10	Add more POCT staff if warranted.
11	Form a POC oversight committee with various members from all departments within the institution.
12	Implement a bar-coded armband system for placement on all floors.
13	Investigate and implement billing for POCT for both inpatients and outpatients.

POC, point of care; POCT, point-of-care testing; NCCLS, National Committee for Clinical Laboratory Standards; QC, quality control.

TABLE 25.5. TOP FIVE REQUIREMENTS FOR POINT-OF-CARE COORDINATORS

1. Connectivity including data management.
2. Low-cost solutions.
3. Instruments that are easy to use.
4. Customer support and service from vendors.
5. Accurate and precise results that correlate with the laboratory.

widely dispersed in the United States. All programs were diverse in scope and volume of POCT testing.

CONCLUSIONS

Every POCT program is different in many ways depending upon the regulatory body, who holds the CLIA number for POCT, and how the medical director oversees the necessary components of the program. Assessing a program is a very time-consuming and detailed process that needs the commitment and dedication from those involved in the POCT arena. Through self-assessment, a program can overcome many of its weaknesses and enhance its strengths by:

- Involving numerous individuals from the hospital, which raises the level of awareness of what POCT is and how it affects all departments.
- Summarizing the test volumes and costs of reagents and supplies, which provides a snapshot for the facility of what testing is currently performed and how much it costs.
- Evaluating the procedures, policy, QC logs, and patient results, which can prepare the institution for the next inspection.
- Involving many different departments to investigate the institution's performance improvement measures, which can help improvement processes.
- Obtaining foundation information for determining revenue generation potential through consideration of payer mix and total volumes and costs of POCT.
- Eliminating redundant forms and unnecessary ordering of supplies, which can lead to greater efficiency.

- Determining the active role of the POCC, which can give this individual more recognition within the hospital setting.

As stated above, the goal of the assessment is to help meet the POCT needs of the institution. Through the assessment process, education, networking, and creative ideas, the world of POCT will continue to grow as an avenue for providing quality patient care.

REFERENCES

1. Kiechle FL, Ingram-Main R. *Workshop for laboratory professionals: point of care testing and the clinical laboratory.* American Society of Clinical Pathologists,1999.
2. Cembrowski GS, Keichle FL. Point of care testing: critical analysis and practical application. *Adv Pathol Lab Med* 1994; :3–26.
3. Cook C, Earnest D, Mann P, et al. Ask the experts. *AACC Turn Around Times* March 2001:5.
4. Keichle FL, Cembrowski G. Quality improvement in the critical care laboratory. *Crit Care Rep* 1991;2:282–294.
5. Kost GJ. The laboratory-clinical interface in point of care testing. *Chest* 1999;115:1150.
6. Sprovieri J. *Tracking the cost of POCT: laboratories look beyond convenience to justify the price of point-of-care testing.* Critical Care Information Center, November 1999. Available at: http://www.cap.org/html/publications/point/cost.html. Accessed on December 6, 2001.
7. Kiechle FL, Ingram-Main R. Quality improvement and point-of-care testing. *J Clin Ligand Assay* 1995;18:14–20.
8. Weilert M, Workman R, Danaye-Elmi M, et al. A cost effective, high performance approach to critical care testing. *Lab Med* 1999;30:601–604.
9. Joint Commission on the Accreditation of Healthcare Organizations. *How to meet the most frequently cited questions: laboratory standards.* Oakbrook Terrace, IL: Joint Commission on the Accreditation of Healthcare Organizations, 1996.
10. College of American Pathologists. *Checklist 30: point of care testing.* Northfield, IL: College of American Pathologists, 2000.
11. Joint Commission on the Accreditation of Healthcare Organizations. *Comprehensive accreditation manual for pathology and clinical laboratory services.* Section 2 Waived Testing WT1-WT10, 2000–2001. Oakbrook Terrace, IL: Joint Commission on Accreditation of Healthcare Organizations, 2001.
12. Connectivity Industry Consortium. *Point of care coordinators workshop summary.* 2000.
13. Logue J. *Are you ready for year 2000?* Audio conference, Clinical Laboratory Management Association, November 1999.
14. Voorhees D. *Coding, billing, reimbursement, and compliance.* DV and Associates, 2000.

26

QUALITY MANAGEMENT AND ADMINISTRATION OF POINT-OF-CARE TESTING PROGRAMS

RONALD H. LAESSIG
SHARON S. EHRMEYER

TOTAL QUALITY PRINCIPLES FOR POINT-OF-CARE TESTING

Total quality management (TQM) refers to a management philosophy in which optimizing "quality" is a primary consideration when organizing, executing, and utilizing a product or service (1,2). At the most basic level, "quality" means "suitability for intended use." For point-of-care testing (POCT), "quality" is focused on improving patient outcomes and processes to meet or exceed customers'—patients, clinicians, and institutions—expectations. The word is used both as a descriptor, as in "high or low quality," and to designate a philosophical idea, as in "quality management." Deming (3) states that improved "quality" leads to better productivity by eliminating "rework." Improved efficiency of the total POCT process is the primary TQM goal. Juran et al. (4) assert that "quality" actually reduces costs. This suggests that timely testing, resulting in improved patient care is, in the long run, less expensive. Improved cost effectiveness along with improved quality of patient care and better outcomes are the major rationales for implementing POCT using a TQM process.

Not surprisingly, healthcare providers most often cite as justification for implementing POCT *the need for reduced test turnaround time to improve patient care* (5). It is deceptively easy to accept this as a valid rationale without further critical analysis (6). This rationale seems to embrace TQM principles. It would be hard to argue against improving clinicians' cost effectiveness by providing rapid, accurate test results that enable them to simultaneously enhance their productivity and make critical decisions resulting in more timely patient treatment (7). However, a true TQM-based justification for implementing POCT requires a demonstrated improvement in the patient outcome (8–10).

Site Neutrality

Prior to the Clinical Laboratory Improvement Amendments of 1988 (CLIA '88), laboratory regulations focused primarily on large, central testing facilities (11,12). CLIA '88 profoundly changed the prevailing U.S. regulatory philosophy by imposing uniform requirements for all laboratory tests regardless of where performed (13). This "site-neutral" approach means that for any

particular test, such as glucose determination, whether it is performed at a large reference laboratory, major clinic, local hospital, small physician-office laboratory, or at the patient's bedside, it is subject to the same uniform regulations. The clear intent of the "site-neutral" CLIA '88 regulations is to ensure that all tests meet a minimum standard of quality. For POCT, this often means that patient-care professionals are forced to deal with a complex set of regulatory requirements and protocols written by and for laboratorians.

Clinical Laboratory Improvement Amendments of 1988

CLIA '88 was signed into law in 1988 and went into effect on September 1, 1992 (13,14). The amendments specifically require every testing site, including point-of-care sites, examining "materials derived from the human body for the purpose of providing information for the diagnosis, prevention, or treatment of any disease" to be regulated (14). CLIA '88 superceded all previous laboratory requirements to become the first national regulations to impose uniform, minimum standards for all clinical laboratory testing (11,12). The requirements for implementing CLIA '88 were developed by the Centers for Medicare and Medicaid Services (CMS) (formerly the Health Care Financing Administration), working with the Centers for Disease Control and Prevention (CDC), and the Food and Drug Administration (FDA). The regulations, encompassing hundreds of pages of rules, criteria, and explanations, mandate the minimum quality standards for all laboratory testing sites. They continue to evolve in response to the changes in technology and the testing environment. Updated rules appear periodically in the *Federal Register* (15–20).

Test Categorization

The CDC originally and now the FDA, as part of their CLIA '88 responsibilities, classifies all test systems and/or methodologies into one of three categories (waived, moderately complex, and highly complex) based on the necessary knowledge, skill, and background required to perform the specific test. CLIA '88 regulations in turn identify specific, minimum quality (procedural) requirements for each test category. For example, the only CLIA '88 requirement for waived tests is to "follow the manufacturer's directions." Other accrediting organizations such as the Joint Commission on Accreditation of Healthcare Organizations (JCAHO), the Commission on Office Laboratory Accreditation (COLA), and the College of American Pathologists (CAP) have developed alternative requirements that typically go beyond the basic CLIA '88 requirements, but may be used by point-of-care test sites to meet the regulations (21,22). Originally, CLIA '88 identified eight simple-to-perform, risk-free tests as being "waived." In essence, this categorization means "not subject to inspection and most CLIA '88 requirements." This category included (a) dipstick/tablet reagent urinalysis, (b) visual ovulation tests, (c) visual urine pregnancy tests, (d) nonautomated erythrocyte sedimentation rate, (e) hemoglobin by copper sulfate,

TABLE 26.1. WAIVED TESTS (JANUARY, 2002)

Category	Name of Analyte
Bacteriology/virology	Helicobacter pylori Group A streptococcus Influenza A and B
Endocrinology	HCG urine Ovulation test (visual color comparison) Urine hCG (visual color comparison) N-telopeptides (for osteoporosis) FSH and LH Estrone-3 glucuronide Semen (for male fertility screen)
General chemistry	Amines Lactic acid Cholesterol Fecal occult blood Fructosamine Gastric occult Blood Glucose (glucose monitoring) Hemoglobin A₁C Microalbumin Triglycerides HDL cholesterol Ketones (blood and urine) Lyme disease antibodies Bladder tumor associated antigen Vaginal pH Alanine aminotransferase (ALT)
General immunology	H. pylori antibodies Infectious mononucleosis
Hematology	Sedimentation rate Hematocrit Hemoglobin Prothrombin time (PT)
Toxicology	Nicotine Ethanol (saliva alcohol) Cocaine Metabolites Cannabinoids Opiates PCP Amphetamines/methamphetamines
Urinalysis	Urine catalase Urine dipstick Urine qualitative dipstick (automated)

hCG, human chroionic gonadotropin; HDL, high-density lipoprotein.

(f) fecal occult blood, (g) spun microhematocrit, and (h) blood glucose meters cleared by the FDA for home use. The list continues to grow and currently includes more than 30 analytes and hundreds of methods or "kits" that are categorized as waived. The current list of analytes for which at least one waived method exists appears in Table 26.1 and on the FDA and CMS websites.

There are roughly 10,000 tests and/or methods that are either classified as moderately or highly complex. A POCT site employing one of these must meet the minimum CLIA '88 "quality" requirements for quality control (QC), quality assurance, personnel competency, proficiency testing, and so on. A waived or moderately complex test methodology, if modified by the user, automatically becomes high complexity and therefore subject to the most stringent performance standards. The most recent information on test complexity can be obtained from the FDA's and CMS' websites (http://www.fda.gov/cdrh/clia/ and http://www.hcfa.gov/medicaid/clia/cliahome.htm) or through the CliaNet link on the American Association for Clinical Chemistry's home page (http://www.aacc.org/links_b2b.stm). The manufacturer of a test system is an excellent source of information regarding a test's complexity and the regulatory requirements relating to its product. The CMS clearly intended that manufacturers play an important, proactive role in helping customers meet the CLIA requirements. Both the CMS and the FDA encourage manufacturers to supply customers with operating protocols, including procedure manuals.

Applying Total Quality Principles to Point-of-Care Testing

Based on recent growth and demand, it is reasonable to assume that POCT will continue to be an important aspect of health care. Incorporating TQM principles into the management and delivery of POCT services is not an option. It has been thoroughly incorporated into the CLIA '88 regulations and accrediting agencies' standards (JCAHO, COLA, and CAP). TQM principles force the healthcare provider to simultaneously focus on three distinct "quality" aspects critical to POCT—customer needs, institutional objectives, and the validity of the testing process.

When Congress created CLIA '88, the legislation clearly espoused the concept of a minimum standard of quality for all laboratory testing sites. Conceptually, all patients are entitled to quality laboratory results, regardless of where, when, and who does testing. No healthcare provider objects to the premise of ensuring universal quality in laboratory testing. The issue is not legislative intent, but rather how to achieve it. The overall goal of POCT is to improve patient care. Integrating total quality principles into the POCT process means empowering and requiring professionals to focus on meeting the customer's true needs. As one part of the TQM approach, each institution must design its own *continuous quality improvement program* for POCT (23). This includes establishing quality indicators, perpetually monitoring process data, and being continuously alert to ways to improve performance. This continuous quality improvement concept is incorporated into all accreditation agencies' standards.

Point-of-Care Testing Coordinator

POCT as implemented in large healthcare organizations has given rise to a new specialty, the POCT coordinator. The formation of two West Coast professional organizations focused on this specialty attests to their increasing numbers (24). The 1999 JCAHO handbook, *Quality Point-of-Care Testing* devotes a chapter to the topic (25). All accrediting organizations—CMS (CLIA), JCAHO, CAP, and COLA—recognize the need for institution-wide laboratory test results of consistent, uniform quality, unambiguous meaning, and in full conformance with the applicable regulations and accreditation standards. Accomplishing this task institution-wide falls to the POCT coordinator. The task of bringing together different departments focused on a common objective is daunting and difficult. In many instances the task involves bridging gaps between parts of the organization that often do not share the same short-term goals. For example, the central laboratory may want to perform or control all tests, while nurses may prefer the convenience of a test when and where they want it. Surgeons may wish to perform tests in real time in the operating room. The coordinator must ensure that all stakeholders are represented in the decision process. Under the CLIA regulations as well as JCAHO, CAP, and COLA voluntary standards, the responsibility for organization-wide functions fall under a coordinator's purview, such as ensuring that results from all sites, including those from the main laboratory, point of care, satellite clinics, and so on, are equivalent; reviewing QC data; setting up a quality assurance plan; and training and assessing continued competency. The key, of course, is selecting the right individual for the job; this must be preceded by a top-level management decision to truly empower the position, to provide a universally accepted job description, and a commitment to meet the standards of practice that characterize a quality POCT program.

Customer-Focused Total Quality Management Principles—Physicians, Patients, and Manufacturers

In an ideal TQM environment, the process of implementing POCT begins with a careful and objective assessment of needs *and* capabilities. The most frequently cited reasons for implementing POCT suggest improved patient outcomes and net cost savings to the entire healthcare system. These anticipated benefits are derived from quicker treatment, faster patient recovery, reduced length of stay, increased efficiency of caregivers, and better utilization of resources (26–28). Many of these benefits are specifically linked to shorter turnaround times—usually defined as the time from ordering the test to receiving or acting on the result. Clinicians are quick to cite decreased turnaround time as a means of enhancing their effectiveness, increasing their efficiency, improving their diagnostic acumen, and therefore, improving patient outcomes. This "zero-turnaround-time" scenario embodies an obvious justification for instituting POCT. It assumes an improved patient outcome as a result of better treatment and a provider benefit—enhanced overall efficiency (cost effectiveness)—through better use of clinician time.

Institutional Point-of-Care Testing Committees

In all of the models, management of POCT processes on an institution-wide basis falls to an interdisciplinary committee or team led by the POCT coordinator. Typically membership includes the medical staff, nursing services, laboratory, respiratory care, and administration. The last group may include records, purchasing, stockroom or pharmacy (maintain and disperse inventory), and a point-of-care coordinator. Utilizing TQM principles, the committee's responsibilities extend to meeting regulatory requirements, implementing the testing program including developing policies and procedures, and overall quality assurance responsibility for the testing process. All of these, under the rubric of quality assurance, are ongoing "continuous improvement processes." The committee's responsibilities include a proactive role in overseeing POCT—in short, implementing a true TQM-based process (29,30). The organizational structure must suit each institution's specific situation. However, even small POCT programs that involve only a few departments benefit from a quality team approach to POCT.

The committee must decide when and where POCT is to be implemented, which tests should be offered, and how oversight and management will be provided (31,32). This is not a trivial task. Many things must be considered in a quality-managed environment: clinicians' (and patients') demands and the justifiable need for POCT, the ability of the central laboratory to perform the requested tests and deliver timely results, staffing to conduct the testing, cost of instrumentation and related supplies, fulfilling training requirements, meeting the regulations, documentation of results in patient records, and providing the coordinator with authority to ensure that a true quality-managed, point-of-care program is established. A point-of-care committee must have the authority to make and enforce policy, assign responsibility for various functions, make recommendations and decisions, resolve problems, provide administrative support, offer advice and informational resources, and build bridges among colleagues and departments.

Hospitals without a coordinating committee are likely to be cited for not integrating POCT into the overall patient-care plan. Typically, the JCAHO requires documentation showing that an institution-wide, total quality loop (which includes all instruments and methods, quality monitors, data review and documentation) is present. Since POCT sites are often widely distributed and quite independent from one another and from the main laboratory, a major coordination of efforts is needed to meet the JCAHO requirements for a seamless testing operation while demonstrating a clear link among all test sites (33).

The POCT committee has two objectives: avoid inspection deficiencies and apply total quality principles, including continuous quality improvement, to ensure successful POCT. Many deficiencies cited in inspections can be avoided through cooperation, common sense, preparation, and ongoing supervision. Regulatory requirements are clear, explicit, and objective: analyze the appropriate type and number of quality controls, record results, remedy and document problems, and review performance. They are not discretionary! Specific requirements may be met in a variety of ways. For example, proficiency testing may or may not be a point-of-care requirement, depending, in part, on whether the committee decides to have the test site apply for independent certification (34). However, proficiency testing, required or voluntary, also can be used to assess personnel competency, as suggested by the JCAHO and CAP, for waived or moderate complexity tests. The POCT committee's greatest potential contribution lies in the area of TQM. This inspector-preferred approach assures that the POCT program focuses on realistic goals, pays proper attention to critical requirements, and obtains the maximum efficiency for the effort expended.

Point-of-Care Testing in Today's JCAHO-Total Quality Management Environment

As noted in the section on the point-of-care coordinator, the JCAHO has led all regulating and accrediting agencies in requiring an organization to employ a TQM approach. At the tactical level, the testing processes at all sites must be able to provide a uniform level of test result quality. This is no small challenge—effectively pitting a handheld, unit-use device against the most sophisticated, costly, and automated laboratory analyzer. The JCAHO, in its comprehensive accreditation standards and in its handbook, goes well beyond tactics to focus on POCT as a true strategic goal (21,25,35). In TQM terms, this begins with a thoughtful assessment of purpose as well as careful planning, design implementation, and evaluation of meaningful performance measures. Change is implemented through the continuous quality improvement process. The cycle repeats endlessly—plan, do, check, and act. This approach, of necessity, makes POCT a true institutional commitment.

Creating the Total Quality Managed Environment

Institutional implementation of a POCT program is a major undertaking (36). The creation of a total quality managed environment for POCT forces the institution to deal simultaneously with two difficult challenges—creating a new testing process as well as creating a new management paradigm. Experience teaches that in spite of the obvious advantages of doing both (when viewed in the abstract), achieving the objectives of both is far from an inevitable outcome. Transformation of a process, much less an organization, to function in a true, total-quality-managed environment requires considerable time and effort.

The regulations governing laboratory testing strongly suggest the wisdom of using the total-quality-managed approach during implementation as well as continuing operation. Those charged with overseeing and managing the POCT process begin by focusing on the basic questions: "What are we trying to accomplish?" and "Who are our true customers?" An investment of effort at this level will begin to assure that a quality-managed POCT process will follow.

Total Quality Managed Point-of-Care Testing—CLIA Creates a Shared Responsibility

The CLIA '88 regulations envision a true quality partnership focused on the patient. In addition to providers (hospitals, clinicians, and laboratories), manufacturers, and regulators, the entire laboratory community is challenged to take an enlightened approach—not just to meet the regulations, but also to address the true quality objective (37–40).

CLIA '88 allows manufacturers of POCT devices to supply laboratories with procedure manuals, design QC protocols, pro-

vide control materials, train operators, devise record-keeping systems, suggest performance standards, and so on. In short, manufacturers are encouraged to actively partner with the customer to creatively meet the regulations. Beginning in 1976, the FDA required manufacturers, through the labeling regulations, to provide essential data such as normal (reference) ranges, performance criteria (expected bias and level of imprecision), and data on interferences, dynamic range, and more (41). CLIA '88 takes this "partnership" to the next level through the "quality alliance" (42). For example, the 1992 CLIA regulations invite manufacturers to propose alternatives to the rigid "two controls per test day" rule heretofore imposed, without exception, on every moderate- and high-complexity test (13). This provision is often cited as the "September 1, 1994 rule," the date the FDA was to implement this CLIA provision.

An example of this alliance at work has been the evolution of "electronic controls." Based on technological advances, manufacturers have proposed using built-in, electronic checks in lieu of actual liquid controls on test systems used at the point of care. Regulators have accepted this radical departure not envisioned in the original CLIA '88 regulations. Clearly no one partner could independently introduce this concept. The other "regulators"—JCAHO, CAP, COLA, and states—have accepted electronic controls under specific conditions, most notably in POCT settings. The underlying assumption in the original CLIA regulations was that alternatives to traditional QC and calibration protocols could be accepted if the product's claimed level of quality, based on real data, was demonstrated. Other than allowing electronic controls, the CMS has repeatedly delayed implementing this approach, citing cost factors (16,18,20,43). There is little optimism among the laboratory testing community that a major revamping of QC will soon emerge. The clear intent of the drafters of the regulation, however, remains.

PERFORMANCE ENHANCEMENT AND ADMINISTRATION OF POINT-OF-CARE TESTING

CLIA '88 regulations have two major objectives. First is the creation of uniform, baseline quality practices, which assure a minimum level of quality for all testing—irrespective of test site. These practices contain objective performance standards such as run two controls per test per day, maintain an up-to-date procedure manual, provide staff training, and participate in proficiency testing, among others. The assumption is that if the test site fulfills certain minimum process requirements, a level of quality will follow. Second, the regulations mandate creation of a "total quality managed" testing environment designed to both oversee and continuously improve the quality of service provided to customers and improve patient outcomes (44). The JCAHO's 1999 handbook effectively combines these two concepts in the POCT context (25).

The challenges are many. The first is to deliver timely and quality results. POCT sites often must use low-cost and less elaborate (by comparison) equipment. They are located outside the traditional controlled laboratory environment and must function without trained laboratory professionals using sophisticated management and control processes. Second, the tests demanded at point-of-care sites continue to grow in complexity and sophistication. The challenge extends to providing an extensive test menu 24 hours a day, 7 days a week, with near zero turnaround time. The testing processes must be in full compliance with a complex set of very technical regulations and overarching professional standards written with the centralized laboratory in mind. Third, POCT must be viewed as part of complex, interconnected entities not focused on testing per se, but rather organized in a total quality managed system to focus on the ultimate customers—the patients.

Point-of-Care Testing—Connectivity Is the Key

In the context of POCT, connectivity simply means integrating the point-of-care test results and supporting data with the patient's record and ultimately incorporating all information into the healthcare organization's database. Discussions of connectivity are often made needlessly complex because of a failure to distinguish between three quite different aspects: (a) the intellectual process of integrating individual test results into a patient's record to permit contextual use of the data, such as monitoring a 48-hour sequence of POCT blood gas results to assess progress (45–48); (b) the process of moving data from point to point, which can be as rudimentary as transcribing information from the POCT device to a sophisticated wireless computer-linked network (46); and (c) the process of integrating the test results and associated data into an institutional database and using it for sophisticated offline analyses. Examples of offline use may include billing, quality assurance (methodology or analyst assessment), utilization review, analysis of ordering patterns, and ultimately, outcome assessment (49).

In the first case, the answer is obvious: unless the test result—properly documented as to time, preanalytical conditions, traceability to quality assurance data, and even interpretation or utilization—is captured in the patient's record, all of the nonimmediate benefits are lost. Worse yet, gaps in documenting changes in the patient's progress are created (49). The consequence of failing to achieve the first aspect of connectivity for POCT results can be best understood by the extreme case—no one would consider providing long-term patient care without creating charts or permanent medical records. A POCT result disassociated from the patient's record is a much less extreme, but nevertheless relevant example. The second case of POCT connectivity relates to data transfer. POCT systems typically provide hardcopy printouts. Minimally, this printout should, in addition to the test result, contain patient identification, date, time, analyst, quality check, reagent lot numbers, and instrument identification. Computer programming screens can assist users (47,48). Docking stations, connecting modules, or wireless systems as fully automated and capable as today's cellular phones, can accomplish the entire downloading process automatically and in real time while eliminating human transcription error (46). Hospital information systems, laboratory computers, terminals at nursing stations, and even individual patient data managers fall under this aspect of connectivity.

Finally, in the third case, POCT data are utilized beyond the immediate treatment of the patient. Dr. James Nichols of Johns Hopkins (now Baystate, MA) uses connectivity to assess patients' medical records and the degree to which the point-of-care tests changed outcomes (47). Visionary perhaps, but connectivity is the first step. For all three cases, point-of-care connectivity is recognized as an emerging discipline (45). Currently, the Connectivity Industry Consortium (http://www.poccic.org) seeks to publish (voluntary) standards for POC devices and to evaluate practical application of the standards at care-provider sites.

Reduction of Preanalytic, Analytic, and Postanalytic Errors

An unexpected benefit of POCT is to reduce some sources of error associated with centralized testing. Two quantitative studies demonstrate that POCT may have an unexpected effect on the total quality of the entire analytical testing process. Ross and Boone (44) in the United States and Plebani and Carraro (50) in Europe independently identified pre- and postanalytical errors as the major sources of error in the testing process. Analytical error associated with the testing process itself amounted to only about 10% of the total error (Table 26.2). Their assessments provide an interesting, if unplanned, justification for POCT. Tests performed at or near the patient, by definition, eliminate many of the preanalytical errors associated with patient identification, sample transport, and processing. Results generated at or near the patient, and immediately available to clinicians, eliminate the postanalytical errors associated with the data handling, transcription, reporting, and communicating results. Pre- and postanalytical errors aside, POCT technologies are expected to provide test results with equivalent levels of quality (accuracy, precision, sensitivity, specificity, etc.) when compared to laboratory-based methodologies. The literature is replete with studies both pro and con. Our assessment is that the "quality gap" associated with POCT has narrowed significantly and POCT quality is continuing to improve.

Conventional Quality Control, Unit-Use Devices, and Electronic Controls

Traditional, centralized laboratory test systems follow daily or more frequent QC protocols using liquid samples that emulate patient specimens. Since the true analyte values of the "controls" are known, the performance of the test system can be assessed. At the time the CLIA '88 rules were promulgated, many of the point-of-care devices we know today were nonexistent. The CLIA '88 rules clearly did not foresee the growth in POCT

TABLE 26.2. DISTRIBUTION OF TOTAL ANALYTICAL ERROR

Source of Error	Ross and Boone[a]	Plebani and Carraro[b]
Preanalytical	46%	68%
Analytical	7%	13%
Postanalytical	47%	19%

[a]From Ross JW, Boone DJ. *Institute on Critical Issues in Health Laboratory Practice symposium proceedings* (Minneapolis, MN: DuPont Press, 1991).
[b]From Plebani M, Carraro P. Mistakes in a state laboratory: types and frequency, *Clin Chem* 1997;43:1348–1351.

technology or the need for new QC paradigms (1,51). For any nonwaived point-of-care test system, the routine, daily use of controls and assessment of the results is not an option; it is a requirement.

Point-of-Care Test Devices with Built-in Controls

Many unit-use, disposable test devices have "built-in" controls that are analyzed concurrently and automatically with each patient sample. The simplest of such devices are urine pregnancy test systems where instructions say in essence, "add sample; if one line appears, it is a negative test; if two lines appear, it is a positive test; and if no lines appear, the test has failed." The "negative line" serves both as a process control (i.e., verifies the testing process has proceeded correctly) and a negative control (demonstrates a negative result). Strictly speaking, for nonwaived tests, running a positive control once a day is also necessary. Some of today's devices include built-in positive and negative controls. If the manufacturer claims the built-in controls meet the regulatory requirements, its literature will so indicate. Accrediting agencies may require additional liquid controls on a periodic basis. The test site should (a) follow the manufacturer's directions exactly, and (b) seek the manufacturer's assistance in addressing any problems encountered during inspection.

Increasingly, today's POCT environment stresses use of onboard controls in test devices to meet the QC requirements with a minimum or zero additional effort by the operator. Capturing the data is another matter. The JCAHO, CAP, and COLA require documentation of the QC activities, recording of control results, and assessment of daily and long-term performance for all test sites including waived sites. Documentation need not be elaborate.

Surrogate Controls

Some POCT instruments use surrogate controls that consist of reusable "reference cassettes" or similar devices such as colored filters and permanently colored dipsticks that simulate a given level of response to the analytes being tested (52). When inserted into the instrument, they engage some parts of the test system to produce a "control" value. If the responses are within acceptable limits, the requirement to run controls is deemed to be satisfied. The results must be recorded and processed as if they were from true controls. The main criticism of surrogate controls is that only some of the electronic-sensing and data-handling circuits of the system are evaluated while bypassing all of the "chemical" and analytical processing steps in the test procedure. Although there are strong philosophical and practical arguments against relying on surrogate controls, they currently are recognized as meeting CLIA, COLA, JCAHO, and CAP QC requirements. The surrogate controls must first be qualified by direct comparison to conventional controls.

Electronic Checks and Electronic Controls

Today's POCT devices often are highly sophisticated digital/electronic instrumental systems that contain many internal, self-adjusting circuits or actual computers that automati-

cally perform multiple function checks concurrent with each analysis. These systems are highly sophisticated, checking for stability in the circuits, battery status, sensor voltage, unwanted gas bubbles, barometric pressure, outdated reagents, computational processes, and more, before accepting the patient specimen and producing a test result. Some systems also apply an electronic signal directly to the sensor, to produce the equivalent of a control result. Dubbed "electronic controls," these devices have set off a firestorm of passionate debate within the laboratory community (53–55). Purists insist that true controls must mimic patient specimens (e.g., are of the same matrix, whole blood, serum, plasma, or urine), contain the true analyte (e.g., cholesterol, glucose, or potassium), and go through the entire analytical measurement process. These arguments contend that the electronic controls measure essentially nothing relevant to testing patients' specimens.

The argument regarding acceptability of electronic controls is, however, moot. CMS (CLIA), COLA, CAP, and JCAHO requirements all now accept electronic controls as meeting the "two controls per test per day" requirement. However, the CAP and JCAHO require a documented, initial inhouse study that verifies that the electronic controls yield results equivalent to conventional controls. Practically, this means that a "once-only" comparison of conventional (liquid) and electronic controls must be made for each instrument. The CAP and JCAHO also require periodic reverification based on less-extensive direct comparisons. Basically, this means that two levels of liquid controls have to be run approximately once per month. Electronic controls can then be used to meet all other, including daily quality control, requirements. The control data must still be recorded and periodically evaluated by a supervisor.

Lock-Out Quality Control Systems

Some computerized point-of-care test devices can be programmed to "demand" that the operator run a control or controls at a predetermined frequency. The onboard computer first evaluates the control result for acceptability ("Is it within tolerance?"), and only then allows patient specimens to be analyzed. If the control result is out of tolerance, the device withholds the patient test result. These systems are characterized as having a "lock-out" QC system. Since these systems have programmable tolerances, the control limits can target a desired level of analytical accuracy at critical levels. For example, such a device testing potassium might be set to a control tolerance of 0.5 mmol/L. If a control is tested and the result is within 0.5 mmol/L of the correct potassium value, the patient's test result is produced. This lock-out system theoretically assures the clinician that the system has been checked for adequate performance and no patient result will be in error by more than the tolerance.

Design and Management of Point-of-Care Proficiency Testing Programs

Proficiency testing or external quality assessment programs under the CLIA regulations serve a dual purpose—an independent, regulatory assessment of performance and/or a means of quality assurance. In either case, proficiency testing is the cornerstone of CLIA '88 and used as a means of evaluating every licensed testing site's proficiency, that is, its ability to produce the "right" answer. Proficiency testing has a documented history as a successful quality assurance tool. For the 40-plus years preceding CLIA '88, it was a major component of professional accreditation programs (56–60). Faced with the need to implement a universal laboratory regulation, the CMS decided that proficiency testing could be provided readily through third parties without significant expense to the federal government. As a result, proficiency testing became a primary means of uniformly regulating test performance in all nonwaived sites under CLIA '88. While proficiency testing is a universal requirement for "regulated" analytes under the CLIA, COLA, and JCAHO, it is a general requirement, when available, for all, including waived analytes, under the CAP. The team responsible for managing the institution's POCT program typically decides on which regulator will inspect the point-of-care test site, and therefore, which set of proficiency testing requirements will be followed.

How Point-of-Care Proficiency Testing Works

Each testing site participating in mandatory proficiency testing receives, from an HCFA-approved proficiency testing provider, three shipments of five "unknown" samples per year for each regulated analyte. The test site analyzes these unknown specimens just as they would patients' specimens (routine analyst, instrument, number of replicates, etc.) and reports the results to the proficiency testing provider. The provider evaluates the results for correctness and then notifies the testing site and the CMS of the composite score ("pass" or "fail" grading system). Once the proficiency testing report is received, it needs to be reviewed by the test site supervisor (point-of-care coordinator) and, when necessary, appropriate corrective actions initiated. This review and the corrective actions must be documented.

When proficiency testing is used for regulatory purposes, the testing site must achieve a minimum frequency of correct results in order to "pass." "Passing proficiency testing" is absolutely essential for the test site to maintain its CLIA certificate and continue to test. In some cases under the CLIA, COLA, and JCAHO, participation in proficiency testing is not specifically required but is a highly recommended quality assurance practice. The CAP essentially requires successful participation in proficiency testing for all analytes the test site offers as part of its certification process.

Proficiency Testing Requirements Are Based on Institutional Certification

The institution has some latitude in selecting the appropriate strategy for meeting the CLIA '88 proficiency testing requirement. Participation in an approved proficiency testing program, once for each regulated analyte identified in the 1992 *Federal Register*, is required for each CLIA certificate (14). For example, in a large hospital where the central laboratory holds the institution's CLIA certificate and also is responsible for POCT, the central laboratory would most likely analyze the proficiency testing samples using high-volume, automated instruments. The point-of-care sites would not be required to participate in profi-

ciency testing. On the other hand, if the POCT site offers blood gas analyses under its own CLIA certificate, the site must participate in a CMS-approved proficiency testing program for blood gases. Because there are multiple management issues to consider including costs, institutional organization, record keeping, personnel, and training, among others, CLIA certification and proficiency testing strategies involving POCT sites require careful institution-wide review. The consequences extend far beyond the testing site itself, impacting, for example, hospital-wide accreditation under the JCAHO. The institution-wide POCT committee must understand regulatory requirements as well as their institutional implications and assimilate a variety of viewpoints in making its decision.

Irrespective of which regulator inspects the test site and the strategy chosen, an overriding TQM principle is that all testing processes within the institution must be evaluated for accuracy and all testing sites within the institution must demonstrate the capability of producing equivalent results. Institution-wide documentation of this site-to-site testing equivalence is required by all inspecting agencies. In particular, the JCAHO institutional accreditation process focuses on achieving one level of care within the entire healthcare organization and specifically requires biannual demonstrated equivalency of test results across all test sites and/or CLIA certificates.

Proficiency Testing Alternatives

Under CLIA '88, regulatory proficiency testing programs are provided by governmental entities such as states or nonprofit-sector professional organizations such as the CAP, American Association of Bioanalysts, and American Thoracic Society. Each program must be approved by the CMS and must follow mandated protocols. Once the CMS approves programs as meeting minimum proficiency testing standards, the programs can be marketed to testing sites.

Currently there are approximately 20 approved proficiency testing providers. Some provide programs geared specifically to POCT sites; others focus on large laboratories. Typically the cost of such programs is tied to the scope of services provided. In selecting a program for a given testing situation, judicious choice translates into cost savings. The POCT coordinator responsible for the selection is strongly urged to discuss the programs with the individual vendors. The most up-to-date listing of proficiency testing providers is available through the CMS' website (http://www.hcfa.gov/medicaid/clia/cliahome.htm).

Practical Uses of Proficiency Testing Data to Address Other Regulatory Requirements

- Waived tests, by definition, are exempt from regulatory proficiency testing. However, CAP requirements strongly recommend that every analyte, including waived analytes, be evaluated by proficiency testing. These data can be used to address a myriad of quality-assurance requirements (competency assessment, training, method comparison, etc.).
- For each CLIA certificate, every nonwaived test system must be evaluated by an approved proficiency testing program. If multiple sites and/or methods test the same analyte under the

same certificate, proficiency testing is required for only one site or method per certificate. All sites must be intercompared as part of quality assurance.

■ Test results from all sites in the same institution must be coordinated. Intercomparison of regulatory or quality assurance-based proficiency testing data is one means by which the POCT committee can address this requirement common to all inspection and accreditation programs.

■ Proficiency testing results also can be used for a variety of regulatory and quality assurance purposes including accuracy assessment, instrument validation, and demonstration of test site and analyst competence.

■ An essential element of successful proficiency testing participation, and means of fulfilling the regulatory requirements, is a documented, thoughtful review of proficiency testing results by the point-of-care coordinator. Failure to comply with this review requirement is a commonly cited inspection deficiency.

Proficiency Testing-Based Intralaboratory Quality Control Requirements

The CLIA '88 requirements enacted on February 28, 1992, not only mandate "universal" proficiency testing participation for nonwaived analytes, but also set minimum intralaboratory performance standards (14). For example, the acceptable proficiency testing result for potassium must be within 0.5 mmol/L of the target (true) value; for sodium, within 4 mmol/L; for PCO_2, 5 mm Hg; and for pH, 0.04 units. In a series of papers, we have demonstrated the link between the proficiency testing requirements and actual intralaboratory QC-performance requirements (61,62). In order to pass proficiency testing consistently, it is critical that the instrument or method, under normal operation, be capable of achieving a minimum level of performance. Obviously, a test methodology with an inherent error of 1.0 mmol/L for potassium would fail proficiency testing on a regular basis and place the test site's CLIA '88 certificate in jeopardy. On the other hand, an instrument with a performance standard of 0.1 mmol/L would easily pass, but probably exceeds medical needs and may be too expensive or impractical for use in a point-of-care setting. This situation gives rise to the TQM approach to POCT. Our statistical modeling studies suggest that an intralaboratory imprecision of 33% of the CLIA '88 standard will ensure passing proficiency testing (63). Clearly, point-of-care instrument selection is not a simple matter of performance, cost, or convenience, but rather a combination of all three as well as other variables. The optimum selection of instruments and proficiency testing providers requires a variety of talents represented on the point-of-care committee.

ORGANIZATION AND SELECTION OF QUALITY MONITORS AND PRACTICE PARAMETERS

CLIA, COLA, JCAHO, and CAP requirements have adopted a TQM-based philosophy implemented through inspection and accreditation. Consequently, when POCT sites are inspected, the site is expected to be managed by, and to adhere to, total quality principles. The responsibility for taking an institution-wide view is vested in the POCT committee. It is expected to develop a suitable, site-specific, quality assurance plan to address both needs and requirements. While inspectors are given latitude in assessing the adequacy of the site's plan, they receive guidance in the form of specific "quality indicators" embodied in the CLIA '88 regulations and incorporated into their agency's inspection guidelines.

Quality indicators or practice parameters are defined as the actual quantitative measures used to assess the adequacy of the test site's performance. For example, in the specific area of QC, the CLIA '88 regulations mandate minimum control frequency, but also empower the testing site to (a) design a process to ensure that appropriate controls are run at the required frequency, (b) define practice parameters (i.e., specify what constitutes acceptable performance), and (c) set criteria to systematically assess control data to ensure that the quality goals are being met.

Monitors Related to Total Quality Management

The CLIA regulations go a step beyond requiring the testing site to design and implement a system to assure the quality of the testing process. In the context of TQM principles, testing sites are mandated to continuously step back and assess their total testing processes. The regulations specifically define ten areas for which quality monitors and associated (measurable) performance parameters must be developed. (The ten areas are listed in Table 27.1.)

The monitors are both specific (performance oriented) and general (process oriented). For routine QC, an example is: "Quality control for the point-of-care test potassium shall be performed once per day (every 24 hours) using two levels of controls; acceptable performance is defined as 95% of results being within ±0.5 mmol/L of the target values." The first half is the monitor; the latter is the performance parameter. In reviewing the control data created, the designee of the POCT committee would have to decide if the method met the criteria or if the method needed improvement or should be abandoned.

Critical Quality Assurance Monitors at Point-of-Care

The CLIA '88 regulations, as well as professional organizations' inspection standards, seek to promote a TQM approach to quality assurance. They enumerate ten specific areas, which affect test quality. The process of deciding what to measure (i.e., "monitor") begins with the critical questions: "What are we trying to accomplish?" "What can we measure to assess it?" "How do we know when we are successful?" The process requires selection of a manageable number (two to four) of the most relevant quality assurance monitors. Not all ten quality assurance areas are evaluated concurrently. If, upon evaluation, the monitor (e.g., the frequency of erroneous potassium control results) is successfully achieved (less than 5% of control results have a deviation that exceeds 0.5 mmol/L), this monitor could be set aside and another selected to evaluate a different area. The selection of a specific monitor often is based on caregivers' feedback (customer complaints). Some monitors—for example, assaying two

TABLE 26.3. EXAMPLES OF QUALITY ASSURANCE MONITORS AND PERFORMANCE PARAMETERS

CLIA Quality Assurance Topics (§493.1703–21)	Critical Question	Quality Monitor	Performance Parameter
Patient test management	Are blood gas data recorded in the patients' charts?	Comparison over 1 month of instrument log to patients' charts.	100% compliance.
Quality control	Are appropriate responses documented for out-of-control situations for potassium?	Monthly review of potassium quality control data and remedial action log.	95% compliance.
Proficiency testing	Are corrective actions for failed tests documented?	Review 1 year of proficiency testing data and corrective action log.	100% out of tolerance test results are investigated.
Test comparisons	Are blood-gas results compared semiannually with the central laboratory?	Review results from point-of-care and the central laboratory on split patient samples or controls.	100% compliance.
Relate results to clinical data	Are the point-of-care results for glucose consistent with the patient's condition?	Review 10 patient charts for evidence of need for glucose testing.	100% compliance.
Personnel	Do personnel performing protimes have documented training?	Review personnel records of all authorized personnel.	100% compliance.
Communications	Does the clinical staff know which tests are available at point of care?	Survey 10 clinicians as to what point-of-care tests are available on their service.	At least 7 of the 10 are able to provide substantially correct information.
Complaints	Has the turnaround time for blood-gas results from the central laboratory generated complaints?	Review point-of-care committee minutes and/or complaint log.	If "yes," investigate possible solutions.
Staff review	Has the policy for annual competency assessment been communicated to the entire point-of-care testing staff?	Review the minutes of the staff meetings and the attendance sheets.	100% compliance.
Records	Is the audit trail complete for glucose test results?	Review five selected patient records for documentation of analyst, instrument, quality control results, and maintenance records.	100% compliance.

controls per test per day for moderately complex tests—are fixed requirements and must be continued indefinitely. Others, such as turnaround time, staff competency, and result reporting, are expected to show improvement and be placed in and out of the total quality assurance activity. The National Committee for Clinical Laboratory Standards has a guideline to assist healthcare institutions in developing a quality system approach (64).

Sample Quality Assurance Monitors for Point-of-Care

Table 26.3 provides an illustrative list of monitors and practice parameters. It is not exhaustive, nor does it include all potential monitors identified in the regulations—its purpose is to suggest to the POCT committee "TQM-type" monitors and practice parameters.

Tracking, Benchmarking, and Improving Performance—Staff and Instruments

Tracking, benchmarking, and process improvement are major tenets of the TQM process. In this context, "tracking" means basically following an indicator used to assess or verify the ongoing quality of a process. The concept of tracking ties to the CLIA '88 required process of selecting and assessing monitors and performance parameters as part of continuous quality improvement. "Benchmarking" is a practice by which one qual-

ity-managed unit (which can be as large as an entire institution or as small as a department, unit, or team) systematically observes the operations of another. The objective is to learn from a peer operation, which is one held in high regard and usually identified by reputation. A point-of-care test site, which has received an excellent report on inspection, might be "benchmarked" by another facing an accreditation inspection. This TQM activity can be very broad or highly specific. It may range from the POCT committee seeking to improve the entire process to learning how QC data can better be monitored, utilized, and recorded. In the context of TQM, process improvement is ongoing. Changes can be global or incremental.

Selecting Monitors—Role of the Point-of-Care Testing Committee

Selecting monitors—simply put as deciding what to measure, when to do it, how much data to collect and how to evaluate the data—is often the most daunting challenge of creating a true total-quality-managed process. It is also the most fundamental requirement envisioned by the regulations. This task falls to the POCT coordinator and the institutional committee. There are many acceptable ways to accomplish this task, but for purposes of an illustrative example, we outline a simple ten-step process.

1. The POCT committee spends 15 minutes in a brainstorming session with "post-its" to create a list of possible monitors.

2. Using an affinity process, combine duplicate or closely related ideas and clarify meanings of the ideas.
3. Using independent, anonymous voting, have each member identify his or her top three choices. The "best" potential monitor gets a value of 3 points, second best 2 points, and third best 1 point. Total the scores.
4. Look at the top five vote items; revote if necessary.
5. Select from one to three potential monitors to implement.
6. The POCT coordinator creates for the next meeting a plan of implementation for each monitor. Note that this proposed plan should include what will be monitored; what is actually measured; the data collection process, including who is responsible; how long the process will continue; and a suggestion of targets so the committee can recognize success or failure.
7. At the next committee meeting, the coordinator presents the plans for discussion, refinement, and authorization to proceed.
8. After the requisite amount of data is collected, the coordinator presents a summary of results to the committee for review and discussion.
9. For each monitor, the committee decides on a course of action, such as the performance meets institutional needs so the monitor can be discontinued and a new one selected; more data are needed or the collection process needs refinement; or the performance data do not meet institutional needs, and thus a plan of correction is created for improvement.
10. When each step in the process is carefully documented, the accrediting agency's inspectors will be very happy, since some version of this process is fundamental to TQM. Put simply, the process involves carefully defining what is intended to be accomplished and then "doing the right thing."

Improving Staff Performance

The qualifications of individuals to perform point-of-care tests are tied to the test-complexity model and related CLIA '88 educational and training requirements as well as professional accreditation standards. Under the principles of TQM, the POCT program is further required to define specific qualifications and training and retraining criteria, and to develop assessment practices commensurate with producing quality results and meeting institutional needs (e.g., its quality objectives). This is an outcome-based approach that focuses on the overall objectives of the testing process.

In practical terms, this means that for each POCT procedure the analyst's as well as the method's performance must be monitored. Obviously, the challenge is to answer the questions: "What is an appropriate level of quality?" followed by "What do we measure to evaluate our performance?" To illustrate, a quality objective, for the trained and competent analyst providing potassium tests at the point of care, is to have 95% of patient test results fall within 0.5 mmol/L of the true value with no deviation greater than 1.0 mmol/L. Periodically reviewing an individual's performance on proficiency testing or split patient samples is a means of assessing and documenting performance against the quality objective.

Like all other aspects of quality management, the four-step process of deciding on what constitutes a quality outcome, deciding what to monitor, assessing performance, and creating documented evidence of the evaluation, is the key to meeting both specific regulatory requirements and TQM-based objectives.

Improving Instrument Performance

At a POCT site, improving instrument performance also uses TQM techniques. Through QC the actual performance is assessed. Through quality management, the POCT committee decides if the instrument's performance meets the institution's quality goals. If the performance is not acceptable, the choice is obvious—improve it or change instrumentation. This assessment is not trivial; it requires significant laboratory expertise in method evaluation and real data. Instrument assessment ideally should precede deployment.

Assessment of an instrument's characteristics is an essential part of the decision to deploy a particular device as well as the design of the training program. However, the reality is that often POCT sites are saddled with decisions made with less-than-optimal data or by the institution's purchasing department or by quasi-independent departments. The POCT committee must be prepared to deal with the result of the decision after the fact.

CONCLUSIONS AND RECOMMENDATIONS FOR THE FUTURE

Ideally, TQM principles should be part of a POCT process from its inception. In a vast majority of cases, POCT is joined with TQM sometime after both have been incorporated into the institution's culture. The regulators and organizations that enforce professional standards are aware of this typical chain of events; they are also adamant that these two concepts must be merged and become the standard of practice in a successful POCT program. The benefits are obvious.

The current regulatory environment prescribes how point-of-care tests are to be provided. We have described the types of basic actions that must be undertaken as well as the approach to empower the POCT committee to tailor the program to the institution's needs.

In our quality alliance proposal, we suggest going a step further. Manufacturers possess extensive data on product performance, only some of which are submitted to the FDA as part of the new product approval or 510(k) process. Most of the data, derived from research, development, and field-testing of a test method, are unpublished. This "profound knowledge" surely enables the manufacturer, in the specific, not the regulator in the abstract, to determine what quality assurance procedures are necessary to ensure quality performance. This concept is particularly applicable to test systems that involve "unit-use" or "single-use" disposable test strips, slides, packs, or cartridges, where traditional quality assurance protocols required by the current regulations yield a minimum of relevant performance data. Manufacturers' data, on the other hand, contain a wealth of information on lot-to-lot characteristics, which actually define the device's performance. Under the concept of the proposed quality alliance, this information could virtually eliminate the need for point-of-care sites to engage in near-meaningless retesting. Adopting such an approach would make POCT processes more efficient and cost effective. Manufacturers, along with regulators and healthcare professionals—all partners in the quality alliance—could focus on the ultimate customer, the patient. This alliance, as it evolves, will change again the face of POCT.

REFERENCES

1. Phillips DL, et al. *Quality management for unit-use testing: proposed guideline EP18-P.* Wayne, PA: National Committee for Clinical Laboratory Standards, 1999.
2. Goldsmith BM, et al. *Point of care in vitro diagnostic (IVD) testing: approved guideline AST2-A.* Wayne, PA: National Committee for Clinical Laboratory Standards, 1999.
3. Deming WE. *Out of crisis.* Cambridge, MA: Massachusetts Institute of Technology, 1982.
4. Juran JM, et al. *Quality control handbook.* New York: McGraw-Hill, 1974.
5. Barr JT, et al. *Blood glucose testing in settings without laboratory support: approved guideline AST4-A.* Wayne, PA: National Committee for Clinical Laboratory Standards, 1999.
6. Harvey, MA. Point-of-care laboratory testing in critical care. *Am J Crit Care* 1999;8:72–83.
7. Barr JT, et al. *Ancillary (bedside) blood glucose testing in acute and chronic care facilities: approved guideline C30-A.* Wayne, PA: National Committee for Clinical Laboratory Standards, 1994.
8. Kost GJ, Hague C. The current and future status of critical care testing and patient monitoring. *Am J Clin Pathol* 1995;104:S2–S17.
9. Kost GJ. Guidelines for point-of-care testing: improving patient outcomes. *Am J Clin Pathol* 1995;104:S111–S127.
10. Nichols JH, Poe SS. Quality assurance, practical management, and outcomes of point-of-care testing: laboratory perspectives (part 1). *Clin Lab Mgmt Rev* 1999;13:341–350.
11. U.S. Department of Health, Education and Welfare, Public Health Service. Clinical Laboratory Improvement Act of 1967. *Federal Register* 1968;33.
12. U.S. Department of Health, Education and Welfare, Social Security Administration. *Federal health insurance for the aged: regulations for coverage of service of independent laboratories.* No. HIR-13. Washington, DC: U.S. Department of Health, Education and Welfare, 1968.
13. Public Health Service Act. §353, 42 USC §263a (1988).
14. U.S. Department of Health and Human Services. Medicare, Medicaid and CLIA programs: regulations implementing the Clinical Laboratory Improvement Amendments of 1988 (CLIA). Final rule. *Federal Register* 1992;57:7002–7186.
15. U.S. Department of Health and Human Services. Medicare, Medicaid and CLIA programs: regulations implementing the Clinical Laboratory Improvement Amendments of 1988 (CLIA) and Clinical Laboratory Act program fee collection. *Federal Register* 1993;58:5215–5237.
16. U.S. Department of Health and Human Services. Medicare, Medicaid and CLIA programs: extension of certain effective dates for clinical laboratory requirements and personnel requirements for cytologists. *Federal Register* 1994;59:62606–62609.
17. U.S. Department of Health and Human Services. Medicare, Medicaid and CLIA programs: categorization of tests and personnel modifications. *Federal Register* 1995;60:20035–20051.
18. U.S. Department of Health and Human Services. Medicare, Medicaid and CLIA programs: extension of certain effective dates for clinical laboratory requirements under CLIA. *Federal Register* 1997;62:25855–25858.
19. U.S. Department of Health and Human Services. Medicare, Medicaid and CLIA programs: simplifying CLIA regulations relating to accreditation, exemption of laboratories under a state licensure program, pro-

20. ficiency testing, and inspection. *Federal Register* 1998;63:26722–26738.
20. U.S. Department of Health and Human Services. Medicare, Medicaid and CLIA programs: extensions of certain dates for clinical laboratory requirements under CLIA. *Federal Register* 1998;63:55031–55034.
21. Joint Commission on Accreditation of Healthcare Organizations. *Comprehensive accreditation manual for pathology and clinical laboratory services.* Oakbrook Terrace, IL: Joint Commission on Accreditation of Healthcare Organizations, 2000.
22. College of American Pathologists. *Point-of-care testing inspection checklist.* Northfield, IL: CAP Commission on Laboratory Accreditation, 1998:Sec 1, 25, 26, 30.
23. Gogola M. A joint hospital/vendor project brings CQI and point-of-care technology to home care. *Computers in Nursing* 1995;13:143–150.
24. Kost GJ. Personal communication. January 2001.
25. Joint Commission on Accreditation of Healthcare Organizations. *Quality point-of-care testing.* Oakbrook Terrace, IL: Joint Commission on Accreditation of Healthcare Organizations, 1999.
26. Despotis GJ, Joist JH, Goodnough LT. Monitoring of hemostasis in cardiac surgical patients: impact of point-of-care testing on blood loss and transfusion outcomes. *Clin Chem* 1997;43:1684–1696.
27. Parvin CA, Lo SF, Deuser SM, et al. Impact of point-of-care testing on patients: length of stay in a large emergency department. *Clin Chem* 1996;42:711–717.
28. Kost GJ. *Point-of-care testing: clinical impact and potential for improving outcomes.* Northbrook, IL: American College of Chest Physicians, 1997.
29. Lamb LS Jr. Responsibilities in point-of-care testing: an institutional perspective. *Arch Pathol Lab Med* 1995;119:886–889.
30. Collier CP, Houlden RL, Rhymer SL. How to develop an effective decentralized laboratory testing program. *Clin Lab Mgmt Rev* 1998;12:418–423.
31. Point-of-Care Working Group of Education and Management Division of International Federation of Clinical Chemistry and Laboratory Medicine. Guidelines for implementation of point of care testing. *Ann Biol Clin (Paris)* 1999;57:232–236.
32. Handorf CR. Assuring quality in laboratory testing at the point of care. *Clin Chim Acta* 1997;260:207–216.
33. Kost GJ. Optimizing point-of-care testing in clinical systems management. *Clin Lab Mgmt Rev* 1998;12:356–363.
34. Ehrmeyer SS, Laessig RH. Check sample—clinical chemistry no. CC 98-7 (CC-293). *Lab Med* 1998;38:107–112.
35. Goldsmith BM. New POCT (point-of-care testing) guide establishes testing uniformity. *Med Lab Observer* 1995;27:50–52.
36. Kost GJ. Planning and implementing point-of-care testing system. In: Tobin MJ, ed. *Principles and practices of intensive care monitoring.* New York: McGraw-Hill, 1998:1297–1328.
37. Carlson DA. Point-of-care testing: regulation and accreditation. *Clin Lab Sci* 1996;9:298–302.
38. Wilkinson DS. The role of technology in the clinical laboratory of the future. *Clin Lab Mgmt Rev* 1997;11:322–330.
39. Belanger AC. Alternate site testing: the regulatory perspective. *Arch Pathol Lab Med* 1995;119:902–906.
40. Ehrmeyer SS, Laessig RH. Regulatory requirements (CLIA '88, JCAHO, CAP) for decentralized testing. *Am J Clin Pathol* 1995;104 [Suppl 1]:S40–S49.
41. U.S. Department of Health, Education and Welfare, Food and Drug Administration. In vitro diagnostic products for human use (labeling regulations). *Federal Register* 1976;21:84–89.
42. Laessig RH, Ehrmeyer SS. Quality: the next six months. *Clin Chem* 1997;43:903–907.
43. U.S. Department of Health and Human Services. Medicare, Medicaid and CLIA programs: extension of certain effective dates for clinical laboratory requirements. *Federal Register* 2000;65:82941–82944.
44. Ross JW, Boone DJ. In: *Institute on Critical Issues in Health Laboratory Practice symposium proceedings.* Minneapolis, MN: DuPont Press, 1991: (abst).
45. Kost GJ. Connectivity, the millennium challenge for point-of-care testing. *Arch Pathol Lab Med* 2000;124:1108–1110.

46. Toffaletti J. Wireless POCT data transmission. *Med Lab Observer* 2000;32:44–49.
47. Check W. Connectivity at core of POC growing pains. *CAP Today* 1999;13:1, 11, 14–24.
48. Southwick K. Electronic data interface puts patient results on fast track. *CAP Today* 1999;13:4, 6.
49. DuBois J. Getting to the point: integrating critical care tests in the patient care setting. *Med Lab Observer* 2000;32:52–56.
50. Plebani M, Carraro P. Mistakes in a state laboratory: types and frequency. *Clin Chem* 1997;43:1348–1351.
51. Ehrmeyer SS, Laessig RH. Point-of-care testing technology: is quality control still relevant? *Med Lab Obser* 1997:10[Suppl]:3.
52. Auxter S. Looking at laboratory quality control in a new light. *Clin Lab News* 1996;22:5.
53. Westgard JO. Strategies for cost-effective quality control. *Clin Lab News* 1996;22:8–9.
54. Auxter S. CDC, CLIAC rethink quality control under CLIA '88. *Clin Lab News* 1996;22:1, 16.
55. Belk WP, Sunderman FW. A survey of the accuracy of chemical analysis in clinical laboratories. *Am J Clin Pathol* 1947;17:853–861.
56. Sunderman FW. The origin of proficiency testing for clinical laboratories in the United States. In: *Proceedings of Second National Conference on Proficiency Testing. Information Services.* Bethesda, MD: , 1975:6.
57. Skendzel LP, Copeland BE. An international laboratory survey. *Am J Clin Pathol* 1975;63:1007–1011.
58. Dorsey DB. The evolution of proficiency testing in the USA. In: *Proceedings of Second National Conference on Proficiency Testing. Information Services.* Bethesda, MD: 1975:8–9.
59. Eilers RJ. Total quality control for the medical laboratory: the role of the College of American Pathologists Survey Program. *Am J Clin Pathol* 1970;54:435–436.
60. Ehrmeyer SS, Laessig RH. An analysis of the use of the 1_{2s} rule to detect substandard performance in proficiency testing. *Clin Chem* 1987;33:788–791.
61. Ehrmeyer SS, Laessig RH. An evaluation of proficiency testing programs' ability to determine intralaboratory performance: peer group statistics versus clinical usefulness limits. *Arch Pathol Lab Med* 1988;112:444–448.
62. Ehrmeyer SS, Laessig RH. Interlaboratory proficiency testing programs: a computer model to assess their capability to correctly characterize intralaboratory performance. *Clin Chem* 1987;33:784–787.
63. Ehrmeyer SS, Laessig RH, Leinweber JE, et al. The 1990 Medicare/CLIA final rules for proficiency testing: minimum intralaboratory performance characteristics (CV-bias) needed to pass. *Clin Chem* 1990;36:1736–1740.
64. Sazama K, et al. *A quality system model for health care: approved guideline GP26-A.* Wayne, PA: National Committee for Clinical Laboratory Standards, 1999.

27

REGULATION, ACCREDITATION, AND EDUCATION FOR POINT-OF-CARE TESTING

SHARON S. EHRMEYER
RONALD H. LAESSIG

ACCREDITATION AGENCIES AND REQUIREMENTS FOR POINT-OF-CARE TESTING

All laboratory testing, including that performed at the point of care, is regulated under the Clinical Laboratory Improvement Amendments of 1988 (CLIA) (1,2). As such, point-of-care testing (POCT) must meet the minimum standards specified in the CLIA regulations. The Centers for Medicare & Medicaid Services (CMS), formerly the Health Care Financing Administration (HCFA), serves as the primary inspection agency for many testing sites; however, inspection of POCT sites in hospitals usually is by "deemed" professional organizations, primarily the Joint Commission on Accreditation of Healthcare Organizations (JCAHO) and the College of American Pathologists (CAP). All three agencies consider the unique nature of POCT (instruments, circumstances, personnel, etc.) when inspecting for compliance with the testing regulations. Therefore, the management of POCT sites must be cognizant of the basic CLIA requirements as well as the applicable professional guidelines, checklists, professional standards. Two areas of particular concern relate to education and quality assurance. Since nonlaboratory personnel often perform testing, training and competency assessment are essential. Quality assurance is important because testing at the point-of-care site often lacks an overall long-term perspective of the entire testing process that is commonplace in the central laboratory. Today's regulations for POCT address these concerns.

Centers for Medicare & Medicaid Services

The CMS, in conjunction with the Centers for Disease Control and Prevention (CDC), developed and promulgated regulations necessary to implement CLIA (2–9). Based on test complexity, or difficulty to perform a test methodology, these regulations govern all laboratory testing and all testing sites, including point of care. Most testing performed at the point of care is classified as waived or moderately complex under CLIA. For waived testing, the only CLIA requirement is to follow the manufacturer's

directions for the tests performed. Obviously, "good laboratory practices" may dictate doing more. For moderately complex testing, CLIA specifies a series of requirements designed to ensure quality of the testing process including the education and training and ongoing competency assessment and responsibilities for four personnel positions—director, technical consultant, clinical consultant, and testing personnel (2–13).

The quality control (QC) requirements for moderate complexity testing are, perhaps, the most confusing. In addition to analyzing QC materials at specified intervals, they include procedure manual, calibration, remedial action for out-of-control situations, and documentation requirements. Like the central laboratory, POCT sites need to *establish and follow written quality control procedures for monitoring and evaluating the quality of the analytical testing process of each method to assure the accuracy and reliability of patient test results and reports*" (2). Section 493.1202(c) of the *Federal Register* identifies the minimum requirements for all moderate complexity testing: (a) follow manufacturer's directions; (b) have a procedure manual that identifies how to perform the testing and report results; (c) perform and document calibration procedures or check calibration at least once every 6 months; (d) assay at least two levels of control materials each day of testing (a run cannot exceed 24 hours) and keep records; (e) perform and document any applicable specialty and subspecialty control procedures, such as blood gases, automated hematology, and coagulation; (f) perform and document remedial actions; and (g) maintain records of all QC activities for 2 years (2,3,10–13).

The Centers for Medicare & Medicaid Services does allow the use of surrogate or electronic controls in place of traditional liquid controls to fulfill the daily QC requirement provided the test manufacturer specifies their use. Point-of-care sites may choose to impose more, but not less, stringent QC requirements on the testing process. For unit-use testing devices often used for POCT, the NCCLS (formerly known as the National Committee for Clinical Laboratory Standards) document EP18-P (14) suggests that test sites consider what the combination of electronic controls and instrument function checks routinely evaluate and then augment these with additional checks to ensure the quality of the entire testing process. Whether liquid or electronic controls are used, the testing site must analyze, at a minimum, two levels of controls per day for most analytes and review and document the results. Documentation of both QC data and specific remedial actions to "out-of-control results" must be available to the inspector.

Written policies and procedures must include protocols for specimen collection, instrument calibration, QC and remedial actions, and how to perform the testing and reporting of results. CLIA allows POCT sites to rely on the manufacturer's performance data to define test sensitivity, specificity, and reportable range and to use the manufacturer's reference range, or normal range, as long as it is suitable to the testing site's clientele.

By integrating the principles of continuous quality improvement as well as total quality management (TQM) into the regulatory process, the quality assurance requirements are perhaps the most innovative part of CLIA. Specifically, *"Each laboratory must establish and follow written policies and procedures for a comprehensive quality assurance program designed to evaluate the ongoing and overall quality of the testing process. The laboratories' quality assurance program must evaluate the effectiveness of its policies and procedures, identify and correct problems, assure reliable and prompt reporting of test reports and assure the adequacy and competence of the staff"* (2). The test site's quality assurance program must monitor and evaluate both the ongoing and overall quality of the total testing process through error detection, corrective actions, review of corrective actions, and the integration of improvements in future policies and procedures. Table 27.1 identifies the ten mandatory elements that must be included in a testing site's quality assurance plan, when the site holds its own CLIA certificate, and suggests monitors to evaluate achievement of the elements (2). When a point-of-care site is under another laboratory's CLIA certificate, test results from different methodologies/instruments performed within the institution and under the same CLIA certificate must be compared to each other at least twice each year and the comparative results reviewed systematically and documented for acceptability. The accuracy of all analytes tested also must be documented at least twice each year. In both cases, the site's director decides "how close is close enough."

The patient test-management section of CLIA is concerned with specimen integrity and maintaining patient identification throughout the entire testing process. While usually not a problem with POCT, the site is responsible for providing documentation that the entire testing process—from issuing the order to recording and interpreting results—is carried out at a level of quality commensurate with the needs of the patient. Policies and procedures must describe how to identify and prepare the patient for specimen collection and maintain sample integrity and positive identification from sample collection through data reporting. Results also need to be promptly reported to the proper medical personnel for optimum patient care. Procedures addressing patient-test-management concerns usually are incorporated into the quality assurance plan.

Under CLIA, regulatory proficiency testing plays a key role in assessing the internal quality for moderate- and high-complexity testing only. Successful participation in proficiency testing is a requirement for maintaining the CLIA certificate of compliance. When the point-of-care site holds its own CLIA certificate, the site must participate in a CMS-approved, proficiency testing program for the CLIA-regulated analytes (2,15). When POCT is under the central laboratory's certificate, the central laboratory, not the POCT site, typically participates in proficiency testing. The interface between the site(s) with the proficiency testing process is through method comparison, which is at least a semiannual quality assurance activity. CLIA identifies the minimum limits for passing the three proficiency testing events that occur yearly and mandates that proficiency testing samples be treated, as much as possible, like patient specimens (2). Testing sites failing the same analyte in two of three consecutive proficiency testing events can be subject to sanctions ranging from being required to submit a plan of correction to mandatory suspension of testing for the failed analyte. The CMS now views proficiency testing as educational and has indicated that its intent is not to revoke CLIA certificates, except in cases of clear danger to patients (9).

TABLE 27.1. CLIA QUALITY ASSURANCE REQUIREMENTS AND POSSIBLE MONITORS

CLIA Quality Assurance Requirement	Federal Register Citation	Possible Monitors
Patient test management	§493.1703	Patient preparation, specimen collection, requisition information, specimen rejection criteria, necessary patient information, turnaround time, data recording and retrieval
Quality control	§493.1705	Frequency of control use, control data, corrective actions, data review, documentation
Proficiency testing	§493.1707	Participation, data review, corrective actions, documentation of review and actions
Test comparisons	§493.1709	Cross-correlations
Relate results to clinical data	§493.1711	Result data consistent with clinical diagnosis
Personnel	§493.1713	Training and competency assessment
Communications	§493.1715	Clinician input into test selection and management
Complaints	§493.1717	Recognition and resolution of complaints
Staff review	§493.1719	Team participation and ownership of point-of-care testing process, dissemination of information
Records	§493.1721	Documentation of test result, audit trail

CLIA, Clinical Laboratory Improvement Amendments.

CLIA requires those sites performing moderate- and high-complexity tests to be inspected every 2 years for compliance to the regulations. The CMS assesses a fee for this process. In 1996, the CMS tested and in 1998 implemented a TQM-based, self-inspection plan called the "Alternate Quality Assurance Survey" (9,16). Relying on quality indicators for continued good test performance, the self-inspection process reflects an outcome-oriented, quality improvement assessment. Eligible testing sites are those passing inspections with few or minor deficiencies and having ongoing, satisfactory proficiency testing performance.

Joint Commission on Accreditation of Healthcare Organizations

The regulations stipulate that the CMS can approve nonprofit, professional organizations having laboratory testing standards that are essentially equivalent to or more stringent than those of CLIA (2). Two principal organizations that have received "deemed" status are the JCAHO and the Laboratory Accreditation Program of the CAP. Testing sites may voluntarily choose to be accredited by a deemed organization and pay the required fees, which are in addition to the ongoing CLIA fees, for this privilege. When these sites meet, as assessed through inspections, the accreditation agencies' testing requirements, they are, in essence, meeting CLIA requirements.

JCAHO is a voluntary organization that accredits over 80% of U.S. healthcare organizations. All POCT sites in a JCAHO-accredited institution need to adhere, at a minimum, to the standards identified in its *Comprehensive Accreditation Manual for Pathology and Clinical Laboratory Services* (17). These testing standards focus on quality improvement and are designed to promote quality outcomes (17–20). Inspection for compliance is conducted every 2 years by inspectors hired and trained by the JCAHO. The JCAHO assesses additional fees for this process. The JCAHO does not accept CMS inspections for compliance, but does accept the CAP's inspection findings for POCT. If the CAP inspects POCT, the JCAHO will reinspect all waived testing at point of care as part of its 3-year hospital accreditation process. The CMS does have the right to reinspect 5% of JCAHO-accredited testing sites. The JCAHO handbook, *Quality Point-of-Care Testing*, provides a good overview of testing outside the central laboratory and includes the rationale for starting POCT, management tactics, quality concerns, training and competency approaches, and regulatory oversight and accreditation options (19).

While the JCAHO recognizes waived test methodologies as defined by CLIA, it requires more than just following manufacturers' directions (10,18–21). The standards identified under waived testing in the JCAHO manual include: (a) defining the use (diagnosis, treatment, or screening, and whether follow-up confirmatory testing is needed); (b) identifying testing personnel and supervisors of the testing activities; (c) documenting testing personnel's initial training and continued competency; (d) having current written procedures; (e) defining QC to meet the minimum manufacturer's recommendations (for each instrument and glucose meter used, at least two levels of control are required each day a test is performed); and (f) maintaining appropriate QC and test records (17). The records must establish an audit trail, which includes a mechanism to link the ana-lysts, QC records, instrument and instrument maintenance records, and individual patient test results. All testing personnel must be authorized to test through training on the test methodologies used and being evaluated at least annually for competency. JCAHO inspectors may look for more frequent assessments for individuals not demonstrating competency and infrequent testers.

The JCAHO's regulations for moderately complex testing parallel, for the most part, CLIA requirements discussed above. The education and training requirements for the four personnel positions are the same. The goal of the JCAHO's approach to QC is to produce the best possible test results and outcomes. For QC, all sites must follow manufacturers' directions. Specifically, the JCAHO requires that each specialty and subspecialty (of testing) have a documented QC program which can include electronic controls (QC.1); the testing site's QC system must include daily surveillance of results by appropriate personnel (QC.1.3); the testing site must initiate remedial action for deficiencies identified through QC measures or authorized inspections and documentation of all actions (QC.1.4); and the site must ensure that QC results meet its criteria for acceptability before it reports patient test results (QC.1.5) (17). The JCAHO, like CLIA, accepts surrogate or electronic controls; however, the JCAHO requires that the manufacturer's claims for these controls be verified before use and that external (usually liquid) controls be run periodically to validate that no change over time has occurred with the testing system.

Documentation for the JCAHO must show at least annual review and evaluation of the procedure manual by the point-of-care site director or appropriate supervisor. This manual must be available to all testing personnel. In addition, the JCAHO requires evidence that each method or system meets the needs of the site's clientele on a consistent basis before being placed into use. For newly introduced methods/systems, this means point-of-care sites need to verify accuracy, precision, and reportable range, and ensure that the reference ranges used are appropriate to the patient population. When implementing the same test method/system elsewhere in the organization, QC data and test performance histories are adequate to confirm test validity.

For proficiency testing, the JCAHO follows CLIA in that only moderate and highly complex regulated analytes need evaluation. The JCAHO requires documented review of the data and corrective actions taken for all proficiency testing failures. As part of ongoing quality assurance and performance improvement, the accuracy of all analytes tested, even those generated from waived methodologies, need to be verified at least twice each year through proficiency testing or some other mechanism. Because the JCAHO mandates only one standard of care for its patients, organizations must establish and document, at least twice each year, the relationship of results among all test methods within the entire accredited organization, even those under different CLIA certificates (17).

Laboratory Accreditation Program of the College of American Pathologists

The CAP also provides a CMS-deemed, voluntary accreditation program. However, the CAP only accredits laboratory testing sites and not the entire healthcare organization. The CAP accredits POCT when it is under the direction of a CAP-accredited central laboratory and its CLIA certificate or when the POCT site has its own CLIA certificate and specifically seeks CAP accreditation. Every 2 years, "peers," or individuals from similar CAP-accredited testing sites, conduct the inspections. Additional fees are assessed for this process. The CAP does not accept CMS or JCAHO inspection in lieu of its own. The CMS does have the right to reinspect 5% of CAP-accredited testing sites.

The CAP's goal is for continuous quality improvement, and to this end, it requires testing sites to comply with specific requirements identified in its checklists. POCT sites need to meet the standards identified in the Laboratory General (section 1) checklist in addition to a specialty checklist that best describes the testing situation: Point-of-Care (POC), Limited Services (SLV) for sites offering a menu of 10 to 20 analytes, or Blood Gas Laboratory (BGL) for sites performing blood gases and related whole-blood analytes (22).

The CAP views all test methods, including those performed at the point of care, in the same light and, consequently, does not adhere to CLIA's test complexity categorization, nor do the testing requirements vary with the level of complexity. In CLIA terms, the CAP's requirements for all testing closely parallel those identified for highly complex tests (2,10–13,22,23). Individuals must be identified and meet the requirements for five personnel categories—director, clinical consultant, technical supervisor, general supervisor, and testing personnel. Because some testing sites may have difficulty finding appropriately qualified staff to fill the testing personnel positions, the CAP does accept individuals meeting CLIA-defined requirements for moderate- or high-complexity testing (GEN) (22). CAP requires a listing of all testing personnel authorized to perform specific tests through documentation of their initial training and continued competence assessment.

The CAP's QC requirements stipulate that point-of-care sites follow manufacturers' directions and have a procedure manual that is in substantial compliance with the NCCLS GP-3A document (POC) (22,24). The CAP requires two levels of QC every 24 hours for most analytes. Blood gases, glucose meters, and automated hematology and coagulation test systems require two levels of controls every 8 hours of testing. The CAP also requires an audit trail for all testing that links patient results to the analyst, instrument, instrument maintenance records, and QC data. In addition, if the analyst does not possess an associate degree, the QC data should include documented review by the supervisor on the next shift, if no supervisor is on site during the testing process. At this time, all QC data for POCT must demonstrate at least a monthly review by the director or director's designee (POC) (22).

The CAP allows instrument and/or electronic controls to fulfill the daily QC requirement for unmodified test systems cleared by the Food and Drug Administration (FDA) and classified by CLIA as either waived or moderately complex as long as these are a "scientifically acceptable alternative . . . that control the entire analytic process (POC)" (22). The testing sites must have data to validate the reliability of the controls before implementation. The CAP also mandates periodic evaluation of the test system with liquid controls. In all cases, at least two levels of controls must be analyzed every 8 or 24 hours, depending on the analyte and method, and the control results must be documented and reviewed to ensure the adequacy of the testing process.

The Laboratory General Checklist (GEN) includes performance verification requirements-accuracy, precision, sensitivity, specificity, reportable range, and reference range—for each test procedure or instrument (22). "Specificity" implies an evaluation of the method's ability to respond correctly to the concentration of analyte in the presence of interfering substances. The CAP now allows a testing site to rely on reagent/instrument manufacturers' evaluations to establish specificity. The CAP does allow test sites to use reference ranges cited in the literature or manufacturer's package inserts as long as the site's director specifies that they are appropriate for the clientele served. For all methods, the CAP requires test sites to establish initially and reverify, at least every 6 months, the reportable range, or the range of values that the point-of-care test site accepts as providing results adequate for the intended use. Technically, values outside the range should not be reported.

Proficiency testing has long been an important component of CAP programs. CAP-accredited laboratories must participate in proficiency testing through CAP or CAP-approved surveys for every analyte tested. When POCT is under the central laboratory's CLIA certificate, the central laboratory will analyze the proficiency testing samples. The semiannual comparison of test results links the point-of-care site's results with those in the central laboratory. The point-of-care site with its own CLIA certificate must participate in proficiency testing as an independent laboratory. In both situations for quality assurance, accuracy of test systems for all analytes must be verified at least twice each year.

Role of Other Agencies

Three federal agencies—the CDC, CMS, and FDA—have a history of dealing with regulatory issues relating to clinical laboratory testing and were involved in the development of the CLIA regulations. The CMS became the lead agency responsible for developing and implementing the final regulations. Until January 2000, the CDC was involved in the classification of testing methodologies according to the complexity model. It now manages the Clinical Laboratory Improvement Advisory Committee, which provides input for potential changes in CLIA regulations. The FDA is responsible for regulating all *in vitro* diagnostic products (test methodologies, reagents, etc.), promulgating regulations covering blood banks, and, since January 2000, classifying test methodologies as to complexity. These three agencies all report to the secretary of the Department of Health and Human Services and operate under an agency-wide mandate to provide a coordinated system of regulations for meeting the legislative intent of CLIA. To date these efforts have been largely successful.

Internet Resources

The regulations for complying with CLIA and requirements for the JCAHO and CAP continue to evolve. CLIA has not been finalized and the JCAHO and CAP update their standards and checklists, which are subject to the CMS' approval, about every

TABLE 27.2. WEBSITE ADDRESSES

Organization	Website Address
Centers for Medicare & Medicaid Services	www.hcfa.gov/medicaid/clia/cliahome.htm
Centers for Disease Control and Prevention	www.phppo.cdc.gov/dls/clia/
Food and Drug Administration	www.fda.gov
College of American Pathologists	www.cap.org
Joint Commission on Accreditation of Healthcare Organizations	www.jcaho.org
American Association for Clinical Chemistry	www.aacc.org
NCCLS	www.nccls.org

2 years. It is essential that managers responsible for point-of-care sites stay current and the web is a useful tool for this purpose. These individual websites (Table 27.2) contain useful information in their own right as well as links to other sites. The CMS' website offers general and regulatory information on CLIA including lists of test methodologies classified according to complexity, approved proficiency testing providers, accrediting organizations, exempt states, statistical information, fee schedules, commonly cited inspection deficiencies, the Alternative Quality Assessment Survey, the application for Certification Form CMS-116, and links to pertinent *Federal Registers*. The CDC's site contains the chronology of CLIA, summaries of the Clinical Laboratory Improvement Advisory Committee meetings, a current listing of the classification (complexity level) of each test methodology by analyte and product name, approved proficiency testing providers, and links to *Federal Register* search engines and other pertinent laboratory information. The FDA website is designed primarily for manufacturers of POCT devices. The CAP's site contains information on the college and its Laboratory Accreditation Program. It is especially valuable in that all current and proposed inspection checklists can be downloaded directly. The JCAHO's site serves the general public by providing a complete directory of all accredited healthcare organizations. It allows the visitor to review accreditation status and performance reports. It serves healthcare organizations and professionals with information on JCAHO initiatives (ORYX/performance measurement), educational programs, conferences, and publications. It does not contain the laboratory standards identified in the organization's *Accreditation Manual for Pathology and Clinical Laboratory Services*. Other professional organizations also have excellent websites that provide a variety of useful information and links to specific regulatory information. The American Association for Clinical Chemistry's home page has a CLIA link (CliaNet) that quickly leads to regulatory resources. The NCCLS's site identifies national consensus standards and guidelines, which are frequently referenced by accrediting organizations (CMS, JCAHO, and CAP) in meeting the requirements and training personnel.

MANAGEMENT AND CONSOLIDATION OF ACCREDITATION

Today's healthcare providers often are faced with a variety of overlapping regulatory and accreditation requirements (25–27).

Table 27.3 shows some similarities and differences among CMS, JCAHO, and CAP testing requirements. In a JCAHO-accredited organization, POCT needs to meet the standards of the JCAHO, and this is ascertained through a JCAHO or CAP inspection. The JCAHO has agreed to accept the results from CAP inspections for those sites specifically seeking additional CAP accreditation. The JCAHO will not reinspect moderately complex POCT, but will inspect all waived testing as part of the 3-year hospital reaccreditation cycle. For POCT performed in an organization not accredited by the JCAHO, the CMS will inspect moderately complex testing for compliance to CLIA or the CAP will inspect all POCT if the CAP's accreditation is specifically sought. When deciding which agency will accredit POCT, healthcare organizations need to decide what accreditation agency's requirements are most appropriate for their situation. This may determine whether a POCT site is under the main laboratory's CLIA certificate or under a separate certificate. Management of a POCT site that is accredited differently than the central laboratory is not as formidable as one might imagine, and may be appropriate in today's healthcare environment. Obviously fewer accreditations and fewer CLIA certificates will lower costs and reduce duplication of records and possible confusion of which regulations are applicable.

Management of Documentation and Quality Assurance Data

All POCT sites must meet, at a minimum, CLIA regulations, which through quality assurance principles, seek to ensure that all patients receive quality test results. In this case the word "quality" is used in the broadest sense and covers all aspects of the testing process from ordering the appropriate test to adequately and promptly reporting the results to the physician. The regulations from the CMS, JCAHO, and CAP share a common TQM approach. They all mandate documentation that establishes the relationships among various elements of the quality process. Without detailing the intricacies of the CLIA regulations and the various accreditation requirements, the POCT site's documentation must demonstrate active management of the entire testing process. The need for documentation has a twofold purpose: (a) to assure the inspectors and managers that the regulations are being followed, and (b) to provide data that enable the POCT site to utilize continuous quality improvement processes.

Each agency empowers and requires the site to design and implement an approach that is most appropriate to best meet

TABLE 27.3. SELECTED POINT-OF-CARE REQUIREMENTS BY CERTIFYING/ACCREDITING AGENCY

Requirement	CMS (CLIA)	JCAHO	CAP
Waived testing			
Daily QC requirement	Follow test manufacturer's directions.	Follow test manufacturer's directions. When none, develop test site policy. Follow JCAHO's waived testing standards.	Does not recognize waived testing. All test methodologies must meet the same testing standards defined in the checklists.
Documented personnel training and annual competency assessment	No	Yes	Yes
Proficiency testing	No	No	Yes
Method performance verification before implementation	No	Yes, accuracy, precision, reportable range, and appropriateness of reference ranges.	Yes, accuracy, precision, reportable range, sensitivity, and appropriateness of reference ranges.
Method verification before implementation for multiple instruments, same model	No	No, instrument performance history and QC data suffice.	Yes, for each instrument.
Assessment of accuracy at least every 6 months	No	Yes	Yes
Moderately complex testing			
QC for most analytes	Two levels of QC per day. More frequent evaluation is required for some analytes.	Two levels of QC per day. More frequent evaluation is required for some analytes.	Two levels of QC per day. More frequent evaluation is required for some analytes.
Accepts electronic controls	Yes, follow manufacturer's recommendation.	Yes, with verification of manufacturer's claims and periodic assessment with liquid controls.	Yes, with verification of manufacturer's claims and periodic assessment with liquid controls.
Method verification before implementation	No, accepts manufacturer's data.	Accuracy, precision, reportable range, and appropriateness of reference ranges.	Accuracy, precision, reportable range, sensitivity, and appropriateness of reference ranges.
Method verification before implementation for multiple instruments, same model	No	No, instrument performance history and QC data suffice.	Yes, for each instrument.
Assessment of reportable range (every 6 months)	No	No	Yes
Participation in regulatory proficiency testing	Only for CLIA "regulated" analytes.	Only for CLIA "regulated" analytes.	For all analytes tested, when proficiency test is available.
Method correlations at least every 6 months as part of quality assurance	For test results from different methodologies under the same CLIA certificate.	For test results from different methodologies across entire . JCAHO healthcare organization	For test results from different methodologies under the same CLIA certificate.
Establishment of accuracy (twice each year) for analytes not in proficiency testing	Yes	Yes	Yes
Documented personnel training and annual competency assessment	Yes	Yes	Yes

CAP, College of American Pathologists; CLIA, Clinical Laboratory Improvement Amendments; CMS, Centers for Medicare & Medicaid Services; JCAHO, Joint Commission on Accreditation of Healthcare Organizations.

the needs of its patients. On one end of the spectrum, the primary element of required documentation is the patient's chart. For example, starting with the patient's name, date, time, and ordering physician, the inspector can trace from data stored by the instrument, the analyst, patient test result, and QC information that validates the result. Other POCT site records must enable the inspector to link a given patient test result with the analyst's training, proficiency testing performance, instrument maintenance, calibration, function checks, and more. In a different POCT situation, the strategy for meeting the requirements may emanate from the instrument's onboard data management systems. For still other situations, the starting point for meeting the documentation requirement may begin with the hospital or laboratory information systems.

Continuous quality improvement strongly implies that a systematic review of test-related documentation, including QC and proficiency testing, must be part of the TQM process. The inspectors will look for evidence that POCT problems are identified, assessments undertaken, solutions designed and implemented, and the information disseminated to concerned parties to prevent the problem from recurring. It is clearly management's responsibility to strive continuously to improve the POCT process by initiating the necessary quality processes.

Accreditation Inspections

On-site inspections verifying compliance with the requirements are an integral part of all agencies' programs. Inspection standards include absolute requirements such as analyzing a minimum of two controls per test per day. In addition to the basic requirements, inspection standards or checklists allow the on-site inspectors considerable latitude to decide whether the outcomes achieved by the site's policies and procedures meet the patients' needs. POCT sites are empowered under the TQM philosophy to create appropriate protocols for their testing situation. With the CMS' self-assessment survey, the TQM approach to meeting CLIA requirements is even more strongly emphasized (7).

The CMS typically administers inspections for compliance with CLIA by contracting with state agencies through a program coordinated by the ten regional CMS offices. The JCAHO hires and trains laboratory professionals to conduct its inspections and the CAP engages "peers" from similar institutions to carry out inspections. Inspectors review POCT sites for compliance with the appropriate regulations, standards, or checklists, and produce, at the end of the process, an inspection report. This report assesses overall compliance with the requirements and identifies specific areas of noncompliance, termed "deficiencies," which may require a plan of correction. The process of identifying and correcting deficiencies is designed to make inspections part of a test site's continuous quality improvement activities. Usually nonlife-threatening deficiencies are followed up in the subsequent 2-year inspection cycle. In practical terms, this means that during the next inspection, the inspectors will review the previous report and the plan of correction and seek documentation that the plan has been implemented and the problem corrected. It is critically important that managers of POCT sites recognize that a deficiency identified in the inspection report must be remedied in a reasonable time frame and that documentation of the remedy is essential. In many cases, "reasonable" means "immediately." All agencies have a process for filing and following-up on inspection reports. A POCT site's failure to correct and document a deficiency can place the entire institution's accreditation or CLIA certification in jeopardy.

Inspections of POCT sites under CLIA, JCAHO, and CAP are repeated on a 2-year cycle. Surprisingly, the most frequently occurring deficiencies reported have remained much the same through three cycles. A composite list of the most frequently cited deficiencies include failure to follow manufacturer's directions, analyze the appropriate number of controls per test per day, document the results, review the data, establish and follow effective quality assurance policies, evaluate the quality of the total testing process, review and document review of proficiency testing results, and initiate appropriate remedial actions for QC and proficiency testing failures (21,28).

Generally, POCT sites encounter deficiencies related to failure to perform specific actions (e.g., run controls), rather than the fundamental principles and goals of TQM. This demonstrates a commitment by these sites to providing quality care and to meeting the patients' needs. Conversely, the deficiencies often represent a failure to understand and carry out the basic tenets of a quality testing process. When such violations are discovered, the inspector is left with no alternative but to cite the institution. POCT managers preparing for inspections are well advised to focus on and adhere to the fundamental requirements defined by the accrediting agencies.

Successful Inspections—Checklists, Preparedness, and Quality Assurance Opportunities

The most common problem associated with inspection of POCT sites is traceable to the fact that regulations and accreditation requirements focus on the central laboratory's perspective of the testing process, not the viewpoint of the caregiver. Therefore, it is essential that all personnel involved in the POCT process understand the nature, philosophy, and rationale of the inspection. On a practical basis, those involved should know the applicable requirements, conduct internal assessments for compliance, review policies and procedures, and ensure that all staff members understand the process and the testing protocols. Most importantly, all documentation should be relevant, up-to-date, in place, and retrievable.

When dealing with a particular instrument or test system, invaluable help can be obtained from the manufacturer, even to the point of providing materials for procedure manuals, defining QC protocols, and assisting with staff training. Accrediting agencies also have help lines. The CAP has technical associates trained to explain the checklist questions. The JCAHO's Department of Standards can be contacted for assistance. And finally, the Laboratory Program Specialists at the CMS' ten regional offices will assist with questions concerning compliance with CLIA.

Selection of Accrediting Agency—Cost-Effective Consolidation of Regulations

All POCT should be carefully coordinated and integrated in order to streamline the time and expense involved with the certification and accreditation process, improve cost effectiveness (minimize duplication of efforts, instrumentation, proficiency testing, reagents, etc), enhance performance, and benefit patient care (29–31). It is the management's responsibility to devise a reasonable certification and accreditation approach to best meet the needs of the institution. There is no universal right way. Many large healthcare organizations have only one CLIA certificate with the main laboratory managing all testing, while other organizations have multiple CLIA certificates, even a separate certification for each testing site. Often the primary reason for the multiple certificate approach is an irrational fear that problems encountered on inspection might jeopardize the entire institution's testing capabilities if all testing was consolidated under a single CLIA certificate. Other reasons cited for separate certificates include remote location of testing sites, different site director, and the desire to have POCT comply with less stringent accreditation standards.

Costs of Accreditation

Each CLIA certificate has associated fees—a one-time registration fee of $100 and a renewal fee (every 2 years) ranging from a minimum of $150 per test site performing fewer than 10,000 tests per year to $7,940 for those sites performing more than 1 million tests of all complexity levels (32). In addition to CLIA registration and certification fees, accreditations, inspections, and proficiency testing have additional costs associated with them. For a typical POCT site performing less than 10,000 tests per year, registration, certification, and inspections could be as low as $0 when POCT is part of and administered by the central laboratory. A "worst case," that is, most expensive, scenario could easily cost several thousand dollars per site when every POCT site has its own CLIA certificate, is accredited and inspected by the CAP, and offers testing in several specialties, each requiring external evaluation through proficiency testing.

Cost issues notwithstanding, the issue of choosing an accreditation/inspection strategy for the institution ultimately focuses on the fundamental question of "who is in charge of the POCT processes?" When the director of the central laboratory is in charge, accreditation by a single agency may be the best practical strategy. While there is no universal truth, failure to address the fundamental issue is a failure of management.

EDUCATION AND TRAINING

Accreditation and Regulatory Requirements for Training and Education

To fulfill the fundamental CLIA tenet to provide quality results regardless of test location, it is essential that those involved in the POCT process be knowledgeable and properly trained. Training must be a carefully planned, ongoing activity. CLIA mandates that all personnel involved in moderate- and high-complexity testing be qualified and competent through education and experience. Personnel must have specific documented training in all methods performed and have their competence assessed twice the first year and once a year thereafter (2). CLIA's procedural requirements include: (a) adhering to policies and following procedures for the entire testing process from specimen handling and process to reporting and maintaining patient test results; (b) performing and documenting QC, proficiency testing, and maintenance activities; (c) following established corrective action policies; and (d) identifying, correcting, and documenting problems that may adversely affect test results. The JCAHO and CAP also mandate these same requirements, but include *all* testing personnel, even those performing only waived tests.

National Committee for Clinical Laboratory Standards and Other Training Guidelines

POCT personnel, at a minimum, need to be trained in patient preparation and identification; sample requirements, collection, and handling; universal precautions; and disposal of biohazardous materials. A current procedure manual containing detailed step-by-step test procedures, QC information, and reporting results is absolutely essential. Reagent handling needs to include proper storage and checking for outdates. Result reporting must address policies for panic or critical values and for documenting the result in the patient's permanent record. A clear and concise QC protocol must be included in the training and describe how to respond to out-of-control situations. Finally, maintenance, troubleshooting, and backup procedures should be detailed.

Training for POCT is conducted typically by manufacturers, designated instructors in the healthcare organization, and/or through self-instructional modules. Training materials for these sessions are available in a variety of forms (web-based, written, videos, and CD-ROMs) and can be obtained from many sources including professional societies, accrediting organizations, consultants, and manufacturers (19,20,33–38). Inhouse studies have demonstrated that formal, instructor-provided training facilitates better learning and that trainees learn more effectively in a group setting (39). Institutional instructors from the laboratory, nursing service, and POCT committee, among others, can provide highly customized, point-of-care training. For instance, nurses may respond best to a nurse trainer who can focus on POCT as a means to improve patient care and respiratory therapists to a trainer who can emphasize patient treatments. Training sessions are most successful with an interested and enthusiastic trainer having a detailed understanding of the whole scope of requirements. Because individuals learn differently, some combination of manufacturer, self-study, and institutional training may be the most effective approach.

Whatever format, clearly stated objectives are critical for successful training. Concepts must be presented in a manner commensurate with the professional objectives of those involved and the training must focus on the needs of the trainee. NCCLS document GP21-A, *Training Verification for Laboratory Personnel*, provides background information related to providing quality training and recommends an infrastructure for developing a training verification program that meets quality and regulatory objectives (40).

Creating and Managing Credentials for Point-of Care Testing Staff

Documentation of training and ongoing competency assessments is mandatory for moderate and high complexity testing under CLIA and for all testing being accredited by the JCAHO or CAP. Records documenting education and experience and establishing the individual's training typically are a mandatory part of the individual's personnel or human resource department files. When evaluating an individual's competence, the inspectors must be granted access to the personnel records. Documentation, while essential, need not be a laborious process. In many situations, a short form or grid may suffice to collect and tabulate the appropriate education, training, and ongoing competency assessments. Other approaches include the NCCLS's Training Verification Tracker database to help testing sites document training and the American Society of Clinical Pathologists' Point of Care Evaluator Program to assist in the development of a competency assessment program and in the documentation of competency (41,42).

CONCLUSIONS

- POCT is governed by CLIA regulations.
- CLIA regulations focus on the quality of the testing process.
- CLIA regulations are site neutral, that is, set minimum performance for all testing.
- Point-of-care test sites can choose to be accredited by the JCAHO or CAP, two CMS-deemed professional organizations.
- CLIA regulations as well as those of the JCAHO and CAP are "quality" based. This empowers POCT managers to be somewhat innovative in the design of the overall approach to meeting regulations.
- Regulators, particularly the JCAHO, define as a function of management, the creation of a comprehensive program focused on the ultimate "customer"—clinician and patient.
- Managers of POCT have a variety of options to create the most effective program.
- There are, depending on the approach chosen, significant cost issues to be considered.

REFERENCES

1. Public Health Service Act. §353, 42 USC §263a (1988).
2. U.S. Department of Health and Human Services. Medicare, Medicaid and CLIA programs: regulations implementing the Clinical Laboratory Improvement Amendments of 1988 (CLIA). Final rule. *Federal Register* 1992;57:7002–7186.
3. U.S. Department of Health and Human Services. Medicare, Medicaid and CLIA programs: regulations implementing the Clinical Laboratory Improvement Amendments of 1988 (CLIA) and Clinical Laboratory Act program fee collection. *Federal Register* 1993;58:5215–5237.
4. U.S. Department of Health and Human Services. Medicare, Medicaid and CLIA programs: extension of certain effective dates for clinical laboratory requirements and personnel requirements for cytologists. *Federal Register* 1994;59:62606–62609.
5. U.S. Department of Health and Human Services. Medicare, Medicaid and CLIA programs: categorization of tests and personnel modifications. *Federal Register* 1995;60:20035–20051.
6. U.S. Department of Health and Human Services. Medicare, Medicaid and CLIA programs: extension of certain effective dates for clinical laboratory requirements under CLIA. *Federal Register* 1997;62:25855–25858.
7. U.S. Department of Health and Human Services. Medicare, Medicaid and CLIA programs: simplifying CLIA regulations relating to accreditation, exemption of laboratories under a state licensure program, proficiency testing, and inspection. *Federal Register* 1998;63:26722–26738.
8. U.S. Department of Health and Human Services. Medicare, Medicaid and CLIA programs: extensions of certain dates for clinical laboratory requirements under CLIA. *Federal Register* 1998;63:55031–55034.
9. U.S. Department of Health and Human Services. Medicare, Medicaid and CLIA programs: simplifying CLIA regulations relating to accreditation, exemption of laboratories under a state licensure program, proficiency testing, and inspection. *Federal Register* 1998;63:26722–26738.
10. Ehrmeyer SS, Laessig RH. Regulatory requirements (CLIA '88, JCAHO, CAP) for decentralized testing. *Am J Clin Pathol* 1995;104 (Suppl):S40–S49.
11. Kost GJ. Planning and implementing point-of-care testing system. In: Tobin MJ, ed. *Principles and practices of intensive care monitoring.* New York: McGraw-Hill, 1998:1297–1328.
12. Kost GJ, Ehrmeyer SS, Chernow B, et al. Laboratory-clinical interface: point of care (POC) testing. *Chest* 1999;115:1140–1154.
13. Ehrmeyer SS, Laessig RH. POCT regulations and inspections. In: *New approaches to point-of-care testing.* Audioconference series. Washington, DC: American Association for Clinical Chemistry, February 25, 1997.
14. Phillips DL, et al. *Quality management for unit-use testing.* Doc. EP18-P. Wayne, PA: NCCLS, 1999.
15. Health Care Financing Administration. *List of proficiency testing (PT) providers.* Available at: http://www.hcfa.gov/medicaid/clia/ptlist.pdf. Accessed on December 6, 2001.
16. Health Care Financing Administration. *Alternate quality assessment survey.* Available at: http://www.hcfa.gov/medicaid/clia/aqas.htm. Accessed on December 6, 2001.
17. Joint Commission on Accreditation of Healthcare Organizations. *Comprehensive accreditation manual for pathology and clinical laboratory services.* Oakbrook Terrace, IL: JCAHO, 2001.
18. Belanger A. JCAHO's perspective on POCT. *Advance Admin Lab* 1997;6:10–1.
19. Joint Commission on Accreditation of Healthcare Organizations. *Quality point of care.* Oakbrook Terrace, IL: Joint Commission on Accreditation of Healthcare Organizations, 2000.
20. Joint Commission on Accreditation of Healthcare Organizations. *Improving performance in the lab: a case study approach.* Video and guide. Oakbrook Terrace, IL: Joint Commission on Accreditation of Healthcare Organizations, 1997.
21. Joint Commission on Accreditation of Healthcare Organizations. *How to meet the most frequently cited laboratory standards.* Oakbrook Terrace, IL: JCAHO, 2001.
22. College of American Pathologists. *Point-of-care testing inspection checklist.* Checklists GEN, LSV, BGL, and POC. Northfield, IL: College of American Pathologists Commission on Laboratory Accreditation, 1998.
23. Ehrmeyer SS, Laessig RH. A guide to waived glucose POCT regulatory requirements. *Advance/Lab* 1998;7:48–52.
24. NCCLS. *Clinical laboratory technical procedure manuals.* 3rd ed. Doc. GP2-A3. Wayne, PA: NCCLS, 1996.
25. Ehrmeyer SS, Laessig RH. *Clinical chemistry check sample.* No. CC98-7 (CC-293). Chicago, IL: American Society for Clinical Pathologists, 1998.
26. Ehrmeyer SS, Laessig RH. POCT regulations and inspections. In: *New approaches to point-of-care testing.* Audioconference series. Washington, DC: American Association for Clinical Chemistry, February 25, 1997.
27. Ehrmeyer SS, Laessig RH. Point of care testing: living with multiple regulators. In: *Education/management.* Audioconference series. Chicago, IL: American Society for Clinical Pathology, September 9, 1998.
28. Health Care Financing Administration. *Top four CLIA deficiencies cited.* Available at: http://www.hcfa.gov/medicaid/clia/stat4def.pdf. Accessed on December 6, 2001.
29. Kost GJ. The hybrid laboratory: shifting the focus to the point of care. *Med Lab Observer* 1992;24:17–28.
30. Kost GJ. Point-of-care testing: the hybrid laboratory and knowledge optimization. In: Kost GJ, ed. *Handbook of clinical automation, robotics, and optimization.* New York: Wiley, 1996:757–838.
31. Kost GJ. *Point-of-care testing: clinical impact and potential for improving outcomes.* Northbrook, IL: American College of Chest Physicians, 1997.
32. U.S. Department of Health and Human Services. Medicare, Medicaid and CLIA programs: fee schedule revision. *Federal Register* 1997;62:45815–45821.
33. Ehrmeyer SS, Laessig RH. Bedside: teaching competency at the point of care. *Advance/Lab* 1996;5:17–21.
34. Commission on Office Laboratory Accreditation. *COLA training guides.* Columbia, MD: Commission on Office Laboratory Accreditation, 1996.
35. *National laboratory training network.* http://ww.phppo.cdc.gov/nlnt/default.asp
36. Barr JT, Betschart J, Bracey A, et al. *Ancillary (bedside) blood glucose*

testing in acute and chronic care facilities. Doc. C30-A. Wayne, PA: National Committee for Clinical Laboratory Standards, 1994.

37. Goldsmith BM, Travers EM, Bakes-Martin R, et al. *Point-of-care in vitro diagnostic (IVD) testing.* Doc. AST2-P. Wayne, PA: National Committee for Clinical Laboratory Standards, 1995.

38. Joint Commission on Accreditation of Healthcare Organizations. *The competent laboratory.* Oakbrook Terrace, IL: Joint Commission on Accreditation of Healthcare Organizations, 2000.

39. American Diabetes Association. Consensus statement on self-monitoring of blood glucose. *Diabet Care* 1987:10;95–99.

40. Nevalainen DE, Berte LM, Bardell SL, et al. *Training verification for laboratory personnel.* Doc. GP21-A. Wayne, PA: NCCLS, 1995.

41. NCCLS. *Training verification tracker database.* Doc. GP21TVT. Wayne, PA: NCCLS, 1997.

42. American Society of Clinical Pathologists. *Point of care evaluator program.* Chicago, IL: American Society of Clinical Pathologists, 1997.

28

POINT-OF-CARE TESTING AND JCAHO

JOANNE M. BORN

The Joint Commission on Accreditation of Healthcare Organizations (JCAHO) is a nonprofit organization that accredits over 19,000 healthcare organizations throughout the world via its accreditation programs. It was established in 1951 through a partnership of the American College of Physicians, the American College of Surgeons, the American Hospital Association, and the American Medical Association (1). The mission of the JCAHO is to continuously improve the safety and quality of care provided to the public through the provision of healthcare accreditation and related services that support performance improvement in healthcare organizations (2).

The JCAHO accredits laboratories, including point-of-care testing (POCT), by evaluating performance in meeting or exceeding requirements of JCAHO standards and intent statements. These standards are professionally developed, with input from several sources, including professional technical advisory committees. Figure 28.1 illustrates the standards refinement process (3).

LABORATORY ACCREDITATION SURVEY

The JCAHO's laboratory accreditation survey is a voluntary process and is conducted every 2 years. It is designed to assist organizations in planning and achieving high-quality performance, to meet requirements set forth by the Clinical Laboratory Improvement Amendments of 1988 (CLIA) and by other regulatory agencies, and to improve the quality of patient care. This is achieved through assessment of demonstrated compliance with performance-focused standards and intent statements during an on-site survey. These standards are functional in nature, cross departments and disciplines within an organization, and address the integration of quality performance with day-to-day activities. Compliance is demonstrated in many ways, including written and electronic documentation, staff interviews, and data collection (4).

The JCAHO's survey focuses on performance, that is, what is done and how well it is done to provide patient care. The level of performance includes the degree to which laboratory services are efficacious and appropriate for the individual patient and the degree to which these services are available in a timely manner

to the patients, effective, continuous with other care, safe, efficient, and caring and respectful of the patient.

The characteristics of what is done and how well it is done are referred to as "dimensions of performance" (3). The dimensions of performance follow:

- Doing the right thing
- Efficacy of the procedure in relation to the patient's condition
- Appropriateness of a test to meet the patient's need
- Doing the right thing well
- Availability of a needed test
- Timeliness with which the test is provided to the patient or customer
- Effectiveness with which the test is provided
- Continuity of services over time
- Safety of the patient and others when the testing is provided
- Efficiency of testing provided
- Respect and caring given to the patient when service is provided

Dimensions of performance are assessed during a survey of POCT by examining the vital link between organizational functions and technical functions. The organizational functions relate to people and processes that cross departmental boundaries and provide support throughout the continuum of patient care. Technical functions include the laboratory-specific processes necessary for accurate and precise test results. Many of these processes are mandated by CLIA. JCAHO functions are summarized below (3).

Organizational functions

- Improving organization performance
- Leadership
- Management of the laboratory environment
- Management of human resources
- Management of information
- Surveillance, prevention, and control of infection
  Technical functions
- Quality control
- Waived testing

One or more laboratory specialists conduct the survey. These specialists, or surveyors, are medical technologists or patholo-

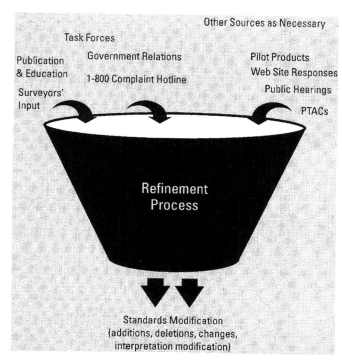

FIGURE 28.1. Joint Commission on Accreditation of Healthcare Organizations' standards refinement process. Information is received from several sources, including public hearings, publications, and professional technical advisory committees. (From Joint Commission on Accreditation of Healthcare Organizations. *Comprehensive accreditation manual for pathology and clinical laboratory services.* Oakbrook Terrace, IL: Joint Commission on Healthcare Organizations, 1999.)

gists with extensive experience in clinical laboratories. Duration of the survey is variable, depending on the complexity of POCT and on the number of testing sites being reviewed.

Categories of laboratory testing are defined by complexity in CLIA (5). Each laboratory test is assigned to one of these categories, with designated requirements for testing personnel, quality control, and directorship. The JCAHO includes review of these requirements in the survey process. The CLIA categories of testing are

- Waived testing
- Moderate complexity
- High complexity

A JCAHO survey of POCT addresses the CLIA requirements of each testing category and includes a review of appropriate laboratory standards linked to organization functions and technical functions. Each standard is accompanied by an intent statement, which describes specific points that must be addressed by the organization for compliance. Computer technology is used to assign a score for each standard. The level of compliance for each standard is based on a point scale of one through five, and the numeric score corresponds to a level of compliance. Any standard not in compliance receives a recommendation for improvement.

The JCAHO process surveys individual standards and their relationship to other standards in the integration and coordina-

tion of services. It is a "system survey," and thus not limited to an inspection of a predetermined checklist of requirements. It is an interactive, consultative process with a focus on patient outcomes, measurement, and performance improvement.

While each survey of POCT is unique, all laboratory surveys share common processes (3). They include the following activities:

- Opening conference
- Document review
- Interview of laboratory leaders
- Visit to POCT and patient units
- Laboratory staff conference (optional)
- Feedback sessions
- Leadership exit conference

Gaining an understanding of survey goals and the process is essential in preparing for a POCT survey.

SURVEY PREPARATION

The application for survey should be completed and submitted 4 to 6 months in advance of the expected date of survey. This allows the JCAHO time to process the application, resolve any issues, and assign a survey date. It also allows the organization time to obtain a copy of the *Comprehensive Accreditation Manual for Pathology and Clinical Laboratory Services*, distribute it to staff members, and establish a track record of compliance with standards. The minimum requirement for an initial survey is a 4-month track record (3).

Each organization should determine the number of POCT sites and should review the testing menu at each. These sites may include departments in a hospital, ambulances, or patient rooms. Attention should be given to the complexity of testing at each site by comparing the test menu to the CLIA categories of complexity and to the CLIA specialties (hematology, chemistry, etc.). This is essential in providing the JCAHO with accurate, complete information on the survey application form. The JCAHO uses this information to assign the appropriate number of days to the survey, so that adequate time is allotted for thorough review.

Once the application for survey is submitted, survey preparation should include an in-depth assessment of all processes relative to POCT. The assessment may be reviewed during the survey process, and therefore should be accurately conducted and well documented (6). It should address the following issues:

- CLIA category of test complexity
- Inventory of tests, methods, and equipment
- Review of state and federal requirements for testing directorship and testing personnel, safety, and infection control
- List of staff members and responsibilities
- Communication pathways within and among testing sites and entire organization
- Information systems used to capture or transmit patient test results or other data
- Problem-solving mechanisms
- Functional links to other service areas in the organization

This assessment then becomes the map that guides the organization through the standards manual to determine which standards are applicable. There are over 250 laboratory standards, but only a limited number are relevant to POCT. The point-of-care (POC) survey will address only the standards that are applicable to the organization.

In general, standards within the organization functions and a limited number of specific standards within the technical functions are always addressed in a survey of moderate- or high-complexity testing. When POCT is limited to waived tests, only the specific standards for waived testing, found in the technical functions, are surveyed. Because of the technical nature of POCT, a substantial portion of any POC survey addresses the technical functions.

Upon review of the standards for relevancy, organizations should develop plans and timelines for compliance. Policies and procedures should be written, staff education needs should be addressed, documentation tools should be developed and distributed, and data should be collected at defined time periods. This data collection encompasses everything from attendance lists at staff education programs to daily documentation of performance of equipment maintenance and quality control.

Probably the most important part of survey preparation is the organization's mechanism to monitor processes for compliance, measure the effect of these processes on patient care, and to obtain performance improvement. To this end, baseline performance expectations should be defined and ongoing data should be collected to monitor effectiveness in achieving desired outcomes. Data aggregation and analysis are an integral part of the JCAHO survey. Performance improvement, demonstrated through measurement, is the goal.

To help prepare for a POCT survey, following some of the suggestions given in this chapter is recommended. As an example, the next section discusses some typical preparation steps and also discusses some of the key standards and functions that are addressed during survey activities. A fictitious organization is used as an example to assist the reader in understanding the JCAHO survey process.

POINT-OF-CARE SURVEY OF COMMUNITY HOSPITAL X

Overview of Testing Sites and Staff

Consider the case of a community hospital that provides acute care services. The hospital has a full-service main laboratory and provides POCT in the surgery and intensive care units. POCT is directed by the chief pathologist of the main laboratory, which has its own separate CLIA certificate. Nursing staff members perform testing in intensive care and surgery. Additionally, bedside glucose monitoring is available throughout all patient-care units, and is performed by nursing staff members and patient-care technicians. A medical technologist from the main laboratory works closely with the nursing directors to oversee testing activities.

Test Menu and CLIA Requirements

An assessment of POCT is performed. Using the list discussed in the previous section, the organization gathers information to use in determining key standards and issues to be addressed for compliance. The information collected from the nursing units, surgery and intensive care unit includes the following specifics: (a) blood gases test, moderate complexity, using blood gas analyzer; and (b) whole-blood glucose test, waived test, using a whole-blood reflectance meter.

Federal CLIA Requirements for Personnel

The pathologist meets the requirements for directorship of moderate complexity and waived testing. CLIA does not mandate specific requirements for testing personnel who perform waived testing; however, staff members who perform the blood gases must meet one of the following requirements for moderate complexity testing:

- MD or DO with state licensure in state where the laboratory is located
- PhD, master of science, or bachelor of science in a chemical, physical, biological, or clinical laboratory science, or medical technology discipline
- Associate of science in a chemical, physical, or biological science, or medical laboratory technology
- High school diploma (or equivalent) with either documentation of training appropriate for testing performed, or successful completion of 50 weeks of medical laboratory courses in the military

Additional questions regarding personnel qualifications can be answered through review of the *Clinical Federal Register* 42.

Safety and Infection Control Concerns

This organization must consider many topics for safety and infection control. Among these are local fire safety codes, electrical safety, chemical exposure and hazardous materials management, bloodborne pathogens, and disaster preparedness.

Staff List and Responsibilities

A complete list of all staff members in the surgery and intensive care units is compiled along with a list of testing or leadership responsibilities for each member. Information regarding educational background and credentials is also gathered.

Communication Pathways

POCT in this organization involves the following communication pathways:

- Each testing site has its own nursing leader who manages the other staff members performing testing.
- The nursing leader works with the medical technologist from the main laboratory on issues related to POCT.
- The medical technologist reports to the pathologist who is the director of the main laboratory and of all POCT.
- Nursing leaders and the medical technologist communicate directly during brief meetings. Information is disseminated to all staff members during meetings held at each POCT site.
- All staff members in the organization have access to the organization's electronic mail system.

Information Systems

Both automated and manual information processes are used for transferring information for POCT.

- The hospital's computer system is used for patient registration data.
- Each blood gas analyzer has a paper instrument printout for patient test results and quality control results.
- Blood gas results are recorded in the patient's medical record by taping the instrument printout to a paper document.
- Glucose meters have a digital readout for results of patient tests and quality control.
- Glucose results are handwritten into the medical record on a paper document.
- Policies and procedures for testing processes, quality control activities, equipment maintenance, and safety are available in written manuals.

Problem-Solving Mechanisms

The organization has a POC committee comprised of medical staff members, the medical technologist, and nursing leaders. They have periodic meetings to discuss issues and collect data. This information is disseminated to staff members at staff meetings and through the electronic mail system and is presented at medical staff meetings. Information is also given to the organization's quality council, which reports directly to the board of directors of the entire organization.

Functional Links, Key Standards, and Survey Activities

Many functional links exist within this organization. The organization has a biomedical engineering department that oversees installation, maintenance, and repair of equipment, including POCT instruments and refrigerators used for storage of test materials. There is a safety officer for the organization and also an infection control chairperson. The human resources department maintains personnel files containing job descriptions, credentialing information, and organizational education programs.

After obtaining specific information about POCT in this organization, the standards manual is thoroughly reviewed. Each JCAHO "function" is reviewed and a list of relevant standards within each function is compiled. For this organization's POCT survey, a list of important functions and standards includes all those standards contained in the organization functions and a limited number of standards contained in the technical functions. For a list of these standards, consult the *Comprehensive Accreditation Manual for Pathology and Clinical Laboratory Services*, Appendix B, and the "Waived Testing" chapter of Section 2.

Within each function, the JCAHO groups the standards into major sections or topics. The organization should consider these major topics and how specific processes within the organization are addressed in each topic. These groupings of related standards are aggregated and scored together on the survey report as grid elements.

Flowcharts of the organizational JCAHO functions that address these major topics may assist the reader in better understanding applicable standards requirements.

The leadership function is addressed in Figure. 28.2. Leadership is divided into four major topics: planning and designing services, directing services, integrating and coordinating services, and improving performance. The organization leaders are given responsibility for needs assessment and development of a mission and vision for the organization. Leaders must

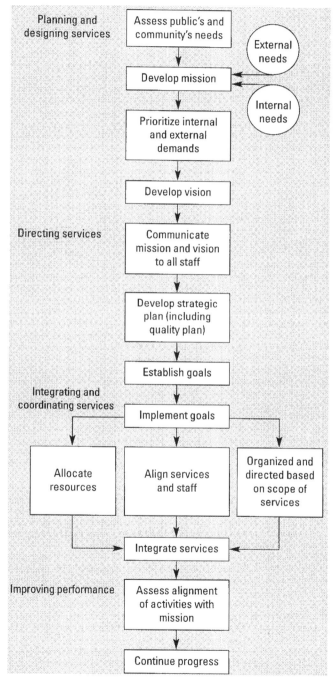

FIGURE 28.2. The four main components of the leadership function: planning and design of services, directing services, integrating and coordinating services, and improving performance. (From Joint Commission on Accreditation of Healthcare Organizations. *Comprehensive accreditation manual for pathology and clinical laboratory services.* Oakbrook Terrace, IL: Joint Commission on Healthcare Organizations, 1999.)

communicate this mission and vision to staff members to develop strategic plans and goals. The implementation of these goals includes integration and coordination of services that are dependent on resource allocation, alignment of service and staff, and direction, which is based on the scope of services. Lastly, the leaders must assess the alignment of activities with the organization's mission in order to achieve performance improvement. Standards within this function include requirements for administrative planning as well as specific requirements for POC laboratory directorship. At Community Hospital X, the leaders include the pathologist from the main laboratory, the technical consultant, nursing leaders, administrative leadership, and the medical staff.

Figure. 28.3 addresses the improving organization performance function. Organization leaders must develop a plan for improvement. The improvement cycle is ongoing and is carried out by leaders, managers, physicians, and other staff members who support services. The essential elements of performance improvement are design, data collection, aggregation and analysis of data, and performance improvement. Improvement efforts may start at any point in the cycle, such as when a new service is designed (e.g., the addition of POCT in surgery) or when problems are identified (e.g., failure of nursing staff to appropriately perform waived testing quality control). The performance improvement function emphasizes outcome measurement and the use of comparative data to evaluate new and existing organization processes. Standards in this function address many activities, including identification, assessment, and response to sentinel events

Management of the laboratory environment is depicted in Figure 28.4. Two key elements for the laboratory environment are design and implementation. When an organization designs the laboratory environment, the planning process includes provisions for safety, security, hazardous materials and waste management, emergency preparedness, life safety, laboratory equipment, utilities needed, and components of the physical work environment such as space and ergonomics. Staff education is included with the implementation of the plan. Process effectiveness is measured and assessed to identify areas for per-

formance improvement. Policies, procedures, and documentation for the laboratory environment include standards that address specifics such as reagent refrigerator temperatures, calibration and equipment maintenance for POC blood gas analyzers, disposal of contaminated needles, staff participation in fire drills, and appropriate provisions for backup electrical power.

Figure 28.5 represents important activities for the management of the human resources function. The organization's mission dictates the necessary qualifications, competencies, and numbers of staff needed to provide service. It is the responsibility of leadership to provide competent staff members and to assess, maintain, and improve the competency of staff. Standards found in the human resources function address CLIA requirements for laboratory testing personnel and laboratory leadership. Documentation reviewed during a POCT survey of Community Hospital X includes job descriptions, personnel files, education records, and technical competency assessments for testing personnel.

The management of information function is very complex, as depicted in Figure 28.6. It begins with a thorough assessment that includes patient needs, services to provide care, provider needs, regulatory needs, and performance improvement. Information needs are then divided into four categories: laboratory specific data, aggregate data, knowledge-based information, and comparative data. Each of these topics defines data sources and this information is transferred across many areas of the organization. These data sources at Community Hospital X may be paper (e.g., a written policy, reference book, or a blood gas instrument tape) or electronic storage via computer (e.g., patient registration data). The data are analyzed, interpreted, transformed into information, and transmitted to the user. The user at Community Hospital X might need this information to make clinical decisions, to educate patients, for research, for performance improvement, or to make organizational decisions such as budget allocation. Standards contained in the management of information function address procedure manuals for POCT, reference ranges for interpretation of test results, formats of test result reports,

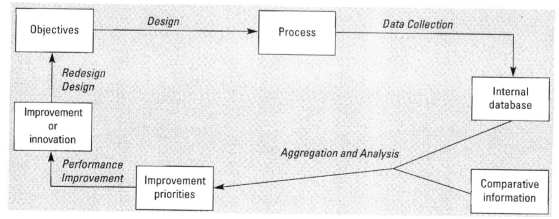

FIGURE 28.3. Improving organization performance function. (From Joint Commission on Accreditation of Healthcare Organizations. *Comprehensive accreditation manual for pathology and clinical laboratory services.* Oakbrook Terrace, IL: Joint Commission on Healthcare Organizations, 1999.)

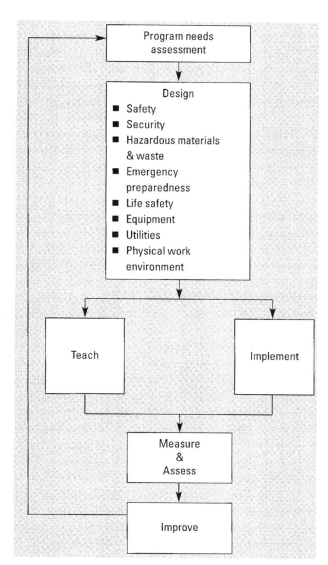

FIGURE 28.4. Management of the laboratory environment. (From Joint Commission on Accreditation of Healthcare Organizations. *Comprehensive accreditation manual for pathology and clinical laboratory services.* Oakbrook Terrace, IL: Joint Commission on Healthcare Organizations, 1999.)

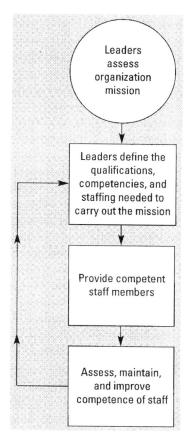

FIGURE 28.5. Management of human resources function. (From Joint Commission on Accreditation of Healthcare Organizations. *Comprehensive accreditation manual for pathology and clinical laboratory services.* Oakbrook Terrace, IL: Joint Commission on Healthcare Organizations, 1999.)

standardized abbreviations used, privacy and confidentiality of information, and planning for records retention and disaster recovery.

Surveillance, prevention, and control of infection are described in Figure 28.7. Infection control is dependent on the organization's ability to identify, analyze, prevent, control, and report infectious processes. Standards in this function address activities for appropriate protection of staff members and patients during collection of blood specimens and storage and transport of biohazardous materials as well as their appropriate disposal.

Using the list of survey activities previously discussed, the organization may choose to develop a survey activity script by compiling a list of discussion topics, pertinent standards, data and other documentation likely to be reviewed during each sur-

vey activity. This allows the organization to develop and determine a baseline for compliance. Functional links among staff, processes, and patient-care sites can be reviewed and a timetable can then be established for additional work on policies, procedures, data collection, and improvement priorities. Many organizations choose to label each document with the appropriate standard(s) it references.

The opening conference is primarily used to set the survey agenda and to introduce key staff members. Surveyors attempt to gain an overview of the organization's leadership structure and the leadership and report mechanisms for POCT. Performance improvement activities may be discussed as well as mechanisms to orient and train staff members. Documentation is generally not reviewed, as this is a time for interviews. At Community Hospital X, the pathologist, nursing leaders, and the technical consultant would attend this conference as well as other leaders.

The document review for Community Hospital X would include review of documentation that supports compliance with the JCAHO standards and the regulatory requirements of CLIA. The list of documents reviewed is lengthy but minimally includes:

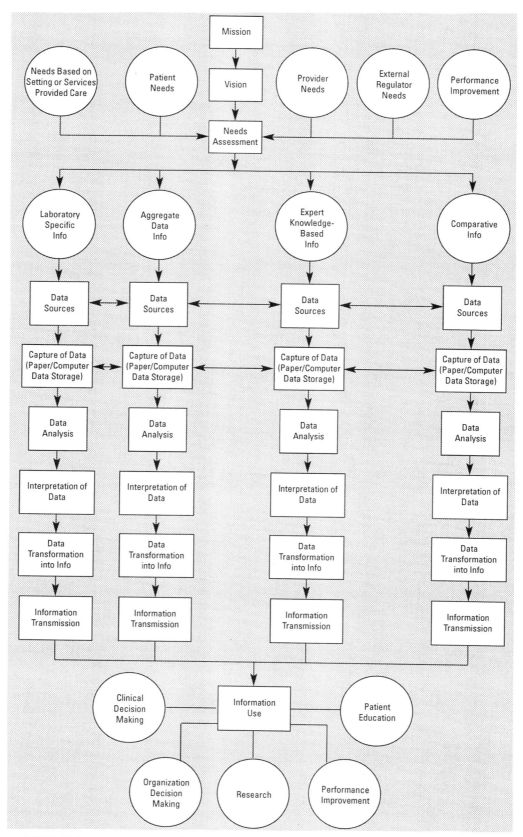

FIGURE 28.6. Management of information. Four types of information are reviewed during a point-of-care survey: laboratory specific, aggregate data, knowledge based, and comparative. (From Joint Commission on Accreditation of Healthcare Organizations. *Comprehensive accreditation manual for pathology and clinical laboratory services.* Oakbrook Terrace, IL: Joint Commission on Healthcare Organizations, 1999.)

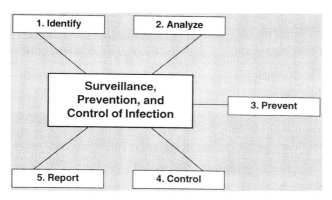

FIGURE 28.7. Surveillance, prevention, and control of infection. (From Joint Commission on Accreditation of Healthcare Organizations. *Comprehensive accreditation manual for pathology and clinical laboratory services.* Oakbrook Terrace, IL: Joint Commission on Healthcare Organizations, 1999.)

- Personnel files
- CLIA certificates
- Technical and administrative policies and procedures
- Proficiency testing for blood gas analysis
- Data collection for performance improvement and risk management
- Departmental meeting minutes and POC committee minutes
- Examples of patient-test report formats
- Quality control and equipment maintenance records including correlation among sites performing blood gas testing

Standards from the organizational functions and technical functions are addressed in this document review. Many of the documents reviewed at this time address CLIA requirements for testing personnel, directorship, competency, and quality control.

The laboratory leadership is interviewed briefly, and standards that relate to directorship and oversight of quality control and competency are reviewed. Meeting minutes from staff meetings and data collection from performance improvement activities may be reviewed and discussed. The pathologist, technical consultant, and nursing leaders of Community Hospital X would respond to questions regarding individual roles in the POC oversight process.

During a visit to POCT areas, the surveyor will interview the staff members who perform blood gas analysis or whole-blood glucose testing and observe infection control and safety practices. Placement of equipment, space, utility needs, and storage of supplies will be reviewed. This process addresses key standards in the management of the laboratory environment and infection control but may include others as well. On-site documentation, such as work logs or patient medical records may be reviewed. The emphasis is on observed practice that supports the planning that was reviewed during document review or discussions with leadership.

Survey result feedback is often provided to the staff during each survey activity, but an end-of-day feedback session may also be conducted. Compliance with standards is discussed as well as any opportunities for improvement. Surveyors may give specific

examples to assist in follow-up activities. These sessions are generally informal.

The survey concludes with a leadership exit conference that is a formal summary of survey findings. A preliminary report and score are determined through surveyor use of computer technology and this report is shared with attendees. Any required follow-up to survey recommendations for improvement is also discussed. This last survey activity is normally open to the leadership and any other staff members who wish to attend.

PROBLEMATIC TOPICS

The JCAHO periodically publishes a book of frequently cited standards (4) and describes various mechanisms to improve performance. It is interesting that many of these problematic standards relate to the technical functions of quality control and waived testing. Standards that address proficiency testing, correlation of results, performance of quality control at required time periods, and remedial action in response to problems all appear on this list.

POCT sites may be numerous in many organizations and may involve large numbers of testing personnel and pieces of equipment. These numbers make good communication difficult and compliance with standards requirements even more so. Add to this varying levels of education and laboratory-specific training, and the leadership and oversight of POCT becomes a key element in performance improvement. Not surprisingly, one of the leadership standards that addresses effective directorship also appears on this list of problematic standards.

CONCLUSIONS

The JCAHO is an accrediting body that strives to improve the quality and safety of health care provided to the public. Through its POCT survey, the JCAHO accredits organizations that provide POCT. This survey process begins with an evaluation of compliance with performance-focused standards during an on-site review. The evaluation examines laboratory technical functions as well as organizational functions throughout the continuum of care. It is a systems survey of applicable standards that examines integration of services throughout an organization, and is therefore not limited to a checklist of requirements. Additionally, it includes an evaluation of compliance with CLIA.

The goal of all JCAHO accreditation surveys is to achieve and improve quality for positive patient outcomes. The survey evaluates this through data collection and performance improvement as demonstrated through measurement. Patient safety is a key focus area.

As the complexity of healthcare organizations evolves, the challenges associated with quality and performance improvement for POCT increase. Good communication, strong leadership, and oversight of quality control processes are key indicators of success.

REFERENCES

1. Brauer CM. *Champions of quality in health care: a history of the Joint Commission on Accreditation of Healthcare Organizations.* Lyme, CT: Greenwich Publishing Group, 2001.
2. Joint Commission on Accreditation of Healthcare Organizations. *Facts about the Joint Commission on Accreditation of Healthcare Organizations.* Available at: http://www.jcaho.org/whatwedo_frm.html. Accessed on December 6, 2001.
3. Joint Commission on Accreditation of Healthcare Organizations. *Comprehensive accreditation manual for pathology and clinical laboratory ser-* *vices.* Oakbrook Terrace, IL: Joint Commission on Accreditation of Healthcare Organizations, 1999.
4. Joint Commission on Accreditation of Healthcare Organizations. *How to meet the most frequently cited laboratory standards,* 2nd ed. Oakbrook Terrace, IL: Joint Commission on Accreditation of Healthcare Organizations, 2001.
5. U.S. Department of Health and Human Services. Medicare, Medicaid and CLIA programs: categorization of tests and personnel modifications. *Federal Register* 1995;60:20035–20051.
6. Joint Commission on Accreditation of Healthcare Organizations. *Quality point of care testing.* Oakbrook Terrace, IL: Joint Commission on Accreditation of Healthcare Organizations, 1999.

29

POINT-OF-CARE TESTING AND THE COLLEGE OF AMERICAN PATHOLOGISTS

THOMAS F. RUHLEN

Point-of-care testing (POCT) may be accredited through several means. The College of American Pathologists (CAP) administers an accreditation program for medical laboratories that is widely regarded by medical laboratorians for its excellence. The CAP accreditation program, the Laboratory Accreditation Program (LAP), can be used to accredit POCT. This chapter describes the history, principles, and process of accreditation of the LAP, as well as details of the requirements of the program as it applies to POCT. This chapter is intended to serve as a resource for anyone striving to improve the quality of POCT, whether or not through CAP accreditation.

DEFINITION OF POINT-OF-CARE TESTING

The CAP definition of POCT is limited to tests performed using portable instruments that are transported to the testing site and that are not performed at a site dedicated to laboratory testing. The central criterion is the absence of a fixed space dedicated to laboratory testing (1). Examples include bedside use of glucometers, occult fecal blood tests used near the patient, and instruments temporarily transported into an operating room or an emergency room. POCT, as defined by this book, overlaps with the CAP definition of limited-service satellite laboratories. Limited-service satellite laboratories are small laboratories, outside of a central laboratory, with limited test menus that have space permanently dedicated for laboratory testing. Examples include blood gas laboratories and small laboratories within emergency rooms, operating suites, and outpatient clinics (Fig. 29.1).

LABORATORY ACCREDITATION PROGRAM

Definition of Laboratory

The LAP has struggled over the years with how to define what comprises a laboratory. Laboratories are organized in a variety of ways that are sometimes quite complex. For example, there may be multiple satellite laboratories within an institution at different addresses or even in different cities. Sometimes there are multiple laboratories within an institution with different laboratory directors. Currently, the LAP essentially uses the laboratory number, assigned by the Centers for Medicare & Medicaid Services (CMS), formerly the Health Care Financing Administration (HCFA), for licensure under the Clinical Laboratories Improvement Amendments of 1988 (CLIA '88) (2) to define the limits of a laboratory (3).

POCT in an institution may be accredited by the CAP either as an individual laboratory or in conjunction with accreditation of other laboratories within the institution. POCT can be accredited as a separate laboratory if it has a CLIA number separate from other laboratories in the institution.

The CAP only accredits entire laboratories and will not accredit only a portion of a laboratory. For example, if a laboratory includes a central laboratory and one or more satellite laboratories under a single CLIA number, then LAP will include all of the laboratories in its inspection and accreditation of the central laboratory. If one of the satellite laboratories has a CLIA number separate from the central laboratory, then the LAP will consider it an individual laboratory and accredit it separately from the central laboratory, if the satellite laboratory also applies for CAP accreditation.

The same principle applies to POCT. If a central laboratory includes POCT in its CLIA number, the LAP will include the POCT activity in the inspection and accreditation of the laboratory. If POCT is not under the laboratory's CLIA number, then the LAP will not inspect and accredit the POCT activity as part of the laboratory's accreditation. It is very important for laboratories to be very specific about what POCT activities are included in their CAP application for accreditation. Failure to clearly identify POCT has led to the need for inspectors to revisit laboratories to complete the inspection process.

History

The CAP first established a program for laboratory inspection and accreditation in 1962 (4). The program, initially called the Inspection and Accreditation Program, operated under the direction of a commission consisting of a chair and ten regional commissioners, one each from ten defined regions of the United

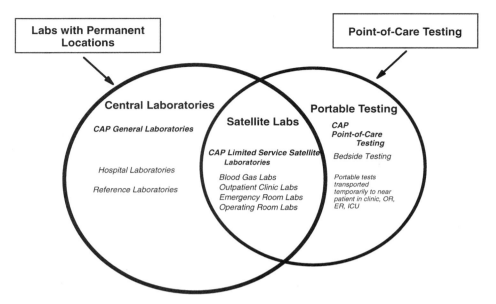

FIGURE 29.1. Laboratory Accreditation Program definition of point-of-care testing.

States. The commission reported directly to the CAP Board of Governors. The commission developed standards for accreditation that covered a laboratory's physical plant, organization, efficiency of service, space, equipment, personnel, quality control, and record keeping. By the fall of 1963, 222 laboratories had been recruited into the program. The LAP became an international program in 1969 with accreditation of the first overseas laboratory in Bombay, India. In 1979, the commission was renamed the Commission on Laboratory Accreditation (CLA) and the name of the inspection program was changed to the Laboratory Accreditation Program (LAP).

The CLA recognized the need to accommodate testing performed outside of a traditional central hospital laboratory as early as 1981. In 1982, a special checklist was developed for inspecting small satellite laboratories and procedures were developed to include these laboratories in the accreditation process. The CLA subsequently extended the accreditation process to include POCT.

In 1988, federal legislation was enacted to update Medicare regulations for laboratory licensure in CLIA '88. This legislation required any clinical laboratory providing test results for the diagnosis and treatment of human disease or establishment of health to be licensed by the federal government. The responsibility for developing regulations and enforcing the new law was assigned to the secretary of the Department of Health and Human Services and thence to the Centers for Disease Control and the CMS. The legislation allowed CMS to approve accrediting organizations to conduct laboratory inspection and accreditation in lieu of inspections conducted by CMS agencies. The CAP Board of Governors decided to seek CMS "deemed status" as an approved accrediting organization. The LAP was recognized as an approved accrediting organization by the CMS in early 1994. As a condition for approval for deemed status, the CAP was required to include several changes in the LAP. Among

these changes were requirements relating to the test complexity model developed by CLIA '88 and CMS oversight approval of Checklist questions.

Currently, the LAP is administered by the CLA with assistance from numerous deputy regional commissioners, state commissioners, and LAP staff in the CAP headquarters in Northfield, Illinois, and accredits over 6,000 laboratories.

Principles

The goal of the LAP is laboratory improvement and is based on the principles of voluntary participation, peer review, and education. Participation in the program is voluntary. Laboratories have the option to achieve accreditation through other agencies.

Peer review and education are absolutely central to the CAP philosophy of laboratory improvement. Inspectors in the program are practicing pathologists, clinical scientists, and medical technologists who bring their own experience and knowledge to the laboratory being inspected. This facilitates exchange of meaningful, practical information between the inspectors and inspectees. Laboratorians are much more likely to obtain useful information from inspectors who perform the same tasks as they do daily. The flow of information is two-way. Inspectors learn new approaches to the problems they encounter in their own laboratories. It is very common for inspectors to leave an inspection with copies of procedures, policies, and forms from the laboratory they inspect for use in their own laboratory.

The approach of the CAP to inspection of POCT rests upon the concept of "site neutrality." The CAP believes all laboratory tests have the potential to affect patient care; therefore, it is essential that all laboratory tests be performed accurately regardless of who is the analyst or where the analysis occurs. The CAP does not subscribe to the CLIA '88 concept of categorizing tests as "waived," "provider-performed microscopy," "moderate com-

TABLE 29.1. ACCREDITATION REQUIREMENTS COMPARISON

Requirements	CAP Point-of-Care Testing	CLIA '88 Waived Testing
Personnel training	Yes	No
Proficiency testing	Yes	No
Quality control	Yes	Follow manufacturer's instructions
Quality improvement plan	Yes	No
Procedure manuals	Yes	No
Routine on-site inspections	Yes	No

CAP, College of American Pathologists; CLIA '88, Clinical Laboratory Improvement Amendments of 1988.

plexity," and "high complexity," with differing requirements for quality control and oversight for each category. The CAP believes all laboratory tests that are performed incorrectly have the potential for causing harm to patients. The CAP maintains the same quality control and oversight requirements for all tests, whether performed in full-service laboratories by medical technologists or at patients' bedsides by nurses (Table 29.1).

Standards

The CAP developed four standards that are the basis for accreditation decisions (5). The standards address broad issues that characterize laboratories of quality. Decisions to revoke or deny accreditation are based on failure to fulfill the requirements of these standards.

Standard I addresses the medical director of the laboratory. The director must be qualified to assume the responsibilities of leadership of a medical laboratory and must have sufficient authority to implement and maintain the standards. The director is expected to fulfill several duties including consultation regarding the medical significance of laboratory data, performance of anatomic pathology, participation as a member of the active medical staff, definition and maintenance or standards of quality control, implementation and maintenance of a quality improvement plan, provision of adequate staffing, performance of strategic planning, provision of educational programs to laboratory and medical staff, selection of reference laboratories, and maintenance of safety standards within the laboratory. The medical director does not need to personally perform all of these duties and may delegate functions to other staff; however, the director is held responsible for the successful performance of all of these duties.

Standard II addresses physical facilities and safety. There must be adequate space and equipment to operate a quality laboratory. Safety of laboratory personnel, patients, and visitors is essential. Safety concerns include fire, chemical, electrical, and infectious hazards. The laboratory must comply with all federal, state, and local fire and safety codes.

Standard III addresses quality control and quality improvement. The laboratory must have a defined and adequate plan for monitoring the quality of laboratory testing including enrollment in proficiency testing (see "Proficiency Testing" section).

There must also be a defined system implemented that strives to monitor and continually improve the quality of the laboratory's operation. This system should be integrated into the institution's overall quality improvement plan and fulfill the requirements of other agencies that accredit the institution.

Standard IV addresses inspection requirements. Each laboratory must undergo an on-site inspection every 2 years and conduct a self-inspection in the interim. Deficiencies identified during on-site inspections must be corrected before accreditation will be issued or renewed. Deficiencies identified during self-inspections must be corrected. A laboratory is expected to provide the results of self-inspection, and corrective actions taken, to the next on-site inspector. Laboratories must submit to additional on-site inspections if required by the CLA. The CLA may require additional inspection when there is a change in directorship, location, or ownership of the laboratory, or if the CLA perceives a possible deterioration of laboratory quality through the results of proficiency testing or complaint investigation. Every laboratory is also required to provide an inspection team every 2 years, if requested.

Checklists

The LAP maintains several checklists, which are the tools that inspectors use during inspections to assess whether laboratories meet the intent of the standards. The checklists are not standards in and of themselves. The checklists are organized by laboratory discipline and include checklists for hematology and coagulation, chemistry, special chemistry, urinalysis and clinical microscopy, toxicology, microbiology, transfusion medicine, immunology and syphilis serology, anatomic pathology, cytology, cytogentics, histocompatibility, flow cytometry, molecular pathology, blood gas laboratory, limited service laboratory, and POCT.

All laboratory inspections include the use of the Laboratory General Checklist (6). This checklist, which addresses global issues of the laboratory, is used for all inspections and is supplemented with the discipline-specific checklists appropriate to the laboratory's test menu. The Laboratory General Checklist includes questions regarding quality improvement, quality control, proficiency testing, personnel, computer services, and safety.

The checklists contain a total of over 3,000 questions. The number of questions in individual checklists ranges from 65 to over 300. An inspector records a laboratory's performance by assessing compliance for each of the questions in the checklists used in an inspection.

There are two categories of questions in the checklists. Phase II questions address items that may seriously impact the quality of patient care or pose serious safety threats to personnel. Phase II questions cited as deficient by the inspector, referred to as phase-II deficiencies, must be corrected before accreditation will be granted or renewed. Failure to properly perform quality control is an example of a phase-II deficiency. Phase I questions address items that do not have the potential to seriously impact the quality of patient care or pose serious safety threats. Minor shortage of space in the laboratory is an example of a phase-I deficiency.

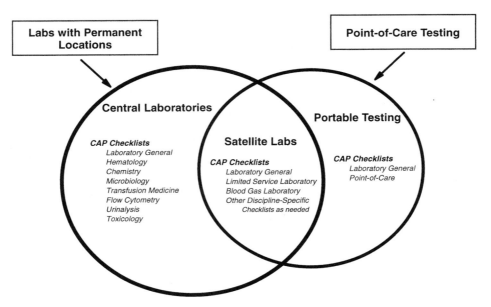

FIGURE 29.2. Laboratory Accreditation Program use of inspection checklists.

POCT is inspected using the Point-of-Care Testing Checklist (Fig. 29.2). This checklist is used when POCT does not take place at a fixed site and instead, involves transport of the testing instrument or material to the patient's location. Examples include the use of glucometers and occult blood testing performed at the bedside and portable instruments taken into an operating room. One Point-of-Care Checklist can be used to inspect multiple POCT activities as long as the oversight and records are centrally maintained in one location. Otherwise, multiple copies of the checklist are required for the inspection. The use of multiple copies of the Point-of-Care Checklist not only complicates the inspection process, but also increases inspection costs as the charge structure for accreditation is based, in part, on the number of checklists used for the inspection (Table 29.2).

POCT occurring in satellite laboratories (fixed space dedicated to testing outside of the main laboratory) is inspected using the Limited Service Checklist (7). This checklist is designed to inspect only one satellite laboratory per checklist.

The contents of the Limited Service Checklist and the Point-of-Care Checklist are essentially the same as the checklists used to inspect all other laboratories. Requirements for oversight, quality control, personnel, documentation, and proficiency testing are uniform throughout all the checklists.

Deficiencies cited from inspections of POCT most commonly involve documentation issues including reagent labeling, quality control records, corrective actions, results reporting, and reference range reporting.

Checklist Updates

Checklists undergo continual revision. Current versions of checklists are posted on the CAP website (http://www.cap.org) and are available for download at no charge. Laboratories can review current versions of the checklists in order to anticipate revisions in advance of their on-site inspections. Checklists are also available in printed form and on computer disks.

Explanatory notes, commentary, and literature references accompany checklist questions. This accompanying information is intended to provide laboratories and inspectors with additional information and resources to understand the intent of the questions.

Inquiries regarding checklist questions can be directed to members of the CLA and to the technical staff of the CAP Central Office. Inquiries can also be submitted online at the CAP website.

The CLA includes the checklist commissioner who oversees maintenance of the checklists. Each checklist is also assigned to a regional commissioner for oversight. Suggestions for new questions and revisions of existing questions are received from many

TABLE 29.2. COLLEGE OF AMERICAN PATHOLOGISTS

Program	2001 Annual Fees
Laboratory accreditation program[a]	
1–4 Checklists	$950
5–8 Checklists	$1620
9 Checklists	$1920
>9 Checklists	$1920 plus $290 per checklist over nine
Proficiency test surveys[b]	
Whole blood glucose (WGB)	$270
Clinical microscopy (CM)	$174
Occult blood (OCB)	$120
Activated clotting time (ACT)	$291
hCG, serum, qualitative (hCG)	$144

[a]From College of American Pathologists, *Laboratory accreditation program: 2001 accreditation fees, application for accreditation* (Northfield, IL: College of American Pathologists, 2000).
[b]From College of American Pathologists, *2001 Surveys & educational anatomic pathology programs* (Northfield, IL: College of American Pathologists, 2000).

sources including CAP scientific resource committees, CLA members and staff, CAP members, and laboratory personnel. Appropriate scientific resource committees of the CAP review suggestions for significant changes. All changes in the checklists must be approved by the CLA. Checklist changes are also subject to approval by the CMS as a condition of the CAP's deemed status under CLIA '88.

Inspection Process

The inspection process begins when a laboratory submits a completed written application to the CLA (Fig. 29.3). The application provides demographic information about the laboratory and includes information on test menus, instrumentation, test volumes, personnel, and floor plans. The appropriate state commissioner is notified and assigns an inspection team leader. Inspection team leaders are usually pathologists from CAP-accredited laboratories who have undergone training in the inspection process and philosophy. The team leader assembles a team of inspectors. The inspection team members can be medical technologists, other pathologists, clinical scientists, pathology residents, and other medical personnel actively involved in laboratory testing. The laboratory's application information is sent to the team leader along with the appropriate checklists. The team leader consults with the laboratory's medical director and sets a date for the inspection. When a laboratory is applying for renewal of accreditation, the inspection date must be within the 30 days before the laboratory's anniversary date of its initial inspection.

On the day of the inspection, the inspection team uses the checklists to record the laboratory's compliance with the standards. Each checklist question is answered "yes," "no," or "not applicable." Checklist questions judged to be not in compliance are listed on the inspector's report. At the end of the inspection,

a summation conference is held in which the inspection findings are reviewed by the inspection team with the laboratory director, staff, and administration. A copy of the inspection report is left with the laboratory and the original copy of the report is sent to the CAP central office.

The laboratory has 30 days from the day of inspection to document corrective action of all phase-II deficiencies and to report what action will be taken to address all phase-I deficiencies. A laboratory may contest a deficiency if it believes it was cited in error. This may occur if an inspector misunderstands the laboratory's response, misunderstands the question, or did not find existing required documentation during the inspection.

The laboratory's documentation of corrective action is sent to the CAP Central Office where it is reviewed for adequacy. If inadequate responses are identified, the laboratory will be requested to provide additional documentation. The inspection results and responses receive final review by one of the regional commissioners. The regional commissioner may communicate further with the laboratory to clarify responses or request additional corrective action or documentation. The regional commissioner will also expunge from the record any deficiencies the laboratory successfully contests.

The regional commissioner recommends the laboratory for accreditation. Accreditation is conferred for a period of 2 years. The laboratory may renew accreditation by undergoing additional on-site inspections every 2 years.

CHECKLIST REQUIREMENTS

This section provides details of the questions from the Point-of-Care Checklist and pertinent questions from the Laboratory

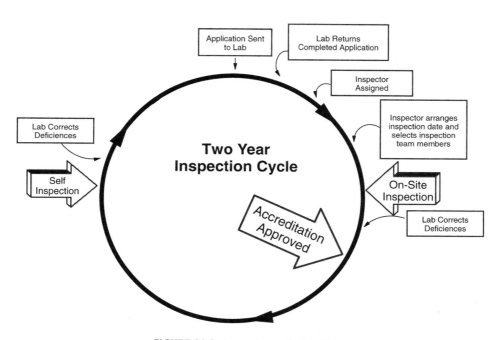

FIGURE 29.3. Inspection cycle time line.

General Checklist. The discussion includes checklist question numbers for reference. The information presented in this section was obtained from the checklists as of October 2001. As the checklists are frequently revised, the reader is encouraged to obtain the most recent versions of the checklists from the CAP website (http://www.cap.org) for review.

Procedure Manuals

Laboratories are required to develop and maintain procedure manuals. Procedure manuals contain detailed written instructions and information for each of the tests performed in a laboratory. Procedures should be written substantially in the format of the National Committee on Clinical Laboratory Standards manual GP2-A3 (8) but do not need to precisely emulate it. Procedures should include the following information: principle of the test method, clinical significance, specimen type, reagents, calibration, quality control, procedural steps, calculations, reference ranges, and interpretation (Checklist question POC:03900). It is acceptable to use procedures or inserts prepared by the instrument manufacturer, provided such information is personalized for the laboratory. Items that might need modification include reference ranges, reporting procedures, and the definition of critical limits. It is also acceptable to maintain procedures entirely electronically without having printed copies if there are provisions for adequate document control, that is, only authorized people may modify procedures. Procedure manuals should be available to the people doing the testing and not sequestered in an office. It is acceptable to use work cards with abbreviated versions of procedures provided the work cards are kept current, correspond to full procedures, and are subject to adequate document control.

Procedures must be reviewed annually by the laboratory director or qualified designee (Checklist question POC:04100). Each procedure must show evidence of annual review. A single signature indicating review of an entire set of procedures in a manual is not sufficient. If the director delegates this function to another qualified person, the delegation should be documented. Documentation of delegation may be accomplished within written job descriptions or as a separate document.

The laboratory must have a system to ensure that personnel are knowledgeable about the contents of the procedures to the extent needed for their level of testing (Checklist question POC:04200). This requirement also encompasses changes made to the procedure. Laboratories often meet this requirement by having personnel sign a statement attesting that they have reviewed the procedure. Another method used is to include evidence of an employee's knowledge of procedures in their annual competency evaluation.

Whenever a procedure is discontinued, a copy of the procedure should be retained for at least 2 years. The initial date of use and the retirement date of the procedure should be recorded (Checklist question POC:04270). This requirement includes procedures that are replaced with new copies of procedures after updates. The intent is to maintain an accurate record of what procedural steps were in place during the past 2 years.

When there is a change in the directorship of the laboratory, the new director must ensure that the laboratory's procedure manuals are well documented and reviewed annually (Checklist question POC:04230). This does not mean that the new director must necessarily sign each procedure; however, the director does need to establish that the laboratory's procedures are current and complete.

Specimen Handling

The laboratory must have a system defined for ensuring adequate identification of patient specimens, including capillary tube specimens and aliquots (Checklist question POC:04300). The identification system should be consistently applied. In POCT settings, the proximity of the patient allows some modifications to patient specimen identification but does not negate the need for a consistent system to be in place. Although the system may not require specific labeling of specimen containers when testing takes place immediately at the patient's side, the system does need to include the steps taken to properly identify the patient.

The laboratory should make an effort to minimize phlebotomy volumes (Checklist question POC:04350). Many point-of-care (POC) test systems require only small volumes of blood for testing, but not all systems do so. Personnel working in POCT sites may also draw blood specimens for a central laboratory with higher specimen volume requirements. The laboratory should attempt to use smaller volume blood specimens, where possible, to help avoid iatrogenic anemia, particularly in pediatric patients.

Reporting of Results

The laboratory must have a defined system for reporting test results that includes creating a permanent record of the results in the patient medical record (Checklist question POC:04400). In POC settings, the test result may be reported immediately to the physician either verbally or through instrument printouts. The test result must be subsequently permanently recorded in the medical record.

Test results should be reported with reference ranges of the tests, when applicable (Checklist question POC:04500). This is one of the most common deficiencies cited in CAP inspections of POCT. POC test results are often recorded manually. Unless the report form already includes the reference ranges for the tests, it is left to the person recording the result to also record reference ranges of the tests. This step is easily missed. Laboratories have devised several solutions to provide the reference range in this circumstance, including the use of preprinted forms and rubber stamps. The use of a computer system for result reporting can greatly facilitate fulfilling this requirement.

In some circumstances, the requirement for reporting reference ranges is not applicable. For example, glucose tests may be reported as part of a clinical protocol used to adjust insulin doses. The clinical protocol provides the interpretative parameters of the test result, obviating the need to also report a reference range. It would also appear to be excessively rigid to insist on reporting reference ranges for fecal occult blood, which universally has a normal reference range of negative.

The laboratory should establish or verify reference ranges for the patient population of the laboratory (Checklist question POC:04525). If the laboratory cannot perform its own study to establish reference ranges, then it should evaluate the use of published reference range studies.

Critical limits are test results that are so abnormal as to require immediate notification of the patient's physician. Critical limits should be established for the tests performed in POCT (Checklist question POC:04525). It is not necessary to establish critical limits if test results are always reported immediately to the physician as, for example, may be the case when POCT takes place in the operating room.

The laboratory should document its notification of a patient's physician when critical limits are encountered (Checklist question POC:04600). The checklist does not specify the manner in which this documentation is made and the documentation does not need to be a part of the test report. I have found this documentation to be invaluable when a physician alleges that the laboratory overlooked a critical value.

The laboratory must establish the analytic limits for the instruments in use (Checklist question POC:04650). Specimen dilution or other specimen pretreatment may, for some instruments, extend the analytic limits. The laboratory should define what procedures are to be taken when test results fall outside of these ranges. These steps might include repeat testing. A result falling outside the limits of the instrument should be reported as "greater than" or "less than" the value of the instrument's limit.

The identity of the analyst performing the test should be recorded (Checklist question POC:04700). This does not need to appear on the test report but should be captured in some retrievable manner in the laboratory's records.

Reagents

The laboratory must verify that new lots of reagents will perform as expected before they are used to report patient results (Checklist question POC:05000). The purpose is to establish whether reference ranges and quality control limits are appropriate for the new reagents. The laboratory should define the manner in which this is done. Laboratories often test new reagents using patient specimens with known results. Reference materials may also be used for this purpose.

The laboratory should also establish what course of action to take when new reagents are found to not perform as expected (Checklist question POC:05020). This may entail obtaining new reagents, modifications of reference ranges, or modifications of quality control tolerance limits.

POCT often uses tests in a kit form. When there are multiple components of reagents in a test kit, the laboratory must not use individual components with test kits from different lots unless the manufacturer specifies this as an acceptable practice (Checklist question POC:05050).

Reagents used in POCT must be adequately labeled. The labeling should indicate what the material is, how it is to be stored, date of preparation or reconstitution (if applicable), and expiration date (Checklist question POC:04800). This requirement is the source of many deficiencies cited during CAP inspections. It is difficult for laboratories to ensure that POC

personnel follow these labeling requirements. The reagent containers in test kits are sometimes too small to allow room for additional labeling. It is acceptable to record the required dates on the reagent kit container provided the individual components of the kit are kept together.

Calibration and Controls

Calibration of instruments must be performed using calibration materials of adequately high quality (Checklist question POC:05150). The procedures used to calibrate instruments must be adequate to ensure accurate test results, and calibration results must be documented (Checklist question POC:05100). Calibration must demonstrate the instrument's ability to produce accurate results throughout the instrument's analytic range, including the low and high ends of the range, using at least three levels. In POCT, calibration procedures are often established by the instrument manufacturer. The laboratory needs to ensure that these procedures encompass the above requirements. For example, the use of only two levels of calibrator material is not adequate. Also, it is not adequate to perform calibrations using the same material used for daily quality control.

CLIA '88 regulations include requirements for verifying accurate calibration through the performance of calibration verification (9). Calibration verification must be performed for each instrument as defined by criteria established by the laboratory, and must be performed, and documented, at least every 6 months (Checklist question POC:05330). The criteria for when to perform calibration verification may include such events as a complete change of reagents affecting the range used to report patient values, failure of quality control to meet established criteria, after major instrument maintenance, and when recommended by the manufacturer. If calibration verification confirms that the instrument is in calibration, then the laboratory does not need to recalibrate the instrument. If calibration verification reveals the instrument has lost calibration, then the instrument must be recalibrated. Regardless of the time that calibration was last performed, calibration verification must be performed at least every 6 months.

Controls are samples with known values that are tested as surrogates for patient specimens in order to demonstrate that the test system is performing as expected. At least two levels of controls must be run at least each day of use for quantitative tests (Checklist question POC:05500). Under current federal law, coagulation, hematology, and blood gas testing systems must run controls during each 8-hour period of testing. Qualitative tests must include positive and negative controls during at least each day of use (Checklist question POC:05800). The use of internal controls for qualitative tests is acceptable provided the laboratory has verified that the internal controls adequately challenge the test system. Many test systems in POCT utilize electronic controls that challenge the system electronically without using liquid control material. The use of electronic controls is acceptable for test systems classified by CLIA '88 as "waived" or "moderate complexity," provided the laboratory documents the classification of the test system and documents their verification of the validity of the electronic control system. The CAP does not specify what steps should be taken to verify the validity of the electronic control system and leaves it to the judgment of the medical director to establish this validity.

The laboratory must establish tolerance limits for quality control results (Checklist question POC:06100) and quality control results must be verified as acceptable before patient results are reported (Checklist question POC:06260). Quality control results should also be reviewed each day to detect instrument trends that indicate potential failure of the test system (Checklist question POC:05900). The laboratory should document any corrective actions taken when quality control results exceed tolerance limits (Checklist question POC:06200). Quality control samples must be run by the same people who use the instrument for patient testing (Checklist question POC:06230). In POCT, it is a common practice for the central laboratory to maintain POC instruments. It is not acceptable for the personnel of the central laboratory to run the daily quality control samples on these instruments if they are not the personnel actually performing the patient tests.

Instruments and Equipment

The Point-of-Care Checklist contains only a few questions regarding instruments and equipment. The instruments and equipment a laboratory uses must be selected with the approval of the laboratory director (Checklist question POC:06300). Selection of instruments and equipment for use in POCT without the approval of the laboratory director may be interpreted as an abdication of the laboratory director's responsibility under Standard I.

Instruments and equipment used in POCT must be on a schedule, or other system, for regular checking of operating characteristics (Checklist question POC:06400). The procedures and schedules of instrument maintenance required will vary considerably depending on the specifics of the equipment and instruments used, but must be performed at least as frequently and as extensively as recommended by the manufacturer. The maintenance records must be documented and must be reviewed at least monthly by the laboratory director or designee (Checklist question POC:06500).

Quality Control and Improvement

The laboratory must have a documented program of quality control and improvement that defines the design of the program and the frequency and mechanism of review (Checklist question POC:03500). The section on calibration and controls describes specific requirements relating to quality control procedures. The laboratory needs to include quality control review results in its quality improvement plan as potential opportunities for quality improvement may be identified through the active review of quality control results. The laboratory's quality control and improvement plan should be documented, as should the findings of the plan. The design of the program should include a description of how the plan's findings will be reviewed and at what frequency. The plan should address preanalytic, analytic, and postanalytic phases of specimen testing. This is accomplished, in part, by having procedures for patient identification, patient preparation, specimen collection, specimen identifica-

tion, specimen preservation, specimen processing, and results reporting (Checklist question POC:03600). The plan should also include review of instrument maintenance and function (Checklist question POC:03650). Review of quality control data and instrument maintenance data, including temperature records if applicable, should be performed at least monthly. More frequent review may be appropriate for individual POCT settings; however, the checklist does not mandate or preclude more frequent review.

The quality control and improvement plan should also include a system to detect and correct significant clerical errors, analytic errors, and unusual test results (Checklist question POC:03700). In POCT, this system may require feedback from physicians to detect unusual patterns of test results that may indicate analytic error. In a POCT setting, the personnel performing the tests may also be responsible for administering medications based on the test results. There should be defined criteria available for the testing personnel to provide guidance on correlating unexpected test results with clinical findings. For example, a patient exhibiting signs and symptoms of hypoglycemia should not be given insulin, based on a POC glucose test result that indicates hyperglycemia, without further investigation.

The Point-of-Care Checklist includes a question that asks whether there is supervisory review of test results obtained in the absence of an on-site supervisor (Checklist question POC:03800). This question is often misinterpreted to mean that there must be supervisor review of all test results, or that there should be supervisor review of all test results obtained when a supervisor is not present. The CAP does not require supervisory review of all test results in POC settings or in the central laboratory. The requirement for supervisor review addressed by this question only applies to CLIA '88 defined "high-complexity testing" performed by trained high school graduates qualified under 42CFR493.1489(b)(5) when a qualified supervisor is not present. It does not apply to tests defined under CLIA '88 as "waived" or "moderate complexity." POC tests are currently nearly always "waived" or "moderate complexity" and the question does not apply when this is the case.

Computer Services

Checklist requirements for computer services are found in the Laboratory General Checklist and cover numerous aspects of information systems including system security, data entry, reports, data storage, data retrieval, system maintenance, interfaces, and networks. Data entry of patient results in POCT may take place through manual entry of results into an information system or through instrument-to-computer interfaces. This section will highlight three aspects of computer systems applicable to POCT: report format approval by the laboratory director, confirmation of data transfer across system interfaces, and backup procedures for when the system is down.

The laboratory director must approve the content and format of computer-generated, printed, patient test result reports at least annually (Checklist question GEN:43500). The format of a computer system's reports must be clear enough for physicians using them to be able to accurately interpret the results and the test reference ranges. Computer systems used for reporting patient results are an integral part of the laboratory testing process and, therefore, are the responsibility of the laboratory director. It is not acceptable to leave the format of result reports to the oversight of information systems personnel without input and approval by the laboratory director.

Test results from POC may pass through one or more computer system interfaces as they travel from the testing instrument to the patient report, whether printed or displayed on a video terminal. The laboratory must ensure that the results are transferred through interfaces without alteration, including any accompanying comments and reference ranges (Checklist question GEN:42500). This requirement applies to results entered manually into a computer system as well as those entered through instrument-to-computer interfaces. The laboratory is required to document its verification of the accuracy of interface data transfer.

The laboratory must have a defined system in place to be able to continue patient testing and results reporting in the event that the computer system is down (Checklist questions GEN:44700, GEN:44800). It is not acceptable to be forced to discontinue patient testing and reporting in the event of scheduled or unscheduled computer downtimes. These backup procedures typically involve the use of manual procedures for test requests and results reporting. The laboratory must anticipate this eventuality and prepare a documented plan to cope with computer downtimes.

Safety

Checklist requirements for safety are found in the Laboratory General Checklist and apply to POCT in addition to the central laboratory. There are several questions regarding written policies and procedures as well as questions addressing physical findings relating to safety. Aspects of safety addressed in the checklists include fire protection, electrical hazards, chemical hazards, microbiologic hazards, waste disposal, radioactive hazards, and disaster preparedness. Generally, the aspects of safety that most prominently apply to POCT, are those addressing microbiologic hazards and can be largely met by following the practices of "universal or standard precautions." The details of checklist questions regarding safety will not be enumerated here and, instead, the reader is encouraged to review the Laboratory General Checklist. POCT personnel should be aware that during a CAP inspection, the safety-related questions found in the Laboratory General Checklist will be reviewed by the inspector in POCT sites as well as in the central laboratory.

Personnel

POCT personnel must have documented training and orientation to perform the testing (Checklist question POC:06700). Some of this training may have occurred as part of a person's education but there will always be a need to provide some additional training regarding the specifics of the testing as performed in an individual institution. For example, a nurse's education may have included how to use glucometers, but that education would not have included how test results are reported in a specific institution.

The laboratory must have a list of personnel who are authorized to perform POCT (Checklist question POC:06800) and the list should be kept current. This allows the laboratory to ensure that the personnel performing POCT have received the necessary training.

The laboratory should ensure maintenance of POC personnel's competency to perform testing (Checklist question POC:06900). This requires periodic assessment of competency and additional training if necessary. Assessment of competency can be performed in a number of ways including direct observation of testing, written or oral examinations, review of performance, performance on challenge specimens, and evaluation of problem-solving skills.

The Point-of-Care Checklist requires that POC technical personnel be tested for color blindness, as applicable (Checklist question POC:07100). Some test systems require visual interpretation of colors, such as visual interpretation of urine dipsticks. The intent of the question is to ensure that personnel with impaired visual color discrimination are not assigned testing responsibilities that require visual color discrimination. If the POCT setting does not include any tests requiring visual color discrimination, then the question is not applicable.

PROFICIENCY TESTING

Proficiency testing is required for accreditation of POCT. Proficiency testing is an exercise in which a laboratory is challenged with test samples containing known concentrations of analytes. The laboratory analyzes these samples without knowing the target values of the analytes and then reports their results to the proficiency test provider. The laboratory's test results are then compared to the target values. This exercise allows a laboratory to spot check performance for accuracy and allows the CLA to monitor laboratory performance between inspections.

The CAP adopted proficiency testing requirements as a part of the LAP in 1979. Laboratories accredited by the CAP are required to enroll in proficiency testing programs approved by the CAP. The results of proficiency tests are received by the LAP, allowing the LAP to monitor laboratory performance between on-site inspections. If a laboratory performs poorly on a proficiency testing event, the LAP will ask the laboratory to provide documentation of their investigation and any needed corrective actions resulting from the failed event.

For years, the CAP only permitted enrollment in the CAP proficiency testing program. Recently, however, the CAP developed a process whereby non-CAP proficiency programs can receive approval for use in the LAP.

Most proficiency tests are of sufficient precision to allow the provider of the proficiency test to grade the results, that is, set statistically valid acceptable ranges for the results. Such proficiency tests are referred to as "graded." For example, proficiency tests for serum electrolytes are graded. Other proficiency tests are not of sufficient precision to allow statistically valid grading of results and are referred to as "nongraded." For example, erythrocyte sedimentation rate is a nongraded proficiency test.

Laboratories are required to enroll in proficiency tests that are graded. Enrollment in nongraded proficiency tests is not required, but may serve as a convenient assessment of interlaboratory accuracy.

For analytes where graded proficiency tests are not available, the laboratory must use other procedures to validate its performance at least twice a year (Checklist question POC:03450). The laboratory can validate performance by enrolling in a nongrade proficiency test or use other procedures including use of split sample analysis with other laboratories, split sample analysis with other inhouse methods, assayed materials, and clinical validation by chart review.

Enrollment in proficiency testing is required on a per analyte basis. If a laboratory uses two instruments or methods to test for an analyte, it is not required to enroll in separate proficiency tests for each instrument unless, in some instances, the specimen matrix is different on the two instruments. For example, serum sodium analyzed on two different instruments in a laboratory does not require enrollment in two separate proficiency tests for sodium. The matrix (serum) and the analyte (sodium) are the same. On the other hand, if a laboratory analyzes serum glucose on one instrument and whole-blood glucose on a second instrument, then it is required to enroll in proficiency tests for each instrument because while the analyte (glucose) is the same, the matrix (serum and whole blood) are different. A laboratory using two or more instruments to test for an analyte should run correlation studies using patient samples twice a year to ensure that the results of the two instruments are comparable (Checklist question POC:05450). This correlation is not reported as part of the proficiency testing process.

Proficiency tests specimens must be tested in a manner similar to actual patient samples. Proficiency testing must be performed on the same instruments and by the same people who normally test patient samples. It is forbidden to run proficiency test samples repeatedly before reporting results, if repeated testing is not the manner in which patient samples are analyzed. It is also forbidden to compare proficiency test results with other laboratories before reporting results.

Proficiency testing is required for POCT. If a laboratory's POC tests include analytes that are not also tested elsewhere in the laboratory, then enrollment in proficiency testing is required. If a laboratory's POC tests are also analyzed elsewhere in the laboratory using the same specimen matrix, then separate enrollment in proficiency testing is not required for those POC tests. Instead, a laboratory would be required, at least twice a year, to validate POC test results by correlation with the laboratory's other instruments. This validation must be performed for each of the individual instruments used in POCT as, for example, when multiple glucometers are in use. Many laboratories use the CAP proficiency test for whole blood glucose, which allows reporting of multiple glucometers.

The results of proficiency tests, whether graded, nongraded, or by alternative methods, must be reviewed by the laboratory director or designee (Checklist question POC:03300). When there are unacceptable proficiency test results, the laboratory must document investigation of the results and document any corrective action taken (Checklist question POC:03400).

MANAGEMENT STRATEGY FOR CAP ACCREDITATION

The principal problems encountered in achieving CAP accreditation of POCT include coordination of multiple POC activities and documentation issues. Management strategies must address these areas in order to succeed. The CLA does not mandate any specific solutions to address these areas; however, I offer the following comments.

CAP accreditation is facilitated when a central coordinator oversees all POCT. A coordinator can more easily stay current with the accreditation requirements than can multiple supervisors. A coordinator can also ensure that consistent and uniform approaches are taken towards documentation throughout the POC activities in an institution and can monitor testing personnel's completion of documentation. The coordinator does not necessarily have to be someone in the institution's central laboratory.

Documentation issues are common in POCT. Often the testing is performed by nonlaboratorians who are not familiar with standard laboratory procedures and do not understand the importance of performing and recording quality control results and quality control corrective actions. They also sometimes fail to record dates on reagents and to report reference ranges with patient results. Many of these requirements are more consistently met when the POC program is computerized. Instruments and information systems are available that require testing personnel to perform quality control, enter required data, and allow transfer of test results into the laboratory information system. These systems greatly facilitate fulfillment of accreditation requirements.

Sometimes testing personnel in point of care feel they are being expected to work with instruments that are cumbersome to operate or that otherwise unnecessarily add to their burden of work. The medical director of POCT is responsible for the selection of test instruments and systems; however, acceptance of testing systems by the testing personnel is greatly enhanced when they have significant input into the selection of the test systems. Their acceptance can significantly reduce problems with personnel fulfilling accreditation requirements.

RESOURCES

The CAP provides several resources on the Laboratory Accreditation Program.

The *Laboratory Accreditation Manual* includes a detailed explanation of the LAP and is a valuable resource for anyone preparing for inspections either as an inspector or as someone to be inspected. It is available in printed form from the CAP (1-800-323-4040) and can be downloaded without charge from the CAP website (http://www.cap.org).

The *Standards for Laboratory Accreditation* contains the four standards as well as explanatory material. This document is available in printed form and on the CAP website.

The checklists contain the checklist questions as well as explanatory notes, commentary, and references. The checklists are available in printed format and on computer disk from the CAP. The current versions are available for downloading at the CAP website.

LAP Inspector Training Seminars are live educational courses presented throughout the United States. These seminars provide current information regarding the inspection process and checklist content. A schedule of dates and locations is available from the CAP and on the CAP website.

LAP Inspector Training Self-Study Modules provide the material from the live inspector training seminars in a self-study format. They are available in printed form from the CAP and can be downloaded from the CAP website.

The CAP presents audio conferences on various aspects of laboratory accreditation periodically. The schedule of conferences is available from the CAP. Past audio conferences are available for downloading at the CAP website and include the printed materials of the conferences as well as the audio presentations.

The *Laboratory Accreditation Newsletter* is published by the CLA and is available in the CAP's publication, *CAP Today*, as well as on the CAP website.

The CAP website (http://www.cap.org) is not only a valuable resource for information on the LAP but also contains a wealth of information on other CAP resources including proficiency testing (surveys) and POCT.

CONCLUSIONS AND FUTURE DIRECTIONS

This chapter presented an overview of the CAP Laboratory Accreditation Program requirements for accreditation of POCT.

Key Points

- CAP accreditation of POCT can be achieved either as part of a central laboratory's testing or as a separate function in an institution.
- Accreditation of POCT is facilitated by use of a central coordinator, information systems, and testing personnel input into selection of test systems.
- The CAP website is an excellent source of current information regarding CAP laboratory accreditation, including checklist updates.
- The accreditation program includes laboratory inspections conducted by peers.
- The *Standards for Laboratory Accreditation* are the basis of accreditation decisions.
- Checklists are the tools that inspectors use to assess laboratory compliance with the standards.

Future Directions

The CLA is currently addressing additional issues in POCT including physician-performed testing and new testing technologies such as specimen-based *in vivo* and transcutaneous testing. Physician-performed testing is POC tests personally performed by a physician in the course of examining or treating a patient. The CLA recently determined it would accredit physician-performed testing when requested by the laboratory, and is developing procedures and checklist questions to do so. Newer technologies offer a host of challenges for accreditation requirements. Many of these new technologies do not involve removal of a specimen from the patient. Traditional methods of performing quality control are not applicable with many of these new technologies. The CLA is currently determining what requirements are reasonable and feasible to ensure high-quality testing using these newer technologies.

Disclaimer

The material in this chapter represents the views and opinions of the author and is not an official statement of the College of American Pathologists.

REFERENCES

1. College of American Pathologists, Commission on Laboratory Accreditation. *Point-of-care testing checklist*. Northfield, IL: College of American Pathologists, October 2001.
2. Public Health Service Act. §353, 42 USC §263a (1988).
3. Merrick T, ed. *Laboratory accreditation manual*. Northfield, IL: College of American Pathologists, October 2001.
4. Hamlin WB, Duckworth JK. Historical perspectives in pathology and laboratory medicine, the College of American Pathologists, 1946–1996: laboratory accreditation. *Arch Pathol Lab Med* 1997;121:745–753.
5. College of American Pathologists. *Standards for laboratory accreditation*. Northfield, IL: College of American Pathologists, 1999.
6. College of American Pathologists, Commission on Laboratory Accreditation. *Laboratory general checklist*. Northfield, IL: College of American Pathologists, September 2001.
7. College of American Pathologists, Commission on Laboratory Accreditation. *Limited service laboratory checklist*. Northfield, IL: College of American Pathologists, October 2001.
8. National Committee for Clinical Laboratory Standards. *Clinical laboratory technical procedure manuals*, 3rd ed. Approved guideline GP2-A3. Wayne, PA: National Committee for Clinical Laboratory Standards, 1996.
9. U.S. Department of Health and Human Services. Medicare, Medicaid and CLIA programs: regulations implementing the Clinical Laboratory Improvement Amendments of 1988 (CLIA). Final rule *Federal Register* 1992 Feb 28;57:7002–7186.

30

FDA REGULATION OF HOME-USE
IN VITRO DIAGNOSTIC DEVICES

STEVEN GUTMAN
KIMBER CREAGER RICHTER

THE FOOD AND DRUG ADMINISTRATION'S REGULATORY PARADIGM FOR *IN VITRO* DIAGNOSTIC DEVICES

In 1976 Congress passed the Medical Device Amendments (1) to the *Food, Drug, and Cosmetic Act*, initiating oversight of medical devices by the Food and Drug Administration (FDA). Since the definition of devices included any device "intended for use in the diagnosis of disease or other conditions" (1), *in vitro* diagnostic devices (IVDs) were included under this new regulation. This law established several requirements including the need for IVD manufacturers to register with the FDA and list their products, to comply with good manufacturing practices, and to report serious device failures. This provided the agency with a listing of tests in the marketplace, mechanisms to assure that medical devices were made using sound manufacturing practices, and a system to identify serious problems related to device failure, so that the FDA could interact with companies in identifying mechanisms for dealing with these problems. In addition to these general controls, the new law also put into place requirements for premarket review of medical devices entering the market for the first time.

Two types of premarket submissions were established. Devices similar to existing marketed devices are "cleared" as premarket notifications if they demonstrate substantial equivalence to the previous device. Because the portion of the law describing this is the 510(k) section, these are referred to as 510(k) submissions. Fundamentally new devices are "approved" as premarket approval applications (PMAs). FDA review of devices, unlike review of drugs, is not associated with user fees and therefore is performed without cost to the manufacturer.

In the semantic framework of FDA language, a determination of whether a device is considered old or new is based on identification of a predicate—a device that was legally marketed prior to May 28, 1976, or a device which has been found substantially equivalent by the FDA to such a previously marketed device—against which the device can be compared. An *in vitro* diagnostic test is essentially a laboratory test.

PREMARKET NOTIFICATIONS

Most IVD submissions are premarket notifications or 510(k)s. The agency currently handles approximately 750 of these per year. The operative term in 510(k) review is "substantial equivalence." The law requires, as noted above, that new versions of existing devices be substantially equivalent to a predicate device. Review of most 510(k) submissions is straightforward and based on an analysis of the fundamental performance of a test including accuracy, precision, analytical sensitivity, and analytical specificity. There are limitations to the review process. The 510(k) review is entirely a paper review; the FDA does not submit these products to direct laboratory evaluation and the agency therefore has no hands-on experience with the vast majority of devices it considers. In addition, the agency is continually challenged by the need to determine appropriate standards for the substantial equivalence decision, since these are not well addressed in either the laboratory medicine or clinical literature. The 510(k) review process has well-established administrative requirements and a targeted FDA review time of 90 days. Information on this type of submission can be obtained on the FDA home page (http://www.fda.cdrh.gov) or by calling the Division of Small Manufacturers Assistance (1-800-638-2041).

PREMARKET APPROVAL APPLICATIONS

The agency reviews far fewer IVD premarket approval submissions—generally one to two dozen are under review in the course of a year. The key factor in a PMA review is "safety and effectiveness." Since no predicate can be defined, it is necessary to establish independently that the product is "safe and effective." In fact, since passage of the *Safe Medical Devices Act of 1990* (2), the FDA has taken a broader interest in the safety and effectiveness of all devices. We now require for 510(k) submissions either a summary of safety and effectiveness or a statement that the company will make available all information in the premarket submission on safety and effectiveness upon request.

For all PMAs and for at least a subset of 510(k)s, the FDA now has data requirements that include not only the analytical performance of a device but clinical performance as well, including clinical or diagnostic sensitivity, clinical or diagnostic specificity, and in some cases information on the expected predictive values of testing. Limitations of the review are again obvious. In evaluating new products there is often a lack of a "gold standard" against which to judge performance. Bias may occur in collection of data to establish safety and effectiveness through problems in the study design or conduct. Finally, as with 510(k) submissions, determining the minimum performance required for approval can be difficult and challenging. The PMA review process, like the 510(k) process, has well-established administrative requirements. Because these submissions are often more complex than 510(k)s, the targeted FDA review time is 180 days. Information on this type of submission can also be obtained on the FDA home page (http://www.fda.cdrh.gov) or by calling the Division of Small Manufacturers Assistance (1-800-638-2041.)

LABELING OF *IN VITRO* DEVICES

IVDs are unique in that they have their own labeling regulations—CFR 809.10. These regulations clearly specify the information required to support device labeling and submissions. The labeling regulation is divided into 15 separate components that are outlined in Table 30.1.

Of these various elements the most important is evaluation of the intended use and the related indications for use. The intended use and indications for use of a product will determine the type of review (whether a product is a 510(k) or PMA), the questions likely to be raised, and the data likely to be required in the course of review.

TABLE 30.1. FOOD AND DRUG ADMINISTRATION LABELING REQUIREMENTS

Proprietary name and established name
Intended use
Summary and explanation of test
Principle of procedure
Information on reagents
Information on instruments (operation manual)
Information on specimen collection and preparation
Procedures
Results
Limitations of procedure
Expected values
Specific performance characteristics
Bibliography
Name and place of business
Date of the last revision of package insert

DEVELOPMENT OF A STANDARDIZED SCIENTIFIC REVIEW MODEL

A central concern of the FDA over the past several years has been development of a strong but pragmatic scientific model to frame the review. The agency believes that while there is not one path to truth in terms of the development of information to support product review, there are several basic tenets for good science. These include the need for the following:

- Up-front design of the study. All submissions, whether simple or complex, require an established design in advance of the study. In some cases all that is needed is referencing the National Committee on Clinical Laboratory Standards (NCCLS) or other voluntary evaluation standards that will be used; in others there may be a need to develop extensive and complex protocols with carefully formulated hypotheses. Design of the study in advance helps prevent bias and assures that the data obtained will address the intended use and advertising claims desired.
- Careful and meticulous collection of data. Careful execution of the study following the protocol is essential to obtain useful data. Each step of testing should be carefully conducted and documented so that any questions regarding the results can be answered later.
- Interpretation of results using sound, preferably referenceable, statistical techniques. A statistical plan for analyzing results should be prepared in advance of testing and included in the protocol. Results must be analyzed according to this plan. Individual product review obviously varies by the type of product and intended use.

REVIEW OF QUANTITATIVE TESTS

For a quantitative test, 510(k) review focuses on information on bias or, if possible, accuracy, comparing the new method by linear regression or other valid statistical techniques to a reference and/or a predicate method; information on precision, ideally studied using an ANOVA analysis to allow comprehensive assessment of components of variation, and experiments designed to evaluate analytical specificity and, if appropriate, sensitivity.

REVIEW OF QUALITATIVE TESTS

For a qualitative test, 510(k) review requirements usually at a minimum require all of the information requested for quantitative tests but in addition seek information on cutoff points established and discrimination or equivocal zones present in the test system.

For certain submissions, clinical as well as analytical data are required to allow test performance to be analyzed within a clinical framework. The FDA prefers when possible that information on clinical performance characteristics be defined in terms of receiver-operator characteristic curves.

THE SCOPE OF FOOD AND DRUG ADMINISTRATION REVIEW REQUIREMENTS

FDA review has historically not required outcome data showing how new tests will impact morbidity or mortality and/or actually change the quality of medical care. The presumption that clinical information is useful usually suffices to support the review process, and the FDA works closely with sponsors of new tests to help them identify appropriate clinical or laboratory endpoints or surrogate endpoints on which to establish test performance and to base test claims. In some instances a new test may have no obvious potential clinical use and no clear measure of effectiveness. In these cases medical literature and/or clinical outcome data may be required to demonstrate safety and effectiveness. Prospective clinical studies are required in only a handful of new tests, most commonly those in which the clinical claim involves a prediction of future endpoints or outcomes. Usually concurrent sample analysis comparing new tests to one or more predicate tests or reference methods can be used to support product review and timely clearance or approval.

FDA review does require meticulous attention to detail in data collection and presentation. Providing a high-quality study and a clear and well-written submission makes the agency's review job simpler and helps assure success for the company in bringing the product to market quickly.

Premarket review by FDA is conducted for the purpose of assuring the safety and effectiveness of *in vitro* diagnostic products. The FDA contributes to quality of marketed IVDs in at least three ways: it provides for oversight and objective review of new laboratory tests, sets minimum thresholds for product safety and effectiveness, and finally, ensures that organized data and appropriate labeling are provided to the users in support of a device's intended use.

THE REGULATION OF HOME-USE *IN VITRO* DIAGNOSTIC DEVICES

Home-use tests have been commercially marketed in the United States for more than 25 years. At the time of passage of the Medical Device Amendments in 1976 at least two important products were being sold over the counter. The first was the urine dipstick for evaluation of glucose and other common analytes. The second was the urine pregnancy test.

Following the passage of the Medical Devices Amendments, the FDA cleared the first home-use test in 1979 (a urine glucose test). Since then the agency has reviewed and cleared more than 300 *in vitro* diagnostic tests for home use in 14 distinct categories (Table 30.2). A comprehensive list of products cleared for home use can be found on the FDA website (www.fda.gov/cdrh/ode/otclist.html).

The FDA's approach toward regulation of this type of product was first outlined in 1988 with the publication of a guidance document entitled "Assessing the Safety and Effectiveness of Home-Use *In Vitro* Diagnostic Devices (IVDs): Draft Points to Consider Regarding Labeling and Premarket Submissions" (3).

TABLE 30.2. CATEGORIES OF *IN VITRO* DIAGNOSTIC DEVICES CLEARED BY FOOD AND DRUG ADMINISTRATION FOR HOME USE

Glucose
Cholesterol
Fecal occult blood
Human chorionic gonadotropin
Luteinizing hormone
Urine dipsticks
Filter paper collection strips for glycohemoglobin
Filter paper collection strips for antibody for HIV
Collection devices for drugs of abuse
Fructosamine
Prothrombin time
Point of care drugs of abuse
Triglycerides
High-density lipoproteins

This document, which was created with input from representatives of industry and professional groups as well as consumers, is designed to assist manufacturers of home-use IVDs comply with existing regulations and premarket clearance requirements. The document outlines the following key parameters of importance in the FDA review of home-use devices:

- When used in the hands of the lay user, the test should produce acceptable results when compared to results performed in the hands of professional users.
- Test results should be interpretable by lay users.
- The benefits of use should be found to outweigh the risks.

EVALUATION OF HOME-USE PERFORMANCE IN THE HANDS OF LAY USERS

Documentation of the first point is usually based on field studies designed to mimic real-world use. Data sets from lay users are used to establish key performance parameters such as accuracy and precision in the hands of these untrained users. The FDA suggests that these studies be done in a population representative of the population likely to purchase the device. Optimally, populations studied should include a broad base so that performance is assessed in individuals from a wide variety of socioeconomic, educational, and cultural backgrounds.

The FDA also suggests that the studies replicate as closely as possible the likely real-world use. Tests are often used by consumers at home without oversight in their normal daily schedules. Instructions for use in a study normally are the same as would be expected in the final labeling. Special training programs or materials may be used as part of a study only if the intention is to make these same materials available during the actual use of the product. The FDA also encourages manufacturers to perform both observational studies of consumers using the product and focus testing with small groups of users to ensure that performance is adequately characterized, design features are understood, and labeling is optimized for correct use.

EVALUATION OF HOME-USE BENEFITS AND RISKS IN THE HANDS OF HOME USERS

The second and third points require a clinical evaluation of the test and an intense review of proposed labeling. The FDA's review of the merit of a home test takes into account the impact of home access to test results. A major issue in this evaluation is whether information can be clearly communicated to lay users and would be expected to lead to actions that promote personal or public health and minimize illness.

At least two questions are posed during FDA review regarding benefits of the device, both outlined in the 1988 home-use document. The first question is focused on the clinical benefit of the test to the patient in terms of screening, diagnosing, or monitoring a particular disease, condition, or risk factor. The second is focused on the benefits to the patient of having the test available for home use as opposed to having the test performed by healthcare professionals.

At least two questions are also posed regarding risks of the device during FDA review. The first is what is the impact on the user of a false-positive or false-negative result? The second is what are the risks to the user in terms of delay in obtaining a professional examination if a proposed home-use IVD that is intended for use on symptomatic subjects gives a false or equivocal result?

REQUIREMENTS FOR HOME-USE PERFORMANCE

In the 1988 guidance document, the FDA outlines three considerations in evaluating the performance of a home-use device. First, the home-use IVD should perform as well as the professional-use equivalent. Second, the home-use device should be designed with a view to ensuring that the device's performance will not be appreciably affected by expected variation in user technique or environment. Finally, the home-use device should include a simple method by which consumers can determine if the test is working properly. Most frequently this involves providing either a user quality control system in the kit or a "built-in" form of quality control.

REQUIREMENTS FOR HOME-USE LABELING

Because of the wide variation expected in education and competency of the home-use operator, the FDA has developed extensive recommendations, which can be followed by manufacturers to develop user-friendly labeling (3). In addition, the agency frequently cites an NCCLS document (4) with advice on home labeling. This document includes information on techniques for evaluating the reading level of a label; the FDA requires these products to be targeted at an eighth-grade reading level. The document also includes information on how test reliability can be reported in a manner understandable by lay users. Finally, the agency encourages use of a monograph published by FDA in 1993 entitled "Write it Right," which provides manu-

facturers with further instructions on the development of user-friendly language for lay consumers (5).

Basic points checked in labeling review are the need for simplicity and brevity, the use of diagrams and pictures to reinforce text, providing information in a question-and-answer format, and the identification of a technical assistance number to provide technical support and advice to individuals using a test.

THE STATUS OF HOME-USE TESTS

Although a large total number of individual devices have been cleared for home use, these represent a relatively small number of test types (Table 30.2). Until the end of 1996, only the first seven categories had been cleared for marketing.

Marketing of urine cups for collecting and sending in samples for drugs-of-abuse testing is the result of a special initiative designed by the agency to reduce barriers to testing for concerned parents. This initiative, which is described in a final rule published on April 7, 2000, allows test collection systems to be sold for home use as long as the sample is sent to a Substance Abuse and Mental Health Services Administration certified laboratory or equivalent, is tested using an FDA cleared or approved product or one recognized as equivalent, and is labeled and processed in a manner to minimize mishandling and generation of incorrect results.

Marketing of filter paper strips for home HIV testing was approved by the Center for Biologics Evaluation and Research after extensive review, public and panel discussion, and determination by the FDA that the product produced results equivalent to professional use results and that the public health benefits of increased access to information on HIV status outweighed potential risks.

INTRODUCTION OF NEW CLASSES OF HOME-USE TESTS—FRUCTOSAMINE AND PROTHROMBIN TIMES

In 1997, FDA cleared two new first-of-a-kind tests for use at home. The first was a test for fructosamine. This product was cleared after extensive review of analytical and clinical data and a formal panel meeting to evaluate issues of performance, labeling, quality control, and potential use. The sponsor provided clinical studies and peer-reviewed scientific literature to help establish user-friendly cutoff points to maximize the chance for proper interpretation by lay users. The fructosamine was an unusual choice for a home-use test because, in spite of a large body of literature supporting its use, healthcare professionals do not commonly request it. This test was viewed as a low-risk addition to those currently in use for monitoring glucose control.

The second type cleared were tests for home measurement of prothrombin times (PTs). These products were also cleared after extensive review of analytical and clinical data, after a panel meeting to discuss the relevant review issues, and with agreements by the involved sponsors to undertake postmarket studies to assess the real-world performance of these devices over time.

Clearance of the PT tests was a milestone for the FDA. We believed that these devices afforded the potential for unique benefits. Clinical experience in Europe with home PT testing had clearly demonstrated improved anticoagulant status and patient outcomes. We also believed that these devices afforded the potential for unique risks in terms of testing or dosing errors.

As a result of this unique set of benefits and risks, our review division suggested, the hematology panel supported, and the device sponsors accepted the use of a special designation for this test category. These devices were cleared for "home use by prescription" rather than direct sale over the counter. The designation of prescription home-use devices is one that has been used on occasion in the past for other medical devices. However, these two new PT tests represent the first application of this restriction for *in vitro* diagnostic products. The obvious significance in this designation is the requirement that a physician be involved in choosing patients who are appropriate candidates for home testing, be responsible for appropriate training of the patient and for oversight of the home-testing system, and be involved in doing dosage changes that might occur as a result of home-test results.

FDA review of these products focused not only on the issues of performance and use but also on the specific user training programs developed by each of the device sponsors.

INTRODUCTION OF HOME-USE SCREENING TEST FOR DRUGS OF ABUSE

In 1998 the home-use market yet again expanded with clearance of the first home drug-screening test for drugs of abuse. This product was also the result of extensive policy and submission guidance development, deliberation by a formal panel meeting to discuss scientific and regulatory issues, and a careful review of risks, benefits, and requisite labeling. Clearance of this product as a 510(k) was based on establishing a framework to maximize benefit and minimize risk of this device. The device is configured to read out results only as inconclusive (requires further testing) or negative. The cost of confirmatory testing for inconclusive results is expected to be built into the cost of the product. Home-use testing results demonstrated the ability of this test to produce negative and inconclusive results with the same performance as that expected for a comparable point-of-care test.

INTRODUCTION OF NEW TESTS FOR LIPID FRACTIONS

In 2000, FDA expanded home-use lipid testing by clearing two new tests for measurement of triglycerides and for HDL. Although these tests represented logical extensions of home testing for cholesterol, they did introduce for the first time more complicated potential combinations of test results for use by lay users. Instructions for test use attempt to clarify results in simple terms that can be easily understood by lay users and strongly emphasize the value for discussion of results with healthcare providers.

FDA RESPONSIBILITY FOR WAIVED TEST APPLICATIONS

In 1999, the responsibility for CLIA-waived test determinations was reassigned from the Centers for Disease Control and Prevention (CDC) to the FDA. Oversight of the program for high- and moderate-complexity determinations was transferred in November 1999; oversight of the program for waiver determinations was transferred in February 2000. Although the CDC model for waiver determinations was in part originally derived from the FDA program historically used for premarket review of home-use devices, the FDA has developed further guidance outlining and clarifying data sets that may be appropriate for use in waiver determinations. The division is currently actively evaluating the similarities and differences between these two review processes and determining if opportunities for harmonization exist. The draft CLIA-waiver document has been posted on the FDA website (www.fda.gov/cdrh/ode/guidance/1147.pdf) and input is actively being solicited.

THE FUTURE OF HOME-USE TESTING

The FDA expects continued growth in the number and scope of products offered for home use. Interest in this market is made possible by improved technologies that allow products to be designed for reliable use in the home setting. The increased health consciousness of the general public, changes in the healthcare system with a focus on preventive care and cost containment, and the need for increased and easier access to health information, including the results of laboratory testing, all will continue to encourage expansion of this new part of the IVD market.

Although the agency is currently initiating a number of reengineering initiatives based on decreasing resources, and a number of review reforms are occurring in response to the new *FDA Modernization Act of 1997* (5), the agency continues to view near-patient testing and home-use testing in particular as devices that deserve continued close regulatory oversight.

Disclaimer

The opinions expressed in this chapter are those of the authors and do not represent official policy of the Food and Drug Administration.

REFERENCES

1. Medical Device Amendments of 1976. Pub L No. 94-295, 90 Stat 539.
2. Safe Medical Device Act of 1990. Pub L No. 101-629, 104 Stat 4523.
3. Food and Drug Administration. *Assessing the safety and effectiveness of home use in vitro diagnostics (IVDs): guidance regarding premarket submissions.* Rockville, MD: Center for Devices and Radiological Health, 1988.
4. National Committee on Clinical Laboratory Standards. *Labeling of home use in vitro testing products: approved guideline.* Doc. GP 14-A. Wayne, PA: National Committee on Clinical Laboratory Standards, 1996.
5. Backinger CL, Kingsley PA. *Write it right.* Rockville, MD: U.S. Department of Health and Human Services, Public Health Service, Food and Drug Administration, Center for Devices and Radiological Health, 1993.
6. FDA Modernization Act. Pub L No. 105-115, 133 Stat 830.

31

REGULATORY QUALIFICATION OF NEW POINT-OF-CARE DIAGNOSTICS

ERIKA B. AMMIRATI

GENERAL PROCESSES FOR REGULATORY QUALIFICATION

In vitro diagnostics (IVDs; see Table 31.1 for list of chapter abbreviations and definitions) are regulated as medical devices by the U.S. Food and Drug Administration (FDA). This means IVD manufacturers must satisfy specific FDA requirements and obtain FDA approval before a product can be legally marketed in the United States. IVDs represent a unique subset of medical devices; therefore, their safety and effectiveness are supported by unique types of data. Further, IVDs specifically designed for POC environments are subject to additional regulatory oversight beyond what is required for IVDs designed for traditional environments, that is, the hospital or reference laboratory. This chapter begins with a review of the regulatory requirements for traditional IVDs and continues with a description of specific requirements for POC IVDs. The chapter continues with a discussion of the time and costs involved with bringing a POC IVD to market, and this is followed by the necessary elements for keeping an IVD on the market (quality and compliance issues).

Food and Drug Administration Premarket Notification Process

Manufacturers desiring to bring an IVD through the FDA most often must prepare and file the necessary documentation via one of two regulatory routes. Recently, new FDA regulation has provided a third option that exempts certain low-risk IVDs from this type of documentation, but all POC IVDs have been classified as "reserved" devices, and therefore the exemption cannot apply (1). (All reserved devices must undergo conventional FDA review).

The first regulatory route is entitled a *premarket notification*, or *clearance*. This document has been given the jargon term of *510(k)* within the industry; the 510(k) is named after the section in Food Drug and Cosmetic Act, where this regulatory path is described (2). The second regulatory route is the premarket approval process, and this document in entitled a *PMA*. The 510(k) is the more streamlined and straightforward submission, and this pathway applies to most IVDs as well as other medical devices. IVD PMAs are reserved for tests that are considered novel in terms of the analyte being measured or the measurement technology or for those tests where the consequences of

TABLE 31.1. LIST OF ABBREVIATIONS AND DEFINITIONS

Abbreviation	Name	Definition (If Applicable)
510(k)	510(k) or premarket notification	Name of regulatory document that must be filed with the FDA by the manufacturer for most laboratory products
CDC	Centers for Disease Control and Prevention	
DMR	Device master record	The manufacturer's official log for a product that includes all manufacturing information
FDA	Food and Drug Administration	
FD&C	Food, Drug, and Cosmetic Act	Name of the law that regulates food, drugs, devices, and cosmetics
IRB	Institutional review board	A committee designed to protect human subjects who are enrolled in clinical studies
IVD	*In Vitro* diagnostic	
NCCLS	National Committee for Clinical Laboratory Standards	
CV	Coefficient of variation	Statistical term to express imprecision of an assay system
PMA	Premarket approval	Name of regulatory document that must be filed with the FDA by the manufacturer for selected laboratory products
QSR	Quality system regulation	Name of the federal regulation (law) that covers device manufacturers to ensure medical devices will be safe and effective, and otherwise in compliance with the FD&C
SOP	Standard operating procedure	

the clinical interpretation are of the highest risk. For example, tests that diagnose cancer are regulated as PMAs. Because most point-of-care IVDs are regulated as 510(k)s, this chapter is limited to that regulatory route.

The manufacturer's primary objective in preparing the 510(k) document is the demonstration of substantial equivalence between the new IVD and a similar product already being marketed domestically (the *predicate device*). In other words, the manufacturer must show that the new device and the predicate device have physical and performance characteristics in common. Substantial equivalence is a relative term for many medical devices, but in the realm of IVDs, substantial equivalence is defined almost exclusively by a test's intended use, its physical and technologic characteristics, its analytical performance characteristics, and its clinical performance characteristics. Each of the aforementioned elements of substantial equivalence is described in the following sections.

Intended Use

An IVD's intended use encompasses the "who, what, where, and why" of the assay or test system. The intended use describes which analyte is measured and in which particular matrix (e.g., calcium in serum or urine, cholesterol in fingerstick whole blood); it also defines whether the test will be used for screening, monitoring, or diagnostic purposes. The intended use describes the environment where the test will be used (e.g., traditional laboratory, emergency room, doctor's office) and also describes the relationship between levels of the analyte and a medical condition or risk factor. For example, elevated levels of cholesterol are associated with coronary risk, and elevated levels of myocardial muscle creatine kinase isoenzyme (CK-MB) are diagnostic of coronary infarction. This last relationship is often referred to as the *clinical utility* of a test, or the test's *indications for use*.

The intended use is an extremely important factor when determining substantial equivalence. The FDA carefully reviews 510(k) applications to ensure that the labeling for the new IVD does not claim uses or indications that exceed those described by the predicate device. For a new IVD to be substantially equivalent to its predicate, the two intended uses must closely relate to one another but do not need to match identically.

Technologic Characteristics

Another element for demonstrating substantial equivalence between the two IVDs is the comparison of the physical and technologic characteristics. Examples of various IVD formats include 96-well plate enzyme immunoassays, classic stoichiometric "wet-chemistry" assays, high-throughput chemistry analyzers, and biosensor-based systems. Many point-of-care devices consist of unitary, disposable units or easy-to-operate "permanent" units with single-use, disposable cartridges or test strips for each patient sample.

Other test system characteristics include the sample type(s) of choice and the procedural steps. An IVD may be designed for only one matrix, or it may be designed for multiple matrices; it may require a high level of technical expertise and manual dexterity, or it may have "walk-away" attributes where there are essentially no procedural steps after sample addition. This last category is often seen with point-of-care devices.

In contrast to the intended use discussion, it is not mandatory that a new IVD be of the same format as its predicate device or share the same technologic characteristics. In fact, one of the most common reasons for developing a new IVD is to modernize a test from a more labor-intensive format to that of a less labor-intensive format. This is quite often the case for many point-of-care devices where internal and external components have been unitized, miniaturized, and procedurally simplified. In terms of substantial equivalence, the FDA requires that the manufacturer describe why the changes in test formats do not raise new issues of safety and effectiveness. For example, if the transformation of an assay from a desktop analyzer to a point-of-care unitary device does not put additional risk burdens on the operator (safety) and the results obtained from the point-of-care device are comparable to the predicate device (effectiveness), it can be claimed that no new issues of safety and effectiveness have been raised, and a substantially equivalent determination can be made.

Analytic Performance Characteristics

An IVD's analytic performance characteristics include the standard laboratory measurements of analytic sensitivity, analytic specificity, linearity, and spike recovery. Other analytic measurements may be added, depending on the test system. The analytic performance characteristics are almost always generated in-house in the manufacturer's laboratory, in contrast to the clinical performance characteristics of accuracy and precision. Accuracy and precision are best supported by field studies (or clinical trials) conducted outside the manufacturer's laboratory in actual clinical settings. (See next section.)

A manufacturer must demonstrate that the analytic performance of the new IVD is comparable to that described in the labeling (package insert) of the predicate IVD. A brief discussion of the experimental objectives and designs for the major analytic components (sensitivity, specificity, linearity, and recovery) follows.

Analytic Sensitivity

The analytic *sensitivity* of an assay is defined as the lowest level of the analyte that can be measured with reasonable precision. This is also referred to as an assay's *limit of detection*. There are various means for establishing analytic sensitivity, and a common method is to assay the test system's buffer matrix or "zero calibrator" in 20 to 30 replicates. From these measurements, a mean value and the standard deviation are calculated. The value of two standard deviations is added to the mean value, and this becomes the lowest limit of detection, or the lowest level that can be distinguished from zero.

Analytic Specificity

The analytical *specificity* of an assay is defined by two sets of requirements. The first requirement is the system's ability to measure a distinct entity, and not compounds that are closely related to the analyte of interest. For example, if the IVD is intended to measure levels of luteinizing hormone (LH), the level of cross-reactivity with beta human chorionic gonadotropin (β-hCG), which shares a common alpha subunit with LH, must be identified and included in the labeling. Another example of two closely related compounds is thyroxine (T_4) and triiodothyronine (T_3) in thyroid testing.

The second specificity requirement is evaluation of interfering substances. *Interfering substances* are those constituents in the blood (or other matrix) that can cause false-positive or false-negative results in qualitative systems or that can cause falsely depressed or falsely elevated results in quantitative systems. Although there is an infinite list of substances that could be tested for interference, it is the manufacturer's responsibility to test a reasonable number of candidate substances. These substances generally fall into one of three categories: elevated levels of biological compounds (e.g., bilirubin, hemoglobin, and lipids), elevated levels of over-the-counter medications, and elevated levels of prescription drugs that are associated with the analyte being measured.

Because many IVD systems use color, or a color change, as the measurement endpoint, substances that impart color changes to the testing matrix need to be evaluated. Elevated levels of bilirubin, hemoglobin, and lipids are routinely included in specificity testing because high levels of these substances can cause subtle color changes of yellow, red (or green), and milky white, respectively. The second category of candidate testing substances are over-the-counter medications. Many patients self-prescribe high doses of analgesics or vitamins, and the effects of these products need to be tested. The third category of potentially interfering substances is prescription medications. Here the manufacturer should try to include the testing of those medications that bear a relationship to the analyte being identified or measured. For example, a test for cholesterol should include in its interference testing some form of lipid-lowering drugs; patients or consumers who have a need to monitor their cholesterol levels often have this class of pharmaceutical prescribed to them. Similarly, a manufacturer of an IVD for the monitoring of bone metabolism would include high levels of calcium in its interference testing because calcium supplements are widely recommended and prescribed.

Interference testing can be accomplished in a number of ways, and a common method is described as follows. Elevated levels of the various potentially interfering substances are added to two pools with known quantities of the analyte (*controls*). The pools are generally "positive" and "negative" for the particular analyte when evaluating qualitative systems and are "low level" and "high level" for the particular analyte when evaluating quantitative systems.

All samples are tested as routine "unknowns," and the difference between the "true results" (controls) and the "on-test results" (samples with interfering substances) are compared. If the differences between the two results are within the imprecision of the assay, then the substance is considered noninterfering. If the differences are large, those substances are considered potentially interfering and are disclosed as such in the "Limitations" section of the product-labeling (package insert). The National Committee for Clinical Laboratory Standards (NCCLS) EP-7 document (3) describes numerous candidate substances, target levels for interfering concentrations, and guidelines for statistical evaluation.

Linearity

Linearity measures the ability of an assay to "read" predictably throughout the reportable range. It also can be an indication of the presence (or absence) of matrix effects from clinical samples. Some systems are susceptible to quantitative biases at the high or low endpoints of the measurement ranges, and linearity experiments are designed to identify these errors. Like specificity testing, the linearity of an assay also can be determined by various testing routes. One well-accepted method is described in the NCCLS EP-6 document (4), and a brief description of that method follows.

Two levels of neat samples are identified: one at, or near, the lower limit of the measurement range, and the other at (or near) the upper limit. From these two extreme samples, three intermediate samples are prepared at the midpoint between the "high" and "low" samples, at an intermediate low point, and at an intermediate high point. The "formulations" of the five levels are presented in Table 31.2.

Once all samples have been prepared, they are analyzed by the new IVD system. The quantitation of samples 1 and 5 at the extremes of the range is used to calculate the expected quantitation of the three intermediate levels. Sometimes an independent reference method is used to assay samples 1 and 5 to achieve the highest level of accuracy. Sample 3 is expected to lie midway between samples 1 and 5, sample 2 is expected to be midway between samples 1 and 3, and sample 4 is expected to be midway between sample 3 and sample 5. The observed values (y) are plotted against the expected values (x), and the data are, at a minimum, visually examined for linearity. In addition, various statistical tests can be used to confirm linearity. The IVD's claimed dynamic range has to be consistent with those limits established by the linearity experiments.

Spike Recovery

Spike recovery is somewhat analogous to linearity. Both measurements are an indication of systematic biases or matrix effects, but the measurement techniques are different. Whereas linearity begins with known levels of the analyte and studies the dilutional effects, spike recovery begins with a zero or very low levels of the analyte in a base pool, and known amounts of the analyte are added and tested.

TABLE 31.2. FORMULATIONS OF SAMPLES FOR LINEARITY TESTING

Sample No.	Level	Preparation
1	Lower limit of range ("low")	Neat[a]
2	Intermediate low	3 Parts 1 and 1 Part 5
3	Midpoint	Equal Parts no. 1 and no. 5
4	Intermediate high	1 Part no. 1 and 3 Parts no. 5
5	Upper limit of range ("high")	Neat

[a]Undiluted, unchanged.

To perform spike recovery, generally four or five samples with varying levels of the analyte are tested. Five "negative" pools (samples) are prepared, and known amounts of increasingly concentrated analyte are added to each sample. All samples are assayed as unknowns, and the observed measurements are compared with the expected measurements based on the amount of analyte added. The percent recovery of each sample is the mathematical calculation of [observed]-[expected] / [expected] × 100. A general guideline is that each level should be within 10% of the expected measurement, with biases being nonsystematic, meaning differences should be both positive (>100% recovery) and negative (<100% recovery).

Clinical Performance Characteristics

The clinical performance characteristics are the next benchmark for the determination of substantial equivalence between the new IVD and the predicate IVD. The clinical characteristics are often considered the "heart and soul" of the premarket notification because here is where precision and accuracy data are presented, and thereby the question of does the test work gets answered.

Precision and accuracy can be established in-house by the manufacturer's laboratories, but over the past 10 years, the FDA has placed an increasingly larger focus on these studies (termed clinical trials, field studies, or method comparisons) being conducted in their eventual settings. This means manufacturers will recruit hospital laboratories for the evaluation of traditional IVDs, and emergency departments, doctor's offices, and even consumers for the evaluation of point-of-care IVDs. The reason for this is to provide the most realistic view of the IVD's precision and accuracy and thereby allow the eventual end user to have an accurate expectation of system performance.

Precision

Precision reflects the IVD's ability to provide reproducible results. The manufacturer's challenge is to optimize the IVD system so that aliquots of the same sample demonstrate very similar results within a "run," from run to run on the same days and from run to run between days and with different operators, as appropriate. The presentation of precision data may include intraassay variation (within-run), and/or inter-assay (between-run) variation, depending on the IVD's technologic format. Precision also can be evaluated on an interlaboratory basis with the same lot of product or may be evaluated lot-to-lot.

Precision is always evaluated at more than one level within the measurement range because precision generally varies depending on concentration. For qualitative systems, precision is usually evaluated with a negative sample, a positive sample, and a low positive sample that has been titered near the cutoff value. For quantitative systems, precision is usually evaluated at two to four levels, depending on the breadth of the measurement range. An IVD with a wider range of reportable results will require more precision samples than an IVD with a narrower reportable range. Further, precision samples for quantitative tests should be targeted at or near medical decision points (5). In this way, the manufacturer can demonstrate precision statistics at those levels associated with clinical diagnoses.

Precision can be evaluated and analyzed in several ways, but it always requires repeat testing of a multilevel precision panel over several runs. The NCCLS EP-5 document (5) describes a well-accepted protocol for precision testing that requires the sampling of two runs per day over 20 days; each run consists of two aliquots of test material for each concentration. From these data, means, standard deviations, and percent coefficients of variation (%CVs) are calculated. The "bottom line" for precision testing is expressed as %CVs, and acceptable %CVs for IVDs range from 2% to 15%, depending on the specific technology. IVDs that are heavily technique dependent, or with multiple internal steps, are expected to reflect greater assay-to-assay variation than the simpler IVDs.

Accuracy

Accuracy is the IVD's ability to report the "right answer." The right answer is defined by the result obtained by an existing IVD (the predicate device) or by a recognized reference method when split; aliquoted samples from the same individual are tested by both methods. Good accuracy is largely achieved by close calibration of the new IVD against its predicate device. Accuracy also must be defined and supported for multiple matrices, as appropriate. If product labeling specifies that multiple matrices may be used, for example, whole blood, plasma, and serum, all claims must be validated.

For IVD clinical trials, the external laboratory performs the analyses using the new IVD, and comparative testing with the existing IVD may be performed either by the external laboratory or by the manufacturer. There is more latitude with the testing of the predicate method because this method is a legally marketed device, and the performance characteristics already have been established. In either case, it is imperative that all testing be performed in a blinded fashion where the operator has no knowledge of the comparative result or the clinical status of the patient from which the sample was collected.

Accuracy can be evaluated and expressed in a variety of ways, and the NCCLS recommends that accuracy be expressed as the percent biases throughout the reportable range. In their EP-9 document (6), it is stated that the manufacturer must collect and analyze comparative data from a minimum of 40 split patient samples, and these samples must cover most of the reportable range. Manufacturers generally include 100 to 200 samples in their comparative testing to obtain more representative data and to characterize fully the effects from different operators and other environmental factors. Also, if samples are being collected and tested prospectively by the participating external laboratory (i.e., stored, banked samples are not being used), it is likely more than 40 samples will be necessary because of the natural tendency of results to cluster around the middle or "normal" range. In the event the majority of the measurement range still is not covered by patient samples, it is allowable to supplement the data set with contrived samples that have been specifically prepared at the high or low ends of the IVD's dynamic range. These samples are prepared by the manufacturer and then sent to the laboratory for blinded comparative testing.

Once the assays have been performed by the laboratory and the results have been sent to the manufacturer, it is the manufacturer's responsibility to summarize and analyze the data. For qualitative tests, data are analyzed as the percentages of true-positive or true-negative results and false-positive or false-negative results. The results from the new method are compared with those obtained with the predicate method. For quantitative tests, the data are analyzed by linear regression statistics (e.g., least-squares, or Deming), where the reference, predicate, or "true" results constitute the x-axis, and the new IVD results constitute the y-axis. Numerous software packages are available for performing these analyses, complete with graphics and calculations of the slope, y-intercept, correlation coefficient, and 95% confidence intervals.

After the linear regression equation is determined, percent biases throughout the new IVD's dynamic range are calculated. The manufacturer has the discretion to choose appropriate levels for bias estimation, but usually the chosen levels include clinical decision points. A good example is provided by cholesterol. The National Cholesterol Education Program (NCEP) has determined that the levels of 200 mg per deciliter and 240 mg per deciliter are the cut points between "desirable" (<200 mg/dL) and "borderline high," (200 – 240 mg/dL) and "high," (>240 mg/dL), respectively. The manufacturer will likely calculate the biases at 150 mg per deciliter (arbitrary low concentration), 200 mg per deciliter, 240 mg per deciliter (the two cutpoints), and at 300 mg per deciliter as an arbitrary high concentration. In this way, data are provided for high and low levels and at the two medical decision points. Results between or beyond the four levels may be interpolated from the calculated data. An example of calculated percent biases from a hypothetical study is presented in the following section.

In our example, the linear regression equation for a 152-sample data set is $y = 1.02x - 12$. From this equation, the percent biases can be estimated at the four quantitation levels, as described earlier. The data are presented in Table 31.3. It is demonstrated from these data that percent biases ranged from −2% at the high end to −6% at the low end. This would be considered a good assay, with a low likelihood of misdiagnosis based on the cholesterol results.

Another statistical tool for expressing accuracy is the measurement of clinical sensitivity and specificity. Clinical sensitivity and specificity differ from their analytic counterparts and have separate definitions. The *clinical sensitivity* of an assay is its ability to identify true positives for a given disease or condition, and the *clinical specificity* is the ability of an assay to identify true negatives. Clinical sensitivity and specificity are used less commonly than regression statistics for determining IVD accuracy, but they can be valuable tools. Examples of appropriate situations are for the evaluation of microbiology systems where an assay is compared with routine culture results and also for tumor marker assays that monitor disease progression. Here assay results are compared to clinical symptoms and other diagnostic tools, e.g., x-rays, magnetic resonance technology.

Using the example of a new IVD immunoassay for Group A *Streptococcus* (Strep A), suppose a clinical study was conducted with 100 throat swab samples where there were 50 positive samples, and 50 negative samples, as determined by routine culture on blood agar plates. The new IVD was evaluated with a second throat swab from the same individuals, and this method identified 52 positive samples, and 48 negative samples. The new IVD would therefore demonstrate a clinical sensitivity of 100% (all true-positive samples were correctly identified) and a clinical specificity of 96% (two false-positive results). This type of accuracy data is most often presented as 2×2 contingency tables as shown in Table 31.4.

Clinical sensitivity and specificity are also useful measures for determining the accuracy of tumor marker assays for monitoring disease progression. If an assay shows that disease is likely to be present above a certain threshold level and that below this level there should be no evidence of disease, then the clinical sensitivity from a particular study would be the percentage of cases in which the threshold value was reached or exceeded in the presence of disease progression (as determined by appropriate clinical markers). The clinical specificity would be the percentage of cases in which the results were below the threshold and there was no evidence of disease. A false-positive result would be described as an assay result above the threshold and no evidence of disease progression and a false-negative result would be, conversely, a non-elevated assay result, but with evidence of disease progression.

These various performance characteristics (analytic and clinical) are provided in the product's package labeling. All labeling is reviewed carefully by the FDA as part of the 510(k) process. With this disclosure of the data, the end user (customer) has an expectation of how the IVD should perform in the particular setting. It is understood that another set of experiments with the same IVD would not produce the exact same statistics, but it would be expected that overall performance would be similar. Further discussion of the FDA's labeling requirements is provided as follows.

TABLE 31.3. ESTIMATED PERCENT BIASES FROM CHOLESTEROL EXAMPLE[a]

"True" Result	Estimated Result	Difference in Clinical Units	Percent Bias
150	141	9	−6
200	192	8	−4
240	233	7	−3
300	294	6	−2

[a]All units mg/dL.

TABLE 31.4. HYPOTHETICAL 2 × 2 ACCURACY DATA

	Culture Positive	Culture Negative	Total
IVD positive	50	2	52
IVD negative	0	48	48

IVD, *in vitro* diagnostic.
Formulae for computing sensitivity and specificity, and positive and negative predictive values:
Sensitivity = True positives/ (true positives + false negatives)
Specificity = True negatives/ (true negatives + false positives)
Positive predictive value = true positives/ (true positives + false positives)
Negative predictive value = true negatives/ (true negatives + false negatives)
From the hypothetical example:
IVD sensitivity = 50/50 + 0 = 50/50 = 100%
IVD specificity = 50/50 + 2 = 50/52 = 96%
IVD positive predictive value = 50/50 + 2 = 50/52 = 96%
IVD negative predictive value = 50/50 + 0 = 50/50 = 100%.

Labeling Requirements

Manufacturers are required to provide package inserts and manuals (as appropriate) along with the IVD systems. The contents of the package inserts are well defined within the Code of Federal Regulations (21 CFR. 809.10), and inserts are reviewed for consistency within and between product lines. Some of the labeling requirements are purely administrative (company's name and address), and some requirements are highly technical. There are 15 required elements for IVD package inserts, and those elements are listed below:

- Proprietary and established test name
- Intended use(s)
- Summary and explanation of why the test is useful (discussion of disease, etc.)
- Principle of the test procedure
- Information on the reagents
- Information on the instrumentation
- Information on sample collection and preparation
- Test procedures
- Test results (e.g., calculations)
- Limitations
- Expected values
- Performance characteristics (both analytic and clinical)
- Bibliography
- Name and place of business
- Date and revision number (if applicable) of the latest version of the package insert

In summary, the 510(k) is a composite of an IVD's description (including the intended use), its performance characteristics (both analytic and clinical), and its labeling. The manufacturer's goal is to demonstrate, via scientific evidence, substantial equivalence between the new IVD and the predicate IVD and thereby show the safety and effectiveness of the new IVD.

Clinical Laboratories Improvement Act of 1988 and Test Categorization

The Clinical Laboratories Improvement Act of 1988 (CLIA '88) is a federal law that regulates laboratories. As such, manufacturers are not directly regulated by CLIA '88, but it has a tremendous impact on manufacturers because it is the laboratories that purchase the IVD products. Other chapters in this book discuss CLIA '88 from the viewpoint of the laboratories, and this discussion is limited to the industry view.

The CLIA '88 regulates laboratories by monitoring their compliance to five standards; these standards are as follows:

- Personnel requirements
- Proficiency testing
- Quality control
- Quality assurance
- Patient test management

All laboratories in the United States (inclusive of traditional and nontraditional sites) must comply with these five standards, but CLIA '88 makes some distinctions among laboratories regarding the level of rigor required to meet the standards. Those distinctions are described in the following section.

There are three classifications of laboratories, namely *waived*, *moderately complex*, and *highly complex*. The decision of which classification is applied to each laboratory depends on the tests performed by each laboratory. All laboratory tests have similarly been categorized as waived, moderately complex, or highly complex, and a laboratory is classified according to its highest "ranking" test. That is to say, if a laboratory performs all moderately complex tests except for one highly complex test, then the laboratory is highly complex. CLIA test categorization originally was performed by the Centers for Disease Control and Prevention (CDC), but this responsibility was transferred to the FDA in February 2000.

There are minimal regulatory differences between moderately complex tests and highly complex tests. Highly complex tests can be performed only by personnel with a higher level of education and training (personnel standards), but the differences in the four remaining CLIA '88 standards are invisible or much subtler. In contrast, there are enormous differences between the requirements for waived tests and the other two categories. Waived tests are, as would be surmised by the name, waived from compliance to all five standards. Functionally, waived laboratories are free to hire personnel with any level of education and training; they do not need to perform routine quality control testing on the IVDs (normally this is specified as two levels of controls for each day patient results are reported), and they do not need to participate in a proficiency testing program. The other two standards (quality assurance and patient test management) deal with global quality issues and are separate from IVD testing.

With this administrative structure, manufacturers see the advantage of commercializing waived tests. Waived tests have a much lower regulatory burden for market entry because these products may be used with less governmental oversight. This is especially beneficial to many point-of-care sites that do not have the advantages of large staffs and other elements of a traditional laboratory's infrastructure. Clearly, a doctor's office using point-of-care IVDs has different CLIA '88 concerns than a critical care unit within a hospital using the same IVD. The critical care unit is most likely operating under the main laboratory's CLIA license and is not impacted by a test's CLIA categorization. In contrast, the doctor's office, as a stand-alone unit, may be reluctant to perform IVD testing of nonwaived tests because of the financial and administrative constraints.

As stated, the FDA now has the responsibility of categorizing IVDs for complexity. If no special request is made, a new IVD generally is assigned the CLIA test categorization of its predicate, assuming the predicate is moderately or highly complex. The request for waived status always requires special considerations.

In vitro diagnostics can become waived by one of three routes: (a) the test system is one of the original eight products that became waived by congressional regulation, (b) the IVD is "down-classified" from moderate complexity or high complexity by petition, or (c) the IVD is waived by virtue of being cleared for home use by the FDA. (Home-use IVDs are automatically CLIA waived.)

The original eight tests waived (by regulation) are the following:

- Dipstick/tablet urinalysis (nonautomated)
- Ovulation test kit (visual color comparison)
- Urine pregnancy test (visual color comparison)
- Erythrocyte sedimentation rate (nonautomated)
- Hemoglobin (copper sulfate)
- Fecal occult blood
- Spun hematocrit
- Blood glucose (FDA-cleared home use device)

If a manufacturer wishes to clear and market these assays (and not all these tests are suitable for assays), nothing more is required for waived status. Similarly, home-use IVDs do not require additional efforts for waived status.

The most common route for a manufacturer to obtain waived status is through the petition process. As of this writing, the FDA has not yet released official guidelines for what the petition process will require, but it has been proposed that petitions must include the following elements:

- Conformance of the IVD to waived criteria
- Lay user field studies for precision
- Lay user field studies for accuracy

The IVD waived criteria were originally defined by the CDC, and it appears the FDA will not be modifying the criteria; they are as follows:

- The system uses direct, unprocessed specimens (only whole-blood and urine assays may be waived).
- The system is fully automated and requires no operator intervention during the analytical phase.
- The system provides a direct readout of results.
- The system includes "fail-safe" mechanisms, in which no result is reported in the event of a malfunction or if result is outside of the reportable range.
- There is no invasive troubleshooting or electronic/mechanical maintenance.
- The labeling provides step-by-step instructions, which has been targeted to no greater than the seventh-grade reading level.

Clearly, many point-of-care IVDs are well suited for waived status based on these criteria. This is especially true of IVDs targeted to the doctor's office.

The second and third criteria for a waived petition are fulfilled by data from field studies with lay (untrained) users. Two separate field studies are required, one study for precision and one study for accuracy.

The precision field study must include the following:

- Three sites and a minimum of 20 testing subjects per site.
- Subjects assay three samples, and samples contain varying analyte concentrations.
- Subjects are untrained in laboratory or medical procedures.
- Subjects can rely only on written instructions.

Data from these field studies are analyzed to determine whether the untrained subjects can achieve the same precision as trained personnel.

Third, the FDA wishes to see comparative accuracy data from 300 lay users; each user tests just one sample. Split aliquots from these 300 samples also are tested by one or more trained persons, and the two data sets (untrained testers and trained testers) are compared. Data are analyzed by various statistical methods, depending on whether the IVD generates qualitative or quantitative results.

FDA REGULATORY PROCESSES UNIQUE TO POINT-OF-CARE

The previous section reviewed the FDA's general requirements for bringing traditional IVDs to market. This section identifies the issues manufacturers must consider when designing the clinical trials and preparing the 510(k) for point-of-care IVDs. The issues center on the clinical trial design and the study's personnel requirements.

Clinical Trial Design

Testing Sites

As discussed, the FDA is currently placing emphasis on clinical trials being conducted in the IVD's eventual setting. For the point-of-care IVD, this means that studies may need to be conducted in doctor's offices, emergency rooms, and critical care units. The FDA's general policy is that these studies need to be conducted at a minimum of three sites, preferably at three sites that are located in different geographic areas of the country (7). This policy is to ensure that regional demographic factors regarding patients and laboratory personnel have been sufficiently addressed.

Rate of Subject Recruitment

One important aspect of any study's clinical design is the rate of patient recruitment and the possible constraints of sample processing. Because it is less likely that samples can be batch tested for point-of-care technology, a point-of-care study often requires more time for completion than does its traditional IVD counterpart. Samples may need to be analyzed "one at a time," with continual replacement of the system's disposable components. Also, if an IVD is targeted for the doctor's office, the office staff may need to specifically recruit certain subjects, or wait for "foot traffic" to enter the office. To assist with this issue, the FDA often allows a percentage of the clinical samples to be banked instead of freshly collected. The manufacturer may collect and store serum, plasma, or urine samples and then deliver the samples to the testing site. These samples may be tested in a batch or over a few days, whereas several more days or weeks may be required to collect fresh samples prospectively.

Sample Matrices

Another aspect of point-of-care clinical design is the stability and volume of the sample matrix. Whole-blood assays are very convenient from the standpoint of not requiring clotting time or centrifugation, but whole blood is not a stable matrix, and therefore arrangements must be made to obtain sample for the comparative method. Further, fingerstick whole blood samples almost always will be of insufficient volume for comparative testing.

To work around the matrix issue, many studies require that a second, more stable sample be collected in addition to the sample for the point-of-care IVD. For example, a study designed for a new fingerstick whole-blood hCG test will need a separate sample for analysis with the predicate IVD. This is because the predicate IVD will most likely be a conventional system that uses venous serum or plasma. In this case, the testing site must be able and willing to obtain a venous draw in addition to the fingerstick sample.

Personnel Requirements

Point-of-care testing quite often is performed by nonlaboratory personnel who have not received applicable education and training. Because of this, the FDA requires that the persons who are performing the testing are representative of the eventual end user. In the case of doctors' offices, the testers are likely to be medical assistants and office staff; in the case of emergency rooms and critical care units, the testers are likely to be nurses and paramedical personnel. The FDA frequently asks that the 510(k) include the resumes of the personnel who performed the testing for the new point-of-care IVD.

COSTS AND TIME REQUIRED FOR MARKET INTRODUCTION

There is a tremendous amount of variation in the amount of time and financial resources required to bring a point-of-care IVD to market. A general rule is the more novel the analyte or the technology, the longer and more costly is the route. This section provides general details on the major components of the product development phase, the clinical trial phase, and the regulatory interaction phase.

Product Development Phase

The *product development phase* is arbitrarily defined here as the time from when a product is an idea to the time it enters clinical trials. This can easily require 1 to 2 years, depending on the "newness" of the technology. Clearly, a manufacturer develops in-house expertise over time concerning a particular test platform, and sequential products reap the benefit of institutional knowledge from their predecessor products. Still, every new IVD brings with it a new set of challenges.

To begin the process, a product in the research stage must be shown to be viable from the marketing point of view; that is, it is believed someone will wish to buy it. A feasibility effort begins to determine whether the test system can perform to predetermined minimum specifications. These specifications should be established by all functional departments within the company (research and development, clinical/regulatory, operations, and marketing), and there should be consensus among the depart-

ments regarding the outcome of the feasibility testing. Feasibility should also take into account the eventual "manufacturability" of the final product, even if feasibility lots were "handmade" on a small scale.

After feasibility has been shown, true development begins with numerous iterative versions of prepilot and pilot lots. Experimentation with various materials and processes is undertaken so that performance is optimized. Modern IVDs (point-of-care and traditional) often include sophisticated software and hardware systems, thereby adding new levels of complexity that were not a part of conventional "wet chemistry" technology.

After there is a high level of confidence with the pilot lots, the IVD is ready for clinical trials. These clinical trials will produce the performance characteristics that will support the 510(k) and will define the product from the marketing point of view (data provided in package insert). Because of the tremendous cost and time associated with the trials, it is best to not begin clinical trials before a product is fully characterized and has been shown to meet preliminary specifications. It is estimated that development costs to this point range from $10 million to $20 million for the first product on a newly developed platform, and then $2 to $3 million are needed for additional assays and applications.

Clinical Trials Phase

Successful clinical trials will show that a point-of-care IVD is substantially equivalent to a predicate IVD. This will be done mostly by the demonstration of accuracy and precision in the hands of the eventual end user. Before this can begin, many administrative tasks need to be completed. These preparatory tasks can require 3 to 6 months and are briefly described in the following section.

Preparatory Tasks for Clinical Trials

The preparatory tasks are as follows:

- Writing the study protocol (inclusive of identifying the predicate device, establishing appropriate inclusion/exclusion criteria for subjects and samples, and developing case report forms and data summary sheets, as appropriate)
- Identifying a minimum of three clinical sites
- Qualifying the clinical sites
- Negotiating budgets with the clinical sites
- Obtaining Institutional Review Board (IRB) approval for the testing of human subjects
- Training the clinical sites with the new IVD procedure, processing steps, and administrative steps
- Coordinating the shipment of samples and supplies to the clinical sites
- Training the clinical sites with the comparative methods, as needed
- Coordinating the shipment of samples and data back to the manufacturer

Once the trials have begun, monitoring is necessary to ensure that the protocol is being followed and data are being recorded correctly. Monitoring of IVD trials is far less complex and time consuming than the monitoring of pharmaceutical trials because of the shorter duration (usually measured in weeks rather than years) and the *in vitro* component of the study objectives. Samples are being withdrawn and tested rather than the subject being required to ingest a pharmacologic compound.

The costs for point-of-care IVD clinical trials can range from $30,000 to $60,000 above the company's general overhead. There are potential expenses for IRB approvals, compensation to the investigational site, compensation to the recruited subjects, purchasing of reagents and instrumentation for the comparative method, shipping costs, copying costs, and travel costs to the three clinical sites.

Regulatory Interactions Phase

Once the clinical sites have completed the testing, the data are summarized and analyzed by the manufacturer. This may require a few weeks to many months, depending on the complexity of the data. The data then are prepared in a logical format, and the balance of the 510(k) is written. There is no mandatory format for the 510(k); along with the performance sections for analytic performance and clinical performance, however, the document includes a section for product description, a comparative chart showing the similarities and differences between the new IVD and the predicate IVD, a brief manufacturing section, and a software validation section, if needed. Preparation of the 510(k) may require a few weeks to a few months, depending on the scope of the data and in-house resources.

When the 510(k) is complete, it is submitted to a specific branch within a specific division at the FDA. The FDA is organized in such a way that like products are reviewed together. There is no charge to the manufacturer for the FDA's review, although there is continual discussion of user fees for all devices. The submission is logged into the FDA's system and the "clock" begins. The FDA makes a good effort to complete its initial review within 60 days, and there is almost always a round of questions asked of the manufacturer for additional information. The manufacturer must supply the information or come to an agreement with the FDA that the information is already present in the document or that the request is not feasible or appropriate. If the FDA believes the additional information cannot be obtained within 30 days, the FDA retains the right to withdraw the document from their system. The manufacturer would then need to resubmit the 510(k) at a later date with the added information.

If the request for additional information is such that it can, and is, submitted within 30 days of its request, then a new FDA cycle begins. The FDA generally tries to complete this review within the next 30 days, but the time limits are nonstatutory, and the FDA may exceed this target. Usually one to two additional minor rounds of questions are presented, and labeling issues are discussed in great detail at this point. Once FDA is satisfied that all policy, statutory, and scientific requirements have been met, a substantially equivalent determination is granted. Only then can the IVD be legally marketed. The time frame for this can be 3 months to 2 years, with most point-of-care IVDs needing 6 to 9 months for clearance. FDA believes a higher level

of scrutiny is required of point-of-care IVDs to protect the public's health. This is due largely to the nontraditional environments where the tests are used.

QUALITY SYSTEMS AND COMPLIANCE ISSUES

Quality System Regulation

After an IVD has been cleared by the FDA, a manufacturer's focus shifts to compliance issues to ensure that the product stays on the market and remains in good regulatory stead. This is accomplished largely through compliance to FDA's Quality System Regulation (QSR). The QSR is an "umbrella" regulation that was designed to ensure consistent product quality for all devices. The regulation was written in general terms to fit a wide array of devices and technologies; so an IVD manufacturer must identify which aspects of the regulation apply to its products and design the company's quality system accordingly. The QSR mostly identifies the goals for product quality, but it also provides some specifics on how to accomplish those goals.

Under the QSR, manufacturers are responsible for ensuring that all purchased goods and services meet established criteria so that the devices meet specifications and perform as expected. The QSR includes provisions for virtually every aspect of a device's design, manufacturing process, and finished acceptance testing; Table 31.5 lists those major provisions.

Clearly a comprehensive discussion of all QSR provisions is beyond the scope of this section, but an abbreviated presentation of manufacturing responsibilities for product lot acceptance activities is provided. The acceptance activities have been categorized by the QSR as receiving, in-process, and finished-device activities.

Receiving Activities

Because a product can be only as good as its starting material, it is important that the manufacturing process begin with quali-

TABLE 31.5. QUALITY SYSTEM REGULATION PROVISIONS

Management responsibilities
Buildings and physical space
Internal audit procedures
Personnel requirements and training
Design controls
Document controls
Purchasing controls
Materials identification and traceability
Production and process controls
Inspection, measuring and test equipment
Process validation
Acceptance activities (receiving, in-process, finished device)
Nonconforming product
Corrective and preventative action
Labeling and packaging control
Product handling, storage, distribution, and installation
Records and records retention
Complaint files
Servicing

fied components, reagents, and other materials. The QSR states that incoming products must be inspected, tested, or otherwise verified as conforming to specified requirements, and that product acceptance or rejection must be documented [21 CFR 820.80(b)]. Before this can be done, however, the manufacturer must decide what specific characteristics of the components will determine their acceptability and must create specific acceptance criteria (via inspection or testing) that will confirm component/reagent acceptability. The tested characteristics may include appearance, dimensions, and performance. For an IVD manufacturer, receiving criteria may be the purity of an antigen or chemical, the affinity of an antibody, or the reliability of hardware components.

In-process Activities

The term *in-process activities* refers to controls that are imposed during the manufacturing process. Manufacturers are given discretion to decide when it is appropriate to establish and to maintain acceptance procedures for in-process product [21 CFR 820.80(c)]. In-process testing is valuable because it can prevent further loss of time and materials when it is clear that a lot of product will fail to meet its final release criteria. As an IVD example, the optical density of an enzyme conjugate may be obtained "off the line" before it is lyophilized to a dried pellet. If the reagent does not meet its targeted range of acceptable values, the manufacturer has the options of "reworking" the conjugate (if this is possible), placing the product in quarantine for further evaluation or discarding the lot. All recourses must be documented.

Final Acceptance Activities

Final acceptance procedures must be established and maintained so that each production run, lot, or batch of finished devices meets the acceptance criteria identified in the device master record [DMR, 21 CFR 820.80(d)]. (The DMR is the "official log" for a product, and it contains the device specifications; production process specifications; quality assurance procedures and specifications; and installation, maintenance, and servicing procedures and methods.) Acceptance criteria should include all parameters that the device must meet to perform its intended use. Manufacturers have the discretion to choose a combination of methods for finished device inspection or testing. The inspection and testing methods should ensure that the finished run, lot, or batch meets specified requirements.

For an IVD manufacturer, final product testing usually includes evaluation of accuracy and precision. Accuracy may be confirmed by means of testing a well-characterized accuracy panel with each lot. The panel may consist of three to ten samples that span the assay's dynamic range. The standard operating procedure (SOP) for this testing specifies how close quantitation needs to be to the "right answers." Accuracy may be expressed as the percent differences between the two sets of data (established panel results and the on-test lot) or by linear regression statistics. These specifications define the accuracy of "pass/fail" for the lot.

Final acceptance testing for precision is conducted in much the same manner. A two- to four-level precision panel may be assayed with the new lot in multiple runs. From this testing, means, standard deviations, and percent coefficients of variation are calculated, and the precision testing SOP provides the limits for the amount of allowable variation. These specifications define the precision of "pass/fail" for the lot. The objective of this combined final acceptance testing is to confirm that each lot of product meets the product's claim for accuracy and precision.

Until the new lots of devices have satisfied the final acceptance procedures and have been released, they must be held in quarantine or controlled by some other means. Finished devices may not be released until the manufacturer completes activities required in the DMR; reviews associated data and documentation; and a designated individual signs, authorizes, and the dates the release.

Compliance Implications: Warning Letter, Seizure, Injunction, and Prosecution

The FDA maintains oversight of manufacturers and the devices they produce by two primary mechanisms: by performing on-site inspections and by monitoring device problems as identified through product recalls (see later). The Food Drug and Cosmetic Act (FD&C) allows inspections for purposes of enforcement, and it permits the FDA to inspect all documents specified in the QSR. Therefore, a company may be cited for violation of any of the provisions discussed in the previous QSR section.

The FDA may routinely inspect a manufacturer as often as every 2 years, although realistically the frequency is much less. Routine inspections will include review of the 510(k) status for each of the company's devices and also will focus on complaint handling, changes manufacturers have made in design and production processes, and a review of records showing in-process or finished device testing failures. This information provides the FDA inspectors with an overview of the company's quality system. An FDA inspector has access to all company records except those dealing with financial matters, customer lists, and personnel issues beyond training and education.

If the FDA inspector finds a serious violation of the QSR, meaning that (a) finished devices are unsafe or ineffective, or (b) conditions exist whereby there is a reasonable probability that unsafe or ineffective devices will be produced, a warning letter may be issued detailing the observation(s) and identifying the provision(s) of the QSR that was violated. The manufacturer must provide a written response to the warning letter within a defined amount of time, and the response must include the steps that will be taken to correct the violation (corrective action) and the estimated amount of time that will be needed. A comprehensive follow-up inspection will re-inspect the condition(s) that led to the original citing plus the balance of the QSR requirements will be reviewed and inspected. The manufacturer may be allowed to continue production of the device while the quality issues are being resolved, depending on the nature of the product and the violation.

If the FDA inspector finds less serious QSR violations or deviations where it is believed there is only a minimal probability that nonconforming product will result if the deviations are not corrected, then a Notice of Inspectional Observations (Form 483) will be issued. The notice will advise the company of the deviations, and the company should respond promptly and thoroughly. Responses should present the manufacturer's views of the facts and their interpretations of the relevant QSR requirements. If the violations alleged in Form 483 are serious, the manufacturer should consider submitting to the FDA a proposal for voluntary corrective action.

The FDA's goal in enforcing the QSR regulation is to bring manufacturers into a "state of control" by eliciting voluntary cooperative efforts. When voluntary cooperation is insufficient, the FDA may initiate further regulatory or judicial action. In the event there is inadequate response to a warning letter, or if initial observations appear to harm public health, the FDA may escalate enforcement activities through seizure, injunction, and prosecution.

Seizure of a product generally is limited to devices that are misbranded or adulterated, not for violations of the QSR. This is an extreme measure where the government can gain control of an allegedly violative product based merely on a complaint (8).

In extreme cases, seizures often are accompanied by injunction orders. An injunction is a remedy against a person, including individuals or corporations, that orders the person to do or not to do something. Typically, injunction orders under FD&C prohibit the conduct of business "unless and until" certain actions are taken and approved by the FDA. The FDA usually pursues injunctions only for the following circumstances: when adequate warning to a defendant has been given, when the FDA believes violations of the FD&C are clear, when the defendant refuses to discontinue the allegedly violative conduct voluntarily, or when a seizure does not appear to protect public health adequately.

The FDA is also more apt to seek injunctions rather than seizures against violations of the QSR regulations because injunctions effectively close a business until the QSR is in place. Injunctions are more applicable when the violation is systemic rather than applying only to one product. Injunctive orders are also the remedy of choice for the FDA when a violation presents a health risk.

As a final resort, persons who violate the FD&C may be subject to criminal prosecution and penalties, including imprisonment or monetary penalties or both. The amount of punishment is determined by the type of violation, namely, whether it is a misdemeanor or a felony. Because felonies are conscious violations of the FD&C, they are subject to greater punishment than misdemeanors. The FDA has used criminal authority sparingly, but these are viable options for the agency.

Product Recalls

Most product recalls are initiated by the manufacturer when it is realized that the device does not meet specifications. The FDA also has the authority to impose mandatory recalls when a device "presents an unreasonable risk of substantial harm to the public health" [Section 518(a) of the FD&C], but these recalls are less common.

Product recalls are categorized into one of three classifications: class I, II, or III. The significance of these classifications relates to the extent of the recall and the effectiveness checks that will be required to consider the recall closed in the FDA's view. Additionally, a correct recall classification is important because it represents the FDA's evaluation of the hazard a device presents to the public and therefore has potential significance to a product liability suit against the recalling firm.

A class I recall represents a situation in which there is "a reasonable probability that using a violative product will cause serious adverse health consequences or death." This is the most significant recall classification and would require the greatest recall depth, the greatest extension of the recall into the product distribution chain, and the greatest degree of follow-up to ensure the effectiveness of the recall (i.e., proof that any remaining product was returned to the company or destroyed). An example of a class I recall would be for a faulty surgical irrigation device that could result in an air embolism during surgery. Additionally, a class I recall may include public notification that is reserved for urgent public health situations.

A class II recall is one in which "a violative product will cause temporary or medically reversible adverse health consequences" and the probability of serious effects is remote. Examples of class II recalls include defective latex gloves, printers not being compatible with alarm driver boards on ventilators, needle tips that may separate from the sheath during a surgical operation, possible inaccurate noninvasive blood pressure measurements, and cracked components that may compromise the sterility barrier.

A class III recall describes a violative product that is unlikely to cause adverse health consequences. Class III recalls commonly result from labeling errors and mixups. Examples of class III recalls include incorrect barcoding, incorrect packaging, control solutions not meeting their target values, and incorrect chemical formulations.

Recalls of IVD products, because of their nature of working outside the body and providing information instead of physical changes to the body, are always class II or III, mainly class III. IVDs can be recalled whenever any portion of the system cannot perform as intended. This includes situations when reagents lose stability or become contaminated, when instruments do not function properly, and when control solutions are mislabeled or erroneously quantitated.

CONCLUSIONS AND BEST APPROACHES FOR THE FUTURE

The regulatory considerations of bringing an IVD to market include interactions with the FDA. The FDA is responsible for the following:

- Granting market clearance via the decision that the product is safe and effective for its intended use
- Determining test categorization under CLIA '88 requirements
- Providing regulatory oversight for quality issues to ensure that the product continues to meet its performance claims

Getting an IVD on the market requires the presentation of scientific data supporting analytic and clinical performance characteristics. Getting a point-of-care IVD on the market requires an increased regulatory burden to ensure that the product will be used appropriately in the nontraditional laboratory environment.

TABLE 31.6. INTERNET CONTACTS FOR REGULATORY AND RELATED ORGANIZATIONS

Organization	Internet Address
Food and Drug Administration (FDA)	www.fda.gov
FDA Center for Devices and Radiological Health	www.fda.gov/cdrh/index.html
Code of Federal Regulations	www.access.gpo.gov/nara/cfr/cfr-table-search-html
Centers for Medicare & Medicaid Services, formerly the Health Care Financing Administration	www.hcfa.gov
Centers for Disease Control and Prevention	www.cdc.gov
Biotechnology Industry Association	www.bio.org
Food and Drug Law Institute	www.fdli.org
Health Industry Manufacturers Association	www.himanet.com
Regulatory Affairs Professionals Society	www.raps.org

Before POC clinical trials are designed, it is very important to open a dialogue with the FDA so that the agency's concerns and questions can be voiced. This is best done by contacting the specific branch that regulates the type of IVD (e.g., clinical chemistry, hematology, microbiology) and speaking with the Branch Chief or a member of the review staff. Whereas FDA regulations are slow to change, FDA policy can change rather quickly; so it is critical that manufacturers be aware of the most current regulatory attitudes toward POCT. Similarly, if a manufacturer is interested in obtaining waived status for an IVD, it is important to open a dialogue early with the FDA (before the field studies are conducted) so that subtle changes in the require-

ments can be addressed. Table 31.6 lists convenient Internet addresses for the FDA and other agencies

Keeping an IVD on the market requires compliance with the QSR and other statutory measures. The FDA keeps surveillance over IVD manufacturers by on-site inspections and by monitoring product recalls. To ensure that the QSR and other requirements are being met, it is critical that persons within the company keep updated on the changes in laws and policy. The FDA has a considerable arsenal of regulatory and judicial remedies for instances when violative product can affect public health.

REFERENCES

1. Federal Register Notice, 63 FR 5387 (2/2/98).
2. Federal Food, Drug, and Cosmetic Act, 21 USC Section 301 et seq.
3. National Committee on Clinical Laboratory Standards (NCCLS). *Interference testing in clinical chemistry: proposed guideline (EP7-P)*, Vol 6. Villanova, PA: NCCLS, 1986.
4. National Committee on Clinical Laboratory Standards (NCCLS). *Evaluation of the linearity of quantitative analytical methods: proposed guideline (EP6-P)*, Vol 6. Villanova, PA: NCCLS, 1986.
5. National Committee on Clinical Laboratory Standards (NCCLS). *Evaluation of precision performance of clinical chemistry devices (EP5-T2)*, Vol 12. Villanova, PA: NCCLS, 1992.
6. National Committee on Clinical Laboratory Standards (NCCLS). *Method comparison and bias estimation using patient samples; approved guideline (EP9-A)*, Vol 6. Villanova, PA: NCCLS, 1995.
7. Center for Devices and Radiological Health. FDA guidance document. Review criteria for assessment of cholesterol *in vitro* diagnostic devices using enzymatic methodology for clinical laboratories, physician's office laboratories, and home use, July 1997.
8. *Guide to medical device regulation*, Vol 1. Washington, DC: Thompson Publishing Group, 1993, p. 77.

CASE
J

THE ART OF MANAGING A POCT PROGRAM

ROBYN MEDEIROS

Managing an effective point-of-care testing (POCT) program is not something they taught us how to do in school. From my 10 years of experience as a medical technologist, only about 30% helped to prepare me for managing a POCT program; the rest I learned by doing. Here I discuss the ways I found most effective for managing the challenges I faced as a POCT coordinator and describe the methods I used to monitor and maintain a strong program.

On a daily basis, POCT coordinators face many challenges. The top three for me are (a) the obligation to provide a continuum of care, (b) the need to comply with all regulatory requirements, and (c) providing effective leadership to other health care professionals. As patients move through a health care system, point-of-care values are mixed in with clinical laboratory values. It is our obligation to certify that POCT results measure up to laboratory standards of accuracy, reliability, and timeliness. Regulatory requirements will vary depending on test complexity and types of licensure and accreditation. Although we are good at regulatory compliance in the clinical laboratory, it takes on new dimensions with POCT. It is critical that we provide effective leadership, and this requires POCT coordinators to play many roles. First, you need to be a trainer who provides education to hospital staff and an internal technical consultant who remains current on all aspects of the program and field. You also must be a project manager who can assess, design, delegate, implement, and reassess all aspects of the program. You are a facilitator who listens and skillfully resolves conflicts. You become a detective to find out what is really going on, asking questions at every opportunity and opening cabinets and drawers to search for errant laboratory tests that have found their way into the nursing unit! Finally, as a motivator, you are the "heart and soul" of the program, the "cheerleader" who keeps the team members on track, sends the right cues to generate enthusiasm, and helps testing personnel stay focused.

Managing a POCT program is an art. In our laboratory, we practice the *ART* of laboratory medicine. Our product is information, and it must be *accurate*, *reliable*, and *timely*. We know how to do this well; but whereas these three parts are vital to running a strong POCT program, managing the program also requires people management skills to foster positive *attitudes*, *relationships*, and *teamwork*. The overall success of a program will improve as this aspect of the ART is incorporated into daily oversight of the program. It will have a positive impact on how each person chooses to approach the process, how staff members treat each other, and how they participate as a team member.

Success did not happen overnight in our hospital. In February 1996, we launched our POCT program after many meetings with a newly formed POCT advisory committee, nursing directors, and managers. We seemed to be off to a good start, but by the end of the year, our program compliance was only 59% for the whole-blood glucose (WBG) testing, despite having just retrained 800 testing personnel on WBG. Something needed to change. I presented this information at a Patient Care Council meeting attended by nursing administration, directors, managers, and educators representing every service line. At the end of my talk, I asked for their help and reminded them that the Joint Commission on Accreditation of Healthcare Organizations (JCAHO) would be visiting our hospital soon. That was the turning point. The nursing vice-president (VP) assigned a clinical nurse specialist to assist the laboratory with improving the hospital's POCT compliance to 90% or better by the JCAHO visit in April 1998. Hence, our first multidisciplinary performance improvement (PI) project was born.

This PI project reinforced how important it is for laboratorians to understand that the nursing perspective of POCT is very different from our own. A Clinical Laboratory Management Association (CLMA) article (1) states: "It is the art of nursing that attracted most nurses to the profession. It is the science of nursing that enables nurses to accomplish their art." Nurses struggle to maintain a balance between the art and the science. They believe POCT devices are beneficial to patient care because they enable clinical decisions to be made more quickly, but the process is also viewed as time and labor intensive. The changes in the nursing field have greatly affected how they practice as well. They have seen an increase in patient acuity and throughput and are continually confronted with the management of new patient-care technologies. They are doing more with less and not getting as much bedside time with their patients. Considering this, and the fact that their training is strongest in the preanalytic and postanalytic aspects of patient care, it is not surprising that analytic concepts of calibration, accuracy, and precision are not so easily accepted. One of the greatest challenges of POCT coordinators is in helping each group understand the other.

To accomplish this, I have found the following approach invaluable in improving regulatory compliance at our hospital:

1. Maintain good personal contacts, and meet as many people as you can across shifts.
2. Work closely with the diabetes educator. In our facility, this person has a huge impact on the staff, who is the first link to POCT when staff members come through training and often the one who answers questions on the floor.
3. Send a monthly report card for quality assurance compliance. Include two types of reporting. A department-specific performance report should include percent compliance in the areas reviewed each week, details of problems encountered, action taken, and manager's signature. A hospital-wide performance report should be sent to nursing directors and VPs. We found it to be effective in fostering healthy competition and stimulating compliance.
4. Meet with clinical nurse managers initially and then annually to define clear expectations. Provide easy-to-read bulleted outlines on how the program is run in their unit. Offer daily log templates for manual documentation tests, and give training and competency guidelines.
5. Provide inspection readiness materials in the form of a "most commonly asked questions" flyer, perform mock surveys, and meet individually with designated point people to help ensure compliance.
6. Use a lot of humor. This may be as easy as incorporating a clip art or cartoon to get a point across or making whimsical flyers for "thank you's" and announcements.
7. Go on "walkabouts" often. This is part of staying visible and connected to what is going on within individual floors. Be prepared to drop into one of the many roles a POCT coordinator plays—detective, consultant, facilitator, cheerleader, and so on.
8. Be easily available by phone, e-mail, or pager. This will decrease frustration levels if people can reach you quickly.
9. Chocolate is very important. We use it during training as an incentive for people to complete recertification and as "thank you's."
10. Use a variety of communication tools. I send memos, flyers, awards, and recognitions, tidbit notes that are small, brightly colored pieces of paper attached to an instrument or log to give quick information, reminders, or alerts. For example, when we change the quality control lockout time on our WBG instruments, we attach one to every analyzer, or when lot numbers are changed, we attach a note to alert people and give reminder instructions.
11. Start a POCT coordinators' group in your area. Our Bay Area POCT group meets twice a year, has more than 70

TABLE J.1. WHOLE-BLOOD GLUCOSE PROGRAM COMPLIANCE, EL CAMINO HOSPITAL POCT PROGRAM, MOUNTAIN VIEW, CA

Quarter	1996	1997	1998	1999	2000
1	NA	73	82	87	92
2	49	87	86	89	91
3	61	87	87	89	NA
4	68	86	87	90	NA
Total	59%	82%	85%	89%	91%

POCT, point-of-care testing; NA, not available.

members, and represents more than 35 hospitals in a 150-mile radius. It is a key way to share ideas, problems, solutions, and inspection highlights.

With these tools, we were able to achieve the program compliance we sought. Nursing managers and staff began to take an active role in reducing variances by assigning "point people" to be responsible for the POCT program in their unit and taking corrective actions after reviewing the monthly POCT reports. The performance improvement project that began in 1997 successfully improved the WBG program compliance from 59% to more than 90% by 2000 (Table J.1). This success is a direct result of using both the approach mentioned earlier and the efforts of persons in each patient care area, who made all the difference in the ways that they motivated their staff. We also saw our manual testing compliance improve from 88% to 96% by 1999. Additional performance improvement projects we have been involved with are neonatal glucose studies, permanent record normal ranges, chart audits for transcription of manual test results, and critical value audits.

Managing an effective POCT program is definitely a multidisciplinary experience. One of the greatest benefits is the building of professional connections throughout your organization. By practicing the ART, an *a*ttitude of mutual respect develops *r*elationships and fosters *t*eamwork between us all.

REFERENCES

1. Poe S, Nichols J. Quality assurance, practical management, and outcomes of point-of-care testing: nursing perspectives, Part II. *Clinical Laboratory Management Association* 2000;14:12–18.

CONTINUOUS QUALITY IMPROVEMENT AND QUALITY MANAGEMENT FOR POINT-OF-CARE URINALYSIS

FREDERICK L. KIECHLE
ISABEL GAUSS

Implementation of a point-of-care testing (POCT) program in a hospital generally requires the formation of a committee empowered to make all decisions related to technique selection, authorization, quality control, quality assurance, and other issues (1). These decisions should be reviewed by another hospital committee that is engaged in monitoring overall patient care. Although the membership of the POCT committee may vary, potential members include individual(s) from laboratory services, nursing service, medical staff, quality assurance, hospital administration, infection control, purchasing, information services, and financial analysis. Requests for a new POCT program or new site for an existing program should include data related to changes in patient care, patient outcome, and cost. A study may need to be conducted to assess these issues. Certainly, each POCT program must be evaluated by each institution for its cost competitiveness compared with that of the central laboratory. The introduction of robotics/automation, pneumatic tube system, bar-code labeling, and improved data management for POCT programs will have a major impact on these cost-analysis exercises (1).

A coordinator should be appointed to facilitate training, quality assurance monitoring, and equipment evaluations. This coordinator must ensure that the hospital programs are in compliance with generic and analyte-specific regulations and guidelines that have been modified to include regulations found in the Clinical Laboratories Improvement Act of 1988 (CLIA '88). Generic guidelines for POCT are issued by the Centers for Medicare and Medicaid Services (formerly the Health Care Financing Administration), the Joint Commission on Accreditation of Healthcare Organizations, the College of American Pathologists, and the National Committee for Clinical Laboratory Standards.

Urinalysis is defined as the physical evaluation, microscopic examination or chemical examination of urine. The chemical examination using a dipstick or reagent tablet is a waived test, whereas microscopy performed by the physician is categorized as physician-performed microscopy (PPM) by CLIA '88. POCT for chemical urinalysis will include dipstick vendor selection, tester training leading to authorization, quality control, competency, and quality assurance (1-3). Table K.1 outlines some of the components of a POCT program for chemical urinalysis. Training should be performed in small groups of six to eight persons and an instructor. Replacement of the instructor with a videotape leads to inferior performance (4). Each trainee must complete a checklist of skills and pass a written examination. Visual confirmation or initial analysis of urine dipstick requires good color discrimination. Two levels of quality control (Quantimetrix Corporation, Redondo Beach, CA, U.S.A.) should be performed at least daily for each open bottle of urine dipsticks. Because urine dipsticks exposed to room air in open vials may generate erroneous results within 7 days of exposure, the number of urine dipstick vials in use should be limited to one or two per nursing unit rather than one vial per patient or patient room (5). This practice may prevent lengthy periods of air exposure for urine dipsticks because a number of testers can use the same vial. A mechanism should be established for assessing operator competency every 6 months for the first year and annually thereafter (1-3). One of at least four methods can be used. The first method requires a supervisor to observe the test performed by the operator. Alternatively, the operator may meet this requirement by performing quality control tests, following up on all quality control failures and using a number of urine dipsticks that compares well with the number of results reported (3).

The POCT coordinator for the chemical urinalysis program must closely monitor which body fluids are being used. The dipsticks are designed for use in urine; however, they have been used to screen for potential bacterial infections in a variety of body fluids for which the dipsticks were not originally designed (6-8). Two of ten urine dipstick reactions (glucose and pH) were markedly decreased in bacterial-contaminated units of platelets (6). Amniotic fluid leukocyte esterase had a sensitivity of 91% and a specificity of 95% in detecting chorioamnionitis but was not a predictor of endometritis in women delivering by cesarean section (8). There is no agreement about whether leukocyte esterase reaction is sensitive enough to detect a clinically significant number of leukocytes in cerebrospinal fluid (7). In addition, a false-negative result may occur for protein if the total protein in cerebrospinal fluid is greater than 3 g per liter. Presumably, synovial fluid has not been evaluated because it is too viscous to penetrate the reaction pad of the urine dipstick. Careful evaluation of any urine dipstick application to another body fluid must precede its introduction to a POCT program.

TABLE K.1. COMPONENTS FOR POCT PROGRAM IN URINALYSIS

Training with skills checklist and written examination
Colorblindness check
Two levels of quality control
Quality control performed once per day per open bottle of dipsticks
Results recorded manually and/or in computer
Operator competency
   How often quality control not performed
   No follow-up of quality control failures
   Strips used/tests reported do not correlate
   Supervisor observes test performance

POCT, point-of-care testing.

For microscopic examination of urine, 12 mL of well-mixed, fresh urine is spun for 400 $\times g$ for 5 minutes. The supernatant is decanted and the sediment is resuspended. A drop of the resuspended sediment is placed on a glass slide and coverslipped. After 30 to 60 seconds, the cellular elements will have settled and microscopic evaluation with a bright-field or phase-contrast microscopy may be performed. Standardization, technical competence, and continuing education must be ensured for accurate assessment of patient samples (3). The POCT coordinator should be familiar with the locations where provider-performed urine microscopy procedures are used to ensure that appropriate CLIA licensure has been obtained for the physician responsible for these procedures. An alternative approach is to include PPM under the POCT program coordinated by the laboratory. Training new residents could be undertaken during their orientation time. Kodachrome images may be used. This same slide file could be used to organize proficiency testing activity, or this goal may be achieved by purchasing the Excel program XL-G from the College of American Pathologists. Quality control materials are not available. Hospitals performing provider-performed urine microscopy, however, are expected to follow good laboratory practices in terms of quality control, quality assurance, and proficiency testing. Competency indicators for urine PPM might include monitoring the number of proficiency testing or testing failures or failed procedural observations (3). Problems encountered in a hospital-based application of urine PPM include difficulty in review of findings by another individual due to specimen lability, lack of quality control in the quality assurance program, no outcome analysis available, and finally whether the data are placed on the chart manually or not at all. The resolution of most of these issues will depend on local policies, procedures, and politics.

REFERENCES

1. Main RI, Kiechle FL. Point-of-care testing: administration within a health system. *Lab Med* 2000;31:453–459.
2. Kiechle FL. Point-of-care testing. In: Rainey P, ed. Washington, DC: American Association for Clinical Chemistry, 1998:1–98.
3. Joint Commission. *Quality point-of-care testing: a Joint Commission Handbook.* Oakbrook Terrace, IL: Joint Commission on Accreditation of Healthcare Organizations, 1999.
4. Kucher MA, Goormastic M, Hoogwerf G. Influence of frequency, time interval from initial instruction and method of instruction on performance competency for blood glucose monitoring. *Diabetes Care* 1990; 13:488–491.
5. Gallagher EJ, Schwartz E, Weinstein RS. Performance characteristics of urine dipsticks stored in open containers. *Am J Emerg Med* 1990;8: 121–123.
6. Burstain JM, Brecher ME, Workman K, et al. Rapid identification of bacterially contaminated platelets using reagent strips: glucose and pH analysis as markers of bacterial contamination. *Transfusion* 1997;37: 255–258.
7. Moosa AA, Quortum HA, Ibrahim MD. Rapid diagnosis of bacterial meningitis with reagent strips. *Lancet* 1995;345:1290–1291.
8. Keski-Nisula L, Katila M-L, Kirkinen PA, et al. Amniotic fluid leukocytes and leukocyte esterase activity in parturients delivered by caesarean section. *Scand J Infect Dis* 1997;29:291–296.

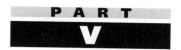

INFORMATION, CONNECTIVITY, AND KNOWLEDGE SYSTEMS

32

INFORMATICS AND DATA MANAGEMENT

DAVID CHOU
RAYMOND D. ALLER

PRINCIPLES OF POINT-OF-CARE TESTING INFORMATION MANAGEMENT

Point-of-care testing (POCT) devices permit users to perform laboratory testing with tremendous freedom from central resource limitations. This individual freedom, however, has conflicted with organizational needs in areas such as the documentation of testing and clinical decisions made from testing results. Cooperation with organizational needs is particularly difficult with a large distributed base of users and instruments, and the cost and effort needed to overcome these problems often exceed the cost of the POCT devices themselves. One particularly challenging area is the entry of POCT results into information systems as institutions implement electronic medical records. To meet this need, a point-of-care device must have a certain minimum level of information management functionality. Regrettably, many devices deployed in the first decades of POCT lack this capability because of cost or complexity constraints. As the importance of integrating this information into the broader information architecture of health care and as technology increases, key elements to support the integration of POCT results must be incorporated into designs. Information connectivity remains one of the major challenges for POCT devices (1).

Broadly defined, three features facilitate the integration of POCT instruments into information management architectures. These include (a) the entry or capture of patient identification, (b) the electronic transfer of test results linked with the patient identifier to host(s) managing test results, and (c) the use of industry-standard protocols and codes to represent that information. Each is considered in detail here.

Patient Identification

Most information systems require a unique patient identifier to which patient results will be linked. Substantial ambiguity is possible with patient names. Even simple variations in the presentation of first names (e.g., John, Jack, Johnny, J.) make it difficult, if not impossible, for an information system to integrate patient information. For a point-of-care instrument to obtain a patient identifier, two options exist. Either (a) the instrument operator enters the patient identifier manually, or (b) the patient identifier is captured through some form of automatic identification. For a patient identifier to be entered manually, a keypad or a touch screen with equivalent functions is needed. New approaches also include handwriting recognition, such as those found on personal data assistants (PDAs), and voice recognition. Once entered, the patient identifier must be validated, either through a check digit or by comparing the captured information with a central database. A check digit is one or more digits added to a patient identifier, computationally derived from other digits or characters in the patient identifier. With a check digit, the point-of-care device then can validate the patient identifier by performing the same computation and comparing the result with the check digit. Most single-digit errors and digit transpositions can be detected by a check digit algorithm, allowing the instrument to detect and notify the operator of many data entry errors. Check digits are particularly useful in a point-of-care instrument where patient numbers cannot be validated against a database. Over the past three decades, many hospitals have eliminated check digits from patient identifiers, in part because they do not understand the cost or frequency of errors preventable by the use of check digits. Often this occurs when the check digit field is used as a short cut to expand the patient number field. A significant obstacle for incorporating check digits in instruments is the large number and complexity of algorithms in use. This requires the instrument manufacturer to support a variety of specialized computations. An example of check-digit validation is shown in Table 32.1.

If the patient identifier contains an alpha character, a means to enter alphanumeric characters is needed. Alpha characters are common for patient identifiers in countries outside of the United States. Check digits are possible but are complicated by alpha characters. Keypad data entry of a patient identifier containing alpha characters is also more difficult and may force the addition of a large keyboard to a small instrument, a difficult design task on most POCT instruments. Exceptions to this, of course, include a point-of-care instrument designed to function in conjunction with a larger device, such as a critical care monitoring system.

If the available patient identifier does *not* have an integral check digit, the availability of two key items of patient demo-

TABLE 32.1. AN EXAMPLE OF A PATIENT NUMBER CHECK-DIGIT SYSTEM

The patient number is 12345676.
The first 7 digits (1234567) represent the patient's number.
The last digit (6) is the check digit computed in the following manner:
  check-digit = $[2*C_1 + 3*C_2 + 4*C_3 + 5*C_4 + 6*C_5 + 7*C_6 + 2*C_7]$ modulo 10
Modulo 10 is the remainder after dividing the result by 10.
Therefore, the result is
  check-digit = $[2*(1) + 3*(2) + 4*(3) + 5*(4) + 6*(5) + 7*(6) + 2*(7)]$
  modulo 10
  = 6

Note: If the clerk types 22345676, the check-digit calculation will result in a 7. Because 6 is expected, the patient number is rejected by the computer. Check digits do not guarantee accuracy but, properly designed, help reduce errors.

graphic information, such as identifier and birth date or identifier and first and last initials, will enable the system to recognize erroneous entries when the data are uploaded to a master database. Unfortunately, such checks are often made after the fact, when it is difficult to correct bad data. Another possibility is a real-time connection with the master patient database, so that the patient name can be immediately fed back to the operator. Unfortunately, experience shows that this is not as reliable as a check digit because an operator often makes errors in verifying the patient name. The ability to maintain a real-time connection to a master database adds complexity to the POCT instrument and is not common with most portable devices. Such a connection typically requires a wireless networking capability.

If feasible, automated capture of the patient identifier is preferable to manual operator entry. At present, the most practical, widely deployed, and least expensive technology is to incorporate a barcode reader into the POCT device. Portable wand-type readers can be built into the corner of a handheld unit for a manufacturing cost of well less than $100. Using a barcoded patient armband, the user is virtually assured of having the correct patient number. Unfortunately, most hospitals today do not use such patient identification armbands; consequently, POCT manufacturers seldom offer such features.

Biometric identifiers can also link POCT results to the proper patient. Fingerprint classifiers are rapidly becoming more available, and iris scanners may well have the specificity to serve as a truly robust identification system. Both approaches are unlikely to be used because of the current costs and difficulties for implementing these technologies. Other technologies, such as radio frequency identification (RFID) or semiconductor chips readable and writeable using radiofrequency (RF) scanners, can be used on armbands. They are attractive because of their robustness and ability to store large amounts of information. RFID chips also have been inserted under the skin for identification purposes in veterinary applications, but this is likely to be a socially unacceptable practice in health care. The Institute of Medicine report has focused on the costs of medical errors (2) and the need to use technologies to reduce the frequency of such errors. Unfortunately, short-term goals often lead to the neglect of simple measures, such as the check digit, which can have profound effects on

reducing patient identification errors. Thus, it may be a long time before such sophisticated patient identification devices are purchased by most institutions.

Electronic Transfer of Testing Results with Linked Patient Identifiers

Once the POCT produces the results, transfer of that information into the patient's permanent medical record is very important. Numerous approaches are being promoted by manufacturers of today's testing devices, including batch transfers (e.g., by plugging the device into a docking station on the nursing unit, often long after the testing has been completed) and real-time connection into the information system through a network connection. The details and technologies for connectivity are discussed elsewhere in this chapter.

Use of Industry-standard Protocols and Codes to Represent Test Information

As information is transferred to the central information system, it is most efficacious if this transfer is implemented by using standard protocols rather than a proprietary format differing from one device to the next. ASTM E1381 (3) and ASTM E1394 (4), developed under the organizational structure of the American Society for Testing and Materials (ASTM), define the low-level and high-level protocols for communications between analytic instruments and the laboratory information system. Logical Observation Identifiers, Names, and Codes (LOINCs) (5–7) provide for unambiguous identification of tests and their results. These standards and their applicability to POCT instruments are discussed later.

The Electronic Medical Record and Data Warehouses

The importance of point-of-care data in an electronic medical record (EMR) was stated previously. For a host of reasons, including economic pressures and better patient care, the EMR has replaced the paper chart in institutions (8), especially as costs have dropped. Large integrated health systems and care networks have uncovered limitations of the paper medical record. The paper chart is particularly inadequate in its ability to meet the needs of practitioners who need access for a patient being treated at multiple centers. To utilize expensive resources, a patient may be moved among institutions. Access to the paper chart by multiple personnel even within a single institution is difficult. Such access may be nearly impossible with two geographically separated institutions. Commercially available EMRs vary in capabilities. Information systems typically send all relevant clinical and administrative data, such as dictated operative notes and discharge summaries. In most EMRs, laboratory data constitute a high proportion of the total data.

An information system collecting and storing large amounts of data, primarily produced from other computer systems, is called a *data warehouse* (9). In contrast to an EMR, which is designed to provide real-time retrieval of patient data for a clinician, most data warehouses are designed to perform data analyses of large databases, a process called *data mining* (10). Data analysis requires knowledge of how the data were collected and its context. A hospital data warehouse might contain only administrative data, such as billing information, for example, or it might integrate both administrative and clinical data. Analyzing the costs of performing a particular surgical procedure (e.g., coronary artery bypass graft) allows a hospital to determine the profitability of that procedure. Analyzing the costs for a health maintenance organization (HMO) allows it to pursue contracts with knowledge of their profitability. In general, data mining of clinical information has been less productive than data mining of administrative data because of the descriptive, textual, and qualitative nature of clinical data and the lack of tools available for performing the analyses on such data.

The principal advantage of data warehouses lies in their ability to support ad hoc queries designed to extract quantitative information and to find relationships among data items. Although relatively few projects are implemented using data warehousing, 84% of these projects are reported to succeed in meeting design goals (11). The cost for data warehouses is decreasing but still requires an average expenditure of several million dollars exclusive of local institutional resources (12). Unfortunately, data warehouses typically require substantial custom software development and technical expertise, even though a few semicustom software systems have emerged, and so the actual costs are much greater. Because of this cost and expertise, the data warehouse may be unavailable except at larger institutions. In a hospital with many departmental systems, a sizable cost of building the data warehouse will be the cost of providing data feeds from other systems into the warehouse. Finally, there are few, if any, tools available for "reading" text found in discharge summaries and similar documents; so it is difficult to analyze clinical information stored in a data warehouse in this format.

CONNECTIVITY

Point-of-care instruments excel in providing the clinician with rapid testing by reducing delays in specimen transport and results reporting. To keep costs down and units compact and because users did not demand such features, manufacturers of these instruments often have sacrificed the ability of these units to send analytic results to information systems. Without an interface, a user must transcribe results onto the patient chart or type results into a computer. Because these tasks can be time consuming, most documentation of results has been erratic, and users are motivated to skip record keeping.

A well-designed interface can reduce the effort required for record keeping. Many handheld POCT instruments interact with a data management station, through which one or more portable instruments interface with a host system. In most cases, the interfaces are based on communications standards in the health care industry. Computer networks, serving as digital information highways, interconnect computers. Interfaces based on wireless and portable computer devices [PDAs and personal computers (PCs)] have made this connectivity even easier. This section covers the issues associated with connectivity, a term that

qualitatively describes the ability of a device or system to communicate digitally with another computer system.

Standards and Objectives

Early clinical laboratory instrumentation utilized divergent hardware and software techniques for interfacing to a laboratory information system (LIS). Idiosyncrasies, vendor secrecy, proprietary software and hardware, and suboptimal instrument designs made the interface task difficult and expensive. Dissatisfactions with this chaotic process led to the formation of an instrument interface standards group under ASTM. By 1991, three standards were approved and issued. These included one to define the low-level protocol for transferring messages standardizing on the RS-232 serial interface (ASTM E1381-95) (4), one to define the format for transferring information between clinical instruments and the LIS (ASTM E1394-97) (4), and one to define the use of barcoding for specimens in instruments (ASTM E1466-92) (13). These protocols were designed for instruments with medium- to high-data volume operating within the clinical laboratory and considerably improved the consistency of instrument interfaces. In particular, the E1466 standard is largely irrelevant to POCT instruments because automated specimen handling is uncommon. These standards evolve as needs change. For example, the National Committee on Clinical Laboratory Standards (NCCLS) and its Area Committee on Automation is developing new standards for laboratory automation. The Subcommittee on Specimen Identification has proposed new barcode standards labeling of patient specimens, which could have applicability in specimens used for POCT and later referred to a central laboratory for additional testing (14).

The normal point-of-care workflow differs significantly from that of the clinical laboratory. The ASTM instrument interface specifications address only some needs of the POCT instrument. For example, LIS test ordering and patient admissions usually are performed in the specimen receiving area of the laboratory, eliminating the need for these at the instrument. In the point-of-care environment, these functions are often required for the entry of results into an information system. The Health Level 7 (HL-7) standard (15) and its subset ASTM E1238-97 (16) cover these functions. Their primary function is to cover the area of interfacing information systems in a health care environment and to cover the aspects of managing and transferring patient data. Unfortunately, the complexity of these protocols, especially the subtleties in the HL-7 dialects, has previously made it unattractive for implementing these in small instruments.

The Connectivity Industrial Consortium (CIC) (17), which consists of POCT instrument manufacturers, users, and information system vendors, was formed in early 2000 to address these deficiencies. The consortium planned a 12- to 15-month process to develop standards better enabling the interfacing of instruments to information systems. The outcome of this process is described in another chapter in this book. Because many vendors were participants in this effort, it is expected that the standards will become widely accepted. Continued support and future development for this standard have been passed to the NCCLS.

Data Downloading Station and Interfacing to Computerized Information Systems

Because features such as a keyboard and larger screen decrease portability, vendors often include minimal inboard data handling in POCT instruments. If the unit has a data interface, it usually is limited to downloading data into an outboard data management station (DMS). Data may be entered into a DMS through the interface or manually. The DMS provides additional data-handling capabilities, such as result editing, quality assurance, data storage, data analysis/management reports, and uploading to a hospital information system (HIS) or LIS. If a single DMS is used for multiple devices, it also can be very cost-effective because costs are not added for each instrument, and the expense of connecting to the LIS or HIS is minimized. Usually, the instrument holds minimal data such as a patient identifier, the time of testing, the test results, and an operator code. The DMS augments these data with information such as the patient name and provides longer-term data storage and data analysis. Lastly, a DMS operator can supplement results with comments such as "IV running." Because users forget, this last capability has minimal utility unless the instrument download to the DMS occurs immediately after testing.

The growth of EMRs has created an extensive dependency on laboratory data in an electronic format. This requires POCT data to be uploaded into an LIS or HIS computer. To facilitate this process, the DMS must perform at least two functions: (a) collect/consolidate data from one or more instruments, and (b) verify and transmit captured data to the LIS or HIS computer. In addition to entering results, the host computer can provide functions such as billing and quality assurance. Traditional LIS instrument interfaces based on ASTM or HL-7 standards are available for some POCT instruments and require the purchase of software from both the instrument and the LIS vendor. The cost of these LIS interfaces can be more than $10,000, and delays are common because cooperation between the LIS vendor, the instrument vendor, and the user are needed for implementation. The low data rates of the POCT instrument also permit alternative techniques using standardized tools as building blocks. Some vendors use screen capture and terminal scripting tools. PC software, such as Microsoft's Visual Basic and Access database operating under Microsoft Windows, can mimic a person performing data entry on a terminal. More sophisticated and comprehensive scripting tools are available from vendors such as Microscript (Danvers, MA, U.S.A.). Scripting capabilities are also built into the capabilities of most commercially available interface engines (New Era of Networks, Pacheco, CA, U.S.A.; Software Technologies Corp., Monrovia, CA, U.S.A.; HCI Cloverleaf, Dallas, TX, U.S.A.). Low initial cost, simplicity, and the ability for the interface to be developed without LIS vendor cooperation are attractive features. To imitate a terminal, the PC either connects to the host through a serial port or operates on a network as a terminal using terminal emulation software.

To perform a download, the DMS starts the screen capture software, and the scripting software imitates a user. If the DMS is on a hospital network, the script attaches to the desired host system and starts the log-in process. If the DMS is attached through a modem on a dial-up telephone line, the script dials the host computer and starts the log-in process. After log-in, the DMS script authenticates the patient. If the patient is not in the host computer, the DMS can hold the result for later transmission, initiate a process to admit the patient into the host, or simply issue an error message. If necessary, the software orders the appropriate tests in the host and the results for the ordered tests. The disadvantage of any scripting software is that any change in the host computer software or hardware that affects the format or sequence of prompts on terminal screens, such as a test name change or a LIS software update, will require a corresponding change in the scripting software. If the scripting software fails and the POCT vendor has the responsibility for making changes, the interface may not be functional for a while. Capture/scripting software can be very difficult to implement and use in an environment where line noise causes an unanticipated response from the host. Most scripts provide users with few error messages when a LIS or HIS download fails.

Data handling can be particularly difficult in POCT environments when a large number of users operate instruments infrequently. Unless the designs are intuitive, unacceptable analytic results and poor record keeping are inevitable. A well-designed human interface requires development time and can be costly to implement. Easy-to-use features are particularly difficult to implement on handheld devices with limited keyboards and small displays in an environment as complex as POCT. This difficulty is compounded by the overhead associated with the *in vitro* diagnostics industry and federal regulations. It is not surprising that a DMS and an instrument interface can only partially resolve many of the data-handling problems associated with POCT. In rare cases, a DMS is designed primarily to satisfy a marketing need.

Computerized Quality Control and Results Tracking

Quality control for POCT systems can be managed in a manner similar to other automated instrumentation. Frequently, the instrument and reagent quality assurance checks are performed under the supervision of the clinical laboratory on a periodic basis. Some instruments also support an electronic checkout, which does not test user competency or detect lot number problems with the reagent/analytic module. In many cases, a disposable analytic module is responsible for its own calibration. This brings additional challenges for quality assurance because there is the potential for more variations than that associated with traditional laboratory instruments where the analytic module is retained.

Quality assurance algorithms may be programmed into a POCT instrument. The instrument enforces the number, frequency, and type of quality assurance samples. For example, a high, low, and midrange control must be run within a 24-hour period. If the samples are not run, or the results are out of range, the instrument locks out patient samples until it has been repaired. Either the DMS or LIS maintains the quality assurance data and allows trending and other analysis of the quality assurance tests.

COMPUTER NETWORKS

The widespread availability of high-speed computer networks through most of the United States and other developed countries has greatly changed the approach to information processing. In many parts of the United States, homes and hospitals alike have access to high-speed networks; this resulted from the rapid proliferation of fiberoptic cables and demand for high-speed data access. The social and technologic impacts of this technology have been and will continue to be significant (18). Networks provide an infrastructure for connecting POCT devices to information systems and provide patients with a communications channel for information about their own disease and treatments.

A POCT instrument may connect directly to the network or, more likely, indirectly to the network through a data management station. A *computer network* or simply a *network* describes a system interconnecting two or more computers or computer devices for the purposes of data interchange. A physically limited network, usually where these devices are all within 2 to 3 miles, is called a *local area network*, or LAN. A network connecting two or more LANs over larger distances is called a *wide-area network*, or *WAN*. WANs are likely to depend on public telecommunications utilities, such as telephone companies, whereas most LANs are owned by the hospital and maintained locally. Most hospitals have LANs. Larger hospital systems operate WANs to interconnect several hospitals and satellite facilities. LANs and WANs allow the creation of structures supporting a decentralized physical and organizational operation (19). Satellite and multihospital operations are becoming increasingly important as laboratories expand in size to increase operating efficiencies. Services provided by public utilities include high-speed data lines (e.g., T-1 or OC-3), analog lines (e.g., dial-up telephone) or lower speed data lines (e.g., digital subscriber line, or DSL).

Small LANs can be inexpensive (<$50 per connection) and can be user installed. To share files and printers and to access the Internet and e-mail, computers installed in the office environment usually require *Ethernet*, the most common LAN. Most computers today can be networked with minimal effort. Depending on the type of Ethernet, the network can carry data at rates from 10 to 1,000 megabits per second or more.

Ethernet connections between the network and the computer usually are made with category 5 unshielded twisted pair wire (CAT 5 UTP). Ethernet using UTP is *10BaseT* for 10 megabits per second twisted pair Ethernet, *100BaseT* for 100 megabits per second twisted pair Ethernet, or *1000BaseT* for 1 gigabit per second twisted pair Ethernet. CAT 5 UTP supports connections up to 100 m for 10BaseT and up to 30 m for 100BaseT. *Thinwire* and *10Base2 Ethernet* (10 megabits and 200 m maximum length), which uses a thin coaxial cable similar to that for cable television and *thickwire* or *10Base5 Ethernet* (for the 500 m maximum for this cable), which uses a thicker coaxial cable, are older and less frequently used today. In many applications, fiberoptic cables (10BaseFi) provide higher speeds and longer distances than UTP cables. These benefits help offset the additional cost of fiber cable.

Because networks can be shared, the speed of data between any two will depend on the amount of competing traffic. Limitations of the hardware, such as the network adapter card in a personal computer, also may result in transfer rates less than the maximum possible. The installation and maintenance requirements for LANs increase greatly with the number of devices. To limit the complexity and to reduce the conflicts of sharing, networks are often divided into *subnets*. Subnets and networks are interconnected through devices called *routers*. These devices control and regulate the types of information being passed and also can serve as a means for controlling unwanted intrusions. A small institution may operate as a single network; larger organizations may possess multiple subnets. Managing networks requires the resolution of conflicting hardware and software and the use of compatible protocols. A connection to the Internet, for example, requires that the networked computer utilize the standard Transmission Control Protocol/Internet Protocol (TCP/IP). The Internet is the name given to the international network interconnecting all smaller networks.

The most common communications protocol used on networks, including the Internet, is TCP/IP. Variations in the user interfaces for TCP/IP include Telnet (for terminal emulation), FTP (file transfer protocol), and HTTP (HyperText Transmission Protocol, for web browsing). In the TCP/IP protocol, each computer or computer device on the network must be assigned a unique IP (Internet protocol) address. An IP address is written as four numbers separated by three periods (e.g., 128.10.11.99); each number ranges between 0 and 255. An IP address or block of addresses also may be assigned a name, or *domain name*. A computer translating the domain name into an IP address is known as a *domain name server* or DNS.

Prior to 1998, IP addresses or blocks of addresses were assigned centrally. After 1998, the U.S. Department of Commerce (DOC) created the Internet Corporation for Assigned Names and Numbers (ICANN) for the purposes of registering addresses and domain names. The Internet Network Information Center (InterNIC) is responsible for providing information about this process (www.internic.net). A user can request a license for a single address with all four numbers assigned. A user also may receive a group of addresses where the first one, two, or three numbers are assigned (20). If only the first number is assigned, the user has a class A license and is responsible for managing the remaining triplet of numbers. If the first two numbers are assigned, the user has a class B license and is responsible for managing the remaining duplex. If three addresses are assigned, the user has a class C license and the responsible for managing the last number. Although many class C licenses are available, most class A and class B licenses have been used. As a result, a new scheme expanding the IP address to a set of six numbers is in the process of being implemented. The exploding Internet has created a management problem for the assignment of IP addresses similar to the problems associated with the rapidly growing use of telephone numbers.

Web Concepts

The current Internet has its roots when the Department of Defense created the Advance Research Projects Agency Network

(ARPANET) project in 1969 for the purposes of interconnecting widely separated computers. The project had changed sufficient in scope that responsibility for the network was transferred to the National Science Foundation in 1987. In 1995, the network was moved to a public and more commercial venue, where it has exploded as the Internet and the World Wide Web (21,22). The Web browser interface has gained tremendous popularity as a method for presenting and receiving information on the Internet. In this approach, a browser client interacts with a Web server via a network. The Web interface permits the use of both graphics and text using hypertext markup language (HTML). Several investigators have demonstrated the usefulness of HTML to display laboratory data stored on a server (23). Browser software can operate on almost any desktop or host computer. A browser also can be incorporated as a part of the hardware in a network terminal, a device dedicated to the browser function. In hospital environments, the Web browser has been particularly popular as a user front-end for patient results.

Along with traditional access through corporate and university facilities, Internet service providers (ISPs) have sprung up, greatly expanding access to the Internet through dial-up telephone lines and modems. With such universal availability, the Web has become a natural tool for providing remote users with laboratory results or for remote users to enter POCT results into a master database. It is even possible for a remote data management station (see later section on these devices) to download its data into a central data repository through the Internet, although the heterogeneity of the Internet makes this less attractive. For example, it may be preferable to bear the costs for long-distance telephone calls rather than incur the costs for developing software to communicate (including security measures to preserve patient confidentiality) through the Internet. The Web has become and likely will increase as a resource for POCT. In many major metropolitan communities, more than half of the families already have access to the Web, making it an excellent mechanism for capturing POCT results performed in the home setting. Likewise, the Web becomes an excellent resource for patients to access information about their own medical needs, for sharing information with other patients, and for the delivery of patient care.

Wireless Communications (Hospital-based and Care Networks)

Most computer networks are constructed from copper or fiberoptic cable. Some health care institutions have augmented hard-wired networks with wireless devices to provide users with mobility. For example, patients can walk around the hospital while being attached to a cardiac monitor. Health care workers can be provided with both computer connectivity and mobility. Wireless networks permit mobile point-of-care instruments to be interfaced to a host computer while being used, freeing the user performing the test from walking to a nursing station to download results (24). Similarly, wireless systems based on cellular telephone technology permit home health care personnel performing testing to be connected to a central computer facility while still in the patient's home. Wireless technologies vary in the distances between the access point and the mobile device.

For example, cellular telephone–based systems can operate over several miles while Infrared Data Association (IrDA) infrared devices, are limited to 1 to 2 meters between mobile and fixed stations. In wireless networks, the fixed station is frequently called the *access point* (AP); the area serviced by the AP is called the *service cell*. For most networks, multiple cells are needed and must be interconnected by a *distribution system* (Fig. 32.1), usually a LAN.

Wireless networks within hospitals have been implemented using one of two techniques: infrared (IR) and spread spectrum radiofrequency (SSRF) (25). The Institute of Electrical and Electronic Engineers (IEEE) 802.11 standard (26) approved in 1997 recognizes a diffused infrared (DFIR) approach and two SSRF approaches. If the device can be maintained within line-of-sight of a transmitter or its reflections, DFIR technology is inexpensive and can be implemented easily. One or more DFIR transmitters flood an area with infrared signals picked up by a detector on the mobile device. The approach may use point-to-point transmission or "sun-and-moon" configuration where signals are reflected off walls and other surfaces. The mobile device has a transmitter broadcasting to the AP. This approach can be used in an intensive care unit where a POCT instrument needs to communicate with a central data management station and where all POCT devices are within line-of-sight of the central transmitter and receiver. Data rates for DFIR technologies are excellent and can range from 50% to 100% of the bandwidth of a 10-megabit Ethernet channel. The major limitation of any IR technology is its inability to penetrate solid objects. Interference and data security are usually not problems because DFIR signals are contained within the room.

Infrared devices also have been developed under the IrDA standard. These IrDA devices have been chosen by the CIC developing standards for connecting POCT devices as a way to communicate between a portable device and a network interface. Because of their low cost ($1-2), multiple IrDA devices can be wired to a single more expensive network interface. IrDA devices are very similar to transmitters and receivers used for home electronics and are limited to data rates up to 115k and distances of 1-2 meters. Even though these data rates and distances are inadequate to support a LAN, they are useful as an alternative for collecting and forwarding data to a network interface.

SSRF networks provide additional flexibility since they are less restricted by physical barriers than IR since they will pass through materials used to construct most common interior walls. Microwave frequencies in the 2.4 GHz band are used to communicate between fixed and mobile stations. Most local radio-frequency techniques limit the distance between the fixed and mobile unit from 100 to 800 feet and coverage up to 50,000 square feet. A large hospital requires many overlapping cells to get complete coverage. A single fixed cell transmitter-receiver access point can cost under $150 and a mobile network connection costs less than $50. Although costs are dropping, a mobile network connection is still more expensive than a fixed network connection, although the elimination of wiring costs can considerably narrow this difference. A network to cover a large hospital may require 50 or more cells and several thousand mobile units, making the total cost of the network significant. These costs, however, may be attractive when compared with the

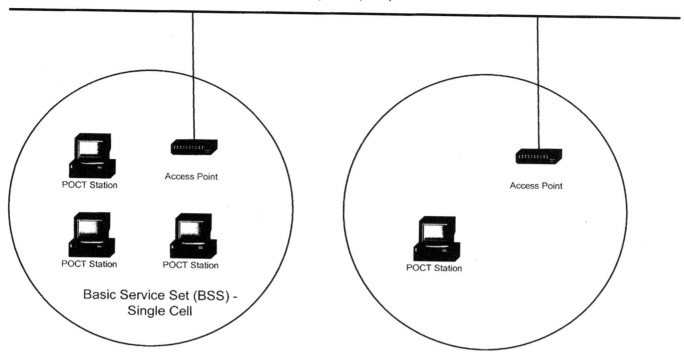

FIGURE 32.1. Topology of a wireless network. (From the Institute of Electrical and Electronic Engineers (IEEE) 802.11.)

costs for updating or installing network cabling in existing buildings. To ensure security and minimize interference, systems incorporate either a complex frequency hopping scheme (FHSS or frequency hopping spread spectrum) or broaden the bandwidth of the signal through a spreading code (DSSS or direct sequence spread spectrum). Data transmission rates are typically 1-2 megabits or 10-20% of a full Ethernet channel. Changes in the 802.11 standard ratified in 1999 modified the DSSS protocol (802.11b) (26) to operate at the theoretical limit of an 11 megabit Ethernet. Unlike more powerful devices such as cellular telephones, the low power of SSRF (<1 watt) minimizes the possibility of interference with other electronic devices in the hospital. Because of its versatility, this is almost an ideal technology for point-of-care instruments. It is likely that instruments will incorporate SSRF as such networks become more widely installed and as portable devices appear which support SSRF. For example, a version of the Palm Pilot has wireless LAN built-in. Wireless networks, however, will always be subject to interference from other RF devices, especially as distances between the access point and the mobile unit increases. This can make the actual data rates of wireless networks much lower than the maximum rated speeds, especially as the number of devices increases.

Cellular telephones, pagers, and other similar public systems provide capabilities for the user to be connected to a hospital network at distances outside the hospital campus. Like WAN,

hospitals usually purchase these capabilities from a local telecommunications supplier. A cellular modem permits a patient or care provider to be connected to a central host computer from nearly anywhere in developed countries, making this technology nearly ideal for home health care providers providing services in communities without other communications. In many metropolitan areas, service providers such as Ricochet (Metricom, San Jose, CA), provide wireless modems to the Internet for less than the cost of cellular telephone service, making this technology attractive for routine use. The data rates for such devices range from 20k to 128k bits per second depending on the location and quality of signal. Generally, data rates are unimportant with most POC data, but interruptions in communications can occur frequently with cellular systems when used under mobile conditions, and privacy can be poor unless encryption is used.

Security and Privacy

The ubiquity of networks in general and their broad accessibility through the Internet has resulted in increased concern for data security. Likewise, the increased use of data warehouses and other computerized databases has resulted in a patient concern for their privacy. Security is defined as the measures taken to keep information safe from unauthorized access or harm. Privacy or confidentiality is defined as a requirement for keeping sensitive information from being disclosed to unauthorized recipients. The Health Insurance Portability and Accountability Act of 1996 (HIPAA) (27) led to the development of regulations on patient privacy, to be enacted in spring, 2003. This law will greatly impact the responsibility of providers to secure and maintain the privacy of patient information.

Networks and information systems facilitate medical care through eliminating barriers for physicians and other patient care providers to access patient results. Unfortunately, the reduction of these barriers also permits unauthorized and malicious use of this data. A POCT device on a hospital network, for example, may be violated through a viruslike software, which changes its calibration or other functional behavior. A data management station may have its data corrupted by a malicious intruder. Messages between a data manager and its LIS host about a celebrity may be intercepted and distributed or sold to a magazine.

Proper management of privacy and security requires substantial attention to policies, procedures, and technology. Particular attention must be paid to appropriate policies and procedures. One of the most common approaches to maintaining security is the use of passwords, but poorly selected and managed passwords can be easily circumvented. Therefore, the effective use of "password technology" requires policies and procedures where users frequently change their passwords and where users select passwords not easily guessed. For example, a POCT instrument cannot protect itself against a nursing unit that decides to share a single password.

Effective privacy and security requires that these capabilities be designed into and incorporated into networks and information systems. In addition to password schemes described in the preceding section, which identify users and their permissions, networks require the use of "firewalls," or electronic barriers to intruders originating from outside. These electronic moats, of course, are less effective to attacks from the inside and add substantial complexities to the management of networks and computer systems. Monitoring systems for unexpected activities can be highly effective but require substantial expertise from skilled personnel. Across the Internet, encryption technologies must be used and are required by HIPAA. Because the Internet is an open forum, it is possible to use it for snooping of private information. In public-key encryption (PKI), the sender scrambles the information in a message before sending it using a public polynomial-based key. On receiving the message, the receiver unscrambles it with a mirrored private key and reverse polynomial. Depending on the sophistication of the polynomial and the length of the key, the effort required to unscramble a message without the key is usually beyond the capabilities of most facilities.

The greatest difficulty associated with security and privacy lies in the ever-changing boundaries of the technology. As computers have become more powerful, security measures require greater levels of sophistication. The availability of automated software on the Internet allows even high school students to penetrate well-managed systems and requires managers to constantly monitor information systems and networks. Software viruses are released daily that can attack office software systems and, incidentally, other computers. All these issues require the POCT instrument to employ technology sufficiently secure and available in most hospital and similar patient care settings and that users of such devices enact adequate policies and procedures to maintain privacy and security.

AUTOMATION, ROBOTICS, AND SYSTEMS

Automated and Robotic Workstations

Felder (28) and others have described a series of automated "near-patient" POCT devices, which may be under limited robotic control and are monitored remotely, usually by skilled technologists within the clinical laboratory. Full robotic function, where an articulated arm introduces the blood specimen into a blood–gas analyzer, has not proven cost-effective, because the robotics adds significant complexity and cost. The approach where care personnel manually inject the sample into a nearby analytical instrument, followed by remote monitoring, and remote release of results, can be implemented more economically. The proximity of the instrument near the patient and the monitoring in the laboratory meets the needs of both and eliminates the need for specimen transport. Systems are now commercially available from Medical Automation Systems (Charlottesville, VA, U.S.A.) as well as from Chiron Diagnostics (Medford, MA, U.S.A.), and Nova Biomedical (Waltham, MA, U.S.A.).

Remote Control and Remote Review

Remote control of a POCT instrument and remote review of the results prior to availability for clinical use are quite important for dealing with more complex analytic systems, such as multiparameter whole-blood chemistry analyzers and hematology cell counters. Unfortunately, most direct patient-care personnel are not attuned to verifying proper instrument function before using the results produced. Trained laboratory personnel, focused on analytic validity rather than the direct clinical application of the results, are more likely to review instrument parameters properly, check for error conditions, and confirm result validity prior to releasing the results to the clinical user. Economics precludes staffing each POCT area directly with a trained laboratory person, but their time can be effectively shared among many areas with electronic transmission of status information to the central laboratory and of authorization to release results back to the point of testing.

MANAGEMENT OF RESULTS

Emergency Notification: Standard of Care, Risks of Notification Failure, and Liability

As POCT is performed, it should be documented properly in the medical record, preferably through a real-time electronic linkage. The physician then will access that information just as he or she would access any other piece of data generated in the normal course of nursing care. Certain results, however, such as critical values, indicate the need for immediate therapeutic intervention. In such cases, the nonlaboratory personnel performing the assay may not recognize the critical nature of results, particularly if the task has been delegated to a secretary or patient care technician who may not be aware of the medical consequences of the test result. Therefore, the POCT device, or the data system to which it is linked, must recognize critical values and alert the testing staff so that they can undertake physician notification. Alternatively, it must electronically convey the results to the physician and confirm that he or she has acknowledged receipt and understanding of the significance of the result. Failure to notify places the patient at great risk and exposes the health care system to liability for failure to act. In this context, the simplest model is to ensure that the POCT device has built-in critical value checks and alerting. Of course, one is then dependent on follow-through by the testing staff actually to notify the physician. Alternatively, one must rely on a more complex, and error-prone, electronic linkage to the hospital information network and the ability of that network to notify the testing personnel with the risks as described or to transmit the alert electronically to the physician.

Protocols for Communication and Prioritization of Information

Once results have been entered into the patient's central database, values requiring immediate action must be communicated immediately to the primary physician, as discussed earlier. Many other results may be relevant for transmission, however, and patient care is facilitated by informing the physician sooner, rather than the next time he or she happens to check the patient's medical record. These benefits pertain to whether the results are produced at the bedside or by the central laboratory.

An interesting application of this approach was developed several years ago by Metriplex (Metriplex, Inc., Cambridge, MA, U.S.A., http://www.metriplex.com), who linked an electronic pager-based text messaging system with the output of the laboratory information system at Boston University Medical Center. Results fitting a profile defined by the individual physician would be transmitted to the pager as they were produced by the laboratory information system. Although this expedited patient care, and presumably permitted faster therapeutic interventions, cost justification was difficult to define and the system was not a commercial success. The product subsequently evolved to LabAlert, a system using a small handheld computer in conjunction with a pager. Other demonstrations of such systems over the years have included systems to alert house staff of probable sepsis in their patients.

The availability of low-cost numeric and alphanumeric pagers has removed some of the constraints encountered by earlier systems. Many alphanumeric paging services now accept messages via e-mail, providing information systems with even greater flexibility. Numeric-only pagers require much simpler equipment and software but are more limited. Even in automated environments, they are best suited for applications where a patient care provider is asked to call back a particular phone number because coded messages can be confusing and error prone. Another problem is that messages may be lost or delayed. With a one-way pager, the sender never knows whether the recipient has received the message. Even with the more expensive 1.5- and 2-way pagers, which acknowledge the delivery of messages, the message can be delayed until the recipient exits one of the many "dead zones" found in the typical hospital.

The greatest problem with pagers is their potential for over utilization. If a pager generates so many alerts that the recipient begins to ignore them, the paging system has lost its effectiveness. It is, therefore, critical to put filters into the messaging system adequate to meet the requirements of the recipient(s). Most notification systems today implement filters designed to support a larger practice group, often with differing requirements. This approach is costly and may result in the practitioner being unresponsive secondary to being overloaded. Setting up notification system filters should be the responsibility of the end-user. If the system operates through an e-mail system, modifications of existing e-mail filters could offer this capability. Filters designed to meet individual needs are critical. For example, a neurologist chooses to dose a particular patient with an anticonvulsant at above the laboratory's critical level and does not want to be paged. He or she, however, desires to be paged if the serum level is 10 mg above the laboratory's critical level. On other patients, the neurologist would like to be paged using the laboratory's critical values. Such a protocol allows notification protocols to be individualized down to a physician–patient combination. Some information systems are able to implement even more notification schemes through rules-based logic (see next section).

Motorola (Schaumburg, IL) and Eclipsys (Delray Beach, FL) are marketing their DocLink software package, which takes a much more comprehensive view of the provider notification task. Built around a detailed database of every provider's calendar, coverage schedule, and details of how to contact each provider at various times of the day, it is fed by alerts originating in a patient care system, which in turn also may have logic filters based on other patient data. The system triages alerts, based on criteria in the message, defined by the organization, and by the individual provider, so that less urgent ones can be communicated to ancillary staff. For urgent alerts, the system repeatedly attempts to contact designated persons until acknowledgment is received. If the primary on-call person has not responded in a defined window of time, the backup person is contacted. The system provides alerts through devices already in common use, such as pagers, faxes, e-mails, telephones, and voice mails. When sending alerts to devices with two-way capability, such as telephones, two-way pagers, and fax machines, receipt acknowledgment and closure of an alert can be monitored automatically. When alerts are sent to one-way devices, such as a typical pager, the recipient can respond to the system via telephone or e-mail to provide receipt acknowledgment and alert closure. The capability to monitor receipt acknowledgment and alert closure has significant benefit in critical cases.

Facilitated Interpretation of Test Results and the Role of Expert Systems

Many information system vendors have incorporated capabilities to execute user-defined algorithms, a series of tasks executed according to a predetermined set of rules. These algorithms can be used to establish best-practice guidelines by providing feedback to the ordering clinician about test utilization, test interpretation, and so on and to perform certain actions, such as follow-up testing or physician notification of results. Most current "rules logic" capabilities are based on the ability to look at one or more previous results and the tests being ordered. Vendors frequently describe the capability of an information system to execute these "best-practice" algorithms as an expert system. LIS reporting also can be augmented by rules logic by adding comments to the clinician based on the results of tests performed by the laboratory.

Rules logic can eliminate unnecessary testing, such as by making previous results available, by informing the clinician of the meaning of test results, or by blocking tests being ordered for improper indications. Most POCT instruments have limited, if any, storage for old results and cannot implement algorithms. Such capabilities could be made available at the POCT instrument through a wireless connection to a server computer programmed with appropriate algorithms. Rules logic also can be used for informing clinicians of unusual or life-endangering conditions through a device such as an alphanumeric pager. Optimally, these rules should be customized to an individual physician's practice patterns. Unfortunately, the maintenance issues associated with managing hundreds of rules can be difficult in a large, dynamic environment. Even a few requests from each resident in a large training facility can overwhelm the staff responsible for entering these rules.

One way to overcome this problem is to allow individual physicians to enter their own rules for notification. Although most current systems require the maintenance to be performed on a large host system, future systems could be designed so that physicians could tailor filters on their own PDAs as the need arises. Maintenance also can be minimized through the development of rules common to a larger practice group. The implementation and management of these computer-based rules are administratively and technically complex. For example, practitioners should not be able to modify rules associated with "guidelines and best practices," but should be allowed to add their own nonconflicting filters. The type of filters permitted also should be coupled to the experience and expertise of the practitioner. It is not clear that a computer can determine these differences. Likewise, the power of such rules-based systems for reducing errors and improving patient care, when coupled with technologies such as wireless networks, are impressive. We are just beginning to explore a rich and highly complex area.

CONCLUSIONS

- Point-of-care instrumentation offers tremendous advantages in providing the end user with the ability to perform testing when and where it is needed and without the constraints of a centralized service.
- Instrumentation often is designed without consideration to information management.
- With the advent of the electronic medical record and record-keeping regulations, users are demanding that POCT data be downloaded to them.
- The availability of portable hand computers and PDAs, evolving wireless data networks, and connectivity standards should help to reduce the difficulty of portable devices to communicate with information systems.
- The ubiquity of the Internet and data networks, the economic pressures for data warehouses, and the need for electronic medical records to improve patient care will strongly conflict with the demand for patient privacy and data security.
- Improving the ability of the point-of-care instrument to link to information systems will ultimately expand its place in the health care arena.

REFERENCES

1. Kost, GJ. Connectivity, the millennium challenge for point-of-care testing. *Arch Pathol Lab Med* 2000;124:1108–1110.
2. Kohn LT, Corrigan JM, Donaldson MS, eds. *To err is human: building a safer health system.* Washington, DC: National Academy Press, 2000.
3. American Society for Testing and Materials. ASTM E1381-95. Standard specification for low-level protocol to transfer messages between clinical laboratory instruments and computer systems. In: *2000 Annual book of ASTM standards: Health care informatics; computerized systems and chemical and material information.* Vol 14.01.West Conshohocken, PA: ASTM, 2000.
4. ASTM E1394-97. Standard specification for transferring information between clinical instruments and computer systems. In: *2000 annual book of ASTM standards, health care informatics; computerized systems and chemical and material information.* Vol 14.01. West Conshohocken, PA: ASTM, 2000.
5. Forrey AW, McDonald CJ, DeMoor G, et al. Logical observation identifier names and codes (LOINC) database: a public use set of codes and names for electronic reporting of clinical laboratory test results. *Clin Chem* 1996;42:81–90. LOINC information is also available at: http://www.regenstrief.org/loinc/. Accessed December 12, 2001.
6. Bakken S, Cimino JJ, Haskell R, et al. Evaluation of the clinical LOINC (Logical Observation Identifiers, Names, and Codes) semantic structure as a terminology model for standardized assessment measures. *J Am Med Inform Assoc* 2000;7:529–538.
7. McDonald C, Overhage JM, Dexter PR, et al. The Regenstrief Medical Record System 1999: sharing data between hospitals. *Proc AMIA Annu Fall Symp* 1999;1–2:1212.
8. Dick RS, Steen EB, Detmer DE, eds. *The computer-based patient record: an essential technology for health care,* revised edition. Washington, DC: National Academy Press, 1997.
9. Sen A, Jacob VS, eds. Industrial-strength data warehousing. *Comm of ACM* 1998;41:28–69.
10. Fayyad U, Uthurusamy R, eds. Data mining and knowledge discovery in databases. *Comm of ACM* 1996;39:24–68.
11. Pickering C. *Survey of advanced technology—1996.* Overland Park, KS: Systems Development, 1996.
12. Meta Group. Survey of 1242 projects in 1996 and 915 projects in 1997. *Computerworld* 1998;32:51.
13. American Society for Testing and Materials (ASTM) E1466-92. Standard specification for use of bar codes on specimen tubes in the clinical laboratory. In: *2000 annual book of ASTM standards, health care informatics; computerized systems and chemical and material information.* West Conshohocken, PA: ASTM, 2000.
14. Chou D, Davis R, Moss PS, et al. *Laboratory automation: bar codes for specimen container identification; approved standard.* Vol 18. Wayne, PA: NCCLS, 2000.
15. Beeler GW, Rishel W, Shakir AMS, et al. and the HL7 Modeling and Methodology Committee. *HL7, version 3: message development framework, 1998.* Available at: http://www.mcis.duke.edu/standards/HL7/pubs/version3/Version3.htm as mdfv3_1.zip. Accessed December 12, 2001.
16. American Society for Testing and Materials (ASTM) E1238-97. Standard specification for transferring clinical observations between independent computer systems. In: *2000 Annual book of ASTM*

standards, health care informatics; computerized systems and chemical and material information. Vol 14.01. West Conshohocken, PA: ASTM, 2000.

17. DuBois JA, Dunka L, Alfred T, et al. Point-of-care connectivity: approved standard, vol. 21. Wayne, PA, NCCLS, 2001.
18. Elevitch FR. Multimedia communications networks: patient care through interactive point-of-care testing. *Clin Lab Med* 1994;14: 559–567.9.
19. Friedman B, Mitchell W. Horizontal and vertical integration in hospital laboratories and the laboratory information system. *Clin Lab Med* 1990;10:627–641.
20. Comer DE. *Internetworking with TCPIP: principles, protocols, and architecture*, 2nd ed. Englewood Cliffs, NJ: Prentice-Hall, 1991.
21. Schatz BR, Hardin JB. NCSA mosaic and the World Wide Web: global hypermedia protocols for the Internet. *Science* 1994;265:895–901.
22. Waldrop MM. Software agents to prepare to sift the riches of cyberspace. *Science* 1994;265:882–883.
23. Connelly DP, Sielaff BH, Willard KE. A clinician's workstation for improving laboratory use: integrated display of laboratory results. *Am J Clin Pathol* 1995;104:243–252.
24. Jacobs E. Information integration for point-of-care and satellite testing. In: Kost GJ, ed. *Handbook of clinical automation, robotics, and optimization.* New York: John Wiley, 1996:620–630.
25. Pahlavan K. Trends in wireless networks. *IEEE Communications* 1995: 99–108.
26. ISO/IEC 8802-11: 1999 (ANSI/IEEE Std 802.11, 1999 ed.). Information Technology - Telecommunications and Information Exchange between Systems—Local and Metropolitan Area Network Specific Requirements Part 11: Wireless LAN Medium Access Control (MAC) and Physical Layer (PHY) Specifications, 1999.
27. Standards for privacy of individually identifiable health information. Final rule (45 CFR, parts 160 and 164). *Federal Register* 2000;65: 82461–82829.
28. Felder R. Robotic automation of near-patient testing. In: Kost GJ, ed. *Handbook of clinical automation, robotics, and optimization.* New York: John Wiley, 1996:596–619.

33

INFORMATION SYSTEMS FOR POINT-OF-CARE TESTING IN CRITICAL CARE

KENNETH E. BLICK
NEIL A. HALPERN

Critical care medicine clinicians consistently seek to diagnose, treat, and monitor acutely ill patients in an efficient and effective manner. Therefore, intensivists focus on the expedient identification and correction of common acute acid–base, electrolyte, hematologic, coagulation, and cardiac disorders observed in the intensive care unit (ICU). This situation places an ever-increasing stress on the central laboratory to facilitate rapid laboratory evaluation of samples sent from critically ill patients. Indeed, most critical care clinicians feel that the therapeutic turnaround-time (TTAT) for urgently needed laboratory results is slow. Furthermore, intensivists perceive that the value of critical care laboratory data depreciates quite rapidly. When ICU receipt of testing results is delayed, the data become "historical" and do not yield immediate diagnostic and therapeutic significance (1–3).

THE INFORMATION AGE OF LABORATORY MEDICINE

Laboratories are entering the "information age" of laboratory medicine. In the past, laboratory testing was technically difficult and was performed only by highly trained technologists. The laboratory focused more on the analytic aspects of the testing process rather than on the true clinical value of laboratory information. Today, using highly automated and computerized laboratory instruments, "doing the test" in many cases has become the easiest, most controlled aspect of the testing process (4). Problems in test performance have been replaced with challenges in improving information management (5).

THE CENTRAL LABORATORY: HIGH-TECHNOLOGY SOLUTIONS

Central hospital laboratories are overwhelmed by the concomitant receipt of routine and STAT ("statim," that is, urgent or emergency) samples from critical care and noncritical care areas. The central laboratory's inability to sort, process, and deliver, effectively and expediently, these results in a predictable and reliable time frame has supported the clinicians' perception that the central laboratory is inefficient. Clinicians attempt to overcome the slow TTAT by "up-coding" most ICU requests to STAT priority, thereby causing the laboratory to encounter further difficulties in identifying and handling the true STAT requests and additionally exacerbating the problem. The central laboratory may not recognize or fully appreciate the need of the clinical caregivers for the rapid availability of testing results. Laboratory staff members are oriented to laboratory analyses and not to clinical imperatives. The central laboratory is also buffered from clinical pressures because it is physically isolated from the patient care areas. The solution to these problems requires a total revamping of the traditional clinical laboratory model and a sophisticated approach to laboratory informatics (6,7) (Table 33.1).

TABLE 33.1. THE RAPID RESPONSE AUTOMATED CENTRAL LABORATORY WITH POCT

Redesign of central laboratory from multisection model to an integrated model

Implementation of "rapid response" system through full computerization and automation of specimen collection, specimen transport, front-end specimen receiving, analyzers, and results reporting

Incorporation of whole blood analyzers for commonly requested STAT testing

Enhancement of the LIS with universal connectivity and interfaces that conform to industry standards and address laboratory and client needs

Integration of the latest advances in wired and wireless communications technology directly into the LIS for near "real-time" results reporting (auto-fax, auto-page, e-mail, PDA)

Decentralize high volume routine type, critical care testing to nonlaboratory clinical locations (POCT) under the auspices of the central laboratory

POCT, point of care testing; STAT, statim; LIS, laboratory information service; PDA, personal data assistant.

THE RAPID-RESPONSE LABORATORY

In many cities, hospital-based laboratory services are being forced to reevaluate their missions as hospitals merge to form health care networks. Such hospital groups are perceived to confer economic advantages on the member hospitals (8,9). As a result of these mergers, large network laboratories have been formed that are designed to serve the entire network of hospitals for noncritical laboratory testing. Individual hospitals are therefore shifting their focus to developing rapid-response laboratories for on-site testing.

Whether a hospital-based central laboratory is encountering network challenges or not, the central laboratory must effectively address the pressing clinical needs of the clinicians. This can be accomplished by either redesigning the entire central laboratory into a rapid response testing facility or by establishing a rapid response area. In the rapid response model, STAT tests are performed expeditiously, with short and predictable TTAT. Importantly, the members of the rapid-response laboratory team develop an understanding of the testing demands of the critically ill and are thus able to accommodate emergent clinical testing circumstances appropriately.

LABORATORY INFORMATION SYSTEM

At the same time that the central laboratory process is being improved, concomitant process enhancements in the laboratory information system (LIS) must be implemented to permit the LIS to manage effectively the reformatted central laboratory and interact with clinical users (10). The LIS must be fully capable of tracking the specimen for the entirety of the testing process and displaying the testing status immediately on request. Improvements in the LIS must be accompanied by the redesign of hospital locations at the sites where testing orders are entered into the hospital information system (HIS) and samples are obtained and prepared for transport. Workstations in these clinical areas must be upgraded to facilitate test ordering, and barcode devices must be installed to generate labels that communicate demographic, test processing, and billing information for laboratory specimens. The LIS always must address patient confidentiality and associated "firewall" security issues especially when the Internet or intranets are used to send and receive specimen orders and patient results.

POINT-OF-CARE TESTING

Regardless of the efficacy and success of the rapid-response laboratory model described in the preceding section, bottlenecks in specimen processing may occur, and the TTAT of STAT critical care specimens still may be considered suboptimal by intensivists. A potential solution is to decentralize the portion of the central laboratory test processing that is routinely ordered and emergently needed for patients in critical care locales (ICU, perioperative settings, and emergency departments) to the patient care area itself (11–14). This paradigm is known as point-of-care testing (POCT). Other terminology used to describe POCT includes near-patient testing, distributed or decentralized testing, point-of-care or immediate-care diagnostics, ancillary testing, and alternate-site testing. In POCT, the local staff (nurses, physicians, and respiratory therapists) will perform the testing at or within the general vicinity of the patient's bedside. POCT provides for real-time testing with immediate availability of the results, thus facilitating diagnosis, therapy, and ongoing monitoring.

A technical revolution has facilitated the development and utilization of POCT. Reliable miniaturized biosensors that analyze whole blood are now economically produced. POCT instruments have become more compact and are operated using configurable, menu-driven, and user-friendly software. Through these advances, bedside clinical staff can be easily educated to operate POCT devices successfully despite a lack of formal laboratory training. Central laboratories themselves have procured POCT-type devices for use within their own rapid-response areas because of their ease of use and ability to process whole blood rapidly. Of course, POCT has been welcomed into critical care settings (15–17).

Point-of-Care Testing Devices

A general overview of the commercially available POCT devices is important both for understanding the intricacies of the devices and for determining their information needs. POCT devices can be described as analyzers or monitors (Fig. 33.1). Analyzers use biosensor technology to measure analytes on whole blood that has been *permanently* removed from the patient. Monitors, in contrast, measure analytes on blood *not permanently* removed from the vascular tree. Typical POCT analytes include blood gases, electrolytes, glucose, hematologic and coagulation parameters, cardiac markers, as well as medication levels. Some emergency departments include POCT for pregnancy evaluation, urine analysis, and toxicology.

Data Management Systems in Point-of-Care Testing

Information management is a crucial component of a successfully planned and implemented POCT program (18–28). Central laboratories interface their laboratory instruments to commercially available LISs. If POCT-type devices are stationed within the central laboratory, these devices are likewise directly interfaced to the LIS.

Commercially available LISs are designed to connect, interface, and manage data for stationary laboratory instruments used by trained technicians. The LIS is not easily capable of connecting, interfacing, and managing data for POCT devices that are located in multiple clinical sites and used by a myriad of clinically focused personnel. Therefore, data management systems (DMS) designed specifically for POCT to address the unique issues that arise with broadly distributed and used POCT devices have been developed.

The DMS must include a tracking system for the POCT devices and their disposable and time-limited components (cal-

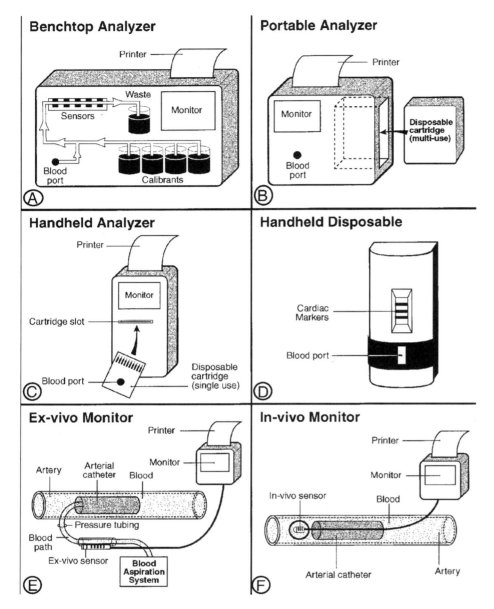

FIGURE 33.1. Point-of-care testing (POCT) analyzers and monitors. Whereas POCT analyzers vary in size and configuration, the essential components of a POCT analyzer are similar. These include a sample port, biosensors, calibration solutions, a waste containment system, and a monitor and printer to display results. The essential components are included in the chassis of the analyzer (benchtop analyzer) (**A**), within a multiuse disposable cartridge (portable/midsize analyzer) (**B**), on a single-use disposable cartridge (handheld analyzer) (**C**), or within a wholly disposable self-contained unit (handheld disposable analyzer) (**D**). The primary analytic component of the POCT monitors is a multi-biosensor array. The biosensor array may be inserted within pressure tubing attached to an indwelling intravascular catheter but external to the patient (extracorporeal or *ex vivo*) (**E**), or it may be inserted through an indwelling intravascular catheter (intracorporeal or *in vivo*) (**F**). (From *Critical Care Clinics.* Philadelphia: WB Saunders, October 2000, pg. 625.)

ibration solutions, biosensors, POCT cartridges) and for maintenance and repair events. DMS software configurations must include connectivity and bidirectional interfacing of the POCT devices to the LIS or HIS (Fig. 33.2), remote supervision of the POCT devices, and maintenance of a consolidated POCT database. Other DMS features must focus on management of the quality control program, generation of reports, and short- and long-term storage of results.

Because many users will be using the POCT devices, the DMS must be able to collect data on the individual users and to help them as needed. The DMS should have configurable programming that proactively assists the users in recognizing and correcting problems that occur during the performance of quality control. Algorithms that rapidly identify highly abnormal results or results that differ greatly from prior trends should prompt corrective actions and should be included in the DMS.

The DMS should also have a user-configured autovalidation (autoverification) feature. DMS can be purchased directly from the POCT vendor or from a third party (Table 33.2).

Point-of-Care Testing Connectivity

The POCT devices can be connected to the DMS, LIS, and HIS using various techniques of connectivity (modem, direct serial, Ethernet wired and wireless). Regardless of the precise connection method used, optimal connectivity relies on the linkage of POCT devices to the DMS and the subsequent DMS connection to the LIS or HIS (29) (Fig. 33.2). The DMS can be located in the POCT area or within the central laboratory. There are several options for longitudinal connectivity (Fig. 33.3).

POCT connectivity using direct cabling is cumbersome and modem connections are slow. A preferred route of data transfer

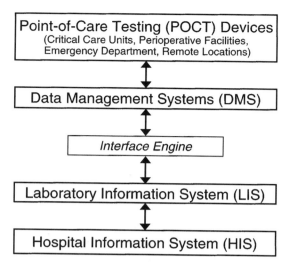

Point-of-Care Testing (POCT) Devices
(Critical Care Units, Perioperative Facilities,
Emergency Department, Remote Locations)

Data Management Systems (DMS)

Interface Engine

Laboratory Information System (LIS)

Hospital Information System (HIS)

FIGURE 33.2. Point-of-care testing (POCT) connectivity and interfaces. The optimal paradigm for POCT devices used in point-of-care environments is to have the POCT devices connected and interfaced with a data management system (DMS). The DMS then forwards the POCT data to the laboratory information system (LIS). These data are subsequently transmitted to the hospital information system. An interface engine (Instrument Manager, Data Innovations, South Burlington, VT, U.S.A., www.datainnovations.com; or ResultsNet System, Dawning Technologies, Fairport, NY, U.S.A., www.dawning.com) may be required to accept data in nonstandard streams from the DMS and convert these data to protocols acceptable to the LIS or hospital information system.

is the hospital intranet with the assignment of Transmission Control Protocol/Internet Protocol (TCP/IP) addresses to POCT devices or DMS workstations. Wireless transmission from the POCT device to the DMS has been used but requires the installation of wireless nodes and transmission hubs that take into account existing wireless frequencies as well as physical barriers that may impede optimal wireless transmission.

Handheld POCT devices pose a special connectivity challenge because of their ubiquitous distribution and continuously moving presence throughout an institution (Fig. 33.4). Device connection and data transfer from handheld devices are facilitated through their placement in docking stations or cradles. There are many methods of linking the docking station to the DMS and transmitting data; one must consult with each vendor for the supported approaches (Table 33.2).

Point-of-Care Testing Interfaces

Beyond successful POCT connectivity, interfacing protocols are required to transmit information from POCT devices or POCT-DMS workstations to the LIS or HIS. Some hospitals choose not to interface their POCT systems to the LIS or HIS. Without this interface, data will not reach the LIS or HIS unless the POCT data are manually entered. Manual data entry is quite personnel intensive, inefficient, time consuming, and fraught with the possibility for serious errors in data entry. In the best of manual-entry circumstances, only an indeterminate quantity of POCT data will ever reach the HIS and electronic medical record (EMR).

There are two levels of POCT interfaces (Fig. 33.2). First, the POCT device must be interfaced with the DMS. This interface usually is not complicated, and the transfer and receipt of information are quite simple if both the POCT device and the DMS are purchased from the same vendor. The challenge for successful data transfer exists in the second level of interfacing, when the DMS of one vendor is connected to the LIS or HIS of second and third parties. Interface protocols include industry standards [American Society for Testing and Materials (ASTM) or Health Level 7 (HL-7)] or proprietary interfaces. Proprietary interfaces are generated by a combined effort of the POCT-DMS, LIS, and HIS vendors and the hospital. All interfaces must be updated periodically.

TABLE 33.2. POCT DATA MANAGEMENT SYSTEMS

POCT and POCT DMS Solution Companies[a]	Data Management Systems	Web Sites
Abbott Diagnostics (Abbott Park, IL)	QC Manager/Precision Net	www.abbottdiagnostics.com
Philips Medical Systems (Andover, MA)	IRMA Data Management System (IDMS)	www3.medical.philips.com
Bayer (Medfield, MA)	Rapidlink Critical Care-POC Information Management System	www.bayerdiag.com
Biosite Diagnostics (San Diego, CA)	Triage Census Data Management Software	www.biosite.com
Diametrics Medical (Roseville, MN)	IRMA Data Management System (IDMS)	www.diametrics.com
Instrumentation Laboratory (Lexington, MA)	IMPACT for Critical Care	www.ilww.com
International Technidyne (Edison, NJ)	Hemochron Response Data Manager	www.itcmed.com
i-STAT (Princeton, NJ)	Central Data Station	www.istat.com
Lifescan (Milpitas, CA)	DataLink Data Management System	www.lifescan.com
Medical Automation Systems[a] (Charlottesville, VA)	RALS-Plus (Remote Automated Laboratory System)	www.medicalautomation.com
Medtronic (Parker, CO)	Interact Data Management	www.medtronic.com
Nova Biomedical (Waltham, MA)	Patient Data Management System	www.novabiomedical.com
PharmaNetics (Raleigh, NC)	Rapidlink Critical Care Information Management System	www.pharmanetics.com
Radiometer America, Inc. (Westlake, OH)	RADIANCE STAT Analyzer Management System	www.radiometer.com
Roche Diagnostics (Indianapolis, IN)	CoaguChek Pro/DM	www.roche.com/diagnostics
Roche Diagnostics (Indianapolis, IN)	Roche DataCare POC Critical Care Information Management System	
Telcor (Lincoln, NE)	Quick-Suite	www.telcorinc.com

POCT, point of care testing; DMS, data management system.

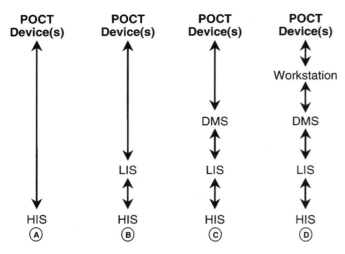

FIGURE 33.3. Longitudinal models of point-of-care testing (POCT) connectivity and interfaces. There are multiple configurations for linking POCT devices to the laboratory information system (LIS) and hospital information system (HIS). These include direct connections and interfaces of POCT to HIS (**A**), POCT to LIS and then to the HIS (**B**), POCT to DMS and then to LIS and HIS (**C**), or attaching multiple POCT devices to a DMS workstation and linking the workstations to the DMS and then subsequently to the LIS and HIS (**D**).

A common approach to the DMS to LIS interface focuses on using a scripted interface, otherwise known as *terminal emulation* (18,30). In the scripted interface, the DMS invokes a program that *imitates* the entire process of test requisitioning (Table 33.3) and passes the POCT data from the DMS into the LIS using prescripted steps and emulating keyboard entry as on a LIS terminal.

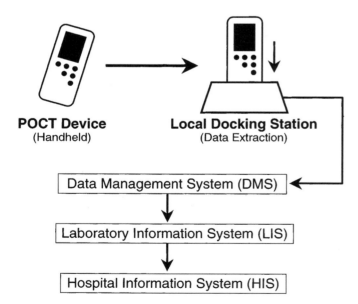

FIGURE 33.4. Handheld point-of-care testing (POCT) devices. Handheld POCT devices usually are connected to the information systems [data management system (DMS), laboratory information system (LIS), hospital information system (HIS)] through placement in a local docking stations. The data then travels from the handheld unit to the local docking station and onto the DMS, LIS, and HIS. Data are transferred within the docking station by wireless or direct connections.

TABLE 33.3. SCRIPTED INTERFACE FUNCTIONS

Identifies the patient
Orders the test
Assigns date and time of POCT
Verifies POCT results
Forwards results to clients in real-time
Reports results on daily cumulative report for review
Transmits results to HIS
Bills and gathers statistical data

POCT, point of care testing; HIS, hospital information system.

The downside to such script emulation interfaces is that changes to the LIS and its data-entry screens during periodic LIS upgrades usually necessitates an update to the scripted interface. Otherwise, script interfaces work very well and are a relatively inexpensive and trouble-free approach to POCT interfacing.

More sophisticated electronic, nonscript-based interfaces between DMS and LIS have been developed as well. These interfaces are bidirectional, with the LIS or HIS supplying patient demographic information and the DMS obtaining a test accession number (or order number) through automatic host query options. The DMS then links the laboratory results obtained from the POCT device with the patients' records and transmits this data to the LIS or HIS.

At times, an interface engine, sometimes known as a *universal translator*, is inserted between the DMS and LIS or HIS. Interface engines accept data from an instrument or DMS in any format or protocol and convert it to standard languages acceptable to the LIS and HIS (ASTM or HL-7) or into a proprietary format (Fig. 33.2). The great advantage to using such products is that they can be modified to work with virtually any laboratory device, DMS, LIS, and HIS. This broad capability adds stability to the POCT data management infrastructure even as individual components are upgraded or replaced. The disadvantage to an interface engine is that interface problems requiring vendor support can result in "finger pointing" between the vendors that support the POCT instruments, the interface engine, and the LIS and HIS.

An institution may have several POCT systems, each with its own DMS. In this scenario, every one of the DMS to LIS interfaces must be separately written and monitored (Fig. 33.5A). A single DMS interface solution that connects and interfaces with the various POCT platforms and the LIS may be far more preferable (Fig. 33.5B). The single DMS–LIS interface facilitates data management and maintenance of a common POCT database and minimizes training and support issues involved in hardware, software, connectivity, and interfaces. Importantly, informatics resources are concentrated on one, rather than on multiple, DMS to LIS or HIS interfaces. Specific POCT vendors may produce DMSs that are compatible with their own POCT products and those of other manufacturers. At present, to our knowledge, there are two independent DMS vendors (RALS-Plus, Medical Automation Systems, Charlottesville, VA, U.S.A.; and Quick Suite, Telcor, Lincoln, NE, U.S.A.) that specialize in POCT-DMS solutions (Table 33.2) that support a vast array of POCT devices and provide for connectivity and interfaces with LIS or HIS (Table 33.2).

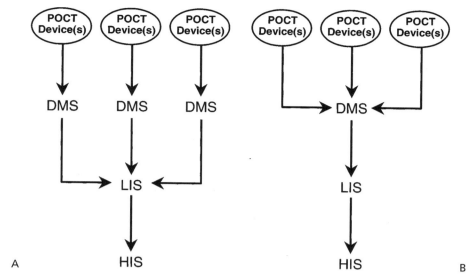

FIGURE 33.5. Point-of-care testing (POCT) and data management system (DMS) integration. POCT devices from different manufacturers each can be linked to the laboratory information system (LIS) through their own proprietary DMSs (**A**). Alternatively, each of the disparate POCT devices can be linked through one DMS that is designed to support, connect, and interface POCT devices from multiple vendors (**B**). The data then are transmitted from the single DMS using one interface to the LIS or hospital information system.

Intensive Care Unit–Point-of-Care Testing Bedside Connectivity and Interfaces

Throughout the hospital, POCT devices may be used in a stand-alone manner without being connected or interfaced, or the POCT devices may be connected and interfaced to the DMS or LIS using standard techniques of connectivity and interfacing. Within the critical care environment, POCT devices also may be directly connected to, or integral components of, the ICU bedside physiologic monitoring system (Fig. 33.6). This scenario offers many technical challenges in connectivity and interfacing (31,32). Monitoring vendors have taken various approaches to integrating their own or third-party POCT devices to bedside physiologic monitoring systems (Fig. 33.6).

Currently, POCT data are displayed on bedside physiologic monitors, provided the POCT devices are directly connected to them. Whether or not the POCT data are subsequently managed, archived, or further transmitted to a DMS, LIS, or HIS depends on the answers to the following questions. Is the bedside physiologic monitoring network connected and interfaced with a POCT-DMS, LIS, or HIS? Has a critical care clinical information system (CIS) been instituted that manages all the monitoring system data, including POCT data? Is the CIS connected to the DMS, LIS, or HIS (33)? The ultimate goal for POCT devices that are connected to the ICU bedside system is for the POCT data to be automatically transmitted to the LIS or HIS; however, this goal is rarely achieved today.

CONNECTIVITY STANDARDS

Over the years, many organizations that develop standards have set out to create standards for POCT network architecture, device connectivity, and data transfer. These include the American National Standards Institute (ANSI, New York, NY, U.S.A.; *www.ansi.org*), International Organization for Standardization (ISO, Geneva, Switzerland; *www.iso.ch*), the Institute of Electrical and Electronic Engineers (IEEE, New York, NY, U.S.A.; *www.ieee.org*), American Society for Testing and Materials (ASTM, West Conshohocken, PA, U.S.A.; *www.astm.org*) and Health Level Seven, Inc. (HL-7, Ann Arbor, MI, U.S.A.; *www.hl7.org*). As standards improve and instrument interfaces become more "plug-and-play," connecting and interfacing POCT systems should become less challenging. The new POCT standard entitled POCT 1-A, Point-of-Care Connectivity, Approved Standard is available at the website of the National Committee for Clinical Laboratory Standards (NCCLS) www.nccls.org.

Point-of-Care Testing Politics and Hospital Policies

Practical and political barriers may exist to the development of an institution-wide POCT informatics infrastructure. These obstacles usually originate in the manner that POCT emerges within an institution. Informatics suffers when POCT is introduced by clinical services because the central laboratory and the information technology department have commonly not participated in the POCT process and a coordinated strategy for information management does not exist. In contrast, when the central laboratory institutes POCT on its own, or partners with clinical services, the related informatics concerns of connectivity and interfacing usually are well addressed (21,29,34). A host of informatics issues that occur in the POCT paradigm are not encountered when samples are sent to and processed in the traditional manner in the central laboratory and the results are transmitted to the LIS and HIS.

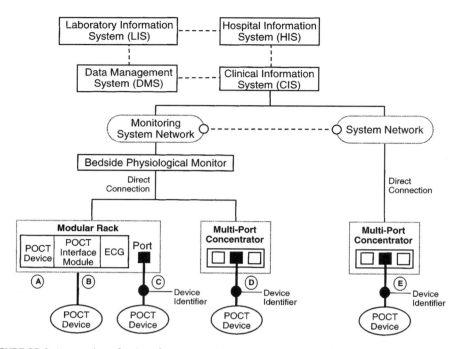

FIGURE 33.6. Integration of point-of-care testing (POCT) devices to bedside intensive care unit monitoring systems. POCT data may be transmitted directly into the bedside psychologic monitor using modular or data port connections. In the first modular option, the POCT device is constructed as a POCT module (**A**) and inserted into the modular rack (BAM Blood Analysis Module, Philips Medical Systems, Andover, MA, U.S.A., www3.medical.philips.com). In the second modular application, the bedside POCT device is attached via cable to a POCT data recipient module (**B**) (VueLink, Philips Medical Systems). POCT devices can be linked directly to the bedside monitor through a data port located on the modular rack (**C**) (Flexport Interface, SpaceLabs Medical, Redmond, WA, U.S.A., www.spacelabs.com) or on a multiport concentrator (**D**) [Octanet, GE Medical Systems (Marquette) Milwaukee, WI, U.S.A., www.gemedicalsystems.com]. A device identifier cable attached to the POCT device alerts the data port to the identification and specifications of the POCT device and its data stream. Alternatively, POCT devices can be linked to multiport concentrators (**E**) [Octacomm, GE Medical Systems (Marquette) or Device Link, Philips Medical Systems] that reside on networks parallel to the standard bedside monitoring networks. The bedside monitoring network may be managed by a clinical information system (CIS) and interfaced to the hospital information system (HIS). The parallel system network of multiport concentrators (not connected to the bedside monitor) may also be linked to the clinical information system. POCT data may flow through the CIS to the laboratory information system (LIS) or HIS. A POCT data management system may exist on the network to facilitate POCT data management and subsequent connectivity and interfaces to the LIS or HIS. The specifics of data flow in each system must be investigated with the monitoring system vendor.

Physicians' Orders for Point-of-Care Testing

Central laboratory testing always requires a physician's order. Practically speaking, however, in POCT, a physician's order is not required to perform the laboratory test and to obtain the result. The physician's order for POCT even may be considered by the clinical staff to be an unnecessary task. Hospital POCT policy must address whether a physician's order will be necessary for POCT. The elimination of the physician's order step does have practical consequences if the data are to be transmitted to the LIS or HIS. If the physician's order is not input into the LIS, an accession number is not issued, and the LIS is not aware that a POCT specimen will be processed and resultant data will be forthcoming. The lack of an order also may cause difficulty in complying with regulatory requirements for medical necessity, reimbursement, and coding. A "no POCT physician's order" policy may function well, as long as the DMS is connected and interfaced with the LIS or HIS, and the order or order equivalent is generated (scripted or electronic), thereby compensating for the "missing" order and creating an accession number for the specimen result.

Data Management and Data Management System Location

Central laboratory testing devices and results are always managed according to accepted laboratory standards using an LIS. Various approaches are used in relation to the management of POCT data. Currently, there are many POCT sites that do not transmit the POCT data to a DMS for management. Optimally, POCT data should be managed in a manner similar to testing data generated by the central laboratory.

Once it is agreed within a hospital community that POCT data must be managed, the next step is to determine the appropriate physical location for the POCT-DMS workstations. Options include placing the DMS workstation within the central laboratory, at the remote POCT sites, or in both locations. If the DMS is placed within the central laboratory, the central laboratory will feel ownership responsibility for POCT. The central laboratory technicians will continuously monitor the POCT network, review and verify results, authorize transmission of POCT data to the LIS or HIS, and inform POCT users of device or quality control problems. Alternatively, if the DMS is located within the remote POCT area, outside the central laboratory, the local users and supervisors should closely follow the POCT program, monitor problems as delineated by the DMS, and oversee transmission of data to the LIS or HIS.

The central laboratory validates (verifies) testing data prior to distribution to the LIS or HIS. This process originated years ago, when testing was technically difficult. The POCT group must decide whether the POCT process is similar to central laboratory analyses and even requires test validation prior to LIS or HIS distribution. Possibly, POCT data may not require validation. POCT systems are considered quite reliable. Moreover, POCT data already were acted on by the bedside caregivers as soon as the data were displayed on the POCT device; so validation may be considered a moot point. The validation issue, however, can be resolved easily using autovalidation algorithms present in most DMSs.

Point-of-Care Testing Result Integration to and Portrayal on the Laboratory Information Systems and Hospital Information Systems

Central laboratory data are transmitted to the LIS, HIS, and EMR and constitute the majority of data within the laboratory sections of the HIS and EMR. Central laboratories also are located away from the patients' bedsides; thus, data distribution to the LIS or HIS is mandatory if the clinicians are to see the testing results. Perhaps POCT data differ from central laboratory testing data in regard to these two issues and do not need to be integrated into the HIS or EMR. First, POCT data, at best, constitute only a small portion of laboratory data during a hospital stay. Second, POCT data are already available and are used within the patient's immediate vicinity without transmission to the LIS or HIS.

Recent nonpublished surveys of hospitals using POCT indicate that less than 10% of the hospitals are even transmitting POCT data to the patient's EMR, where it can be integrated with laboratory data generated in the central laboratory. We believe that the HIS or EMR is incomplete without containing all the laboratory data that were used to decide patient care, regardless of whether the data were produced by the central laboratory or POCT (18–20,24–27). Occasionally, there are objections by the central laboratorians to integrating POCT data into the LIS because they note that the POCT data were not generated directly by their own carefully supervised and regulated central laboratory personnel. Our suggestion is that the central laboratory should expand its base of operations to include control and monitoring of all POCT to alleviate these problems.

Attention also must be placed on the manner in which POCT data are portrayed in the LIS and HIS display screens and printouts. Should POCT data be identified distinctly as POCT in origin, or should the POCT data not be differentiated from data submitted by the central laboratory? If the POCT data are specifically identified as POCT, then the POCT test location and possibly the clinical service affiliation of the POCT testing personnel (nursing, respiratory therapy, and physicians) should be noted. POCT-specific reference ranges also should be appended to the POCT results because these results may differ from traditional central laboratory testing ranges. POCT data can be longitudinally integrated among the other central laboratory data to allow for trending views. Alternatively, POCT data can be grouped separately under a POCT banner.

Point-of-Care Testing Data from the Intensive Care Unit Bedside Monitoring System

Central laboratory instruments are not integrated into the equipment at the patient's bedside. POCT devices, however, can be fully integrated into the ICU bedside physiologic monitoring system. This POCT bedside relationship engenders a whole host of complexities in the handling of POCT laboratory data. What, in fact, happens with data generated by POCT devices integrated into the ICU bedside? Are the POCT data managed and transmitted further to the LIS or HIS? As discussed earlier, there are significant challenges to tracking the flow of data from the bedside physiologic monitors and subsequently integrating these data into hospital-wide information systems (Fig. 33.6). A concerted effort must be undertaken to develop an approach for handling POCT data that originate from POCT devices that are directly integrated into bedside systems.

Data from Point-of-Care Testing Monitors

Central laboratory analyzers are subject to the Clinical Laboratory Improvement Act of 1988 (CLIA '88) and state and local regulations. Data from POCT monitors (Fig. 33.1), however, are not subject to the federal CLIA '88 regulations. Such data are considered by many to be "monitored" data, no different from heart rate or blood pressure (19,20,35,36), even though data from the POCT monitor both "look and feel" just like traditional laboratory data. The categorization and regulation of POCT monitor data are far from resolved. Compounding the question of how to classify or regulate data from a POCT monitor are the issues of data management and transmission to the LIS or HIS. Unfortunately, at present, DMS for POCT monitors are in the earliest stages of development. Thus, data from POCT monitors cannot be easily managed or transmitted to the LIS or HIS.

POINT-OF-CARE TESTING REGULATORY REQUIREMENTS

The POCT model presented herein suggests that the central laboratory is best suited to coordinate a comprehensive POCT informatics program. Through such oversight, the central laboratory will be in a position to ensure that the POCT program remains in compliance with regulatory requirements. A detailed discussion of quality control and regulatory issues is beyond the scope of this chapter (35,36). Information on point of care can be obtained from the point of care website (*www.pointofcare.net*).

CONCLUSIONS

Point-of-care testing has the potential to revolutionize laboratory testing by facilitating diagnostic and therapeutic interventions, especially for critically ill patients. Our preference is that all laboratory data, including POCT data, should be treated with the same high standards. Thus, POCT data should be managed and transmitted to the LIS or HIS. The successful implementation of POCT in general, and POCT informatics specifically, requires a multidisciplinary team approach, including POCT clinicians, hospital laboratorians, information technology experts, and representatives of the POCT, DMS, LIS, and HIS vendors. Optimally, the central laboratory should lead the effort in partnership with the end users, the clinical advocates for POCT. This collaborative effort will advance laboratory care throughout and ensure quality and compliance with standards; it also will permit POCT data integration into the LIS. POCT informatics should be seamless, transparent, helpful, and, most importantly, painless to the clinicians.

REFERENCES

1. Castro H, Oropello J, Halpern N. Point-of-care testing in the intensive care unit: the intensive care physician's perspective. *Am J Clin Pathol* l995;104:S95–S99.
2. Drenck N. Point of care testing in critical care medicine: the clinician's view. *Clin Chim Acta* 2001;307:3–7.
3. Kilgore ML, Steindel SJ, Smith JA. Evaluating stat testing options in an academic heath center: therapeutic turn around time and staff satisfaction. *Clin Chem* 1998;44:1597–1603.
4. Wilkinson DS. The role of technology in the clinical laboratory of the future. *Clin Lab Manage Rev* 1997;11:322–330.
5. Blick KE. Decision making laboratory computer systems as essential tools for achievement of total quality. *Clin Chem* 1997;43:908–912.
6. Markin RS, Whalen SA. Laboratory automation: trajectory, technology, and tactics. *Clin Chem* 2000;46:764–771.
7. Boyd JC, Felder RA, Savory J. Robotics and the changing face of the clinical laboratory. *Clin Chem* 1996;42:1901–1910.
8. Seaberg RS, Stallone RO, Statland BE. The role of total laboratory automation in a consolidated laboratory network. *Clin Chem* 2000; 46:751–756.
9. Takemura Y, Beck JR. Laboratory testing under managed care dominance in the USA. *J Clin Pathol* 2001;54:89–95.
10. Emergency Care Research Institute (ECRI). Information systems, laboratory. In: *Healthcare product comparison.* Plymouth Meeting, PA: ECRI, 2000.
11. Kost GJ. Planning and implementing point-of-care testing systems. In:

12. Kost GJ. Point of care testing in intensive care. In: Tobin MJ, ed. *Principles and practice of intensive care monitoring.* New York: McGraw-Hill, 1998:1267–1296.
13. Emergency Care Research Institute (ECRI). Point-of-care analyzers, clinical laboratory. In: *Healthcare product comparison*, Plymouth Meeting, PA: ECRI, 2000:1–51.
14. DuBois JA. Getting to the point: integrating critical care tests in the patient care setting. *Medical Laboratory Observer* 2000;6:52–56.
15. Harvey MA. Point of care laboratory testing in critical care. *Am J Crit Care* 1999;8:72–83.
16. Kost GJ, Ehrmeyer SS, Chernow B, et al. The laboratory–clinical interface: point-of-care testing. *Chest* 1999;115:1140–1154.
17. Shapiro BA. Point of care testing: more than simply changing venue. *Chest* 1999;115:917–918.
18. Clarke B, Cederdahl M. Connectivity: point-of-care solutions. *Advance Adm in Lab* 1998;7:34–37.
19. Halpern N, Brentjens T. Point of care testing informatics: the critical care-hospital interface. *Crit Care Clin* 1999;15;577–591.
20. Halpern NA. Point of care diagnostics and networks. *Crit Care Clin* 2000;16:623–639.
21. Montoya ID, Carlson JW. Point-of-care systems, informatics and health care delivery. *Health Care Supervisor* 1996;15:17–26.
22. Bernard D, Vanhee D, Blaton V. Implementation of an integrated instrument control and data management system for point-of-care testing. *Clin Chim Acta* 2001;307:169–173.
23. Auerbach D. Alternate site testing: Information handling and reporting issues. *Arch Pathol Lab Med* 1995;119:924–925.
24. Quigley L. POCT data management: a problem-solving approach. *Medical Laboratory Observer* 1995;27:12–15.
25. Laessig R, Ehrmeyer S. Data management of POCT: the vision. *Med Lab Observer*1995;27:1–6.
26. Palenick JA. A developmental perspective on POCT data management. *Medical Laboratory Observer* 1995;27:25–27.
27. Brooks JD. Fundamentals of POCT data management: a perfusionist's perspective. *Medical Laboratory Observer* 1995;27:20–24.
28. Parker J. LIS vendor, POCT manufacturer, laboratorian: who's responsible for POCT data management? *Medical Laboratory Observer* 1995; 27:8–11.
29. Kost GJ. Connectivity: the millennium challenge for point-of-care testing. *Arch Pathol Lab Med* 2000;124:1108–1110.
30. Anderson D, Belzberg H. POCT data management by terminal emulation in a paperless ICU. *Medical Laboratory Observer* 1995;27:16–19.
31. Medical Products Group. Technology white paper. *Communication standards in the clinical setting: an introduction.* Andover, MA: Hewlett Packard, 1998.
32. Medical Products Group. Technology white paper. *Communication standards in the clinical setting: a closer look at the details.* Andover, MA: Hewlett Packard, 1998.
33. Clinical Information Systems for the ICU. *MEEN Cardiology Critical Care Technology* 2001;41:34–37. Available at: http:www.C3Tonline.net. Accessed December 14, 2001.
34. Felder RA. The distributed laboratory: point-of-care services with core laboratory management. In: Price CP, Hicks JM, eds. *Point-of-care testing.* Washington, DC: AACC Press, 1999;99–118.
35. St-Louis P. Status of point-of-care testing: promise, realities and possibilities. *Clin Biochem* 2000;33:427–440.
36. Laessing RH, Ehrmeyer SS. *The new poor man's (person's) guide to the regulations (CLIA '88, JCAHO, CAP, & COLA),* 5th ed. Madison, WI: R & S Consultants, 2001.

Tobin MJ, ed. *Principles and practice of intensive care monitoring.* New York: McGraw-Hill,1998:1297–1328.

34

POINT-OF-CARE TESTING INTEGRATION AND CONNECTIVITY

JEFFREY PERRY
BOB ANDERS
DIRK BOECKER

Over the last decade, advances in microfluidics and other miniaturization technologies have enabled a new class of diagnostic device. This new device class supports a wide diversity of diagnostic testing directly at the *point of care* (POC). Tests previously limited to the domain of central laboratory analyzers are now available near the patient in a variety of care settings. Sophisticated tests are possible at the hospital bedside, during patient encounters in primary and secondary care clinics, and even in the home. This new POC device class offers the advantages of fast therapeutic turnaround time and quite possibly cost reduction for some types of tests. Indeed, approximately 10% of all diagnostic tests now are performed at the POC (1).

These POC devices present new challenges for health care information management systems. Typically, these devices are portable and are not directly connected to communication infrastructures. This complicates the task of extracting patient test result information for reporting, charting, and billing purposes.

In addition, from a regulatory perspective, a diagnostic test is not differentiated based on where the test is performed. Someone in the institution must be able to show that the test was performed in compliance with the policies of an overall diagnostic testing quality system for the institution. It is thus incumbent on POC device vendors to offer mechanisms by which their devices can be integrated into an institution's diagnostic information management system. These requirements for integration drive the need for connectivity standardization.

To date, POC device and information system vendors have faced this integration problem individually and have derived unique solutions. Any institution embarking on incorporating multivendor POC devices into their diagnostic testing facilities has had to face the equipment and management costs of multiple integration solutions. In fact, the cost and disjointedness of multivendor POC diagnostic integration are seen as significant barriers to adoption of this new and exciting class of diagnostic device (2).

This chapter describes technical details of the POC diagnostic connectivity problem, presents an overview of currently available commercial offerings, and discusses the connectivity-enabling standards developed by the POC Connectivity Industry Consortium (CIC). Readers of this chapter will understand the principal systems and roles involved in POC information management and will learn how standardized connectivity can reduce the cost and complexity of POC diagnostic integration.

CURRENT CONNECTIVITY LANDSCAPE

Figure 34.1 illustrates common problems with current POC integration solutions. This figure depicts the typical systems and linkages deployed at institutions that choose several POC devices from several different vendors (Fig. 34.1). The following problems characterize this situation: too many computers/boxes, too many cables, too many system interfaces, and too many different software systems

THE CONNECTIVITY INDUSTRY CONSORTIUM

In February 2000, a group of 49 health care institutions, POC device vendors, diagnostic test system vendors, and system integrators formed the CIC to create standards for POC diagnostic integration. The consortium's membership, governing principles, guidelines, and timelines, can be found at the Website of the CIC (www.poccic.org). The board of directors of the CIC created the following vision statement to guide the CIC work teams:

> The vision of the CIC is to expeditiously develop, pilot, and transfer the foundation for a set of seamless 'plug and play' POC communication standards ensuring fulfillment of the critical user requirements of bi-directionality, device connection commonality, commercial software interoperability, security, and QC/regulatory compliance.

The deliverable from this vision is a set of standards that form the foundation for POC connectivity across the health care continuum. To meet this vision, the resulting standards are self-sustaining and utilize practical, cost-effective, user-focused solutions. The desired outcome of this vision is broad-based vendor and provider adoption of the CIC standards (Table 34.1).

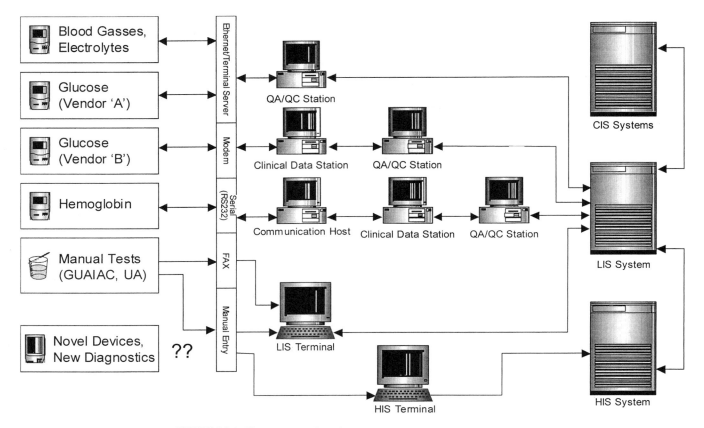

FIGURE 34.1. The current point-of-care diagnostic connectivity landscape.

TABLE 34.1. CIC MEMBERSHIP

Core vendors
Abbott Laboratories
Agilent Technologies
Bayer Diagnostics
BD
Instrumentation Laboratory
Lifescan
Medical Automation Systems
Radiometer Medical
Roche Diagnostics
Sunquest Information Systems
Supporting vendors
Abaxis
Avocet Medical
Cerner
Clarinet Systems
Comtrol Corporation
First Medical/Sigma Diagnostics
GE Medical Systems Information Technologies
HemoCue
HemoSense
InterComponentWare
i-STAT Corporation
International Technidyne Corporation (ITC)
Lantronix
Medtronic
Motorola

Orasure Technologies
Pharmacia & Upjohn
SMS/Siemens
TELCOR
Core providers
Banner Health System
Bradford Royal Infirmary
Geisinger Healthcare System
Johns Hopkins Medical Institutions
Kaiser Permanente
Mayo Clinic
Profil GmbH
St. Vincent Mercy Medical Center
The Mount Sinai Hospital
University of Iowa Healthcare
Individual Providers
Maurice Green, PhD
Neil Halpern, MD
Georg Hoffmann
LTC Forrest Kneisel
Gerald Kost, MD, PhD
Petrie Rainey, MD PhD
Liaisons
AACC
COLA
IFCC Scientific Division
Medical Devices Agency

The CIC worked within a "fast-track" model and developed the POC connectivity specification within its planned 12- to 15-month lifetime. Having met its objectives, the CIC then "sunset" and handed the connectivity specification to the National Committee for Clinical Laboratory Standards (NCCLS; www.nccls.org), Health Level 7 (www.hl7.org), and the Institute of Electrical and Electronics Engineers (IEEE; www.ieee.org) organizations for subsequent maintenance and extension. In July 2001, the NCCLS published a "for review" consensus POC diagnostic connectivity standard, based on the work of the CIC. The IEEE and HL-7 organizations will also publish standards in 2001 that are derived from the CIC's specifications to enable seamless POC connectivity. By using these standards, it will be possible in a few years to reduce the myriad cables, computers, and software interfaces currently required to integrate POC diagnostic devices to a few standard interfaces.

SOLUTION OVERVIEW

The CIC specification covers two broad areas of POC device behavior: application integration and physical integration.

Application Integration

The CIC specification defines the dialogues in which POC devices and participating systems engage. Ultimately, these dialogues manifest as a set of messages that pass between participants via well-defined interfaces in a CIC-compliant system. The CIC has sought to define a sufficient set of dialogues to meet the integration and regulatory requirements imposed on a diagnostic test system that includes POC devices. The CIC has been careful to not overspecify such dialogues. Such overspecification would leave the specification brittle in response to change and could impede innovative development in the relatively young POC industry.

Physical Integration

There are significant costs in multivendor POC diagnostic integration that cannot be reduced unless there is some standardization of the physical and link-level interfaces used by POC devices and associated systems. The CIC specification therefore also defines a set of physical connections and associated protocols. The CIC has sought to prescribe a minimal set of physical definitions so as to reduce the cost of POC diagnostic integration and yet not restrict vendors in their delivery of POC innovation.

The CIC defined two standard interfaces: a device interface and an observation reporting interface. Figure 34.2 overlays these interfaces on the "boxes and wires" that constitute typical solutions for POC information management (Fig. 34.2).

Boxes and Wires

It is best to start by describing the devices and networks typically found in CIC-enabled POC testing (POCT) systems. It should be easier to understand the abstract parts of the interface specifications with a good image of a physical system in mind.

The Point-of-Care Device

The emerging new diagnostic test technologies are packaged in a variety of instruments. The devices within the scope of the CIC specification include handheld instruments, test modules that are part of other instrumentation (a patient monitor, for example), or small bench-top analyzers.

The bench-top analyzers support the concept of a remote or "satellite" laboratory located close to patients in the hospital or in a clinic setting. Some bedside instruments, such as vital signs monitors, support "plug-in" POC diagnostic modules. These modules may thus leverage the electrical power and connectivity infrastructure provided by host instrumentation at the bedside. Handheld analyzers are portable. These devices are used in a variety of settings that range from the hospital room to the home as well as the clinic.

Although there is considerable diversity in device type and role, the CIC specification attempts to support all POC diagnostic instruments. Accommodation is made in the specification to recognize the typically limited computing power and user interface facilities of these devices. In addition, the specification recognizes that handheld devices are not continuously con-

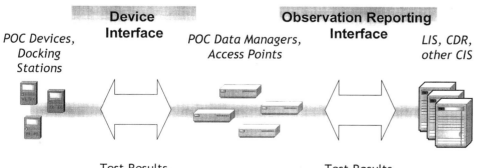

FIGURE 34.2. The two Connectivity Industry Consortium-specified interfaces.

nected to a network, whereas the bedside monitor POC diagnostic modules and the bench-top analyzers typically are.

The Point-of-Care Data Manager

The primary role of a POC data manager is to host one or more services to which POC devices will connect when they connect to the network. These services facilitate the collection of test and quality assurance/quality control data from POC devices as well as the management of POC instruments. In addition, services hosted by a data manager may exchange data with existing clinical information systems (CIS) that already exist in the hospital or laboratory. In particular, data manager services may interact with laboratory information systems (LIS), order communication systems, and electronic medical record (EMR) systems.

Today, single-purpose computer systems typically serve as data managers; however, in the future, other systems concerned with observation management and reporting (e.g., LIS) may host the role of data manager. It is important to keep in mind that the CIC connectivity standard does not require the existence of a stand-alone data manager. Instead, it requires only that some system fill the role and responsibilities of a data manager.

Data managers usually are implemented in conventional information technology (IT) hardware with conventional IT software. Data managers typically reside within the IT spaces of the institution with fixed connections to the hospital's network. There may be more than one data manager in a health care system. There may be some specialization of services in any given data manager. A data manager may host CIC-compliant or proprietary services.

The Observation Recipient

Although outside the scope of the CIC specification, observation recipient systems play an important role in POC diagnostic systems. In many cases, the final destination of a POC test observation is an observation recipient system.

Typically, LIS or clinical data repository (CDR) systems fill the role of observation recipient. The CIC specification does not describe observation recipient behavior. CIC-specified services, however, do facilitate interaction with observation recipient systems (e.g., to exchange test results and ordering information).

Interfaces

One goal of the CIC is to develop standards that can support a wide variety of POC information management implementations, including existing "legacy" systems as well as all reasonably conceivable future developments and topologies.

Two interfaces constitute the heart of the CIC specification (Fig. 34.2). In general, the *device interface* governs the flow of information between devices and data managers and the *observation reporting interface* (sometimes referred to as the *EDI interface*) describes messaging between data managers and observation recipients. The character, nature, and attributes of the device messaging layer (DML) and access-point specifications are described in more detail in the following subsections.

The Device Interface

In general, devices and data managers are very tightly coupled systems. Devices with limited user–interface capabilities must rely on configuration and management services provided by data managers. In turn, data managers need strict control of devices to fulfill their responsibility to manage the quality and reporting of POCT results. The fact that this tight coupling must be deployed and maintained across large geographic areas and over a variety of telecommunication infrastructures [local area network (LAN), phone, Internet, wireless] presents additional complexity to the design of this interface.

The CIC device interface addresses these requirements and challenges with a two-part specification. The DML specification describes the structure, content, and flow of messages between a device and a data manager. The device and access point (DAP) specification defines a low-cost, flexible means to communicate these messages reliably. Figure 34.3 illustrates how these two specifications are layered atop one another. Separating the specifications for messaging and for network access allows great flexibility for the future evolution of this interface. For example, one needs only to update the DML to add support for additional application-level services, such as POC ordering or result review.

Likewise, whereas the DAP specification defines a transport optimized for current technology and market economics today (Infrared Data Association, or IrDA, infrared and cable-connected), it is important to allow for the future use of other lower-level transport and physical layers (e.g., Bluetooth or IEEE 802.11 wireless networking). Figure 34.4 illustrates how other robust reliable transports could be used in the future to carry device messages.

Device Messaging Layer Specification

The DML specification describes the dialogue between a device and a data manager. This protocol is a pure application-layer messaging scheme, assuming the existence of a robust, reliable lower-level transport. The terms *robust* and *reliable* have formal meanings. In a nutshell, a transport with these attributes guarantees that messages will not be corrupted in transit and that the sender will always be informed if a message cannot be delivered. The DML allows for bidirectional data exchange on the topics outlined in Figure 34.5.

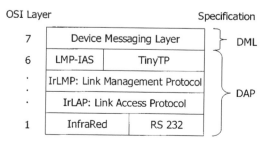

FIGURE 34.3. Layers of the device interface specification.

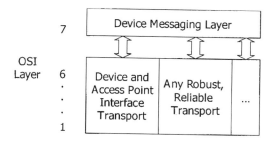

OSI Layer 7 6 . . . 1

Device Messaging Layer

Device and Access Point Interface Transport | Any Robust, Reliable Transport | ...

FIGURE 34.4. Device interface evolution.

The POC devices on the market today encompass a wide range of capabilities and complexities. For example, "simple" analyzers, like some handheld glucose meters, need only to (and indeed only are able to) report their status and stored observations. Other more complex handheld instruments may be able to handle the entire range of topics listed in Figure 34.5. Devices also differ in how they connect to download data. Most handheld devices require a user periodically to "dock" the instrument to initiate the data exchange. In some cases, this docking involves placing the device in a special cradle. In other cases, it involves pointing the instrument's infrared port at a fixed transceiver. No matter what the mechanism, the following general observations apply to these docking systems:

1. The operator initiates the establishment of a physical connection.
2. The operator initiates the start of a "data download" sequence.

1. Device Status
2. Observations
    2.1. Patient Tests
    2.2. Calibration Tests
    2.3. Quality Tests
        2.3.1. Liquid QC
        2.3.2. Electronic QC
        2.3.3. Calibration Verification
        2.3.4. Proficiency Test
3. Device Events
    3.1. Test Denied
    3.2. Uncertified Operator
    3.3. Vendor-specific
4. Update Lists
    4.1. Operator List
    4.2. Patient List
5. Directives
    5.1. Set Time
    5.2. Lockout (with explanation)
    5.3. Remove Lockout
    5.4. Vendor-specific
6. Vendor-specific Data Exchange

FIGURE 34.5. Device messaging layer data topics.

3. The physical connection may be interrupted (e.g., when the device is "undocked").

In contrast to this *intermittent* connection model, some more complex bench-top instruments have built-in network connectivity. Because these devices are not routinely portable, they can remain *persistently* connected to network-located data management services. Consequently, there is no need for users to initiate download sequences. Typically, these devices automatically report new status, configuration, or observation information whenever it becomes available.

This variability presents several challenges for the messaging layer. To address these issues, the DML allows some flexibility in how devices implement data exchange. The following are key aspects of this approach:

1. Minimum topic requirements: All devices are required to support at least the status and observation topics. An exchange covering only these topics is sufficient to support test result reporting processes.
2. Scalable conversation topics: Beyond the minimum topic requirement, devices may support any number or combination of the additional topics listed in Figure 34.5. The DML specification provides a mechanism by which a device informs a data manager of the topics it supports.
3. Dialogues tailored to device capabilities: The data manager bears the responsibility of tailoring the conversation to only those subjects that are relevant to the device.
4. Separate dialogue for intermittent and persistently connected devices: The characteristics of the device connection determine the nature of the device and data manager message exchange. *Intermittently* connected devices use a message flow that is designed rapidly to exchange all data required to synchronize the device and data manager. *Persistently* connected devices maintain a long-term message flow, reporting new information as it becomes available.

To get a feeling for the DML's data flow, consider the following example of a dialogue between an intermittently connected device and a data manager, described in terms of a dialogue between two actors. The following "script" outlines how this dialogue proceeds between a device and a data manager (Fig. 34.6).

<u>DEV</u>: Hello Data Manager, I'm device 'xyz'. I'm on-line
<u>DM</u>: Hello 'xyz'. You are a registered device. Please proceed...
<u>DEV</u>: Here is my Device Status. What else would you like me to do?
<u>DM</u>: Device 'xyz', please report your Observations
<u>DEV</u>: Here are my Observations. What else would you like me to do?
<u>DM</u>: Device 'xyz', please report your Device Events
<u>DEV</u>: Here are my Device Events. What else would you like me to do?
<u>DM</u>: Device 'xyz', please accept this Directive: 'xxx'
<u>DEV</u>: I can perform Directive 'xxx'. What else would you like me to do?
<u>DM</u>: Device 'xyz', please accept this Vendor-specific Communication: 'yyy'
<u>DEV</u>: I have received Vendor-specific Communication 'yyy'. What else would you like me to do?
<u>DM</u>: Device 'xyz', please terminate this conversation.
<u>DEV</u>: Goodbye, Data Manager.

FIGURE 34.6. Device messaging dialogue.

```xml
<?xml version="1.0" encoding="UTF-8"?>
<OBS.R01>
    <HDR>
        <HDR.msg_type V="OBS^R01"/>
        <HDR.control_id EX="10000001"/>
        <HDR.version_id EX="1.0" AAN="CIC"/>
        <HDR.msg_time V="2001-02-12T10:00:00-08:00"/>
    </HDR>
    <SVC>
        <SVC.role V="OBS"/>
        <SVC.time V="2001-02-12T08:00:00-8:00"/>
        <OPR>
            <OPR.id EX="OP777-88-9999"/>
            <OPR.name V="Pat Operator"/>
        </OPR>
        <ORD>
            <ORD.service_id V="12345" SN="LOINC" DN="POC Glucose"/>
            <ORD.ordering_provider_id EX="ORD555-12-1212"/>
            <ORD.order_id EX="ORD567891234"/>
        </ORD>
        <SPC>
            <SPC.id EX="SPC89012345678"/>
            <SPC.time V="2001-02-12T06:00:00-8:00"/>
            <SPC.source NULL="LLFA"/>
        </SPC>
        <PT>
            <PT.id EX="PT222-55-7777"/>
            <PT.name V="Jane Patient"/>
            <PT.birth_date V="1960-08-30"/>
            <PT.gender V="F"/>
            <PT.location V="ICU-4"/>
            <PT.weight V="120" U="lbs"/>
            <PT.height V="5.5" U="ft"/>
        </PT>
        <RGT>
            <RGT.id>glu_strip</RGT.id>
            <RGT.lot_nbr>GL78901</RGT.lot_nbr>
            <RGT.exp_date V="2002-7-31"/>
        </RGT>
        <OBS>
            <OBS.value V="6.2"/>
            <OBS.method V="M"/>
        </OBS>
    </SVC>
</OBS.R01>
```

FIGURE 34.7. Sample of glucose test result message.

The individual messages in this conversation are encoded in extensible markup language (XML). The CIC-weighed the merits of many different encoding schemes and determined that an XML-based approach best met the requirements of flexibility, robustness, simplicity, and widespread, cross-industry support. Rather than developing a completely new language in XML, the DML leverages existing work done by the HL-7 organization. Principally, the CIC specification leverages the rules for encoding data types and elements of the information model defined for version 3 of the HL-7 standard. Figure 34.7 shows an example of the observation message used to report a glucose test result.

Device and Access Point Specification

The DAP specification describes a low-cost, flexible, reliable means to connect devices to data managers located on a network. This standard describes low-level communication protocols and physical interfaces used to connect to POC devices. It

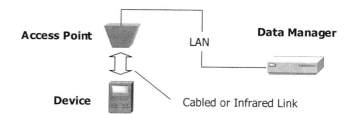

FIGURE 34.8. Example of access point use.

specifies the use of a single transport protocol (TinyTP) running over either of two physical layers: infrared or cable connected.

To keep the implementation cost low (less than a dollar per device), this specification leverages widely deployed, commercially available standards. The infrared link is based on the connection standard developed by the IrDA. Transceivers using this standard are found in more than 100 million laptops, cell phones, and personal digital assistants. The IrDA port is that small semitransparent red window you might have wondered about on one of these devices. The cable-connected link is based on the IEEE Medical Information Bus (MIB) lower-layers standard commonly used to connect acute-care patient management devices (such as infusion pumps, ventilators, electrocardiographs) to bedside patient monitors. Figure 34.8 illustrates how an access point can be used to provide an infrared or cable-connected device access to a data manager located on a network (Fig. 34.8).

An added benefit of this proposal is that it should be possible to build a *common access point* that can support CIC POC, MIB, and PDA devices, regardless of any differences between their upper-layer protocols and applications. The availability of a common access point infrastructure that can support POC, MIB, and handheld PDA devices in all patient-care areas would be a major benefit to all care providers.

The Observation Reporting Interface

The observation reporting interface facilitates communication of test results and order information between data managers and observation recipients. The interface provides bidirectional information flow between these services. Data managers use this interface to report test results and associated order information. Observation recipients use this interface either to inform the data manager when results have been successfully reported or to communicate error information when a result or order cannot be stored (Fig. 34.9).

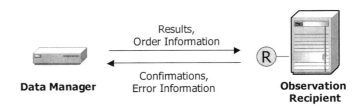

FIGURE 34.9. Observation reporting interface.

```
<VT>
MSH|^~\&|CICDMS|OBSREV|CICLIS|OBSRCPT|20000610010355||ORU^Ryy|20000610010355:023|P|2.4|||AL|AL<CR>
PID|||MR12345678^^^1||||||||||||||ActID135792468^^^1<CR>
ORC|RE<CR>
OBR||OrdIDA24680||1234-5^GLU^LN|||||||O|||||5555^Smith^John^J^Dr<CR>
OBX||ST|1234-5^GLU^LN||120|mg/dl|||||F|||||User9876||CICDEV-111^SINGRES|20000609102135<CR>
NTE|||Stat~Physician Notified<CR>
<FS><CR>
```

FIGURE 34.10. Example of observation reporting interface message.

The clinical workflow surrounding POC measurement and ordering processes is quite complex, dynamic, and flexible. The data manager and observation recipient bear the principal responsibility for making and managing the connection between orders and results. Thus, the observation reporting interface is designed to handle the three most common result-and-ordering use cases:

1. Unordered observation, place an order— A test is performed prior to the issuance of an order. An order must be automatically generated. One example of this use occurs when a doctor verbally instructs a nurse to perform a test. From an information management perspective, it would be best if the nurse electronically entered an order before performing the test. In the real world, however, there usually is no time for order entry in these situations. In fact, it is highly desirable for the POC measurement process to become automated. Then the only action a user needs to take is to make a measurement on the POC analyzer, with all other processes for generating an order, and tying it in to the observation handled by the "machines."
2. New observation, search for an order—A test is performed that may or may not have an order previously placed. In this case, the data manager does not know whether an order has been placed. It instructs the observation recipient to search for an existing order for the associated results. The institution's business rules will determine what the observation recipient does if it cannot find a matching order. Possibilities include automatically placing an order (as in use case 1) or logging an exception rather than recording the result.
3. Preordered observation—A test is performed that was previously ordered. From a traditional central laboratory perspective, this use case is probably the predominant (if not exclusive) one. In the POC environment, however, it is actually uncommon to have an order already generated when a test is done.

The observation reporting interface heavily leverages the messages defined for laboratory instrument communication as defined in Chapter 13 of HL-7's version 2.4 specification. In fact, the CIC specification is an implementation guide for using HL-7 version 2.4 messages to support POCT. As such, the CIC specification does not define any new messages, segments, or fields. Instead, it simply provides a strict set of rules to define which messages are used and how each message is constructed. These rules increase the likelihood that separate implementations of this interface will easily interoperate.

For illustration purposes, Figure 34.10 shows a hypothetical message from a data manager reporting a new result from a glucose meter (120 mg/dL) that is associated with a previously placed order (e.g., "OrdIDA24680") (Fig. 34.10).

EXTENSIBILITY AND FLEXIBILITY

In an unrealistically perfect world, the CIC specification would support all system diversity. For example, a data manager would be able to interact with a heterogeneous collection of devices without the necessity of understanding the particular behavior of each device. Certainly, there would be diversity in the analytes supported, but this diversity would be accommodated in the specification. The data manager could rest assured that it could handle any device without special attention as long as that device complied with the CIC specification.

In the real world, however, such complete encapsulation is not possible (or desirable, as we shall see). For example, it is far outside the scope of the CIC specification to make any statements with regard to device installation and configuration behavior. Each vendor will develop its own processes for code updates, diagnostics, and so on. In addition, there are aspects of quality control and quality assurance behavior that cannot be codified by the CIC specification. Thus, data managers must deal with device diversity. For example, a data manager will need to understand that the concept of "lot identification (ID)" for vendor Z's cartridge-based glucose meter is different from the ID for the liquid reagents used in vendor Q's blood gas analyzer. The figure of merit for data manager vendors will be their ability to hide this device diversity from operators. In the best case, the POC coordinator should not need to know the vendor of a particular device for normal day-to-day operation of a CIC-supported system.

This exposed diversity is not a failure of the specification. First, the CIC common access point specification allows this variety of devices to use the same CIC-compliant connectivity infrastructure. This extraordinary success removes all the vendor-specific cabling and boxes that drive up the price of integration. Second, the CIC specification successfully defines common core concepts like *calibration verification* and objects like *lot ID*. The fact that the representation of these concepts is diverse among devices can be hidden by good data manager design. This major success will allow operators to perceive and deal with a common conceptual model for these objects without having to know intimate particulars of the diverse representations.

Finally, if the CIC were able to encapsulate all variability in current systems, the result would likely be brittle and quickly become obsolete. Advancements in instrument capability would require an accompanying elaboration in the CIC specification. If the level of detail in the CIC specification were too fine, the pace of the specification's evolution would limit the rate of deployment of novel POC diagnostic features and devices. Data manager design is complicated by device diversity, but not to an unworkable degree. On the other hand, this diversity offers an area for data manager vendors to add value to POC diagnostic information management systems.

CONCLUSIONS

The current state-of-the-art of POC diagnostic connectivity solutions does not meet health care providers' needs to support a range of diagnostic instruments from multiple vendors. This shortcoming is not a failure of technology; rather, it reflects the isolated evolution of vendor-specific information management solutions. The consequent high cost of integration has retarded the growth of the POC marketplace. In response, industry, academic, and health care institutions banded together in the CIC to develop standards based on modern technologies that would lower the cost and complexity barrier to multivendor integration.

Just as it took the combined effort of commercial vendors and POC customers (health care institutions and providers) to develop the POC connectivity standards, it will take a combined vendor–customer effort to ensure that these standards are realized in the marketplace. Device and information system vendors must make the internal investment required to adapt and redesign their products to use the CIC interfaces. In a market driven by cost pressures, this investment must be justified by customer demand. Thus, the key success factor for the commercial realization of the CIC standards is for health care providers and institutions to begin to build investment and purchasing strategies around easily integrated, standard POC offerings. In important ways, this challenge parallels the early days of the Internet. The value of the standard Internet interfaces and protocols (e.g., Transmission Control Protocol/Internet Protocol (TCP/IP) and hypertext markup language (HTML)] has grown as an exponential function of the number of nodes connected: the so-called network effect. So, too, will POC customers realize dramatic returns on their investment in POC devices and data management solutions that adhere to standard connectivity protocols.

GLOSSARY

Access Point   A subsystem that consolidates data from one or more POC devices onto another communication link. One example is a multiport concentrator or a dedicated single-port access point, typically connected to a local-area network (LAN). An access point also can be part of a multifunctional device such as a patient monitor or personal computer.

Clinical Information System (CIS)   Any health care information system responsible for housing clinical information.

Laboratory information systems (LIS), clinical data repositories (CDR), and electronic medical record (EMR) systems are examples of CIS systems.

Data Manager   Typically, a network-connected computer that performs such functions as point-of-care test results review and forwarding, quality assurance and quality control enforcement and reporting, and other point-of-care instrument and data management functions.

Device   A point-of-care *device* performs diagnostic tests in collaboration with an operator. As part of a connectivity framework, a device connects to one or more data manager services to transfer test observations, to participate in the correlation of test results with test orders, and to behave in compliance with the local point-of-care quality system.

Device and Access Point (DAP) Interface   The DAP interface specifies the link between a device and an access point.

Device Messaging Layer (DML)   The DML specification defines a bidirectional messaging protocol to exchange results and quality information between devices and data managers.

Docking Station   A mechanical and electrical interface that a point-of-care device uses to connect to exchange data and configuration information with a data manager.

Extensible Markup Language (XML)   A meta-language widely used on the web and for business-to-business data exchange. XML is to data and information as HTML is to documents and presentation.

Health Level 7 (HL-7)   An American National Standards Institute–accredited standards development organization focused on messaging to support the exchange of clinical and administrative healthcare data (www.hl7.org).

The Institute of Electrical and Electronics Engineers (IEEE)   Among its many roles, the IEEE sets standards for the electronics industry, such as IEEE Std 1073 for medical device communications and IEEE Std 802.3, which forms the lower-layer foundation for the Internet (www.ieee.org).

Infrared (IR)   A band of electromagnetic radiation that is often used for wireless communication. An IR communication port can be found behind the small oval window found on most cell phones and laptop and palmtop computers.

Infrared Data Association (IrDA)   *IrDA* is an organization that creates and promotes interoperable, low-cost infrared data interconnection standards (www.irda.org).

Medical Information Bus (MIB)   The common name given to IEEE Std 1073 and lower-layers IEEE Std 1073.3.2. MIB is a medical device connectivity standard optimized for real-time acute care settings and other areas that use similar devices (e.g., patient monitors, intravenous pumps, ventilators, pulse oximeters).

Observation Recipient   A system that is the principal authority for clinical test result information within a healthcare institution. In hospitals, the laboratory information service and electronic medical records systems frequently play this role.

Personal Digital Assistant (PDA) A portable electronic device that typically handles various functions such as calendaring and managing contact lists and to-do lists.

Point-of-care (POC) The environment immediately surrounding a patient.

Point-of-Care Coordinator A person who has overall responsibility for assuring that the operation of all point-of-care (POC) devices in the institution is compliant with the institution's POC quality system. The services provided by data manager systems are key tools used by the POC coordinator to ensure compliance.

Quality Assurance (QA) Part of quality management focused on providing confidence that quality requirements will be fulfilled (ISO 9000, 3.2.1) (3).

Quality Control (QC) Part of quality management focused on fulfilling quality requirements (ISO 9000 3.2.10) (3).

Tiny Transport Protocol (TinyTP) An Infrared Data Association (IrDA) transport protocol that provides multiple, concurrent, reliable, bidirectional communication streams on an IrDA link with robust flow control.

Transmission Control Protocol/Internet Protocol (TCP/IP) *TCP/IP* is a transport protocol that provides reliable, bidirectional, stream-oriented communication on the Internet.

REFERENCES

1. *In vitro diagnostics, pharmaceutical companies and medical informatics.* Decision Resources, 1999:7–1.
2. *1999 EAC US hospital POC survey.* Enterprise Analysis Corporation, 1999.
3. International Organization for Standardization (ISO) 9000. *Quality management systems—fundamentals and vocabulary.* American Society for Quality, 2000.

35

INTERNET-BASED DISEASE MANAGEMENT FOR HOME CARE AND SELF-TESTING

HOLLY B. JIMISON
JUDY KIRBY

A CHANGING ENVIRONMENT FOR THE PRACTICE OF MEDICINE

There are many social, economic, and technologic trends that are having a profound effect on the way medicine is practiced today. In the United States, we see that the population is aging fairly dramatically and that most health care dollars are being spent on chronic disease and conditions associated with aging. People with chronic disease are now living longer and participating in their care to a much greater degree. In general, there is an increase in consumerism that has affected medical care. Patients are taking more interest in their health, obtaining information from books, magazines, newspapers, television, and now the Web. They are also more interested in participating in decisions about their medical care. For treatment decisions for chronic diseases, it is important to incorporate patient preferences on health outcomes into the decision-making process.

Economic pressures on health care providers have been enormous in the past decade. The membership in managed care programs has increased dramatically. Capitation and global payment methods have put health care providers in the position of being accountable for financial as well as clinical outcomes. It is now critical for providers to integrate and manage services effectively.

Additionally, the government has become less of a provider of medical services and more of a purchaser of medical services (1). With the growth in managed care and an increase in government contracts for medical care, insurers and medical organizations have found that they now must manage the care of higher-risk members than they have traditionally served. Often, in response to market pressures, providers have formed networks to negotiate directly with purchasers and thus to assume financial risk. The early response to the new economic pressures created a competitive environment focused on price. With purchaser demand for quality information as well as price, the field of outcomes measurement grew, and the current model for competition is based much more on value, which includes quality as well as price.

Concurrently, there has been a strong movement toward evidence-based medicine and guidelines for clinical practice (clini-cal protocols, clinical pathways). The effort has been to standardize care on the most proven and effective methods. Economic pressures encouraged first considering the high utilizers and most expensive diseases. The management of chronic illness, characterized by a lack of integration and coordination among services and providers, was a prime target for change. Disease management has emerged as a method to coordinate care and reduce costs for members with a chronic illness. Rapidly improving information and communications technology facilitated disease management efforts by enabling in-home monitoring and feedback, automated feedback, outcomes information, service coordination, and communication between the provider and the patient.

THE PRACTICE AND GROWTH OF DISEASE MANAGEMENT

Amidst efforts in the health care community to produce optimal health outcomes through improved quality of care and simultaneously to control costs, the approach of disease management is distinct in focusing on providing more appropriate combinations of health care resources through a coordinated, system-level approach (2). Bernard defines disease management as follows:

> A comprehensive integrated system for managing patients...by using best practices, clinical practice improvement information technology, and other resources and tools to reduce overall cost and improve measurable outcomes in the quality of care (3).

Disease management programs are used to target populations with a specific chronic illness and are also distinct from traditional medical care in that the interventions occur across the continuum of care (including home care), not just during discrete episodes. Although the overall goal is to improve the quality and efficiency of care, most often, early efforts focus on a subset of patients with a specific condition that utilizes a disproportionate amount of resources, with an effort at preventing costly future interventions. In analyses of large administrative

TABLE 35.1. CHRONIC DISEASES SUITABLE FOR DISEASE MANAGEMENT PROGRAMS

Disease Management Programs with Highest Potential Payoff	Other Chronic Diseases Suitable for Disease Management Programs
Diabetes	Arthritis
Congestive heart failure	Chronic obstructive pulmonary disease
Asthma	Depression
	Gastroesophageal reflux disease
	Hypertension
	Hypercholesterolemia
	HIV/AIDS
	Low back pain
	Migraine headache

HIV, human immunodeficiency virus; AIDS, acquired immunodeficiency disease.

databases, it is often found that as few as 10% of members with severe or chronic illnesses consume approximately 70% of the health care resources (4).

Chronic illnesses that are most appropriate for disease management should have several characteristics. They should be common, costly, have an effective treatment that prevents expensive events (e.g., emergency department visits), and have measurable cost and quality outcomes. Additionally, for practical implementation reasons, there must be a potential for a rapid return on investment. In the current economic climate, a program with any significant cost outlay and only long-term benefits probably will not be considered.

By most analyses, diabetes, congestive heart failure (CHF), and asthma most closely fit the requirements for a successful disease management program. In each case, focused interventions that include patient education and monitoring in the home can be used to anticipate and prevent expensive emergency visits or later complications of the disease. Table 35.1 also lists other chronic illnesses for which disease management programs may be effective.

A disease management intervention program may be set up between a health care system and an outside group, such as a pharmaceutical company or an independent service company. Alternatively, a managed care organization may institute a disease management program completely within its own organization, using its own data to identify patients, and intervening with patient education or nurse advice independently of the patient's health care provider. In either case, the interventions are population based and include patient-specific therapy and behavior-modification strategies. The results of early disease management programs have been encouraging, although not all have shown near-term cost savings.

EXTENDING CARE FOR CHRONIC DISEASE TO THE HOME

For most disease-management programs, a large part of the intervention involves extending the care and monitoring of chronic illness to include the patient and the patient's family in the home. Although it has always been true that out of necessity, the large part of the care and management of chronic illness has occurred in the home at the hands of the patient, disease management programs have formalized efforts to make that self-management more effective and to provide a greater coordination with professional care.

Diabetes, as a chronic disease, offers the most compelling motivation for self-management and care in the home. Glycemic regulation is key to slowing the progression of microvascular complications. Cross-sectional and retrospective studies have repeatedly shown that poor glycemic control [high hemoglobin A1C (HbA1C) levels] correlate with retinopathy, nephropathy, neuropathy, and cardiovascular disease. Prospective studies, such as the Diabetes Control and Complications Trial (DCCT), have shown that intensive glycemic management will slow the progression of these complications. This intensive management may require from one to four or more blood glucose measurements per day. This degree of monitoring can be practical and effective only through patient self-monitoring of blood glucose. Patients are routinely taught to perform these tests, and when they are done accurately, the blood glucose readings correlate well with HbA1C levels (5).

CARING FOR CHRONIC DISEASE IN THE HOME

Chronic diseases have a timeliness of care that entails frequent interventions and monitoring. Diabetes, CHF, hypertension, and asthma, for example, all require daily interventions and decisions by the patient. There is medication to be taken at prescribed times, specific dietary interventions, and treatments to be done, sometimes several times daily. For a system of intensive diabetes management to be successful, the patient must learn to understand and manage his or her own disease and its treatment (6). Patient self-management includes daily decisions about care, including diet and exercise, that may influence health outcomes, such as blood glucose values. The patient is taught to monitor and regulate these effects and factor them into other aspects of life. Attention to detail and disciplined repetition of tasks makes compliance a challenge. Successful management requires awareness, on some level, of the fact that their chronic disease is an ever-present component of life.

Self-management may sometimes include decisions on medications, from a provider directed algorithm, such as determination of insulin doses based on blood glucose values. Frequent insulin adjustment is an essential component of intensive insulin regimens (7). This means more decisions, more thinking about how life will be lived that day. This daily monitoring, problem solving, and decision making by the patient enable the effective management of this chronic disease. It is impossible to imagine the health care team participating in such an active daily way. Caring for chronic disease in the home necessitates the full partnership of the patient as a member of the team. Communication about the results of patient self-management is imperative to ensure successful outcomes from the plan. The patient and the health care team must have mutual, frequently communicated treatment goals and an unimpeded flow of information to and from the patient and the team. The frequency of these communications will be determined based on individual patient needs.

Patient education is as an extremely important component of self-management. Any attempt to control chronic disease through patient self-management must necessarily include the thorough education of the patient as disease manager, including access to both group and individual education sessions. As an example, the 1999 Clinical Practice Recommendations of the American Diabetes Association (6) recommends an education plan, based on an individualized assessment of needs, that includes making changes in nutrition and exercise habits leading to improved metabolic control. The educational program must include appropriate nutrition, exercise, medication, record-keeping systems, and self-monitoring of blood glucose (SMBG) (8). Because of the complexity and potentially progressive nature of the disease, additional education after the initial program may be necessary. As the patient begins to understand the rationale for intensive control of blood glucose, the regimen can be modified and the patient exposed to some of the clinical practice guidelines that provide reasons for modification. Disease management is meant to foster the consistent application-of-care guidelines in a cost-efficient manner (9). A more collaborative atmosphere might pave the way for greater autonomy for the patient, with the health care team assuming a more global management role.

NEW TECHNOLOGY APPLIED TO DISEASE MANAGEMENT

The management of patients by the use of computers has been limited in the health care community. The potential is there, however, to use computers in many areas: databases to store patient data; statistical and graphical packages to assist the clinician; expert systems for use by clinicians; patient education packages; dietary programs to examine food composition, as the dietary regimen relates to diabetic food exchanges, and to help devise meal plans; handheld insulin dosage computers to advise patients; and even games for children (10). Many avenues are available to explore for disease management. The telephone, the oldest telecommunications system, can be a less costly alternative for communication in home care through telemedicine. Interactive voice response systems can be used to manage routine communications. Telemedicine, the delivery of health care over a distance using a telecommunications system, usually refers to interactive televideo, "store-and-forward" image transmission, medical record transmission via computer, and remote monitoring (11). In home care, televideo equipment that runs over regular phone lines allows providers to increase the level of care and frequency of visits without incurring the total cost of a home visit. Direct interaction between the patient and the provider is possible with the video monitor, and various medical devices allow remote monitoring of heart and lung sounds, blood pressure (BP), and fetal heart monitoring. Pulse oximetry and respiratory flow data can be electronically transmitted, blood glucose values can be monitored, and visual observation of the insulin syringe prior to injection can ensure that visually impaired patients with diabetes draw up the correct insulin dose.

Some legal issues remain unresolved, however, primarily concerning the security and confidentiality of patient records, liability, practitioner licensing, and insurance payment.

Another use of the telephone has been to facilitate the task of glycemic control through an electronic case manager (ECM). An ECM is a customized microcomputer system located at a clinic that can be accessed by touch-tone telephone 24 hours a day. Patients typically use the system every 2 weeks to report daily self-measured glucose levels, hypoglycemic symptoms, and associated lifestyle events. The ECM also provides online assistance in adjusting daily insulin or tablet therapy. Results of a study of the system (12) showed an approximate threefold (p <0.05) decrease of diabetes-related crises (hyperglycemia or hypoglycemia) and a statistically significant decrease in HbA1C at 6 months ($n = 45$, $p = 0.024$) and at 12 months ($n = 30$, $p = 0.044$). Knowing that their data entries are monitored and reviewed by a health care professional regularly can increase feelings of satisfaction and security for a patient. Using phones and computers in this way also can improve access to health care for patients living in underserved localities.

Electronic mail, or e-mail, can be applied to disease management and can both monitor and encourage patient self-management in the home. The technology is available to anyone with Internet access and is easy to use. Patient-to-physician communication, although there are issues to be resolved, can be used efficiently, legally, and privately. The American Medical Informatics Association has published e-mail guidelines available online (13) that address "effective interaction between the clinician and patient, and observance of medicolegal prudence." E-mail communications, unlike the telephone, become a part of the patient's chart and therefore can give a precise and accurate record of communications. With the use of appropriate headings, such as appointment request, refill request, or advice request, the e-mail can be efficiently directed to an appropriate person for response, thereby saving time and an overload of e-mail messages. The tools, processes, and plans to manage the flow will mature as e-mail acceptance levels rise. A benefit of e-mail is that it is an asynchronous method of communication that will be used at a time that is convenient for both the patient and the physician; it cannot and must not be used if an immediate answer is needed. It is, however, an excellent way to transmit complex information such as blood glucose values sent from the patient or a list of acceptable and not acceptable foods sent from the dietitian, or the specifics of a complex medication regimen sent by the physician or nurse practitioner. Sending test results, without an accompanying clear and understandable explanation, via e-mail could be problematic, however. The patient could become unduly worried because of a lack of understanding of the results, and the physician would not be available to answer questions by telephone. Another concern of e-mail use relates to the uncertainty of whether an e-mailed message was actually received, but services are available that can ensure receipt. The sender can request a receipt, automatically delivered after the recipient opens the mail that verifies that the message was received.

The World Wide Web is another resource that is now being used for disease management, providing a new way for health care professionals to reach or interact with patients (14). The

Web enables easy access to disparate data sets, software, and communication devices. This integration enables and facilitates a new mode of patient care, even beyond disease management in the home. The technology will challenge the health care community to create partnerships with patients. Consumers appear to be positively disposed toward online solutions (15,16). Using the Internet as an information resource can be an effective adjunct to patient education. Much more breadth, depth, and timeliness of information can be provided than is typically available during a physician–patient interaction. Just-in-time medical information is seldom available at the point of care, but high-quality resources in the form of patient education or disease-specific support networks can be provided (17). Care must be taken to ensure valid information for patients. The overall quality of information available on the Web has been notoriously poor. There is no "gold standard" of quality assessment, but there are online versions of traditional information sources. Patients are turning to the Internet on their own to validate suggested therapies or to seek alternative therapies; so it is up to the medical community to provide pointers to reliable health care information.

Jenkins and Erdman (18) describe Web-based computerized information systems for home care that are both cost and quality effective while providing security and easy access. Applications include Web-based scheduling, patient records, remote point-of-care data capture, complete clinical assessment and care-plan generation, as well as the more usual billing, payroll, and integrated financial reporting. They also describe a system for consumers that provides medication reminders, access to educational information, and an ongoing health record that would provide more complete outcomes management.

MONITORING DEVICES IN THE HOME

Technology applied to disease management also includes monitoring devices available for use by patients in their homes. These include meters for testing the blood glucose levels of people with diabetes, peak flow meters used for monitoring patients with respiratory conditions such as asthma, BP testing devices for use in managing hypertension as well as other conditions, and scales for measuring weight gain or loss for patients with CHF. Teaching patients how to use equipment properly, accurately, and effectively is of paramount importance. Favorable outcomes depend on the proper use of the various machines. Issues include accuracy as well as proper cleaning, maintenance, and calibration, if necessary. Evaluation of the patient's technique in using the various machines should be done periodically by a health care professional. Patient acceptance and willingness to use the machines are, of course, critical. The following sections describe accuracy and use issues with representative home monitoring devices used in disease management to the home.

Home Glucose Meters

Management decisions for the treatment of diabetes are based both on monitoring done in the home and on testing done in a physician's office. Self-monitoring enables patients to under-stand and take control of their diabetes. When monitoring blood glucose, a number of factors should be considered: the supplies and equipment, monitoring methods, and correct data entry. Accurate results of SMBG have been shown to be technique and user dependent. Teaching patients how to use equipment is extremely important; positive outcomes depend on the proper use of the meters and strips and on patient motivation.

Blood glucose meters designed for home uses have come under close scrutiny for their accuracy in many studies. Recent findings (19) state that the evaluation of SMBG systems can be more effective using the percentage of values within the 10% interval of the reference value according to the American Diabetes Association consensus statement and the error grid analysis. These two methods consistently classified meters as to their accuracy with a high degree of reproducibility.

In one study, six SMBG machines were examined for performance using venous blood samples from 88 patients (20). The machines were Accutrend, Reflolux S, Companion 2, Glucometer GX, Glucometer IV, and One Touch II. Four machines from each brand were tested. Machine-generated whole-blood glucose (BG) values were corrected before comparison with laboratory plasma glucose values, measured by using a glucose oxidase method. Most of the corrected machine-generated BG values were clinically acceptable based on error grid analysis. Accutrend, Glucometer IV, and Companion 2 showed the greatest consistency between machines of the same brand. More than 80% of corrected BG values generated by Glucometer IV fell within ±10% of the reference values. SMBG machines are clinically accurate, but, again, patients using the machines must be taught to use the machines correctly to ensure accurate measurements at home.

Although physicians and patients both expect that BG monitoring machines will provide reliable results, some of the issues of reliability are the environmental, physiologic, and operational factors that can affect system performance and yield inaccurate or unpredictable results. For example, in a test of temperature effects, four BG meters (Accutrend, ExacTech Companion, Medisense Companion 2, and Glucometer III) were tested at temperatures ranging from 4° to 44°C (control solutions) and 8°C, 24°C, and 36°C (venous blood) and at humidities of 60% and 80% (21). Low and high temperatures resulted in a number of statistically significant changes in glucose readings with all meters. Accutrend, Medisense Companion 2, and Glucometer III were 100% clinically accurate at all temperatures. With the ExacTech Companion, only 70.8% of control solution and 55.6% of venous blood results were clinically accurate. The main errors occurred when (a) cold temperatures lowered the result so that euglycemic levels erroneously read in the hypoglycemic range and hyperglycemic levels gave a better than actual result and (b) hot temperatures increased the result whereby hypoglycemic levels falsely gave a euglycemic result. Weather conditions at which BG meters may be operated can affect results and potentially lead to errors in clinical decisions.

Because patients are encouraged to keep their BG values as near normal as possible, there is greater risk of hypoglycemic events. When meters were tested for accuracy at normal and hypoglycemic ranges in two studies (22,23), there were substantial differences between the blood glucose meters during hypoglycemia, and none of the devices met the latest criteria recommended by the American Diabetes Association.

Another source of potential error of glucose measurement in the home relates to errors in patient data entry. In an analysis of videotaped interactions between subjects and the Diabetes Home Monitoring Module (24), the most common error made during the process of data entry was that of entering information on the wrong date. Patient education must include instruction on accurate data entry and the reason why this is important. Data entry is sometimes done by hand in a paper-based system, or it can be done by telephone in a computerized system. The Vista 350 telephone (25) is a product that allows data to be entered to a central databank from home using technology that is at about the same level of complication as the standard telephone. Menus allow the input of BG levels, time, date, and "unusual events," such as exercise, stress, or intake of carbohydrates that may have affected the BG. Current insulin doses can be displayed and changes entered. Hypoglycemic events and their severity can be recorded. In addition, feedback summaries are also available to the user. This system also relies, however, on the patient entering correct data. Most glucose meters now have data transmission capabilities, and, with the appropriate disease management technology and software to make use of the automation capabilities, many of the patient entry errors will be eliminated.

Overall, it is important to recognize the possible types of errors that may occur in the measurement of glucose in the home; however, point-of-care measurement of glucose is essential for diabetics, and treatment decisions and management must be made with the information available.

Other more recent developments for home diabetes monitoring include devices that allow the self-testing of glycated protein. These are home versions of the fructosamin test, which has previously been available only in laboratories. Often, a weekly home test of fructosamine is advised to complement a patient's recommended regimen of daily BG testing and quarterly or semiannual HbA1c measurement. The recent research evaluating the benefits of this additional home monitoring has yet to show a differential improvement in glycemic control (26); however, this development could be particularly helpful for patients with type 2 diabetes, who traditionally show poor monitoring adherence. Fructosamine monitoring in the home is more sensitive to recent changes in glucose control than HbA1c; so this home monitoring can enable patients and their physicians to intervene earlier with new recommendations for diet, exercise, and medication levels.

An additional new development that promises to relieve some of the burden of daily testing for blood glucose levels is the new wristwatch-like device that measures glucose levels every few minutes through the skin. The device uses electroosmosis to draw glucose molecules from the patient's skin into a dermal patch, where the contents are measured and interpreted by an integrated circuit within the device. Currently, these devices are not considered to be sufficiently accurate to replace completely the fingerprick blood tests; however, these types of advances that dramatically reduce the burden of diabetes monitoring in the home offer the potential for improved diabetes management and health outcomes.

Home Peak-Flow Meters

Peak-flow monitoring is used as part of an asthma treatment plan to assist in establishing a diagnosis of asthma, to measure asthma severity, to assess the response to treatment, and to recognize deteriorating asthma. The peak expiratory flow rate is an objective measure of airflow obstruction that patients can learn with proper instruction and that provides physicians with objective information for assessing a patient's condition. Accurate results depend on the patient's ability to use the meter correctly. Usefulness to the clinician then also depends on the patient recording the results accurately. Typically, patients are instructed to measure peak flow at least every morning on awakening and to record the best of three tries each time. Patients also are instructed to find personal-best peak-flow numbers and the highest peak-flow number achievable over a 2- to 3-week period when asthma is under good control. Based on the peak-flow readings and patient symptoms, the physician may write a medication algorithm for patient use.

A portable electronic peak-flow meter combined with an asthma monitor (AM1, Jaeger, Germany) was found to measure peak expiratory flow and forced expiratory volume in 1 second, which matched the accuracy criteria of the American Thoracic Society standards for monitoring devices (27). Accuracy of the instruments is not the only criterion in home monitoring, however. In a prospective 1-year study in asthma clinics from three tertiary-care hospitals (28), 26 patients with moderate to severe asthma took part in an asthma education program. They were asked to measure morning and evening peak expiratory flow (PEF) using an electronic peak-flow meter with a 3-month memory, unaware that the device recorded the values found. Results showed good short-term compliance with PEF measurements, but even with regular reinforcement, compliance fell to 50% at 6 months and to 33% at 12 months. These investigators suggested using PEF measuring devices for those showing a strong personal interest in using them and limiting use to short periods. In a similar study (29), 65 children were randomized to receive a simple mini-Wright (SM) or an electronic recording meter (ERM), unaware that the ERM recorded the measurements electronically. Findings resembled the Cote study, and these researchers suggested that initiating and maintaining peak-flow recordings is difficult. In a third study (30) using similar methods, the researchers concluded that compliance with daily PEF is generally poor in chronic stable asthmatic subjects assessed on two visits separated by a 3-month period. Also, a substantial number of values (22%) are invented.

An accepted way of testing peak-flow meters is by comparison with values from a pneumotachograph. Folgering and colleagues (31) compared 11 peak-flow meters in two test series. In the first test, the meter being tested was connected downstream in series with a Fleisch no. 4 pneumotachograph. One subject performed 50 partial forced expiratory maneuvers through this ensemble. In the second series, 50 adult patients and 25 healthy children performed sequential maximal forced expiratory maneuvers on each peak-flow meter and on the pneumotachograph. Differences in the quality of the meters were found, but meters could be found that were in close agreement with the pneumotachograph. The accuracy of peak-flow meters can be tested, and accurate meters are available, but the main issue in peak flow meters appears to be patient compliance with use. A more interactive disease management program could greatly improve compliance behaviors.

Home Blood Pressure Devices

Home BP monitoring devices and patient self-readings have been examined for accuracy in several studies. Screening BPs (measured at health examinations) were compared with BPs measured at home (32). Measurements were taken 1 year apart, and the correlations between the readings were significantly higher for the home BP measurements (systolic, $r = 0.844$; diastolic, $r = 0.830$) than for the screening BP measurements (systolic, $r = 0.692$; diastolic, $r = 0.570$). In another study (33), 946 subjects measured home BP readings twice daily for 7 days. A baseline BP was also measured at the clinic and was repeated by 735 of the subjects 3 years later. The home BP readings on both examinations were reproducible and proved predictive of subsequent BP trends. A home BP of 128 and 83 mm Hg or higher detected "sustained" hypertension with 48% sensitivity and 93% specificity. Readings of 120 and 80 mm Hg or lower predicted future normotension with 45% sensitivity and 91% specificity. These investigators concluded that home monitoring of BP was useful in the management of borderline hypertension. Santilli and English (1990) (34) also found that home BP monitoring can be useful in the management of borderline hypertension. Their study compared office and home BP measurements in 36 borderline hypertensive subjects to determine the accuracy of the home monitoring units used. Again, the monitors were found to be accurate and useful in the management of hypertension. In a somewhat larger and more recent study (35), volunteers who used BP-monitoring devices were studied to see how the devices were used and to assess their accuracy. A BP reading was considered accurate if the differences between the volunteers' and technicians' systolic and diastolic readings were both 10 mm Hg or less. Of the 91 patients, 31 (34%) obtained inaccurate readings. The inaccuracy could not be attributed to the type, cost, or age of the instrument or to the educational level of the user. The researchers concluded that supervision of the use of BP-monitoring devices needs to be incorporated into the physician follow-up to ensure that there is a reasonable correlation between values obtained using the mercury sphygmomanometer and the BP-monitoring device.

Home Measurement of Weight

Congestive heart failure is the most common discharge diagnosis for Medicare beneficiaries (36). CHF is a frequent reason for hospital admission, often results in unplanned readmissions, and has a high mortality rate (37). The importance of avoiding recurrent admissions is clear. A program of intensive case management may reduce the burden attributable to CHF. The impact of treatment on prognosis of patients with chronic CHF depends not only on pharmacologic therapy but also on nonpharmacologic aspects of patient management. Patient compliance, lifestyle changes, salt and fluid restriction, detailed patient information, and measures of self-control greatly affect thera-

peutic efficacy. Many patients with chronic heart failure frequently have inadequate knowledge about necessary lifestyle changes or do not remember the instructions on key issues of necessary lifestyle changes and diet. Many patients gain weight from retained fluid before decompensation, a condition that could be detected by self-monitoring of weight and improved by changes in medication.

Bathroom scales, measuring devices typically used by patients, can be affected by moisture and temperature changes. Scales found at the physician's office are usually the most accurate kind. Patient instruction to monitor weight at the same time every morning (right after getting out of bed and emptying the bladder), dressed in the same weight of clothes (or no clothes), can increase the reliability of weights measured on a home scale. Additionally, there are now electronic scales with modem connections to report the weights automatically. This can offer a great improvement in data accuracy, given that many heart failure patients also suffer from a degree of confusion and cognitive impairment from their disease. The task of writing and recording their weight information and relaying the data are difficult tasks for some. Patient education to monitor and report weight gain in a timely fashion can affect prognosis and prevent disease exacerbation. Patient education must be ongoing to reinforce the necessity for nonpharmacologic aspects of disease management.

A disease management approach to patient care combines patient education, provider use of practice guidelines, appropriate consultation, and supplies of drugs and ancillary services. A disease management system in home care could have a profound effect on the care and outcomes of the growing population with long-term health concerns.

Home Monitoring of Prothrombin Time

Warfarin (Coumadin) is a commonly used anticoagulant that is effective in treating and preventing venous and arterial thrombosis. The therapy often requires periodic monitoring of the prothrombin time (PT) to ensure that the drug levels remain within the therapeutic range. The PT usually is measured every 1 to 4 weeks in an outpatient laboratory, and often the therapy is expected to continue for a period of 6 months or longer. In addition, warfarin has a narrow therapeutic range that is greatly affected by an individual's metabolism, diet, and other medications; therefore, it is important to monitor the dosage carefully and frequently. In-home testing has the potential to improve the control of anticoagulant therapy by making these frequent and ongoing measurements more feasible.

In 1997, the U.S. Food and Drug Administration cleared the use of fingerstick monitors for PT testing in the home. In a study of patient use of a portable PT measurement device, researchers found that patient self-testing measurements were fairly accurate (38): 66% of the home results matched the reference laboratory's range classification. When a mismatch occurred, the home result was more likely to be low compared with the reference laboratory result. These findings are very similar to the in-hospital point-of-care use of a portable PT device. An additional important finding is that patients overwhelmingly reported satisfaction with the procedure and a willingness to perform the self-testing of PT (38).

There has been a recent trend to manage anticoagulant patient care through specialty anticoagulant clinics. Typically, these are staffed by nurses who track patients taking warfarin through their therapy. The nurses access electronic patient databases with patient diagnoses, previous procedures, therapeutic goals, and previous laboratory results (specifically PT reported in the format of the international normalized ratio, or INR). The nurses are typically responsible for a set group of patients, whom they contact and manage by phone. The information systems often classify the patients as high risk, medium risk, and low risk, and in addition report deviations of INRs from the target range for a patient's condition. This type of complex management is highly amenable to Internet-based management in addition to phone management.

WEB-BASED INFORMATION AND COMMUNICATIONS SYSTEMS DESIGN

Using Web interfaces to integrate clinical databases is certainly a growing trend for hospitals, clinics, and managed care organizations. There are many compelling reasons for this in clinical settings. For example, Web access to clinical databases provides easy access from home computers for physicians and other professionals, a unified interface to disparate data sets and software, and the ability to have an overlay of security and access definitions that would not need to be repeated for each task. Currently, however, many clinics have only their practice management functions automated and encoded electronically. Many still rely primarily on paper charts for clinical information in the medical record.

For disease management that involves day-to-day care and monitoring, computer applications and new capabilities for clinical databases become more than desirable; they are essential to the process. Disease management systems consist of a mix of communications and information management components. Figure 35.1 illustrates the software, devices, and personnel required for disease management to the home. Contact with the patient and the management of disease through the system may be accomplished from the perspective of either a specialty clinic or an organization with an interest in the management of the patient's disease but without the normal channels of direct clinical care (e.g., managed care organizations and pharmaceutical companies). The database of disease management information is usually kept separate from existing organizational databases, such as the practice management systems and electronic medical records that might be found in a clinic or the claims data that a managed care organization might have. It is important, however, that the databases be able to query each other and have compatible standards and terminology, for example, the use of Health Level 7 (HL-7) or International Classification of Diseases (ICD9) codes. A disease management database should contain the following types of information for each patient:

- Name, phone, e-mail (if available), address, caregiver or family information
- Security information (password, level of access to data)
- Assigned case manager, physician

- Diagnosis and stage or level (e.g., type 2 diabetes, 2 years since diagnosis)
- Summarized history (e.g., age, gender, risk factors)
- Current medications
- Current treatment plan (very specific, based on home-care management)
- Record of previous laboratory results
- Record of home monitoring data
- Record of messages to and from the patient
- User preferences (e.g., phone versus e-mail, time-of-day for reminders)

The disease management database will also likely contain identity, security, and preference information for the health care professions using the system as well. Most typically, there will be a custom Web interface to this data. Patients using the Web will see screens that contain only their data and will not have access to information about other patients. Patients will be able to download their monitoring information, access patient education information, and communication with their case manager. The Web interface for the case manager, on the other hand, will show summary statistics, identify patients with urgent needs, and enable efficient communication with patients.

The disease management database and the accompanying control software usually reside on a highly secured server (with appropriate backup capabilities). This server may be located in the host clinic (or health maintenance organization) or may physically be kept at the location of a service organization that would manage the technology. It is also typical for the software that controls the monitoring and communications functions to be located on the same server. Software modules include the following:

Algorithms that encode treatment guidelines, trend detection, comparisons of patient-specific normal values and alarm conditions with monitored data

Communications message control

- Tailored further questions to ask the patient when data is outside normal limits
- When and how quickly to alert the case manager or physician
- Broadcast messages to groups of similar patients (e.g., patient education tips for those patients with recent high blood glucose values) by phone or e-mail
- Protocols for handling personal patient messages (immediate answer versus research question and reply later)
- Interactive voice response systems for messaging via the phone in the patient's home
- Moderated chat room protocols for Internet support groups
- Security checking algorithms

Summary statistics for clinician review of patient population or subgroups

This sophisticated software enables ongoing timely care to the home for a variety of disease management programs. Case managers can track patient progress on a large number of similar patients and intervene when necessary. Tailored messages can be generated automatically through a predetermined protocol based on current and past patient data. These messages then can

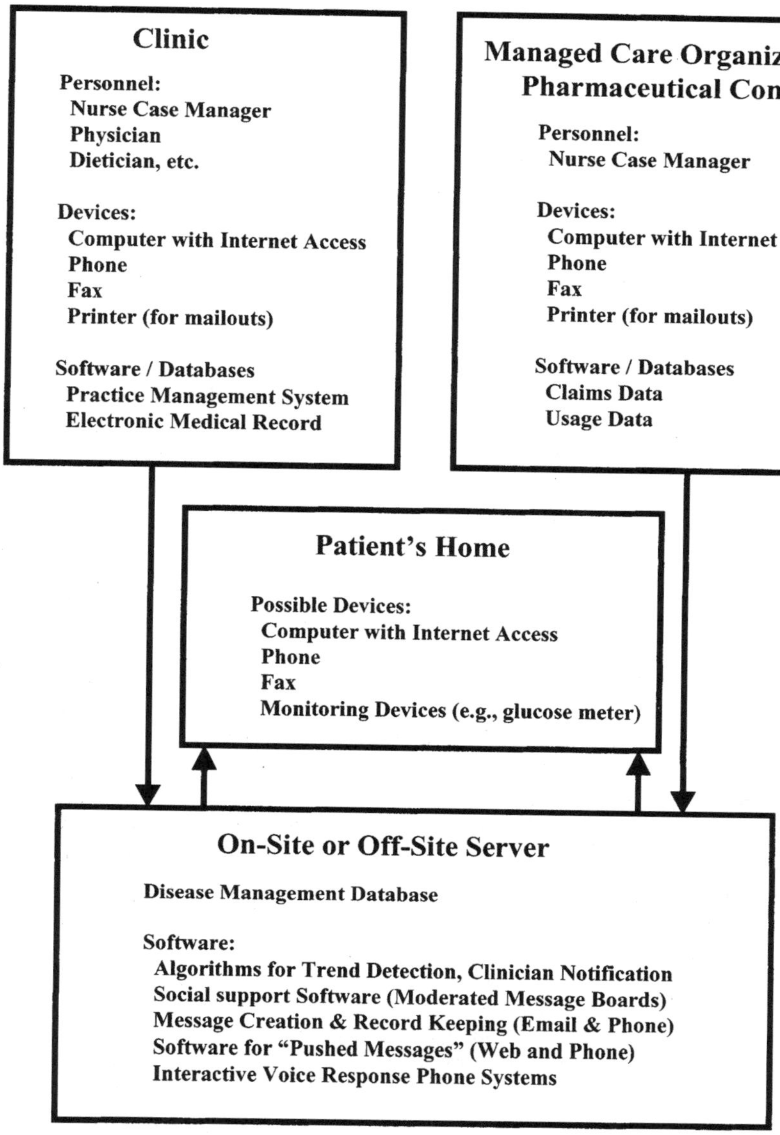

```
┌─────────────────────────────────┐      ┌─────────────────────────────────┐
│            Clinic               │      │  Managed Care Organization or   │
│                                 │      │    Pharmaceutical Company       │
│  Personnel:                     │      │                                 │
│    Nurse Case Manager           │      │    Personnel:                   │
│    Physician                    │      │      Nurse Case Manager         │
│    Dietician, etc.              │      │                                 │
│                                 │      │    Devices:                     │
│  Devices:                       │      │      Computer with Internet Access │
│    Computer with Internet Access│      │      Phone                      │
│    Phone                        │      │      Fax                        │
│    Fax                          │      │      Printer (for mailouts)     │
│    Printer (for mailouts)       │      │                                 │
│                                 │      │    Software / Databases         │
│  Software / Databases           │      │      Claims Data                │
│    Practice Management System   │      │      Usage Data                 │
│    Electronic Medical Record    │      │                                 │
└─────────────────────────────────┘      └─────────────────────────────────┘

              ┌───────────────────────────────────┐
              │           Patient's Home          │
              │                                   │
              │  Possible Devices:                │
              │    Computer with Internet Access  │
              │    Phone                          │
              │    Fax                            │
              │    Monitoring Devices (e.g., glucose meter) │
              └───────────────────────────────────┘

┌───────────────────────────────────────────────────────┐
│           On-Site or Off-Site Server                  │
│                                                       │
│  Disease Management Database                          │
│                                                       │
│  Software:                                            │
│    Algorithms for Trend Detection, Clinician Notification │
│    Social support Software (Moderated Message Boards) │
│    Message Creation & Record Keeping (Email & Phone)  │
│    Software for "Pushed Messages" (Web and Phone)     │
│    Interactive Voice Response Phone Systems           │
└───────────────────────────────────────────────────────┘
```

FIGURE 35.1. Information flow in a disease management system from the point of view of a specialty clinic or from an independent organization, such as a health maintenance organization or pharmaceutical company.

be sent by e-mail or by an interactive voice response (IVR) phone system. Most Internet-based disease management programs to the home also offer a phone component. The interactivity provided through a Web page and e-mail for monitoring and "pushed" messages can be partially replicated with an IVR phone system, where automated messages deliver tailored reminders, messages of encouragement, or news but in addition allow the patient to input responses to questionnaires or monitoring values. Clinical algorithms for disease management are activated by updated patient information. These then alert the nurse case manager and, if sufficiently urgent, the managing physician to intervene in the management of the patient. Several of these types of systems have been designed and tested for various chronic disease applications (39–41).

Data security is an important concern in all medical databases, but it is especially important for disease management systems where there are multiple users with varying access capabilities and the data may not even reside on site. All users must be authenticated and must maintain authentication throughout the encounter. Currently, this is usually accomplished with a password, but in the future biometric authentication (fingerprint or iris pattern sensing) or sophisticated voice recognition systems will be more common. A great deal of recent work in the Internet industry has focused on making Internet transactions secure for e-commerce. Current security measures include firewalls, encryption, and digital signatures. Security systems are continually being developed to scramble and unscramble messages; to verify the source and destination of information; and to ensure that the information is not stolen, tampered with, or viewed along the way. Although not all the communications in disease management are highly sensitive, the whole picture of information on a patient with a chronic disease is sensitive. Privacy and security need to be handled with the best methods available.

CHALLENGES TO THE EFFECTIVE IMPLEMENTATION OF HOME-BASED DISEASE MANAGEMENT

Computer applications have been notoriously slow in making inroads in clinical care (compared with other industries). Quite often, systems with expert-level diagnostic performance are not seen to be commercially viable; conversely, very simple systems may have a large effect. Historically, computer inroads in clinical areas have started through billing and administrative functions. Also, isolated departments, such as clinical laboratories and pharmacies, have made early use of specific software and databases. The electronic medical record, with important clinical information necessary for quality disease management, has been much slower to follow. The most important barriers seem to be in the areas of workflow analysis and user interface design.

Similarly, with disease management systems, the largest challenges are making the technology and information an integral and seamless part of the workflow of the health care professionals as well as for the patients in the home. Many disease management systems have failed, or at least have been underused, because not enough care was taken to integrate and change workflow habits in the clinic. The following are common barriers to success:

- Asking nurses who are already working full time to serve as case managers in addition to their normal responsibilities (giving the impression that this should be done over their lunch hour or at the end of a long day): The workflow has to be integrated and save time overall.
- Requiring use of a separate computer system (and, worse yet, in a separate location): Disease management software should be an always-on function that is easy to access and easy to use.
- Having a cumbersome user interface: The system should minimize data entry and minimize the number of mouse clicks and time to get to the needed information.

Communications should be streamlined and effective. For the patient Web interface, it is critical that the displays be simple and understandable. Long training periods are not an option. For patients who are communicating by phone only, the messages must be clear, succinct, and of perceived value to the patient. Keypunching and data entry by phone are cumbersome.

Generally, system users are willing to put more effort into using a new system if there is perceived value to them directly and fairly soon. Patients will give up quickly if they perceive that their case manager or health care provider is not looking at the information they submit. From the case manager's point of view, the system must save time and effort, not just create extra work. It is also important to obtain the "buy-in" of the physicians early on because doing disease management right requires a fundamental reorganization and standardization of clinical care. There must be agreement on guidelines and an understanding of the quality-of-care benefits. Doctors are averse to imposed systems that appear to be "cookbook" solutions. The solution here is to involve physicians in the program, to align incentives, to emphasize that it is an evidence-based approach, and to provide them with feedback on the quality of care outcomes of disease management.

CONCLUSIONS AND FUTURE TRENDS

The medical care environment and rapid technologic advances are leading to dramatic new ways of practicing medicine. Internet-based disease management in the home, enabled by point-of-care devices for patient use, has become one of the most significant results of these trends. It is likely that home-based disease management will become a standard part of clinical care in the future. In addition, the techniques associated with collaborative goal setting for health behavior change and self-monitoring will expand to the areas of disease prevention and health maintenance. Given that health care dollars are being spent increasingly on chronic diseases and diseases associated with aging, this care-to-the-home model also will become standard in nursing homes and assisted living situations.

The key technologies that will enable further developments for this new approach to care include the following:

- A growing variety of point-of-care monitoring devices for the home, such as BG meters for diabetes, peak-flow meters for asthma, portable PT meters for anticoagulation management, automated weight records, and transmission for heart failure patients, and others
- An integration of phones, pagers, Internet, television, and computing capabilities, thus offering consumers a great deal of functionality required for care to the home through their day-to-day routine technology
- High-bandwidth Internet available over cable lines and viewable on home televisions with the use of new set-top boxes
- Video that is easily available for two-way communication between advice nurses and patients, doctors and patients, as well as for social support among patients themselves
- Software algorithms and intelligent systems that will integrate health care and disease management activities into patients' daily lives. Web-based interfaces and calendars will coordinate personal management functions that include medication reminders; action plans for exercise, diets, etc.; tailored menu planning, pantry availability, and automated food shopping; and messages from one's health care provider, which will be a seamless part of the overall personal information and communications functions.

These new forms of disease and health management, enabled by the Internet, point-of-care devices, and newly developed technology, will likely become ubiquitous and integrated into both clinical workflow and home activities. These systems that enable patients to be active partners with clinicians in managing their care in a timely and interactive fashion offer promise for substantial improvements in quality of care and health outcomes.

REFERENCES

1. Taylor R, Lessin L. Restructureing the health care delivery system in the United States. *Journal of Health Care Finance* 1996;22:33–60.
2. Coons SJ. (1996). Disease management: Definitions and exploration of issues. *Clinical Therapeutics* 1996;18:1321–1326.
3. Bernard S. Disease management: pharmaceutical industry perspective. *Pharm Exec* 1995;1:48–50.

4. Meyer LC, Rohl B. An innovative approach to treating chronic disabling asthma. *Case Manager* 1993;4:54–69.

5. Bennett BD. Blood glucose determination: point of care testing. *South Med J* 1997;90:678–680.

6. American Diabetes Association (ADA*). Physician's guide to non-insulin-dependent (type II) diabetes: diagnosis and treatment,* 2nd ed. Alexandria, VA: American Diabetes Association, 1989.

7. Diabetes Control and Complications Trial Research Group. The effect of intensive treatment of diabetes on the development and progression of long-term complications in insulin-dependent diabetes mellitus. *N Engl J Med* 1993;329:977–986.

8. American Association of Clinical Endocrinologists (AACE). AACE clinical guidelines. http://www.aace.com/clin/guides/diabetes_guide.html. American Diabetes Association. Clinical practice recommendations 1999. *Diabetes Care* 1999;22(Suppl 1).

9. Smith SA, Murphy ME, Huschka TR, et al. Impact of a diabetes electronic management system on the care of patients seen in a subspecialty diabetes clinic. *Diabetes Care* 1998;21:972–976.

10. Chiarelli F, DiRocco L, Catino M, et al. Modern management of childhood diabetes: a role for computerized devices? *Acta Paediatr Jpn* 1998;40:299–302.

11. Strode SW, Gustke S, Allen A. Technical and clinical progress in telemedicine. *JAMA* 1999;281:1066–1068.

12. Meneghini LF, Albisser AM, Goldberg RB, et al. An electronic case manager for diabetes control. *Diabetes Care* 1998;21:591–596.

13. Kane B, Sands DZ. 1998. Guidelines for the clinical use of electronic mail with ptients. *J Am Med Inform Assoc* 1998;5:104–111.

14. Lewis D. The Internet as a resource for healthcare information. *The Diabetes Educator* 1998;24:627–630,632.

15. Tetzlaff L. Consumer informatics in chronic illness. *J Am Med Inform Assoc* 1997;4:285–300.

16. Trajanoski Z, Brunner GA, Gfrerer RJ, et al. Accuracy of home blood glucose meters during hpoglycemia. *Diabetes Care* 1996;19:1212–1215.

17. Hubbs PR, Rindfleisch TC, Godin P, et al. Medical information on the Internet. *JAMA* 1998;280(1363).

18. Jenkins J, Erdman K. Web-based documentation systems. *Home Health Care Management and Practice* 1998;10:52–61.

19. Poirier JY, Prieur N, Campion L, et al. Clinical and statistical evaluation of self-monitoring blood glucose meters. *Diabetes Care* 1998;21:1919–1924.

20. Chan JC, Wong RY, Cheung CK, et al. Accuracy, precision and user-acceptability of self blood glucose monitoring machines. *Diabetes Research Clinical Practice* 1997;36:91–104.

21. King JM, Eigenmann CA, Colagiuri S. Effect of ambient temperature and humidity on performance of blood glucose meters. *Diabetes Med* 1995;12:337–40.

22. Glasmacher AG, Brennemann W, Hahn C, et al. Evaluation of five devices for self-monitoring of blood glucose in the normoglycaemic range. *Exp Clin Endocrinol Diabetes* 1998;106:360–364.

23. Trajanoski Z, Brunner GA, Gfrerer RJ, et al. Accuracy of home blood glucose meters during hypoglycemia. *Diabetes Care* 1996;19:1412–1215.

24. Cytryn KN, Patel VL. Reasoning about diabetes and its relationship to the use of telecommunication technology by patients and physicians. *International J Med Informatics* 1998;51:137–151.

25. Edmonds E, Bauer M, Osborn S, et al. Using the Vista 350 telephone to communicate the results of home monitoring of diabetes mellitus to a central database and to provide feedback. *Int J Med Inform* 1998;51:117–125.

26. Petitti DG, Contreras R, Dudl J. Randomized trial of fructosamine home monitoring in patients with diabetes. *Eff Clinical Practice* 2001;4:18–23.

27. Richter K, Kanniess F, Mark B, et al. Assessment of accuracy and applicability of a new electronic peak flow meter and asthma monitor. *Eur Respir J* 1998;12:457–462.

28. Cote J, Cartier A, Malo JL, et al. Compliance with peak expiratory flow monitoring in home management of asthma. *Chest* 1998;113:968–972.

29. Redline S, Wright EC, Kattan M, et al. Short-term compliance with peak flow monitoring: results from a study of inner city children with asthma. *Pediatr Pulmonol* 1996;21:203–210.

30. Verschelden P, Cartier A, L'Archeveque J, et al. Compliance with and accuracy of daily self-assessments of peak expiratory flows (PEF) in asthmatic subjects over a three month period. *Eur Respir J* 1996;9:880–885.

31. Folgering H, Brink W, Heeswijk O, et al. Eleven peak flow meters: a clinical evaluation. *Eur Respir J* 1998;11:188–193.

32. Sakuma M, Imai Y, Nagai K, et al. Reproducibility of home blood pressure measurements over a 1-year period. *Am J Hypertens* 1997;10(7 Part 1):798–803.

33. Nesbitt SD, Amerena JV, Grant E, et al. Home blood pressure as a predictor of future blood pressure stability in borderline hypertension: the Tecumseh Study. *Am J Hypertens* 1997;10:1270–1280.

34. Santilli GM, English JC. Home blood pressure readings in borderline hypertensive patients. *Fam Pract Res J* 1990;10:97–103.

35. Merrick RD, Olive KE, Hamdy RC, et al. Factors influencing the accuracy of home blood pressure measurement. *South Med J* 1997;90:1110–1114.

36. Krumholz HM, Parent EM, Tu N, et al. Readmission after hospitalization for congestive heart failure among Medicare beneficiaries. *Arch Intern Med* 1997;157:99–104.

37. Lowe JM, Candlish PM, Henry DA, et al. Management and outcomes of congestive heart failure: a prospective study of hospitalised patients. *Med J Aust* 1998;168:115–118.

38. Oral Anticoagulation Monitoring Study Group. Prothrombin measurement using a patient self-testing system. *Am J Clin Pathol* 2001;115:280–287.

39. Piette JD. Interactive voice response systems in the diagnosis and management of chronic disease. *American Journal of Managed Care* 2000;6:817–827.

40. Gilbert JA. Disease management hits home. *Health Data Management* 1998;6:58–60.

41. Finkelstein J, Hripcsak G, Cabrera MR. Patients' acceptance of Internet-based home asthma telemonitoring. *Proceedings of the AMIA Symposium,* 1996:336–340.

AN INTERNET-BASED EXTERNAL QUALITY-ASSESSMENT SCHEME FOR POCT

A. DOUGLAS HIRST

The problems associated with external quality assessment (EQA) in point-of-care testing (POCT) are very different from laboratory-based schemes and include data handling by the laboratory, data presentation to nonscientific staff, and establishing a laboratory-type quality culture for testing in nonlaboratory areas. Choice of specimen also is a difficult area.

One of the main laboratory problems is to provide the resources to operate an EQA scheme because, unlike laboratory proficiency testing, there is often no income stream to finance the operation. The main labor costs are in specimen preparation and distribution and in data processing and report distribution. To address this problem, we have produced an EQA system for POCT that reduces the data processing labor costs by using Internet technology. This allows the users to enter their own data and, following statistical analysis, to receive an automatic e-mail message informing them of their performance. Participants then can examine their performance on the Web site with real-time graphical presentations derived from the database.

The system comprises a Microsoft Access database running on a Windows NT 4.0 Web server with an SMTP e-mail gateway (http://Elab.org.uk). Each participant in the scheme is allocated an identification (ID) code and password, which is required for the Web site log-in screen and allows entry and viewing of the individual's data. The participant's e-mail address also is stored for transmission of reports.

As each distribution is prepared, the pool data for the QA material are entered into the database. This consists of target value (preferably by reference method), allowable error (standard deviation), e-mail limits (see later), and deadline date (date after which the Web entry is disabled). When participants log in, they can select the distribution, chemistry, and instrument (e.g., glucose meter) and enter their result. The system will redisplay the data for the participant to confirm before acceptance. Results that have been entered in this way do not go directly into the database but are stored in a temporary Web results file. This file is inspected manually before statistics calculation, but to assist this process, the database flags each field for credibility, and it is a very quick process to scroll through the file. After checking, the statistics calculation is initiated, and the participant's performance becomes available for viewing on the Web site.

The final step is to initiate the e-mail routine. This is accessed through an active server page on the Web site by a standard Web browser, which is also password protected. The routine operates by checking each participant's result against the e-mail limits defined for the quality assurance material. As the system steps through the returned results, it creates and builds four mailing lists: acceptable performance, suboptimal performance, unacceptable performance, and no return. The e-mail address for each participant is added to one of the four lists according to their performance, together with their ID and result. A standard simple message then is generated for each list: laboratory ID, scheme, distribution date, results, message: "Your result is acceptable/suboptimal/unacceptable/no return." If the result is suboptimal or unacceptable, the system adds the message, "Please inspect your performance on the Web site."

Participants are able to view their performance on the Web site. Confidentiality is maintained through the same password-protected log-in screen used for data entry, and users have a choice of data entry or performance review. The performance review offers two choices: (a) display of the results statistics and histogram for any chosen distribution or (b) a trend display of the last ten distributions comprising a Levy-Jennings chart and a linearity plot. These displays are generated by first calling a database search routine to extract the data and then downloading the data plus JAVA graphing tools to the users' PC to display the data. This can be a slow process, especially for the first graphics display.

Operation started in January 1999 with a blood-glucose EQA scheme for the hospital comprising 50 wards with Roche Advantage (Roche Diagnostics) blood-glucose meters. The e-mail function was added in autumn 1999. Recently, a group of general practitioners joined the scheme, and a neighboring hospital also is testing the system, raising the number of participants to 102.

Matrix is a major problem because the different glucose measurement systems react differently to different materials, particularly aqueous material. We have tried using freshly donated blood stabilized with Iodoacetate. This gives remarkable stability for the Roche Advantage system, but other systems, such as MediSense and Glucotrend, significantly underestimate after storage for a few days. This may be a matrix problem related to the rate at which the sample soaks into the test strip. Because of these problems, we have returned to using horse blood with added glucose, stabilized with fluoride oxalate. This material seems to have good stability in most glucose measurement systems for 5 days, which is sufficient for a local scheme, and most systems produce comparable results.

The laboratory supervises the use of 21 DCA 2000 analyzers for hemoglobin A1c (HbA1c) analysis in the local community. These analyzers are shared by 50 general-practice surgeries in rotation to coincide with their diabetic clinics. We have found daily internal quality control on these instruments to be very expensive and ineffective and have replaced this with a regular EQA scheme using the same Internet technology system.

Because material was again a problem, we used diabetic blood stabilized with EDTA donated from another EQA provider (WEQAS, Cardiff, UK). This material was stable for 4 weeks at +4°C, but it was prone to causing the DCA analyzers to give error messages. We also tried our own fresh donated diabetic blood, which we analyzed within 1 week, and this reduced the error messages. We had hoped to use the same material for both HbA1c and blood glucose EQA schemes, but the problems with different blood-glucose systems have prevented this for the present.

Our laboratory has operated an EQA scheme for POCT blood-gas analyzers for several years. In mid-1999, this scheme also was added to the EQA Internet technology platform, which currently comprises 30 hospitals and 65 blood-gas analyzers. Originally, the scheme was only for pH, partial pressure of carbon dioxide (PCO_2) and partial pressure of oxygen (PO_2), and an aqueous fluorocarbon matrix was used. We have since added ions, lactate, and glucose, which require a protein-based matrix, and will need to progress to a hemolysate to add heme pigments.

All the other analyses have been quantitative, but in 2000 we started a pilot EQA scheme for fecal occult blood (FOB) for colorectal cancer screening, which now comprises 30 hospital laboratories. This test generates a result that is qualitative (±) and is a challenge to data processing. We devised a method for converting these results to scores (the subject of a separate publication), and this scheme has been operating successfully for 6 months. We are facing a major challenge with the choice of cutoff limit, however. We have taken a view from the literature that 1 mL of blood per 100 g of feces is the appropriate cutoff, but most laboratories use commercial kits with a cutoff of around 0.5 mL of blood per 100 g of feces and therefore do not perform well in the borderline area, causing a degree of consternation among some participants.

The development of this database has been a valuable experience, and we have learned a number of important lessons. First, the choice of database is the most important aspect because it must be able to handle complex calculation routines for large numbers of records. In our experience, Microsoft Access starts to slow down significantly when the system exceeds 8,000 records. Second, an EQA scheme for POCT requires a complex database design for displaying multiple meters per site or multiple chemistry measurements per meter or both. There is also a need at data entry for entry of multiple results (chemistries) for a single sample, for which the current database is not designed (it was designed originally for blood glucose EQA). Third, for graphics displays, we used JAVA graphing tools linked to SQL database searches. This system worked very well for real-time data display, but we found that display functions are complex and limited and require considerable expertise in JAVA programming, and that display is slow and difficult to speed. We believe that alternative, server-based graphing routines would be a better approach. Finally, for nonnumeric data (e.g., FOB schemes) that must be manually converted to scores in the laboratory, we recommend using a database that can be programmed with a front-end routine for preprocessing nonnumeric results for participant data entry to work.

AN INTRANET-BASED TUTORIAL FOR WARD-BASED BLOOD GLUCOSE TESTING

A. DOUGLAS HIRST

Point-of-care testing (POCT) is widely used in a number of clinical situations, particularly in critical care cases requiring prompt therapeutic intervention. One of the most common applications is for testing blood glucose, which is used for the diagnosis, stabilization, and monitoring of patients with diabetes. For the best quality of care, it is important that medical staff are trained in the proper use of the test to prevent errors leading to inappropriate therapy. Several studies involving nursing staff have shown that they need to be trained to obtain accurate results and that the quality of glucose testing is improved by the introduction of quality control, training, and periodic retraining. In the United Kingdom, the Department of Health issued hazard notices following fatalities caused by the misuse of glucose meters.

The meters and strips are usually very reliable, and most problems arise from operator error, for which the most likely cause is poor or nonexistent training. Few hospitals provide structured training on a continuing basis. Training for POCT devices has a major resource implication that is usually overlooked when POCT systems are introduced. For this reason, training often is provided by the instrument's company representative or is passed on from one staff member to another. In the latter case, this practice often fosters a belief that the meters always give a correct answer.

In our hospital, a single system—the Roche Advantage system—was adopted recently for blood glucose testing. This involved retraining the nursing staff, which in turn led to development of a training package based on the hospital intranet and accessible by personal computers (PCs) on all wards to address the resource issue of providing continuing training. Use of intranet technology is a very effective way of addressing both the training quality and the resource issues.

The tutorial was designed for training nursing and other medical staff and was based on a standard Web browser design, with photographs or diagrams for every stage and process, accompanied by text explaining the process. The tutorial was produced using Asymetrix Toolbook (a commercial package specifically designed for tutorials) and includes several features, including page links and scoring, which make this an ideal medium for producing programmed-learning systems. The tutorial was designed as a linear progression, split into eight sections consisting of three to ten pages. At the end of each section, there is a multiple-choice question that must be answered correctly before the trainee can proceed to the next section. A programmed learning approach was adopted, whereby if the reader selects the wrong answer to a question, the page where the correct answer can be found is displayed. The reader cannot progress until the correct answer has been given, and marks are deducted for each wrong answer. Psychological education techniques (e.g., use of color and appropriate wording) can be used to indicate right and wrong answers, such that it will stimulate careful study of the tutorial.

Operation of the tutorial was kept simple with a choice of arrow icons for moving to the next page or for indicating the answer to the questions. Nurses with no Web-browsing experience picked up this method of operation without any difficulty. The first section presents the theory and mechanism of glucose measurement (e.g., electrochemical reaction) and the theory of electrochemistry, followed by sections on clinical indications for performing the test, patient preparation, instrument calibration, quality control checks, strip and meter care, performing the blood test, recording results, action on abnormal results, and troubleshooting.

An audit of the tutorial was performed on a typical medical ward with every grade of nurse on the ward. The audit form consisted of seven questions and was completed immediately after the tutorial. Eleven nurses participated in the audit. The results of the questionnaire showed that (a) nursing staff enjoyed using the intranet and preferred it to traditional teaching; (b) the tutorial was not considered too complex; (c) the tutorial was found to be very relevant; and (d) the length of the tutorial was just right. In addition to this questionnaire, the senior nurses were asked for their impression of the intranet approach to training. The main response was that it was a very useful learning tool and was preferable by far to the traditional didactic teaching provided by instrument company representatives. The tutorial also was found to be a convenient mode by which training could be arranged to fit in with other ward activities.

One of the major problems with POCT in a large hospital is that the number of staff who need teaching and the hours they work mean that there are major resource implications in providing personal training over a short or continuing period. If nonhospital staff provide the training, there is a loss of control over the content of the training package. To avoid errors in diagnosis and treatment, it is important to ensure that staff members understand all aspects of the test they are performing, including the mechanism, causes of errors, and clinical consequences. For this reason, it is important that professional laboratory staff manage the content of any POCT training program. An effective way of addressing the resource problems associated with using laboratory staff is to use intranet-based training packages.

Programmed learning has been shown to be a very successful educational technique because it can be used to respond to individual learning problems. It was not widely adopted as a teaching technique because it is difficult and expensive to plan in printed form. This form of teaching is easy to construct using intranet technology, however, particularly commercial packages such as Toolbook

This project has established that an intranet-based tutorial designed by expert laboratory staff was well received by nursing staff. It achieved the objectives of teaching how to measure blood glucose with accuracy and confidence and was available to all nursing staff at all hours. The intranet approach also should be considered as a very cost-effective alternative to traditional training on a long-term basis. Clearly, the best outcome for improved training is improved patient care.

ECONOMICS, OUTCOMES, AND OPTIMIZATION

36

BILLING AND PAYMENT OF POINT-OF-CARE TESTING

JOAN LOGUE

POINT-OF-CARE BILLING SYSTEMS AND PROCESSES

The growth of point-of-care testing (POCT) devices and applications, coupled with comparatively low acquisition costs and favorable federal and private third-party payment rates, has resulted in a growing acceptance and integration of POCT in both traditional and nontraditional clinical settings. Evaluating the true costs of POCT in hospital settings has not been possible because the individual test charges frequently are not captured. This has limited the opportunity to measure cost against revenues. Electronic capturing of POCT charges appears to depend on:

- complexity of the clinical setting,
- availability of efficient communication technology, and
- an understanding of the various payment criteria.

As the payment environment becomes more restrictive, developing systems to ensure that all revenue is captured becomes more critical. Typically hospitals have not billed point-of-care (POC) services because the POC devices lacked the connectivity capability. This has now changed, and it is time to re-evaluate the decision not to bill POCT. Analyzing the test volume by department for each POC test can quickly identify the level of potential outpatient and non-Medicare inpatient revenue.

Figure 36.1 illustrates the monthly revenue billed and not billed for a hospital that performs 2000 billable point-of-care glucose tests per month. The off-site waived laboratory serves as a collection station and performs POCT. It averages 100 POC glucose tests per month. The laboratory bills the POC glucose tests performed by this site because the collection station orders the glucoses directly into the laboratory information system (LIS) terminal located at the site.

The monthly glucose POC revenue from the Emergency Department, diabetic clinic, and for non-Medicare inpatients averages $10,298 per month or $123,576 annually in lost revenue. When this type of analysis is done for each POC procedure performed on outpatients, including urine dipstick and occult blood tests, the annual lost revenue is usually significant.

Clinical Setting

Non-Hospital Setting

Capturing the charge in most freestanding ambulatory settings is less problematic than in the hospital setting. In the physician office, freestanding urgent care center, or clinic, the POCT charge is captured, either manually or electronically, when the POCT is ordered. However, in the busy hospital emergency department (ED), hospital clinic, or inpatient unit, the charge often is not captured in the hospital financial system unless the

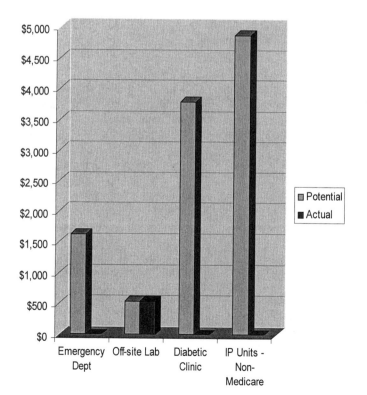

FIGURE 36.1. Potential vs. actual revenue.

results are uploaded into the laboratory information system (LIS) and the test is simultaneously ordered, received, and resulted, or manually charged in the hospital information system (HIS).

Hospital Outpatient Setting

The ability to electronically segregate for billing purposes outpatient clinical laboratory POCT from other patient services provided in the hospital ED or hospital outpatient clinics is particularly important in light of the Medicare Hospital Outpatient Prospective Payment System (PPS). Under hospital outpatient PPS, certain related outpatient services are grouped into Ambulatory Payment Classifications referred to as APCs. Packaged or bundled services are those services that are recognized as being similar both clinically and in use of resources (1). The majority of services provided during a visit to a hospital clinic or ED are grouped and paid under PPS at a fixed APC rate. The APC capitated payment rates for clinic and emergency visits take into account the variation in service intensity and levels of resources consumed.

Certain services that are currently paid according to existing fee schedules, such as outpatient clinical laboratory tests, are not bundled into the APC (1). Therefore, payment for outpatient clinical laboratory services remains as it has been since the implementation of the clinical laboratory fee schedule in 1984.

Having the ability to capture billings for services excluded from APCs requires having appropriate electronic systems and processes in place that will ensure separate billing for these services. If the clinical laboratory POCTs are buried in the ED or clinic medical visit protocol and not separately ordered, the hospital is billing only for the visit, payment is at the APC rate only, and the revenue for the clinical laboratory POCT is lost.

Hospital Inpatient Setting

Capturing the charges for high-volume POCTs provided to non-Medicare patients on the inpatient units also is difficult. In many hospitals, charges are initiated for lower-volume POCTs administered by respiratory or laboratory staff. However, high-volume POCTs administered by the nursing units often are not billed because of the time required to manually enter the test order into the hospital information system. For this reason, many hospitals are including the cost of certain POCTs, such as glucose in the facility routine services charge rather than under the laboratory cost center.

When the cost of the point-of-care test is included in the facility routine service charge, it is not separately billed and the revenue not captured can be significant. The amount of lost revenue depends on the hospital's payer mix and the status of the Medicare patient. Revenues lost from the non-Medicare population will be less significant in those areas with high Medicare populations. Generally, POCTs furnished to Medicare inpatients in a Part A stay are included in the diagnosis-related group (DRG) and not reimbursed separately. However, for Medicare inpatients who have exhausted their Part A coverage, inpatient

laboratory tests are covered under Medicare Part B and will be reimbursed separately when correctly reported to Medicare (2).

Hospital Revenue Centers

Incorporating a clinical laboratory test into the routine service revenue center is contrary to the *Medicare Hospital Manual* and Medicare's cost reporting instructions. Point-of-care glucose is not routinely furnished to hospital patients. It is performed only when medically necessary and when specifically ordered by a physician. Under Medicare policy, the revenue code for routine services should include only nursing services, which are generally provided to all patients and which ordinarily are not billed separately. Placing the point-of-care glucose test or other laboratory test in the routine service charge also is in conflict with Medicare's cost reporting instructions. These instructions state that the cost accumulated in the nursing and other service cost centers is applicable to general routine care in a hospital and does not include incurred costs applicable to any cost centers that are treated separately. Ancillary services (i.e., clinical laboratory) in a hospital or skilled nursing facility are treated separately on the Medicare cost report (3).

Medicare has defined specific numeric revenue center codes to identify each cost center for which a separate charge is billed (type of accommodation or ancillary)(4). The revenue code explains the inpatient charge to Medicare. If the revenue code is listed for some other department, the Medicare payer is unable to identify the charge as a laboratory ancillary service charge. Revenues are lost for any Medicare inpatients that have exhausted their Part A coverage and should have their laboratory services covered under Part B. Also, using the appropriate revenue center codes when reporting services on the Medicare 1450 (UB92) claim form is critical for the proper apportionment of allowable costs in the Medicare cost report.

Allotting POC charges to the laboratory revenue center code is consistent with the structure of most hospital POC programs. For the most part, the laboratory incurs much of the costs of these services. The point-of-care coordinator (POCC) is nor-

TABLE 36.1. CLINICAL LABORATORY REVENUE CENTER CODES

30X Laboratory	
Subcategory	Standard Abbreviation
300—General classification	Laboratory
301—Chemistry	Lab/chemistry
302—Immunology	Lab/immunology
303—Renal patient (home)	Lab/renal home
304—Nonroutine dialysis	Lab/NR dialysis
305—Hematology	Lab/hematology
306—Bacteriology & microbiology	Lab/bact-micro
307—Urology	Lab/urology
309—Other laboratory	Lab/other

From U.S. Department of Health and Human Services, Health Care Financing Administration, *Medicare Intermediary Manual,* part III, chapter VII, section 3604. Available at: http://www.hcfa.gov/pubforms/ 13_int/a3604.htm#_1_1. Accessed on December 9, 2001.

mally on the laboratory staff and purchasing POC supplies is often the responsibility of the laboratory. Also, some payers will deny outpatient claims if the CPT code submitted is not consistent with the revenue code.

Clinical laboratory tests are to be recorded under the 300 series revenue codes assigned to laboratory services for reporting charges for the performance of diagnostic and routine clinical laboratory tests. The 300 series is broken down by major laboratory clinical disciplines to meet the needs of the hospital and third-party billing requirements. The clinical laboratory revenue center subclassifications are described in Table 36.1.

Hosptial Financial System

Hospital charges are captured using the hospital charge description master file. This is an electronic file residing in the HIS that lists all revenue producing services provided by the hospital. The file format generally contains the procedure charge code assigned by the hospital for the service, department code identifying where the service is provided, description of the service, the revenue center code, the CPT code and the price. As mentioned earlier, the revenue center code should be consistent with the CPT code (i.e., laboratory CPT code and laboratory revenue center code).

Hospitals frequently list POC laboratory tests on the charge description master with the revenue center code of the hospital department providing the service, rather than the appropriate ancillary cost center. This is done because of concern in crediting the department that incurred the cost with the associated revenue. However, department generated revenue data can be identified in the hospital information system by the department code listed in the charge description master file rather than the revenue center code.

The ability to communicate the point-of-care test charge information to the hospital charge description master is the key to capturing the POCT revenues. The issues surrounding the billing for a POC laboratory test are similar to those concerning capturing the test result on the patient's electronic record, as discussed in Chapter 35. Both require an understanding of the electronic systems and their relationship to each other and an assessment of the performing department's electronic capability to integrate the test result and charge into the patient's electronic medical record and the patient's electronic account record.

Electronic data transfer or wireless local area network technology, as discussed in Chapters 33 and 35, enhances the opportunity for the busy clinical setting to capture the POCT order, thus generating a charge in addition to the test result as is done in the main laboratory. Resulting and charging through the LIS system appears to be the most efficient method for electronically capturing both the point-of-care laboratory test result and the associated charge.

Charges for tests performed in the main hospital laboratory are billed either at the time the specimen is received in the laboratory or when the LIS compiles a raw billing data file comprised of charges for the preceding twenty-four hours and sends the file to the HIS financial system. In either case, the billing data communicated to the HIS financial system depend on the test being ordered in the LIS and the specimen indicated as being received in the LIS. When test results are uploaded into the LIS, the system automatically triggers the specimen-received function, thus allowing a charge to be generated.

POC laboratory test systems capable of electronic data transfer or hospitals that have wireless local area network technology should be able to capture both the result and the charge in the LIS for all point-of-care laboratory tests performed at sites outside the main laboratory. Once the patient demographics and the test results are in the LIS, the LIS bill code associated with the POCT crosses the interface to the HIS system. The LIS bill code maps to the HIS charge code in the charge description master file, which is linked to the CPT billing code, test description, revenue center code, and price. The LIS bill code and the HIS charge code must be identical for each test procedure listing in both files. The billing data are compiled, posted to the patient's account, and pass to the Medicare 1450 (UB92) for billing to the third-party payer. Figure 36.2 shows the billing data flow and the mapping of the LIS bill code to the HIS charge code.

The POCT procedure charge code is the key to ensuring that the department responsible for administering the point-of-care test is credited with the POC revenue. Laboratory tests are electronically ordered via the hospital procedure charge code and billed via the hospital procedure charge code. The LIS test directory or billing file must contain a listing for each point-of-care laboratory test as shown in Figure 36.2. The number of listings depends on the number of sites performing the POC laboratory test. Each listing contains the procedure charge code assigned by the hospital, department code unique to the performing department, and the test description. The download in the LIS reads to the department's procedure charge code listed in the LIS file. This initiates the bill data function as described previously and allows for the charge to be identified with the department performing the service.

PAYMENT SYSTEMS

Designing the electronic systems and the file formats is only the first step in billing for POC laboratory tests. Receiving appropriate payment for POCT also requires understanding the various payment programs and the conditions under which laboratory services are paid. Billing rules for POCT services must address the same regulatory requirements and payment restrictions as billing for tests performed in the traditional clinical laboratory. The Medicare regulatory requirements and payment system are the driving force in today's health-care payment environment. Services for the non-Medicare patient in the hospital or outpatient setting are paid based on the contractual arrangement of the plans, but payment restrictions often mirror those of the Medicare program. Both government and private payers are focusing on compliant laboratory billing and developing billing systems and processes that meet the Medicare regulatory requirements will ensure compliant billing for all payers.

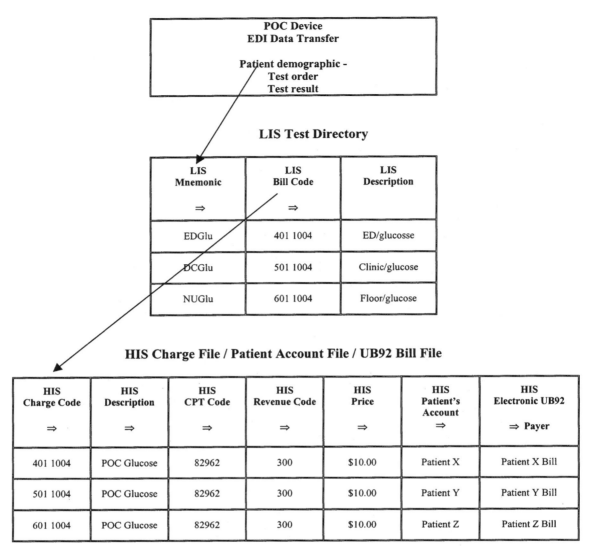

FIGURE 36.2. POC test order and billing data flow model.

Medicare Program

The Medicare programs are funded by two trust funds. The Hospital Insurance Fund, Medicare Part A, covers services furnished to hospital inpatients, patients in post-hospital skilled nursing facility stays, home health agencies, hospice care, and services provided by end stage renal disease (ESRD) dialysis facilities. Outpatient services are funded under the Supplementary Medicare Insurance for the Aged and Disabled, Medicare Part B. The majority of beneficiaries receive benefits through the traditional Medicare fee-for-service program, but an increasing number of beneficiaries are selecting one of the Medicare risk-based plans. These plans, known as Medicare+Choice or Part C, include coordinated care plans, private, unrestricted fee-for-service plans and the medical savings account plan (MSA). The Medicare Part C programs have complex financing, depending on the plan chosen, but basically funding comes from both the Hospital Insurance Fund, Part A, and the Supplemental Medical Insurance fund, Part B (5).

Medicare Program Administration

The Centers for Medicare & Medicaid Services (CMS), formerly the Health Care Financing Administration (HCFA), a federal agency within the Department of Health and Human Services, has primary responsibility for administering the Medicare programs. CMS formulates national Medicare regulatory policies and guidelines, provides contractor oversight, and is responsible for the use of Medicare resources and program integrity. To assist with program administration at the local level, CMS contracts with insurance companies to serve as fiscal agents between the healthcare provider and the federal government. The insurance company contracted to process Medicare Part A claims is termed an "intermediary." The intermediary processes all inpatient hospital claims and hospital outpatient Part B claims for clinical laboratory and other outpatient services. Intermediaries also process claims submitted by other Part A providers, such as skilled nursing facilities and home health agencies (5).

The Medicare insurance contractors responsible for processing physician services, independent laboratory services and physician office laboratory services and other non-physician supplies and services are called "carriers." Unlike intermediaries, carriers process only Part B claims. Each state is assigned a carrier and an intermediary. Providers of Part A and Part B services must submit Medicare claims to their designated intermediary or carrier. Both the carriers and intermediaries have the responsibility of ensuring only medically necessary services are paid for under the Medicare program (5). However, their payment policies may differ.

Although hospitals and other Part A providers must follow the payment policies of the intermediary, physician offices, independent laboratories, and other Part B providers must follow the payment policies of their carriers. Differences in policies occur because CMS has given considerable discretionary authority to local intermediaries and carriers to develop local coverage policies based on the utilization patterns of the providers whose claims they process (6–8).

Medicare National Coverage Policy

Certain clinical laboratory payment policies are communicated as national policies through the CMS central office. Prior to 2001 the national policies for clinical laboratory tests only addressed payments mandated by federal legislation for screening tests, such as the screening Pap test, the screening occult blood test, or the screening prostatic-specific antigen test. However, this changed as a result of the Balanced Budget Act of 1997 (BBA). BBA directed the use of a negotiated rule-making committee to develop national coverage and administrative policies for clinical laboratory services. The resulting national coverage policies that became final in November 2001 address twenty-three high-volume clinical laboratory tests. The policies are designed to promote Medicare program integrity and national uniformity, and to simplify administrative requirements for clinical laboratory services paid under Medicare Part B. Table 36.2 lists twenty-three tests that now fall under national coverage decisions, four of which have POC capability.   These policies define the medical conditions by ICD-9-CM diagnosis code for which the test is considered reasonable and necessary and therefore eligible for reimbursement under the Medicare program. The coverage criteria are defined for each test in each of the national coverage decisions, and apply whether the test is performed in the traditional clinical laboratory or at point of care.

In addition to the national coverage policies for the twenty-three tests, the final rule addresses basic billing policies such as:

- patient information required to be submitted with each claim
- record keeping requirements including physician's obligation regarding such requirements
- procedures for filing claims and for providing remittances by electronic media

TABLE 36.2. CLINICAL LABORATORY TESTS UNDER NATIONAL COVERAGE POLICIES

Urine culture
Human immunodeficiency virus testing (prognosis, including monitoring)
   HIV-1 or HIV-2 quantification / viral load
Human immunodeficiency virus testing (diagnosis)
   HIV, HIV-1, HIV1/2, HTVL III, Human T-cell lymphotrophic virus, AIDS
Blood counts
Partial thromboplastin time
Prothrombin time
Iron studies
Blood glucose
Glycated hemoglobin/glycated protein
Thyroid testing
Collagen crosslinks
Lipids
Digoxin
Alpha-fetoprotein
Carcinoembronic antigen
Human chorionic gonadotropin
CA 125
CA 15-3/CA27.29
CA 19-9
Total prostate specific antigen
Gamma glutamyltransferase
Hepatitis panel
Fecal occult blood

- limitations on frequency of coverage for the same services performed on the same individual (9).

The final rule applies to all laboratory services billed to Medicare Part B regardless of the location of the entity furnishing the laboratory service (e.g., physician office, hospital, skilled nursing facility, independent laboratory, ESRD facility), or of the type of Medicare contractor (carrier or intermediary) processing the claim. All carriers' and intermediary local medical review policies (LMRP) that are in conflict with the national coverage decisions for the twenty-three tests must be changed to conform to these policies. However, a carrier or intermediary may have an LMRP that supplements a national coverage decision, thus making it more restrictive than the national policy (9).

This final rule can be obtained at http://www.access.gpo.gov/su_docs/fedreg/a011123c.html. It is an excellent review of regulatory requirements for billing clinical laboratory services and recommended reading for those responsible for billing compliance of POC laboratory services.   National coverage decisions apply nationwide and are binding on all Medicare carriers and fiscal intermediaries and Medicare prepaid health plans (9).

Medicare Local Medical Review Policy

Coverage policies for clinical laboratory services are also developed at the local level. When a local carrier or intermediary develops a local medical review policy, it only applies within the area that the carrier or intermediary services. LMRP payment restrictions on laboratory tests are communicated to the provider through the local intermediary or carrier bulletin.

Local medical review policies are developed based on the local providers' utilization of services. For example, prior to the development of the national policy for glucose, most Medicare payers had a local medical review policy that limited the payment for blood glucose to specific ICD-9-CM diagnosis codes. Glucose test claim data have demonstrated high utilization of the glucose test and this indicated to the local Medicare payer that the claims submitted for glucose tests may not have been medically necessary in all cases. The development of a local medical review policy ensures that claims submitted without an acceptable ICD-9-CM code will not be paid. The local carrier or intermediary has the option to supplement a national coverage decision to make a local policy for a clinical laboratory test more stringent than the national coverage decision (9).

Hospital and other providers providing point-of-care laboratory testing in outpatient settings should educate the ordering physicians to both the national coverage policies and the local medical review policies currently in effect.

Medicare Prospective Payment Systems

Medicare inpatient hospital services are paid under a Prospective Payment System (PPS) or the contractual terms of one of the Medicare Part C risk-based plans. Under PPS, services are bundled and paid at a capitated rate based on a diagnosis-related group (DRG). As discussed earlier, most hospital outpatient services also are to be paid under an Outpatient Prospective Payment System as mandated by the Balanced Budget Act of 1997. Hospital outpatient clinical laboratory tests are excluded from PPS because all outpatient clinical laboratory services are paid according to a fee schedule, regardless of the ambulatory setting, and the government did not wish to interrupt this uniformity of payment across all provider settings.

The Balanced Budget Act of 1997 also mandated the implementation of a *per diem* prospective payment system for skilled nursing facilities covering all costs (i.e., routine, ancillary, and capital) related to the services furnished to Medicare beneficiaries in a Part A stay. The transition to PPS went into effect with the cost reporting periods beginning on or after July 1, 1998. Payment for point-of-care laboratory tests provided to beneficiaries in a Part A stay is included in the PPS rate (9,10).

Skilled nursing facility patients who are not in Part A stays continue to have medically necessary medical clinical laboratory services covered under Part B. The BBA had also mandated a separate payment system for Part B services known as "consolidated billing." Under consolidated billing, payment for laboratory services was to be made only to the skilled nursing facility at the fee schedule amount. However, the Benefits Improvement and Protection Act of 2000 (BIPA), rescinded the consolidated billing provisions for Part B services. Outside clinical laboratories providing laboratory services for skilled nursing facility long-term care patients may continue to third-party bill for these services. BIPA 2000 retained PPS provisions for services furnished to Medicare beneficiaries in a Part A stay (9,11).

Clinical Laboratory Fee Schedule

Medicare pays for clinical laboratory services according to a laboratory fee schedule authorized by section 1833 of the Social Security Act. The fee schedule amounts for payment of Part B clinical laboratory services are set on a local carrier-wide basis. The fee schedule, as we know it today, has it roots in major pieces of legislation enacted in 1984. The method for establishing the fee schedule rate is defined in statute and used clinical laboratory charge data for the year 1983. Because the fee schedule method is defined in statute, pricing for tests cannot change even though it is well recognized that inequities existed in the 1983 charge data.

The fee schedule payment rates may be adjusted annually based on the Consumer Price Index (CPI). However, over the years Congress has dictated frequent freezes for the CPI update to reduce the cost of the Medicare program. CMS has the responsibility to maintain the fee schedule and set pricing for new codes. The method for pricing new codes is not clearly defined in the legislation giving CMS significant latitude in this area. Currently, CMS determines pricing for new codes either by a "gap fill" or a "cross-walk" method.

Gap Fill Pricing

Fee schedule pricing for new CPT codes may be established through a process called "gap fill." Once the FDA approves a new test procedure, the American Medical Association's (AMA) CPT Editorial Panel may establish a new code if a current code does not exist. The local carrier determines the amounts charged by the local providers for the new code on claims received for a specified period of time defined by the CMS central office. The carrier is instructed by CMS to consider the charge for the test in its area as well as the cost of performing the test in a laboratory with adequate volume to ensure cost efficiencies. The local carrier establishes a local prevailing rate. At the end of the gap fill time period, carriers report their local payment amounts to CMS. The national median rate is determined and a national limitation amount (NLA) is established for the new code.

The NLA is 74% of the median of the local fees for all codes that had NLA amounts established before January 1, 2001. The Benefits Improvement and Protection Act of 2000 mandates that the NLA must be set at 100% of the median for new clinical laboratory test codes for which no NLA has previously been established. Carrier areas that have established a local prevailing amount below the NLA will continue to pay for the new procedure at the local prevailing rate. Carrier areas that established a local prevailing amount above the NLA will lower the payment amount to that of the NLA. Since there is no defined method for the gap fill process as it relates to clinical laboratory tests, the local prevailing pricing determinations may not always be representative of local reasonable charges for the service.

Cross Walk Pricing

CMS also establishes clinical laboratory test pricing by mapping new codes to existing codes. The decision to establish a new code price by "cross walk" rather than gap fill is made based on CMS' judgment that the test is similar to an existing test and the prevailing charge level for the existing test is acceptable for the new test. However, cross walk decisions appear to be very subjective and often without any scientific basis, resulting in inappropriately low payment levels. The cross walks also perpetuate state inequities for existing codes that were originally underpaid owing to errors in the original 1983 payment data.

For example, in 2001 the new code 83663 for "fetal lung maturity assessment by fluorescent polarization" was mapped to the "foam stability test," code 83662, with a NLA of $13.07 (13,14). The cross walk was not only technically inappropriate but resulted in payment levels as low as $1.99 in one carrier area. The cross walk process, like the gap fill process, should be well defined and allow for review and comment from the laboratory community to ensure fair and equitable payment rates.

QW Modifier

Waived POCTs are indicated on the fee schedule with a "QW" after the numeric CPT code. CLIA-approved waived laboratories must report a waived test with the CPT code and the QW modifier on the claim. In some cases, the waived test listed on the fee schedule may have been down coded by CMS to a code with a lesser payment amount. Providers may disagree with the code designated by CMS, but are required to report the waived test using the Medicare-designated code for Medicare claims. CMS periodically publishes a "Program Memorandum" listing the current approved waived test procedures with the required reporting CPT codes. A provider may obtain the current listing from the CMS web site at *www.hcfa.gov/stats/pufiles.htm*

Providers should compare the fee schedule payment amounts to their own internal fee schedules. It is not unusual to find some laboratory services billed below fee schedule amounts. Medicare pays the lesser of (a) the bill amount, (b) the local prevailing fee schedule amount, or (c) the national limitation amount. The current clinical laboratory fee schedule listing the fee schedule amounts for each state or carrier area also may be obtained from the CMS web site listed previously. Each December, CMS posts the new fee schedules for the coming year.

Coding Point-Of-Care Tests

Medical services are reported to government and private third-party payers using coding systems. The Medicare and other federal programs have adopted the HCPCS (pronounced *hic piks*) coding system. HCPCS is an acronym for <u>H</u>ealth <u>C</u>are <u>P</u>rocedural <u>C</u>oding <u>S</u>ystems and collectively describes three groups of codes. The first group consists of the CPT codes for physician services defined in the American Medical Association *Current Procedural Terminology (CPT)*. The AMA CPT designates a separate code series for each medical, surgical, radiology, laboratory, and anesthesiology physician service. The CPT codes are five digit numeric codes, and laboratory services are reported using the 80,000 series codes in the "Pathology and Laboratory Medicine" section of the CPT (14).

The second group consists of national codes that are five digit alphanumeric codes developed by CMS to describe non-physician procedures, services, and supplies that are covered by the Medicare program but are not described in CPT. These codes are often referred to as HCPCS codes. CMS may assign a national HCPCS code to a laboratory service. For example, the venipuncture draw and certain Medicare approved screening tests, such as the screening of occult blood, PAP smear, and prostatic-specific antigen (PSA), when performed at a defined frequency for Medicare patients, are reported to government payers using HCPCS codes rather than the CPT codes.

The third group of codes consists of local codes assigned by the carrier. CMS is phasing out the local codes and those remaining do not apply to laboratory services. Both the AMA and CMS update the codes each year to include new codes, to delete obsolete codes, and to revise definitions to be current with technology and medical practice.

Clinical laboratories place great emphasis on correctly coding their services to ensure accurate and compliant billing. The laboratory CPT codes and revenue codes listed on the hospital charge description master are normally updated annually. In many hospitals the coding for POCT procedures is not reviewed annually. Therefore, incorrect CPT codes are often not corrected or updated once assigned. Coding errors commonly encountered for POCTs include urine dipstick test coded to the complete urinalysis, Mantoux test coded to the tuberculosis tine test, and arterial blood gases coded to include direct measurement rather than calculated O_2 saturation.

The assignment of CPT codes to point-of-care glucose is also somewhat confusing for sites performing bedside glucose testing, because the AMA CPT lists four glucose codes. A quantitative blood glucose test is reported using the quantitative blood glucose CPT code 82947. In 2001, the CPT added a new quantitative glucose code, 82945, to be used for reporting glucose determination on body fluids other than blood. The AMA Coding Department clarified that the glucose blood reagent strip, CPT code 82948, is used when the blood glucose level is determined by reagent strip method and visually compared to a color chart (14,15).

CPT code 82962 is used when the glucose is determined by devices cleared by the FDA for home use (14,15). Several payers have listed this code as noncovered. Most of the point-of-care glucose test devices on the market today provide a quantitative determination, and it is unclear why CPT code 82962 was added to the CPT. Its presence in CPT appears to imply that a device approved for home use may be less precise, when, in fact, this is not always the case.

Prior to the transfer of responsibility for classifying *in vitro* diagnostic products from CDC to the FDA, many manufacturers found it more expedient to obtain home use approval through the FDA, as this automatically classifies the instrument as waived, rather than going through the longer process of applying for waived status through the Centers for Disease Control.

The "approved for home use" label has, in some cases, resulted in negative payment consequences. CMS may arbitrarily assign a lower payment amount when a device is approved for home use than for a waived device not approved for home use.

This occurred in year 2000 with the waived BTA stat test for qualitative detection of bladder tumor antigen in urine. CMS assigned this "approved for home use" waived POC procedure a nonspecific immunoassay method code, 83518 QW, that paid considerably less than the generic immunoassay tumor antigen code 86316, which prior to the 2001 CPT was not designated as a quantitative code. CMS appears to be of the opinion that all waived procedures should be priced lower than nonwaived procedures. However, the method for establishing payment amounts under the clinical laboratory fee schedule limits CMS' ability to set lower amounts for waived tests except by down coding as described in the case of the bladder tumor antigen test. However, the pricing for this code was corrected when the new 2001 qualitative tumor antigen code, 86294, was priced by the gap fill method.

CMS, also in 2001, established lower pricing for code 82962, point-of-care glucose determinations by devices cleared by the FDA for home use. This code has been in the CPT and on the clinical laboratory fee schedule since 1993. The 1993 payment amount for this code was established by cross walking it to the CPT code 82948, which is used for reporting qualitative glucose determinations by reagent strip (14,15). From 1993 through 2000, both codes 82962 and 82948, had the identical payment level.

Because of a significant increase in the number of claims submitted to intermediaries for point-of-care glucoses coded as 82962, CMS made a decision to re-price code 82962. The agency believes that a glucose monitoring service with a home-use device is substantially different from a glucose test by reagent strip. CMS stated that the original mapping was in error. To correct what CMS considers an error and to lower the payment amount, CMS gap filled this code for the year 2001 (16). The resulting 2002 national limitation amount for a point-of-care glucose test performed by an instrument approved by the FDA for home use was lowered from the previous fee schedule amount of $4.37 to $3.23.

The clinical laboratory community should be vigilant as to CMS' method for determining payment amounts for waived point-of-care technology. The fee schedule amount established in 2001 for the CPT code 88400, transcutaneous total bilirubin, was cross walked to the non-waived total bilirubin code and arbitrarily priced at one half the fee schedule amount for the total bilirubin code, 82247 (13,14). The resulting Medicare NLA listed on the 2001 clinical laboratory fee schedule is $3.47 with four states, Louisiana, Ohio, Washington, and West Virginia paid below this at the state's local prevailing level.

Should this price remain at this level it could stifle the widespread use of the test and the development of similar non-invasive technology for other analytes. This test is used primarily for neonates in the hospital setting and in the clinic or home care environment, which tends to serve a high Medicaid population. The low Medicare allowance will affect the state Medicaid allowance that by law must be lower than that of the Medicare fee schedule. Unreasonably low payment amounts that do not adequately cover point-of-care procedures may slow the growth and acceptance of point-of-care technology. Once payment amounts are determined and published in the Medicare clinical laboratory fee schedule it is very difficult to obtain a pricing change.

AMA Modifier 91

Certain POCTs, such as glucose or activated clotting time, are often ordered by the physician to be performed at multiple intervals on the same date of service. Each test performed may be billed when there is documentation in the patient's chart of the physician's order. When the same POCT is performed multiple times within the same date of service, the test is reported to Medicare with the AMA modifier 91, "repeat clinical diagnostic laboratory test" (14) to indicate that the test is a separate physician order. Modifier 91 may not be used for a test performed as a recheck of the initial result, which is not billable, or where a CPT code exists for a series of tests, such as the glucose tolerance tests.

The modifier 91 should not be confused with the AMA modifier 59 "distinct procedural services" (14). Modifier 59 is used for reporting the same code for separate services performed for the same patient during a twenty-four hour period. For example, modifier 59 would be used for reporting separate cultures taken from different parts of a patient's body on the same day. Each culture is considered a distinct procedural service although it is reported with the same CPT code.

Medical Necessity

Point-of-care outpatient laboratory tests, like tests performed in the traditional laboratory, must meet certain medical necessity criteria to be billed to the Medicare program. The definition of "medical necessity" has evolved and been refined over time by CMS, but the definition of paying only for services that are "reasonable and necessary" for the diagnosis and treatment of an illness or injury still remains the basis for coverage. However, the definition of "reasonable and necessary" is not stated in regulation and, therefore, the term may be interpreted differently by CMS or its contractors than by physicians. In many cases, one must look to the national coverage policy or the local payer's medical review policy to identify conditions under which a laboratory test is considered reasonable and necessary and thus a covered service.

Generally, a noncovered laboratory service is a test performed for screening purposes. For example, a glucose determination performed on a patient who has a strong family history of diabetes, but who shows no sign of disease, would be considered a screening test and consequently not payable under the Medicare fee-for-service program. However, as discussed earlier, Congress has legislated certain screening tests to be covered at defined frequencies. Screening tests approved for payment are Pap smears once every two years, or at more frequent intervals for women at high risk, occult blood once a year, and PSA once a year. These tests, when performed as screening tests, must be billed to Medicare with a designated HCPCS code rather than the CPT code.

In a program memorandum issued in December 2000, CMS addressed medical necessity for point-of-care glucoses but the medical necessity criteria cited apply to all clinical laboratory tests. CMS states that according to the Section 42 *Code of Federal Regulations* (CFR) 410.32 and 411.15, "for a laboratory service to be reasonable and necessary, it must not only be ordered by the physician but the ordering physician must also use the result in the management of the beneficiary's specific medical problem" (16).

CMS is now interpreting this regulation for point-of-care glucoses to mean that the laboratory result must be reported to the physician promptly in order for the physician to use the result and provide instructions on patient care, which includes the physician order for another laboratory service. This program memorandum states, "a standing order is not usually acceptable documentation for covered laboratory services." It also instructs the local Medicare payers to clarify in their glucose test coverage policy that glucose monitoring must be performed according to criteria that include the clear use of the laboratory result by the physician before a repeat order to qualify for separate Medicare payment (16).

Another area of government concern is the use of custom panels designed for the convenience of the ordering physician. The various combinations of i-STAT tests are custom panels and may result in the physician ordering tests that may not be medically necessary. Medicare requires that each test billed must be medically necessary and will deny payment for those services within the custom panel that are not medically necessary. Some of the individual tests included in the i-STAT grouping may be under national coverage decisions, or local medical review policies, and payment will be denied if the diagnosis submitted is a noncovered diagnosis.

A number of payers have LMRPs for ionized calcium and chloride, and glucose is under a national coverage decision. At least one of these analytes is included in six i-STAT cartridges. The tests included in the i-STAT cartridges are separately billed by the individual CPT code and will require medical necessity documentation in the patient's chart. Ordering physicians need to be made aware of the coverage limitation for the I-STAT tests.

The design of the hospital claim form (UB92) does not allow for the diagnosis code to be tied to the specific CPT code. However, the payer audit functions allow for provider billing profiles to be developed that may indicate overutilization by CPT code or diagnosis code. The government clearly views custom panels as promoting unnecessary testing. The Office of Inspector General (OIG) has reaffirmed its position on custom panels in numerous OIG publications.

Certain panels place the provider at higher risk. An automated panel, such as the comprehensive metabolic panel containing fourteen tests may be difficult to medically justify. Medicare requires that the patient record indicate that each test within the panel is medically necessary. A fourteen-test panel may appear to Medicare to be a screening or a wellness panel and if overutilized, the Medicare payer may require the physician and the laboratory to medically justify all analytes within the panel. The OIG is concerned that panels and profiles desensitize physician concern about the medical necessity of tests they are ordering. Encouraging the physicians to order i-STAT tests individually, rather than by groups, affirms the provider's concern for compliant billing.

Diagnosis-Related Group Payment Window

The DRG payment window, also referred to as the 72-hour rule, must be considered for point-of-care tests performed in the hospital Emergency Department or clinics. The 72-hour rule requires that any laboratory test performed within 72 hours of admission must be included in the DRG if the patient is admitted within this time period. Most hospitals have set up electronic processes that compare daily admissions to outpatient services provided within the three-day window. This process allows them to effectively capture outpatient laboratory charges that need to be reclassified as inpatient charges and included under the DRG. If there are delays in uploading the point-of-care test charges into the system, charges for outpatient testing that should be converted to an inpatient charge may be missed and incorrectly billed to Medicare.

Future Payment Of Clinical Laboratory Services

The clinical laboratory community effectively communicated to Congress that the payment method for setting pricing based on a system developed in the early 1980s was inadequate for keeping payment up to date with technology. As a result Congress mandated that the Department of Health and Human Services commission a study to assess current Medicare payment policy. The Institute of Medicine was commissioned to establish a committee to examine the laboratory industry, evaluate payment policies, and make recommendations to improve the system. The study was completed in 2000 and a report was issued that called for some very specific changes that could improve the payment for all clinical laboratory services (17).

The committee reached consensus on twelve recommendations for improving Medicare's payment system for outpatient clinical laboratory service (17). Several of the recommendations address some of the issues raised in this chapter such as:

- developing an open process for establishing fees for new tests,
- discontinuing the use of diagnosis codes as the basis for determining the medical necessity and therefore payment, and
- in the interim, while a more equitable system is studied, basing all payments on the NLAs rather than the 56 separate fee schedules.

The full report is a valuable planning tool for the clinical laboratory community and especially important for the POC industry considering CMS' apparent desire to lower the payment amount for waived procedures. Although not all recommendations will be acted upon, the report has influenced on how future payment decisions will be made and allows for input from the laboratory community. Congress responded to the recommendations in the Institute of Medicine report by mandating that CMS establish procedures for coding and payment determinations for new clinical diagnostic laboratory tests that permit public consultation conducted in a manner consistent with the procedures established for implementing coding modification for ICD-9-CM (12). The full Institute of Medicine report is available online and can be obtained at *www.nap.edu*.

CONCLUSIONS

Electronic data transfer and mobile computing devices with wireless networks appear to offer the potential to capture not only the POCT result in the patient's electronic record, but also to capture the charge. As the payment environment becomes more restrictive, the provider must develop systems to ensure that all revenue is captured. With this capability comes the responsibility to develop an effective internal system and processes that will ensure compliant billing of POCT services. The physician's written order in the chart, documentation of medical necessity, current and correct coding, and an understanding of the payment systems are as critical with POCTs as they are with tests provided in the traditional laboratory. Developing a compliant POC billing system requires a considerable amount of time and commitment, but the return on investment will quickly be realized in the form of additional revenues.

REFERENCES

1. U.S. Department of Health and Human Services, Health Care Financing Administration. 42-CFR Part 419, Medicare Program; Prospective Payment for Hospital Outpatient Services; Interim Final Rule. *Federal Register* 2000:67798–68020.
2. U.S. Department of Health and Human Services, Health Care Financing Administration. *Medicare Hospital Manual,* Section 2002: 228.B;415.6.B.
3. U.S. Department of Health and Human Services, Health Care Financing Administration. *Medicare Provider Reimbursement Manual,* Section 2002: 2202.5, 2202.8, 2203.
4. U.S. Department of Health and Human Services, Health Care Financing Administration. *Medicare Intermediary Manual,* 2002: Chapter VII, section 3604.
5. U.S. Department of Health and Human Services, Health Care Financing Administration Bulletin Board. *http://www.CMS.gov/medicare/pub-forms/actuary/ormedmed.htm.*
6. Logue J. Federal reimbursement to laboratories. *Clin Chem* 1996;42. 5:817–821.
7. Logue, J. Medicare 101. *Proceedings of the Clinical Laboratory Management Association Annual Meeting 1998.* Audio recording. Palm Desert, CA, Convention Cassettes Unlimited.
8. Logue, J. Point-of-care billing. University Health Systems Consortium Laboratory Meeting. 1999. Dallas, Texas.
9. Department of Health and Human Services, Health Care Financing Administration. 42-CFR Part 410, Medicare Program; Negotiated Rulemaking: Coverage and Administrative Policies for Clinical Diagnostic Laboratory Services; *Federal Register* 2001;66(226):58787-58836.
10. 1997 Medicare and Medicaid Legislation: Law and Explanation. *Title IV and Selected Provisions of Title V of the Balanced Budget Act of 1997.* Chicago, IL:CCH, Incorporated 60646, 800/835-5224, www.cch.com.
11. U.S. Department of Health and Human Services, Health Care Financing Administration. *Program Memorandum Intermediaries.* Transmittal No. A-98-16. May 1998. Subject: Coverage and Claims Processing for Prospective Payment for Skilled Nursing Facilities—The Balanced Budget Act of 1997.
12. Medicare, Medicaid and SCHIP Benefits Improvement and Protection Act of 2000 H.R.5661. *Text of Bill.* Chicago, IL: CCH, Incorporated, 60646, 800/835-5224, www.cch.com.
13. U.S. Department of Health and Human Services, Health Care Financing Administration. *Program Memorandum Intermediaries.* Transmittal No. AB-00-109. November 29, 2000. Subject: 2001 Clinical Laboratory Fee Schedule and Laboratory Costs Subject to Reasonable Charge Payment Methodology.
14. American Medical Association. *Current Procedural Terminology CPT 2001.* Professional Edition. Section Pathology and Laboratory. 333, Chicago, IL.
15. American Medical Association. *CPT Assistant* 1999;9:1:10–11.
16. U.S. Department of Health and Human Services, Health Care Financing Administration. *Program Memorandum Intermediaries.* Transmittal No. AB-00-108. December 1, 2000. Subject: Glucose Monitoring.
17. National Academy of Science, Institute of Medicine. *Medicare Laboratory Payment Policy Now and In The Future.* Washington, DC: National Academy Press, 2000.

37

THE ROLE OF POINT-OF-CARE TESTING IN CARE PATHS

ALEXANDER J. INDRIKOVS

Over the past decade healthcare providers have witnessed an evolutionary change in efforts to improve the quality of health care in the United States (1). In an effort to identify substandard care delivery systems and practices and take corrective actions, providers have shifted from retrospective analysis of patient records to statistical analysis of the outcomes of care based on these systems and practices. This outcomes-focused approach seeks to identify a "best practices" standard by learning which interventions can be incorporated into day-to-day practices and have a positive impact on patient outcomes. As the importance of utilization, quality, and outcome issues has expanded, care paths have emerged as an important strategy to improve clinical practice. Healthcare professionals, delivery systems, regulatory bodies, accrediting organizations, and governmental agencies have promoted the use of care paths. These initiatives have a significant impact on clinical laboratories and clinical laboratory specialists.

Care paths address a wide range of clinical issues, and almost universally include laboratory issues. Pathways often include recommendations regarding which laboratory tests should be provided for which patients. For many pathways, laboratory issues are the primary focus. Furthermore, laboratory issues are also addressed in many pathways that focus primarily on other clinical issues. Care paths are clinical tools for communication and for achieving better quality and cost outcomes by outlining and sequencing the usual and/or desired care for particular groups of patients. They are developed for specific patient populations defined by diagnosis, procedure, or condition, including high-volume, high-cost, and high-risk groups.

The practice of medicine is best described as "fragmented." The reasons for this descriptive word are easily understood when one considers the diversity of physician practice patterns and the influence of government, insurance companies, managed care, business demand for reduced costs, and last but not least, extreme paranoia about malpractice suits (2). Attempts to reduce this fragmentation have resulted in the production of varying protocols for standardizing care so that payers, physicians, hospitals, and patients have a model for cost-effective medical practice. Care paths and practice guidelines are two terms commonly used to describe these attempts to standardize

practice. Some authors establish a distinction between care paths and practice guidelines.

Practice guidelines (Fig. 37.1) are diagnostic and treatment guides or algorithms developed by experts in a specialized field of medicine for other physicians serving patients in the same field. The intended goals of practice guidelines are to reduce inappropriate care and to improve patient outcomes. Practice guidelines are also cited as potential tools for reducing the costs of health care, for enhancing quality assurance, and for improving medical education (3). Care paths (Fig. 37.2) may be described as a preoperative, operative, and postoperative time-line protocol of a disease process that involves services and personnel responsible for the patient's care. Included are the primary care physician, specialists, clinic resources, clinic and hospital nursing, physical therapy, occupational therapy, laboratory, radiology, and facilities to which the patient may be transferred following complete or partial recovery.

EVOLUTION OF PRACTICE GUIDELINES

Some may argue that practice guidelines are as old as medical textbooks or even as old as clinical training itself (4). Practice guidelines have grown into a more prominent national health policy issue in the last ten years. Three major factors played a role in the swift turn of events.

1. Rising healthcare costs. By 1990, healthcare expenditures had increased to more than $600 billion per year, or about 12% of the gross national product. Of particular concern to the federal government was the increased cost of the Medicare program. Major political and economic pressures provided a strong incentive for Congress to determine whether services provided under Medicare were necessary and could be eliminated.
2. Practice variations. Many studies have documented large inconsistencies in the rate with which physicians in different geographic areas perform specific procedures. The perception of many is that at least some of the variation reflects excessive or inadequate use of procedures by physicians in

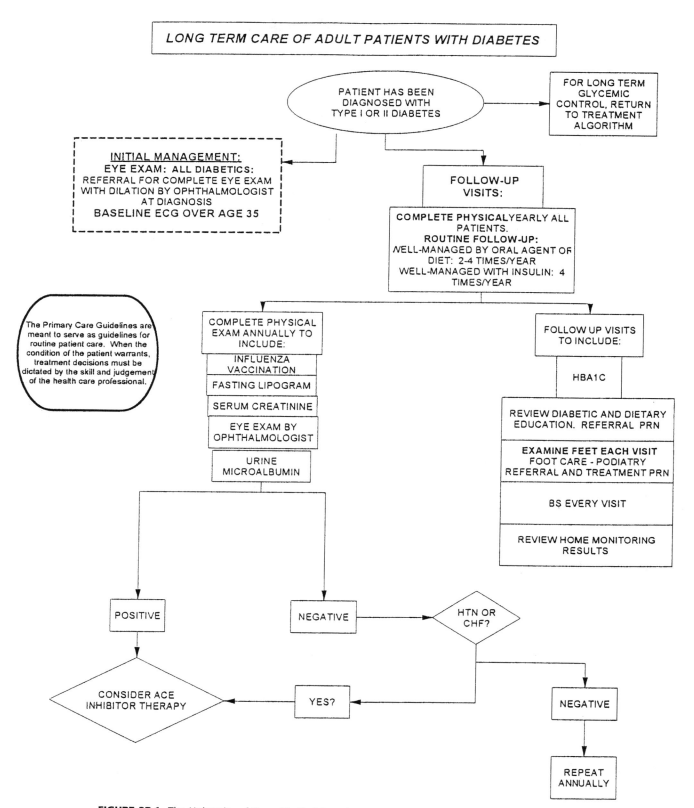

FIGURE 37.1. The University of Texas Medical Branch at Galveston primary care management guidelines.

DKA-Critical Pathway

<u>Note:</u>	The Critical Pathway is meant to serve as a guideline for routine patient care. When the condition of the patient warrants, treatment decisions must be dictated by the skill and judgement of the health care professional.
	Seek advice of the pediatric endocrine/diabetes and/or PICU faculty when managing a Patient with DKA.
<u>Inclusion Criteria:</u>	Clinical symptoms of DKA accompanied by vpH < 7.3, serum bicarbonate <15, blood sugar > 250 mg.dL, ketonemia/ketonuria.
<u>Note:</u> with	Some patients, most of them known diabetics, may present with significant acidosis but Blood sugar values < 250 mg/dL.
<u>Initial Assessment:</u>	History - Symptoms, insulin regimen and precipitating factors in known diabetics, associated conditions. Physical - Vital signs, weight, degree of dehydration, hemodynamic and respiratory status, Abdomen, neurological status, level of consciousness, search for occult infection. Laboratory - *Blood*: vpH (ABGs if indicated by clinical picture), Na, K, Cl, CO_2, blood sugar (fingerstick and laboratory). CA, P, BUN, creatinine, osmolality. *Urine*: ketones, glucose (test strip), UA. Other test as indicated by clinical picture. Calculate osmolality, anion gap, corrected NA. *Estimated osmolality = (NA x2) + Glucose/18 + BUN/2.8
<u>Initial Treatment(ER Management):</u>	Give 10-20 ml/kg of 0/9% NaCl over 1 hour or faster if warranted. This may need to be repeated in case of hemodynamic compromise. Avoid administering bicarbonated bolus or infusion unless respiratory depression and/or cardiovascular compromise (hypotension, arrhythmias) are present in the setting of severe acidosis. Withhold treatment with insulin until after completion of initial fluid bolus treatment.
<u>Admit to PICU:</u>	If any of the following is present: severe dehydration, hemodynamic or respiratory compromise, altered neurological status/level of consciousness, significant acidosis (vpH < 7.12), age $\leq$ 2 years.
<u>Admit to Floor:</u>	If the above signs/symptoms are absent at the initial presentation.

NOTE: The Clinical Practice Guideline/Critical Pathway is meant to serve as a guideline for routine patient care. When the condition of the patient warrants, treatment decisions must be dictated by the skill and judgment of the health care professional.	
IF PT CARD OR LABEL NOT AVAILABLE, WRITE DATE, NAME AND UH# IN SPACE BELOW	**DKA Critical Pathway** **Pediatric** **Endocrine**
Appendix B	Medical Record Form 5629-03/11/1999 **The University of Texas Medical Branch Hospitals** **Galveston, Texas** Original - Medical Record QCC approved 02/20/97

FIGURE 37.2. The University of Texas Medical Branch at Galveston DKA-Critical Pathway.

certain areas, and that providing clinicians with guidelines might be useful in reducing the magnitude of practice variation and inappropriate care.

3. Inappropriate care. Evidence suggested that the proportion of medical procedures performed unnecessarily by physicians was large. In one study, more than 5,000 medical records were reviewed to measure the appropriateness of three procedures: coronary angiography, carotid endarterectomy, and upper gastrointestinal (GI) tract endoscopy. A substantial proportion appeared to be inappropriate. Some healthcare leaders suggest that one-fourth to one-third of all medical care may be unnecessary.

These observations stimulated interest among health services researchers and the federal government in obtaining better information on the effectiveness of practice guidelines (5). An effectiveness initiative was launched by the Department of Health and Human Services to stimulate governmental and academic programs to obtain this information. By 1988, federal health officials were receiving repeated advice to consider practice guidelines as a means of reducing physician practice variations and unnecessary or ineffective services. This was specifically suggested in a March 1988 report to Congress by the Physician Payment Review Commission, which advises Congress on physician payment reform under Medicare. The establishment in 1989 of the Agency for Health Care Policy and Research (AHCPR) carried important implications for medicine. It placed the government in the role of promoting the development and dissemination of practice guidelines on how physicians should evaluate and manage medical conditions. The AHCPR was also charged with conducting and supporting pilot testing and evaluations of the impact of practice guidelines on medical practice, to include describing the extent to which practice guidelines influence the quality, effectiveness, and appropriateness of care.

Federal involvement in practice guidelines for physicians has been followed carefully by organized medicine. National medical-specialty societies have been issuing practice guidelines for many years. For example, the American Academy of Pediatrics began publishing its guidelines for the treatment of infectious diseases in 1938, and the American College of Obstetricians and Gynecologists issued its first practice standards in 1959. According to a 1989 survey, more than 35 physician organizations and national medical-specialty societies reported having developed some form of practice guidelines (4). For many years, the American Medical Association has issued practice recommendations as part of its Diagnostic and Therapeutic Technology Assessment program.

Guidelines have always been prominent in the quality assurance and peer-review activities of hospitals. Insurance companies and other payers were using practice guidelines well before the current surge of activity, but their objectives differed. Insurers were mainly using guidelines initially as a basis for making claims decisions, utilization assessments, and selecting providers for plans. A number of businesses provide practice guidelines commercially to insurers, employers, health maintenance organizations, and other entities. Some organizations provide purchasers of care with information on practice variations and outcomes data that are then used to assess appropriateness.

DEVELOPMENT OF PRACTICE GUIDELINES
Methods

Only a few attempts have been made to classify development methods of practice guidelines. Methods used vary among organizations, and individual methods often draw elements from more than one approach.

For decades, developers of practice guidelines have created guidelines almost entirely on the basis of expert opinion. These guidelines emerge from meetings of expert panels in which agreement is reached through open discussion, sometimes producing recommendations in a single meeting. This type of approach, in which participants simply decide what to recommend, can be described as informal consensus development, because the criteria by which decisions are made are often poorly defined. The guideline documents generally provide only recommendations and little background on the process by which they were developed. Scientific evidence is often cited in the discussion, but generally little methodologic information is provided to assure users that the science was reviewed without bias and that the recommendations were actually influenced by the evidence. This method is a common approach for developing practice guidelines. It has the appeal of being relatively easy, fast, and free of complex analytic procedures. Panel members who are unfamiliar with formal analytical methods easily adopt this method.

The problem with this approach is that practice guidelines are often of poor quality for several reasons. First, there are fundamental limitations to the validity of expert opinion as a basis of defining appropriateness. The fact that a group of individuals think that a practice is beneficial does not ensure that it actually is. Second, the lack of explicit methods raises questions about how consensus was reached. Guidelines that are produced in group meetings without systematic procedures are easily influenced by group dynamics, dominant and outspoken personalities, and organizational and specialty politics. Third, the absence of documented methods makes it difficult for readers to judge whether the guidelines were influenced by scientific evidence or whether the evidence was overlooked due to panel biases.

More formal methods of reaching consensus on practice guidelines were introduced in the United States in the 1970s. In 1977, the National Institute of Health Consensus Development Program introduced its approach, in which an expert panel reaches consensus on recommendations in a structured two-and-a-half-day conference (3). Guidelines are developed in closed sessions and, after a plenary session and open discussion, are presented to an audience and press conference on the third day. Although this method provides greater structure to the analytic process than informal consensus development, the absence of explicit criteria and the requirement to produce recommendations quickly in a single meeting have been criticized.

Another formal approach to consensus development was introduced by the Rand Corporation in the 1980s. An expert panel is provided with background articles that review existing scientific evidence for a procedure, as well as a list of potential indications for performing the procedure. A two-step Delphi technique follows. Before the first panel meeting, panel members are asked to assess the appropriateness of the procedure for each indication. When the panel meets, members consider each indication on the list, review the distribution of the scores submitted by the group, compare the group scores with their own judgments, and discuss reasons for disagreement. Panel members then repeat the scoring process, revising their scores on the basis of the discussion at the meeting. The final list of appropriateness ratings reflects the extent of agreement of the panelists about the appropriateness of the procedure for each indication. A limitation of this approach is that its product, a long list of appropriateness scores, is often difficult for clinicians to apply in practice. The approach also retains many of the fundamental limitations of consensus development: opinion is used as the basis for defining appropriateness. Furthermore, the method does not provide an explicit linkage between recommendations and the quality of the scientific evidence.

Other approaches link recommendations to the quality of the underlying evidence. These approaches may develop guidelines over a period of years on the basis of evaluations of supporting evidence by expert consultants. Although the evidence-based approach has been credited with enhancing the scientific rigor of practice guidelines development, the problem with this approach is that it is often unable to produce recommendations in the absence of acceptable evidence. Neutral recommendations, neither for nor against the procedure, are often issued. Critics argue that strict adherence to an evidence-based approach excludes a large proportion of modern medical practice, since only a small number of current interventions have been validated through clinical studies.

Many guideline development panels have adopted a methodology that combines a detailed evidence-based approach with a process that accommodates expert opinion as a source of input. This approach promotes the use of more explicit methods of guideline development to help clarify the rationale. In this approach, guideline developers specify the benefits, harms, and costs of potential interventions and derive explicit estimates of the probability of each outcome. Whenever possible, scientific evidence and formal analytic methods (e.g., mathematical modeling) are used to generate the estimates. Estimates are also generated by expert opinion, but the source of the estimate is documented. The assumptions are tabulated in a "balance sheet" that allows patients, clinicians, and policymakers to review the potential benefits, harms, and costs of each choice. Critics argue that this complex analytic task may be too impractical for busy developers with limited time and resources.

Steps in the Development of Practice Guidelines

Regardless of which approach is used, certain steps are central to guideline development. These tasks are almost universal, although groups differ in how much emphasis is given to each step and in the sequence in which they are performed. For example, scientific evidence is generally considered in most guidelines, but the level of sophistication can range from simple references (e.g., a citation at the end of a sentence) to complex analyses (e.g., meta-analysis). Some groups may perform only some of the steps before reaching closure on a guideline.

The steps in practice guidelines development can be broadly categorized as follows:

- Introductory decisions
- Assessments of clinical appropriateness
- Assessments of public policy issues
- Guideline document development and evaluation

Introductory Decisions

Guidelines produced by an expert panel are influenced greatly by the size and composition of its members. Panel members generally (and sometimes exclusively) include physicians, but they can also include other health professionals (e.g., nurses or dentists), methodologists (e.g., epidemiologists, statisticians, or healthcare economists), and members of other disciplines. Some panels include patients and consumer representatives. Once the panel is established, it needs to define its topic carefully. This includes specification of the target condition, the type of patients and clinical presentations for which the guidelines are intended, and the interventions to be considered. The panel should reach agreement on the setting for which the practice guidelines are intended, including the type of providers (e.g., physicians, nonphysicians, specialists, or primary care providers) and practice settings (e.g., hospital, office, or operating room). The topics of practice guidelines are generally either *conditions*, such as diseases (e.g., acute appendicitis) or presenting complaints (e.g., chest pain), or *procedures* (e.g., upper GI endoscopy). They can focus on prevention, diagnosis, treatment, or rehabilitation.

Assessment of Clinical Appropriateness

The principal analytic task in developing practice guidelines is to define appropriate clinical practices based on what is best for the patient. Thus, the proper starting point is to determine which practices produce the best clinical outcomes. The two principal sources of information about clinical benefits and harms are scientific evidence and expert opinion. Panels vary in the comprehensiveness of their literature reviews. The review of the evidence involves three steps: (a) retrieval of evidence; (b) evaluation of individual studies; and (c) synthesis of the evidence.

Expert opinion is important in assessing clinical benefits and harms because reliable scientific evidence is lacking for many clinical practices. The opinions and rationale of the experts should be documented explicitly so that readers are aware that the recommendations are based on opinion. Scientific evidence and expert opinion provide the basis for summarizing the potential benefits and harms of each option. Decision analysis can play an important role in comparing the benefits and harms associated with different choices. This technique allows guideline developers to simulate the effects of different treatment strategies on specific outcomes based on available data on the natural course of the disease and the effectiveness of treatment options. Information about benefits and harms is used to determine which practices are appropriate, which are inappropriate, and which are in the "gray zone" of uncertain appropriateness.

A large number of clinical practices fall into this "gray zone" category because of uncertainties about the benefits and harms of interventions, variability in patients and their responses to treatments, and differences in patient preferences about the desirability of outcomes.

Assessment of Public Policy Issues

Practice guidelines intended for large numbers of patients are public policies and can have broad societal impact. They often cannot be based exclusively on clinical criteria, without attention to important resource limitations and feasibility issues. Practice guidelines may be unrealistic if recommended services cannot be paid for by patients or society. The same concerns apply to other limited resources, such as equipment and personnel. Opportunity costs must also be considered; recommended practices may displace resources away from more effective healthcare services. Although a significant number of practice guidelines developers include assessments of costs in their analyses, groups differ in how much they allow costs to influence their recommendations.

Recommendations based exclusively on research findings may not be applicable to "real-world" practice conditions. Important factors that need to be considered include constraints faced by practitioners (e.g., time pressures and conflict between the practice guidelines and local standards of care); the concerns of patients (e.g., access to care, and perceived right to health services, even if not recommended in practice guidelines); and the limitations of the healthcare system (availability of personnel, supplies, and follow-up care).

Guideline Document Development and Evaluation

Practice guidelines are written to provide clear recommendations for practitioners and to document the rationale on which the recommendations are based. Practice guidelines have always been expected to provide clear information about *what to do* — the proper method of performing procedures and administering treatments. Draft guidelines are reviewed by relevant content experts to ensure scientific and clinical validity, as well as by relevant organizations and agencies to provide broad input on content and policy issues. Some groups perform pretesting by asking a small sample of practitioners to use the practice guideline for a brief period and by collecting their suggestions on ways to improve the document. The process of practice guidelines development must not end with the publication of the document, since this step alone is unlikely to change practice behavior. A diffusion plan must be adopted to ensure dissemination of the guidelines to the target audience, to build consensus, and to achieve behavior change. Evaluation research is necessary to determine whether guidelines alter practice patterns and improve health outcomes. Practice guidelines must also be updated as new evidence and new technologies become available.

The process of developing practice guidelines often calls attention to important gaps in scientific evidence. The clarification of research needs may be the most important outcome of practice guidelines, and it may help promote a rational research agenda that defines the key issues that are most in need of study.

CARE PATHS

Many studies have demonstrated the potential benefit of practice guidelines in improving clinical practice. Practice guidelines provide a basis for the development of care paths used in patient management, and also provide a foundation for review criteria used in quality and utilization management (5). Care paths have been developed for a wide variety of clinical populations in multiple acute- and critical-care settings. They serve as collaborative guidelines that identify, time, and provide a sequence for the major interventions of healthcare providers for a particular case type. Care paths provide a framework for care and reflect the collaboration required among many disciplines to treat patients.

Care Path Development, Implementation, Routine Use, Ongoing Evaluation and Revision

In general, there are five steps in care path development: development, implementation, routine use, ongoing evaluation, and revision. In the development and implementation of care paths, a number of issues require thoughtful planning, collaborative teamwork, and an understanding of the evolutionary nature of this work. The initial step in the creation of any care path is building a strong team of professional healthcare providers from key disciplines or departments. Most commonly, team members include physicians from various medical services, and individuals from nursing, social services, the pathology department, nutrition, and hospital administration. A pathway's success depends on implementation. The initial step in implementation is the educational process whereby the house staff, other relevant physicians, nurses, case managers, and ward secretaries are informed about all aspects of the pathway, including the specific role each will play.

In many centers, the care paths are a part of the medical record. The printed problems, goals, outcomes, and activities replace other nursing documentation. Charting by exception is the premise behind the documentation. It is understood that the goals, outcomes, and activities on the pathway are met or occur unless they are marked or circled (5). Data coding, analysis, and feedback are a vital part of a care path program. Theoretically, analysis of process variance should identify patterns of clinical practice that are associated with outcomes (desired or undesired), and therefore should allow for objective forecasting of process changes that should improve care. In practice, however, variance tracking may prove to be extremely resource intensive, frustrating, and of limited value if the use and goals of the data are not carefully considered prospectively. It is important to limit data presentation to critical elements or key events to prevent data paralysis.

The first step in planning for variance analysis is an identification of the variances that will be documented. In other words, what information will be collected? Some of these variances may be positive, that is, those that occur when a patient's progress toward anticipated outcomes is faster than anticipated, or when the patient progresses more quickly on the care path. Negative variances are those that identify an activity or goal that has not occurred within the time frame identified on the pathway, has not occurred at all, or has occurred in addition to what is on the pathway. Variance data reporting is a key component of the care path initiative. Variance data offer caregivers the opportunity to evaluate what works and what must be refined. Variances from care processes on the pathway are correlated with patient outcomes and cost. Process variance may or may not affect the quality of care a patient receives, and may increase, decrease, or have no effect on cost.

The pathway is considered a dynamic tool and is altered to reflect changes in practice that occur as a result of team decisions, research, case studies, or outcomes for the patient group. Teams must take action concurrently for individuals and retrospectively for the population as a whole. At the time the pathway, physician orders, patient version, and variance-tracking form are ready for implementation, the team determines the length of time needed for implementation before collecting variance data. This is the learning period when capturing data may not be very accurate because everyone is learning the system. The team also identifies the patients who shall be selected for initiation of care paths. Exclusion criteria can be developed to help determine patients for whom it is inappropriate to initiate the pathway.

When evaluating the impact of a care path, it is important to consider the effect the pathway has on patient outcomes such as cost, patient satisfaction, health status, and employment. Reporting of outcome data, in conjunction with variance data, provides an opportunity for providers to see how processes of care are linked with patient outcomes. Patient outcomes are the end results of care processes. Outcomes of care are best managed through improvement in care processes. Unless outcomes are measured simultaneously or in conjunction with care path implementation, it is difficult to assure (a) that quality of care is maintained or improved; (b) that cost of care and length of stay decline, and (c) that patient satisfaction with care is optimal.

Role of the Clinical Laboratory in Care Paths

The clinical laboratory should get involved in all five steps in care path development. Clinical laboratory specialists have an opportunity to play an influential leadership role (6). Laboratorians should (a) provide recommendations for optimal laboratory use, (b) become familiar with the potential impact of care paths on the clinical laboratory, (c) understand the benefits and limitations of care paths, (d) evaluate care paths that address laboratory issues, (e) develop strategies to participate in initiatives to develop and improve care paths, (f) provide assistance to the developers and users of care paths that relate to laboratory issues, and (g) assist in efforts to link laboratory databases with other administrative and clinical databases. A good way to become familiar with the purpose, development, and implementation of pathways is to read the recent relevant literature. Who is the person in charge of pathway development in your healthcare facility and who are the pathway members? Find out to what extent the laboratory has or has not been involved in this process,

specifically who has been involved and the nature of the department's commitment. Pathologists, laboratory managers, section supervisors, and bench technologists all have been members on different hospital pathway teams.

The attitude that laboratories have only a peripheral role in the process needs to be challenged. Laboratories should be an integral part of every care path. Laboratory personnel are expected to be advocates for the laboratory's role in care paths, and thus, they should be as knowledgeable as possible about the laboratory-related aspects of the condition addressed by the pathway. In addition, they will need to assess what the impact of the pathway will be on the laboratory. Make sure that the laboratory can deliver on agreed-upon services, as pathways cannot optimally function if expected services fail to materialize. An essential part of planning includes continuing discussions with the other parties in the laboratory (7). These individuals need to know how the pathway is developing and what, if any, their roles will be in the plan's implementation. Team members may request specific testing to be performed by the laboratory. The laboratory should determine if it can or cannot be done and present alternatives as necessary. Expect to help with the educational process of the pathways. Laboratory personnel involved in care paths will be responsible for educating other laboratory personnel about the process. In addition, the laboratory may be called upon to assist nursing, social services, or other departments. Different ideas from different members of the team should be expected. Care paths are working documents and may need to be altered to work properly. As new laboratory techniques become available, laboratory personnel can introduce them to the team and they may be used to modify the original pathway. This process provides a unique opportunity for laboratorians to improve the quality of patient care.

For most pathways, the laboratory's involvement includes performing a small number of crucial laboratory tests (7). The number of crucial tests may be small, but these tests often determine treatment decisions. Therefore, we must be aware of the crucial tests and structure the laboratory to provide the testing. In the case of routine orders, the laboratory can play a facilitating role in changing systems to assure that the laboratory can meet the pathway's needs. Some healthcare conditions are highly dependent on the laboratory as a major resource for either diagnosis or treatment. The laboratory's most important role is to understand the impact of testing on the pathway and to structure its services to fulfill that role. To understand its role, laboratorians must review pathways in the development stages, explain any limitations to the development team, and structure the laboratory to deliver timely test results.

LABORATORY TESTS AND CARE PATHS

The number of clinical laboratory tests performed has increased greatly in recent years in nearly all health centers in the United States. This rise in laboratory use has been a major factor contributing to escalating healthcare costs. The need for such a large number of laboratory tests has quite reasonably been questioned. Reasons offered for the increased number of tests include overzealous documentation, medico-legal considerations, building of personal databases, and profit, in addition to valid clinical indications (8). Little hard data are available to document why physicians order laboratory tests or to indicate what percentage of tests is ordered for these various reasons.

The purpose and function of clinical pathologists and laboratory medicine specialists are to assist clinicians in (a) confirming or rejecting a diagnosis, (b) providing guidelines in patient management, (c) establishing a prognosis, (d) detecting disease through case finding or screening, and (d) monitoring follow-up therapy (9). The operation of the clinical laboratory and effective delivery of service to clinicians, patients, and the public requires a complex interdigitation of (a) expertise in medical, scientific, and technical areas; (b) resources in the form of personnel, laboratory and data processing equipment, supplies, and facilities; and (c) skills in organization, management, and communication. All laboratory personnel, especially those in leadership and management, must be aware of current accreditation and governmental regulations and evolving practice guidelines and care paths that relate to laboratory services. Clinically useful data generated by the laboratory must be reported promptly and accurately to optimize patient management. Delay in reporting can make data useless.

A study by Wertman et al. (8) indicates that three reasons contribute almost equally to the ordering of laboratory tests: diagnosis, screening, and monitoring. Actions brought about by the test reports show that by far the most common action is a change in therapy. Other contributions of laboratory tests include change in diagnosis, prognosis, and understanding of disease. Testing and monitoring are distinct acts with approaches that have important clinical implications (10). They differ in technologies used, time required for performing tests, and in some cases, sites in which the assessment takes place. Testing determines the presence of an abnormality, substance, or disease by measuring a parameter at a fixed point in time. Monitoring, on the other hand, examines a parameter continuously or at frequent intervals. The results can warn caregivers when undesirable limits are being approached. The term "monitor" applies, among other things, to discrete measuring devices used at the point of patient care to provide clinical data in real time. The clinical team uses this information in formulating immediate therapeutic decisions. A parameter that changes continuously, such as blood gases in a patient with compromised cardiopulmonary function, is best assessed via monitoring. For a parameter that changes slowly, such as serum bilirubin in a patient with advanced cirrhosis, testing is more appropriate.

Laboratory turnaround times may be considered from three perspectives. *Laboratory time* refers to the time required to perform a test after the specimen has arrived in the clinical laboratory. *Testing time* involves the interval elapsed in obtaining the specimen, transporting it to the laboratory, performing the analysis, and deriving results. The more comprehensive *therapeutic turnaround time* is defined as the time from test ordering to treatment. It consists of two intervals: (a) the time from test ordering based on diagnostic hypotheses to receipt of results by the clinical team, plus (b) the time needed for the clinical team to initiate (change or discontinue) medical or surgical treatment. For critically ill patients, early treatment generally helps to improve patient outcomes. It also helps to decrease the third

time interval, or at least diminish complications and unforeseen problems that delay favorable outcomes, prolong critical care, and waste medical and financial resources (11).

Most lab tests now performed on hospitalized patients are used to monitor the course of treatment for known conditions (12). In medical intensive care units, more than three-fourths of admissions may be for monitoring rather than for immediate major therapeutic interventions. Monitoring tests performed in the central laboratory have the advantage of having one instrument in one location, which minimizes quality control and cost issues. Its disadvantages include the need to have the patient travel to the central facility and, subsequently, to have a second interaction with the patient to report the results. Furthermore, the objective of monitoring therapeutic drug effects is to detect a change in steady state, and long-term routine testing in the central laboratory at a frequency of more than once a month is not practical.

How could the central laboratory best provide test results to physically separated locations? Four options could be considered: (a) operating a satellite laboratory, (b) installing a pneumatic tube system, (c) using couriers to transport samples, and (d) using point-of-care testing (POCT). To make a sound decision, administrators, clinicians, and laboratorians must review anticipated capital and operating costs, and consider expected turnaround time for each option.

POINT-OF-CARE TESTING IN CARE PATHS

POCT is defined as "testing at or near the site of patient care whenever the medical care is needed." The purpose of POCT is to provide immediate information to physicians about the patient's condition, so that this information can be integrated into appropriate treatment decisions that improve patient outcomes, that is, reduce patients' criticality, morbidity, and mortality. POCT can be performed in different environments, such as in the hospital, at home, or at other locations (13). The increase in POCT during the last ten years has been made possible by a number of factors, including advances in computer technology. Because POCT methods and instruments require less sample, are easy to use, are smaller and more portable, and produce results on a variety of analytes more quickly than traditional laboratory instruments, their use appeals to both the medical and the nursing staffs (14).

There is growing debate about the cost effectiveness of POCT. While it appears that POCT may be more expensive than laboratory testing, some argue that other attributes of POCT could shorten the length of patient stay or offset the costs of POCT, or both. In the operating room, POCT is cost effective for hemostasis evaluation and transfusion management (15). In some cases, such as rapid parathyroid hormone (PTH) testing for parathyroid surgery, speed alone is crucial in saving operating room time and reducing the length of hospitalization (16). Wians et al. (17) report that the value is well established for intraoperative PTH testing using a rapid assay for reducing the time spent under anesthesia by patients undergoing outpatient parathyroid gland surgery for hyperparathyroidism and in reducing the reoperative rate due to a failed initial surgery. However, the authors conclude that the cost effectiveness of intraoperative PTH-guided parathyroid gland surgery and whether or not this testing should be performed entirely intraoperatively or in a central laboratory are less firmly established.

Prolonged therapeutic time, inevitable when the primary physician is busy or leaves the patient's area, delays therapy, thereby increasing hospital stay and cost. Reduction in turnaround times provides timely data about the patient to the clinical staff, improving their therapeutic decisions. Higher productivity, fewer repeat tests, and shorter hospital stays consequently result in lower costs.

At the Johns Hopkins Hospital, more than 1,000 adult cardiac surgeries are performed each year, with the majority of patients receiving either coronary artery bypass graft (CABG) surgery or valve replacement (18). The CABG course of care consists of a preoperative workup, an intraoperative period, a postoperative period, and a 6-week postdischarge period. Laboratory testing is an integral part of the entire CABG pathway, starting with the preoperative evaluation. The combination of laboratory tests and other clinical parameters assist in determining the health status and suitability of patients for the procedure, identifying high-risk patients, and predicting the likelihood of blood transfusion. The majority of testing in the CABG pathway takes place during the surgical procedure itself and in the subsequent stay in the intensive care unit. Because intraoperative testing requires short turnaround times, surgical tests are performed in a satellite laboratory located near the operating suites, and using POCT in the operating room itself. By implementing the CABG pathway, the Johns Hopkins Hospital realized financial savings in reduced length of stay for cardiac surgery patients and lower utilization rates for laboratory tests. Activated coagulation time has been used for many years to monitor heparinization during cardiopulmonary surgery and vascular catheterization and in the coronary care unit and is useful for monitoring heparin during renal dialysis. The immediate availability of test results can significantly improve clinical care (19). In a study by Scott (20), patients receiving point-of-care (POC) coagulation monitoring in the cardiothoracic operating room required fewer blood component transfusions, had shorter operative times, and had less chest-tube drainage volume. Rapid evaluation of quantitative and qualitative platelet disorders, and coagulation factor deficiencies can facilitate the optimal administration of pharmacologic and transfusion-based therapy (21,22).

In recent years, there has been a dramatic increase in the need for monitoring resulting from significantly expanded use of drugs with narrow therapeutic indexes. One excellent example is the expanded use of anticoagulation, especially in the areas of atrial fibrillation and coronary artery disease. It has been documented that as many as 75% of patients are not receiving appropriate therapy, in many cases due to the problems with monitoring chronic anticoagulant therapy. Slight changes in the dose of Coumadin can shift prothrombin time (PT) values outside the therapeutic range. There are exponential rises in thrombotic and bleeding complications when the PT, reported as the international normalized ratio (INR), drops below 2.0 or rises above 5.0, respectively. It is clear from this example that there is little margin for error, resulting in the need for frequent monitoring. POCT at the site of patient visit (i.e., outpatient clinic) offers

much promise. The results can be reported and the patient counseled during the one visit. Self-testing has also shown significant improvements. One longitudinal study in Germany with more than 200 patient-years of follow-up (20), found the anticoagulant therapy to be in the therapeutic range 92% of the time with patient home testing, compared to 60% in a well-managed anticoagulant clinic. This resulted in a significant decrease in both thrombotic and hemorrhagic complications.

Control of anticoagulation therapy has been plagued with a high incidence of adverse reactions, either hemorrhage or thrombosis. A number of innovations have emerged in response to these problems. In some clinical settings, the desire for immediate results of coagulation testing has been met with the placement of coagulation analyzers at the POC. A variety of technologies have been developed for POCT, depending on the application. Satellite anticoagulation control clinics have been organized specifically to initiate and monitor anticoagulation therapy, either with heparin or warfarin, and are staffed by physicians and nurse practitioners with special expertise. The immediate availability of test results makes patient care much more efficient (23). Home PT testing was initiated several years ago in Germany and has been used successfully by more than 35,000 patients. An anticoagulation program that includes self-management of anticoagulation therapy results in improved accuracy of anticoagulation control and in treatment-related quality of life (24). In a 1996 report, Ansell and Hughes (25) described 40 patients with a variety of indications for oral anticoagulation who were followed for 7 years. Doing testing at home and adjusting their oral anticoagulation dosages according to treatment guidelines resulted in improved anticoagulation. It is important to ensure that POCT done by patients receiving anticoagulants or by technologists provides results comparable with those of the central laboratory (26).

People with diabetes can suffer potentially serious physical effects from their disease. Total healthcare expenditures attributed to all types of diabetes in 1995 in the United States were $47.9 billion (27). Glucose level determinations are a routine activity in the clinical laboratory and part of many care paths for the diagnosis and monitoring of patients with diabetes. Evidence indicates conclusively that when blood glucose is maintained at a level near normal, the onset and progression of microvascular changes, especially in the retina and kidneys, are delayed (28). Revised guidelines for diagnosing and classifying diabetes mellitus have been recently published (29). The goal of these new parameters is to identify asymptomatic patients with undiagnosed diabetes at an early stage of illness to avoid the consequences of a chronically elevated blood-sugar level. Most patients with diabetes can be instructed to self-monitor blood glucose successfully to maintain control of their glycemia (30). Portable glucose devices have improved in precision and accuracy with each generation. As with many other clinical conditions, the usual justification for the use of POC glucose testing is to decrease turnaround time and improve patient care. The average turnaround time for a point-of care glucose test is 5 minutes. In a major teaching hospital with a 21-bed diabetic unit using a sliding-scale, insulin-dose clinical protocol, failure to complete glucose determination in the central laboratory and to make the result available to the diabetic unit 26% of the time resulted in annual costs of $45,100 (31). A variety of noninvasive, blood-glucose monitoring techniques are currently under evaluation. Noninvasive methods will permit real-time bedside and/or home glucose monitoring without the requirement of skin puncture (32).

Minimally invasive or noninvasive POCT has the potential to become an integral part of numerous care paths. It relieves the anxiety patients feel about needles, lowers the risk of exposing laboratory professionals to bloodborne diseases, and reduces the turnaround time for test results (33). A noninvasive method that measures the concentration of bilirubin in the forehead skin of 1- to 8-day-old newborns costs 20% to 25% of what it costs to do a serum bilirubin level. Furthermore, it produces results in 15 seconds and improves customer (parent) satisfaction. Other minimally invasive POCTs currently available include a test for PT and a breath test for *Helicobacter pylori*.

When someone requests POCT, two important questions to ask are: Why can't the central laboratory provide the service? What is the anticipated benefit to the patient? The first component required for successful POCT is a description of the medical use of test results. Next is an itemization of the conditions under which a patient may perform his or her own POC measurement if appropriate. There should also be periodic comparisons with the central laboratory. Last but not least, before initiating a POCT program, each institution must evaluate its true costs.

CONCLUSIONS

Over the past decade, the increase in healthcare costs has outdistanced increases in both wages and the cost of living. In 1998, national health expenditures amounted to $1.1 trillion, and the Centers for Medicare & Medicaid Services (CMS), formerly the Health Care Financing Administration (HCFA), predicts that amount will increase by 37.6% in the next 5 years. Among the tools used by hospitals for cost management are cost data, interdisciplinary approaches, benchmarks, care paths, physician profiles, and case management. Care paths, as discussed in this chapter, are useful tools in identifying unneeded tests, successful forms of treatment, and overutilization of resources by physicians (34). In today's world of heightened interest in healthcare costs, it is important not to lose sight of the impact cost reduction may have on patient outcomes and overall healthcare quality (35). The true emphasis should not be on lowering the cost of laboratory testing or other diagnostic testing, but on using appropriate testing to lower the cost of an episode of care and the costs of managing disease. Traditionally, hospitals have managed their resources by specialties or cost centers. Individual departments tried to minimize the cost of each component of care. The laboratory, for example, would look at the most cost-effective testing strategy to assess chest pain, while the cardiology department might develop its own assessment system. Managed care and capitated reimbursement systems focus on lowering the cost of an episode of care, and laboratories are learning how to work with other departments to control overall costs.

Use of care paths promotes laboratory involvement in the development of clinical protocols, facilitates implementation of systems to ensure appropriate use of laboratory tests, and provides mechanisms to track financial and quality outcomes of tests used in this standardized way. Through active participation in these pathways, laboratorians can have a significant impact on the quality of care for patients. Moreover, it is a unique opportunity to demonstrate the added value that knowledgeable and motivated laboratory professionals can provide to assist in the diagnosis and management of clinical conditions. Laboratorians play an important role in care paths, not only in the design of new pathways and modification of existing pathways, but also through clinical consultations and, most importantly, in providing efficient and timely service to meet the defined pathway goals and requirements.

POCT has emerged as a powerful tool in healthcare delivery (36). The big difference today is that POCT methods are generally user friendly and rapid (37). Whether POCT is performed in the main hospital or in the physician's office, the ultimate mission is to generate accurate and reliable laboratory testing that meets the quality standards our patients expect and deserve.

As more traditional diagnostic tests are done with the use of microchips (biochips), tests should become easier to do, less expensive, faster, and more likely to be done at the POC rather than a centralized laboratory (38). Telemedicine, one of the communications technologies that will figure significantly in healthcare delivery in the future, uses electronic information and communications technologies to provide medical diagnoses and/or patient health care when distances separate the participants. Home health care is expected to most fully exploit the advantages of telemedicine. Physicians and other healthcare professionals will be able to deliver effective noninvasive care over standard telephone lines and cable television infrastructures. These advances in communications, paired with the use of low-cost, POC home testing, will enable physicians to monitor chronic health conditions such as diabetes and high blood pressure. Because many home health visits do not require direct contact between patient and physician, the use of telemedicine technology can reduce the cost of home health care significantly. It also can reduce hospital stays because follow-up convalescent care can be provided in the home (39).

REFERENCES

1. Spath PL, ed. *Clinical paths: tools for outcomes management.* Chicago: American Hospital Publishing, 1994.
2. Weiland DE. Why use clinical pathways rather than practice guidelines? *Am J Surg* 1997;174:592–595.
3. Woolf SH. Practice guidelines, a new reality in medicine. II. Methods of developing guidelines. *Arch Intern Med* 1992;152:946–962.
4. Woolf SH. Practice guidelines: a new reality in medicine. *Arch Intern Med* 1990;150:1811–1818.
5. Ibarra V, Titler MG, Reiter RC. Issues in the development and implementation of clinical pathways. *AACN Clin Issues* 1996;7:436–447.
6. Kelly JT. Role of clinical practice guidelines and clinical profiling in facilitating optimal laboratory use. *Clin Chem* 1995;41:1234–1236.
7. Howard B, Keiser JF. Critical pathways: an introduction. *Critical pathways: probe module 8.* Clinical Laboratory Management Association, August 1997:1–12.
8. Wertman BG, Sostrin SV, Pavlova Z, et al. Why do physicians order laboratory tests? A study of laboratory test request and use patterns. *JAMA* 1980;243:2080–2082.

9. Henry JB, ed. *Clinical diagnosis and management by laboratory methods,* 19th ed. Philadelphia: Saunders, 1996.
10. Zaloga GP. Monitoring versus testing technologies: present and future. *Med Lab Observer* 1991;23:20–31.
11. Kost GJ. Point-of-care testing: clinical impact and potential for improving patient outcomes. Paper presented at Clinical Laboratory Management Association Annual Conference and Exhibition, 1997.
12. Rock RC. Why testing is being moved to the site of patient care. *Med Lab Observer* 1991;23:2–5.
13. Louie RF, Tang Z, Shelby DG, et al. Point-of-care testing: millennium technology for critical care. *Lab Med* 2000;31:402–408.
14. Ingram Main R, Kiechle FL. Point-of-care testing: administration within a health system. *Lab Med* 2000;31:453–459.
15. Despotis GJ, Santoro SA, Spitznagel E, et al. Prospective evaluation and clinical utility of on-site monitoring of coagulation in patients undergoing cardiac operation. *J Thorac Cardiovasc Surg* 1994;107:271–279.
16. Scott MG. Is faster better? An outcomes approach to POCT implementation decisions. In: *Managing your POCT program for success.* Audio conference. Washington, DC: American Association of Clinical Chemistry, January 20, 2000.
17. Wians FH, Balko JA, Hsu RM, et al. Intraoperative vs central laboratory PTH testing during parathyroidectomy surgery. *Lab Med* 2000; 31:616–621.
18. Sokoll LJ, Li DJ, Dawson PB, et al. Critical pathways: the laboratory's role in coronary artery bypass surgery. *AACC Clinical Laboratory News* Apr 1997.
19. Doty DB, Knott HW, Hoyt JL, et al. Heparin dose for accurate anticoagulation in cardiac surgery. *J Cardiovasc Surg* 1979;20:597–604.
20. Scott FI. Integrating point-of-care testing with continuity of care. Part 4: Case studies in anticoagulant therapy, cardiac markers and blood gases. *Am Clin Lab* 1998;17:4–9.
21. Despotis GJ. Prospective evaluation and clinical utility of on-site monitoring of coagulation in patients undergoing cardiac operation. *J Thorac Cardiovasc Surg* 1994;107:271–279.
22. Despotis GJ, Joist JH, Goodnough LT. Monitoring of hemostasis in cardiac surgical patients: impact of point-of-care testing on blood loss and transfusion outcomes. *Clin Chem* 1997;43:1684–1696.
23. Koepke JA. Point-of-care coagulation testing. *Lab Med* 2000;31: 343–346.
24. Bernardo A. Experience with patient self-management of oral anticoagulation. *J Thromb Thrombolysis* 1996;2:321–325.
25. Ansell JE, Hughes R. Evolving models of warfarin management: anticoagulation clinics, patient self-monitoring and patient self-management. *Am Heart J* 1996;132:1095–1100.
26. Koepke JA. Technologies for coagulation instruments. *Lab Med* 2000; 31:211–215.
27. Hodgson TA, Cohen AJ. Medical care expenditures for diabetes, its chronic complications, and its comorbidities. *Prev Med* 1999;29: 173–186.
28. Diabetes Control and Complications Trial Research Group. The effect of intensive treatment of diabetes on the development and progression of long-term complications in insulin-dependent diabetes mellitus. *N Engl J Med* 1993;329:977–985.
29. Report of the Expert Committee on the diagnosis and classification of diabetes mellitus. *Diabet Care* 1999;22[Suppl 1]:S5–S19.
30. Burton L. Diagnosing and monitoring patients with diabetes. *Lab Med* 2000;31:84–90.
31. Cembrowski GS, Kiechle FL. Point-of-care testing: critical analysis and practical application. *Adv Pathol Lab Med* 1994;7:3–26.
32. Kiechle FL, Ingram Main R. Blood glucose: measurement in the point-of-care setting. *Lab Med* 2000;31:276–282.
33. Wilson F. Minimally invasive testing expands beyond glucose. *Lab Med* 2000;31:436–441.
34. Ramsey C, Ormsby S, Marsh T. Performance-improvement strategies can reduce costs. *Healthcare Financial Management Resource Guide* 2001:2–6.
35. Bowie LJ. Implementing appropriate testing practices: the role of the laboratory in critical pathways. *AACC Clin Lab News* 1997.
36. Boyle SM. At the bedside: meeting the challenges of point-of-care coordinators. *Adv Adm Lab* 1998;7.
37. Chapman B. Glucose tests at the point of care. It's a tough task to maintain a quality program for near-patient glucose testing. What the central lab can do to make sure it's sound—and stays that way. *CAP Today* 1998;12:24–26.
38. Yox SB. The laboratory on a chip: the future of miniaturization and automation. *Lab Med* 1999;30:456–461.
39. Charles BL. Telemedicine can lower costs and improve access. *Healthcare Financial Mgmt* 2000;54:66–69.

38

POINT-OF-CARE DIAGNOSIS AND MANAGEMENT OF MYOCARDIAL INFARCTION AND CONGESTIVE HEART FAILURE

ALAN S. MAISEL

CARDIAC MARKERS IN AN ACCELERATED DIAGNOSTIC ALGORITHM

In the United States each year, 6 million people present to emergency healthcare facilities with chest pain. Of the 4 million admitted, 1.5 million have acute myocardial infarction (AMI) by World Health Organization (WHO) criteria, and 1 million have unstable angina. Each year AMI is responsible for more than half a million deaths in the United States alone (1).

"Underdiagnosis," or failing to diagnose AMI, results in increased morbidity and mortality (2–6) as well as significant potential for litigation. If fact, one-fifth of the malpractice awards against emergency department (ED) physicians are associated with treatment of myocardial ischemia and AMI (7).

The consequences of "overdiagnosis" are equally significant. A recent estimate (8) (Fig. 38.1) suggests that many patients admitted to the myocardial intensive care unit (MICU) with chest pain either have no significant disease, a nonacute condition, or unstable angina. The annual expense for these admissions approaches $1 billion. In addition, patients admitted to

the MICU become anxious when the wires, IV, and medications are administered. Many become "cardiac cripples," overly concerned with meaningless chest pain and making numerous unnecessary visits to the ED of a hospital. Their lifestyles and careers may be compromised, and the records of admission to MICU may affect their ability to obtain insurance.

Current Guidelines for Care

The American College of Cardiology (ACC) and the American Heart Association (AHA) have published guidelines (9) for the diagnosis of AMI. A patient has AMI if at least two of the following three criteria are consistent with the condition:

- Clinical history of chest discomfort
- Changes in electrocardiogram (ECG) tracings
- Temporal changes in the concentrations of cardiac markers in blood

The ACC/AHA also recommends that an initial patient evaluation be performed within 20 minutes of arrival to the ED to ensure that the "door to needle time" for cardiac markers will be less than 30 minutes, and that, if necessary, percutaneous transluminal coronary angioplasty or other intervention (such as administration of a thrombolytic agent) occurs within 60 to 90 minutes.

Testing at presentation is only the first stage in the evaluation of patients for chest pain. According to a 1993 report (10), the levels of creatine kinase (CK) and CK-MB (an isoenzyme of CK) combined with the ECG tracings still miss 28% of AMIs (Fig. 38.2). The ECG pattern alone misses nearly half of AMIs because the ST elevations are not always present, or, if they are present, may be caused by a non-AMI condition such as a bundle-branch block, electrolyte abnormality, or concomitant use of digitalis. As for CK and CK-MB, these tests alone at presentation miss more than half of AMIs.

The benefits of early and accurate diagnosis of AMI are shown in Figure 38.3 (11). As the graph clearly shows, the quicker the diagnosis is made, the greater the benefit to the

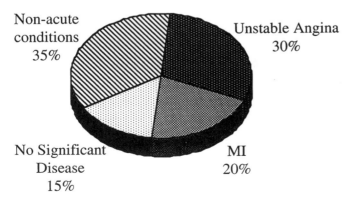

FIGURE 38.1. Estimates of unnecessary chest pain admissions. (From HCIA, Inc., 1999, with permission.)

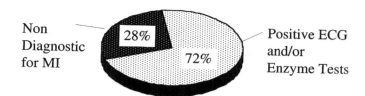

FIGURE 38.2. Initial testing misses 28% of acute myocardial infarction patients. (From Young GP, Green TR. The role of single ECG, creatinine kinase, and CKMB in diagnosing patients with acute chest pain. *Am J Emerg Med* 1993;11:444–449.)

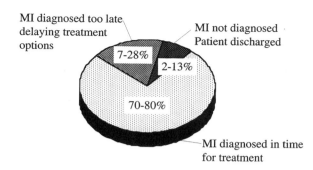

FIGURE 38.4. Diagnosis is made too late for 40% of myocardial infarction patients to receive timely treatment.

patient. Unfortunately, according to a 1994 estimate (12) (Fig. 38.4), diagnosis is made too late for 40% of myocardial infarction (MI) patients to receive timely treatment. This is consistent with the results of a recent survey (13) which shows that 80% of physicians believe that more rapid turnaround times for cardiac marker test results would improve the clinical decision-making process.

Traditionally, blood samples for cardiac marker measurements were taken at certain time intervals and transported to a central laboratory for centrifugation and distribution to testing systems for analysis. When results were available they were communicated to the physician as promptly as possible. Of prime importance was accurate documentation of the sampling time for each measurement so that the physician could correctly interpret the pattern of events revealed by the temporal behavior of the cardiac markers.

With so many steps involved, the potential for error was significant and the turnaround time for cardiac marker levels was several hours, which is often too long for the physician to take the results into consideration when deciding whether to admit a patient to MICU. Diagnosis and treatment were either delayed

or made empirically, which produced unnecessary anxiety for both the patient and the physician, not to mention the expense of unnecessary admission.

With the appearance of whole-blood analyzers for point-of-care testing (POCT), however, results are available immediately, and the physician can incorporate the cardiac marker behavior into a diagnostic and treatment algorithm for rapid triage of chest pain patients according to risk. In effect, the physician is "captured" (14) so that he or she can interpret the results and make decisions based on them before leaving the clinical unit. The result is rapid diagnosis, prompt treatment, and a reduction in unnecessary delays, admissions to MICU, relapses, and tests that prolong length of stay and increase morbidity (15–18). If cardiac marker results are quantitative, the physician can establish cutoff values at the point of care rather than relying on values obtained by a central laboratory or documented values of the literature.

POCT is particularly advantageous for measuring an analyte that changes rapidly or unexpectedly; results are current rather than hours old, and the clinician can act immediately to provide maximum benefit to the patient (19). Whole blood is often used because centrifugation, specimen transport and processing, and delays in communication of results to the physician are eliminated, and fewer people are involved (14).

Cardiac Markers

Although none of the currently available markers have all the characteristics of the ideal cardiac marker (Table 38.1), serial testing of these markers in whole blood offers a promising approach for the rapid and accurate diagnosis of AMI. Current studies support a panel approach to diagnose AMI, and the use of cardiac markers in combination for risk stratification of

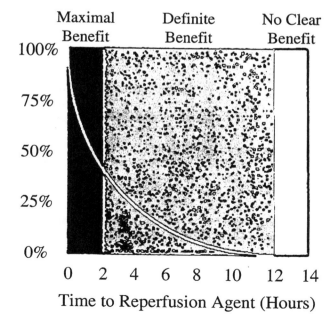

FIGURE 38.3. Benefits of early acute myocardial infarction diagnosis.

TABLE 38.1. ATTRIBUTES OF IDEAL CARDIAC MARKER

Found in high concentration in the heart
Not found in other tissues, even in trace amounts or under
  pathologic conditions
Low molecular weight and thus released early in the course of acute
  myocardial infarction
Remains elevated for several days

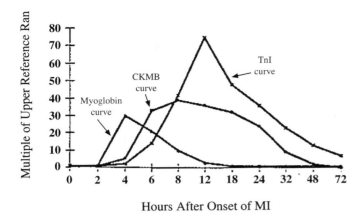

FIGURE 38.5. Appearance of cardiac markers in blood after myocardial infarction.

patients presenting with chest pain has been reviewed (20). The times at which cardiac markers—CK-MB, myoglobin, and cardiac troponin I (cTnI)—appear after the onset of chest pain are shown in Figure 38.5.

Creatine Kinase-MB

Although considered the "gold standard" in the ACC/AHA guidelines, the universally recognized CK-MB, even with its time-honored value in AMI diagnosis, may be unreliable when skeletal muscles are also involved, such as in accidents, trauma, cardiac surgery, severe burns, and extreme exercise. In addition, the CK-MB level may be only slightly elevated and therefore difficult to interpret during the early stages of AMI. Finally, the narrow temporal window of CK-MB elevation precludes its use in diagnosis of AMI in patients arriving days after the onset of chest pain. For example, if a patient presents to the ED 4 to 5 days after the MI has occurred, the CK-MB level would have returned to normal. If this patient also has pulmonary edema and a history of heart failure, these symptoms combined with the normal level of CK-MB might lead the physician to inappropriately prescribe diuretics. As discussed later, a measurement of the cTnI level would have indicated that AMI had caused the heart failure, thus resulting in a more appropriate treatment pathway for the patient.

Troponins

Cardiac troponins exist primarily in two forms, cTnI and cTnT. In contrast to CK-MB, troponins are highly specific to the heart and exist in cardiac tissue at much higher concentrations than CK-MB (21,22). Because troponins are not normally present in blood, their appearance in blood clearly indicates myocardial damage. Troponin levels increase within 3 hours after MI and remain elevated for up to 14 days (23), which is longer than the period of CK-MB elevation (24,25). Skeletal muscle involvement does not interfere with AMI diagnosis based on troponin levels. With serial sampling, blood concentrations of this marker provide 100% sensitivity for AMI.

Because levels of cTnI remain elevated so long, they provide an excellent tool for the retrospective diagnosis of AMI and are a superior prognostic indicator for acute coronary syndromes (ACSs) (26,27). Troponin measurements also offer more sensitivity for unstable angina than CK-MB levels (27–29), and increased cTnI and cTnT concentrations show equal predictive values for MI during hospital stays and within 30 days of discharge for patients with unstable angina (30). In a multicenter study of patients with unstable angina or non–Q-wave infarction, increasing cTnI levels were associated with increased risk of death (27).

Cardiac troponin I is absent from skeletal muscle, even during muscle development and regenerative muscle diseases such as Duchenne muscular dystrophy or polymyositis (in which CK-MB is elevated) (31). As a result, concentrations of cTnI may be used to differentiate between patients with increased CK-MB associated with MI and those with skeletal muscle injury (32,33). Elevated levels of cTnI are also seen in patients with congestive heart failure (CHF) (34). Malignant diseases may cause small increases in troponin as well (35). In addition, CTnI may be used as a marker for minor myocardial injury arising from radio-frequency catheter ablation (36) and as a predictor of mortality 30 days after presentation with ACSs (37). Other potential uses for troponin levels are shown in Table 38.2.

Like CK-MB, troponins are not "early" markers (Fig. 38.5) and they exist in various free and complex forms that challenge their measurement by existing methods. Commercially available assays for cTnI have biases that are compared in Fig. 38.6 (38). Although the alternative form, troponin T, has been advocated for the diagnosis of AMI (39), other investigators (40–42) have reported its lack of cardiac specificity. Recent studies indicate that cTnT is elevated in Duchenne muscular dystrophy, polydermatomyositis (43), rhabdomyolysis (44), and renal failure (29,45–49), thus raising questions of its cardiospecificity compared with cTnI (23). In addition, cTnT has a larger cytosolic pool (6% to 8%) than cTnI (3%), and cTnT has been demonstrated in the fetal skeletal muscle.

Although not necessarily 100% specific for assessing cardiac damage (50), the cardiospecificity of cTnI measurements has been shown in various studies (31,51–55). Its use in assessment of coronary reperfusion after thrombolytic therapy (56), risk stratification of patients with ACSs (27), and long-term prognosis of patients with ACSs without ST-segment elevation (57) has also been reported. One recent study (37) presented evidence that the concentration of cTnT was more accurate in pre-

TABLE 38.2. POTENTIAL USES FOR TROPONIN LEVELS AS MARKER

Reperfusion
Reinfarction
Infarct sizing
Congestive heart failure with concomitant ischemia
Risk stratification
Transplant rejection
Identification of cardiac toxicity from drugs

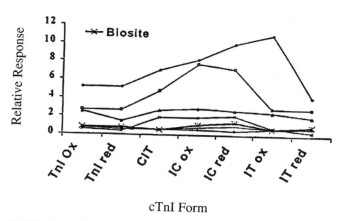

FIGURE 38.6. Biases in measurement of cTnI due to differing responses of immunoassay systems to cTnI forms.

dicting 30-day mortality after presentation with ACS. Table 38.2 lists potential uses for troponin levels as a marker.

In summary, troponin levels have many advantages over CK-MB measurements. First, CK-MB has reduced specificity and sensitivity in detecting microinfarcts, or "infarctlets," because the diagnostic cutoff values are usually set above the upper limit of the reference range, which may obscure the small increase in concentration caused by a microinfarct. Second, the signal-to-noise ratio in troponin measurements is much more favorable than in CK-MB assays. For troponins, as long as the analysis system detects a value above the reference level, the heart is surely involved because troponin is not normally present in blood. Finally, minimally elevated CK-MB could be confounded by coexisting illness.

Myoglobin

Myoglobin is present in high concentration in both cardiac and skeletal muscle. When MI occurs, the myoglobin level in serum rises within 1.5 hours (58), several hours earlier than that of CK, CK-MB, or troponin. The myoglobin concentration may also be elevated in trauma, burns, renal failure, and muscular disorders (58,59), as well as minor muscle injuries (60).

Although present methods provide different values in serum (61), myoglobin has received much recent attention because its nonspecificity can be overcome by making serial measurements. In addition, patients presenting to the ED no longer receive so many injections into muscle, which is known to increase the level of circulating myoglobin. Perhaps most important, immediately available myoglobin values can also be used in conjunction with measured concentrations of the more cardiac-specific troponins to more precisely delineate cardiac events as they occur.

The value of myoglobin as an early detector of MI has been shown in a variety of studies (54,55,62–69). This marker is especially useful when assayed serially (60,70,71) with established reference ranges and decision points and as part of a diagnostic algorithm (70). In the absence of skeletal muscle damage, a greater than 90% sensitivity for AMI was obtained when the myoglobin level either increased by more than 100 ng/mL or

doubled (and exceeded 100 ng/mL) within 2 hours of presentation (60). This is corroborated by the results of Tucker et al. (72), which showed that the incremental myoglobin level of 21 of 22 MI patients doubled within 1 to 2 hours over the baseline value, showing high specificity for MI even when the second myoglobin concentration fell within the reference range. In a study by Davis et al. (69), myoglobin levels were measured at presentation, 1 hour, and 2 hours. A myoglobin level exceeding 100 ng/mL or a change of 50% or more was considered a positive test for MI. With this protocol, the sensitivity of myoglobin was 93% for 14 patients with a diagnosis of AMI. In another study (73), the myoglobin level revealed AMI in 56% of patients at admission and 100% of patients after 2 hours.

Myoglobin levels also offer high negative predictive values for MI (70,73) and two myoglobin levels negative for AMI measured 2 hours apart rule out AMI in more than 90% of patients without complicating conditions (60). In another study (74), the negative predictive value of the myoglobin level for MI reached 89% in a group of patients, which was greater than that of cTnT and CK-MB from 3 to 6 hours after the onset of pain.

The myoglobin level reaches a peak value within 4 hours and returns to a normal level within 6 to 12 hours of MI. With these rapid kinetics, myoglobin provides a good noninvasive marker of coronary perfusion in patients undergoing thrombolysis or percutaneous transluminal coronary angioplasty. Myoglobin levels can also be used to monitor an extension or recurrence of myocardial necrosis.

The ACC/AHA recommends that no more than 30 minutes should elapse from admission to the ED to treatment for patients to derive maximum benefit. Although myoglobin levels provide an early diagnostic marker for MI in many patients, their value is reduced when assay results are not available for 3 to 4 hours. With bedside testing of cardiac markers, however, the turnaround time for measurements is significantly reduced, speeding up diagnosis and maximizing the benefit achieved with early reperfusion. In addition, bedside testing lowers the cost of staffing a laboratory for 24 hours and using analytical equipment on a stat basis (1).

A recent survey (75) shows that the cardiac marker of choice in the United States in the last quarter of 1998 (annualized) was troponin (56%), followed by CK-MB (34%) and myoglobin (10%), and that use of troponin had grown dramatically during the year whereas myoglobin use remained constant. The low usage of myoglobin measurements is surprising, given its potential value in the prompt and accurate triage of patients presenting with chest pain.

Cardiac Markers in Diagnostic Algorithms

In a 6-month prospective study (76) of 505 consecutive patients presenting with chest pain suggestive of MI, serial measurements of cTnI, CK-MB, and myoglobin were incorporated into a diagnostic algorithm to rule in and to rule out patients for MI. Cardiac markers were quantitatively assayed with a point-of-care (POC) system (Opus Plus Analyzer, Behring Diagnostics, Westwood, MA). At presentation (time 0), samples were drawn to obtain baseline values for all three markers. At 2 hours, a sample for myoglobin level was taken, and, at 6 and 12 hours, blood for cTnI was taken and CK-MB measurements were drawn. A positive test for MI could occur with either an elevated cTnI concentration (less than 1.5 ng/mL) at any time or a doubling of the myoglobin level at 2 hours over its baseline value. A subsequent elevation in CK-MB concentration provided further substantiation for MI.

Using our panel of three markers, 37 of 49 infarcts were uncovered at the time of admission (76% sensitivity; confidence intervals, 64% to 88%). The addition of the 2-hour myoglobin added six more infarctions, so that within 2 hours of presentation, 43 of 49 infarctions were detected (88% sensitivity; confidence intervals 77% to 100%). The algorithm required that samples be drawn at least through the 12-hour study period. By 6 hours of presentation, however, the algorithm detected all 49 infarctions (100% sensitivity). The negative predictive value of our combination of markers was 97% (68% to 90%) at 0 hours and 99% (98% to 100%) at 2 hours.

At the time of presentation, elevations of cTnI were seen in 37 of 49 patients subsequently proved by other criteria to have MIs (76% sensitivity confidence intervals, 64% to 88%). This compares to only 24 patients whose infarction was detected by an elevated CK-MB (49% sensitivity; confidence intervals, 36% to 62%; $p < 0.001$). Of the 13 patients ruled in by cTnI but not CK-MB at 0 hours, 10 were due to delayed patient presentation. The other three patients were ruled in by CK-MB at a later time point. The specificity and negative predictive values for cTnI and CK-MB combined exceeded 90% at 0 and 6 hours. The negative predictive value cTnI at 6 hours was 100%.

There were 27 patients who had elevated cTnI levels but normal CK-MB. Ten were late presentations of MI. The other 17 patients were classified as "minor myocardial damage," and were characterized by prolonged chest pain, often at rest; persistent ST changes; and high-grade eccentric stenoses at coronary angiography. The 6-month follow-up revealed ten deaths, many of which were directly or indirectly cardiac related, including three coronary artery–bypass graft procedures, and one subsequent MI.

In patients presenting with less than 6 hours of chest pain, and in whom a 0-hour cTnI or CK-MB was negative, a myoglobin was drawn again 2 hours after the initial presentation. A doubling of myoglobin at 2 hours was seen in six of the remaining 12 infarcts (50% sensitivity; confidence intervals, 22% to 78%). Most of these "false negatives" had elevated 2-hour myoglobin that had not quite doubled from the original value, which were in themselves often greater than normal. These patients had a slightly longer time until presentation (5 to 6 hours versus 2 to 5 hours). All patients who subsequently ruled in for MI and who presented within 6 hours of chest pain and a normal baseline myoglobin had subsequent doubling at 2 hours. The specificity of the 2-hour myoglobin was 100%, with a negative predictive value of 99%.

Cost savings were estimated on the basis of a conservative 3-day hospital stay for each patient—1 day each in MICU, telemetry, and a ward. Resident ED physicians completed surveys designed to show what steps would have been taken had only CK-MB levels been available for evaluation of each patient. The survey results showed that 50% of the patients admitted to telemetry, the ward, or discharged would have been admitted to

TABLE 38.3. ESTIMATED COST SAVINGS WITH PANEL TESTING

Setting	Bed Cost/Day ($)	Savings in Bed Utilization (6 Mo.) ($)
MICU	2,160	—
Telemetry	1,400	66,440
Ward	650	61,020
Home	—	391,530

Total savings: $518,990
MICU, myocardial intensive care unit.

the MICU had the full panel of cardiac markers not been available. The estimated cost savings associated with the 50% reduction in admissions to MICU are shown in Table 38.3.

Cardiac Markers in an Accelerated Diagnostic Algorithm

In a more aggressive effort to reduce the time for diagnosis and treatment of MI, an accelerated diagnostic algorithm (Fig. 38.7) that requires measurements of marker concentrations more frequently than the earlier algorithm was developed (77). As in the first algorithm, the first step is to establish baseline (time 0) values for each of the three markers. If the cTnI level exceeds the decision point for myocardial damage, the physician makes a diagnosis of ACS, regardless of the CK-MB or myoglobin results. (Patients in this group have probably had a heart attack or sustained minor myocardial damage, and most will be admitted to the MICU.) If less than 6 hours have elapsed since the onset of chest pain and the cTnI level falls within the reference range, blood samples are redrawn at 30, 60, and 90 minutes for immediate assay. If the myoglobin concentration increases over its baseline value by 150% during the 90-minute period, the physician makes a diagnosis of ACS. If myoglobin is not increasing during this time, the physician may continue to observe trends in marker levels by taking blood samples at 3 and 6 hours. If the level of CK-MB or cTnI is positive for myocardial injury, the physician admits the patient to MICU. If CK-MB or cTnI results are negative for MI, the probability of MI is low. If suspicion is low for ischemia after 90 minutes, the physician may either discharge the patient or send him or her to a non-MICU setting.

Using the critical pathway in this study, all patients who "ruled in" with an AMI were identified within a 90-minute time period. The negative predictive value of early repetitive cardiac marker testing in this setting was 100% using a combination of three markers. Although not all patients were discharged at 90 minutes, the results of this study indicate that rapid triage of all patients, including high- and low-risk patients, is possible within 90 minutes of presentation. This critical pathway decreased cardiac care unit (CCU) admissions by 40%, while still triaging the sickest patients to the CCU. This decrease, along with its likely associated cost savings regarding ICU costs, may even be underestimated due to the fact that at several time points during our study a shortage of double-occupancy unit (DOU) beds may have falsely elevated the CCU admission rate. It is nearly impossible to account for this number, although we

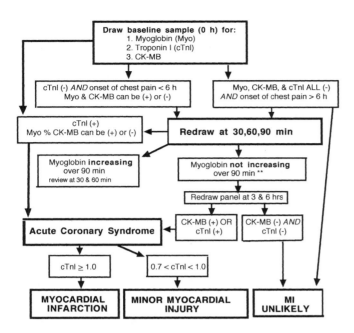

FIGURE 38.7. Accelerated diagnostic algorithm of the San Diego Veterans Affairs Hospital.

estimate that approximately 10% of the CCU patients would have been sent to the DOU, had space been available. In nearly 90% of cases where patients were ultimately discharged home, the decision for discharge was made by evaluating physicians within 90 minutes of presentation. In the 30-day follow-up period, only one patient who was discharged home returned to the ED with an acute non–Q-wave MI on day 12. Twelve others were admitted for "unstable angina." Admission is the standard practice at this veterans hospital whenever a patient returns with chest pain within 1 month of an ED visit.

While multiple cardiac markers can be of tremendous value in the early and accurate diagnosis of MIs, there is also dismay about the cost of performing multiple biochemical tests as part of the routine workup for an MI. Clinicians have aimed efforts at finding alternative cost-effective strategies to exclude MIs aimed at low-risk patients (78–83). In our study, we hypothesized that using a cardiac panel that simultaneously tests for all three markers using a small POC instrument with rapid turnaround time facilitates the diagnose of acute MI. Our results are in agreement with the recent CHECKMATE study (84), which prospectively compared bedside quantitative marker testing versus local laboratory results in 1,005 patients in six chest pain units. They found that rapid analysis of the same markers used in this study identifies positive patients earlier and provides better risk stratification for mortality than a local–laboratory-based, single-marker approach. Other studies using multiple markers support this idea (85–87) and underlie the recommendations of the National Academy of Clinical Biochemistry (88–90).

The ability to differentiate among true positives, false positives, and sporadically elevated cardiac troponin levels has grown in importance as cardiac troponins assume an increasingly dominant role in the diagnosis of coronary syndromes. In a population sample of 1,000 patients who presented consecutively to a

large urban hospital emergency room, 50 of 112 patients who had elevated troponin levels during evaluation for myocardial injury were subsequently found to have had an isolated, spurious elevation of cardiac troponin (what we have termed "troponinosis"), and not a diagnosed MI (91). Logistic regression analysis shows that by hierarchically analyzing electrocardiographic changes with concurrent creatine kinase MB and myoglobin levels at the time of the troponin elevation, one may predict with 91% accuracy whether the troponin elevation is actually indicative of a MI in a patient. "Troponinosis" may be a common occurrence, and if not detected, may result in an increased number of falsely diagnosed MIs. Frequent early sampling with multiple markers was the best way to detect "troponinosis."

Case Study 1

A 61-year-old diabetic man with a history of hypertension presented to the San Diego Veterans Affairs Healthcare System with discomfort in breathing and progressive shortness of breath. The patient denied having chest pain. The ECG revealed evidence of ST-segment elevation. The heart rate was 121 beats per minute, respiratory rate was 22 per minute, and blood pressure was 127/79.

The patient was entered into the accelerated diagnostic algorithm. The serial marker levels (Table 38.4) were determined using the Triage Cardiac Panel (Biosite Diagnostics, San Diego, CA). The initially elevated CK-MB and cTnI levels corroborated the ECG finding that an AMI had occurred, and the marker levels placed the time at more than 6 hours before presentation. Thirty minutes later, however, myoglobin had nearly doubled, strongly suggesting that a new AMI had occurred.

Emergency cardiac catheterization showed that the patient had high-grade lesions of the left anterior descending and right coronary arteries with a fresh clot in the proximal right coronary artery. Emergency angioplasty was performed without complications. The patient was discharged home 5 days later and was doing well 1 month later. In this case, serial testing of all three cardiac markers and the immediate availability of results allowed for rapid detection of the new AMI. The protocol also prevented the inappropriate administration of thrombolytic agents and paved the way for a positive clinical outcome. With traditional testing requiring transport of blood to a central laboratory for testing, the new infarction would not have been detected for hours, thus delaying treatment.

TABLE 38.4. CARDIAC MARKER DATA FOR CASE STUDY

Time	Concentration (ngmL)		
	CK-MB	cTnI	Myoglobin
11:30 p.m.	31	11	150
12:00 a.m.	32	11	257
12:30 a.m.	50	8	>510
3:30 a.m.	>125	13	>510

CK-MB, creatine kinase MB; cTnI, cardiac troponin I.

Case Study 2

A 66-year-old man (a physician) with no history of coronary artery disease presented with occasional burning pain on the right side of his chest. The pain radiated to his right arm and persisted for 2 weeks. Although the patient had found relief by taking an antacid, he came to the ED after 12 hours of continuous pain accompanied by shortness of breath and nausea. The ECG showed ST-segment elevations and Q waves in leads V_2 through V_4.

Because the MI-like symptoms had continued for 12 hours (thus precluding thrombolytic agent administration), the patient was treated with heparin and a nitroglycerin drip. The pain was not affected.

It was decided to apply the accelerated diagnostic algorithm to the treatment of this patient. Analysis of blood samples taken on admission showed normal cTnI and myoglobin levels (less than 1.0 ng/mL and 24 ng/mL, respectively). A sample taken 2 hours later, however, showed a myoglobin concentration greater than 500 ng/mL, indicating that a new infarction had occurred. The patient underwent coronary catheterization that revealed three-vessel disease. The patient was given tissue-type plasminogen activator and the chest pain subsided in 30 minutes. He underwent a triple bypass procedure without complications, was discharged 7 days later with a normal ejection fraction, and was doing well at 30-day follow-up. Had the panel of marker levels not been immediately available, the patient would not have received the aggressive therapy.

Determining Diagnosis

The following guidelines are offered to physicians applying the accelerated diagnostic algorithm.

1. Measure marker levels until the cTnI concentration is positive for MI. If this occurs at 0, 30, 60, or 90 minutes, or 3 or 6 hours, admit the patient to the MICU.
2. Use clinical judgment—MI-negative marker levels alone do not necessarily mean that the patient should not be admitted to the MICU.
3. Suspect AMI if myoglobin concentration increases with time.
4. If myoglobin levels have not increased over 90 minutes and chest pain began less than 6 hours ago, retest myoglobin at 3 and 6 hours if symptoms raise suspicion. If you do not suspect coronary artery disease, consider discharging the patient or admitting him or her to a nonmonitored bed.
5. Consider placing low-risk patients in a ward or discharging home.
6. Admit patients to the MICU if they have one or more of the following: (a) chest pain with ST elevations, (b) chest pain with ST depressions, (c) chest pain not relieved by standard measures, (d) a cTnI concentration positive for MI at any time, (e) a CK-MB level positive for MI at 3 or 6 hours, and (f) a myoglobin level increasing over a 90-minute period.
7. While a patient is in the MICU with an ACS, the three-marker panel must be performed every 6 hours until the enzyme levels taper off.

Point-of-Care Method for Measuring Cardiac Markers

The ACC/AHA has issued the following statement: "Some markers may be more efficient in detecting MI in patients presenting early (e.g., myoglobin), while others are useful for detecting patients who present late (e.g., cardiac-specific troponin T and troponin I)" (9). In addition, the use of myoglobin, troponin I, and CK-MB has been recommended for the diagnosis of AMI (66). It has also been stated that biochemical markers must be available, if required, in less than 20 minutes (92).

To meet these requirements, whole-blood analyzers should (a) be easy to operate, (b) generate reliable results rapidly, and (c) have minimal calibration drift. They should also have streamlined requirements for reagents, maintenance, biohazard disposal, and quality control. Results should compare with those of well-established instruments and the system should interface with a laboratory information system (14).

The Triage Cardiac Panel used in the San Diego Veterans Affairs Hospital algorithm studies meets these requirements. The operator simply adds several drops of whole blood to the Triage Cardiac Panel and inserts it into the battery-powered Triage meter. The self-processing device provides quantitative measurements of troponin I, myoglobin, and CK-MB within 15 minutes. The meter monitors the reaction and displays the concentrations of all three markers on a liquid crystal display screen. Results can be printed and stored in meter memory for downloading to a laboratory information system. A user ID, lock-out functions (to guard against unauthorized use), and warning messages ensure the reliability of the results.

The system measures cardiac markers by fluorescence immunoassay, in which stable fluorescent dyes absorb and emit radiation at wavelengths (670 and 760 nm, respectively) not subject to interference from the whole-blood matrix (93,94). The system can be used in either a POC setting or central laboratory.

When whole blood is added to the sample port, a built-in filter separates blood cells from plasma and capillary action facilitates contact of plasma with dried immunoassay reagents in the reaction chamber. Microcapillaries regulate the flow of fluid throughout the device and a microcapillary time-gate feature controls incubation time. The predetermined amount of plasma reacts with premeasured fluorescence antibody that conjugates to form a reaction mixture. When the incubation is completed, the reaction mixture flows through microcapillaries to the detection lanes that contain three discrete, immobilized antibody zones in which binding of fluorescent reagents occurs and is detected by the meter. The intensity of the resulting fluorescence is directly proportional to the concentration of analyte.

Each device is equipped with quality control zones (low and high) to check that enough sample was applied, reagents are active, and the meter is functioning correctly. The low control is set to generate a fluorescence signal like that at the analyte cut-off point and the high control is set to approximately 75% of the maximum signal of the dose-response curve. The test must be repeated if the results of either control do not fall within predetermined limits (87). A software algorithm uses numerous parameters to accept or reject each test to meet all regulatory requirements.

TABLE 38.5. DETECTION LIMITS, IMPRECISION, AND DECISION POINTS OF BIOSITE TRIAGE SYSTEM

Cardiac Marker	Detection Limit (ng/mL)	Imprecision[a] (%)	Decision Level[b] (ng/mL)
Myoglobin	2.7	9.9	107
CK-MB	0.75	12	4.3
Troponin I	0.19	12	0.4

[a]Upper reference limit/decision point.
[b]Receiver-operated characteristic analysis.
CK-MB, creatine kinase MB.
From Gibler WB, Runyon JP, Levy RC, et al. A rapid diagnostic and treatment center for patients with chest pain in the emergency department. *Ann Emerg Med* 1995;25:1–8, with permission.

The Triage Cardiac System has been evaluated in a multicenter study using 192 patients admitted to the ED for symptoms of AMI (87). The measurements of the Triage Cardiac Panel compare well with those of existing immunoassays (87,95). Detection limits, imprecision, and cutoff values are shown in Table 38.5. According to the authors of the multicenter study, "The Triage Panel offers clinicians a whole-blood, POC analysis of multiple cardiac markers that provides excellent clinical sensitivity and specificity for the detection of acute MI."

CONCLUSIONS

These studies show conclusively that use of the San Diego Veterans Affairs Healthcare System's accelerated algorithm results in rapid and accurate detection of AMI. Critical to application of the algorithm is the POC availability of instrumentation for rapid, quantitative, and accurate measurements of all three cardiac markers. The algorithm allowed for effective screening, less hospitalization, and substantial yearly cost savings.

B-TYPE NATRIURETIC PEPTIDE LEVELS: DIAGNOSTIC AND THERAPEUTIC POTENTIAL

Finding a simple blood test that would aid in the diagnosis and management of patients with CHF would clearly have a favorable impact on the staggering costs associated with the disease. Imagine the difficulty of diagnosing and then managing a life-threatening infection without the use of a white-blood-cell count—or the problems associated with the diagnosis and treatment of prostate cancer without the benefit of a PSA level. Yet, there is no currently accepted blood test to aid in the diagnosis and management of patients with CHF.

B-Type Natriuretic Peptide

B-type natriuretic peptide (BNP) is a 32-aa polypeptide containing a 17-aa ring structure common to all natriuretic peptides (96). Unlike A-type natriuretic peptide (ANP), whose major storage sites include the atria and ventricles, the major source of plasma BNP is cardiac ventricles, suggesting that BNP may be a more sensitive and specific indicator of ventricular disorders

than other natriuretic peptides (97). BNP release appears to be directly proportional to ventricular volume expansion and pressure overload (98). BNP is an independent predictor of high left-ventricular, end-diastolic pressure, and is more useful than ANP or norepinephrine for assessing the mortality in patients with chronic CHF (99).

B-Type Natriuretic Peptide Levels in Normals and Inpatients with Congestive Heart Failure

BNP levels rise with age. Mean BNP levels are 26.2±1.8 pg/ml in the 55 to 64 age cohort; 31.0±2.4 pg/ml, 65 to 74; and 63.7±6 pg/ml, 75 and older (*p*<0.001) (data on file with the Food and Drug Administration, Biosite Diagnostics). Additionally, women without CHF tend to have somewhat higher BNP values than men of the same age group, with women 75 years and older having a mean BNP level of 76.5±3.5 pg/ml. Although the reason is unknown, it is possible that aging women have stiffer left ventricles than age-matched men.

B-Type Natriuretic Peptide and New York Heart Association Classification

While the New York Heart Association (NYHA) classification correlates with symptoms as well as mortality in patients with heart failure, the fact that such a subjective classification is still the major means we use to describe the clinical condition of patients with heart failure underlies the need for more objective surrogates. Because BNP levels correlate to elevated end-diastolic pressure, and since end-diastolic pressure correlates closely to the chief symptom of CHF, dyspnea, it is not surprising that BNP correlates closely to NYHA classification (Fig. 38.8).

What Should the Cutoff for B-Type Natriuretic Peptide Be to Diagnose Congestive Heart Failure?

Receiver-operated characteristic (ROC) curves (data on file, Biosite Diagnostics) suggest that a BNP cutoff point of 100 pg/ml allows for the increased levels seen with advancing age

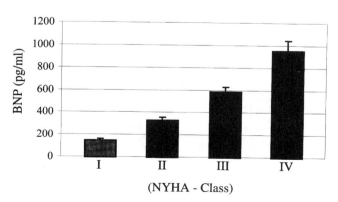

FIGURE 38.8. B-type natriuretic peptide levels in patients with congestive heart failure.

and provides an excellent ability to discriminate CHF subjects from non-CHF subjects. This level shows sensitivity from 82.4% for CHF in general up to over 99% for NYHA class IV. The BNP test specificity exceeds 95% when comparing non-CHF to all CHF patients, and 93% in all subsets studied. A level of 100 pg/ml is high enough to avoid "BNP disease," that is, a group of patients who are mistakenly said to have heart failure because of falsely elevated BNP levels. In practice, though, it is likely that both a high and a low cutoff will be used—a high one (likely around 100 pg/ml) for its specificity and positive predictive value, and a low one (40 to 60 pg/ml) for its high sensitivity and negative predictive value.

Point-of-Care Testing of B-Type Natriuretic Peptide in the Emergency Department Setting

POCT allows diagnostic assays to be performed in locations such as the ED or ICU where treatment decisions are made and care is delivered based on results of the assays. We completed a pilot study using a recently approved, rapid BNP immunoassay (Triage Cardiac, Biosite Diagnostics, San Diego, CA) to assess 250 patients presenting to the San Diego Veterans Affairs Healthcare System urgent care area with the chief complaint of dyspnea (100).

Patients diagnosed with CHF (N=97) had a mean BNP concentration of 1076±138 pg/ml while the non-CHF group (N=139) had a mean BNP concentration of 38±4 pg/ml (Fig. 38.9). The sicker the patient was (severity and admission to the hospital), the higher the BNP level. Of crucial importance was that patients with the final diagnosis of pulmonary disease had lower BNP values (86±39 pg/ml) than those with a final diagnosis of CHF (1076±138 pg/ml, *p*<0.001).

BNP at a cutoff point of 80 pg/ml was found to be highly sensitive (98%) and specific (92%) for the diagnosis of CHF. The negative predictive value of BNP values under 80 pg/ml was 98% for the diagnosis of CHF. Multivariate analysis revealed that after all useful tools for making the diagnosis were taken into account by the ED physician (history, symptoms, signs, radiological studies, and lab findings), BNP levels continued to provide meaning-ful diagnostic information not available from other clinical variables. Thus, the measurement of the BNP concentration in blood appears to be a sensitive and specific test for identification of patients with CHF in acute care settings. At the very minimum, it is likely to be a potent, cost-effective addition to the diagnostic armamentarium of acute care physicians.

B-Type Natriuretic Peptide as a Screen of Left Ventricular Dysfunction

While echocardiography, the most commonly utilized method to diagnose left ventricular (LV) dysfunction, is one of the fastest growing procedures in cardiology, the expense of echocardiography and its limited access in community settings where it may be needed most may not make it the best screening test for patients, especially in those with low probability of left ventricular dysfunction.

We have recently characterized patients who had both echocardiography and BNP levels (101). Among the patients with no documented history of CHF and no past determination of LV function, 51% had abnormal echocardiographic findings. In this group BNP levels were significantly higher (328±29 pg/ml) than the 49% of patients with no history of CHF and a normal echocardiogram (30±3 pg/ml, *p*<0.001). In patients with a known history of CHF, with previously documented LV dysfunction, all had abnormal findings (*n*=102), with elevated BNP levels (545±45 pg/ml). BNP levels were elevated in both systolic and diastolic dysfunction, with the highest values being reported in patients with systolic dysfunction plus a decreased mitral valve deceleration time.

Among patients with diastolic dysfunction, those with a restrictive filling pattern had higher BNP levels (428 pg/ml) than patients with impaired relaxation (230 pg/ml). The area under the ROC curve for BNP to detect diastolic dysfunction by echocardiography in patients with CHF and normal systolic function was 0.958. A BNP value of 71 pg/ml was 96% accurate in the prediction of diastolic dysfunction in this setting. BNP levels below 57 pg/ml gave a negative predictive value of 100% for the detection of clinically significant diastolic dysfunction. Additionally, multivariate analysis showed that in patients with clinical CHF and normal LV function, BNP was the strongest predictor of diastolic abnormalities seen on echocardiography.

Thus, BNP may be an excellent screening tool for left ventricular dysfunction. Low BNP levels may preclude the need for echocardiography in some patients, especially those who, even though at high risk, have no symptoms of heart failure. Elevated BNP levels, on the other hand, clearly indicate the presence of LV dysfunction, whether the patient has symptoms or not, warranting further cardiac workup. It is clear that BNP should not replace imaging techniques in the diagnosis of CHF because these methods provide complementary information.

Can B-Type Natriuretic Peptide Serve as a Surrogate Endpoint for the Treatment of Heart Failure?

Affecting 2% of the population, CHF is the fourth leading cause of adult hospitalizations in the United States and the most fre-

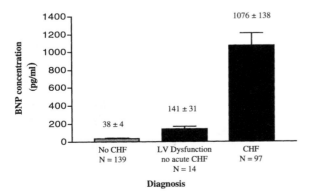

FIGURE 38.9. B-type natriuretic peptide levels in patients whose dyspnea was due to congestive heart failure (CHF), non-CHF causes, or baseline left-ventricular dysfunction but non-CHF causes.

quent cause of hospitalization in patients over the age of 65 (102). While patients who are admitted to the hospital with decompensated heart failure often have improvement in symptoms with the various treatment modalities available, there has been no good way to evaluate the long-term effects of the short-term treatment. Indeed, in-hospital mortality and readmission rate for CHF patients is extremely high. The conventional tests for cardiac function take time and often do not correlate well with symptomatic changes in the patient's conditions. Therefore, most patients are discharged when they "feel better," which might then preclude further titration of medical therapy.

B-Type Natriuretic Peptide in Patients Admitted for Decompensated Congestive Heart Failure

In a pilot study, we followed the course of 72 patients admitted with decompensated NYHA class III to IV CHF, measuring BNP levels on a daily basis (103). We then determined association between initial BNP measurement and the predischarge or premoribund BNP measurement and subsequent adverse outcomes (defined as death and 30-day readmission).

Of the 72 patients admitted with decompensated CHF, 22 endpoints occurred (death, $n=13$; readmission, $n=9$). In these 22 patients, BNP levels increased during hospitalization (mean increase, 233 pg/ml, $p<0.001$; Fig. 38.10). In patients without endpoints, BNP decreased during treatment (mean decrease 215 pg/ml). Patients who had good outcomes were characterized by decreases in both their NYHA class and BNP levels during hospitalization, while those patients who were readmitted within 30 days of discharge had only minimal decreases in their BNP levels during hospitalization, despite improvement in NYHA classification. Finally, subjects who died in the hospital had rising BNP levels and little change in symptoms.

While both admission BNP levels and the change in BNP levels over the period of hospitalization were significant predictors of outcomes, the last measured BNP level was the single variable most strongly associated with patients experiencing one of the prespecified endpoints. The mean BNP concentration was significantly greater in patients experiencing endpoints

(1,801±273 pg/ml versus 690±103 pg/ml) in patients with successful treatment of CHF ($p<0.001$). Patients whose discharge BNP level fell below 430 pg/ml with treatment had a reasonable likelihood of leaving the hospital in good condition and not being readmitted within the following 30 days.

B-Type Natriuretic Peptide Correlations with Falling Wedge Pressures in Patients Being Treated for Congestive Heart Failure

In a pilot study, hemodynamic measurements (pulmonary capillary wedge pressure, cardiac output, right atrial pressure, and systemic vascular resistance) along with BNP levels were recorded every 2 to 4 hours for the first 24 hours and every 4 hours for the next 24 to 48 hours in patients admitted for decompensated CHF (104). Patients were treated at the discretion of the ICU physicians in standard fashion with combinations of intravenous diuretics, vasodilators, and inotropic drug agents. The initial BNP level in the 15 responders (patients with a decrease in wedge pressure to less than 20 mm Hg over the first 24 hours) was 1472±156 pg/ml. Twenty-four hours after treatment, BNP levels had dropped 55% to 670±109 pg/ml. We found a significant correlation between percent change in wedge pressure from baseline per hour and the percent change of BNP from baseline per hour ($r=0.73$, $p<0.05$) with an average fall of BNP of 33±5 pg/ml per hour. The correlation between BNP levels and other indices of cardiac function—cardiac output (thermodilution), mixed venous oxygen saturation, and systemic vascular resistance—was not significant. In the five nonresponders there was little change in wedge pressure and only an 8% drop in BNP levels.

Tailored Treatment of Heart Failure—Is There a Role for B-Type Natriuretic Peptide in the Clinic?

The correlation between the drop in BNP level and the patient's improvement in symptoms (and subsequent outcome) during hospitalization suggests that BNP-guided treatment might make "tailored therapy" more effective in an outpatient setting such as a primary care or cardiology clinic. Recently, Troughton et al. (105) randomized 69 patients to N-BNP guided treatment versus symptom-guided therapy. Patients receiving N-BNP–guided therapy had lower N-BNP levels along with reduced incidence of cardiovascular death, readmission, and new episodes of decompensated CHF.

Thus, while studies have been limited, it appears that BNP levels may be helpful in guiding therapy in the outpatient setting. Further research is needed in this area.

CONCLUSIONS

Finding a simple blood test that would aid in the diagnosis and management of patients with CHF would clearly have a favorable impact on the staggering costs associated with the disease. BNP, which is synthesized in the cardiac ventricles and correlates with LV pressure, amount of dyspnea, and the state of neuro-

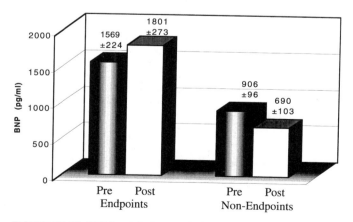

FIGURE 38.10. BNP levels before and after treatment for decompensated congestive heart failure based on whether the patients were a subsequent endpoint (death or readmission within 30 days).

hormonal modulation, makes this peptide the first potential "white count" for heart failure. The fact that a POC rapid assay for BNP has recently been approved by the Food and Drug Administration gives the clinician an opportunity to explore its potential usefulness. Our data and data from others suggest that serial POCT of BNP will be of immense help in patients presenting to urgent care clinics with dyspnea. Additionally, BNP might serve as a screen for patients referred for echocardiography. A low BNP level makes echocardiographic indices of LV dysfunction (both systolic and diastolic) highly unlikely. BNP might also be an effective way to improve the in-hospital management of patients admitted with decompensated CHF. In some instances, BNP levels may obviate the need for invasive hemodynamic monitoring, and in cases where such monitoring is used, may help tailor treatment of the decompensated patient. And finally, the role of BNP in the outpatient cardiac or primary care clinic may be one of critical importance in titration of therapies as well as in assessing the state of neurohormonal compensation of the patient. BNP and cardiac injury marker (see conclusions on page 561) testing represent important POC opportunities to improve patient outcomes.

REFERENCES

1. Dadkhah S, Fisch C, Zonia C, et al. Accelerated coronary reperfusion through the use of rapid bedside cardiac markers—case reports. *Angiology* 1999;50:55–62.
2. Lee TH, Rouan GW, Weisberg MC, et al. Clinical characteristics and natural history of patients with acute myocardial infarction sent home from the emergency room. *Am J Cardiol* 1987;60:219–224.
3. McCarthy BD, Beshansky JR, D'Agostino RB, et al. Missed diagnoses of acute myocardial infarction in the emergency department: results from a multicenter study. *Ann Emerg Med* 1993;22:579–582.
4. Puleo PR, Meyer D, Wathen C, et al. Use of a rapid assay of subforms of creatine kinase MB to diagnose or rule out acute myocardial infarction. *N Engl J Med* 1994;331:561–566.
5. Rusnak RA, Stair TO, Hansen K, et al. Litigation against the emergency physician: common features in cases of missed myocardial infarction. *Ann Emerg Med* 1989;18:1029–1034.
6. McCallion WA, Templeton PA, McKinney LA, et al. Missed myocardial ischaemia in the accident and emergency department: a need for audit? *Arch Emerg Med* 1991;8:102–107.
7. Gibler WB, Runyon JP, Levy RC, et al. A rapid diagnostic and treatment center for patients with chest pain in the emergency department. *Ann Emerg Med* 1995;25:1–8.
8. HCIA, Inc., Baltimore, MD.
9. Ryan TJ, Anderson JL, Antman EM, et al. ACC/AHA guidelines for the management of patients with acute myocardial infarction. A report of the American College of Cardiology/American Heart Association Task Force on Practice Guidelines (Committee on Management of Acute Myocardial Infarction). *J Am Coll Cardiol* 1996;28:1328–1428.
10. Young GP, Owen TP. *Am J Emerg Med* 1993;11: – .
11. National Heart Attack Program Coordinating Committee. *Emergency department: rapid identification and treatment of patients with acute myocardial infarction.* Washington, DC: National Heart, Lung and Blood Institute, National Institutes of Health, September 1993.
12. Cardiology roundtable, 1994.
13. NFO Migliara/Kaplan. CRS research, cardiology survey, American College of Cardiology, April 1997.
14. Kost GJ. New whole blood analyzers and their impact on cardiac and critical care. *Crit Rev Clin Lab Sci* 1993;30:153–202.
15. Kost GJ. Guidelines for point-of-care testing: improving patient outcomes. *Am J Clin Pathol* 1995;104[Suppl 1]:S111–S127.
16. Mair J, Schmidt J, Lechleitner P, et al. Rapid accurate diagnosis of acute myocardial infarction in patients with nontraumatic chest pain within 1 h of admission. *Coron Artery Dis* 1995;6:539–545.
17. Collinson PO, Ramhamadamy EM, Stubbs PJ et al. Rapid enzyme diagnosis of patients with acute chest pain reduces patient stay in the coronary care unit. *Ann Clin Biochem* 1993;30:17–22.
18. Wu AH, Clive JM. Impact of CK-MB testing policies on hospital length of stay and laboratory costs for patients with myocardial infarction or chest pain [Comments]. *Clin Chem* 1997;43:326–332.
19. Kost GJ. Planning and implementing point-of-care testing systems. In: Tobin MJ, ed. *Principles and practice of intensive care monitoring.* New York: McGraw-Hill, 1998:1297–1328.
20. Maisel A. Cardiac markers in the assessment of patients with acute coronary syndromes. *Top Emerg Med* 1998;20:14–22.
21. Adams III JE, Schechtman K, Landt V, et al. Comparable detection of acute myocardial infarction by creatine kinase MB isoenzyme and cardiac troponin I. *Clin Chem* 1994;40:1291–1295.
22. Katus HA, Remppis A, Scheffold T, et al. Intracellular compartmentalization of cardiac troponin T and its release of kinetics in patients with reperfused and nonreperfused myocardial infarction. *Am J Cardiol* 1991;67:1360–1367.
23. Jaffe A. Troponin, where do we go from here? Recent advances in myocardial markers of injury. *Clin Lab Med* 1997;17:737–752.
24. Keffer JH. The cardiac profile and proposed practice guideline for acute ischemic heart disease. *Am J Clin Pathol* 1997;107:398–409.
25. Mercer DW. Role of cardiac markers in evaluation of suspected myocardial infarction. *Postgrad Med* 1997;102:113–122.
26. Ohman EM, Armstrong PW, Christenson RH, et al. for GUSTO IIa Investigators. Cardiac troponin T levels for risk stratification in acute myocardial ischemia. *N Engl J Med* 1996;335:1333–1341.
27. Antman EM, Tanasijevic MJ, Thompson B, et al. Cardiac-specific troponin I levels to predict the risk of mortality in patients with acute coronary syndromes. *N Engl J Med* 1996;335:1342–1349.
28. Galvani M, Ottani F, Ferrini D, et al. Prognostic influence of elevated values of cardiac troponin I in patients with unstable angina. *Circulation* 1997;95:2053–2059.
29. Lindahl B, Venge P, Wallentin L. Relation between troponin T and the risk of subsequent cardiac events in unstable coronary artery disease. *Circulation* 1996;93:1651–1657.
30. Olatidoye AG, Feng Y, Wu A. Do troponin T and I have equal prognostic significance in the same population of unstable angina patients? *Circulation* 1997;96[Suppl]:1-333.
31. Bodor GS, Porterfield D, Voss EM, et al. Cardiac troponin-I is not expressed in fetal and healthy or diseased adult human skeletal muscle tissue. *Clin Chem* 1995;41:1710–1715.
32. Adams JE, Bodor GS, Dávila-Román VG, et al. Cardiac troponin I: a marker with high specificity for cardiac injury. *Circulation* 1993;88:101–106.
33. Adams III JE, Dávila-Román VG, Bessey PQ, et al. Improved detection of cardiac contusion with cardiac troponin I. *Am Heart J* 1996;131:308–312.
34. Missov E, Calzolari C, Pau B. Circulating cardiac troponin I in severe congestive heart failure. *Circulation* 1997;96:2953–2958.
35. Missov E, Pau B, Calzolari C. Increased circulating levels of troponin I in anthracycline-treated patients. *Circulation* 1996;94:4283(abst).
36. del Rey JM, Madrid AH, Valiño JM, et al. Cardiac troponin I and minor cardiac damage: biochemical markers in a clinical model of myocardial lesions. *Clin Chem* 1998;44:2270–2276.
37. Christenson RH, Duh SH, Newby K, et al. Cardiac troponin T and cardiac troponin I: relative values in short-term risk stratification of patients with acute coronary syndromes. *Clin Chem* 1998;44:494–501.
38. Wu AH, Feng YJ, Moore R, et al. Characterization of cardiac troponin subunit release into serum after acute myocardial infarction and comparison of assays for troponin T and I. American Association for Clinical Chemistry Subcommittee on cTnI Standardization. *Clin Chem* 1998;44:1198–1208.
39. McErlean ES, Deluca SA, van Lente F, et al. A prospective study of troponin T as an alternative to CK-MB in suspected coronary syndromes. *Circulation* 1997;96[Suppl]:1-332(abst).
40. Apple FS, Wu AH, Valdes Jr R. Serum cardiac troponin T concentra-

tions in hospitalized patients without acute myocardial infarction. *Scand J Clin Lab Invest* 1996;56:63–68.

41. Baum H, Obst M, Huber U, et al. Cardiac troponin T in patients with high creatinine concentration but normal creatine kinase activity in serum. *Clin Chem* 1996;42:474–475.

42. Fitzgerald RL, Frankel WL, Herold DA. Comparison of troponin-T with other cardiac markers in a VA hospital. *Am J Clin Pathol* 1996; 106:396–401.

43. Bodor GS, Porterfield D, Voss E, et al. Immunohistochemistry of damaged skeletal muscle: cardiac troponin T composition in normal and regenerated human skeletal muscle. *Clin Chem* 1997;43:476–484.

44. Löfberg M, Tähtelä R, Härkönen M, et al. Cardiac troponins in severe rhabdomyolysis. *Clin Chem* 1996;42:1120–1121.

45. Hafner G, Thome-Kromer B, Schaube J, et al. Cardiac troponins in serum in chronic renal failure [Letter]. *Clin Chem* 1994;40:1790–1791.

46. Bhayana V, Gougoulias T, Cohoe S, et al. Discordance between results for serum troponin T and troponin I in renal disease. *Clin Chem* 1995;41:312–317.

47. Frankel WL, Herold DA, Ziegler TW, et al. Cardiac troponin T is elevated in asymptomatic patients with chronic renal failure. *Am J Clin Pathol* 1996;106:118–123.

48. Wu AH, Feng YJ, Roper L, et al. Cardiac troponins T and I before and after renal transplantation [Letter]. *Clin Chem* 1997;43:411–412.

49. Collinson PO. To T or not to T, that is the question [Editorial]. *Clin Chem* 1997;43:421–423.

50. Sacks DB, Wright SA, Sawyer DB, et al. Increased concentrations of cardiac troponin I in patients without myocardial injury. *Clin Chem* 1998;44[Suppl]:A-133(abst).

51. Sasse S, Brand NJ, Kyprianou P, et al. Troponin I gene expression during human cardiac development and in end-stage heart failure. *Circ Res* 1993;72:932–938.

52. Trinquier S, Flécheux O, Bullenger M, et al. Highly specific immunoassay for cardiac troponin I assessed in noninfarct patients with chronic renal failure or severe polytrauma. *Clin Chem* 1995;41:1675–1676.

53. Wu AHB, Feng YJ, Contois JH, et al. Comparison of myoglobin, creatine kinase-MB, and cardiac troponin I for diagnosis of acute myocardial infarction. *Ann Clin Lab Sci* 1996;26:291–300.

54. Mair J, Genser N, Morandell D, et al. Cardiac troponin I in the diagnosis of myocardial injury and infarction. *Clin Chim Acta* 1996;245:19–38.

55. Zaninotto M, Altinier S, Lachin M, et al. Strategies for the early diagnosis of acute myocardial infarction using biochemical markers. *Am J Clin Pathol* 1999;111:399–405.

56. Apple FS, Henry TD, Berger CR, et al. Early monitoring of serum cardiac troponin I for assessment of coronary reperfusion following thrombolytic therapy [Comments]. *Am J Clin Pathol* 1996;105:6–10.

57. Collinson PO, Stubbs PJ, John C, et al. Cardiac troponin I to predict long-term outcome in patients with suspected acute coronary syndromes. *Clin Chem* 1998;44:A-132(abst).

58. Grenadier E, Keidar S, Kahana L, et al. The roles of serum myoglobin, total CK, and CK-MB isoenzyme in the acute phase of myocardial infarction. *Am Heart J* 1983;105:408–416.

59. Vaidya HC. Myoglobin: an early biochemical marker for the diagnosis of acute myocardial infarction. *J Clin Immunoassay* 1994;17:35–39.

60. Gornall DA, Roth SNL. Serial myoglobin quantitation in the early assessment of myocardial damage: a clinical study. *Clin Biochem* 1996; 29:379–384.

61. Plebani M, Zaninotto M. Diagnostic strategies in myocardial infarction using myoglobin measurement. *Eur Heart J* 1998;19[Suppl]:N12–N15.

62. Gibler WB, Gibler CD, Weinshenker C, et al. Myoglobin as an early indicator of acute myocardial infarction. *Ann Emerg Med* 1987;16:851–856.

63. Ohman EM, Casey C, Bengtson JR, et al. Early detection of acute myocardial infarction: additional diagnostic information from serum concentrations of myoglobin in patients without ST elevation. *Br Heart J* 1990;63:335–338.

64. Zimmerman J, Fromm R, Meyer D, et al. Diagnostic marker cooperative study for the diagnosis of myocardial infarction. *Circulation* 1999;99:1671–1677.

65. Hartmann F, Kampmann M, Frey N, et al. Biochemical markers in the diagnosis of coronary artery disease. *Eur Heart J* 1998;19[Suppl]:N2–N7.

66. Kost GJ, Kirk JD, Omand K. A strategy for the use of cardiac injury markers (troponin I and T, creatine kinase-MB mass and isoforms, and myoglobin) in the diagnosis of acute myocardial infarction. *Arch Pathol Lab Med* 1998;122:245–251.

67. Kontos MC, Anderson FP, Schmidt KA, et al. Early diagnosis of acute myocardial infarction in patients without ST-segment elevation. *Am J Cardiol* 1999;83:155–158.

68. Polanczyk CA, Lee T II, Cook EF, et al. Value of additional two-hour myoglobin for the diagnosis of myocardial infarction in the emergency department. *Am J Cardiol* 1999;83:525–529.

69. Davis CP, Barrett K, Torre P, et al. Serial myoglobin levels for patients with possible myocardial infarction. *Acad Emerg Med* 1996;3:590–597.

70. Woo J, Lacbawn FL, Sunheimer R, et al. Is myoglobin useful in the diagnosis of acute myocardial infarction in the department setting? *Am J Clin Path* 1995;103:725–729.

71. Bushnell A, Woo J, Sunheimer R, et al. Utility of myoglobin in the evaluation of chest pain in the ED [Letter]. *Am J Emerg Med* 1999;17:216–217.

72. Tucker JF, Collins RA, Anderson AJ, et al. Value of serial myoglobin levels in the early diagnosis of patients admitted for acute myocardial infarction. *Ann Emerg Med* 1994;24:704–708.

73. Montague C, Kircher T. Myoglobin in the early evaluation of acute chest pain. *Am J Clin Pathol* 1995;104:472–476.

74. de Winter RJ, Koster RW, Sturk A, et al. Value of myoglobin, troponin T, and CK-MB mass in ruling out an acute myocardial infarction in the emergency room. *Circulation* 1995;92:3401–3407.

75. Selected cardiac markers, 1998. *Diagnostic Market Report 1998.* Westport, CT: IMS Health, 1991.

76. Maisel AS, Templin K, Love M, et al. A prospective study of an algorithm using cardiac troponin I and myoglobin as adjuncts in the early diagnosis of acute myocardial infarction and intermediate coronary syndromes in a veterans hospital. *Clin Cardiol* 2000;23:915–920.

77. Ng SM, Krishnaswamy P, Morissey R, et al. A simple critical pathway for chest pain patients allows accurate triaging within 90 minutes of presentation to the emergency room. *Am J Cardiol* 2001;88:611–617.

78. Colon PJ 3rd, Mobarek SK, Milani RV, et al. Prognostic value of stress echocardiography in the evaluation of atypical chest pain patients without known coronary artery disease. *Am J Cardiol* 1998;81:545–551.

79. Radensky PW, Hilton TC, Fulmer H, et al. Potential cost effectiveness of initial myocardial perfusion imaging for assessment of emergency department patients with chest pain. *Am J Cardiol* 1997;79:595–599.

80. Romano S, Varveri A, Aurigemma G, et al. Echocardiography in the coronary care unit: diagnostic and prognostic impact in comparison with clinical and other indicators. *Am J Cardiol* 1998;81:13G–16G.

81. Gibler WB, Runyon JP, Levy RC, et al. A rapid diagnostic and treatment center for patients with chest pain in the emergency department. *Ann Emerg Med* 1995;25:1–8.

82. Stark ME, Vacek JL. The initial electrocardiogram during admission for myocardial infarction: use as a predictor of clinical course and facility utilization. *Arch Intern Med* 1987;147:843–846.

83. Savonitto S, Ardissino D, Granger CB, et al. Prognostic value of the admission electrocardiogram in acute coronary syndromes. *JAMA* 1999;281:707–713.

84. Newby LK, Storrow AB, Gibler WB, et al. Bedside multimarker testing for risk stratification in chest pain units. *Circulation* 2001;103:1832–1837.

85. Maisel AS. Cardiac markers in the assessment of patients with acute coronary syndromes. *Top Emerg Med* 1998;20:14–22.

86. Zimmerman J, Fromm R, Meyer D, et al. Diagnostic marker cooperative study for the diagnosis of myocardial infarction. *Circulation* 1999;99:1671–1677.

87. Apple FS, Christenson RH, Valdes Jr R, et al. Simultaneous rapid measurement of whole blood myoglobin, creatine kinase MB, and cardiac troponin I by the Triage Cardiac Panel for detection of myocardial infarction. *Clin Chem* 1999;45:199–205.

88. Wu AH, Apple FS, Gibler WB, et al. National Academy of Clinical Biochemistry Standards of Laboratory Practice: recommendations for the use of cardiac markers in coronary artery diseases. *Clin Chem* 1999;45:1104–1121.

89. Braunwald E, Antman EM, Beasley JW, et al. ACC/AHA guidelines for the management of patients with unstable angina and non-ST-segment elevation myocardial infarction: a report of the American College of Cardiology/American Heart Association Task Force on Practice Guidelines (Committee on the Management of Patients with Unstable Angina). *J Am Coll Cardiol* 2000;36:970–1062.

90. Antman EM, Fox KM. Guidelines for the diagnosis and management of unstable angina and non-Q-wave myocardial infarction: proposed revisions. International Cardiology Forum. *Am Heart J* 2000;139:461–475.

91. Ng SM, Krishnaswamy P, Morissey R, et al. Mitigation of spurious troponin I elevations in settings of coronary ischemia using serial testing of multiple cardiac markers. *Am J Cardiol* 2001;87:994–999.

92. Henderson AR, Gerhardt W, Apple FS. The use of biochemical markers in ischaemic heart disease: summary of roundtable and extrapolations. *Clin Chim Acta* 1998;272:93–100.

93. McPherson PH, Anderberg JM, Lesefko SM, et al. A rapid, quantitative point-of-care system for simultaneous measurement of CKMB, troponin I and myoglobin in blood. *Clin Chem* 1998;44:A-116(abst).

94. Buechler KF, Dwyer BP, Noar B, et al. A fluorescence energy transfer detection system for immunoassays of biological samples. *Clin Chem* 1997;43:S-136(abst).

95. *Clinical Laboratory Products*, May 1998;27.

96. Grantham JA, Burnett Jr JC. BNP: increasing importance in the pathophysiology and diagnosis of congestive heart failure. *Circulation* 1997;96:388–390.

97. Yandle TG. Biochemistry of natriuretic peptides. *J Intern Med* 1994;235:561–576.

98. Maeda K, Takayoshi T, Wada A, et al. Plasma brain natriuretic peptide as a biochemical marker of high left ventricular end-diastolic pressure in patients with symptomatic left ventricular dysfunction. *Am Heart J* 1998;135:825–832.

99. Tsutamoto T, Wada A, Maeda K, et al. Attenuation of compensation of endogenous cardiac natriuretic peptide system in chronic heart failure: prognostic role of plasma brain natriuretic peptide concentration in patients with chronic symptomatic left ventricular dysfunction. *Circulation* 1997;96:509–516.

100. Dao Q, Krishnaswamy P, Kazanegra R, et al. Utility of B-type natriuretic peptide (BNP) in the diagnosis of CHF in an urgent care setting. *J Am Coll Cardiol* 2001;37:379–385.

101. Maisel AS, Koon J, Hope J, et al. A rapid bedside test for brain natriuretic peptide accurately predicts cardiac function in patients referred for echocardiography. *Am Heart J* 2001;141:374–379.

102. Stevenson LW, Braunwald E. Recognition and management of patients with heart failure. In: Goldman L, Braunwald E, eds. *Primary cardiology*. Philadelphia: Saunders, 1998:310–329.

103. Cheng VL, Krishnaswamy P, Kazanegra R, et al. A rapid bedside test for B-type natriuretic peptide predicts treatment outcomes in patients admitted with decompensated heart failure. *J Am Coll Cardiol* 2001;37:386–391.

104. Kazanagra R, Cheng V, Garcia A, et al. A rapid test for B-type natriuretic peptide (BNP) correlates with falling wedge pressures in patients treated for decompensated heart failure: a pilot study. *J Card Failure* 2001;7:21–22.

105. Troughton RW, Frampton CM, Yandle TG, et al. Treatment of heart failure guided by plasma amino terminal brain natriuretic peptide (N-BNP) concentrations. *Lancet* 2000;355:1126–1130.

39

USING POINT-OF-CARE LACTATE TO PREDICT PATIENT OUTCOMES

JAN BAKKER
SELMA S.J. SCHIEVELD
WILLEM BRINKERT

Time is crucial in the care of the acutely ill patient. Several authors have underlined the importance of early diagnosis and treatment using terms like "the golden hour" and "where every second counts" in the care of emergency patients (1,2).

Point-of-care testing (POCT) is a rapidly evolving area of patient monitoring. It quickly provides the clinician with key variables that otherwise would have a considerably longer turnaround time. In addition, point-of-care (POC) devices usually require a smaller blood sample (3), improving blood conservation in these patients (3–5). POCT could therefore speed up triage, admission, diagnosing, and treatment strategies in emergency patients (5). In these patients, POCT is most advantageous when focusing on vital parameters associated with significant immediate and long-term morbidity and mortality.

Increased blood lactate levels have been related to inadequate oxygen supply of the tissues in both experimental and clinical conditions (6–8). Several investigators have shown that a single blood lactate measurement can identify patients with hospital mortality above 80% (9,10). In addition, prolonged hyperlactatemia has been associated with irreversible circulatory shock, the development of multiple organ failure and ultimate survival (11,12). Lactate could therefore well be one of these vital parameters.

This chapter reviews the use of POC blood lactate levels in emergency patients in and outside the hospital.

BIOCHEMISTRY OF INCREASED BLOOD LACTATE

Lactate is a normal end product of glycolysis. It can only be converted from pyruvate mediated by the enzyme lactate dehydrogenase. All cells are capable of producing lactate; however, lactate metabolism primarily occurs in the liver and kidney. Normal blood lactate levels in healthy adults are 1.3±0.04 (13) with a normal range from 0.5 to 1.6 mmol/L (14,15) (Table 39.1). Arterial blood lactate levels above 2 are considered clinically important (12).

As lactate can only be metabolized by the conversion to pyruvate, blood lactate levels depend on pyruvate metabolism. Molecular oxygen is required for the conversion of pyruvate to acetyl-CoA that is subsequently metabolized in the tricarboxylic acid cycle to produce 36 mmol of adenosine triphosphate (ATP) per mmol glucose/pyruvate metabolized. When oxygen is lacking, pyruvate concentration increases and is converted to lactate. Glucose metabolism during hypoxia produces only 2 mmol of ATP. Although limited, this trickle is extremely important during cellular hypoxia as it maintains the cell viability three to four times longer than if no ATP were produced. Other processes result in increased lactate production. Dysfunction of the pyruvate dehydrogenase complex and increased glycolysis and glucose metabolism have been associated with nonhypoxic increases in blood lactate levels (16–20). In conditions associated with pyruvate dehydrogenase dysfunction (i.e., sepsis), increasing pyruvate dehydrogenase activity using dichloroacetate decreases blood lactate levels (21,22). However, clinically the most relevant cause of limited pyruvate utilization is cellular hypoxia.

Three pathways are involved in the transport of lactate across the cell membrane (23). The most important pathway is an H(+)-linked transporter in the cellular membrane. By this mechanism, lactate uptake by the cell (e.g., skeletal muscle and cardiac myocytes) is increased during acidosis. In contrast, lactate efflux will occur during alkalemia resulting in an increase in lactate levels in these conditions (24,25).

TABLE 39.1. REFERENCE RANGES OF BLOOD LACTATE USING DIFFERENT SAMPLE SITES IN HEALTHY VOLUNTEERS

Sample	Reference Range	Literature Reference
Arterial blood	0.5–1.6 mmol/L	Westgard et al. (14), Huckabee (15)
Capillary blood	0.4–1.5 mmol/L	Wandrup et al. (74)
Venous blood	0.3–1.5 mmol/L	Huckabee (15), Wandrup et al. (74)

HYPERLACTATEMIA AND METABOLIC ACIDOSIS

Lactic acidosis is a relatively frequent condition in acutely ill patients. Incidence has been reported to be up to 3.8% of all patients admitted to the hospital with internal diseases. The mortality associated with this condition is high, ranging from 30% to 88% (9,10). The relationship between blood lactate levels and metabolic acidosis has been the subject of many reviews during the past 2 decades (19,26–31). This persisting interest in the association between and the significance of acidosis and hyperlactatemia is related to several aspects. First, the mechanisms involved in the development of acidosis during tissue hypoxia and hyperlactatemia remain a matter of debate. The production of lactate does not result in net hydrogen ion—H(+)—production as the H(+) ions are reutilized in the production of ATP from adenosine diphosphate and adenosine monophosphate. The inability of the cells to reutilize H(+)-ions generated by the hydrolysis of ATP during hypoxia has been suggested to be an important mechanism in the development of metabolic acidosis (19,32). More recently, changes in protein concentration and shifts in strong ions (i.e., chloride) have also been implicated in the development of the metabolic acidosis (33,34). Second, the cellular effects of a decrease in pH or an increase in lactate concentration differ markedly. Recently, several investigators have shown that an increase in intracellular lactate concentration results in myocardial dysfunction irrespective of the intracellular pH (35,36). In addition, where the effect of acidosis on myocardial dysfunction seems to be reversible, the effects of hyperlactatemia are not (36). These effects of increases in lactate levels as such, fuel the debate on whether the lactate molecule is harmful, and attempts to decrease lactate levels by increasing lactate metabolism could thus be beneficial (22,37, 38). Lastly, as the combination of markedly increased blood lactate levels and a decreased arterial pH or base deficit carries a

very poor prognosis with hospital mortality exceeding 80% (39), early diagnosis of acidosis and increased lactate levels could be of value in the treatment of emergency patients.

However, as the mechanisms involved in the production and clearance of hydrogen ions and lactate are not always related, the relationships between arterial pH base excess and blood lactate are weak (Fig. 39.1). Therefore, in clinical practice blood lactate levels cannot be estimated by measuring arterial pH or base excess.

RELATIONSHIP BETWEEN TISSUE OXYGENATION AND LACTATE LEVELS

When global oxygen delivery decreases, extraction of oxygen is increased to maintain global oxygen consumption at baseline levels. However, when a critical point is reached, the increase in oxygen extraction is insufficient and oxygen consumption starts to decrease. Together with this decrease in oxygen consumption blood lactate levels start to rise. This relationship among oxygen delivery, oxygen consumption, and blood lactate levels has been demonstrated in many experimental models using a progressive limitation in oxygen transport, not only at a global level (6,40,41) but also at the regional (42–44) and organ level (45).

In emergency patients, persistent tissue hypoxia has been associated with increasing organ failure and ultimate death in both surgical and medical emergency patients (46–49). However, parameters reflecting the presence and resolution of tissue hypoxia have been poorly defined in emergency conditions. Traditionally, hemodynamic parameters (e.g., heart rate and blood pressure) and physical examination (e.g., skin color and temperature, Glasgow Coma Scale) have been used to identify patients at risk and to initiate and adjust treatment. Recently, several authors have shown that normal hemodynamics do not guarantee adequate tissue oxygen delivery (9,50,51). In addition, nor-

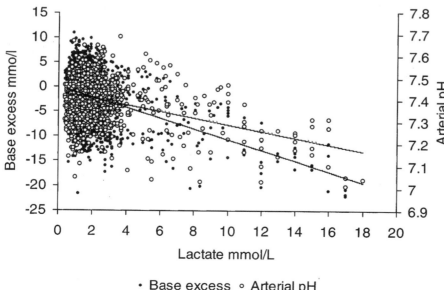

FIGURE 39.1. Relationship between arterial blood lactate, base excess (filled circles) and pH (open circles) in 1754 measurements in critically ill patients. Lines represent the linear regression for lactate vs. base excess (solid line, R(2)=0.18, p<0.01) and lactate vs. arterial pH (dotted line, R(2)=0.12, p<0.01)

malization of hemodynamics does not necessarily resolve tissue hypoxia (52).

Huckabee (18) was one of the first to describe the relationship between increased blood lactate levels and clinical shock. From later experiments it is clear that blood lactate levels rapidly increase when oxygen delivery to the tissues fails to meet the oxygen demand of these tissues (6,8). The excess of lactate has been found to reflect the severity of the oxygen debt (53,54) and the reversibility of shock (11). In addition, therapeutic interventions aimed to increase tissue oxygen delivery have been associated with decreases in lactate levels (55). Also, therapeutic schedules to increase oxygen delivery by use of fluids and inotropes that subsequently decrease/normalize lactate levels have been associated with improvement in morbidity and mortality (56–58).

Recently however, the causality between tissue hypoxia and increased blood lactate levels has been challenged (19,59). Especially in patients with sepsis, other factors could contribute to an increase in blood lactate levels in the absence of tissue hypoxia. At first, increased glucose metabolism will result in increased lactate production, as lactate is a normal end product of glucose metabolism. Increased glucose metabolism could be related to increased metabolic demand (fever, hyperventilation, etc.) or increased epinephrine levels (60). Second, dysfunction of the pyruvate dehydrogenase complex in sepsis results in a decrease in pyruvate utilization causing pyruvate to be metabolized to lactate (61). Dysfunction of pyruvate dehydrogenase could also result in impaired lactate clearance following hemodynamic stabilization of patients with sepsis (62). Third, respiratory alkalosis, frequently associated with early sepsis, decreases cellular lactate uptake and increases cellular lactate release into the circulation, thus increasing blood lactate levels (25). Nevertheless, increased lactate levels in early septic shock, before circulatory resuscitation, seem to be related to an imbalance between tissue oxygen demand and oxygen supply (63). These aspects should be taken into account when evaluating hyperlactatemia in sepsis and septic shock. When the existence of an imbalance between oxygen demand and oxygen supply is unclear, a simple oxygen flux test using limited doses of dobutamine can help to evaluate this relationship (64).

POINT-OF-CARE LACTATE: MEASUREMENT TECHNIQUES

The first lactate measurement described in the literature (1886) took several days and required a withdrawal of at least 200 ml of blood (65). In 1964, Broder and Weil (66) were the first to use a photospectrometric method to measure lactate levels in whole blood. With this they set a trend in the monitoring of blood lactate levels in critically ill patients. The labor intensiveness of the early measurement technique limited its widespread use, as results were usually available long after therapeutic decisions had been made.

The availability of a substrate-specific electrode now enables the clinician to measure lactate concentrations rapidly (within 2 minutes) in a minimal amount (± 130 μL) of plasma or whole blood. These lactate analyzers are based on an electrochemical sensor. Lactate oxidase converts lactate to pyruvate and hydrogen peroxide. The oxidation of hydrogen peroxide to molecular oxygen produces electrons creating a current proportional to the lactate concentration in the sample. If dilution of the sample is necessary due to membrane technology, an analytical error is introduced that increases with increasing hematocrit (67). This causes an underestimation of blood lactate levels when wholeblood samples are used (68). Several devices now available have been validated in emergency medicine and critical care medicine (13,69–71).

As most of these POC instruments are also capable of measuring blood gases and electrolytes, they are often bulky. When used in the emergency department (ED), rapid access to the device is usually more important than portability. However, when used outside the hospital or on general wards in emergency conditions, portability becomes critically important.

Recently a handheld device using a reflective photometry method has been introduced. This handheld lactate analyzer (Accusport®, Roche Diagnostics, Mannheim, Germany) is a small, battery-powered, reflectance photometer. It uses drychemistry-coated test strips on which a drop of blood is applied. In the test strip, red blood cells are trapped in a glass fiber filter before reaching the reaction layer. In this layer, lactate oxidase converts lactate to pyruvate and reduces the mediator. The reduced mediator reacts with phosphomolybdaze to form molybdenum blue. Changes in light absorption are then measured at 660 Nm. As the glass fiber filters cells, the actual measurement is thus carried out in the fluid component of whole blood. The instrument uses empirically determined correction factors for estimating plasma or whole blood values. The turnaround time is approximately 60 seconds and test results are displayed on a liquid crystal display. Data are automatically stored and can be recalled from the memory but not linked to an external computer. The instrument's range is 0.7 to 26 mmol/l for serum lactate concentrations.

We validated this device in 39 intensive care unit (ICU) patients using the plasma values of the device (72). In these patients, 50 convenience measurement cycles were carried out. Each cycle consisted of three paired measurements at a 30-minute interval taken from an indwelling artery catheter. The laboratory's use of the Hitachi 917 (Roche Diagnostics, Mannheim, Germany) served as the reference method. After centrifugation of blood samples, lactate concentrations were measured in plasma. In 129 cases, measurements with the handheld POC instrument were done in duplicate. We found an excellent correlation between the handheld lactate analyzer and the laboratory (slope=1.01, intercept=−0.38, R(2)=0.97, $p<0.001$). Simultaneous handheld POC and laboratory measurements showed a mean difference of −0.32 mmol/l (limits of agreement, −1.34 to 0.70 mmol/l). Precision of the handheld POCI was calculated from 129 duplicate measurements. The overall mean difference was 0.08 mmol/l (limits of agreement, −0.48 to 0.64 mmol/l). The mean of the two measurements did not correlate with the difference between the two measurements.

From this we concluded that this handheld device could adequately measure blood lactate levels in critically ill patients. Similar findings were reported using the device in ED patients (73).

BLOOD LACTATE: SAMPLING SITE

In the hospital, blood lactate levels are usually measured using arterial blood samples. However, in emergency situations on the ward or in the ED, arterial lines are usually not readily available. No studies are available comparing blood lactate measurements in venous, arterial, and capillary blood samples in these conditions. In normal adults at rest or during minor exercise, capillary, venous, and arterial blood samples yield similar lactate concentrations (74,75). However, during heavy exercise significant differences in lactate concentrations can occur using different sampling sites (75–77).

In a small number of patients (*n*=12), Weil et al. (78) showed that in hemodynamically stable patients, lactate measurements sampled either from a central venous line or pulmonary artery catheter resulted in lactate concentrations similar to those in arterial blood. Recently, Jackson et al. (79) confirmed these findings in 48 critically ill patients and 100 patients before percutaneous transluminal coronary angioplasty.

In patients with lung injury, pulmonary lactate production could contribute to the difference between pulmonary artery and arterial blood lactate concentrations (80,81). Several investigators have shown that the amount of lactate released by the lung is related to the severity of the lung injury (80,81). Although no data are available in emergency medicine patients, arterial blood lactate levels could be influenced by severe lung injury. However, differences between mixed venous and arterial blood lactate levels are usually small. In addition, even in these circumstances, the release of lactate by the lung probably reflects tissue hypoxia. Therefore, arterial blood lactate levels still reflect the imbalance between oxygen delivery and oxygen demand in the global circulation.

Local-regional disturbances in oxygen delivery and oxygen demand can limit the use of peripheral or capillary blood samples in critically ill patients. Therefore, when capillary or peripheral venous blood is used, damming of blood and muscle activity should be avoided (82). Recently, Lavery et al. (83) reported an excellent relationship between arterial and venous lactate levels in trauma patients. Although limits of agreement were not reported, the standard error and 95% confidence interval of the linear relationship suggest that venous lactate levels can be used to estimate arterial levels in these patients. As in other studies, venous lactate levels—like arterial lactate levels—discriminate between survivors and nonsurvivors (83,84).

Collected blood samples should be stored on ice and measurements of blood lactate levels should be performed immediately when metabolism of red and white blood cells is not stopped by the addition of, for example, fluoride to the sample. Also, the medium in which the blood samples are collected should not be used interchangeably, as citrate anticoagulant lowers lactate concentrations as compared with heparin or EDTA (85). As lactate concentrations are different in plasma, serum, and whole blood, the compartment of measurement should also remain stable when monitoring lactate levels in an individual patient (85). When using lactate Ringer's solution in fluid resuscitation, the sampling line should be completely cleared as only a small amount of this solution can falsely increase blood lactate concentration (79).

TREATMENT OF HYPERLACTATEMIA

Clinically, blood lactate levels are frequently used to monitor tissue hypoxia. Tissue hypoxia is best described as the presence of an imbalance between oxygen demand and oxygen delivery (DO_2). Global DO_2 is a function of the arterial oxygen content and the cardiac output:

$$DO_2 = CaO_2 \times CO = Hb \times SaO_2 \times CO_{XK} \quad (1)$$
$$CaO_2 = \text{Arterial oxygen content}$$
$$Hb = \text{Hemoglobin level}$$
$$SaO_2 = \text{Arterial oxygen saturation}$$
$$CO = \text{Cardiac output}$$

Although a decrease in each of the components can cause a decrease in DO_2, decreases in hemoglobin levels and arterial oxygen saturation are usually accompanied by compensatory increases in cardiac output so that DO_2 can be maintained to meet oxygen demand (86). When oxygen demand is increased due to agitation or increased oxygen demand of respiratory muscles, sedation and mechanical ventilation can help to restore the balance between oxygen delivery and oxygen demand (87–91). However, these interventions usually do not completely resolve tissue hypoxia in these conditions. The mainstay of treatment in patients with increased blood lactate levels is improvement of tissue oxygen delivery. This is usually accomplished by increases in DO_2. Hemoglobin substitution and oxygen administration are frequently used to improve tissue oxygen delivery. However, the effectiveness of these interventions is usually limited (92–95). Fluid resuscitation and inotropes to increase cardiac output have consistently been found to improve tissue oxygen delivery in patients with tissue hypoxia (64,94–97). Correction of hyperlactatemia by increasing the metabolism of pyruvate could have beneficial effects on myocardial function and thus cardiac output (35,36). Dichloroacetate enhances the activity of the pyruvate dehydrogenase complex thus decreasing blood lactate levels. Both experimental and clinical studies have shown that administration of dichloroacetate decreases blood lactate levels during sepsis and septic shock (21,37). However, in a recent controlled clinical trial (252 patients), administration of dichloroacetate in critically ill patients with hyperlactatemia and metabolic acidosis had no significant effect on hemodynamics and survival (22). In addition, correction of the metabolic acidosis accompanying hyperlactatemia with bicarbonate administration has not been shown to improve hemodynamics, tissue hypoxia and survival in critically ill patients (98,99) and has even been associated with detrimental hemodynamic effects (100).

Thus, treatment of hyperlactatemia should be directed first at the principal cause of tissue hypoxia (ongoing blood loss, tension pneumothorax, cardiac tamponade, etc.). If these measures do not result in the restoration of the balance between oxygen delivery and oxygen demand, global oxygen delivery should be increased. Fluids and, if necessary, inotropes are the principal components of the latter intervention. Few clinical studies have shown that a similar approach is associated with improvement in morbidity and mortality in critically ill patients (56–58,101).

Following adequate resuscitation, blood lactate levels rapidly decrease within 20 minutes (102). Although an increase in blood lactate levels is a relatively late marker of decreasing tissue oxygen delivery, rapid resolution of hyperlactatemia following treatment is indicative of a restoration of tissue oxygenation.

Blood Lactate Levels and Outcome

Cellular hypoxia results in cellular dysfunction and cell death if not quickly corrected. Therefore the duration of cellular hypoxia is critical in the occurrence of ultimate organ dysfunction and failure and finally patient death. Many studies have shown that a single lactate measurement can identify patients at risk of developing multiple organ failure or death (9,10).

Normalization of increased blood lactate levels depends, however, on several factors. First, and probably most importantly, rapid resolution of tissue hypoxia by increasing oxygen delivery stops increased production of lactate and could facilitate lactate metabolism by the liver (45), resulting in rapid resolution of hyperlactatemia. Second, increased lactate production in critically ill patients could result from nonhypoxic cellular processes as has been suggested recently (59,103). Third, as the magnitude of the initial hyperlactatemia has been found to be related to the resolution of hyperlactatemia (9) during intensive care treatment, metabolic clearance of lactate could be an important factor in the duration of hyperlactatemia. Indeed, in patients with sepsis without tissue hypoxia, clearance of lactate is limited (62). In addition, liver dysfunction, as in patients with cirrhosis, is associated with decreased lactate clearance not related to tissue hypoxia (104). Therefore, in critically ill patients prolonged hyperlactatemia could be related to increased production due to tissue hypoxia or nonhypoxic cellular processes or decreased clearance. These factors complicate the interpretation of increased blood lactate levels and the changes in blood lactate levels following initiation of treatment.

Despite the complex etiology of increased blood lactate levels, persistently increased blood lactate levels following treatment have been related to organ failure, increased use of resources, and high mortality in many clinical studies (11,56,105). A favorable outcome is usually associated with a decrease in blood lactate levels within the first 24 hours of admission to the ICU. In trauma patients rapid resolution of increased blood lactate levels (within 12 hours of admission) is associated with a significantly lower incidence of infectious episodes (12.7%) when compared to patients requiring up to 24 hours (40.5%) or more than 24 hours (65.9%) to normalize blood lactate levels (40.5%) (57). In the latter study, the incidence of infectious episodes in patients without increased blood lactate levels was similar to the incidence in patients with rapid resolution of increased blood lactate levels. In addition in major trauma patients, failure to normalize blood lactate levels within 24 hours of admission is related to poor survival (58).

Also in septic shock patients, a decrease in blood lactate levels during the first 24 hours of admission to the ICU is associated with improved survival (12,106). In septic shock patients, we found the time required to normalize blood lactate levels to be the best predictor of survival (12). In addition, the integrated lactate response has been associated with organ damage and death (12). In this latter study we showed that nonsurvivors had a prolonged time to normalize blood lactate levels and an increased area under the lactate-versus-time curve (Fig. 39.2). In addition, in this study, increasing levels of organ failure were related to longer times to normalize lactate levels and increased areas under the lactate-versus-time curve. The interpretation of the relationship between time and lactate levels is however complicated as patients with higher initial lactate levels require more time to normalize their lactate levels (Fig. 39.3). As discussed before, persistent production and decreased clearance can both result in an increased area under the time-lactate-curve without presence of profound tissue hypoxia.

Despite these difficulties in the interpretation of persistently increased blood lactate levels, in the literature a consistent association between increased morbidity and mortality and prolonged hyperlactatemia has been reported, whereas a rapid normalization (within the first 24 hours of admission) usually predicts a favorable outcome. Several factors could contribute to these findings. First, despite hemodynamic stabilization and increases in global oxygen delivery, occult regional tissue hypoperfusion and hypoxia could persist due to microcirculatory derangement leading to organ damage (107–109). Second, per-

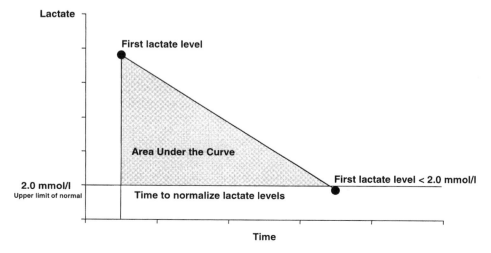

FIGURE 39.2. Time-vs-lactate curve with estimation of the area under the curve.

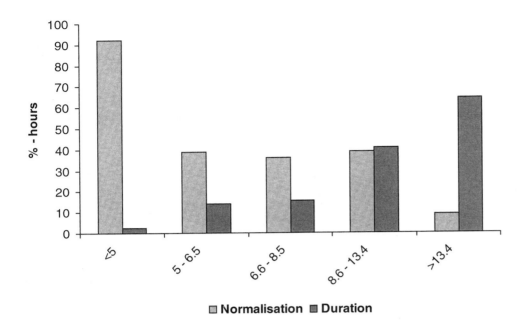

FIGURE 39.3. Time to normalize blood lactate levels and percentage of patients achieving normalization in 126 patients with lactic acidosis. (Adapted from Stacpoole PW, Wright EC, Baumgartner TG, et al. Natural history and course of acquired lactic acidosis in adults. DCA-Lactic Acidosis Study Group. *Am J Med* 1994;97:47–54.)

sistent hyperlactatemia following restoration of tissue oxygen delivery could be a marker of ongoing metabolic derangement related to the primary disease or an underlying disorder, such as liver dysfunction (104), that compromises survival. Finally, prolonged hyperlactatemia could have harmful effects by itself (36,110), although decreasing lactate levels by enhancing lactate metabolism using dichloroacetate administration has failed to show clinical benefit (22).

Lactate Levels in Emergency Medicine

In a general population of ED patients, Aduen et al. (13) showed that blood lactate levels in ultimate nonsurvivors were significantly higher than in survivors (5.14±0.84 versus 2.22±0.12, *p*<0.001). In a population of ED patients and ICU patients with either hypotension or normotension, lactate levels discriminated survivors from nonsurvivors (13). In a recent study (83), arterial and venous lactate levels within 10 minutes after arrival in the ED were related to severity of injury, use of resources and survival. In addition, in this study venous lactate levels had more predictive power of injury severity, morbidity, and mortality than standard triage criteria. Monitoring of lactate levels to guide therapy in trauma patients or critically ill patients in the ED has been shown to improve outcome (111,112). In the latter studies, therapeutic interventions during persistent hyperlactatemia where directed to increase tissue oxygen delivery. In a recent study, Smith et al. (113) showed that lactate levels on admission to the intensive care were excellent predictors of morbidity and mortality. Therefore, admission to the ICU should be considered in critically ill patients with increased blood lactate levels (114).

In patients admitted with internal diseases, Luft et al. (10) showed that a single blood lactate measurement could identify patients with a highly increased mortality ratio. In a later study, Stacpoole et al. (9) showed that a single blood lactate concen-

tration at or above 5 mmol/l in combination with a metabolic acidosis carried a very poor hospital survival rate (17%). Although infrequently used in diabetic patients, biguanides can result in the development of lactic acidosis (115–117). Measurements of blood lactate levels in these patients could thus help to reveal drug toxicity.

Protein markers of myocardial damage are released in the circulation within 1 to 2 hours following the onset of acute chest pain. However, as the heart starts to produce lactate instead of consuming lactate in these conditions, lactate levels increase earlier (within 1 hour). Therefore, increases in blood lactate levels could be an early indicator of myocardial damage. In a recent study, Schmiechen et al. (118) showed that lactate levels above 1.5 mmol/L had a high sensitivity (96%) for the presence of an acute myocardial infarction in 128 patients with acute onset of chest pain. Specificity in this group of patients was, however, low (37%). In addition, increased blood lactate levels are associated with the development of cardiogenic shock and ultimate survival in patients with acute myocardial infarction (119,120). In patients with out-of-hospital circulatory arrest, blood lactate levels correlate poorly with the estimated duration of the arrest and the neurologic outcome (121).

In trauma patients, hypovolemia—usually resulting from major blood loss—is a major cause of tissue hypoxia. At first, global hemodynamic parameters show minor abnormalities despite significant blood loss and the presence of tissue hypoxia. In these situations, blood lactate levels provide a better index of the severity of tissue hypoxia than traditional hemodynamic parameters (122). Several clinical studies have shown that initial blood lactate levels, the duration of hyperlactatemia, and changes in blood lactate levels following fluid resuscitation have important prognostic significance in trauma patients (13,111,123–125). In these patients blood lactate levels have more prognostic value than cardiac output, DO_2, and oxygen consumption (126) or central venous oxygenation (112). In

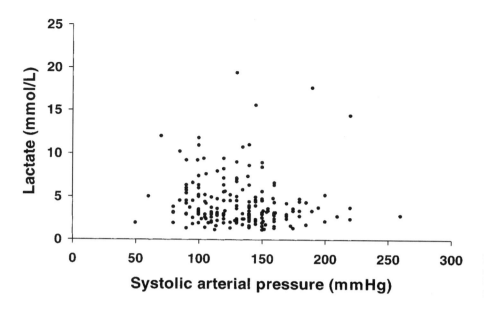

FIGURE 39.4. Relationship between systolic arterial pressure and capillary blood lactate level in 135 out-of-hospital emergency patients.

addition, in neurotrauma patients, blood lactate levels have been shown to better predict intracranial pressure than heart rate, blood pressure and cardiac output (127).

In a recent study in trauma patients (*n*=47), Slomovitz et al. (73) measured arterial or venous blood lactate levels on admission to the emergency room. In this study, lactate levels in patients requiring admission were significantly higher than in patients who could be discharged following treatment (4.7±4.1 versus 1.8±0.6, respectively; *p*<0.001). Others have reported similar findings (128). In patients with blunt liver trauma, Siegel et al. (51) showed that blood lactate levels on admission to the hospital were significantly related to survival.

As patients with grand mal seizures have major increases in blood lactate concentrations (102,129) (frequently more than 10 mmol/L), lactate measurements could help in diagnosing patients with or without a known history of seizures found unconscious. Although markers of airway obstruction are probably a better indicator of the severity of asthma attacks, patients with increased blood lactate levels are at great risk of developing respiratory failure and should be closely monitored (130).

In the ED, measurements of either arterial or venous blood lactate levels could thus help to identify patients at risk of developing significant morbidity or mortality. In these acutely ill patients, increased blood lactate levels should always be considered a serious sign and the underlying pathological disturbances should therefore be explored vigorously.

Preclinical Setting: A Case Study

Although some studies have reported on the use of out-of-hospital blood gas analysis (131), no studies are available assessing the value of blood lactate measurements outside the hospital. We therefore studied the value of out-of-hospital blood lactate measurements in a mixed group of 135 patients. Preliminary results have been reported in abstract form only (132). Lactate measurements were done in capillary blood using a handheld device (Accusport, Roche Diagnostics, Mannheim, Germany) recently validated in ED and ICU patients (72,73). Immediately following arrival at the scene, ambulance personnel collected capillary blood and measured blood lactate levels. Also, heart rate, blood pressure, and pulse oxyimetry data were recorded. The ultimate diagnosis was taken from hospital charts. In this study, we confirmed that blood lactate levels are a better indicator of the severity of injury and illness than traditional clinical assessment and hemodynamic parameters. No significant relationship between systolic arterial pressure and lactate levels was found in these patients (Fig. 39.4). In addition, blood lactate levels were clearly discriminating ultimate survivors from nonsurvivors despite apparently normal hemodynamics (Table 39.2). In eight patients with general seizures, blood lactate levels were significantly increased (9.9±4.0 mmol/L). In one patient without a known history of seizures, the diagnosis was suspected and subsequently confirmed using the high initial lactate level (14.4 mmol/L). Patients admitted to the hospital had significantly higher blood lactate levels than patients who could be discharged following treatment (4.1 ±2.5 versus 2.7 ±0.9, respectively; *p*<0.01).

In out-of-hospital emergency medicine, capillary blood lactate levels could thus help in the process of diagnosing and identifying patients at risk. Also, blood lactate levels could be a bet-

TABLE 39.2. OUT-OF-HOSPITAL HEMODYNAMICS AND BLOOD LACTATE LEVELS IN 135 ACUTELY ILL PATIENTS

Parameter	Mean (SD)
Heart rate b/min	95 (26)
Systolic arterial pressure mm Hg	131 (33)
Pulse oxymetry %	92 (8)
Lactate mmol/L	4.4 (3.1)
Glasgow coma scale	12 (5)
Mortality	24%

SD, standard deviation.

ter parameter to initiate and change treatments than clinical assessment and traditionally measured hemodynamics. Further studies are, however, needed to confirm the value of blood lactate measurements in these conditions.

CONCLUSIONS

In recent decades, blood lactate levels have been related to significant morbidity and mortality in many groups of acutely ill and trauma patients. Even a single blood lactate level can already identify preclinical and clinical patients at increased risk. In addition, response to therapy aiming at improving tissue oxygen delivery clearly separates ultimate surviving patients from nonsurviving patients. Significant changes in blood lactate levels already occur in the first 20 minutes following resuscitation. Lactate levels can be accurately measured using a small battery-powered, handheld device with a turnaround time of 60 seconds. Therefore, lactate measurements represent a rapid assessment of the severity of disease and injury (133) and could thus be used in triaging and treating acutely ill patients in emergency conditions inside or outside the hospital.

REFERENCES

1. McNicholl BP. The golden hour and prehospital trauma care. *Injury* 1994;25:251–254.
2. Hudson T. Telemedicine: where every second counts. *Hosp Health Netw* 1996;70:61.
3. Chernow B. Blood conservation in critical care—the evidence accumulates. *Crit Care Med* 1993;21:481–482.
4. Chernow B, Salem M, Stacey J. Blood conservation—a critical care imperative [Editorial]. *Crit Care Med* 1991;19:313–314.
5. Salem M, Chernow B, Burke R, et al. Bedside diagnostic blood testing: its accuracy, rapidity, and utility in blood conservation. *JAMA* 1991;266:382–389.
6. Cain SM. Appearance of excess lactate in anesthetized dogs during anemic and hypoxic hypoxia. *Am J Physiol* 1965;209:604–608.
7. Lynn J, Teno JM, Phillips RS, et al. Perceptions by family members of the dying experience of older and seriously ill patients. SUPPORT Investigators. Study to understand prognoses and preferences for outcomes and risks of treatments [Comments]. *Ann Intern Med* 1997; 126:97–106.
8. Ronco JJ, Fenwick JC, Tweeddale MG, et al. Identification of the critical oxygen delivery for anaerobic metabolism in critically ill septic and nonseptic humans. *JAMA* 1993;270:1724–1730.
9. Stacpoole PW, Wright EC, Baumgartner TG, et al. Natural history and course of acquired lactic acidosis in adults. DCA-Lactic Acidosis Study Group. *Am J Med* 1994;97:47–54.
10. Luft D, Deichsel G, Schmulling RM, et al. Definition of clinically relevant lactic acidosis in patients with internal diseases. *Am J Clin Pathol* 1983;80:484–589.
11. Broder G, Weil MH. Excess lactate: an index of reversibility of shock in human patients. *Science* 1964;143:1457–1459.
12. Bakker J, Gris P, Coffernils M, et al. Serial blood lactate levels can predict the development of multiple organ failure following septic shock. *Am J Surg* 1996;171:221–226.
13. Aduen J, Bernstein WK, Khastgir T, et al. The use and clinical importance of a substrate-specific electrode for rapid determination of blood lactate concentrations. *JAMA* 1994;272:1678–1685.
14. Westgard JO, Lahmeyer BL, Birnbaum ML. Use of the Du Pont automatic clinical analyzer in direct determination of lactic acid in plasma stabilized with sodium fluoride. *Clin Chem* 1972;18:1334–1338.
15. Huckabee WE. Abnormal resting blood lactate. *Am J Med* 1961;30:833–839.
16. Kreisberg RA. Glucose-lactate inter-relations in man. *N Engl J Med* 1972;287:132–137.
17. Vary TC. Sepsis-induced alterations in pyruvate dehydrogenase complex activity in rat skeletal muscle: effects on plasma lactate. *Shock* 1996;6:89–94.
18. Huckabee WE. Relationships of pyruvate and lactate during anaerobic metabolism. I. Effects of infusion of pyruvate or glucose and of hyperventilation. *J Clin Invest* 1958;37:244.
19. Gutierrez G, Wulf ME. Lactic acidosis in sepsis: a commentary. *Intensive Care Med* 1996;22:6–16.
20. Hurtado FJ, Gutierrez AM, Silva N, et al. Role of tissue hypoxia as the mechanism of lactic acidosis during E. coli endotoxemia. *J Appl Physiol* 1992;72:1895–1901.
21. Curtis SE, Cain SM. Regional and systemic oxygen delivery/uptake relations and lactate flux in hyperdynamic, endotoxin-treated dogs. *Am Rev Respir Dis* 1992;145:348–354.
22. Stacpoole PW, Wright EC, Baumgartner TG, et al. A controlled clinical trial of dichloroacetate for treatment of lactic acidosis in adults. The Dichloroacetate-Lactic Acidosis Study Group. *N Engl J Med* 1992;327:1564–1569.
23. Poole RC, Halestrap AP. Transport of lactate and other monocarboxylates across mammalian plasma membranes. *Am J Physiol* 1993; 264:C761–C782.
24. Gutierrez G, Hurtado FJ, Gutierrez AM, et al. Net uptake of lactate by rabbit hindlimb during hypoxia. *Am Rev Respir Dis* 1993;148: 1204–1209.
25. Druml W, Grimm G, Laggner AN, et al. Lactic acid kinetics in respiratory alkalosis. *Crit Care Med* 1991;19:1120–1124.
26. Stacpoole PW. Lactic acidosis. *Endocrinol Metab Clin North Am* 1993; 22:221–245.
27. Alberti KG, Nattrass M. Lactic acidosis. *Lancet* 1977;2:25–29.
28. Oliva PB. Lactic acidosis. *Am J Med* 1970;48:209–225.
29. Zilva JF. The origin of the acidosis in hyperlactataemia. *Ann Clin Biochem* 1978;15:40–43.
30. Krebs HA, Wood HF, Alberti KGMM. Hyperlactataemia and lactic acidosis. In: Marks V, Hales CN, eds. *Essays in Medical Biochemistry*. London: Biochemical Society and Association of Clinical Biochemists, 1975:81–103.
31. Mizock BA. Controversies in lactic acidosis: implications in critically ill patients. *JAMA* 1987;258:497–501.
32. Laine GA, Allen SJ. Left ventricular myocardial edema: lymph flow, interstitial fibrosis and cardiac function. *Circ Res* 1991;68:1713.
33. Stewart PA. Modern quantitative acid-base chemistry. *Can J Physiol Pharmacol* 1983;61:1444–1461.
34. Kellum JA. Recent advances in acid-base physiology applied to critical care. In: Vincent J-L, ed. *Yearbook of intensive care and emergency medicine*. Berlin: Springer, 1998:577–587.
35. Cross HR, Clarke K, Opie LH, et al. Is lactate-induced myocardial ischaemic injury mediated by decreased pH or increased intracellular lactate? *J Mol Cell Cardiol* 1995;27:1369–1381.
36. Samaja M, Allibardi S, Milano G, et al. Differential depression of myocardial function and metabolism by lactate and H$^+$. *Am J Physiol* 1999;276:H3–H8.
37. Stacpoole PW, Harman EM, Curry SH, et al. Treatment of lactic acidosis with dichloroacetate. *N Engl J Med* 1983;309:390–396.
38. Preiser JC, Moulart D, Vincent JL. Dichloroacetate administration in the treatment of endotoxin shock. *Circ Shock* 1990;30:221–228.
39. Stacpoole PW, Wright EC, Baumgartner TG, et al. Natural history and course of acquired lactic acidosis in adults. DCA-Lactic Acidosis Study Group. *Am J Med* 1994;97:47–54.
40. Nelson DP, Beyer C, Samsel RW, et al. Pathological supply dependence of O$_2$ uptake during bacteremia in dogs. *J Appl Physiol* 1987; 63:1487–1492.
41. De Backer D, Zhang H, Vincent JL. Models to study the relation between oxygen consumption and oxygen delivery during an acute reduction in blood flow: comparison of balloon filling in the inferior vena cava, tamponade, and hemorrhage. *Shock* 1995;4:107–112.
42. Cain SM, Curtis SE. Whole body and regional O$_2$ uptake/delivery

and lactate flux in endotoxic dogs. *Adv Exp Med Biol* 1992;316: 401–408.

43. Zhang H, Rogiers P, De Backer D, et al. Regional arteriovenous differences in PCO$_2$ and pH can reflect critical organ oxygen delivery during endotoxemia. *Shock* 1996;5:349–359.

44. Zhang H, Smail N, Cabral A, et al. Hepato-splanchnic blood flow and oxygen extraction capabilities during experimental tamponade: effects of endotoxin. *J Surg Res* 1999;81:129–138.

45. Samsel RW, Cherqui D, Pietrabissa A, et al. Hepatic oxygen and lactate extraction during stagnant hypoxia. *J Appl Physiol* 1991;70:186–193.

46. Henao FJ, Daes JE, Dennis RJ. Risk factors for multiorgan failure: a case-control study. *J Trauma* 1991;31:74–80.

47. Bakker J, Gris P, Coffernils M, et al. Serial blood lactate levels can predict the development of multiple organ failure following septic shock. *Am J Surg.* 1996;171:221–226.

48. Shoemaker WC, Appel PL, Kram HB. Tissue oxygen debt as a determinant of lethal and nonlethal postoperative organ failure. *Crit Care Med* 1988;16:1117–1120.

49. Shoemaker WC, Appel PL, Kram HB. Role of oxygen debt in the development of organ failure sepsis, and death in high-risk surgical patients. *Chest* 1992;102:208–215.

50. Davis JW, Shackford SR, Mackersie RC, et al. Base deficit as a guide to volume resuscitation. *J Trauma* 1988;28:1464–1467.

51. Siegel JH, Rivkind AI, Dalal S, et al. Early physiologic predictors of injury severity and death in blunt multiple trauma. *Arch Surg* 1990; 125:498–508.

52. Shoemaker WC, Montgomery ES, Kaplan E, et al. Physiologic patterns in surviving and nonsurviving shock patients: use of sequential cardiorespiratory variables in defining criteria for therapeutic goals and early warning of death. *Arch Surg* 1973;106:630–636.

53. Weil MH, Afifi AA. Experimental and clinical studies on lactate and pyruvate as indicators of the severity of acute circulatory failure (shock). *Circulation* 1970;41:989–1001.

54. Siegel JH, Fabian M, Smith JA, et al. Use of recombinant hemoglobin solution in reversing lethal hemorrhagic hypovolemic oxygen debt shock. *J Trauma* 1997;42:199–212.

55. Menzel M, Doppenberg EM, Zauner A, et al. Increased inspired oxygen concentration as a factor in improved brain tissue oxygenation and tissue lactate levels after severe human head injury. *J Neurosurg* 1999;91:1–10.

56. Polonen P, Ruokonen E, Hippelainen M, et al. A prospective, randomized study of goal-oriented hemodynamic therapy in cardiac surgical patients. *Anesth Analg* 2000;90:1052–1059.

57. Claridge JA, Crabtree TD, Pelletier SJ, et al. Persistent occult hypoperfusion is associated with a significant increase in infection rate and mortality in major trauma patients. *J Trauma* 2000;48:8–15.

58. Blow O, Magliore L, Claridge JA, et al. The golden hour and the silver day: detection and correction of occult hypoperfusion within 24 hours improves outcome from major trauma. *J Trauma* 1999;47:964–969.

59. James JH, Luchette FA, McCarter FD, et al. Lactate is an unreliable indicator of tissue hypoxia in injury or sepsis. *Lancet* 1999;354: 505–508.

60. Halmagyi DF, Irving MH, Gillett DJ, et al. Effect of adrenergic blockade on consequences of sustained epinephrine infusion. *J Appl Physiol* 1967;23:171–177.

61. Vary TC, Siegel JH, Nakatani T, et al. Effect of sepsis on activity of pyruvate dehydrogenase complex in skeletal muscle and liver. *Am J Physiol* 1986;250:E634–E640.

62. Levraut J, Ciebiera JP, Chave S, et al. Mild hyperlactatemia in stable septic patients is due to impaired lactate clearance rather than overproduction. *Am J Respir Crit Care Med* 1998;157:1021–1026.

63. Friedman G, De Backer D, Shahla M, et al. Oxygen supply dependency can characterize septic shock. *Intensive Care Med* 1998;24: 118–123.

64. Vincent JL, Roman A, De Backer D, et al. Oxygen uptake/supply dependency: effects of short-term dobutamine infusion. *Am Rev Respir Dis* 1990;142:2–7.

65. Gaglio G. Die milchsaure des blutes un ihre ursprungsstatten. *Arch Anat Physiol* 1886;10:400–414.

66. Sheperd AP, Granger HJ, Smith EE, et al. Local control of tissue oxy-

gen delivery and its contribution to the regulation of cardiac output. *Am J Physiol* 1973;225:747–755.

67. Toffaletti J, Hammes ME, Gray R, et al. Lactate measured in diluted and undiluted whole blood and plasma: comparison of methods and effect of hematocrit. *Clin Chem* 1992;38:2430–2434.

68. Detry B, Nullens W, Cao ML, et al. Assessment of the lactate biosensor methodology. *Eur Respir J* 1998;11:183–187.

69. Noordally O, Vincent JL. Evaluation of a new, rapid lactate analyzer in critical care. *Intensive Care Med* 1999;25:508–513.

70. Godje O, Fuchs A, Dewald O, et al. [On-site laboratory monitoring on the intensive care unit: blood gas, electrolyte, glucose, hemoglobin and lactate determination with the CIBA Corning 865 Analysis System]. *Anasthesiol Intensivmed Notfallmed Schmerzther* 1997;32:549–556.

71. Frankel HL, Rozycki GS, Ochsner MG, et al. Minimizing admission laboratory testing in trauma patients: use of a microanalyzer. *J Trauma* 1994;37:728–736.

72. Brinkert W, Bakker J. Lactate measurements in critically ill patients with a hand-held analyser. *Intensive Care Med* 1999;25:966–969.

73. Slomovitz BM, Lavery RF, Tortella BJ, et al. Validation of a hand-held lactate device in determination of blood lactate in critically injured patients. *Crit Care Med* 1998;26:1523–1528.

74. Wandrup J, Tvede K, Grinsted J, et al. Stat measurements of L-lactate in whole blood and cerebrospinal fluid assessed. *Clin Chem* 1989;35: 1740–1743.

75. Buono MJ, Yeager JE. Intraerythrocyte and plasma lactate concentrations during exercise in humans. *Eur J Appl Physiol* 1986;55:326–329.

76. Harris RT, Dudley GA. Exercise alters the distribution of ammonia and lactate in blood. *J Appl Physiol* 1989;66:313–317.

77. Foxdal P, Sjödin B, Rudstam H, et al. Lactate concentration differences in plasma, whole blood, capillary finger blood and erythrocytes during submaximal graded exercise in humans. *Eur J Appl Physiol* 1990;61:218–222.

78. Weil MH, Michaels S, Rackow EC. Comparison of blood lactate concentrations in central venous, pulmonary artery, and arterial blood. *Crit Care Med* 1987;15:489–490.

79. Jackson EVJ, Wiese J, Sigal B, et al. Effects of crystalloid solutions on circulating lactate concentrations. Part 1. Implications for the proper handling of blood specimens obtained from critically ill patients [Comments]. *Crit Care Med* 1997;25:1840–1846.

80. Brown SD, Clark C, Gutierrez G. Pulmonary lactate release in patients with sepsis and the adult respiratory distress syndrome. *J Crit Care* 1996;11:2–8.

81. Kellum JA, Kramer DJ, Lee K, et al. Release of lactate by the lung in acute lung injury. *Chest* 1997;111:1301–1305.

82. Foxdal P, Sjödin A, Ostman B, et al. The effect of different blood sampling sites and analyses on the relationship between exercise intensity and 4.0 mmol.l-1 blood lactate concentration. *Eur J Appl Physiol* 1991;63:52–54.

83. Lavery RF, Livingston DH, Tortella BJ, et al. The utility of venous lactate to triage injured patients in the trauma center. *J Am Coll Surg* 2000;190:656–664.

84. Cady LDJ, Weil MH, Afifi AA, et al. Quantitation of severity of critical illness with special reference to blood lactate. *Crit Care Med* 1973; 1:75–80.

85. Wiese J, Didwania A, Kerzner R, et al. Use of different anticoagulants in test tubes for analysis of blood lactate concentrations. Part 2. Implications for the proper handling of blood specimens obtained from critically ill patients [Comments]. *Crit Care Med* 1997;25:1847–1850.

86. Weiskopf RB, Viele MK, Feiner J, et al. Human cardiovascular and metabolic response to acute, severe isovolemic anemia. *JAMA* 1998; 279:217–221.

87. Kaufman BS, Griffel MI, Rackow EC, et al. Resolution of lactic acidosis after sedation of a patient with acute myocardial infarction and left ventricular failure. *Crit Care Med* 1991;19:120–122.

88. Rouby JJ, Eurin B, Glaser P, et al. Hemodynamic and metabolic effects of morphine in the critically ill. *Circulation* 1981;64:53–59.

89. Boyd O, Grounds M, Bennett D. The dependency of oxygen consumption on oxygen delivery in critically ill postoperative patients is mimicked by variations in sedation. *Chest* 1992;101:1619–1624.

90. Aubier M, Viires N, Syllie G, et al. Respiratory muscle contribution

to lactic acidosis in low cardiac output. *Am Rev Respir Dis* 1982;126: 648–652.

91. Hussain SNA, Simkus G, Roussos C. Respiratory muscle fatigue: a cause of ventilatory failure in septic shock. *J Appl Physiol* 1985;58: 2033–2040.

92. Hebert PC, Wells G, Tweeddale M, et al. Does transfusion practice affect mortality in critically ill patients? Transfusion Requirements in Critical Care (TRICC) Investigators and the Canadian Critical Care Trials Group. *Am J Respir Crit Care Med* 1997;155:1618–1623.

93. Hebert PC, Wells G, Blajchman MA, et al. A multicenter, randomized, controlled clinical trial of transfusion requirements in critical care. Transfusion Requirements in Critical Care Investigators, Canadian Critical Care Trials Group [Comments]. *N Engl J Med* 1999;340:409–417.

94. Reinhart K, Bloos F, Konig F, et al. Reversible decrease of oxygen consumption by hyperoxia. *Chest* 1991;99:690–694.

95. Marik PE, Sibbald WJ. Effect of stored-blood transfusion on oxygen delivery in patients with sepsis. *JAMA* 1993;269:3024–3029.

96. Haupt MT, Gilbert EM, Carlson RW. Fluid loading increases oxygen consumption in septic patients with lactic acidosis. *Am Rev Respir Dis* 1985;131:912–916.

97. Shoemaker WC, Appel PL, Kram HB, et al. Comparison of hemodynamic and oxygen transport effects of dopamine and dobutamine in critically ill surgical patients. *Chest* 1989;96:120–126.

98. Cooper DJ, Walley KR, Wiggs BR, et al. Bicarbonate does not improve hemodynamics in critically ill patients who have lactic acidosis: a prospective, controlled clinical study. *Ann Intern Med* 1990; 112:492–498.

99. Mathieu D, Neviere R, Billard V, et al. Effects of bicarbonate therapy on hemodynamics and tissue oxygenation in patients with lactic acidosis: a prospective, controlled clinical study. *Crit Care Med* 1991;19: 1352–1356.

100. Gramm J, Smith S, Gamelli RL, et al. Effect of transfusion on oxygen transport in critically ill patients. *Shock* 1996;5:190–193.

101. Crowl AC, Young JS, Kahler DM, et al. Occult hypoperfusion is associated with increased morbidity in patients undergoing early femur fracture fixation. *J Trauma* 2000;48:260–267.

102. Vincent JL, Dufaye P, Berre J, et al. Serial lactate determinations during circulatory shock. *Crit Care Med* 1983;11:449–451.

103. James JH, Fang CH, Schrantz SJ, et al. Linkage of aerobic glycolysis to sodium-potassium transport in rat skeletal muscle: implications for increased muscle lactate production in sepsis. *J Clin Invest* 1996; 98:2388–2397.

104. Almenoff PL, Leavy J, Weil MH, et al. Prolongation of the half-life of lactate after maximal exercise in patients with hepatic dysfunction. *Crit Care Med* 1989;17:870–873.

105. Suistomaa M, Ruokonen E, Kari A, et al. Time-pattern of lactate and lactate to pyruvate ratio in the first 24 hours of intensive care emergency admissions. *Shock* 2000;14:8–12.

106. Bernardin G, Pradier C, Tiger F, et al. Blood pressure and arterial lactate level are early indicators of short-term survival in human septic shock. *Intensive Care Med* 1996;22:17–25.

107. Creteur J, De Backer D, Vincent JL. A dobutamine test can disclose hepatosplanchnic hypoperfusion in septic patients. *Am J Respir Crit Care Med* 1999;160:839–845.

108. De Backer D, Creteur J, Noordally O, et al. Does hepato-splanchnic VO_2/DO_2 dependency exist in critically ill septic patients? *Am J Respir Crit Care Med* 1998;157:1219–1225.

109. Ince C, Sinaasappel M. Microcirculatory oxygenation and shunting in sepsis and shock. *Crit Care Med* 1999;27:1369–1377.

110. Jensen JC, Buresh C, Norton JA. Lactic acidosis increases tumor necrosis factor secretion and transcription in vitro. *J Surg Res* 1990; 49:350–353.

111. Rady MY, Rivers EP, Nowak RM. Resuscitation of the critically ill in the ED: responses of blood pressure, heart rate, shock index, central venous oxygen saturation, and lactate. *Am J Emerg Med* 1996;14: 218–225.

112. Bannon MP, O'Neill CM, Martin M, et al. Central venous oxygen saturation, arterial base deficit, and lactate concentration in trauma patients. *Am Surg* 1995;61:738–745.

113. Smith I, Kumar P, Molloy S, et al. Base excess and lactate as prognostic indicators for patients admitted to intensive care. *Intensive Care Med.* 2000.

114. Bakker J. Lactate: may I have your votes please? *Intensive Care Med.* 2001;27:6–11.

115. Gan SC, Barr J, Arieff AI, et al. Biguanide-associated lactic acidosis: case report and review of the literature. *Arch Intern Med* 1992;152: 2333–2336.

116. Goo AK, Carson DS, Bjelajac A. Metformin: a new treatment option for non-insulin-dependent diabetes mellitus. *J Fam Pract* 1996;42: 612–618.

117. Luft D, Schmulling RM, Eggstein M. Lactic acidosis in biguanide-treated diabetics: a review of 330 cases. *Diabetologia* 1978;14:75–87.

118. Schmiechen NJ, Han C, Milzman DP. ED use of rapid lactate to evaluate patients with acute chest pain. *Ann Emerg Med* 1997;30: 571–577.

119. Mavric Z, Zaputovic L, Zagar D, et al. Usefulness of blood lactate as a predictor of shock development in acute myocardial infarction. *Am J Cardiol* 1991;67:565–568.

120. Henning RJ, Weil MH, Weiner F. Blood lactate as prognostic indicator of survival in patients with acute myocardial infarction. *Circ Shock* 1982;9:307–315.

121. Müllner M, Sterz F, Domanovits H, et al. The association between blood lactate concentration on admission, duration of cardiac arrest, and functional neurological recovery in patients resuscitated from a ventricular fibrillation. *Intensive Care Med* 1997;23:1138–1143.

122. Delashaw J, Duling BR. A study of the functional elements regulating capillary perfusion in striated muscle. *Microvasc Res* 1988;36: 162–171.

123. Sauaia A, Moore FA, Moore EE, et al. Multiple organ failure can be predicted as early as 12 hours after injury. *J Trauma* 1998;45: 291–301.

124. Oda S, Hirasawa H, Sugai T, et al. Cellular injury score for multiple organ failure severity scoring system. *J Trauma* 1998;45: 304–310.

125. Manikis P, Jankowski S, Zhang H, et al. Correlation of serial blood lactate levels to organ failure and mortality after trauma. *Am J Emerg Med* 1995;13:619–622.

126. Abramson D, Scalea TM, Hitchcock R, et al. Lactate clearance and survival following injury. *J Trauma* 1993;35:584–588.

127. Scalea TM, Maltz S, Yelon J, et al. Resuscitation of multiple trauma and head injury: role of crystalloid fluids and inotropes. *Crit Care Med* 1994;22:1610–1615.

128. Shirey TL. *Interpreting lactate in critically ill patients*. Waltham, MA: Nova Biomedical, 1997.

129. Brivet F, Bernardin M, Cherin P, et al. Hyperchloremic acidosis during grand mal seizure lactic acidosis. *Intensive Care Med* 1994;20: 27–31.

130. Appel D, Rubenstein R, Schrager K, et al. Lactic acidosis in severe asthma. *Am J Med* 1983;75:580–584.

131. Prause G, Kaltenböck F, Doppler R. [Preclinical blood gas analysis. 2. Experience with three blood gas analyzers in emergency care]. *Anaesthesist* 1998;47:490–495.

132. Schieveld SJM, Bakker J. Prehospital blood lactate levels in emergency medicine. *Intensive Care Med* 1997;23:S183(abst).

133. Kost GJ. Point-of-care testing ⇒ The hybrid laboratory ⇒ Knowledge optimization. In: Kost GJ, ed. *Handbook of clinical automation, robotics, and optimization*. New York: John Wiley and Sons, 1996; 757–838.

40

CONTROLLING ECONOMICS, PREVENTING ERRORS, AND OPTIMIZING OUTCOMES IN POINT-OF-CARE TESTING

GERALD J. KOST

This chapter explains how to use point-of-care testing (POCT) to create value and improve both medical and economic outcomes. The first section summarizes economic principles, cost-benefit evidence, and controlling measures, and explains the need for a macroeconomic perspective. Economic efficiency and medical efficacy depend, in part, on the prevention of medical errors. Therefore, the second section introduces error reduction systems and safeguards based on a U.S. national survey and consensus process. The third section explains the concepts, logic, and tools of outcomes management and optimization for POCT. The chapter concludes with future goals and practical plans for POCT and patients.

CONTROLLING ECONOMICS

Microeconomic Principles

Microeconomics deals with unique factors that affect economic functions, while macroeconomics considers behavior, interrelationships, and overall economic outcomes (1–12). Table 40.1 summarizes principles of economic analysis for POCT (13–60). Innovating, restructuring, and reengineering POCT programs entail designing alternatives, assessing benefits, and determining costs. Ideal alternatives improve outcomes without any additional expenditure. Good alternatives yield the greatest improvement for the least cost. They also grant ownership of point-of-care (POC) information directly and immediately to the caregiver since value depends on timeliness in relation to the physiological half-life of test results.

Economic analysis of POCT alternatives balances the sum of tangible benefits, such as reduced length of stay (LOS), and intangible benefits, such as physician satisfaction and convenience, against the marginal or total economic costs of diagnostic testing, to arrive at informed decisions. POCT alternatives include strategic combinations of test clusters, instrument formats (transportable, portable, or handheld), modalities (*in vitro*, *ex vivo*, or *in vivo*), and testing sites, plus connectivity (i.e., bidirectional communication between computerized information systems and

POC devices), security, and other operational factors. Even if expenses increase, one should select POCT alternatives that most cost effectively improve patient care.

POCT is justified, in part, by *value-added clinical benefits and productivity* that offset the marginal costs of equipment, consumables, labor, and space (50). Managed care diminishes clinical laboratory economies of scale, and downsizing and regionalizing reduce high fixed costs. Outpatient, urgent care, and ambulatory surgery centers economize health system services. For POCT, undue emphasis on costs per test will "miss the forest for the trees." Cost-benefit judgments regarding selection of the most viable POCT alternatives depend heavily on need, site, and schedule, as well as on variables not readily apparent, such as hidden, downstream, and external failure costs. Do not assess the economic value of POCT in isolation without considering all clinical ramifications.

Cost-Benefit Evidence

Appendices I and II in this text summarize POCT studies, their objectives, and medical and economic outcomes. The findings help decision makers solve problems, set priorities, and select alternatives, but represent individual institutional experiences and a guide for inquiry and planning, not a prescription for action. Generalizations invite trouble. Cost-effectiveness analysis, consideration of marginal costs of competing alternatives, and other means of economic assessment must be individualized to the institution and setting. Managed care requires continual improvement in marginal costs. The POCT director, POCT coordinator, and clinical colleagues should customize objectives, design fiscal criteria, engage in economic analysis (see Table 40.1), and then, make business choices, even if based on "fuzzy" data when clear-cut knowledge of economic consequences or actual outcomes is lacking.

Factors such as physician time spent waiting for testing ("dwell"), finding results, calling if results are not found, identifying the date of collection versus report, remembering the pertinent history of each patient's clinical course, possibly reorder-

TABLE 40.1. PRINCIPLES OF ECONOMIC ANALYSIS FOR POINT-OF-CARE TESTING

Method	Principle
1. Activity-based costing (39)	Assignment of costs to activities required to produce POCT by linking activities to continuous or discrete cost drivers
2. Benchmarking (43)	Surveying comparable settings, institutions, or databases for standards of cost effectiveness and performance used to develop action plans and milestones for POCT efficiency
3. Contingent valuation (42)	Survey-based hypothetical and direct monetary determination of the effects of healthcare technologies, based in part on willingness to pay as a measure of longitudinal benefits
4. Cost basis and marginal analysis (54)	Calculation of POCT basis in the form of cost per test or other metric and for marginal analysis, the additional cost of performing one more test versus benefits derived from that test
5. Cost-centered management (52,58)	Management based on fixed, variable, step-function, and other costs, but often limited to the perspective of a single cost center
6. Cost-impact projection (14,15,36–38)	Quantitative costs recording using standardized forms, accounting ledgers, and task/time tables, and analysis of savings from displacing inefficient testing with POCT and transferring less critical testing to core areas
7. Defect rate-inclusive analysis (18,35,52)	A business enterprise approach that assesses preventative, appraisal, internal failure, and external failure costs, the components of total cost management, ideally with consideration also of hidden and downstream costs
8. Net present value analysis (26)	Comparison of life-cycle costs using rates of inflation for equipment, service contracts, and consumables, and a money discount rate for present value calculation, with consideration of the number of devices, volume of testing, quality control, and other expense factors
9. Opportunity cost analysis (40)	Analysis of the substitution of one testing process for another to determine the costs associated with the next best alternative based on actual (marginal) expenditures with consideration of projected volume of testing and test failure rate
10. Relative value analysis a. Cost benefit (CBA) (19,56,58)	Measure of maximum benefits relative to costs with both generally expressed in monetary or occasionally other terms
b. Cost effectiveness (CEA) (19,20,44,45,54,58–60)	Relationship between the additional cost and the outcome of one intervention ranked with another, expressed in quantitative terms, such as dollars per year of life saved, with consideration of time and preference discounting, uncertainty, and sensitivity to projections over time
c. Cost minimization (CMA) (20,59,60)	Limited comparison of only the costs of interventions, given that the benefits of the interventions are equal or equivalent
d. Cost utility (CUA)	Quantitative relationship between the additional cost and the additional health outcome of one intervention compared with another, expressed in terms of a utility index, such as the ratio of incremental cost to quality-adjusted life year (QALY)
11. Synergy analysis (47)	Identification of full fixed, variable, and overhead costs, and of units of production using a 5-year (or other term) cash flow and net present value to find benefit from combining activities
12. Value chain analysis (16)	Continuous improvement in supply chain processes by defining the customer-expected value of each step and then exceeding expectations for all process steps with appropriate quality at the lowest total cost

POCT, point-of-care testing.

ing and redrawing blood for repeat testing, and reconstructing thoughts on individual patient needs ("switching"), should be figured into the economic analyses. Labor costs for the several small processing steps required by handheld devices should not be overlooked. Numerous processing steps performed by individual caregivers may add up to a large financial burden for the health system, depending on the excess capacity of labor. Investigators often omit these factors because of difficulty measuring their effects. Opportunity costs (the value of alternative interventions performed with the same resources) challenge full assessment as well, but when analyzed, point to the cost effectiveness of POCT (40).

Use of Table 40.1 principles will enhance future POCT research studies. Cost-effectiveness analysis (CEA) allows reasonable and reproducible comparisons of competing alternatives as a basis for funding decisions. The robustness of CEA lends itself to evaluation of POCT (54). For example, using simulation modeling of oral anticoagulant therapy programs, Lafata and colleagues (45) applied CEA and found that on-site clinic monitoring improved health outcomes and was cost effective from the perspective of the provider organization. Self-testing further decreased the financial burden on patients and caregivers and was the most cost-effective alternative. Table 40.1 methods include variables that assess patient function, such as health-years-equivalent (HYE). However, studies in Appendices I and II usually omit these endpoints because disease prevalence, case mix, clinical circumstances, and limited funding can render complex analyses impractical. Nonetheless, POCT programs benefit from some form of cost-benefit evaluation of alternatives.

Collaborative decisions regarding POCT should be based on explicitly assigned values, correctly assessed costs, and clearly defined evidence—the best available, even if imperfect (59,60). The heterogeneous settings and multifarious objectives of studies in Appendices I and II make extrapolation of the microeconomic utility of alternatives to other health systems hazardous, if not impossible. Multicenter studies are important and should be considered, but might not be applicable to individual settings. Usually by default, decisions hinge on intuitive insight, team assessment, and good judgment, all tempered by budgetary constraints. After fulfilling immediate clinical needs, POCT coordinators can make fine-tuning microeconomic adjustments to incrementally decrease high variable expenses over time. This common-sense approach is enhanced by an understanding of economic controls.

Economic Controls

POCT leadership must provide critical thinking and assert economic control of POCT (61–68). For example (7), for bedside glucose testing, the leadership team can (a) limit glucose meters to sites with high testing volumes to achieve local economies of scale (48); (b) decrease the number of meters at each site to reduce daily checks, backup, and maintenance; (c) use existing labor and increase its productivity; (d) secure purchase volume discounts from use of only a limited number of meter systems; (e) distribute uniform lists of cost elements and oversight schedules to help focus efforts to reduce expenses (24,33,37,38); and (f) standardize glucose meters, test strips, and normal ranges to decrease training, inventory, and monitoring costs. (See "Case A. Standardization of Point-of-Care Testing in an Integrated Health Care System" at the end of Part I for an illustration of standardization.) These initiatives require frequent review, process reevaluation, and cost calculation per unit of service provided, in order to determine whether inefficiencies are causing budgetary excesses (47).

Strong leadership for handheld glucose testing also helps galvanize economically valuable initiatives (7) designed to (a) select user-friendly instruments that minimize repeat testing; (b) minimize lot changes and maximize expiration terms; (c) streamline the use of quality control (QC) and proficiency testing (PT) materials; (d) systematize test strip identity to avoid theft; (e) implement QC lock-out and other security measures (see second section); (f) centralize purchasing, join buying groups, and bid competitively; (g) obtain vendor support for personnel training, evaluations, and other functions; and (h) help nursing enhance the management of handheld testing programs (see chapter 13). These initiatives apply generally to POCT programs and to instruments other than handheld glucose meters. Harmonization of test clusters, devices, methods, sample matrices, QC, and other factors increases efficiency and cost effectiveness.

POCT-associated strategic controls with potential economic gain include (a) patient-centering of multiple-analyte test clusters in the most costly acute care situations (69,70) (e.g., organ transplantation, burns, leukemia, trauma, surgery, prematurity, and intensive care), in critical procedures (e.g., cardiopulmonary resuscitation, cardiac catheterization, and hemodialysis), in conditions with the highest cumulative transfusion costs (71,72) (e.g., cardiothoracic procedures, bone marrow transplant, liver transplant, and acute leukemia), and in situations where there are test volume break-even points (31); (b) accelerating decision cycles with POCT to decrease therapeutic turnaround time (TTAT), operative time, and LOS (61–68); (c) creating proximity of testing to the patient to avoid expensive courier or pneumatic transportation of specimens; (d) restructuring, reengineering, and redesigning processes, work flow, and human

resources with POCT to reduce costs in episodes of care (73); (e) analyzing the cost impact of POCT as a mechanism for displacing inefficient testing and transferring less critical testing from satellite sites and stat areas to core facilities (14,15); (f) cutting clinical laboratory fixed costs (24); (g) identifying potential synergy in laboratory services to produce benefits from combining testing activities (47) [e.g., through modular stepwise automation (74,75)]; (h) eliminating standing orders and reducing tests per decision cycle, care episode, and follow-up encounter; (i) relocating underutilized specialized labor during patient census fluctuations and making up for critical labor shortages among medical technologists (28); (j) not adding POCT to existing layers of traditional methods, but instead removing slow, duplicative, and unnecessary testing in the conventional laboratory (51); and (k) surveying physician, nurse, and patient satisfaction to enhance performance across administrative and functional boundaries.

Fiscal control-analytic tools (Table 40.1) applied to POCT include (a) net present-value analysis, which determines POCT instrument and reagent life-cycle costs based on competitive quotes of pricing data from suppliers (26); (b) cost-based accounting (14,15,37,38) and cost-centered management (24, 52), which operate on fixed (typically low), variable (usually high), step-function (discrete, volume-dependent), and indirect POCT costs, and also may include analysis of hidden (e.g., blood transfusion to replace phlebotomy losses), downstream (e.g., transfusion infections), and marginal or incremental costs; (c) activity-based costing, which assigns POCT costs to required activities based on resource consumption and cost drivers within an organization (39); (d) defect rate-inclusive analysis, which encompasses preventive (e.g., QC), appraisal (e.g., PT), internal failure (e.g., lost specimens), and external failure (e.g., late results that delay treatment) costs (18,35,52); and (e) explicit billing for POCT services to speed payment and reduce bad debt (see chapter 36).

Broader systems-oriented initiatives with economic benefits include (a) "ABC analysis," a type of medical needs-based assessment (adapted from inventory control) where tests are ranked according to priorities as, A, critical tests needed on site, B, less critical tests that can be moved, and C, routine tests for which response time allows performance elsewhere (47); (b) transitioning to outpatient services with minimal fixed costs, such as self-monitoring of blood glucose and near-patient and self-monitoring of prothrombin time for ambulatory patients (76,77); (c) use of *ex vivo* and *in vivo* monitoring (and closed-loop technologies when available); (d) annual diagnosis-related group (DRG) analysis to determine where POCT can help manage the most expensive or longest-duration conditions prevalent in the health system and community; (e) competitive positioning in the medical marketplace through screening, monitoring, and well-patient care for better patient-customer satisfaction; and (f) connectivity to facilitate POCT-generated knowledge transfer for time savings and informatics efficiencies.

Fiscal Judgment

Several of the controlling measures above extend beyond simple POCT device evaluations, method comparisons, and isolated applications. The interdepartmental hybrid team should challenge the notion of strictly fiscal boundaries for POCT. Generally, conventional testing has lower marginal costs compared to the fully loaded incremental costs of POCT. However, singular microeconomic maneuvers motivated by comparisons of relative costs per test without consideration of broader economic effects in terms of cost per episode, intermediate outcome, or covered life result in unproductive actions. Management of multidimensional facets in a POCT program inherently requires an intuitive approach and multidisciplinary economic cooperation to trim the bottom line for survival in fast-paced medicine characterized currently by a shrinking resource base.

POCT program leaders should exercise caution. Trade-offs of accuracy and speed, if allowed at all in diagnostic testing, must be assessed carefully to avoid loss of scientific excellence and prevent medical errors. Commercial competitors quickly are introducing new POC devices, often birthed by venture capital, nursed to maturity by public stock offerings, and then consolidated by acquisitions. The recent plethora of POC instruments, even though more accurate, precise, and analytically faster than prior generations, encourages redundant testing and feeds economic waste. High clinical potential may be counterbalanced by weak evidence of medical efficacy, cost effectiveness, or offsetting savings. As investors recoup start-up costs and POC devices saturate the marketplace, costs inevitably will decrease, making some deployment decisions obvious (40), but if POCT is not controlled sensibly, ubiquitous access and increased volume of testing could drive up overall national healthcare expenditures.

The value of POCT must transcend everyday microeconomics. When viewed as a collective body of evidence, numerous research studies (see Appendices I and II) show that fast, POCT-driven, decision making produces economic savings from improved clinical efficiency, conserved blood volume, reduced transfusions, decreased time in critical care, shorter length of hospital stay, prevention of complications (e.g., diabetes), and other efficiencies that lower overall healthcare costs. Intramural and extramural risk-adjusted comparisons of economic outcomes help strategic planning (69,78). Sound economic management presents the laboratorian with challenges and opportunities for partnering with health system leaders. Collective judgment, consensus decisions, and coordinated actions outweigh fiscal uncertainty and enhance benefits.

For example, POCT studies in the emergency department (ED) have yielded equivocal results. Three papers (79–81) showed that POCT did not improve endpoint outcomes. Meanwhile, ED response time has stagnated nationwide, and emergency physicians are dissatisfied with sluggish laboratory testing (82). POCT has merit because on-site testing facilitates fast TTAT, rapid decision making, and expedient therapy of the most pressing medical problems (see chapter 7). Newly reimbursed hourly expenses for patient observation in chest pain evaluation units means that even small accelerations in TTAT improve efficiency. If, in the opinion of ED physicians, conventional laboratory testing is deemed inadequate, then POCT should be integrated into ED protocols to help take diagnostic testing off the critical path (83) and meet the high demands of emergency medicine. Successful healthcare systems adapt and integrate fast TTAT delivery processes. Hence, fiscal judgment must balance changing practices and competing priorities.

"Syntegration"

Systems integration requires process integration. The evidence in Appendices I and II weighs in favor of integrated economic and medical outcomes management. The POCT coordinator and director can frequently rework the POCT program to optimize bedside practice strategies (67). Collaborative leadership, visionary planning, and clinical champions factor heavily into success, especially in critical care settings that require rapid response and systems integration. While prime advantages of POCT include immediacy, flexibility, and simplicity, a different and *higher conceptual level* of strategic planning is needed to reap the full economic benefits of POCT.

POCT yields its greatest overall economic benefits and value to patients when *fully integrated* into clinical services (see the illustrations in the third section of this chapter). If integrated, POCT consistently produces important process changes. After restructuring, reengineering, redesigning, and carefully integrating POCT, investigators have documented valuable cost reductions through process simplification and labor savings, even without undertaking cost-effectiveness, cost-minimization, or other formal analyses. As a partial paradigm, the conventional laboratory lacks direct bedside engagement and cannot achieve the integration naturally inherent in POCT.

Much current effort is being expended appropriately on POCT connectivity, computer interfacing, networking, and data management (84–103). However, physical and electronic integration alone fall short of the clinical need for high-level synthesis of crucial medical data. Simultaneous integration and synthesis ("syntegration") create greater value than either alone (Fig. 40.1). That is, mechanistic integration and heuristic synthesis at the bedside multiply the total yield of POCT as a knowledge tool, and in terms of the economic perspective, help garner multiple benefits for the entire critical care unit, acute care center, and healthcare system.

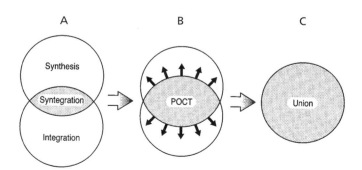

FIGURE 40.1. Dynamic syntegration. Simultaneous **(A)** integration and synthesis ("syntegration") help improve outcomes. Point-of-care testing expands **(B)** syntegration for union **(C)** of integration with synthesis, that is, knowledge optimization (see Chapter 2).

Summary—Macroeconomic Perspective

Resource constraints demand valuation in the clinical context, especially in critical care, where relatively high inelastic expenses (104–115) strain already tight budgets. LOS correlates with overall costs, and for many DRGs, shorter LOS can reduce laboratory costs, which at academic medical centers, for example, constitute approximately 9% of total costs for medical, and 6%, for surgical conditions (69,70). Therefore, targeting POCT to reduce LOS can achieve budgetary savings, both in the conventional laboratory and at the POC. The economic perspective must not be limited to just one site or the other.

Economic analysis (Table 40.1), cost-benefit evidence (see Appendix II), and economic controls should be considered together when implementing POCT. If undertaken by the POCT leadership team, collaborative economic planning by means of cost-effectiveness analysis (CEA) has the potential to preserve high quality while achieving organization-specific priorities for patient care. Laboratorians who adopt a broad holistic view will discover a refreshingly new and rewarding role as outcomes managers in their health systems.

When *well-directed POCT* reduces morbidity and mortality or provides other clinical benefits, such as fast TTAT, by fitting naturally into patient work flow, physicians and nurses will adopt POCT, even if it costs more than conventional laboratory testing. Escalating healthcare costs, an aging population, more critically ill patients, managed care, capitated reimbursement, and national priorities call for reassessment of missions. A *macroeconomic perspective* will balance microeconomic analysis, POCT resources, and medical professionalism.

PREVENTING ERRORS

National Priority

The Committee on Quality of Health Care in America of the Institute of Medicine (IOM) recently published two guidelines intended to reduce excessively high rates of patient deaths caused by medical errors (116,117). Errors in laboratory testing, which often occur preanalytically, can contribute to inappropriate care or modification of therapy (118,119). POCT solves the problem of slow response during the preanalytic phase of testing and also reduces preanalytic error. Although exact error rates challenge quantitation, bedside diagnostic testing, by generating immediately actionable results, may contribute to serious medical errors (67,120–122) if results are not accurate.

As more testing shifts to the POC (62,64) and is performed by increasing numbers of physicians, nurses, and nurse practitioners, there should be adequate safeguards to prevent medical errors and reduce risk. Incorrect results that trigger the wrong treatment may generate more harm than no results at all. POCT should not increase risk, uncertainty, or liability. Personnel participating in the POCT program should enculturate safety (116,117,123) to make error prevention a primary concern and responsibility. Responsibility also rests with industry to provide POCT systems that are validated as safe for each intended clinical application. Current regulatory oversight and QC routines do not meet needs for error reduction in POCT programs.

This section presents new systems and safeguards that will improve the performance, quality, and safety of POCT (124,125). These systems, based on expert specifications, extensive review, and consensus opinion, are intended for error prevention on POC instruments. Prevention of errors in POCT will avoid patient harm, and indirectly, will improve patient outcomes. Hence, error prevention systems should be part of each POCT program. A systems approach positions POCT at the vanguard of an important national priority, rather than disadvantaging POCT to "catch up" at the expense of practice standards and patient welfare.

Consensus Process

The consensus error prevention systems evolved in three steps. Forty-six POCT experts were surveyed in the United States. The experts were selected for geographic diversity and professional leadership. Experts were asked: (a) to state whether lock-out of nonvalidated operators was needed; (b) to list the five most important objectives for security, validation, and performance; and (c) to describe unique aspects of error prevention used or needed in their local POCT programs. Open-ended survey questions encouraged creative responses and original design specifications. The 37 responding experts (37 of 46, an 80.4% response rate) came from a broad range of disciplines in academic health systems and health maintenance organizations distributed geographically in 19 states.

From the tabulated survey responses, three mutually compatible parallel systems were designed for security, validation, and performance functions on POC instruments in order to fulfill the error prevention objectives stated by the experts. An additional emergency system was added to meet expert and professional requirements for medically needed POCT during crises and disasters. A safeguards category specified expert requirements for protecting critical information and patients.

The four error prevention systems and safeguards were critiqued and rated quantitatively (125) by groups of professional managers, specialists, clinicians, and researchers in POCT to whom I presented the concepts in five venues at national and state meetings. Feedback helped improve the system designs and safeguards incrementally until they stabilized in the form of the final consensus configurations presented here. Stabilization occurred after the fourth public presentation and feedback iteration. A total of 260 professionals participated in the national survey and consensus process.

Error Reduction Systems

Three systems (Table 40.2A–C) yield several flexible combinations with which a POCT director and coordinator can adjust risk, limit access, and improve performance according to individual institutional objectives. The security system (Table 40.2A) prioritizes methods of instrument operational security versus risk trade-offs. The validation system (Table 40.2B) for operator access has three levels. The standard level allows the user to review and download QC and patient test results, but excludes actual testing. The intermediate level allows the POC

TABLE 40.2. SYSTEMS TO PREVENT MEDICAL ERRORS IN POINT-OF-CARE TESTING (125)

A. Security System for Point-of-Care Instruments

Tier	Protection Feature	Potential Risk
Low	Require key entry of personal identification number (PIN) or password; becomes *basic* level if *both* PIN and matching password are required	High risk because the PIN or password may be shared or entered incorrectly, and somewhat inconvenient, but the least expensive
Basic	Use badge bar-code reader, magnetic button or strip scan, radio-frequency badge, or digital certificate/signature (with password)	More secure since users are less likely to swap bar codes, buttons, cards, badges, or certificates
High	Identify operator biometrically using optical fingerprint, digits angle, iris pattern, voice or face recognition, or retinal scan	Least risk but the most expensive and may be impractical for portable or small handheld devices

B. Validation System for Access to Results, Testing, and Functions

Level	Access
Standard	Review and/or download (transfer) test results
Intermediate	Above, plus operator enabled to perform patient testing, quality control (QC), and proficiency testing
Master	Access to all testing, performance, setup, and instrument functions

C. Performance System for Quality Control

Priority	Action
Routine	QC required at timed intervals (e.g., day of use, each shift, or defined period) or when use of the device triggers a QC check
Advanced	Above, plus QC check demanded if range exceeded, result rejected, or error detected
Critical	All of the above, but instrument use released only with a physical maintenance key following correction of serious problems

D. Emergency Override System

Emergency personnel must be trained and certified periodically in POCT.
Hospital defines conditions for emergency access to testing, which is flagged and tracked, following mandatory entry of operator's PIN.
  Password (i.e., basic security level) or special emergency code (e.g., in a "break box") also may be required.
During emergencies, operator is warned, initiates testing, and is accountable for recovery actions.
For instruments with override capability and those used during disasters, QC is performed in advance as part of daily work flow to assure that
  each instrument is prepared for critical patient testing.

operator to perform testing. The master level grants access to all testing, performance, setup, and instrument functions, including calibration, reportable ranges, linearity, critical limits, and user-defined functions.

The performance system (Table 40.2C) has three priority levels for QC process interrupts. Mandatory performance of QC helps minimize analytic error, which can adversely affect outcomes. Experts recommended that the POCT coordinator be notified of critical problems and that instrument operation be released (i.e., cleared after the problems are solved) only with a physical maintenance key held by the POCT coordinator or director. The emergency system (Table 40.2D) enables the POCT coordinator or director to define the conditions for partially overriding the other three systems, but if done, demands tracking of the sequence of actions, recovery, and follow-up.

Experts also recommended several important safeguards, which were refined during the consensus process to arrive at the final form shown in Table 40.3. These safeguards include (a) identifying the patient; (b) reporting and documenting critical results; (c) assuring the integrity of the specimen, formats, test results, and statistical process control; (d) preventing inappropriate use of tests, reagents, calibrators, code keys (device chip inserts with test strip lot and calibration), parameters, and settings; and (e) capturing legally and financially necessary information. Safeguards also address detection and tracking of pre-

analytic (e.g., hemolysis), analytic (e.g., measurement errors), and postanalytic (e.g., lost data) problems.

Prevention Principles

Recognized methods of error reduction include (a) decreasing reliance on memory and vigilance, (b) improving information access, (c) structuring critical tasks with constraints and "forcing functions" (required actions), (d) simplifying key steps and systems, (e) standardizing processes and procedures, (f) using reminders and checklists, (g) training in small groups by means of problem simulation to develop skills in failure mode analysis, (h) providing timely information, and (i) error proofing devices (116,126,127). For example, some POC instruments have internal parallel QC and mechanisms for detecting interfering substances (see chapter 6). Identification of error modes, prediction of error expression, training and design for self-detection, and interdiction before transformation into harmful accidents represent helpful actions for protecting patients (126) and achieving the IOM goal of a 50% reduction of medical errors.

To fulfill IOM guidelines, *Health Insurance Portability and Accountability Act of 1996* regulations (128), and other sound advice (126,127,129,130), manufacturers should proactively incorporate the consensus security, validation, performance, and emergency systems into instruments (124,125) so that users will

TABLE 40.3. SAFEGUARDS FOR PATIENTS AND CRITICAL INFORMATION (125)

Identify the patient
 Use bar-coded wristband or radio-frequency badge (magnetic strip reader for outpatients).
 Verify patient identification against an electronically downloaded list (if available).
 Cross-check patient against bed location (e.g., for critically ill patients in an intensive care unit).
 Lock out testing if patient identification is invalid or unavailable.
Report and document critical results (critical, panic, or alert values)
 Build in a list of relevant critical limits and store critical results for easy access.
 Annotate, report, and flag test results that are critical immediately.
 Record individual obtaining or clinician receiving critical results.
 Request verification of critical test results (user-defined option).
Assure the integrity of specimens, formats, test results, and statistical process control
 Signal sample quantity not sufficient, volume inadequate, or wrong anticoagulant.
 Alert hemolysis, out-of-range hematocrit (or P_{O2}, pH), and interferences (e.g., bilirubin, drugs, or lipids).
 Report qualitative "<" or ">" if the test result is out of the reportable range.
 Format storage of patient and sample identification, test results, and quality control/proficiency testing (QC/PT) data.
 Track and record measurement errors, interinstrument variations, and process interrupts.
Prevent inappropriate use of tests, reagents, calibrators, code keys, parameters, and settings
 Lock out use of unnecessary tests and of invalid or unapproved reagent or calibrator lots.
 Disallow use of expired reagents, test strips, or QC materials.
 Stop use if test strips (if used) and code key do not match.
 Lock down calibration, linearity, reportable range, time, date, and other parameters.
 Embed preventative maintenance, downloading protocols, operating rules, and biohazard controls.
Capture legally and financially necessary information
 Record operator identification in prescribed data fields and append to test result record.
 Automate entry of responsible clinician or ordering physician.
 Archive time of specimen collection, results reporting, and system failures.
 Prepare to verify (for inspectors) that test and matching QC/PT results are acceptable.
 Integrate accounting, costing, charging, billing, and inventory information.

have the tools necessary to improve the safety of POCT and to test objectively manufacturers' claims of accurate and precise performance. Table 40.4 outlines the practical use of lock-out functions. The Food and Drug Administration (116,129), which reviews and approves manufacturers' claims, does not, but could, require nonvalidated operator lock-out, noncertified operator lock-out, error reduction options (e.g., lock-out if no QC performed, no data transfer done, or no PT performed), and software-based safeguards (e.g., lock-out if no patient identification) on instruments when licensing new devices and tests for POCT. Availability of these options would allow systems managers and POCT coordinators to track and analyze error-to-injury translation sequences.

Instrument access constitutes a critical gateway point for control of POCT. Human factor problems increase in likelihood with poorly trained operators and technologically complicated instruments, especially when cumulative opportunities for errors exist (131). One hundred percent of the responding experts and virtually all participants who critiqued the systems recommended that only trained, certified, and validated operators should be allowed to operate hospital-based instruments for POCT, and that security standards should be made equivalent to those used for access to other hospital systems, such as computerized medical records. Leadership should assure at least a minimum level of safety and proactively support the error prevention systems.

Selection of Options

To reduce risk, the basic (or higher) tier of security features (see Table 40.2A) should be employed. Use of a personal identification number (PIN) plus a password (alphanumeric) combina-

TABLE 40.4. LOCK-OUT OPTIONS FOR POCT PROGRAM INTEGRITY

Acronym	Lock-Out Function	Significance in Error Reduction
NCO	Noncertified operator	Prevents testing if the operator lacks education, experience, or current skills appropriate for the setting, as required by the collaborative agreement of the POCT director, POCT coordinator, and hybrid team
NVO	Nonvalidated operator	Protects the POCT program from unauthorized and inappropriate use of POC instruments
NQC	No quality control performed	Prevents testing if the QC protocol for the instrument is not followed or if QC is not performed in a timely fashion
NPI	No patient identification	Prevents testing if the patient has not been positively identified and avoids patient misidentification
NDT	No data transferred	Assures the integrity of the medical electronic record and facilitates several other functions, such as monitoring patient data, checking QC compliance, and tracking instrument errors
NPT	No proficiency testing	Prevents testing if PT requirements have not been fulfilled

POC, point of care; POCT, point-of-care testing; PT, proficiency testing; QC, quality control.

tion is preferred because of the potential for sharing a PIN. The password should be changed periodically. In systems that require only a PIN, difficulties arise in tracking the origin of test results, determining if results were produced by competent users, and correcting deficiencies. For flexibility, all three operator access levels (Table 40.2B) should be included as options on instruments. The master level should be limited to the director and/or coordinator in charge of the POCT program.

Figure 40.2 illustrates how the security, validation, and performance systems can overlap, possibly causing increased workload, process delays, and higher costs. Thus, these key elements should be managed efficiently and professionally by a hybrid team who set and enforce the rules in conjunction with the POCT director and coordinator. For example, a transportable whole-blood analyzer with several biosensor-based tests could incorporate radio-frequency badges for definitive, but fast operator identification; three levels of access control; and a physical maintenance key to release fatal quality failures once corrected.

In contrast, a consumer meter for self-monitoring of blood glucose could use PIN-gated access and remind the user to perform a QC check each new day of testing. Except for patient training in self-monitoring (e.g., glucose or pro-thrombin time) prior to discharge, the use of "open" access consumer meters that anyone can use in hospital settings invites errors. Protection features, access levels, and QC interrupts in conjunction with tracking, monitoring, and auditing of the rate of nonvalidated operator use and other compliance metrics will help identify errors by function, correct them promptly, and reduce occurrence rates. On simple instruments, "pass/fail" QC results avoid the abuse of QC routines being used for patient testing.

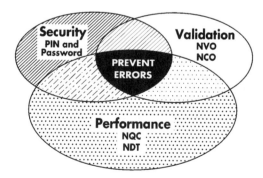

FIGURE 40.2. Selecting security, validation, and performance options. Implementing combinations of the security, validation, and performance systems help prevent errors. For example, a nurse assigned an intermediate access level performs testing (validation system) after accessing instrument operation with a PIN and password (security system), but also must follow quality control (QC) protocols (performance system) before testing patient samples (overlap in the Venn diagram center). In contrast, a validated assistant who *only* reviews results enters a PIN for access, but omits QC testing since no patient testing is performed (overlap of two systems toward the top). System options allow the point-of-care testing coordinator to select and set criteria for operator lock-out, such as nonvalidated operator, noncertified operator, no QC performed, and no data transferred (see Table 40.4).

Emergency Access

Users cannot bypass the security, validation, and performance systems, except in emergencies (see Table 40.2D). Following emergencies, the same users are held accountable within 24 hours for actions by tracking their PIN- and/or password-gated entry to instrument use. All such operators should be trained on site-specific instruments made available for emergencies and disasters. Emergency override allows testing in critical situations when failure to test could harm patients and expose a hospital to excess liability. Emergency override potentially creates problems because of (a) possible errors in clinical decisions based on erroneous test results, (b) management difficulties controlling emergency access, and (c) resulting inconsistent testing practices. Viable options include sending emergency specimens to the core laboratory by courier or calling laboratory personnel to perform testing on site.

However, during a rapidly evolving disaster, communications may be interrupted or sites of emergency care may become physically inaccessible, necessitating testing by available clinical personnel. Therefore, the operation of the emergency override system includes requirements for (a) formal planning of staff who will have access, (b) training and certifying of these individuals, (c) documenting written attestations that PINs and passwords will not be shared, and (d) performing QC in advance as part of daily work flow so that emergency-designated instruments remain perpetually ready. Backup instruments provide additional security. Social security numbers can be used temporarily for patient identification. Immediately after the incident, data should be entered into computerized systems and scrutinized. Staff members periodically conduct surveillance for overrides during nonemergent conditions. With this conservative approach, security features will not obstruct rapid response testing and teamwork (132) during emergencies and disasters.

Training, Competency, Certification, and Validation

Training helps eliminate preanalytic errors resulting from incorrect sampling, specimen mishandling, inconsistent technique, and possibly also distraction and inattention, which produce random errors. Competency assures the operator's ability to perform all phases of POCT correctly. A competency continuum can be documented through certifications and recertifications that assure individual operators meet standards for training and experience. Competency was deemed crucial by consensus participants, a position similar to that of the Joint Commission on Accreditation of HealthCare Organizations (JCAHO) (133,134) and other accreditation agencies. Accreditation agencies want proof of a quality team. Each health system must define its own goals for operator training, certification, and recertification and its own criteria for operator validation. "Validated operator" means that the individual meets all the legal and institutional requirements for instrument operation in a particular clinical setting.

Training and certification alone will not prevent errors. Repeated errors require isolation to the POCT operator responsible for them. Periodic human contact and communication encourage resolution of problems. For example, monthly e-mail notification of QC compliance and within-control scores improves operator performance (135). Real-time QC interrupts (Table 40.2C) should be carefully designed to match clinical needs, fulfill manufacturers' specifications, and encompass accreditation requirements (e.g., no patient results if QC moves out of the control range). Automated internal QC ("wet" reagent and/or "dry" electronic) performed concurrently in parallel with patient testing enhances process efficiency. Accreditation agencies require periodic review of QC results and documented correction of problems.

Safeguards

Safeguards (Table 40.3) can be implemented through instrument system software. The most important safeguards include identifying the patient (preferably by bar-coded armband), integrating critical limits (136–139), and assuring the integrity of specimens, formats, test results, and statistical process control. Some safeguards, such as verifying the sequence and timing of patient test results, QC, and PT for JCAHO accreditation inspections, require a combination of "smart" instruments, data archiving, and collaborative management of the hospital-based POCT program to complete the "quality loop" (133,134). The clinical laboratory enjoys an integral position in the loop and may elect to maintain QC and instrument logs, design split samples surveys, conduct internal PT, and confirm critical value results.

Fulfillment of other requirements, such as alerting interference from confounding variables (140–143) and drugs (144) requires bidirectional connectivity with hospital computerized databases. Root-cause analyses show that serious adverse events frequently are attributed to drug accidents (116). If a drug regimen interferes with test methods, physicians making rapid bedside decisions should be informed of possible analytic errors with a viewable comment when analyte results are displayed. Frantic activity and the rapid flow of POCT data during resuscitations or other crises highlight the importance of these drug therapy safeguards.

Connectivity

Immediately useful information represents a unique value of POCT. Previously rate limiting, connectivity (145) now is revolutionizing POC information capture. Information capture will (a) enable POCT to drive Dx-Rx processes more accurately and efficaciously, (b) improve the efficiency and efficacy of error prevention systems, (c) facilitate safeguards through shared software and information, (d) diminish postanalytic error, (e) help track error and accident episodes for identification and accountability of serious patient effects, (f) integrate POCT data in the health system, and (g) link clinical data repositories to decrease systematic risk and enhance outcomes management. Instruments should be pre-prepared for connectivity by having options to screen for bad patient and QC data and, if found, prohibit testing and downloading (see Chapter 34). Connectivity saves time and effort in management tasks and improves the overall cost effectiveness of POCT.

Summary—Preventive Cure

There is disagreement as to whether medical error rates are over- or underestimated (146–151). The frequency of serious medical errors caused by POCT eludes our current capability to track and document them (130). However, the rapid growth of POCT warrants investment in error prevention and detection, even if only a fraction of the sentinel events or errors actually progress to harmful accidents.

Some errors can be prevented by calibration standardization and improved QC routines and reagents (152–154). However, a broad systems approach will be required to prevent errors where a multitude of human factors are involved. Research in cognitive psychology shows that most errors result from defects in the design, organization, or environment of processes, tasks, training, equipment, and work flow (155). Elimination of unnecessary complexity decreases risk. Meaningful reduction of errors requires anticipation and correction of systems failures.

Systems approaches to error prevention allow people to work smarter and more productively (116,117,126,156–158). Methods focusing on repeated discipline of personnel and punitive measures are not acceptable. Planning, problem-solving, management, and connectivity options on POC instruments will facilitate teamwork (132). Systems-based detection and quantification of errors enable smooth development and implementation of new POC technologies.

POC systems should be designed with respect for human limitations. Timely discovery, recognition, and correction of potential injury-producing errors through the consensus systems for error prevention presented here will help improve patient outcomes. Borrowing from ancient wisdom, "An ounce of prevention is worth a pound of cure!"

OPTIMIZING OUTCOMES
Optimization Principles

This section focuses on fundamental concepts (159–168) and specific principles (169–192) of outcomes optimization for POCT (Table 40.5). Optimization techniques range in scope from broad, such as adaptive learning (168), artificial intelligence (186), and integrative strategies (62–68,73), to specific, such as decision-analysis modeling (45,180), quantitative weighted scoring (170), and unit-use protocols (191). Optimizing outcomes means managing outcomes. Managing outcomes requires specialized knowledge, customized planning, and unique insight. The art of outcomes management cannot be practiced from a distance. Success depends on POC leadership, nursing collaboration, and physician interaction.

The strategies in Table 40.5 help reveal areas of efficiency and efficacy. For example, based on a theoretical framework, decision-analysis modeling (180) shows that clinical outcomes for postoperative coronary artery bypass graft patients primarily depend on response time, and that POCT consistently is linked with positive economic impact. Application of outcomes principles depends on a conceptual understanding of the processes that build favorable intermediate outcomes and of how POCT affects those processes and their temporal distribution through rapid TTAT. A series of good intermediate outcomes improves overall patient care and function.

TABLE 40.5. PRINCIPLES OF OUTCOMES OPTIMIZATION FOR POINT-OF-CARE TESTING

Strategy	Principle
1. Adaptive learning (168)	Systems improvement through the learning organization
2. Artificial intelligence (186)	Expert systems and knowledge structures
3. Care paths and practice guidelines (181,182,188)	Systematic written protocols for patient care, often based on clinical practice guidelines and clinical decision libraries
4. Decision-analysis modeling (45,180)	Expert-based incidence, outcome, and value applied to different clinical scenarios in an explicit, possibly probabilistic, decision-analysis model that allows state transitions
5. Error tolerance limits (140)	Determination of POCT error tolerance limits based on statistical analysis of clinical data from multicenter studies
6. Evidence-based medicine (167)	Analysis based on case-control, cross-over, randomized controlled, treatment effect, or other robust clinical studies
7. Feedback systems (171,172,192)	(a) Automated alerting of critical comments about the rationality of physician test requests drawn from guidelines and knowledge bases, (b) closed-loop therapy, and (c) others
8. Internet (135)	Teaching, monitoring, and notifying via e-mail, Internet, LAN, or WAN to improve POCT performance
9. Integrative strategies (62–68,73)	Maximum clinical value through optimal restructuring and reengineering of process flow using POCT integration to remove delays on the critical path of patient diagnosis, monitoring, and treatment
10. Knowledge optimization (64,65)	Union of integration and synthesis (syntegration) to optimize knowledge (Integration $\cup$ Synthesis $\Rightarrow$ Knowledge Optimization) applied to POCT in a collaborative model
11. Meta-analysis (160)	Quantitative analysis that synthesizes evidence to estimate outcomes of different clinical actions, usually derived from collections of published studies
12. Network analysis (162,164,165,184,185)	Critical path method (CPM), program evaluation and review technique (PERT), influence diagram, intelligent decision system, neural network, and other optimizing approaches
13. Outcomes software (78)	Outcomes management and prediction through software and archiving programs, such as Project IMPACT and the APACHE III Critical Care Series
14. Patient focusing (83)	Team-oriented, patient-centered POCT and other services
15. Pattern recognition (161,187)	Fingerprinting analysis, systems testing quality control (FAST-QC) and visual recognition techniques
16. Performance mapping (65,83)	Quality paths (sequences of activities and performance indicators) optimized in a network system consisting of temporal sequences, diagnostic-therapeutic processes, decision nodes, critical paths, and feedback loops
17. Performance monitors (35,122,159,169,174,179,189,190)	Patient specifications, process improvement, quality assessment, compared replicates, downstream event monitor, and other primarily quantitative approaches to enhance POCT results
18. Quantitative weighted scoring (170)	Weighting of bedside glucose testing evaluation criteria (from a NCCLS standards document) based on a modified two-stage Delphi process, systematically applied to score the relative quality of different POCT programs
19. Root-cause analysis	Successive interrogation until the ultimate cause of an accident is discovered and understood in anticipation of remedy
20. Satisfaction survey (183)	Survey of clinical client satisfaction from use of POCT
21. Simulation (39,173)	Use of Monte Carlo or other simulation approaches to model "real-world" conditions and determine POCT performance measured against clinical and technical benchmarks
22. Surrogates of adverse outcomes (65)	Focal points of detection, correction, prevention, and optimization linked fundamentally to pathophysiological events projecting forward to sublethal and lethal events that significantly affect medical and economic outcomes
23. Treatment algorithm (175–178)	Integrated POCT and treatment options in an agreed instruction set or systematic method for solving a specific clinical problem, represented graphically in a flowchart with decisions pivoting in part on on-site test results
24. Unit-use protocols (191)	Evaluation methods based on qualitative and quantitative factors in an error matrix for unit-use (disposable single-use) test devices.

POCT, point-of-care testing.

Diagnostic-Therapeutic (Dx-Rx) Processes

Progressive Dx-Rx processes (Fig. 40.3) evolve more smoothly and quickly when diagnostic testing provides flexible and fast results. Process delays result commonly from factors such as scheduling tests, waiting for results, and physician decision making (193). The immediacy of POCT helps optimize the patient's clinical course by eliminating delays and by facilitating medical decision making. Handheld, portable, and transportable instruments, as well as custom modalities (*in vitro, ex vivo,* and *in vivo*), provide diagnostic data quickly during crises in the ED, operating room, and ICU, and during field or airborne rescues (194,195). Moving testing closer to the patient means that critical changes in analytes are detected earlier while clinically relevant.

Favorable intermediate outcomes exit the patient from potentially dysfunctional cycles (number 4 in Fig. 40.3) that consume time and money. Each day, whether intuitive or conscious, physicians optimize important medical tasks that efficiently move the patient through Dx-Rx processes (steps 1 through 5) along the trajectory of decreasing patient criticality. These finite processes represent pathophysiologic episodes and

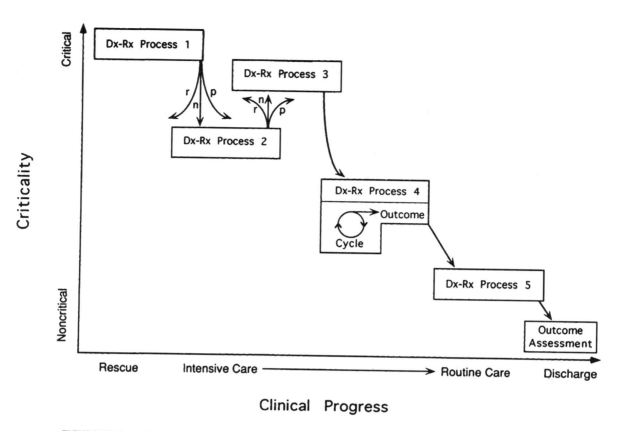

FIGURE 40.3. Optimizing diagnostic-therapeutic processes and intermediate outcomes. Optimization helps speed the successful completion of several process steps each day to quickly and efficiently move the patient through intermediate outcomes along the trajectory of decreasing criticality. One intermediate outcome cycle (number 4) is shown, but each care strategy has several, which should be counted, tracked, and improved. Optimized intermediate outcomes represent the building blocks of successful patient care and the keys to economic savings.

medical problems (e.g., an arrhythmia due to hypokalemia). Optimized solutions to specific medical problems help focus operational strategies for POCT. In the Dx-Rx process model, the interaction, integration, and summation of intermediate outcomes, like building blocks, construct overall clinical success.

Therapeutic Turnaround Time

POCT decreases therapeutic turnaround time (TTAT), the time from test ordering to treatment (see chapter 2) (64,65,67,68, 121), by eliminating time-consuming processes, rate-limiting steps, and other inefficiencies. Fast TTAT improves satisfaction, clinical performance, and patient care (196,197). TTAT reflects the useful life cycle of test cluster results in decision making, and in effect, is a measure of the temporal proximity of information and intervention. Temporal and Dx-Rx process optimization (64,65) depend on rapid clinical decision making, and hence, on fast TTAT. Rapid and accurate decisions generate efficacious care and good outcomes.

In successful POCT applications, such as performance maps (see chapter 2), treatment algorithms (chapter 8), and integrative strategies (see examples below), TTAT provides a clear pic-

ture of the context in which rapid response actions take place through access to actionable diagnostic information. Whether or not investigators document outcomes metrics explicitly, TTAT strategically connects diagnostic test results to clinical decision making. Accreditation agencies may ask hospitals to document adequate TTAT whether or not POCT is being used. Therefore, TTAT forms a fundamental, highly intuitive, and practical concept that guides successful outcomes management.

Outcomes Management

The following clinical examples show how to improve the efficiency of Dx-Rx processes using POCT and illustrate how clinical integration of POCT improves intermediate outcomes. Articulation of highly sensitive intermediate outcomes linked explicitly and tangibly to overall outcomes helps direct POCT toward clinically significant decision making and therapeutic action. The approaches below provide credible alternatives to conventional testing for consideration by administrators who want to optimize the use of POCT.

The first example demonstrates, from an institutional perspective, that whole-blood analysis performed at or near the site of patient care decreases turnaround time and blood volume required for diagnostic testing. The second example shows that POC hemostasis testing speeds decision making. The third example illustrates how an integrated protocol with POCT improves response time and conserves patient blood volume on a surgical ICU and in critical care. Conservation of blood volume represents an important standard of care for all patients, especially newborns and premature infants.

All three clinical examples illustrate how POCT enhances performance at intermediate steps in a series of Dx-Rx processes. Improved *intermediate outcomes* optimize overall outcomes. Therefore, the character and number of intermediate outcomes should be tracked and documented in POCT applications. Clever organizational strategy for optimizing intermediate outcomes produces success. These cases show how to implement POCT, while simultaneously improving intermediate, and hence long-term outcomes, through integration of testing, services, staff, and therapy.

Illustration A: Conserving Blood Volume

The first example is based on a 1-year prospective study of 850 patients in a large university teaching hospital and a university-affiliated community hospital (198). The study confirms a basic axiom (62–64) of the hybrid laboratory: For a critical care test cluster, optimum response time, t_r, is achieved when the combination of total analysis time (t_a) and transit time (t_t, a function of the distance, x, of the measurement from the patient) is minimized: $t_r = \min \{f_k[t_a, t_t(x)]\}$.

Figure 40.4 compares the efficiency of whole-blood analysis performed in a conventional laboratory, a near-patient satellite laboratory, and at the POC in an ICU. The left frame shows the incremental decrease in response time as testing shifted closer to

the patient. The right frame shows that, in addition, POCT decreased the blood volume required for diagnostic tests. Elimination of iatrogenic blood loss and decreased need for transfusions rank as high priorities in critical care (199–206). This example shows the importance of capturing multiple synergistic benefits.

Illustration B: Facilitating Decision Making

Systemic anticoagulation becomes necessary for patients with pulmonary embolism, deep venous thrombosis, and other serious conditions, and for patients undergoing life-saving interventional cardiology procedures (207–209). The second example illustrates how POCT enables rapid decision making for therapeutic monitoring (207) of anticoagulants, which, if not properly controlled, is associated with high risk of hemorrhage and other sequelae. Bedside activated partial thromboplastin time (aPTT) testing was compared to conventional laboratory aPTT testing in a group of 120 patients (272 aPTT determinations) with active venous or arterial thromboembolic disease who were admitted to a coronary care unit and were receiving continuous intravenous infusion of heparin.

Turnaround time was defined as the time from sample acquisition to aPTT result availability, decision time as the time from aPTT determination to heparin titration adjustment, and time to achieve therapeutic state (separate study of 33 patients with 264 aPTT determinations) as the time to achieve an aPTT of at least 65 seconds (Fig. 40.5) (207). All three time intervals were significantly decreased by the use of POCT ($p \leq 0.005$). Bedside testing delivered aPTT results within 3 minutes. The decision time was 14.5 minutes versus 3 hours, and the time to achieve a therapeutic state was 8.2 hours versus 18.1 hours, for bedside versus conventional testing, respectively. Thus, POCT decreased decision time.

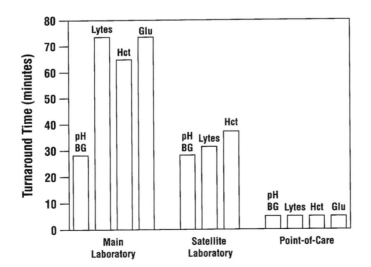 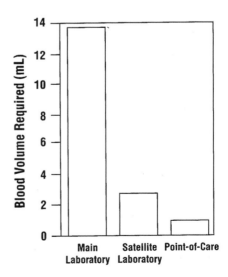

FIGURE 40.4. Point-of-care testing (POCT) improves turnaround time and conserves blood volume. In intensive care, near-patient testing in a satellite laboratory and POCT improved **(left)** turnaround time and required less blood volume **(right)** compared to main laboratory testing. (Drawn from research results published in ref. 198.)

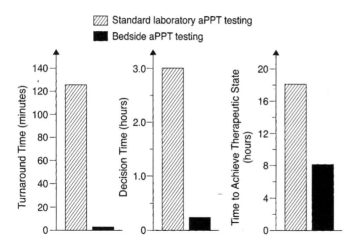

FIGURE 40.5. Point-of-care hemostasis testing improves decision making. Compared to standard laboratory testing, bedside testing of activated partial thromboplastin time improved turnaround time **(left frame)**, decision time for heparin dosage changes **(middle)**, and the time needed to achieve a therapeutic state **(right)**. (Drawn from research results published in ref. 207.)

The investigators noted that for conventional laboratory test results, 30 additional minutes typically elapsed between data availability on the laboratory computer system and clinical decision making, and that a nurse or physician would have to wait patiently by the computer display to avoid further delay. However, this extra time lag was not included in the data shown in Fig. 40.5. In general, if laboratory turnaround time occupies too large a fraction of clinical decision time, then POCT should be implemented (210).

Subsequently, a multicenter study using a weight-adjusted heparin dosing protocol at seven medical centers documented similar benefits of bedside hemostasis testing in facilitating decision making and rapidly achieving a therapeutic range of anticoagulation (113 patients) (209). However, patient-specific strategies are needed to effectively sustain the therapeutic state of anticoagulation. In a study of 1,713 patients receiving intravenous heparin after thrombolysis treatment for acute myocardial infarction, patients monitored at the bedside had significantly fewer bleeding complications as reflected in lower rates of moderate or severe bleeding, smaller mean decrease in hematocrit, and fewer transfusions ($p \leq 0.01$). While recurrent ischemia was observed more frequently (22% versus 20%, $p=0.01$), there were no significant differences in the frequency of death, reinfarction, heart failure, shock, or stroke observed in bedside monitored versus conventional laboratory monitored patients at 30 days or at 1 year (211). These studies demonstrate the practical and medical advantages of POCT-enabled decision making in more quickly achieving therapeutic goals.

Illustration C: Integrating Critical Care

The third example comes from a prospective study designed to assess the merits of POCT integrated with an ordering protocol versus the use of conventional laboratory testing without whole-blood analysis in a surgical ICU in a tertiary-care university teaching hospital (73). The surgical ICU census averaged 14 patients, and the LOS, 2.9 days. In response to mandated cost reduction, the surgical ICU, pediatric ICU (nine patients, 4.7 days average LOS), and medical ICU (nine patients, 3.9 days average LOS) were integrated by means of a protocol that delivered testing services to all three ICUs more promptly and efficiently.

Reengineering included (a) a new on-site surgical ICU laboratory positioned to serve all three ICUs and eliminate 10 to 20 minutes of transport time for most specimens; (b) implementation of whole-blood analysis; (c) user-focused, service-specific order forms with very few ordering steps; (d) mandatory daily renewal of test orders; (e) temporal test sequences patterned for different problems (e.g., interval testing for glucose during insulin infusion in diabetic ketoacidosis); (f) placement of whole-blood analytes toward the top of the order form; (g) a limited array of additional tests indicated by service; (h) alternating testing schedules for work flow optimization; (i) dynamic patient-focused test clusters (e.g., schedules for adult parenteral nutrition and modular enteral feeding); (j) anticipation of test orders over 24-hour intervals and preparation of order entry, labels, and specimen containers in advance; (k) preprinted minimum volume of blood required; (l) transcription-free triplicate forms for the bedside care plan, laboratory, and medical record; and (m) continuous interaction between nursing and laboratory staff.

The patient-focused, integrated approach decreased the number of procedural steps by 33%, allowed all routine tests to be performed at scheduled times, reduced the number of records or forms by 80% or more, and reduced the chance of mislabeling specimens (73). On the medical ICU, the number of tests per patient per 24 hours decreased. Figure 40.6 shows the impact of the integrated protocol on surgical ICU turnaround time (routine and emergency orders), sample volume, and blood removed, all of which improved significantly. The total amount of blood taken from the patient per 24 hours decreased by 63%, reflecting the use of 1-mL syringes and instructing nurses to match the minimum volumes preprinted on laboratory-generated labels when obtaining blood specimens. Preprinted labels improved efficiency. Whole-blood analysis facilitated small sample volume. ICU personnel often combined separate blood collections into one.

Medical technologists who performed the testing could work more efficiently. They found added value and satisfaction. Physicians felt they saved time. Based on preanalytic, analytic, and postanalytic time saved, the investigators attributed substantial financial savings to the integrated strategy. These savings derived primarily from reduced stat and routine blood collections, streamlined order and specimen processing, decreased transport and transfusions, and enhanced personnel efficiency in both the clinical laboratory and the ICUs. First published in 1996, the integrated POCT approach has been expanded to serve a pediatric ICU (73). After several years of experience, supervisors feel that face-to-face interactions and communications save time not only at the POC, but also in the conventional laboratory, and that these two elements represent pivotal attributes of hybrid staff and POCT integration in critical care.

■ **Integrated Protocol with Point-of-Care Testing**
□ **Conventional Approach**

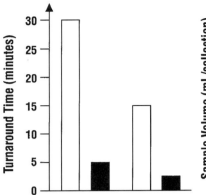
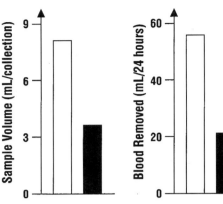

FIGURE 40.6. Integrated point-of-care testing streamlines routine and emergency intensive care unit (ICU) processes. An integrated protocol in conjunction with near-patient and on-site testing using whole-blood analysis decreased response time for both routine and emergency test orders **(left)** and conserved blood volume per collection and per day **(right)** for patients in a surgical ICU. All changes were statistically significant. (Drawn from research results published in ref. 73.)

Outcomes Surrogates

The concept of surrogates allows one to better focus POCT and design outcomes research. Table 40.6 lists soft, metric, and medical outcomes surrogates. Select medical surrogates, such as the contextual analytes, lactate (see chapter 39) and parathyroid hormone (PTH), provide logistics for temporal optimization (64,65) that can be extended, in concept, to other medical surrogates. For example, rapid intraoperative PTH levels facilitate confirmation of removal of diseased gland in surgical parathyroidectomy following preoperative ^{99m}Tc-sestamibi scanning (Fig. 40.7) (212). Temporal optimization through on-site PTH testing leads to fewer frozen sections, minimal anesthesia, and shorter LOS. (See also "Case D. Point-of-Care Parathyroid Hormone Testing" at the end of Part II.) Metric surrogates (Table 40.6), which form a basis for optimizing intermediate outcomes, include LOS, process steps, and other quantitative variables and parameters. POCT leadership should focus on *both* metric and medical surrogates to optimize Dx-Rx processes using quantifiable endpoints. Improvements achieved through "hard" metric and medical surrogates lend credence to "soft" surrogate benefits of POCT, such as convenience and satisfaction.

Surrogates drive medical and economic outcomes. *Directed POCT* facilitates prevention and optimization by accelerating the detection and correction of changes and abnormalities in surrogates of adverse outcomes (Fig. 40.8). Typical medical surrogates include glucose, potassium, ionized calcium, sodium, blood gases, creatinine, hemostasis parameters, cardiac injury markers, infectious agents, sepsis indicators, and lactate. Sudden changes or abnormalities in these surrogates signal, identify, or predict pathophysiologic conditions and acute problems in a *specific context*, such as (the parallel) diabetes, arrhythmia, cardiac dysfunction, encephalopathy, respiratory failure, renal failure, coagulopathy, acute myocardial infarction, infectious disease, shock, and hypoperfusion that lead to sublethal and lethal episodes and to poor medical and economic outcomes. Starting, stopping, switching, or changing therapy based on timely POCT results for these contextual analytes (medical surrogates) avoids poor outcomes.

TABLE 40.6. THE OUTCOMES SURROGATES TOOLBOX

Soft surrogates
  Comfort
  Convenience
  Patient motivation and compliance (self-monitoring)
  Physician capture
  Public image and perception
  Risk (intangible)
  Satisfaction (clinicians, laboratorians, and patients)
Metric surrogates
  Bed utilization (especially critical care)
  Delay (dwell, switching, and waiting)
  Discharge, readmission, referral, and outpatient encounter
  Drug changes, costs, and errors
  Economic analysis derivatives (numerous, see Table 40.1)
  Length of stay (emergency department, operating room, intensive care unit, and hospital)
  Liability and malpractice expense or savings
  Marginal, factor, expected, and total costs per event or episode
  Observation time and hourly cost (e.g., chest pain evaluation unit)
  Operating room and extracorporeal bypass time
  Organ failure scoring, severity, and prediction
  Patient throughout
  Process steps, transport, and work flow
  Stat testing inefficiencies, redraws, and requests
  Testing errors (preanalytic, analytic, and postanalytic)
  Treatment costs (episode and total)
Medical surrogates
  Blood volume removed per patient, time interval, or care episode
  Communications and interactions
  Co-morbidities
  Complications and tangible risk
  Contextual analytes (see text for explanation)
  Critical results (critical limits, critical values)
  Decision making
  Function (patient)
  Infection rates, control, and intrusion
  Intermediate outcomes (number, type, sequence, and significance)
  Morbidity (e.g., arrhythmias) and mortality
  Surgical outcome and reexploration
  Therapeutic efficacy
  Therapeutic turnaround time (TTAT)
  Transfusions (number, type, total exposure, and risk)
  Triage and stratification pivots
  Ventilator time and weaning

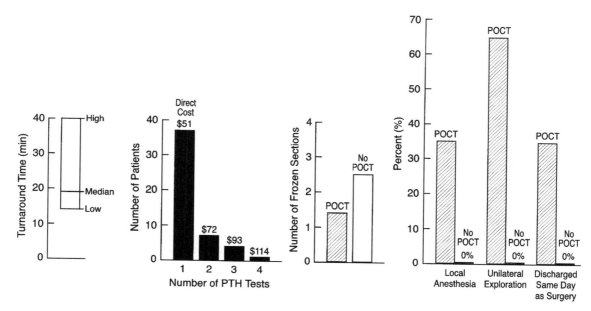

FIGURE 40.7. Point-of-care parathyroid hormone (PTH) testing improves outcomes. Patients were screened first with ^{99m}Tc-sestamibi imaging, and then parathyroidectomy was guided by two to five intraoperative PTH assays, available on site in 19 minutes (median). Savings from significantly fewer frozen sections ($p<0.0001$), more frequent local anesthesia ($p<0.001$), and shorter hospital stays ($p<0.0001$) offset the costs (shown above the bars) of point-of-care testing (POCT). Median PTH decreased 88% (range 33% to 99%) from baseline. A decrease of 50% or more in the PTH level within 10 minutes confirmed concise parathyroidectomy. Both metric (length of stay) and medical (frozen sections, local anesthesia, and unilateral exploration) surrogates were improved significantly compared to the control group, for whom POCT was not used. (Drawn from research results published in ref. 212.)

Medical surrogates provide multidimensional data that require proactive, timely, and astute clinical interpretation in the *relevant medical context*. For example, in unstable angina, elevated POC cardiac troponin T(cTnT) from microinjury is associated with more severe coronary artery disease and poorer left ventricular function, and cTnT-positive patients have a higher frequency of coronary bypass grafting (although no difference in event-free survival following percutaneous coronary interventions) (213). For patients undergoing thrombolysis for acute myocardial infarction with ST-segment elevation, POC cTnT allows risk stratification, and an elevated baseline cTnT predicts higher 30-day mortality (214).

Combined cTnI, creatine kinase-MB, and myoglobin testing helps identify spurious elevations in cTnI (215), provides better risk stratification for mortality than a single-marker approach (216) and algorithmically identifies myocardial injury early (217). POC cTnI peaks detect myocardial injury soon after open-heart surgery and predict patient outcome (218). POCT enhances relevance of both the processes and outcomes (219) and enables contextual application (220). For example, consensus guidelines suggest use of two cardiac injury markers, but instrument designs, test clusters, and algorithmic strategies may make use of multiple simultaneous markers more timely, cost effective, and efficacious.

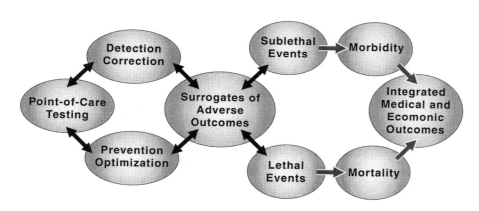

FIGURE 40.8. Medical surrogates of adverse outcomes. Point-of-care testing targets pathophysiologic surrogates of adverse outcomes through early detection and correction, which facilitate prevention and optimization. Timely actions on medical surrogates decrease sublethal and lethal events. Reduced morbidity and mortality feed forward to improve integrated medical and economic outcomes.

Medical surrogates derive value from links to patient outcomes through fundamental cellular and molecular mechanisms of disease. Ideally, POCT would reveal disturbances in homeostasis before they manifest clinically. For example, self-monitoring of blood glucose and careful glucose control at home can help prevent the deleterious side effects of hyperglycemia, now known to lead to nephropathy, retinopathy, and neuropathy, and to increase cardiovascular risk. In cardiac surgery patients, preoperative hypokalemia is associated with increased incidence of perioperative arrhythmia and cardiopulmonary resuscitation (221), which might justify POC screening and potassium repletion prior to surgery, a hypothesis that merits testing. Thus, tracking important medical surrogates creates opportunities to improve patient outcomes.

Good medical surrogates provoke thought and stimulate action. Surrogates for renal failure (creatinine (222)), venous thromboembolic disease (D-dimer (223–227)), multiorgan dysfunction (endotoxin (228)), hemodialysis effects (hemoglobin (229)), and cancer (prostate specific antigen (230)) alert physicians to urgent problems in critical care and other specialties. B-type natriuretic peptide (BNP), a surrogate for left ventricular dysfunction (and possibly ischemia), may eliminate the need for expensive diagnostic evaluations, such as echocardiography, in congestive heart failure in EDs and elsewhere (231–237). POC detection of respiratory syncytial virus before admission of infants enables segregation of infected patients to avoid spread of hospital-acquired infection (238–240). Decisive action is warranted because infectious diseases spread quickly in children. Physicians will "shotgun" antibiotics less frequently and therefore, may not incur antibiotic resistance. A new POC whole-blood spot test for insulin (241) will aid epidemiologic studies of diabetes to augment POC approaches already proven to improve patient and health system outcomes in this disease (242). Optimally planned POCT should be designed to target pertinent medical surrogates pivotal to individual clinical problems, cost-effective evaluation, healthcare utilization, and patient welfare.

When a patient's status changes quickly, timely knowledge of medical surrogates adds value to POCT. In turn, the timeliness of POCT adds value to dynamic patient care. The faster the pace, the higher the stakes, but time, per se, is not necessarily a valid surrogate of adverse outcomes. Conversely, improving turnaround time will not necessarily eliminate the need for POCT. Availability of test results does not ensure action. Physicians not "captured" may not be aware of test results. Each year these errors of omission and lack of subsequent action lead to heavy malpractice losses, which POCT potentially can eliminate. POCT will be recognized increasingly for its dynamic value in optimizing metric surrogates, discovering and quickly scrutinizing medical surrogates, and thereby allowing anticipatory management of medical outcomes at the bedside.

Nursing Outcomes

Nurses have a direct role in POCT outcomes and, conversely, POCT directly affects nursing outcomes (243–273). POCT assists nurses in their pivotal role by triaging patients, moderating interventions, and shortening LOS. When nurses have responsibility for POCT, POCT increases the value of nursing to patients. The speed of POCT helps nurses to compensate for case overload and professional shortages. Managed care increasingly challenges nurses to be accountable and responsible for the results of their interventions and also to contribute to a positive health system image (260). POCT helps nurses meet these challenges by quickly detecting changes in medical surrogates of adverse outcomes that may precipitate serious problems and by improving patient care, potentially without increasing costs (247,248,253).

Nursing professionals find POCT both necessary and useful in patient management (258,259). They cite fast TTAT, immediate informed decision making, blood conservation, avoidance of mistakes, saved time and steps, improved efficiency and quality, monitoring therapeutic results, patient comfort, and quicker discharge as some of the most important POCT advantages that help improve outcomes (39,243–245,248,255,261–264,272, 273). For example, Kilgore et al. (39,197) in a study of TTAT found that more nursing time was consumed in preparing blood gas specimens for transport than in conducting the test at the bedside. Hence, nurses favored the latter.

POCT facilitates evidence-based nursing interventions, especially in critical care, by increasing the number of useful diagnostic tests and eliminating less useful ones (253). Nurses perform a substantial portion of hospital-based POCT and have accepted the approach if familiar with the technology (257–259). One of the most important multidisciplinary nursing goals is the merging of POC test results and information management (252). Connectivity of POCT and blending of test results in the patient's bedside medical electronic record will simplify nursing information capture.

Nurses weigh heavily in the selection and purchase of POCT systems (261–264). As the use of POCT increases, hospitals will rely heavily on nurses for bedside testing (240,246,249–251, 254,265,268,270). Some professional organizations are seeking statutory authority for nurses to perform a broad range of diagnostic testing (including any complexity level). The nursing profession recognizes the value of collaborative teamwork in the design and operation of successful POCT programs and the importance of POCT to patient outcomes in the future (169, 256,259,260,266,267,269,271).

Outcomes Topology: Project IMPACT

Problems arise because of difficulties tracking multidimensional quantitative metric and medical surrogates when assessing integrated patient outcomes (Fig. 40.9). Practical management of outcomes requires user-friendly, sophisticated systems for ongoing optimization (Fig. 40.10). The Society of Critical Care Medicine (SCCM) developed Project IMPACT (PI) (78) in response to reductions in medical reimbursement, the need for preserved quality of patient care, and the desire for a peer-oriented national registry of outcomes data. Following over a year of beta-site testing, in 1996 PI software became available for outcomes management. The PI program now has over 100 ICUs enrolled. Data are entered into a national database at Tri-Analytics (Bethesda, MD), where regular reports are prepared for peer comparisons.

PI peer-review comparisons identify opportunities to improve outcomes, target excessive resource consumption,

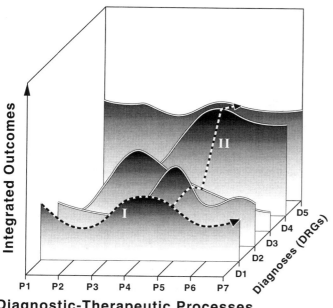

Diagnostic-Therapeutic Processes

FIGURE 40.9. Multidimensional outcomes topology. Heterogeneous diagnoses complicate the topology of outcomes. In comparison to outcomes management for a single diagnosis **(trace I)**, tracking problems occur when simultaneously optimizing outcomes for several diagnoses **(trace II)**. Integrative strategies, treatment algorithms, performance maps, and other collaborative approaches alleviate these problems by allowing the clinical team to anticipate, track, and evaluate outcomes. (*P1-P7*, diagnostic therapeutic (Dx-Rx) processes; *DRGs*, diagnosis-related groups.)

enhance management, validate patient protocols, and benchmark performance. The PI database has been validated with fairly good results. Diagnostic test data in PI may be suitable for research, which the SCCM hopes to promote and expand (78). Critical analysis of LOS data may help POCT investigators to sort out the most efficacious uses of POCT in intensive care. PI meets the criteria of the JCAHO for a performance measurement system that can be included in accreditation processes.

Clinical decision support systems have significant advantages in resource utilization and performance enhancement. Outcomes management software packages, such as the APACHE III Critical Care Series, provide a different perspective for outcomes prediction (78). Organizations such as the University Health-System Consortium are developing and qualifying performance measurement systems. POCT staff can explore these software tools to track practice parameters relevant to diagnostic testing and to participate in measurement systems that simultaneously enhance performance, compare the performance of peer groups, and allow risk-adjusted comparison of actual outcomes with predicted outcomes. POCT outcomes management software, if available, could help sort out implementation priorities.

Summary—Multidimensional Optimization

The whole multidimensional system should be optimized. Integrative strategies that enhance both medical and economic outcomes are embodied in (a) the macroeconomic approach to POCT (first section); (b) the consensus systems for error prevention (second section), and (c) the blending of POCT with clinical services (third section). Chapter 8 describes how on-site testing and a treatment algorithm marry integration and synthesis (syntegration) to improve medical and economic outcomes in the operating room by simultaneously increasing the efficiency and efficacy of transfusion decisions that conserve transfused blood products. Other chapters provide excellent examples of how POCT improves *both* medical and economic outcomes.

The microeconomic principles in Table 40.5 can be combined with the optimizing principles in Table 40.1. For example, severity of illness scoring systems in combination with economic analysis of relative value may help identify patients most likely to benefit from expensive therapies in critical care (19). Hence, strategic planning should combine analysis of both medical and economic outcomes. A productive multidimensional approach to the implementation of POCT starts by evaluating benefits comprehensively from a macroscopic, macroeconomic perspective with all measurable benefits counted, and simultaneously focuses on optimizing medical outcomes for improved patient care.

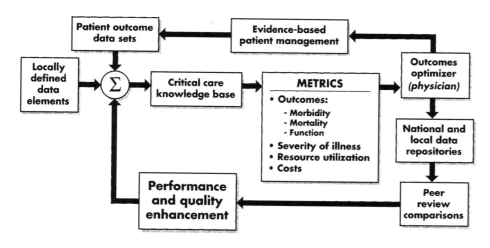

FIGURE 40.10. Outcomes management feedback system. An outcomes management feedback system employs defined outcomes, metrics, evidence-based patient information, and local optimization, and then incorporates performance and quality review based on comparisons with comparable peer institutions. Local data are sent to a national repository for analysis. Local and national assessments feed back into the critical care knowledge for continuous improvement of performance. An example of this type of approach is Project IMPACT (see text).

CONCLUSIONS

Ultimate Goals of Point-of-Care Testing

POCT finds its mission and moment in the 21st century. When navigating superior outcomes, the art of optimization lies in applying a worthy knowledge companion, POCT, to best advantage in adaptive clinical systems. The journey ahead leads to significant milestones: (a) immediate integration and synthesis of medical data to enable intelligent and accurate decision making that will prevent significant medical errors; (b) simultaneous bedside biochemistry, physiology, and monitoring (274–281) to facilitate temporal and Dx-Rx optimization that will improve outcomes; and (c) evidence-based diagnosis and treatment with feedback-molecular and POC-sensor systems (280,281) that will decipher complex critical problems. Each health system has specialized objectives. Customers expect excellent outcomes. Leaders who are well informed in POCT, aware of its potential, and prepared for its future will increase chances of achieving these goals and ultimately, success.

Practical Business Plan

The marginal expenses of new efficient systems ramp up diminishing returns until expenses hit a cost-effectiveness barrier (8). At that point, savings from the displacement of older approaches can lower costs, thereby tunneling through the cost barrier and enabling even bigger savings. For example, POCT connectivity, despite initially ramping up expenses, ultimately will save time, effort, and money as test results are integrated electronically.

The unique benefits of new POC tests and markers mean that relatively high costs need not constrain implementation. Practical success derives from integrating a package of design measures to achieve multiple benefits or from combining measures with improvements already being made. Sagacious leadership will optimize patient care first, since decreased overall costs secondarily increase return on POCT investment. This approach reflects whole-system engineering (8), that is, optimization of the entire care package to capture multiple beneficial outcomes.

Health systems initiating or expanding POCT programs should consider the following pragmatic approach. Based on the feedback concepts (Fig. 40.10) exemplified by clinical decisions systems, Project IMPACT, and outcomes optimization principles (Table 40.5), the POCT committee should preselect whole-systems outcomes and performance targets, design measurement and tracking metrics, monitor results over defined time intervals, and conclude or continue the POCT initiative based on assessment of the total or relative value of medical and economic outcomes.

The POCT director and clinician should challenge the device manufacturer to indemnify the health system against economic losses incurred during POCT implementation in the event that outcomes milestones and thresholds are not met. Investment in POCT outcomes research makes sense because industry increasingly will profit. Quantitative measurements using activity-based metric surrogates, such as waiting time, number of procedures, transfusion exposure, and LOS can form the basis, along with medical surrogates, for decisions regarding continuation of the POC initiative. Soft metrics, such as convenience and satisfaction, weigh in the final balance.

Success produces a "win-win" situation. Failure means recovery of hospital costs from the industrial sponsor. Wishful thinking? POCT represents a "cash cow" of new monetary investment in diagnostics research and development, and companies will assume risks in proportion to rewards in order to prove clinical practice principles. Well-designed piloting of new POCT initiatives using this practical business model allays anxiety, instills accountability, and in the event of failure, cuts health system costs, even without indemnification. Risk control appeals to managed care administrators who operate on a short programmatic cycle.

Principles, Practice, and Patients

Cost effectiveness, error reduction, and superior outcomes remain the common denominator of health care worldwide (Fig. 40.11). Outcomes optimization is achieved best through collective judgment by selecting principles from Tables 40.1 and 40.5 and adapting them in combinations appropriate to individual medical settings. Think globally at a local level. Consider total costs. POCT costs may be overcompensated by reduced treatment costs, with the additional benefit of improved sequences of intermediate outcomes aggregating to enhance patient function on discharge.

The national standard of care, which now requires POCT in several critical care settings and medical circumstances, should be met or exceeded. Each opportunity to improve care with POCT should be explored objectively. To do otherwise would not serve patients well and may increase an institution's liability. In developing countries unable to afford sufficient numbers of large, complex, and expensive diagnostic instruments to serve burgeoning populations, POCT can provide crucial medical data that may not be available otherwise.

Few people return to old ways that they find inconvenient, inefficient, or time consuming. This behavior is characteristic of POCT, which has met with quiet success and widespread endorsement. Ultimately, POCT will "partner" the physician and patient symbiotically for site-independent monitoring (45,282–284) and treatment from critical care to the home. POCT not only is improving outcomes locally when tailored to the individual medical needs of health systems and patients, but also is changing practice patterns and medical delivery globally with the prospect of more equitable care and improved quality of life for patients worldwide.

Acknowledgments

I am indebted to the creative students and colleagues who contributed to this work. I sincerely thank Christopher Kost for his insights and Claudia Graham for her artistry. Figure and table concepts are used courtesy of Knowledge Optimization (Davis, CA).

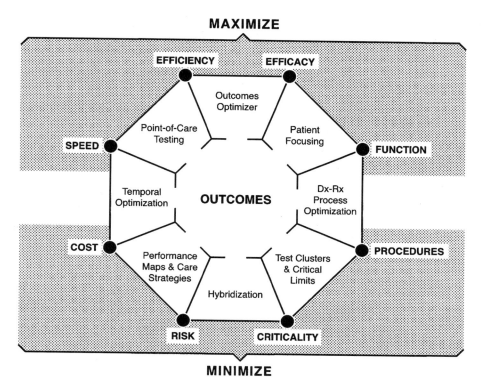

FIGURE 40.11. Adjusting nodal objectives in the outcomes port. The holistic objectives of the health system are to maximize speed, efficiency, efficacy, and function, and simultaneously, to minimize cost, risk, criticality, and procedures, in order to improve medical and economic outcomes. The operators within the octagonal sectors allow physicians to adjust the web appropriately. Outcomes are the product of syntegration in the knowledge optimization model (see Fig. 40.1 and chapter 2).

REFERENCES

1. Bourlier KM. *The hitchhiker's guide to point-of-care testing.* Washington, DC: American Association for Clinical Chemistry Press, 1998.
2. Bozzo P, ed. *Cost-effective laboratory management.* Philadelphia: Lippincott-Raven Publishers, 1998.
3. Cummings JP. *POC tests for cardiac injury markers.* Oak Brook, IL: University HealthSystem Consortium, December 2000.
4. Eastaugh SR. *Health care finance.* Gaithersburg, MD: Aspen Publishers, 1998.
5. Fuchs VR. *Who shall live? Health, economics, and social choice.* River Edge, NJ: World Scientific, 1998.
6. Gold MR, Russell LB, Siegel JE, et al., eds. *Cost-effectiveness in health and medicine.* New York: Oxford University Press, 1996.
7. Horton GL. *Handbook of bedside glucose testing.* Washington, DC: American Association for Clinical Chemistry Press, 1998.
8. Hawken P, Lovins A, Lovins LH. *Natural capitalism: creating the next industrial revolution.* New York: Little, Brown and Company, 1999.
9. Jacobs P. *The economics of health and medical care.* Gaithersburg, MD: Aspen Publishers, 1997.
10. Johansson PO. *Evaluating health risks: an economic approach.* New York: Cambridge University Press, 1995.
11. Parsons ML, Murdaugh CL, Purdon TF, et al. *Strategies for improving patient care: guide to clinical resource management.* Gaithersburg, MD: Aspen Publishers, 1997.
12. Rovin S. *Medicine and business: bridging the gap.* Gaithersburg, MD: Aspen Publishers, 2001.
13. Asimos AW, Gibbs MA, Marx JA, et al. Value of point-of-care testing in emergent trauma management. *J Trauma* 2000;48:1101–1108.
14. Bailey TM, Topham TM, Wantz S, et al. Laboratory process improvement through point-of-care testing. *Joint Commission J Qual Improvement* 1997; 23:362–380.
15. Bailey TM. Understanding the economics of bedside diagnostic testing. In: Price CP, Hicks JM, eds. *Point-of-care testing.* Washington, DC: American Association for Clinical Chemistry Press, 1999: 213–232.
16. Barocci TA. *The value chain applied to critical care testing: a hospital financial perspective.* Atlanta, GA: American Association for Clinical Chemistry National Meeting, 1997.
17. Battelle Medical Technology Assessment and Policy Research Program. The economic and clinical efficiency of point-of-care testing for critically ill patients. *Med Lab Observer* 1996;27:12–16.
18. Cembrowski GS, Kiechle FL. Point of care testing: Critical analysis and practical application. *Adv Pathol Lab Med* 1994;7:3–26.
19. Chalfin DB, Cohen IL, Lambrinos J. The economics and cost-effectiveness of critical care medicine. *Intensive Care Med* 1995;21: 952–961.
20. Collison PO. Economic aspects of new biochemical markers for the detection of myocardial damage: role of biochemical markers in the management of patients with chest pain. In: Kaski JC, Holt DW, eds. *Myocardial damage: early detection by novel biochemical markers.* Boston: Kluwer Academic Publishers, 1998:173–187.
21. Collison PO. Testing for cardiac markers at the point of care. *Clin Lab Med* 2001;21:351–362.
22. Cox CJ. Acute care testing: blood gases and electrolytes at the point of care. *Clin Lab Med* 2001;21:321–335.
23. Craig TM. The economics of near-patient testing. In: Marks V, Alberti KGMM, eds. *Clinical biochemistry nearer the patient.* London: Churchill Livingstone, 1985:162–167.
24. De Cresce RP, Phillips DL, Howanitz PJ. Financial justification of alternate site testing. *Arch Pathol Lab Med* 1995;119:898–901.
25. ECRI. Guidance article. "Point-of-care" laboratory testing: is decentralized testing the best alternative for your hospital? *Health Devices* 1995;24:173–207.
26. ECRI. Whole blood coagulation analyzers. *Health Devices* 1997;26: 296–332.
27. Fiallos MR, Hanhan UA, Orlowski JP. Point-of-care testing. *Pediatr Clin North Am* 2001;48:589–599.
28. Foster K, Despotis G, Scott MG. Point-of-care testing: cost issues and impact on hospital operations. *Clin Lab Med* 2001;21:269–284.
29. Garrison CB. Economics of health care policy. In: Stahl MJ, Dean PJ, eds. *The physician's essential MBA: what every physician leader needs to know.* Gaithersburg, MD: Aspen Publications, 1999:23–44.

30. Gafni A, Birch S. Preferences for outcomes in economic evaluation: an economic approach to addressing economic problems. *Soc Sci Med* 1995;40:767–776.

31. Herpichboehm B. Point of care analyzer systems in hospitals: contributors to cost-efficiency? *J Lab Med* 1999;23:93–96.

32. Heyland DK, Kernerman P, Gafni A, et al. Economic evaluations in the critical care literature: do they help us improve the efficiency of our unit? *Crit Care Med* 1996;24:1591–1598.

33. Howanitz PJ. College of American Pathologists Conference XXVIII on alternate site testing: what must we do now? *Arch Pathol Lab Med* 1995;119:979–983.

34. Hunter L. POCT: costly or cost-effective? *Med Lab Observer* 1996;27:2–3.

35. Jacobs E. Point-of-care (near-patient) testing. In: Kaplan LA, Pesce AJ, eds. *Clinical chemistry: theory, analysis, and correlation.* New York: Mosby, 1994:313–322.

36. Keffer JH. Economic considerations of point-of-care testing. *Am J Clin Pathol* 1995;102[Suppl 1]:S107–S110.

37. Keffer JH. The economic aspects of new delivery options for diagnostic testing. In: Kost GJ, ed. *Handbook of clinical automation, robotics, and optimization.* New York: John Wiley and Sons, 1996:577–595.

38. Keffer J. Health economics aspects of point-of-care testing. In: Price CP, Hicks JM, eds. *Point-of-care testing.* Washington, DC: American Association for Clinical Chemistry Press, 1999:233–247.

39. Kilgore ML, Steindel SJ, Smith JA. Estimating costs and turnaround times: presenting a user-friendly tool for analyzing costs and performance. *Clin Lab Management Rev* 1999;13:179–187.

40. Kilgore ML, Steindel SJ, Smith JA. Cost analysis for decision support: the case of comparing centralized versus distributed methods for blood gas testing. *J Healthcare Management* 1999;44:207–215.

41. Kipp RA, Towner C, Levin HA. Financial and actuarial issues. In: Todd WE, Nash D, eds. *Disease management: a systems approach to improving patient outcomes.* Chicago: American Hospital Publishing, 1997:87–136.

42. Klose T. The contingent valuation method in health care. *Health Policy* 1999;47:97–123.

43. Kreider C, Walsh BA. Benchmarking for a competitive edge. *Med Lab Observer* 1997;29:26–29.

44. Kuffer H, Carlyle JE, Statland BE. Cost analysis. In: Vonderschmitt DJ, ed. *Laboratory organization automation.* New York: Walter de Gruyter, 1991:65–79.

45. Lafata JE, Martin SA, Kaatz S, et al. Anticoagulation clinics and patient self-testing for patients on chronic warfarin therapy: a cost-effectiveness analysis. *J Thromb Thrombolysis* 2000;9:813–819.

46. Laupacis A, Feeny D, Detsky AS, et al. How attractive does a new technology have to be to warrant adoption and utilization? *Can Med Assoc J* 1992;146:473–481.

47. Lautaret NR, Bozzo P. Cost analysis in the laboratory. In: Bozzo P, ed. *Cost-effective laboratory management.* Philadelphia: Lippincott-Raven Publishers, 1998:85–98.

48. Lee-Lewandrowski E, Lewandrowski K. Point-of-care testing: an overview and a look into the future. *Clin Lab Med* 2001;21:217–239.

49. Linz WJ, Gillum R. Assessing the productivity component of cost: the College of American Pathologists laboratory management index program for alternate site testing. *Med Lab Observer* 1996;27:17–18.

50. McDonald JM, Smith JA. Value-added laboratory medicine in an era of managed care. *Clin Chem* 1995;41:1256–1262.

51. Mor M, Waisman Y. Point-of-care testing: a critical review. *Pediatr Emerg Care* 2000;46:45–48.

52. Nash DB, Fernandez AM, Ryan NR, et al. Point of care testing. In: Bozzo P, ed. *Cost-effective laboratory management.* Philadelphia: Lippincott-Raven Publishers, 1998:163–179.

53. Perkins SE. Managing point-of-care testing. In: Snyder JR, Wilkinson DS, eds. *Management in laboratory medicine.* Philadelphia: Lippincott Williams &Wilkins, 1998:423–431.

54. Popper C. Using cost-effectiveness analysis to weigh testing decisions. *Med Lab Observer* 1992;24:29–35.

55. Price CP. Point-of-care testing: impact on medical outcomes. *Clin Lab Med* 2001;21:285–303.

56. Rabbitts DG. Point-of-care testing: needs and cost-benefit analysis. *Clin Lab Sci* 1993;6:228–230.

57. Rapoport J, Teres D, Lemeshow S, et al. A method for assessing the clinical performance and cost-effectiveness of intensive care units: a multicenter inception cohort study. *Crit Care Med* 1994;22:1385–1391.

58. Travers EM. *Clinical laboratory management.* Philadelphia: Williams and Wilkins, 1997.

59. Weinstein MC, Stason WB. Foundations of cost-effectiveness analysis for health and medical practice. *N Engl J Med* 1977;296:716–721.

60. Weinstein MC, Siegel JE, Gold MR, et al. Recommendations of the panel on cost-effectiveness in health and medicine. *JAMA* 1996;276:1253–1258.

61. Kost GJ. The hybrid laboratory: the clinical laboratory of the 1990's is a synthesis of the old and the new. *Arch Pathol Lab Med* 1992;116:1002–1003.

62. Kost GJ. The hybrid laboratory: shifting the focus to the point of care. *Med Lab Observer* 1992;24(9S):17–28.

63. Kost GJ. New whole blood analyzers and their impact on cardiac and critical care. *Crit Rev Clin Lab Sci* 1993;30:153–202.

64. Kost GJ. Point-of-care testing ⇒ the hybrid laboratory ⇒ knowledge optimization. In: Kost GJ, ed. *Handbook of clinical automation, robotics, and optimization.* New York: John Wiley and Sons, 1996:757–838.

65. Kost GJ. Point-of-care testing in intensive care. In: Tobin MJ, ed. *Principles and practice of intensive care monitoring.* New York: McGraw-Hill, 1998:1267–1296.

66. Kost GJ. Planning and implementing point-of-care systems. In: Tobin MJ, ed. *Principles and practice of intensive care monitoring.* New York: McGraw-Hill, 1998:1297–1328.

67. Kost GJ, Ehrmeyer SS, Chernow B, et al. The laboratory-clinical interface: point-of-care testing. *Chest* 1999;115:1140–1154.

68. Kost GJ. Point-of-care testing. In: Meyers RA, ed. *Encyclopedia of analytical chemistry: instrumentation and applications.* New York: John Wiley and Sons, 2000:1603–1625.

69. Young DS, Sachais BS, Jefferies LC. The costs of disease. *Clin Chem* 2000;46:955–966.

70. Young DS, Sachais BS, Jeffries LC. Laboratory costs in the context of disease. *Clin Chem* 2000;46:967–975.

71. Jefferies LC, Sachais BS, Young DS. Blood transfusion costs by diagnosis-related groups in 60 university hospitals in 1995. *Transfusion* 2001;41:522–529.

72. Wallace EL. Blood service costs and charges. *Transfusion* 2001;41:437–439.

73. Steffes MW, Gillen JL, Fuhrman SA. Delivering clinical laboratory services to intensive care units. *Clin Chem* 1996;42:387–391, and personal communication, Sept. 28, 2001.

74. Felder RA, Kost GJ. Modular stepwise automation and the future of diagnostic testing, part I. *Med Lab Observer* 1998;30(4):22–77.

75. Kost GJ, Felder RA. Modular stepwise automation and the future of diagnostic testing, part II. *Med Lab Observer* 1998;30(6):46, 48, 56.

76. Andrew M, Ansell JL, Becker DM, et al. Oral Anticoagulation Monitoring Study Group. Prothrombin measurement using a patient self-testing system. *Am J Clin Pathol* 2001;115:280–287.

77. Andrew M, Ansell JL, Becker DM, et al. Oral Anticoagulation Monitoring Study Group. Point-of-care prothrombin time measurement for professional and patient self-testing use. *Am J Clin Pathol* 2001;115:288–296.

78. Sakallaris BR, Jastremski CA, Von Rueden KT. Clinical decision support systems for outcome measurement and management. *AACN Clin Issues* 2000;11:351–362.

79. Parvin CA, Lo SF, Deuser SM, et al. Impact of point-of-care testing on patients' length of stay in a large emergency department. *Clin Chem* 1996;42:711–717.

80. Kendall J, Reeves B, Clancy M. Point of care testing: randomised controlled trial of clinical outcome. *BMJ* 1998;316:1052–1057.

81. van Heyningen C, Watson ID, Morrice AE. Point-of-care testing outcomes in an emergency department. *Clin Chem* 1999;45:437–438.

82. Steindel SJ, Howanitz PJ. Physician satisfaction and emergency department laboratory test turnaround time: observations based on College of American Pathologists Q-Probes studies. *Arch Pathol Lab Med* 2001;125:863–871.

83. Kost GJ, Lathrop JP. Designing hybrid laboratories, performance maps, and quality paths for patient-focused care. *Med Lab Observer* 1993;25(9S):16–26.

84. Anderson DW, Belzberg H. POCT data management by terminal emulation in a paperless ICU. *Med Lab Observer* 1995;27:16–19.

85. Bernard D, Vanhee D, Baton V. Implementation of an integrated instrument control and data management system for point of care blood gas testing. *Clin Chim Acta* 2001;307:169–173.

86. Blick KE. The essential role of information management in point-of-care/critical care testing. *Clin Chim Acta* 2001;307:159–168.

87. Brooks JD. Fundamentals of POCT data management: a perfusionist's perspective. *Med Lab Observer* 1995;27:20–24.

88. Brown R. Point-of-care integration—our experience. *Med Lab Observer* 1998;30:22–25.

89. DuBois JA. Getting to the point: integrating critical care tests in the patient care setting. *Med Lab Observer* 2000;32:52–56.

90. Elevitch FR. Multimedia communications networks: patient care through interactive point-of-care testing. *Clin Lab Med* 1994;14:559–567.

91. Emons MF. Integrated patient data for optimal patient management: the value of laboratory data in quality improvement. *Clin Chem* 2001;47:1516–1520.

92. Halpern NA, Brentjens T. Point of care testing informatics: the critical care-hospital interface. *Crit Care Clin* 1999;15:577–591.

93. Halpern NA. Point of care diagnostics and networks. *Crit Care Clin* 2000;16:623–639.

94. Harris CM. Integrated delivery system, informatics, and the laboratory: managing patient service and clinical quality in a complex and evolving health care environment. In: Bozzo P, ed. *Cost-effective laboratory management*. Philadelphia: Lippincott-Raven Publishers, 1998:181–186.

95. Humbertson SK. Management of a point-of-care program: organization, quality assurance, and data management. *Clin Lab Med* 2001;21:255–268.

96. Jacobs E, Laudin AG. The satellite laboratory and point-of-care testing: integration of information. *Am J Clin Pathol* 1995;104[Suppl1]:S33–S39.

97. Jacobs E, Hinson KA, Tolnai J, et al. Implementation, management and continuous quality improvement of point-of-care testing in an academic health care setting. *Clin Chim Acta* 2001;307:49–59.

98. Laessig RH, Ehrmeyer SS. Data management of POCT: the vision. *Med Lab Observer* 1995;27:2–6.

99. Nichols J. Management of remote laboratory data. *Lab Med* 2001;32:532–534.

100. Okorodudu AO, Jacobs E, Fogh-Anderson N. Critical care testing in the new millennium: the integration of point-of-care testing. *Clin Chim Acta* 2001;307:1–1.

101. Palenick JA. A developmental perspective on POCT data management. *Med Lab Observer* 1995;27:25–27.

102. Parker JD. LIS vendor, POCT manufacturer, laboratorian: who's responsible for POCT data management? *Med Lab Observer* 1995;27:8–11.

103. Quigley L. POCT data management: a problem-solving approach. *Med Lab Observer* 1995;27:12–15.

104. Practice expense costs in pulmonary and critical care practices: is providing patient care still economically feasible? *Am J Respir Crit Care Med* 2001;163:1524–1527.

105. Dominguez TE, Chalom R, Costarino AT. The impact of adverse patient occurrences on hospital costs in pediatric intensive care unit. *Crit Care Med* 2001;29:169–174.

106. Halpern NA, Bettes L, Greenstein R. Federal and nationwide intensive care units and healthcare costs: 1986–1992. *Crit Care Med* 1994;22:2001–2007.

107. Jacobs P, Noseworthy TW. National estimates of intensive care utilization and costs: Canada and United States. *Crit Care Med* 1990;18:1282–1286.

108. Jacobs P, Edbrooke D, Hibbert C, et al. Descriptive patient data as an explanation for the variation in average daily costs in intensive care. *Anaesthesia* 2001;56:643–647.

109. Kantor RK. Post-intensive care unit pediatric hospital stay and estimated costs. *Crit Care Med* 2000;28:220–230.

110. Kramer DJ. Intensive care unit frequent fliers: morbidity and cost. *Crit Care Med* 2001;29:207–208.

111. Mirski MA, Chang CW, Cowan R. Impact of a neuroscience intensive care unit on neurosurgical patient outcomes and cost of care: evidence-based support for an intensivist-directed specialty ICU model of care. *J Neurosurg Anesthesiol* 2001;13:83–92.

112. Park CA, McGwin G, Smith DR, et al. Trauma-specific intensive care units can be cost effective and contribute to reduced length of stay. *Am Surg* 2001;67:665–670.

113. Rogowski J, Horbar J, Plesk P, et al. Collaborative quality improvement in neonatal intensive care: effects on outcomes, treatment costs and institutional expenditures for improving the quality of NICU care. *Assoc Health Services Res* 1999;16:369–370.

114. Shanmugasundaram R, Padmapriya E, Shyamala J. Cost of neonatal intensive care. *Indian J Pediatr* 1998;65:249–255.

115. Sznajder M, Aegerter P, Launois R, et al. A cost-effectiveness analysis of stays in intensive care units. *Intensive Care Med* 2001;27:146–153.

116. Kohn LT, Corrigan JM, Donaldson MS, eds. *To err is human: building a safer health system*. Washington, DC: National Academy Press, 2000:287.

117. Richardson WL, Berwick DM, Bisgard JC, et al. *Crossing the quality chasm: a new health system for the 21st century*. Washington, DC: National Academy Press, 2001:337.

118. Plebani M, Carraro P. Mistakes in a stat laboratory: types and frequency. *Clin Chem* 1997;43:1348–1351.

119. Witte DL, VanNess SA, Angstadt DS, et al. Errors, mistakes, blunders, outliers, or unacceptable results: how many? *Clin Chem* 1997;43:1352–1356.

120. Bickford GR. Decentralized testing in the '90s. *Clin Lab Management Rev* 1994;8:327–330, 332, 333, 336–338.

121. Kost GJ. Guidelines for point-of-care testing: improving patient outcomes. *Am J Clin Pathol* 1995;104 [Suppl 1]:S111–S127.

122. Kilgore ML, Steindel SJ, Smith JA. Continuous quality improvement for point-of-care testing using background monitoring of duplicate specimens. *Arch Pathol Lab Med* 1999;123:824–828.

123. Sirota RL. The Institute of Medicine's report on medical error: implications for pathology. *Arch Pathol Lab Med* 2000;124:1674–1678.

124. Kost GJ. *Using operator lockout to improve the performance of point-of-care blood glucose monitoring*. Milpitas, CA: LifeScan, 2000.

125. Kost GJ. Preventing medical errors in point-of-care testing: security, validation, performance, safeguards, and connectivity. *Arch Pathol Lab Med* 2001;125:1307–1315.

126. Leape LL. Error in medicine. *JAMA* 1994;272:1851–1857.

127. Wolff AM, Bourke J. Reducing medical errors: a practical guide. *Med J Aust* 2000;173:247–251.

128. Ballam H. HIPAA, security and electronic signature: a closer look. *J Am Health Info Mgmt Assoc* 1999;70:26–30.

129. Witte DL, Astion ML. Panel discussion: how to monitor and minimize variation and mistakes. *Clin Chem* 1997;43:880–885.

130. Witte DL, Van Ness SA. Frequency of unacceptable results in point-of-care testing. *Arch Pathol Lab Med* 1999;123:761.

131. Nanji AA, Poon R, Hinberg I. Decentralized clinical chemistry testing: quality of results obtained by residents and interns in an acute care setting. *J Intensive Care Med* 1998;3:272–277.

132. Risser DT, Rice MM, Salisbury ML, et al. The potential for improved teamwork to reduce medical errors in the emergency department. The MedTeams Research Consortium. *Ann Emerg Med* 1999;34:373–383.

133. Joint Commission on Accreditation of Healthcare Organizations. *Quality point of care testing: a Joint Commission handbook*. Oakbrook Terrace, IL: Joint Commission on Accreditation of Healthcare Organizations, 1999.

134. Joint Commission on Accreditation of Healthcare Organizations. *How to meet the most frequently cited laboratory standards*. Oakbrook Terrace, IL: Joint Commission on Accreditation of Healthcare Organizations, 2001.

135. Louie RF, Tang Z, Shelby DG, Kost GJ. Point-of-care testing: millennium technology for critical care. *Lab Med* 2000;31:402.

136. Kost GJ. Critical limits for urgent clinician notification at US medical centers. *JAMA* 1990;263:704–707.

137. Kost GJ. Critical limits for emergency clinician notification at United States children's hospitals. *Pediatrics* 1991;88:597–603.

138. Kost GJ. Using critical limits to improve patient outcome. *Med Lab Observer* 1993;25:22–27.

139. Kost, G.J. Designing critical limit systems for knowledge optimization. *Arch Pathol Lab Med* 1996;120:616–618.

140. Kost GJ, Vu HT, Lee J. Multicenter study of oxygen insensitive hand-held glucose point-of-care testing in critical care/hospital/ambulatory patients in the United States and Canada. *Crit Care Med* 1998;26:581–590.

141. Louie RF, Tang Z, Sutton DV, et al. Point-of-care testing: effects of critical care variables, influence of reference instruments, and a modular glucose meter design. *Arch Pathol Lab Med* 2000;124:257–266.

142. Tang Z, Louie RF, Payes M, et al. Oxygen effects on glucose measurements with a reference analyzer and three handheld meters. *Diabetes Technol Ther* 2000;2:349–362.

143. Tang Z, Louie RF, Lee JH, Kost GJ. Oxygen effects on glucose meter measurements with glucose dehydrogenase- and oxidase-based test strips for point-of-care testing. *Crit Care Med* 2001;29:1062–1070.

144. Tang Z, Du X, Louie RF, et al. Effects of drugs on glucose measurements with handheld glucose meters and a portable glucose analyzer. *Am J Clin Pathol* 2000:113:75–86.

145. Kost GJ. Connectivity: the millennium challenge for point-of-care testing. *Arch Pathol Lab Med* 2000;124:1108–1110.

146. McDonald CJ, Weiner M, Hui SL. Deaths due to medical errors are exaggerated in Institute of Medicine report. *JAMA* 2000;284:93–95.

147. Leape LL. Institute of Medicine medical error figures are not exaggerated. *JAMA* 2000;284:95–97.

148. Sox HC, Woloshin S. How many deaths are due to medical error? Getting the number right. *Effective Clin Pract* 2000;3:277–283.

149. Bell CM, Redelmeier DA. Mortality among patients admitted to hospitals on weekends as compared with weekdays. *N Engl J Med* 2001;345:663–668.

150. Halm EA, Chassin MR. Why do hospital death rates vary? *N Engl J Med* 2001;345:692–694.

151. Hayward RS, Hofer TP. Estimating hospital deaths due to medical errors: preventability is in the eye of the reviewer. *JAMA* 2001;286:415–420.

152. Fogh-Andersen N, D'Orazio P. Proposal for standardizing direct-reading biosensors for blood glucose. *Clin Chem* 1998;44:655–659.

153. Jenny RW, Jackson-Tarentino KY. Causes of unsatisfactory performance in proficiency testing. *Clin Chem* 2000;46:89–99.

154. Johnson RN, Baker JR. Error detection and measurement in glucose monitors. *Clin Chim Acta* 2001;307:61–67.

155. Leape LL. A systems analysis approach to medical error. *J Eval Clin Pract* 1997;3:213–222.

156. Kost GJ, Hague C. *In vitro, ex vivo,* and *in vivo* biosensor systems. In: Kost GJ, ed. *Handbook of clinical automation, robotics, and optimization.* New York: John Wiley and Sons, 1996:648–753.

157. Kost GJ. Optimizing point-of-care testing in clinical systems management. *Clin Lab Management Rev* 1998;12:353–363.

158. Kern DA, Bennett ST. Quality improvement in the information age. *Med Lab Observer* 1999;31:24–28.

159. Bissell MG, ed. *Laboratory-related measures of patient outcomes: an introduction.* Washington, DC: American Association for Clinical Chemistry Press, 2000.

160. Eddy DM, Hasselblad V, Shachter R. Meta-analysis by the confidence profile method: the statistical synthesis of evidence. New York: Academic Press, 1992.

161. Evans BD. Pattern recognition "fingerprinting" for continuous quality improvement of point-of-care whole blood testing. Master's thesis, University of California-Davis, 1991.

162. Holtzman S. *Intelligent decision systems.* New York: Addison Wesley, 1989.

163. Isenberg SF, Gliklich RE, eds. *Profiting from quality: outcomes strategies for medical practice.* San Francisco: Jossey-Bass, 1999.

164. Oliver RM, Smith JQ, eds. *Influence diagrams, belief nets and decision analysis.* New York: John Wiley and Sons, 1990.

165. Pearl J. *Probabilistic reasoning in intelligent systems: networks of plausible inference.* San Mateo, CA: Morgan Kaufmann Publishers, 1988.

166. Todd WE, Nash D, eds. *Disease management: a systems approach to improving patient outcomes.* Chicago: American Hospital Publishing, 1997.

167. Sackett DL, Straus SE, Richardson WS, et al. *Evidence-based medicine: how to practice and teach EBM.* New York: Churchill-Livingstone, 2000.

168. Senge PM. *The fifth discipline: the art and practice of the learning organization.* New York: Doubleday/Currency, 1990.

169. Bain OF, Brown KD, Sacher RA, et al. A hospital-wide blind control program for bedside glucose meters. *Arch Pathol Lab Med* 1989;113:1370–1375.

170. Barr JT, Otto CN. Development of a quantitative weighted scoring instrument to evaluate bedside blood glucose testing programs. *Clin Lab Management Rev* 1998;12:70–79.

171. Bindels R, de Clercq PA, Winkens RA, et al. A test ordering system with automated reminders for primary care based on practice guidelines. *Int J Med Informatics* 2000;58–59:219–233.

172. Bindels R, Winkens RA, van Wersch JW, et al. Comparing assessment of appropriateness of diagnostic tests between a human expert and an automated reminder system. *Stud Health Technol Informatics* 2000;77:239–243.

173. Boyd JC, Bruns DE. Quality specifications for glucose meters: assessment by simulation modeling of errors in insulin dose. *Clin Chem* 2001;47:209–214.

174. Connelly LM. Past, present, future: a continuous cycle of improvement for ancillary glucose testing. *Clin Lab Management Rev* 1997;11:171–180.

175. Despotis GJ, Santoro SA, Spitznagel E, et al. Prospective evaluation and clinical utility of on-site monitoring of coagulation in patients undergoing cardiac operation. *J Thorac Cardiovasc Surg* 1994;107:271–279.

176. Despotis GJ, Grishaber JE, Goodnough LT. The effect of an intraoperative treatment algorithm on physicians' transfusion practice in cardiac surgery. *Transfusion* 1994;34:290–296.

177. Despotis GJ, Joist JH, Goodnough LT. Monitoring of hemostasis in cardiac surgical patients: impact of point-of-care testing on blood loss and transfusion outcomes. *Clin Chem* 1997;43:1684–1696.

178. Despotis GJ, Skubas NJ, Goodnough LT. Optimal management of bleeding and transfusion in patients undergoing cardiac surgery. *Sem Thorac Cardiovasc Surg* 1999;11:84–104.

179. du Plessis M, Ubbink JB, Vermaak WJH. Analytical quality of near-patient blood cholesterol and glucose determinations. *Clin Chem* 2000;46:1085–1090.

180. Halpern MT, Palmer CS, Simpson KN, et al. The economic and clinical efficiency of point-of-care testing for critically ill patients: a decision-analysis model. *Am J Med Qual* 1998;13:3–12.

181. Harris JS. Development, use, and evaluation of clinical practice guidelines. *J Occup Environ Med* 1997;39:23–34.

182. Keffer JH. Guidelines and algorithms: perceptions of why and when they are successful and how to improve them. *Clin Chem* 2001;47:1563–1572.

183. Kilgore ML, Steindel SJ, Smith JA. Using patient satisfaction as an indicator of the quality of laboratory services: applying social science methods to evaluate outcomes in laboratory medicine. *Clin Lab Management Rev* 1997;11:93–102.

184. Kost GJ. Theory of network planning for laboratory research and development. *Am J Clin Pathol* 1983;79:353–359.

185. Kost GJ. Application of program evaluation and review technique (PERT) for laboratory research and development. *Am J Clin Pathol* 1986;86:188–192.

186. Kost GJ. Artificial intelligence and new knowledge structures. In: Kost GJ, ed. *Handbook of clinical automation, robotics, and optimization.* New York: John Wiley and Sons, 1996:149–193.

187. Kost GJ. Understanding and preventing medical errors in point-of-care testing. In: Nichols JH, ed. *Point-of-care testing: performance improvement and evidence-based outcomes.* New York: Marcel Dekker, (in press).

188. Kost GJ. National Guideline Clearinghouse. *Clin Chem* 2000;46:141–142.

189. Lewandrowski E, MacMillan D, Misiano D, et al. Process improvement for bedside capillary glucose testing in a large academic medical

center: the impact of new technology on point-of-care testing. *Clin Chim Acta* 2001;307:175–179.

190. Skeie S, Thue G, Sandberg S. Patient-derived quality specifications for instruments used in self-monitoring of blood glucose. *Clin Chem* 2001;47:67–73.

191. Whitley RJ, Santrach PJ, Phillips DL. Establishing a quality management system for unit-use testing based on NCCLS proposed guideline (EP 18-P). *Clin Chim Acta* 2001;307:145–149.

192. Winkens RA, Ament AJ, Pop P, et al. Routine individual feedback on requests for diagnostic tests: an economic evaluation. *Med Decis Making* 1996;16:309–314.

193. Selker HP, Beshansky JR, Pauker SG, et al. The epidemiology of delays in a teaching hospital: the development and use of a tool that detects unnecessary hospital days. *Med Care* 1989;27:112–129.

194. Herr DM, Newton NC, Santrach PJ, et al. Airborne and rescue point-of-care testing. *Am J Clin Pathol* 1995;104:S54–S58.

195. Burritt MF, Santrach PJ, Hankins DG, et al. Evaluation of the i-STAT portable clinical analyzer for use in a helicopter. *Scand J Clin Lab Invest* 1996;56[Suppl 224]:121–128.

196. Mohammad AA, Summers H, Burchfield JE, et al. STAT turnaround time: satellite and point-to-point testing. *Lab Med* 1996;27:684–688.

197. Kilgore ML, Steindel SJ, Smith JA. Evaluating stat testing options in an academic health center: therapeutic turnaround time and staff satisfaction. *Clin Chem* 1998;44:1597–1603.

198. Salem M, Chernow B, Burke R, et al. Bedside diagnostic blood testing: its accuracy, rapidity, and utility in blood conservation. *JAMA* 1991;266:382–389.

199. Foulke GE, Harlow DJ. Effective measures for reducing blood loss from diagnostic laboratory tests on intensive care unit patients. *Crit Care Med* 1989;17:1143–1145.

200. Dech ZF. Blood conservation in the critically ill. *AACN Clin Issues Crit Care Nurs* 1994;5:169–177.

201. Cooley DA. Conservation of blood during cardiovascular surgery. *Am J Surg* 1995;170[Suppl 6A]:53S–59S.

202. Dech ZF, Szaflarski NL. Nursing strategies to minimize blood loss associated with phlebotomy. *AACN Clin Issues* 1996;7:277–287.

203. Wilson JR, Gaedeke MK. Blood conservation in neonatal and pediatric populations. *AACN Clin Issues* 1996;7:229–237.

204. Chernow B, Jackson E, Miller JA, et al. Blood conservation in acute care and critical care. *AACN Clin Issues* 1996;7:191–197.

205. von Ahsen N, Muller C, Serke S, et al. Important role of nondiagnostic blood loss and blunted erythropoetic response in the anemia of medical intensive care patients. *Crit Care Med* 1999;27:2630–2639.

206. Eckardt KU. Anemia in critical illness. *Wien Klin Wochenschr* 2001;113:84–89.

207. Becker RC, Cyr J, Corrao JM, et al. Bedside coagulation monitoring in heparin-treated patients with active thromboembolic disease: a coronary care unit experience. *Am Heart J* 1994;128:719–723.

208. Becker RC. Exploring the medical need for alternate site testing: a clinician's perspective. *Arch Pathol Lab Med* 1995;119:894–897.

209. Becker RC, Ball SP, Eisenberg P, et al. A randomized, multicenter trial of weight-adjusted intravenous heparin dose titration and point-of-care coagulation monitoring in hospitalized patients with active thromboembolic disease. *Am Heart J* 1999;137:59–71.

210. Collison PO. The need for a point of care testing: an evidence-based appraisal. *Scand J Clin Lab Invest* 1999;59[Suppl 230]:67–73.

211. Zabel KM, Granger CB, Becker RC, et al. Use of bedside activated partial thromboplastin time monitor to adjust heparin dosing after thrombolysis for acute myocardial infarction: results of GUSTO-I. Global Utilization of Streptokinase and TPA for Occluded Coronary Arteries. *Am Heart J* 1998;136:868–876.

212. Johnson LR, Doherty G, Lairmore T, et al. Evaluation of the performance and clinical impact of a rapid intraoperative parathyroid hormone assay in conjunction with preoperative imaging and concise parathyroidectomy. *Clin Chem* 2001;47:919–925.

213. Frey N, Dietz A, Kurowski V, et al. Angiographic correlates of a positive troponin T test in patients with unstable angina. *Crit Care Med* 2001;29:1130–1136.

214. Ohman EM, Armstrong PW, White HD, et al. Risk stratification

with a point-of-care cardiac troponin T test in acute myocardial infarction. *Am J Cardiol* 1999;84:1281–1286.

215. Ng SM, Krishnaswamy P, Morrisey R, et al. Mitigation of the clinical significance of spurious elevations of cardiac troponin I in settings of coronary ischemia using serial testing of multiple cardiac markers. *Am J Cardiol* 2001;87:994–999.

216. Newby LK, Storrow AB, Gibler WB, et al. Bedside multimarker testing for risk stratification in chest pain units: the chest pain evaluation by creatinine kinase-MB, myoglobin, and troponin I (CHECK-MATE) study. *Circulation* 2001;103:1832–1837.

217. Ng SM, Krishnaswamy P, Morrisey R, et al. Ninety-minute critical pathway for chest pain evaluation. *Am J Cardiol* 2001;88:611–617.

218. Greenson N, Macoviak J, Krishnaswamy P, et al. Usefulness of cardiac troponin I in patients undergoing open heart surgery. *Am Heart J* 2001;141:447–455.

219. Tierney WM. Improving clinical decisions and outcomes with information: A review. *Intl J Med Informatics* 2001;62:1–9.

220. Kost GJ, Omand K, Kirk JD. A strategy for the use of cardiac injury markers (troponin I and T, creatine kinase-MB and mass, and myoglobin) in the diagnosis of acute myocardial infarction. *Arch Pathol Lab Med* 1998;122:245–251.

221. Wahr JA, Parks R, Boisvert D, et al. Preoperative serum potassium levels and perioperative outcomes in cardiac surgery patients. *JAMA* 1999;281:2203–2210.

222. Kollef MH. The identification of ICU-specific outcome predictors: a comparison of medical, surgical, and cardiothoracic ICUs from a single institution. *Heart Lung* 1995;24:60–66.

223. Kollef MH, Eisenberg PR, Shannon W. A rapid assay for the detection of circulating D-dimer is associated with clinical outcomes among critically ill patients. *Crit Care Med* 1998;26:1054–1060.

224. Kollef MH, Zahid M, Eisenberg PR. Predictive value of a rapid semi-quantitative D-dimer assay in critically ill patients with suspected venous thromboembolic disease. *Crit Care Med* 2000;28:414–420.

225. Dempfle C, Schraml M, Besenthal I, et al. Multicentre evaluation of a new point-of-care test for quantitative determination of D-dimer. *Clin Chim Acta* 2001;307:211–218.

226. Kline JA, Israel EG, Michelson EA, et al. Diagnostic accuracy of a bedside D-dimer assay and alveolar dead-space measurement for rapid exclusion of pulmonary embolism: a multicenter study. *JAMA* 2001;285:761–768.

227. Rodger MA, Jones G, Rasuli P, et al. Steady-state end-tidal alveolar dead space fraction and D-dimer: bedside tests to exclude pulmonary embolism. *Chest* 2001;120:115–119.

228. Kollef MH, Eisenberg PR. A rapid qualitative assay to detect circulating endotoxin can predict the development of multiorgan dysfunction. *Chest* 1997;112:173–180.

229. Agarwal R, Heinz T. Bedside hemoglobinometry in hemodialysis patients: lessons from point-of-care testing. *ASAIO J* 2001;47:240–243.

230. Piironen T, Nurmi M, Irjala K, et al. Measurement of circulating forms of prostate-specific antigen in whole blood immediately after venipuncture: implications for point-of-care testing. *Clin Chem* 2001;47:703–711.

231. McDonagh TA, Robb SD, Murdoch DR, et al. Biochemical detection of left-ventricular systolic dysfunction. *Lancet* 1998;351:9–13.

232. McDonagh TA. Asymptomatic left ventricular dysfunction in the community. *Curr Cardiol Rep* 2000;2:470–474.

233. Cheng V, Kazanagra R, Garcia A, et al. A rapid bedside test for B-type peptide predicts treatment outcomes in patients admitted for decompensated heart failure: a pilot study. *J Am Coll Cardiol* 2001;37:386–391.

234. Dao Q, Krishnaswamy P, Kazanegra R, et al. Utility of B-type natriuretic peptide in the diagnosis of congestive heart failure in an urgent care setting. *J Am Coll Cardiol* 2001;37:379–385.

235. Maisel A. B-type natriuretic peptide levels: a potential novel "white count" for congestive heart failure. *J Card Failure* 2001;7:183–193.

236. Maisel AS, Koon J, Krishnaswamy P, et al. Utility of B-natriuretic peptide as a rapid, point-of-care test for screening patients undergoing echocardiography to determine left ventricular dysfunction. *Am Heart J* 2001;141:367–374.

237. Vogeser M, Jacob K. B-type natriuretic peptide (BNP)—validation of an immediate response assay. *Clin Lab* 2001;47:29–33.

238. Krilov LR, Lipson SM, Barone SR, et al. Evaluation of a rapid diagnostic test for respiratory syncytial virus (RSV): potential for bedside diagnosis. *Pediatrics* 1994;93:903–906.

239. Mackenzie A, Hallam N, Mitchell E, et al. Near patient testing for respiratory syncytial virus in paediatric accident and emergency: prospective pilot study. *BMJ* 1999;319:289–290.

240. Mackie PL, Joannidis PA, Beattie J. Evaluation of an acute point-of-care system screening for respiratory syncytial virus infection. *J Hosp Infection* 2001;48:66–71.

241. Butter NL, Hattersley AT, Clark PM. Development of a bloodspot test for insulin. *Clin Chim Acta* 2001;310:141–150.

242. Grieve R, Beech R, Vincent J, et al. Near patient testing in diabetes clinics: appraising costs and outcomes. *Health Technol Assess* 1999;3:1–74.

243. Adams DA, Buus-Frank M. Point-of-care technology: the i-STAT system for bedside blood analysis. *J Pediatr Nurs* 1995;10:194–198.

244. Bayne CG. Point of care testing: testing the system? *Nurs Mgmt* 1997;28:34–36.

245. Bayne CG. Pocket-sized medicine: new POC technologies. *Nurs Mgmt* 1997;28:30–32.

246. Cachia PG, McGregor E, Adlakha S, et al. Accuracy and precision of the TAS analyser for near-patient INR testing by non-pathology staff in the community. *J Clin Pathol* 1998;51:68–72.

247. Dirks JL. Innovations in technology: continuous intra-arterial blood gas monitoring. *Crit Care Nurs* 1995;15:19–27.

248. Dirks JL. Diagnostic blood analysis using point-of-care technology. *AACN Clin Issues* 1996;7:249–259.

249. Fitzmaurice DA, Hobbs FD, Murray ET. Primary care anticoagulant clinic management using computerized decision support and near patient international normalized ratio (INR) testing: routine data from a practice nurse-led clinic. *Fam Pract* 1998;15:144–146.

250. Fitzmaurice DA, Hobbs FD, Murray ET, et al. Oral anticoagulation management in primary care with the use of computerized decision support and near-patient testing: a randomized, controlled trial. *Arch Intern Med* 2000;160:2343–2348.

251. Foley SM, Sommers MS. Molecular genetics: from bench to bedside. *AACN Clin Issues* 1998;9:491–498.

252. Granneman SA, Cochran JE, Ross LP, et al. Improving technology: blood glucose testing. *Nurs Mgmt* 1994;25:36–38.

253. Harvey MA. Point-of-care laboratory testing in critical care. *Am J Crit Care* 1999;8:72–83.

254. Hilton S, Rink E, Fletcher J, et al. Near patient testing in general practice: attitudes of general practitioners and practice nurses and quality assurance procedures carried out. *Brit J Gen Pract* 1994;44:577–580.

255. Hutsko GM, Jones JB, Danielson L. Using point-of-care testing to speed patient care: one emergency department's experience. *J Emerg Nurs* 1995;21:408–412.

256. Kreitzer MJ, Marko M, Nettles A. Implementation of a quality improvement program for a bedside blood glucose testing system: a collaborative endeavor. *J Nurs Care Quality* 1992; [Suppl]:1–11.

257. Krenzischek DA, Tanseco FV. Comparative study of bedside and laboratory measurements of hemoglobin. *Am J Crit Care* 1996;5:427–432.

258. Lamb LS. Responsibilities in point-of-care testing: an institutional perspective. *Arch Pathol Lab Med* 1995;119:886–889.

259. Lamb LS, Parrish RS, Goran SF, et al. Current nursing practice of point-of-care laboratory diagnostic testing in critical care units. *Am J Crit Care* 1995;4:429–434.

260. Lamb-Harvard J. Nurses at the bedside: influencing outcomes. *Nurs Clin North Am* 1997;32:579–587.

261. McConnell EA. Point-of-care testing. *Nurs Mgmt* 1998;27:50.

262. McConnell EA. Hold the lab in the palm of your hand. *Nurs Mgmt* 1999;30:57–59.

263. McConnell EA. POC: testing on the move. *Nurs Mgmt* 2000;31:50–51.

264. McConnell EA. Myths and facts about point-of-care testing. *Nursing* 2000;30:73.

265. Metheny NA, Smith L, Stewart BJ. Development of a reliable and valid bedside test for bilirubin and its utility for improving prediction of feeding tube location. *Nurs Res* 2000;49:302–309.

266. Miller CM, Niznik C, Springer J, et al. Decentralized lab testing: a collaborative approach to point of care testing. *Hosp Top* 1995;73:23–27.

267. Miller KA, Miller NA. Joining forces to improve point-of-care testing. *Nurs Mgmt* 1998;28:34, 36–37.

268. Neil-Urban S. The devil is in the details: body fluid testing regulation and the erosion of nursing practice. *Nurs Forum* 1998;33:11–15.

269. Nichols JH, Poe SS. Quality assurance, practical management, and outcomes of point-of-care testing: laboratory perspectives, part I. *Clin Lab Mgmt Rev* 1999;13:341–350.

270. Osborn DA, Lockley C, Jeffrey HE, et al. Interobserver reliability of the click test: a rapid bedside test to determine surfactant function. *J Paediatr Child Health* 1998;34:544–547.

271. Poe SS, Nichols JH. Quality assurance, practical management, and outcomes of point-of-care testing: nursing perspectives, part II. *Clin Lab Management Rev* 2000;14:12–18.

272. Schallon L. Point of care testing in critical care. *Crit Care Nurs Clin North Am* 1999;11:99–106.

273. Zeler KM, McPharlane TJ, Salamonsen RF. Effectiveness of nursing involvement in bedside control of coagulation status after cardiac surgery. *Am J Crit Care* 1992;1:70–75.

274. Jastremski M, Jastremski C, Shepherd M, et al. A model for technology assessment as applied to closed loop infusion systems. Technology Assessment Task Force of the Society of Critical Care Medicine. *Crit Care Med* 1995;23:1745–1755.

275. Kost GJ, Hague C. The current and future status of critical care testing and patient monitoring. *Am J Clin Pathol* 1995;104[Suppl 1]:S2–S17.

276. Kalogeropoulos D, Carson ER, Collison PO. Clinical-HINTS: integrated intelligent ICU patient monitoring and information management system. *Stud Health Technol Informatics* 1997;43:906–910.

277. Tamada JA, Garg S, Jovanovic L, et al. Noninvasive glucose monitoring: comprehensive clinical results. *JAMA* 1999;282:1839–1844.

278. Webster NR. Monitoring the critically ill patient. *J R Coll Surg Edinb* 1999;44:386–393.

279. Gross TM, Bode BW, Einhorn D, et al. Performance evaluation of the MiniMed continuous glucose monitoring system during patient home use. *Diabetes Technol Ther* 2000;2:49–56.

280. Kohli-Seth R, Oropello JM. The future of bedside monitoring. *Crit Care Clin* 2000;16:557–578.

281. Javanov E, Raskovic D, Price J, et al. Patient monitoring using personal area networks of wireless intelligent sensors. *Biomed Sci Instr* 2001;37:373–378.

282. Bernardo A. Experience with patient self-management of oral anticoagulation. *J Thromb Thrombolysis* 1996;2:321–325.

283. Koepke JA. Point-of-care coagulation testing. *Lab Med* 2000;31:343–346.

284. Laposata M. Point-of-care coagulation testing: stepping gently forward. *Clin Chem* 2001;47:801–802.

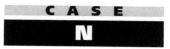
COST–BENEFIT ANALYSIS FOR BLOOD GAS POCT

FREDERICK L. KIECHLE

Blood gas determinations may be performed in the central laboratory, in a satellite laboratory, or by respiratory therapists assigned to a critical care unit such as the neonatal intensive care unit (NICU). We evaluated the processes and costs associated with these three models to determine their cost-to-benefit ratio (1). Current laboratory processes, including turnaround time, process steps, the total number of handoffs, and equipment maintenance time, were monitored. Also, a variety of parameters such as test volume/shift, percent utilization of personnel, utilization costs, labor costs, supervision costs, phlebotomy material, reagent costs, and equipment depreciation were considered. Handoffs included transfer of sample from one person to another, either directly or via a pneumatic tube system, as well as transfer of information regarding a particular order or test from one person to another. Flow diagrams were constructed from the total number of process steps from test request to result availability for the central laboratory and satellite laboratories.

For the satellite laboratory model, there was a 20% to 30% reduction in the total number of specimen handoffs added to information handoffs per specimen compared with the central laboratory. Moreover, the time required to perform process steps such as test order, phlebotomy, transport, paper/computer processing, and result release from the laboratory was decreased by 35 to 45 minutes. Utilization rate was calculated by determining the time to perform daily workload (test/d x min/test) added to maintenance time/d, then divided by the total time the laboratory was open. Finally, the result was converted to a percentage. Personnel utilization rate demonstrated that the satellite laboratory was extensively underutilized compared with the central laboratory or NICU (Table N.1). The satellite laboratory is staffed by a medical technologist who is not performing laboratory procedures 80% of the time and yet accounted for 50% of the total cost for the laboratory. Therefore, the satellite laboratory provided a blood gas value of $4.93 and $6.78 greater cost per procedure than the central laboratory or NICU, respectively. In the future, this satellite laboratory will be closed and replaced by a rapid-response laboratory located in the central laboratory and equipped with several whole-blood analyzers. Only two or three panels of tests using whole blood will be performed in this new laboratory.

In contrast, the NICU laboratory performed a blood gas analysis for $1.85 less than the central laboratory. This savings is achieved by using respiratory therapists to perform the blood gas analysis and occupy their non–laboratory testing time performing other duties. This efficient use of labor and reduction in process steps and handoffs are the primary reasons for the cost reduction in the NICU satellite laboratory model. If a medical technologist had been placed in the NICU to operate the blood gas analyzer, the underutilization of labor would drive the cost per test to a value greater than the central laboratory. This outcome was documented by Winkelman and Wybenga (2), who reported that a medical technologist operating a blood gas satellite laboratory in a NICU generated a total cost per reportable result of $8.98 compared with $3.54 for the central laboratory. Bailey and colleagues (3) demonstrated substantial cost savings by closing three underutilized satellite laboratories and introducing POCT by nursing personnel in the units formerly served by the satellite laboratories. Alternatives to satellite laboratories include rapid specimen transport systems, quality improvement process to reduce preanalytic and postanalytic turnaround time, and mobile carts.

TABLE N.1. LABOR UTILIZATION AND COST PER TEST FOR THREE BLOOD-GAS ANALYSIS MODELS

	Central Lab	Satellite Lab	NICU Lab
Average volume of specimens/d	705[a]	36	30
Hours of operation	24	12	24
Labor utilization	97%	20%	98%
Blood gas[b]	$8.76	$13.69	$6.91

NICU, neonatal intensive care unit.
[a]Stat blood gases and complete blood counts.
[b]Blood gases in NICU are performed by respiratory therapists; satellite lab is staffed by medical technologists.

In conclusion, although satellite laboratories reduce the number of process steps and handoffs and the total turnaround time, they are generally more costly than the central laboratory, primarily because of low staff utilization. Cost–benefit analysis provides a method for evaluating which model for blood gas analysis will generate both the lowest cost per procedure and the best clinical outcome. Each model should be evaluated individually, and alternative strategies for improvement in therapeutic turnaround time should be explored before a final decision is made.

REFERENCES

1. Kiechle FL, Aulakh V. Satellite laboratories: a cost-benefit study. *Medical Laboratory Observer* 1998;30:44–50.
2. Winkelman JW, Wybenga DR. Quantification of medical and operational factors determining central versus satellite laboratory testing of blood gases. *Am J Clin Pathol* 1994;102:7–10.
3. Bailey TM, Topham TM, Wantz S, et al. Laboratory process improvement through point-of-care testing. *Journal of Quality Improvement* 1997;23:262–280.

CASE

O

COST ANALYSIS OF POINT-OF-CARE GLUCOSE TESTING

FREDERICK L. KIECHLE

The cost attributed to point-of-care testing (POCT) programs in a hospital can be determined by two different methods: cost center–based analysis or defect-rate inclusion analysis (1) (Table O.1). Any evaluation of costs applies to current practices, and new calculations are required following any change in volume, reagent costs, methods, salary, and so forth. In general, the cost of performing a POCT glucose is indirectly related to the volume of procedures per nursing unit (2). Units that perform a low volume of glucose analyses should arrange to have their tests performed in the central laboratory (3).

The cost center–based analysis recorded all direct and indirect costs associated with performing a glucose measurement in two locations: in the clinical chemistry laboratory or on the nursing unit using POCT. This method has been used in numerous cost comparisons between POCT and the central laboratory. The conclusion that a POCT program on a nursing unit will be more expensive (by $7.85 and $3.92, respectively) for total and incremental costs than the central laboratory is inevitable when cost center–based analysis is used (Table O.1). Total costs include direct and indirect costs. Direct costs include the personnel time to prepare and perform the test, reagents, quality control, and equipment depreciation. Indirect costs include reporting costs (computer) and hospital overhead. Incremental costs include only the direct costs and not the indirect costs. Therefore, incremental costs demonstrate what it would cost to perform one more glucose test, assuming the equipment and facility are already available (Table O.1). This analysis of direct costs for the central laboratory does not include the cost of the collection tube or labor required to obtain the specimen. It includes only the direct cost assigned to the cost center (clinical chemistry laboratory) that performs the assay. This traditional approach to cost analysis is not ideal for evaluating POCT programs because it fails to quantify the effect of defects (4,5).

The defect-rate inclusion analysis moves beyond the narrow cost-center approach and includes the total cost related to failure to provide a central laboratory or POCT result in a reasonable time. The *defect rate*, or failure to achieve a reasonable turnaround time, may be defined as internal or external failure rates. As a result of delay in the usual turnaround time, the receiver of the test results incurs external failure costs. Internal failure costs are incurred by the testing center as a consequence of a defect in

the testing system. The cost of performing glucose testing in the central laboratory or POCT site was compared using defect-rate inclusion analysis by Cembrowski and Kiechle (1). In this study, the internal failure rate was attributed to the repeat rate: 3% in the central laboratory and 5% in the POCT unit plus requests for the central laboratory to confirm high and low extreme values. The POCT unit contributed approximately six times as much of the internal failure costs as the central laboratory (Table O.1). The central laboratory contributed more than 22 times the cost of the POCT unit for external failure costs. This disproportional distribution is directly related to the central laboratory's failure 27% of the time to provide a glucose value within 15 minutes of the time the food tray was delivered to the POCT unit. Each delay in turnaround time for a glucose value resulted in 16 minutes of a registered nurse delaying insulin treatment and searching in the computer or on the phone for the glucose result. Although defect-rate inclusion analysis does not include all costs related to glucose analysis, it includes the effect of defects on the laboratory and POCT unit when delays in obtaining results are secondary to repeat analysis or other problems.

In conclusion, the evaluation of costs for a POCT program versus central laboratory requires more detail than the cost center-based analysis can provide. Effort should be made to look at the financial consequence of defects, especially internal failure and external failure costs, during cost comparisons between central laboratory and POCT application.

TABLE O.1. COST ANALYSIS FOR EVALUATING POCT GLUCOSE

	Central Lab	POCT Program
Cost-center analysis		
Total cost/glucose	$1.22	$9.07
Incremental cost/glucose	$0.87	$4.79
Annual defect-rate inclusive analysis		
Annual cost/21-bed diabetic unit	$105,045.00	$73,524.00
Internal failure costs	$776.00	$4,525.00
External failure costs	$45,100.00	$2,000.00

POCT, point-of-care testing.

REFERENCES

1. Cembrowski GS, Kiechle FL. Point-of-care testing: critical analysis and practical application. *Adv Pathol Lab Med* 1994;7:3–26.
2. Lee-Lewandrowski E, Laposata M, Eschenbach K, et al. Utilization and cost analysis of bedside capillary glucose testing in a large teaching hospital: implications for managing point-of-care testing. *Am J Med* 1994;97:222–301.
3. Kiechle FL, Main RI. Blood glucose: measurement in the point-of-care setting. *Lab Med* 2000;31:276–282.
4. Kiechle FL, Aulakh V. Satellite laboratories: a cost-benefit study. *Medical Laboratory Observer* 1998;30:44–50.
5. Handorf CR. POC testing: must quality cost more? *Medical Laboratory Observer* 1993;25(Suppl):28–33.

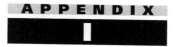

APPENDIX
I

EFFECTS OF POINT-OF-CARE TESTING ON TIME, PROCESS, DECISION MAKING, TREATMENT, AND OUTCOME

GERALD J. KOST
NAM K. TRAN

APPENDIX I. EFFECTS OF POINT-OF-CARE TESTING ON TIME, PROCESS, DECISION MAKING, TREATMENT, AND OUTCOME

Ref.	Condition or Setting	Metric or Medical Surrogate	P (for metric)	Finding(s)
1	ED	TAT Discharge time Admission	0.0001 NA NA	POCT median TAT for cardiac injury markers (cTnI, CK-MB, & myoglobin) was 17 vs. 82.5 min for central stat lab. Discharge time reduced for 5% (normal ECG). Inappropriate admission in 2%–5% depended on cTnI diagnostic threshold.
2	ICU	TAT Cost	NA NA	Handheld/ near-patient TAT was 1–10 min vs. mean of 85 (range, 45–168) for central lab testing. The total cost was lowest for the handheld lactate device.
3	OR	LOS FS, UNE Anesthesia	0.0001 0.0001, 0.001 0.001	Intraoperative PTH POCT had 17/49 vs. 0 discharged day of surgery, 1.4 vs. 2.5 frozen sections (FS), 33% vs. 0% local anesthesia, & 65% vs. 0% unilateral neck explorations (UNE) compared with control group using conventional testing.
4	Bedside	Analysis time Cost	NA NA	Third-generation POC glucose meters give results in a fraction of the time compared with first-generation systems that give results in about 2 min, but POCT costs were higher than conventional lab testing costs.
5	Hospital-acquired infection	RSV positivity	NA	Near-patient testing provided a rapid answer & ensured that infants could be segregated according to RSV infection status, resulting in <1% hospital-acquired infections in planned, accident, & emergency admission patients.
6	ED	TAT, triage Bed utilization Morbidity	NA <0.001 NA	POCT (cTnI, CK-MB, & myoglobin) triaged chest pain patients accurately within 90 min of presenting to the ED, & with algorithm, decreased CCU bed utilization ≥ 40%. POCT & ECG negatives sent home had 0.2% MI in 30 d.
7	Evaluation	TAT	NA	TAT was about 10 min for the POC assay of B-type natriuretic peptide (BNP) vs. longer TAT for other methods.
8	Lung function laboratory	Time difference	NA	Mean time difference between faster POCT & clinical lab results was 13.3 min for a lung function lab, & was 20.2 min for the wards for blood gases. Bubbles in 68% of tube-transported ward samples caused errors, esp. for 100% O_2 test.
9	Trauma	Bubbles Management change Morbidity	NA NA NA	In severe blunt injury within 30 min, POC Hgb (3.5%), ABG (3%), lactate (2.5%), & glucose (0.5%) results yield morbidity-reducing or resource-conserving management changes in prospective, noninterventional study.
10	ED OR	Whole-blood analysis Operators	NA NA	Performance of whole-blood analysis (<2 min) vs. plasma analysis (–5) by nonlab personnel vs. medical technologists, respectively, was equivalent in the OR & ED for Na^+, K^+, Cl^-, glucose, UN, creatinine, TCO_2, & hematocrit.
11	CVDL elective procedures	Wait time: Coagulation Renal	0.014 0.023	POCT decreased wait times for invasive cardiac & radiologic procedures. Coagulation mean 109 ± 41 vs. 171 ± 76 min for central lab; renal, 141 ± 52 vs. 188 ± 54. The percentage of patients meeting scheduled appointments did not improve.
12	Bedside Stat lab	TAT Process steps Decision cycle	NA NA NA	POCT improved TAT: 5:42 min for handheld bedside & 16:13 for stat lab vs. 20:56 for central lab testing. Restructuring with POCT eliminated 12 process steps (6 POCT vs. 18 lab) & improved the efficiency of clinical decision cycles.
13	Active thrombo-embolic patients in 7 hospitals	TTAT Elapsed time Target time	<0.0001 0.0001 0.24	aPTT POCT decreased TTAT for heparin dose adjustment (0.47 vs. 1.60 hr), total elapsed time (1.35 vs. 6.42 hr), & time to reach target aPTT (16.1 vs. 19.4 hr) compared to lab-based coagulation monitoring in multicenter study.
14	District general hospital	TAT Non-CCU LOS Hospital LOS Decision time	<0.0001 0.05 0.0256 NA	Prospective randomized controlled trial showed median TAT for POCT was 20 min vs. 72 for clinical lab testing. In low risk patients, POCT significantly reduced non-CCU (79.5 vs. 145.25) & hospital (149.88 vs. 209.26) LOS. "If the lab TAT exceeds 25% of the decision time, then POCT will be required."
15	General practice	TAT/TTAT Utilization Consultations Cost	0.0161 <0.0001 0.0001 NA	Randomized crossover trial showed near-patient CRP subjects had antibiotics earlier (CRP >50 mg/L), decreased lab services use (CRP, blood samples forwarded), & reduced follow-up phone consultations. Cost effectiveness from reduced services would save $111,160 per yr. TAT 3 min for POCT vs. 1–2 days for lab.
16	Diabetes clinics	Visits, process, costs, control, outcomes	(see the reference)	Controlled trial showed near-patient (NP) $HgbA_{1c}$ led to more management changes for patients who have poor control & mean level was lower in NP cohort. Hospital & clinic visits decreased. Improved process & satisfaction.
17	ED	LOS LOS-discharge LOS-admit	0.02 <0.001 0.25	POCT group LOS was 3:38 (median, hr: min) vs. 4:22 for central lab testing. LOS for POCT patients discharged was 3:05 vs. 4:17 for the control group. The time saving in the POCT group was realized only among the discharged patients.
18	ED	TAT	<0.05	TAT: a) POCT median 5 min; 25–75th percentile, 4–6 min (n = 130) vs. b) porter system: 58 & 47–77 (n = 191), & c) tube transport system: 49 & 37–65 (n = 192). Wait times: a) POCT median, 219 min vs. b) 212, & c) 258 (P NS).

#	Setting	Metric	p-value	Findings
19	ICU	TAT Cost	NA NA	TAT was shorter for POCT: aPPT-CC 6.5 ± 1.9 min, aPPT-TAS 9.6 ± 2.7 vs. 130 ± 38 for central lab coagulation testing. POCT methods cost $4.34–4.84 vs. transportation cost ($3.77) added to central lab direct cost ($1.59) to total $5.36.
20	ED ICU	TAT Cost	NA NA	TAT for POCT was 30 s vs. 60 min for conventional laboratories. Costs of service modalities were considered in implementing POCT.
21	OR CPB	Analysis time	NA	Near-patient hematology analyzer produced 8-parameter CBC results in 2 min; platelet aggregation results were produced after CBC & 5-min incubation. Both deemed feasible for CPB & cardiac catheterization.
22	Bedside	Process steps Nursing time	NA NA	Bedside glucose testing process steps were 6 vs. 15 for central lab testing. Survey of 50 nurses showed less time to perform test than send the sample to the central central lab.
23	ED	DT-hematology DT-biochemistry DT-blood gases	<0.0001 <0.0001 0.09	Decision time (DT) shorter (74 min, hematology; 86, biochemistry; & 21, blood gases) for POCT vs. central lab. Faster changes in treatment deemed critical in 7% of patients. No effect on clinical outcome or time in ED.
24	Intensive care units	Therapeutic TAT (TTAT)	<0.00001	Therapeutic TAT for bedside & CICU satellite lab POCT was significantly shorter vs. TTAT for central lab testing. Principal components showed improved patient care, labor saved, & convenience correlated with higher satisfaction.
25	Bedside Laboratory	TAT	NA	POCT program for whole-blood aPTT was developed because 77 min TAT for laboratory results was inadequate for clinical decision making.
26	AMI patients after thrombolysis	TAT Clinical metrics	NA (see findings)	In GUSTO-I ~3 min TAT aPTT POCT patients had less bleeding (P <0.01), transfusions (P <0.001), & hematocrit decrease (P <0.001), but more recurrent ischemia (P = 0.01) without increased mortality vs. central lab testing group.
27	Bedside Stat lab	TAT Process steps Cost	NA NA NA	POCT TAT demonstrated average reduction of 15:14 min vs. TAT for traditional central lab testing, & 10:52 min vs. stat lab testing. Changes improved decision cycles & decreased process steps. Hospital saved $392,336 annually.
28	ICU NICU CCU	TAT	NA	Areas of high test volume have advantages due to ease of use & shorter time to obtain results with POCT TAT of 60 s vs. 3.5 min without POCT.
29	Laboratory	TAT Cost	NA NA	POCT TAT was 5.5 min & stat lab, 11.5, vs. 52.4 for central lab with a second site blood gas analysis. Total annual savings with POCT was $23,889.
30	CCU ER	TTAT TAT Cost	NA NA NA	Mean TTAT for CCU was 8 vs. 27 min & for ER, 40.6 vs. 72 min, after implementing 2 satellite near-patient labs. Stat TAT improved. Changes made with no workforce increase, net cost decrease, & improved physician satisfaction.
31	Outpatient center in HMO	TAT Length of visit Availability Decisions	0.002 0.145 0.01 NA	CBC TAT for POCT was 34 min vs. central lab, 62. Length of visit for POCT was 108 min vs. central lab, 118 (P NS). Patients left less often before POCT results were available (10.3%) vs. before central lab results available (22.2%). POCT increased the likelihood of medical decisions during outpatient visits.
32	ED	LOS TAT	NS NA	Use of handheld POCT (with limited test cluster) in the ED did not significantly decrease LOS during experimental vs. control period for patients admitted or sent home. POCT TAT was <5 min.
33	Bedside	TAT Cost	NA NA	At two institutions, POCT decreased TAT: institution no. 1 had a TAT of 5.9 min vs. 6.2 for a stat lab. Institution no. 2 had a TAT of 5.0 min vs. 35 for the central lab. Costs/specimen ($) were: 1) 11.03 vs. 4.55, & 2) 8.14 vs. 15.24.
34	ICU Postop CABG	TAT Cost model	NA NA	POCT TAT 5.5 min vs. 11.5 for stat lab & up to maximum of 52.4 for central lab. Modeled 9 scenarios based on 25-hospital survey. POCT savings ranged from $21,508 to $42,438 annually. Deemed suitable for post-op CABG patients.
35	ICU	Blood collection Blood volume Cost TAT	0.002 <0.001 NA NA	Reengineering for ICU POCT reduced process steps up to 80% & saved >$400,000/yr. Blood collected fell from 8.1 to 3.5 mL. Blood volume taken per patient decreased from 56 to 21 mL/24 hr. TAT decreased from 30 to 5 min for routine, & from 15 to 2–3 min for stat test requests.
36	Critical care unit	TAT	<0.05	TAT for portable whole-blood analyzer was 2 min vs. 16.5 for a near-patient lab in a large tertiary critical care unit.
37	Thoracic cardiovascular unit	TAT Ventilator & nursing time	NA NA	Remote automated laboratory system TAT for whole-blood analysis was 4.2 ± 0.3 min at the point of care vs. 20 ± 10 min for lab testing. Ventilator hours for DRG 106 were decreased with POCT, which also saved nursing time.
38	OR Recovery UCL	TAT Cost	NA NA	TAT for a POC satellite lab & an urgent care lab equipped with a rapid transport system (pneumatic tube) were comparable. Savings were estimated at over $45,000 per yr for satellite lab vs. normally staffed lab.

(continued)

APPENDIX I. (continued)

Ref.	Condition or Setting	Metric or Medical Surrogate	P (for metric)	Finding(s)
39	Inpatient substance abuse center	Nursing time	NA	Median time for nurses to perform drugs of abuse POCT was 20 (range 10–60) min. Median number of days before negative
		Days to negative test result	NA	specimens observed varied for lab vs. POCT, for which accuracy improvement measures are necessary.
40	ED	TAT	NA	POCT results were available 31 min (mean) sooner than central laboratory results for Hct; 43 for Na$^+$, K$^+$, & Cl$^-$; & 44 for
		POC decisions	NA	BUN & glucose. Different or earlier Rx in 9.5%, & release or admit decision in 10.7% of patients, if POCT.
41	CCU	TAT	<0.001	TAT for bedside testing of aPTT was less than 3 min vs. 126 ± 84 for conventional lab testing. Time to achieve therapeutic
		TTAT	<0.005	state of systemic anticoagulation was 8.2 vs. 18.1 hr. Decision time (DT) for heparin titration was 14.5 min vs. 3 hr.
		DT	<0.001	
42	CCU	TAT	NA	CCU bedside K$^+$ testing TAT was 2 min vs. 24 for conventional lab testing; number of process steps was 9 at bedside vs. 13 for
		Process steps	NA	conventional lab cycle.
43–45	OR	Blood products	0.0006–0.02	TAT for on-site OR coagulation tests was 4 min vs. 44 for standard lab. FFP, PRBC, platelet use, microvascular bleeding, &
		Bleeding	0.003	operative time decreased significantly. Reexplorations decreased (P NS). First treatment changed in 25%. On-site testing &
		TAT	NA	algorithmic treatment savings worth $1,504 per patient.
		Cost	NA	
46	ED	TAT	NA	TAT with POCT was 6 ± 1 min. vs. 64 ± 3 for standard analysis. POCT helped trauma triage & had the potential to reduce costs
		Triage	NA	substantially.
		Cost	NA	
47	PACU	TAT	NA	ABG TAT average for POCT was 2 min vs. 26 without POCT. LOS was 192.2 min with POCT vs. 209.8 min without POCT. POCT
		LOS	NA	estimated to save $101,376 per yr.
		Cost	NA	
48	Surgical center	TAT	<0.01	On-site satellite vs. central lab, 17 vs. 35 (CBC), 20 vs. 64 (K$^+$), 16 vs. 77 (urinalysis), & 20 vs. 57 (pregnancy) min TAT; 0 vs.
		Delays	0.11	4 surgeries delayed; & 0 vs. 18 surgeries begun without test results, respectively. OR delay time lost would constitute a
		Disjoint results	<0.01	$35,360 annual loss for the hospital.
		Cost	NA	
49	Medical center	LOS	NS	Retrospective study of bedside glucose testing showed no significant difference in LOS (days) for acute diabetics before (10.1 ± 7.5) vs. after (8.8 ± 6.1), & for complicated cases, before (91 ± 77.2) vs. after (85.2 ± 64.8), implementation.
50	Hospital	TAT	NA	Bedside capillary glucose testing decreased TAT, reduced the need for phlebotomy, & facilitated patient training. POCT service
		Phlebotomy	NA	costs depend on test volume. POCT cost in 7 high-volume units was lower that the cost of central lab testing.
		Cost	NA	
51	Cardiac surgery	TAT	NA	TAT for open heart profile testing in a surgical support lab was 5 min vs. 30 for testing provided by the main clinical
		Cost	NA	lab. Combined blood gas & electrolyte testing has potential to reduce costs.
52	VAMC Mobile lab	TAT	NA	Average TAT was 18 min for mobile lab vs. 83 for main lab. Mobile lab saved 467 nursing & clinician man-hrs & changed the
		Man-hours effort	NA	way patient care is delivered by allowing common test results to be reviewed quickly by physicians & nurses.
		Cost	NA	
53	ED	TAT	NA	POCT TAT mean was 8 min (time from blood drawn to results display on device), & central lab, 59 (blood drawn to results
		Cost	NA	entry to mainframe computer). POCT would have resulted in earlier therapeutic action in 19% of patients.
		Decisions	NA	
54	NICU Satellite lab	TAT	NA	NICU satellite lab TAT was 4.5 min vs. 6 for central lab. Difference attributable to pneumatic tube transit & accessioning for
		Cost	NA	central lab. Satellite lab cost was $5.44 higher per reportable result. Weigh medical utility vs. extra cost.
55	ED	TAT	NA	Median within-lab TAT was 61 (chemistry) & 70 (CBC) min, but 45-min delay in physician review was longest component of
		Cost	NA	overall TAT. Second phase TAT was 36 (chemistry) & 55 (hematology), confounded by preanalytic delays.
56	Day-stay department	TAT	NA	POCT vs. lab-based system had faster TAT (3 min vs. 1–2 h) & fewer process steps (4 vs. 11). Quick Hct check before discharge
		Process steps	NA	saved patient wait time. POCT improved lab relations, workflow, immediate therapy, & patient care capacity.
		Waiting time	NA	
57	Bedside glucose testing	Performance time	NA	Total performance time (specimen collection to data entry) was 5 min. Bedside glucose testing cost was $11.50 per test vs.
		Cost	NA	$3.19 for conventional lab testing. Extra cost for 172 VA hospitals estimated to be $3,000,000 per yr.

Ref	Setting	Measure	P-value	Findings
58–60	CAP Q-Probe ED National Survey	TAT Process analysis	NA NA	Median TAT for lab within ED was 30 & 18 min vs. 36 & 26 (25) for K+ & Hgb, respectively, overall. Type of personnel collecting specimen & transport affected TAT. F/U showed ED physicians are not satisfied with lab services.
61	Bedside ICU	TAT Blood volume	— —	Significant time & blood conservation were realized by the use of bedside microchemistry instruments in the ICU.
62–64	ICU	ICU LOS Hospital LOS Hospital cost Ventilator wean/optimize, TT	<0.05 <0.05 <0.05 NA	Average ICU LOS for DKA with a) bedside glucose testing was 1.4 day vs. b) clinical lab testing, 2.5. Average hospital LOS was a) 5.0 vs. b) 8.0. Total hospital costs were a) $2,380 vs. b) $3,925, while testing costs were a) $16.20 vs. $126. Pulse oximetry decreased number of ABG/day, ventilator optimize & wean times, & ICU LOS (1.2 d with vs. 2.1 without). POCT improved therapeutic time (TT).
65	Anticonvulsant clinic critical path method	Throughput Clinic duration Cost	NA NA NA	Near-patient (NP) therapeutic drug monitoring increased productivity 23%. NP vs. pre-NP patients seen, 246 vs. 200; average patients/clinic, 9.5 vs. 7.7; average consultation time, 16 vs. 17 min, clinic duration, 90 vs. 180 min; & clinician time, 45 vs. 180 min. Costs were reduced 18.3% (system) & 34% (patient visit).
66	Satellite Lab National Survey	TAT	NA	Actual TAT for blood gases performed in a satellite lab was 8 min vs. 19 in the routine lab, & 10 vs. 38 for chemistry tests.
67	National Survey	TAT Whole-blood analysis	NA NA	TAT for whole-blood analysis of K+, Ca2+, glucose, & Hct or Hgb ranged from 2 to 20 min. Majority of sites surveyed reported 5 min TAT. POCT electrolytes & blood gases performed most frequently at cardiac transplant centers.
68	Hospital-based anticoagulation clinic	RN time Patient time Cost	<0.02 <0.02 <0.02	Total registered nurse (RN) time per visit averaged 12.4 min for capillary PT vs. 8.3 for standard lab PT, but 16.2 min vs. 20 for mean patient time per visit. Increased costs associated with RN time overweighed by lower costs of POC capillary PT.
69	OR CAB surgery	TAT	<0.05	Mean TAT was 2.5 ± 0.02 min for POCT vs. 8.5 ± 1.0 for results from the OR stat lab. Large changes in ionized calcium (18%) & potassium (38%) levels were noted during cardiac surgery. Arrhythmias responded to KCI administration.
70	Epilepsy center clinic	Therapeutic management Drug assays	<0.01 to <0.05 <0.01	On-site anticonvulsive drug testing (<15 min) vs. not, optimized time to optimal therapy (4.5 vs. 22.9 wk), consultations (1.8 vs. 4), referral letters (2.2 vs. 5.5), drug dose changes (1.5 vs. 2 [NS]), drug assays (2.5 vs. 4.8), & satisfaction.
71	OR Liver transplantation	TTAT Decision time Observation cycle	NA NA NA	Ca2+, K+, & Na+ POCT with TTAT of 2 min decreased Dx-Rx decision time to 5 min needed for rapid changes during liver transplantation where the minimum length of time between analyte observations averaged 10.5 ± 3.5 min. Direct whole-blood analysis was needed for Dx-Rx process optimization.
72	Bedside glucose testing	LOS Cost	NA NA	Bedside glucose testing decreased average LOS from 8.9 (1983) to 7.1 (1985) days in patients with diabetes mellitus & decreased the net average cost for monitoring to 55% of the original cost per admission.
73	Stat lab ICU, CCU, ED, PARU, OR	TAT Cost	NA NA	Within stat lab TAT was 11 min. Results alert immediately life-threatening disturbances, allow the clinician to avoid invasive & injurious interventions, & enable more predictable lifesaving care at the bedside of the critically ill.

ABG, arterial blood gas; BUN, blood urea nitrogen; CAB, coronary artery bypass; CABG, coronary artery bypass graft; CAP, College of American Pathologists; CCP, critical care profile; CCU, coronary care unit; CICU, coronary intensive care unit; CPB, cardiopulmonary bypass; CRP, C-reactive protein; CVDL, Cardiovascular Diagnostic Laboratory; DKA, diabetic ketoacidosis; DT, decision time; Dx-Rx, diagnostic-therapeutic; ED, emergency department; ER, emergency room; FFP, fresh frozen plasma; F/U, follow-up; GUSTO-I, global utilization of streptokinase & TPA for occluded coronary arteries; Hct, hematocrit; Hgb, hemoglobin; ICU, intensive care unit; LOS, length of stay; MI, myocardial infarction; NA, not available; NICU, neonatal intensive care unit; NS, not significant; OR, operating room; PACU, postanesthesia care unit; PARU, postanesthesia recovery unit; PCA, portable clinical analyzer; POC, point-of-care; PRBC, packed red blood cell; PTH, parathyroid hormone; P-value, level of statistical significance; RSV, respiratory syncytial virus; Rx, treatment; TAT, turnaround time; TTAT, therapeutic turnaround time; TT, therapeutic time; UCL, urgent care laboratory; UN, urea nitrogen; VAMC, Veterans Affairs Medical Center.

REFERENCES

1. Altinier S, Zaninotto M, Mion M, et al. Point-of-care testing of cardiac markers: results from an experience in an emergency department. *Clin Chim Acta* 2001;311:67–72.
2. Boldt J, Kumle B, Suttner S, et al. Point-of-care (POC) testing of lactate in the intensive care patient. *Acta Anaesthesiol Scand* 2001;45:194–199.
3. Johnson LR, Doherty G, Lairmore T, et al. Evaluation of the performance and clinical impact of a rapid intraoperative parathyroid hormone assay in conjunction with preoperative imaging and concise parathyroidectomy. *Clin Chem* 2001;47:919–925.
4. Lewandrowski E, Millan DM, Misiano D, et al. Process improvements for bedside capillary glucose testing in a large academic medical center: the impact of new technology on point-of-care testing. *Clin Chim Acta* 2001;307:175–179.
5. Mackie PLK, Joannidis PAM, Beattie J. Evaluation of an acute point-of-care system screening for respiratory syncytial virus. *J Hosp Infect* 2001;48:66–71.
6. Ng SM, Krishnaswamy P, Morissey R, et al. Ninety-minute accelerated critical pathway for chest pain evaluation. *Am J Cardiol* 2001;88: 611–617.
7. Vogeser M, Jacob K. B-type natriuretic peptide (BNP): validation of an immediate response assay. *Clin Laboratorio* 2001;47:29–33.
8. Zaman Z, Demedts M. Blood gas analysis: POCT versus central laboratory on samples sent by a pneumatic tube system. *Clin Chim Acta* 2001;307:101–106.
9. Asimos AW, Gibbs MA, Marx JA, et al. Value of point-of-care testing in emergent trauma management. *J Trauma* 2000;48:1101–1108.
10. Kost GJ, Vu HT, Inn M, et al. Multicenter study of whole-blood creatinine, total carbon dioxide content, and chemistry profiling for laboratory and point-of-care testing in critical care in the United States. *Crit Care Med* 2000;28:2379–2389.
11. Nichols JH, Kickler TS, Dyer KL, et al. Clinical outcomes of point-of-care testing in the interventional radiology and invasive cardiology setting. *Clin Chem* 2000;46:543–550.
12. Bailey TM. Understanding the economics of bedside diagnostic testing. In: Price CP, Hicks JM, eds. *Point-of-care testing*. Washington, DC: AACC Press, 1999:213–232.
13. Becker RC, Ball SP, Eisenberg P, et al. A randomized, multicenter trial of weight-adjusted intravenous heparin dose titration and point-of-care coagulation monitoring in hospitalized patients with active thromboembolic disease. *Am Heart J* 1999;137:59–71.
14. Collison PO. The need for a point of care testing: an evidence-based appraisal. *Scand J Clin Lab Invest* 1999;59(Suppl 230):67–73.
15. Dahler-Eriksen BS, Lauritzen T, Lassen JF, et al. Near-patient test for C-reactive protein in general practice: assessment of clinical, organization, and economic outcomes. *Clin Chem* 1999;45:478–485.
16. Grieve R, Beech R, Vincent J, et al. Near patient testing in diabetes clinics: appraising the costs and outcomes. *Health Technol Assess* 1999;3:1–74.
17. Murray RP, Leroux M, Sabga E, et al. Effect of point of care testing on length of stay in an adult emergency department. *J Emerg Med* 1999; 17:811–814.
18. van Heyningen C, Watson ID, Morrice AE. Point-of-care testing outcomes in an emergency department. *Clin Chem* 1999;45:437–438.
19. Boldt J, Walz G, Triem J, et al. Point-of-care (POC) measurement of coagulation after cardiac surgery. *Intensive Care Med* 1998;24:1187–1193.
20. Brown R. Point of care integration—our experience. *Medical Laboratory Observer* 1998;30:22–25.
21. Carville DGM, Schleckser PA, Guyer KE, et al. Whole blood platelet function assay on the ICHOR point-of-care hematology analyzer. *Journal of Extra-Corporeal Technology* 1998;30:171–177.
22. Hortin GL. Comparing processes of bedside and central laboratory testing. In: *Handbook of bedside glucose testing*. Washington, DC: AACC Press, 1998:41–42.
23. Kendall J, Reeves B, Clancy M. Point of care testing: randomised controlled trial of clinical outcome. *BMJ* 1998;316:1052–1057.
24. Kilgore ML, Steindel SJ, Smith JA. Evaluating stat testing options in an academic health center: therapeutic turnaround time and staff satisfaction. *Clin Chem* 1998;44:1597–1603.
25. Solomon HM, Mullins RE, Lyden P, et al. The diagnostic accuracy of bedside and laboratory coagulation: procedures used to monitor the anticoagulation status of patients treated with heparin. *Am J Clin Pathol* 1998;109:371–378.
26. Zabel KM, Granger CB, Becker RC, et al. Use of bedside activated partial thromboplastin time monitor to adjust heparin dosing after thrombolysis for acute myocardial infarction: results of GUSTO-I. *Am Heart J* 1998;136:868–876.
27. Bailey TM, Topham TM, Wantz S, et al. Laboratory process improvement through point-of-care testing. Joint Commission. *Journal of Quality Improvement* 1997;23:362–380.
28. Toffaletti J. Blood gas testing in the laboratory and at the point of care: finding the right mix. *Medical Laboratory Observer* 1997;29:14–17.
29. Battelle Medical Technology Assessment and Policy Research Program. The economic and clinical efficiency of point-of-care testing for critically ill patients. *Medical Laboratory Observer* 1996;28:12–16.
30. Mohammad AA, Summers H, Burchfield JE, et al. STAT turnaround time: satellite and point-to-point testing. *Lab Med* 1996;27:684–688.
31. O'Brien T, Griffiths R, Eisenberg P, et al. Impact of point of care STAT CBC on turnaround time for test results and duration of visit in a managed care outpatient center: evidence from a randomized, controlled trial. Presented at: Annual Meeting of the International Society of Technology Assessment in Health Care, 1996:53 (abst).
32. Parvin CA, Lo SF, Deuser SM, et al. Impact of point-of-care testing on patients' length of stay in a large emergency department. *Clin Chem* 1996;42:711–717.
33. Seamonds B. Medical, economic, and regulatory factors affecting point-of-care testing: a report of the conference on factors affecting point-of-care testing, Philadelphia, PA, 6–7 May 1994. *Clin Chim Acta* 1996;249:1–19.
34. Simpson KN, LaVallee R, Halpern M, et al. Is POCT cost effective for coronary bypass patients in ICUs? *Medical Laboratory Observer* 1996; 28:58–62.
35. Steffes MW, Gillen JL, Fuhrman SA. Delivering clinical laboratory services to intensive care units. *Clin Chem* 1996;42:387–391.
36. Zaloga GP, Roberts PR, Black K, et al. Hand-held blood gas analyzer is accurate in the critical care setting. *Crit Care Med* 1996;24:957–962.
37. Felder RA. Robotics and automated workstations for rapid response testing. Path Patterns, *Am J Clin Pathol* 1995;104 (Suppl 1):S26–S32.
38. Fleisher M, Schwartz MK. Automated approaches to rapid-response testing: a comparative evaluation of point-of-care and centralized laboratory testing. Pathology patterns. *Am J Clin Pathol* 1995;104:S1–S25.
39. Kranzler HR, Stone J, McLaughlin L. Evaluation of a point-of-care testing product for drugs of abuse: testing site is a key variable. *Drug Alcohol Depend* 1995;40:55–62.
40. Sands VM, Auerbach PS, Birnbaum J, et al. Evaluation of a portable clinical blood analyzer in the emergency department. *Acad Emerg Med* 1995;2:172–178.
41. Becker RC, Cyr J, Corrao JM, et al. Bedside coagulation monitoring in heparin-treated patients with active thromboembolic disease: a coronary care unit experience. *Am Heart J* 1994;128:719–723.
42. Bishop MS, Husain I, Aldred M, Kost GJ. Multisite point-of-care potassium testing for patient-focused care. *Arch Pathol Lab Med* 1994; 118:797–800.
43. Despotis GJ, Santoro SA, Spitznagel E, et al. Prospective evaluation and clinical utility of on-site monitoring of coagulation in patients undergoing cardiac operation. *J Thorac Cardiovasc Surg* 1994;107:271–279.
44. Despotis GJ, Grishaber JE, Goodnough LT. The effect of an intraoperative treatment algorithm on physicians' transfusion practice in cardiac surgery. *Transfusion* 1994;34:290–296.
45. Despotis GJ, Santoro SA, Spitznagel E, et al. On-site prothrombin time, activated partial thromboplastin time, and platelet count: a comparison between whole blood and laboratory assays with coagulation factor analysis in patients presenting for cardiac surgery. *Anesthesiology* 1994;80:338–351.
46. Frankel HL, Rozycki GS, Ochsner MG, et al. Minimizing admission laboratory testing in trauma patients: use of microanalyzer. *J Trauma* 1994;37:728–736.
47. Goodwin SA. Point-of-care testing in a post anesthesia care unit. *Medical Laboratory Observer* 1994;26:15–18.
48. Johnson KF. Does an on-site satellite laboratory reduce surgical delays?

A study of delays in a same day surgical center. *AORN J* 1994;59:1275–6,1279–1282,1285–1290.

49. Kwak YS, Hartfield J, Naito HK, et al. Does bedside testing shorten patient length of stay? *Am J Clin Pathol* 1994;102:553–554.

50. Lee-Lewandrowski E, Laposata M, Eschenbach K, et al. Utilization and cost analysis of bedside capillary glucose testing in a large teaching hospital: implications for managing point of care testing. *Am J Med* 1994;97:222–230.

51. McPeck M. A BG & E program for cardiac surgery. *Medical Laboratory Observer* 1994;26:20–25.

52. Travers EM, Wolke JC, Johnson R, et al. Changing the lab medicine is practiced at the point of care. *Medical Laboratory Observer* 1994;26:33–35,38–40.

53. Tsai WW, Nash DB, Seamonds B, et al. Point-of-care versus central laboratory testing: an economic analysis in an academic medical center. *Clin Ther* 11994;16:898–910.

54. Winkelman JW, Wybenga DR. Quantification of medical and operational factors determining central versus satellite laboratory testing of blood gases. *Am J Clin Pathol* 1994;102:7–10.

55. Saxena S, Wong ET. Does the emergency department need a dedicated stat laboratory? Continuous quality improvement as a management tool for the clinical laboratory. *Am J Clin Pathol* 1993;100:606–610.

56. Thiebe L, Vinci K, Gardner J. Point-of-care testing: Improving day-stay services. *Nursing Management* 1993;24:54,56.

57. Greendyke RM. Cost analysis: bedside blood glucose testing. *Am J Clin Pathol* 1992;97:106–107.

58. Howanitz PJ, Steindel SJ, Cembrowski GS, et al. Emergency department stat test turnaround times: a College of American Pathologists' Q-Probes study for potassium and hemoglobin. *Arch Pathol Lab Med* 1992;116:122–128.

59. Steindel SJ, Howanitz PJ. Changes in emergency department turnaround time performance from 1990 to 1993: a comparison of two College of American Pathologists Q-Probes studies. *Arch Pathol Lab Med* 1997;121:1031–1041.

60. Steindel SJ, Howanitz PJ. Physician satisfaction and emergency department laboratory test turnaround time: observation based on College of American Pathologists Q-Probe studies. *Arch Pathol Lab Med* 2001;125:863–871.

61. Salem M, Chernow B, Burke R, et al. Bedside diagnostic blood testing: its accuracy, rapidity and utility in blood conservation. *JAMA* 1991;266:382–389.

62. Zaloga GP. Monitoring versus testing technologies: present and future. *Medical Laboratory Observer* 1991;23:20–31.

63. Zaloga GP. Evaluation of bedside testing options for the critical care unit. *Chest* 1990;97:185S–190S.

64. Zaloga GP. Bedside reagent testing: blood, CSF, and bacterial cultures. *J Crit Illness* 1988;3(1):85,86,92–94.

65. Elliot K, Watson ID, Tsintis P, et al. The impact of near-patient testing on the organisation and costs of an anticonvulsant clinic. *Ther Drug Monit* 1990;12:434–437.

66. Fleisher M, Schwartz MK. Strategies of organization and service for the critical-care laboratory. *Clin Chem* 1990;36:1557–1561.

67. Kost GJ, Shirey TL. New whole-blood testing for laboratory support of critical care at cardiac transplant centers and US hospitals. *Arch Pathol Lab Med* 1990;114:865–868.

68. Ansell JE, Hamke AK, Holden A, et al. Cost effectiveness of monitoring warfarin therapy using standard versus capillary prothrombin times. *Am J Clin Pathol* 1989;91:587–589.

69. Strickland RA, Hill TR, Zaloga GP. Bedside analysis of arterial blood gases and electrolytes during and after cardiac surgery. *J Clin Anesth* 1989;1:248–252.

70. Patsalos PN, Sander JWAS, et al. Immediate anticonvulsive drug monitoring in management of epilepsy. *Lancet* 1987;2(8549):39.

71. Kost GJ, Jammal MA, Ward RE, et al. Monitoring of ionized calcium during human hepatic transplantation: critical values and their relevance to cardiac and hemodynamic management. *Am J Clin Pathol* 1986;86:61–70.

72. Trundle DS, Weizenecker RA. Capillary glucose testing: a cost-saving bedside system. *Laboratory Management* 1986;24:59–62.

73. Weil MH, Michaels S, Puri VK, et al. The stat laboratory: facilitating blood gas and biochemical measurements for the critically ill and injured. *Am J Clin Pathol* 1981;76:34–42.

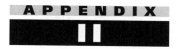

THE ECONOMICS OF
POINT-OF-CARE TESTING

GERALD J. KOST
NAM K. TRAN

APPENDIX II. THE ECONOMICS OF POINT-OF-CARE TESTING

Ref	Clinical Setting	Clinical Objective [Test, Method, or Type]	Economic Outcomes
1	ICU	Study the reliability & costs of two POC lactate devices when compared with central lab method (lactate)	Study costs for measuring lactate were lower for handheld POCT ($248) vs. benchtop ($536) vs. central lab ($493), & transportation cost ($3.61/specimen) must be added if not POC.
2	Hospital	Identify barriers to improving care for individuals with diabetes in community health centers (glucose & $HgbA_{1c}$)	>25% of providers & administrators agreed that a significant barrier involved affordability of home blood glucose & HgA_{1c} monitoring. Better health delivery systems, lower cost, & higher efficiency will help improve healthcare delivery.
3	Near-patient OR	Determine cost effectiveness of a strategy of near-patient H. pylori testing & endoscopy for managing dyspepsia (H. pylori)	Cost effectiveness was based on improved symptoms & use of resources. NPT costs were less than conventional method costs. NPT increased endoscopy rate, which was offset by benefits in symptoms & quality of life.
In 4	Hospital	Estimation of variable costs for glucose in a 1,000-bed hospital (Europe)	Testing volume was 111,000 (1992) & 191,000 (1998), & combined cost of lab & 160 POCT sites was 151,900 (1992) & 613,900 (1998) Euros. Factors other than POCT increased volume.
4	Children's hospital	Recommendations & opinions for use of POCT for hospital & primary care (test cluster)	Cost per test using i-STAT POCT system was $6.07 vs. $7.28 when testing was performed in the central lab, and labor reengineering saved ~$225,000 per year.
5	OR	Determine whether combination of ^{99m}Tc-sestamibi scan & intraoperative parathyroid hormone (PTH) improves outcomes (imaging–PTH synthesis)	Preoperative scan & on-site PTH in OR decreased number of frozen sections, hospital stay, general anesthesia, & the number of bilateral neck explorations. (See Chapter 40.)
6	Academic medical center	Process improvement for bedside capillary glucose testing in a large academic medical center (bedside glucose)	Implemented 3rd-generation bedside glucose testing for efficiency. POCT cost ranges from $4.20 to $13.49 per test, but must fully take into account nursing service efficiency.
7	Pediatric hospital ED	Decrease the risk of children contracting hospital-acquired infection (respiratory syncytial virus)	Near-patient testing of RSV provided a rapid answer & ensured that infants could be segregated according to infection status. Costs far lower than alternatives without RSV POCT.
8	VAMC ED CCU	Evaluate the performance of an accelerated critical pathway for patients with suspected coronary ischemia (cTnI, myoglobin, CK-MB)	Cost of cardiac injury marker testing (2.2 times average) justified compared with savings associated with 40% reduction in CCU admissions, shorter ED LOS, & accurate triage.
9	Near-patient Bedside ED	Evaluate a new POCT device for urine drugs of abuse screening (evaluation)	POCT costs more than lab testing for drugs of abuse. Lab instruments offer a larger menu. POCT is faster. Must consider the impact of POCT on the overall cost of care event.
10	ED	Evaluate POCT for cardiac injury markers (general POC cardiac injury markers)	Use of cardiac markers to reduce inappropriate admissions & therapies can reduce unnecessary hospital & patient costs. Hospitals must consider cost effectiveness in the context of their own patient populations & available resources.
11	Hospital Near-patient Bedside	Negotiate payment for in-house testing for managed care plans & demonstrate the value of NPT (general)	When justifying POCT, use reasons that demonstrate lower cost to the health care system or higher quality of care, as evidenced by better patient outcome or satisfaction.
12	Hospital	The effects of fetal fibronectin testing on admissions to a tertiary maternal-fetal medicine unit & cost savings (fetal fibronectin)	POC fibronectin testing identified patients not in danger of preterm labor, thereby reducing transfers to a major hospital for admission allowing savings of $153,120 (58 patients).
13	Hospital Near-patient	Evaluating POCT for its cost effectiveness vs. the central lab (bedside glucose)	POCT program cost $7.85 per test (total) & $3.92 (incremental) more compared to the lab. However, must consider the financial consequences of internal & external failure costs.
14	Home	A cost-effectiveness analysis for patients on chronic warfarin therapy (capillary INR monitoring)	Patient self-testing is the most cost-effective alternative & yields 8.6/100 patients/5 yrs fewer adverse events, usually nonfatal, as well as net cost savings. Moving only to clinic testing has a cost-effectiveness ratio of $31,327 (all costs).
15	Hospital Near-patient ICU CVU ED, OR	Evaluate the rise & fall of i-STAT POC blood gas testing in an acute care hospital (test cluster)	Fiscal analysis predicted that the i-STAT POC device saved about $225,000 annually. However, P_{CO_2} discrepancies required the cessation of use & use of Opti-CCA instead.
16	ICU CVU ED, OR	Adoption of POCT in an effort to provide faster, more efficient, & higher quality service while reducing costs (multisite RALS)	Use of whole-blood analyzer yielded labor costs of $36,000 vs. $132,000 prior to POCT ($96,000 reduction), & consumable costs of $40,000 vs. $115,000 ($75,000 reduction).
17	OR	Study of clinical & analytical performance of rapid response PTH analysis with preoperative sestamibi imaging (intraoperative PTH)	Cure rate & morbidity similar vs. conventional surgical routine, but significant reductions were observed in both hospital LOS (0.3 vs. 1.8 d) & total charges ($3,174 vs. 6,328). (See case D.)
18	OR	Cost analysis of rapid response PTH testing vs. the central lab (intraoperative PTH)	Intraoperative POC PTH testing during surgery costs $760 per surgery vs. $360 for the central lab. Intraoperative PTH test provides faster, more reliable rapid response & other benefits.
19	Hospital Near-patient	Understand the economics of bedside diagnostic testing (process reengineering)	Restructuring with POCT saved $392,336 annually. Average cost per panel was $8.03 with POCT saving $7.30 vs. $15.33 when the total operating cost of the STAT labs is considered.

No.	Setting	Purpose	Findings
20	Hospital / Near-patient	Assessment of clinical, organizational, & economic outcomes of a near-patient test for C-reactive protein in general practice (CRP)	NPT was cost effective mainly on the basis of reduction in the use of services in the hospital lab by GPs. NPT CRP saved $111,160/yr for 340,000 Danish country inhabitants.
21	Hospital	Cost analysis of arterial blood gas testing using the remote automated lab system (RALS) (remote control & automation)	Total cost with RALS was $3.64 vs. $7.09 for conventional methods, including equipment, labor, supplies, overhead, & other miscellaneous costs.
22	Hospital / Near-patient	Determine when a rapid test might be more cost effective in initiating treatment of more infections (*Chlamydia* POC 1- & 2-step PCR algorithm)	Rapid test, alone or combined, may be preferred for screening or diagnosis of infections in women when communicating results & initiating therapy is delayed.
23	Diabetes clinic	Compare the costs & consequences of providing NPT compared with conventional testing ($HgbA_{1c}$)	Mean $HgbA_{1c}$ was significantly lower for the NPT cohort vs. conventional testing. NPT patients made fewer clinic & hospital visits. NPT improved care process & patient satisfaction.
24	ITU / ED	Cost analysis & exploration of financial incentives to use POCT in the hospital & the accident & emergency department (test cluster)	Introducing i-STAT POCT into ITU & AED replacing existing processes would yield hospital savings from £8,332 to £20,000 with £3.78/test average cost lower.
25	Satellite lab / Bedside	Opportunity cost analysis by substitution modeling comparing centralized vs. distributed blood gas testing (ABG)	A mix of POCT alternatives generated an annual savings of between $250,000 & $300,000. Therefore, technology that appears superficially more costly can deliver better service (faster test results) with lower overall costs.
26	Inner-city hospital	Compare the reliability & relative costs of INR NPT	There were no statistically or clinically significant differences between results from three POCT systems. Costs varied. INR differences in 19%–24% vs. lab could change management.
27	OR	POCT assist for parathyroidectomy in the OR (intraoperative PTH)	PTH POCT increases the surgery success rate & decreases the time of surgery, morbidity, & overall cost by as much as $4,000 per patient.
28	ED	Comment on POCT outcomes in the ED (test cluster)	POCT in the ED was not efficient use of resources. Because of central laboratory funding structure, there were no transferable savings, & there was a substantial additional capital cost.
29	CCU / ICU	A cost-effective, high-performance approach to critical care testing (multisite RALS)	POCT for ICU & CCU improved turnaround time substantially & generated nearly 75% savings compared to costs of previous critical care lab testing.
30	Hospital / Near-patient	Comparisons to clarify costs of POCT vs. central lab (general bedside glucose)	Place the greatest weight on reducing the cost of the episode of care & preventing the progression of illness in the future.
31	ICU	To evaluate different systems for monitoring of coagulation variables at the bedside regarding practicability, accuracy, & costs (aPTT & PT)	The direct costs for measuring aPTT & PT were significantly higher using both POC systems (aPTT-TAS: $4.84; aPTT-CoaguCheck: $4.34) vs. cost for tests done in the central lab ($1.59). However, costs for transportation increased lab-based monitoring costs considerably ($3.77).
32	Hospital ED	Analysis of POCT use in a hospital (general)	Implementation of POCT requires a $255,000 increase in annual operating budget. Must balance need for quick information, immediate action on data, & reduction in LOS.
33	Hospital / Near-patient	NPT for serum cholesterol: attitudes of general practitioners & patients, appropriateness, & costs (cholesterol)	NPT appears to be of benefit to both GPs & patients & to provide cost savings. GPs felt that registration & quality assurance fees were unreasonably high.
34	ED / CCU	Economic aspects of new biochemical markers for the detection of myocardial damage (CEA, CMA, CUA, & CBA; see Chapter 40)	When applied as part of an integrated decision making strategy, cardiac injury markers identify both high risk & low risk patients in a cost-efficient manner.
35	Practice / Nurse-led clinic	Evaluate primary care model of oral anticoagulation monitoring with computerized decision support & NPT (INR)	NPT costs to the practice for 29 patients & 208 appointments were £1,751 for NPT & £2,290 if the patients had been seen at the hospital with the same frequency.
36	ICU	Decision-analysis model of the economic & clinical efficiency of POCT for critically ill patients (decision-analytic model)	The positive clinical impact of using POCT was consistently associated with a positive economic impact. Costs of stat blood analysis are more personnel-related than equipment-related.
37	Hospital / bedside	Develop a guide for bedside glucose testing (general bedside glucose)	Most published analyses report higher costs for bedside testing. Estimated direct costs for bedside glucose testing ranged from about $4–14 per test, while central lab costs are estimated at about $3–4 per test.
38	Hospital / NICU / OR	Cost-benefit study of satellite labs (satellite lab)	Cost of a CBC in satellite labs (2 sites) was $11.79 & $8.91, & in central lab, $8.13. ABG in NICU lab was $6.91, in OR lab, $13.69, & in central lab, $8.76. Satellite labs are fast with fewer process steps, but underutilize labor increasing costs.
39	Bedside / Near-patient	To assess the cost effectiveness of PT self-testing for managed care (5-year state transition decision analytic model)	Moving from usual care to PT self-testing results in a cost-effectiveness ratio of $11,982 per avoided event ($79,263 per QALY), & $31,300 ($231,888), when costs to patients & caregivers are included, & is suitable for managed care.
40	ED	Impact of POCT on patient care units (general review of POCT studies)	According to results, POCT proves to be a more expensive way of delivering rapid lab results compared with the central lab. However, the ability to minimize turnaround time speeds decisions for admissions & discharge, & may shorten LOS.

(continued)

Ref	Clinical Setting	Clinical Objective [Test, Method, or Type]	Economic Outcomes
41	Bedside Stat lab	Improvement in lab processes through POCT (process reengineering)	POCT costs vs. traditional costs showed annual savings of $392,336 compared with the total annual costs of traditional methods. Cost per test panel was $8.03 for POCT & $15.33 for traditional model. POCT saved 4 steps in care.
42	Hospital	Analysis of value chain when applied to critical care testing (economic analysis)	New POCT vs. central lab total costs per test were $7.34 vs. $10.37. Clinical cycle & patient cost were 5–7 min & $13.33/test for old POCT, 5 min & $9.34/test for the new POCT, & 15 min to 24 hr & $10.78/test for the central lab.
43	OR	Impact of POCT on blood loss & transfusion outcomes (aPTT, PT, & platelets)	POCT reduces transfusion requirements, microvascular bleeding, operative time, & reexplorations. Prevention of post-CPB bleeding can reduce expenditures substantially for an annual savings of $267,658. (See Chapter 8 for details.)
44	Hospital	Identify ways to check costs & quality for POCT (QC)	Traditional QC for POCT is costly, ineffective, & often a major hurdle limiting POCT availability. Improvements will result from electronic & internal QC & from error detection.
45	Hospital Near-patient	Cost analysis for POCT (test cluster)	Lab cost comparison shows a savings per test of $1.09, & $135,340 savings annually when using POC i-STAT system at a large university hospital. (Additional cases in ref.)
46	Hospital	Using patient satisfaction as an indicator of the quality of POCT services (methods of social science research, PT)	Preliminary results showed no significant effects from the use of PT POCT on inpatient evaluations of care, but a significant difference in costs vs. the central lab.
47	Neonatal unit	Analyze use of Hemocue portable blood glucose analyzer in a neonatal unit (portable glucose)	Hemocue may overestimate glucose by as much as 2.5 mmol/L. Hemocue also is costly to run & may be more useful on the general wards than the special care baby unit.
48	Primary health care center	Compare costs of decentralized testing vs. centralized (hospital) testing (general)	Cost per procedure was 5% lower in primary care setting. POCT had quicker results, fewer lost samples, & fewer visits for the patient. Largest cost item is personnel.
49	Children's hospital	Evaluate the POC i-STAT system in the NICU & PICU (test cluster)	Analysis showed that blood gas, electrolyte, & glucose testing costs for the i-STAT were approximately the same as the lab.
50	ICU	Compare cost of POCT vs. lab-based testing in ICU & role of the respiratory care practitioner (RCP) (respiratory care management)	Fully loaded POCT costs are high, but in myocardial infarction or suspected MI, immediate blood gases may be a first priority & RCP is well-suited to perform the bedside tests.
51	ICU CCU	Analysis of POCT costs & clinical efficiency for blood analysis in critical care (clinical decision analysis model)	Treatment avoided by POCT & marginal costs yield a total annual savings of $23,889 vs. alternative testing. Rapid results are important in preventing adverse critical clinical events.
52	ICU	A study in the ICU concerning bedside testing of gastric contents (gastric analysis)	The cost of the fecal occult blood slide tests plus the litmus paper were comparable to Gastroccult slide tests. In addition, less nursing time was needed when using the Gastroccult slide test because the tool was easier to use & results easily interpreted.
53	Hospital Near-patient	Rationale for a novel technique of automating POCT with remote oversight (test cluster)	RALS method of providing near-patient testing costs $3.64 for whole-blood analysis vs. $7.09 when performed in the core lab, while offering several features of quality management.
54	Hospital Near-patient	Cost effectiveness in utilizing remote control testing concepts (multisite remote oversight)	Savings from remote controlled tests were due to faster messenger & nursing times, as well as reduced supply & maintenance costs, which provided total savings of $38,650.
55	Dialysis unit	Evaluate i-STAT portable clinical analyzer in a hemodialysis unit (test cluster)	Cost for individual i-STAT E3⁺ cartridges was $6.50 which includes Na⁺, K⁺, & Hct. The EC8⁺ cartridge includes urea, glucose, pH, & P_{CO_2} at a cost of $11.70 per unit. Health plan reimburses $17.05 (Canadian). Special value in hemodialysis.
56	Hospital Near patient	Compare the cost effectiveness of monitoring vs. POC blood gas testing (patient monitoring)	For certain DRGs, average number of tests ranges from 30–50 per stay. With costs from $9–$19 per test, monitoring provides an economical alternative to *in vitro* testing for high risk, low blood-volume patients, such as premature infants.
57	Hospital	Evaluate primary care anticoagulant clinics managed by a pharmacist (devolved management)	Costs to a GP of a pharmacist-led anticoagulant clinic were less than costs charged to the practice for each hospital clinic appointment. Patients like reduced waiting & traveling costs.
58	ED, CCU Satellite lab STAT lab	Evaluate TTAT for redesigned POCT testing & associated lab services (restructuring)	Decrease in TTAT generated physician satisfaction. Achieved with redesigned stat labs, no increase in the workforce, maintained quality, & decreased operating costs.
59	Near-patient Bedside	Cost analysis of POC lab testing (general)	POCT costs exceed central lab costs. However, the ability to obtain improved patient outcomes with economic efficiency depends on the clinical setting & efficient use of test results.
60–62	ED	Evaluate the impact of POCT on patient LOS in a large ED (test cluster)	Handheld testing using a limited menu without a care path or treatment algorithm may produce little economic benefit in a busy ER. Study found no significant change in ED LOS.
63	Bedside	Conference report on medical, economic, & regulatory factors affecting POCT (general)	At two institutions, POCT decreased turnaround time. Institution no. 1, cost/specimen ($) for POCT vs. stat lab was 11.03 vs. 4.55, & at no. 2, POCT vs. central lab was 8.14 vs. 15.24.

	Setting	Objective	Findings
64	OR ICU	Determine costs of POCT for CABG patients (cardiac specialty)	Study of 25 randomly selected hospitals showed POCT for cardiac patients reduced the cost of care annually by $21,508 to $42,438.
65	Hospital	Compare costs of traditional lab testing vs. POCT (general)	POCT increased labor productivity by using existing hospital personnel already performing other functions, not lab FTE, & eliminated central management & office labor components.
66	ICU OR	To integrate POCT in critical care & improve ICU services (integration, see Chapter 40)	NPT decreased process steps & response time by up to 80%, permitting reductions in personnel exceeding $400,000/yr. NPT conserved blood volume & improved main lab operation.
67	Prehospital Ambulance ED	Identify implications of the precision & accuracy of handheld POCT in hostile environment (test cluster)	To justify the additional cost of analysis cassettes, the information obtained in the field must affect patient treatment or disposition (triage) in a managed care setting.
68,69	Hospital	Evaluate POCT whole-blood clinical analyzers (general instrumentation)	A U.S. survey by the University Health System Consortium reported positive tangible & intangible benefits of POCT for integrated health systems.
70	OR Special care Recovery	Comparative evaluation of POCT & central lab testing with transport system (transport system)	Dedicated centralized lab equipped with a rapid specimen transport system provides better comprehensive lab service than a POC facility with limited capability, & costs less.
71	VAMC	Analyze benefits of a mobile lab in alternate site testing (transportable instruments)	Total costs of defects (e.g., delays, calls, and orders) in central lab process is $12.83 per defect. Mobile lab would reduce defect cost, & enhance MT as a hands-on clinical caregiver.
72	Home care	Joint hospital-vendor project team to bring continuous quality improvement & POC technology to home care (aggregate home innovations)	POC technologies in the home increased productivity 20%, with potential to increase revenue $876,000/yr with same staff level. Anticipate future support of critical pathways.
73	Pediatrics NICU	Evaluate the APEC analyzer for whole-blood glucose (glucose devices)	APEC vs. the YSI technical comparison was excellent. APEC cost $0.22 vs. $0.26 per test for the YSI & is somewhat less expensive than the YSI.
74	ED	Analyze use of POCT to speed patient care in the ED (nursing)	Cost of 6-test & 3-test i-STAT cartridges was $8 & 6.75, respectively. Hospital pays a premium in supply costs for POCT. Often, 2-min turnaround time justifies the expense.
75	Hospital Bedside	Identify cost savings & convenience generated by POC glucose testing (glucose meters)	Instrument evaluation, performance enhancement, & careful training can decrease the number of glucose test strips wasted because of technical or QC failures, & produce cost savings.
76	OR	Study whether more precise control of therapy & patient response would effect blood loss & transfusion requirements (hemostasis)	Cost of drugs & tests estimated to add $50 to $60 if hemostasis instruments are used, but is offset by decreased bleeding & transfusion, & is 3% to 10% of estimated cost of aprotinin therapy.
77	Hospital Bedside	Analysis of the use of bedside glucose testing (fiscal-clinical optimization)	Bedside glucose testing is not inherently more expensive than testing performed within the clinical lab. Increased cost is minimized with fewer operators on units with testing >5/day.
78–81	Bedside Near-patient	Cost analysis of POC lab testing in a community hospital (general)	POCT costs exceed central lab stat costs 1.1 to 4.6 times. The more POCT is used, the greater the excess costs compared with the central lab. Urge fiscal caution before indiscriminate use.
82,83	ED	Evaluate a portable clinical blood analyzer for use in emergency medicine (test cluster)	i-STAT showed fast results that might have reduced LOS in 17.3% of patients, but other factors (e.g., results availability & process flow) affect translation into economic savings.
84	Diabetic care unit	Critical analysis & application of POCT (reflectance glucose meters)	Incremental (marginal) POCT cost is $3.92 more than central lab, but inclusion of production, quality, appraisal, & internal & external failure costs shows lab is 1.4 times more costly.
85	OR	On-site testing & algorithmic treatment for control of intra-operative bleeding during cardiovascular surgery (hemostasis)	POCT provided the equivalent of $1,504/patient, or $267,658/yr savings & improved intermediate outcomes (e.g., less blood loss & reduced total transfusion exposure). (See Chapter 8.)
86	ED Trauma	Minimize admission lab testing in trauma patients through the use of a microanalyzer (triage)	Fast microanalysis is accurate & expedient, & conserves blood volume. Routine use can reduce costs substantially by $16,000 per 100 patients.
87	PACU	Evaluate the effectiveness of POCT in the PACU (ABG)	POCT improved LOS & turnaround time, & since each 15 min interval was billed, POCT saved $64/patient. Savings times patients (132) is $8,448/mo or $101,376/yr.
88	Same-day surgical center	Assessment of the reduction of surgery delays by the use of NPT in the OR (nursing)	OR suite charged approximately $5/min. A 7,072 min delay would be a $35,360 annual loss for the hospital. On-site testing reduces time delays & thereby, reduces costs.
89–91	Academic medical center	Study the use & cost of bedside capillary glucose testing in a large teaching hospital (bedside glucose)	POCT was cost effective in high-volume units. Therefore, implementation on inefficient units with low utilization can add substantially to cost. POCT is not inherently more costly.
92	OR	Analysis of POCT program for cardiac surgery (test cluster)	Providing combined blood gas & electrolyte testing to cardiac surgery patients in a controlled environment will reduce costs.
93	Cardiac surgery ICU	Evaluate cost effectiveness of three lab test production processes for management of cardiac surgery ICU patients (clinical decision modeling)	Test costs & the cost effectiveness of testing is heavily influenced by the type of technical production process used. Timely test data impact outcomes.

(continued)

APPENDIX II. (continued)

Ref	Clinical Setting	Clinical Objective [Test, Method, or Type]	Economic Outcomes
94	Hospital Near-patient	Evaluate changing the way lab medicine is practiced at the POC (mobile lab)	Mobile lab eliminates the need for non-test production tasks thereby relieving high-salaried technologists from nonproductive duties, such as waiting for accumulation of batch to run.
95	ED	Economic analysis in an academic medical center for POCT vs. centralized testing (test cluster)	Cost per test for POC analysis ranged from $14.37 to $16.67 depending on test volume. Selective POCT in the ED can result in long-standing cost savings to the hospital.
96	NICU	Quantify medical & operational factors determining central vs. satellite lab testing for blood gases (ABG)	Cost of performing a blood gas analysis in the NICU satellite vs. central lab was $3.54 vs. $8.98. Must weigh medical utility criteria vs. cost in cost-benefit analysis for small time savings.
97	Hospital	Evaluate the fiscal consequences of central vs. distributed testing (bedside glucose)	Turnaround time was 1–2 min shorter with POCT. No significant adverse outcomes were associated with difference. Bedside testing cost was twice that of central lab testing.
98	Hospital	Consideration of whether quality in testing must cost more (general glucose)	Testing by nurses, by phlebotomists, & in central lab cost/yr are $344,864, $255,626, & $366,143, respectively. All costs must be considered when weighing alternatives.
99	Hospital Near-patient	Analysis of experience using POCT for blood gases & electrolyte testing (general)	Lab expenditures for ancillary testing in 1992 totaled $237,606. Costs were calculated by dividing expenditures by 67,000 tests, giving a figure of $3.55 per patient specimen.
100, 101	Primary care	Impact of introducing NPT for standard investigations in general practice (timed crossover study design)	Primary care NPT costs were higher for all tests except mid-stream urine analysis, which was cost effective. Cholesterol gave better recording of coronary heart disease risk factors.
102	ED	Assess if the ED requires a dedicated stat lab (satellite lab)	Hospitals must carefully assess medical need & benefit when making decisions to allocate scarce resources. Requests for expensive additional services must be evaluated critically.
103	ED	Evaluate the use of a portable clinical analyzer in the ED (test cluster)	Use of i-STAT device is $10/panel cost vs. $3/panel cost for the central lab. Potential cost savings may result from quicker decisions, earlier diagnosis, fewer tests, & shorter LOS.
104	Hospital Near-patient	Control error in POCT (general)	POCT reduces preanalytic, analytic, & postanalytic errors in testing, & reduces costs.
105	VAMC	Cost analysis of bedside glucose testing (bedside glucose)	Bedside testing cost/test was $11.50 vs. conventional lab at $3.19. Extra cost/yr estimated to be in excess of $3,000,000.
106	ICU OR ED	Evaluation of consolidation of critical care stat labs (restructuring)	Consolidation of stat lab services produced significant savings (>$500,000) with increase in productivity from 9.4 to 13.8 tests/paid work hour & decrease in cost/test from $2.41 to $1.41.
107	OR	Cost analysis of OR lab vs. main hospital lab. (Na^+-K^+, ABG)	Cost per test for OR vs. main lab was $1.79 & $2.11 vs. $2.86 & $1.66 for ABG & Na^+ & K^+, respectively. OR satellite lab substantially improved patient care at no net true cost increase.
108	ICU	Analyze the advantages & disadvantages of bedside technologies (ABG, glucose, oximetry)	Bedside oxyhemoglobin saturation monitoring with pulse oximeter vs. central lab blood gases in postoperative patients provided a savings of $750 for 15 patients ($50/patient).
109	Hospital Near-patient	Identify the impact of NPT on the organization & costs of an anticonvulsant clinic (critical path analysis)	NPT increased productivity 23%, & decreased testing costs 18.3% (£470 annual difference) & cost per patient visit, 34% (£4.31), saving staff time & improving patient throughput.
110	Stat lab Bedside	Evaluate stat testing alternatives by calculating annual costs (general)	Total annual operating costs were $211,382 for bedside testing & $364,664 for stat lab, including overhead. Need to consult with clinical staff to develop the best testing alternative.
111	Bedside ICU	Evaluate bedside testing options for the critical care unit (ABG, glucose, oximetry)	Bedside testing allows for earlier & more specific diagnosis, faster & more frequent monitoring, & the opportunity to improve patient care & reduce hospital costs.
112	Hospital Near-patient	Assess cost effectiveness of monitoring warfarin therapy by standard plasma PTs from venipuncture vs. capillary samples from fingerstick (PT)	Total labor cost per test for capillary whole-blood PT ($7.55) was significantly (P <0.02) less than standard PT ($15.64). Immediate results provide potential for improved healthcare.

113	Same-day surgery	Analyze the expense of a satellite lab in support of a same-day surgery program (satellite)	Cost/test was $9.89 for satellite lab vs. $7.69 in central lab, but OR overtime ($675) & rescheduling ($75) costs added $750, resulting in $747.80 cost benefit to use satellite lab.
114	ED	Cost effectiveness of an accurate & rapid assay for serum human chorionic gonadotropin in suspected ectopic pregnancy (β-HCG)	Cost of $2.90/test would save the hospital approximately $123,000 annually from decreased culdocentesis ($P <0.001$), ultrasound ($P <0.025$), & admissions ($P <0.01$).
115	ICU	Evaluate Gemstat blood gas, electrolyte, & Hct portable analyzer in the critical care setting (test cluster)	Assuming 25 tests/d, total cost (labor, consumables, service) for Gemstat was $61,000 annually vs. $101,000 for testing in the lab. If 50 tests/d, total cost was $116,000 vs. $123,000.
116	ICU	Analyze bedside reagent testing of blood, CSF, & bacteria (blood, CSF)	Total cost/patient of hospitalization was $2,380 for bedside testing vs. $3,925 for central lab testing, due to decreased ICU (1.4 vs. 2.5 d) & hospital (5 vs. 8 d) LOS (diabetic ketoacidosis).
117	Hospital OR	Cost implications & benefits of decentralized testing (general)	Decentralized testing can eliminate $1.75 in transportation, preparation, & handling costs/request. Modified OR process value of $5/specimen makes cost of testing inconsequential.
118	Bedside	Laboratorian's view of the costs of decentralized testing (glucose)	Cost/result was $1.98 for POCT & $1.07 for lab testing for 400 tests/d with 50% POCT & 50% lab.
119	Bedside	Evaluate capillary glucose testing at the bedside as a cost-saving system (lab management)	Bedside capillary glucose testing saved $1.84 vs. venous blood glucose assay performed in lab. Average cost for admitting a diabetic patient to the hospital was $1,646.
120	Hospital Near-patient	Analysis of the costs of biochemical NPT (general)	NPT is more expensive on a direct-charge basis, but is economically feasible due to improved turnaround time, shorter LOS, discharge, decreased hospital costs, increased physician efficiency, & improved patient competitive position.
121	Home	Compare the accuracy & estimate the costs for home glucose testing (comparison study)	Dextrometer, Eyetone, StatTek, & Chemstrip bG glucose cost/test were $0.71-1.32, $0.51-0.71, $0.72-$1.01 & $0.53, respectively, with least expensive offering additional advantages.
122	Stat lab	Facilitate blood gas & biochemical measurements for the critically ill & injured (test cluster)	Cost of 750 stat panels for 297 patients each month had unit cost of $19.92, & abbreviated panels, $13.01. Costs justified by instantaneous insight into mechanisms of disease states.

AED, accident & emergency department; ABGT, arterial blood gas test; aPTT, activated partial thromboplastin time; CABG, coronary artery bypass graft; CBC, complete blood count; CCU, coronary care unit; CK, creatine kinase; CPB, cardiopulmonary bypass; CSF, cerebral spinal fluid; cTnI/T, cardiac troponin I/T; CVU, cardiovascular unit; EKG, electrocardiogram; ER, emergency room; GP, general physician; Hct, hematocrit; ICU, intensive care unit; INR, international normalized ratio; ITU, intensive therapy unit; LOS, length of stay; MT, medical technologist; NICU, neonatal intensive care unit; NPT, near-patient testing; OR, operating room; PACU, postanesthesia care unit; PCR, polymerase chain reaction; PICU, pediatric intensive care unit; POC, point-of-care; POCT, point-of-care testing; PT, prothrombin time; PTG, parathyroid gland; PTH, parathyroid hormone; QALY, quality-adjusted life year; QC, quality control; RALS, remote automated laboratory system; TTAT, therapeutic turnaround time; VAMC, Veterans Affairs Medical Center; YSI, Yellow Springs Instruments.

REFERENCES

1. Boldt J, Kumle B, Suttner S, et al. Point-of-care (POC) testing of lactate in the intensive care patient: accuracy, reliability, and costs of different measurement systems. *Acta Anaesthesiol Scand* 2001;45:194–199.
2. Chin MH, Cook S, Jin L, et al. Barriers to providing diabetes care in community health centers. *Diabetes Care* 2001;24:268–274.
3. Delaney BC, Wilson S, Roalfe A, et al. Randomized controlled trial of helicobacter pylori testing and endoscopy for dyspepsia in primary care. *BMJ* 2001;322:898–901.
4. Hicks JM, Haeckel R, Price CP, et al. Recommendations and opinions for the use of point-of-care testing for hospitals and primary care: summary of a 1999 symposium. *Clin Chim Acta* 2001;303:1–17.
5. Johnson LR, Doherty G, Lairmore T, et al. Evaluation of the performance and clinical impact of a rapid intraoperative parathyroid hormone assay in conjunction with preoperative imaging and concise parathyroidectomy. *Clin Chem* 2001;47:919–925.
6. Lewandrowski E, Millan DM, Misiano D, et al. Process improvement for bedside capillary glucose testing in a large academic medical center: the impact of new technology on point-of-care testing. *Clin Chim Acta* 2001;307:175–179.
7. Mackie PLK, Joannidis PAM, Beattie J. Evaluation of an acute point-of-care system screening for respiratory syncytial virus infection. *J Hosp Infect* 2001;48:66–71.
8. Ng SM, Krishnaswamy P, Morissey R, et al. Ninety-minute accelerated critical pathway for chest pain evaluation. *Am J Cardiol* 2001;88:611–617.
9. Yang JM, Lewandrowski KB. Urine drugs of abuse testing at the point-of-care: clinical interpretation and programmatic considerations with specific reference to the Syva Rapid Test (SRT). *Clin Chim Acta* 2001;307:27–32.
10. Cummings JP. POC Tests for cardiac injury markers. Clinical Improvement and Effectiveness. Oakbrook, IL: University Health System Consortium, 2000:29–30.
11. Dunn S. Negotiating payment for in-house testing from managed care plans. *Outpatient Care* 1999/2000;15:8,52–54.
12. Giles W, Bisits A, Knox M, et al. The effect of fetal fibronectin testing on admissions to a tertiary maternal-fetal medicine unit and cost savings. *Am J Obstet Gynecol* 2000;182:439–442.
13. Kiechle FL. Comparing cost: point-of-care vs. central lab. *Clin Lab Products* 2000;Jan:24.
14. Lafata JE, Martin SA, Kaatz S, et al. Anticoagulation clinics and patient self-testing for patients on chronic warfarin therapy: a cost-effectiveness analysis. *J Thromb Thrombolysis* 2000;9:S13–S19.
15. Ng VL, Kraemer R, Hogan C, et al. The rise and fall of i-STAT point-of-care blood gas testing in an acute care hospital. *Am J Clin Pathol* 2000;114:128–138.
16. NOVA Biomedical. Successful point-of-care testing solutions. Waltham MA: NOVA Biomedical, 2000:16 pp.
17. Sokall LJ, Drew H, Udelsman R. Intraoperative parathyroid hormone analysis: a study of 200 consecutive cases. *Clin Chem* 2000;46:1662–1668.
18. Wians FH, Balko JA, Hsu RM, et al. Intraoperative vs. central laboratory PTH testing during parathyroidectomy surgery. *Lab Med* 2000;31:616–621.
19. Bailey TM. Understanding the economics of bedside diagnostic testing. In: Hicks JM, Price CP, eds. *Point-of-care testing*. Washington, DC: AACC Press, 1999:213–232.
20. Dahler-Eriksen BS, Lauritzen T, Lassen JF, et al. Near-patient test for c-reactive protein in general practice: assessment of clinical, organizational, and economic outcomes. *Clin Chem* 1999;45:478–485.
21. Felder RA. The distributed laboratory: point-of-care services with core laboratory management. In: Hicks JM, Price CP, eds. *Point-of-care testing*. Washington DC: AACC Press, 1999:99–118.
22. Gift TL, Pate MS, Hook EW, et al. The rapid test paradox: when fewer cases detected lead to more cases treated. *Sex Transm Dis* 1999;26:232–240.
23. Grieve R, Beech R, Vincent J, et al. Near patient testing in diabetes clinics: appraising the costs and outcomes. *Health Technol Assess* 1999;3:1–74
24. Kendall JM, Bevan G, Clancy MJ. Point of care testing in the accident and emergency department: a cost analysis and exploration of financial incentives to use the technology within the hospital. *Journal of Health Service Research and Policy* 1999;4:33–38.
25. Kilgore ML, Steindel SJ, Smith JA. Cost analysis for decision support: the case of comparing centralized versus distributed methods for blood gas testing. *Journal of Healthcare Management* 1999;44:207–215.
26. Murray ET, Fitzmaurice DA, Allan TF, et al. A primary care evaluation of three near patient coagulometers. *J Clin Pathol* 1999;52:842–845.
27. Remaley AT, Woods JJ, Glickman JW. POCT for parathyroid hormone. *Medical Laboratory Observer* 1999;31:20–27.
28. van Heyningen C, Watson ID, Morrice AE. Point-of-care testing outcomes in an emergency department. *Clin Chem* 1999;45:437–438.
29. Weilert M, Workman RD, Danaye-Elmi M, et al. A cost-effective high-performance approach to critical care testing. *Lab Med* 1999;30:601–604.
30. Baer DM. Point-of-care versus central lab costs. *Medical Laboratory Observer* 1998;30(Suppl 9):46–50.
31. Boldt J, Walz G, Triem J, et al. Point-of-care (POC) measurement of coagulation after cardiac surgery. *Intensive Care Med* 1998;24:1187–1193.
32. Brown SR. Point-of-care integration—our experience. *Medical Laboratory Observer* 1998;30(Suppl 9):22–25.
33. Cohen J, Piterman L, McCall LM, et al. Near-patient testing for serum cholesterol: attitudes of general practitioners and patients, appropriateness and costs. *Med J Aust* 1998;168:605–609.
34. Collison PO. Economic aspects of new biochemical markers for the detection of myocardial damage: role of biochemical markers in the management of patients with chest pain. In: Kaski JC, Holt DW, eds. *Myocardial damage: early detection by novel biochemical markers*. Boston: Kluwer Academic, 1998:173–187.
35. Fitzmaurice DA, Hobbs FDR, Murray ET. Primary care anticoagulant clinic management using computerized decision support and near patient International Normalized Ratio (INR) testing: routine data from a practice nurse-led clinic. *Fam Pract* 1998;15:144–146.
36. Halpern MT, Palmer CS, Simpson KN, et al. The economic and clinical efficiency of point of care testing for critically ill patients: a decision-analysis model. *Am J Med Qual* 1998;13:3–12.
37. Hortin GL. *Handbook of bedside glucose testing*. Washington, DC: AACC Press, 1998:39.
38. Kiechle FL, Aulakh V. Satellite laboratories: a cost-benefit study. *Medical Laboratory Observer* 1998;30:44–50.
39. Lafata JE, Martin S, Kaatz S, et al. Monitoring alternatives for patients on anticoagulation therapy: a cost-effective analysis. *Association of Health Services Research* 1998;15:191–192.
40. Nash DB, Fernandez AM, Ryan NR, et al. Point of care testing. In: Bozzo P, et al. *Cost-effective laboratory management*. Philadelphia: Lippincott-Raven, 1998:163–179.
41. Bailey TM, Topham TM, Wantz S, et al. Laboratory process improvement through point-of-care testing. *Joint Com J Quality Improvement* 1997;23:362–380.
42. Barocci TA. *The value chain applied to critical care testing: a hospital's financial perspective*. Presented at: AACC National Meeting, Atlanta, GA, 1997.
43. Despotis GJ, Joist JH, Goodnough LT. Monitoring hemostasis in cardiac surgical patients: impact of point-of-care testing on blood loss and transfusion outcomes. *Clin Chem* 1997;43:1684–1696.
44. Hortin GL. Beyond traditional quality control: how to check costs and quality of point-of-care testing. *Medical Laboratory Observ* 1997;29:31–37.
45. i-STAT. *Comparing traditional blood analysis process costs to point-of-care testing: case studies*. Princeton, NJ: i-STAT Corporation, 1997:1–9.
46. Kilgore ML, Steindel SJ, Smith JA. Using patient satisfaction as an indicator of the quality of laboratory services. *Clin Lab Manage Rev* 1997;11:93–102.

47. Leonard M, Chessal M, Manning D. The use of a Hemocue blood glucose analyzer in a neonatal unit. *Clin Biochem* 1997;34:287–290.

48. Mengal AC, Dahlgren H, Fremner E, et al. Decentralized vs. central laboratory testing – a cost comparison. Presented at: Annual Meeting of the International Society of Technological Assessment of Health Care 1997:138.

49. Murthy JN, Hicks JM, Soldin SJ. Evaluation of i-STAT portable clinical analyzer in a neonatal and pediatric intensive care unit. *Clin Biochem* 1997;30:385–389.

50. Smith I. Defining the elephant. *Journal of Respiratory Care Practitioners* 1997; April-May: 25–33.

51. Battelle Medical Technology Assessment and Policy Research Program. The economic and clinical efficiency of point-of-care testing for critically ill patients. *Medical Laboratory Observer* 1996;28:12–16.

52. Eisenberg P, Muhs SMJ. QI study in the ICU: bedside testing of gastric contents. *Nursing Management* 1996;27:48K–48M.

53. Felder RA. Cost-justifying laboratory automation. *Clin Lab News* 1996;22:10,11,17.

54. Felder RA. Robotic automation of near-patient testing. In: Kost GJ, ed. *Handbook of clinical automation, robotics, and optimization.* New York: Wiley, 1996:596–619.

55. Gault MH, Harding CE. Evaluation of i-STAT portable clinical analyzer in a hemodialysis unit. *Clin Biochem* 1996;29:117–124.

56. Kost GJ, Hague C. *In vitro, ex vivo,* and *in vivo* biosensor systems. In: Kost GJ, ed. Handbook of clinical automation, robotics, and optimization. New York: Wiley, 1996:681–753.

57. Macgregor SH, Hamley JG, Dunbar JA, et al. Evaluation of a primary care anticoagulant clinic managed by a pharmacist. *BMJ* 1996;312:560.

58. Mohammad AA, Summers H, Burchfield JE, et al. STAT turnaround time: satellite and point-to-point testing. *Lab Med* 1996;27:684–688.

59. Nichols JH. Cost analysis of point-of-care laboratory testing. *Adv Path Lab Med* 1996;9:284–297.

60. Parvin CA, Lo SF, Deuser SM, et al. Impact of point-of-care testing on patients' length of stay in a large emergency department. *Clin Chem* 1996;42:711–717.

61. Auerbach PS. Impact of point-of-care testing on healthcare delivery. *Clin Chem* 1996;42:2052–2053.

62. Scott MG, Lo SF, Parvin CA. Reply [to ref 61]. *Clin Chem* 1996;42:2053.

63. Seamonds B. Medical, economic, and regulatory factors affecting point-of-care testing. A report of the conference on factors affecting point-of-care testing, Philadelphia, PA, 6–7 May 1994. *Clin Chim Acta* 1996;249:1–19.

64. Simpson KN, LaVallee R, Halpern M, et al. Is POCT cost effective for coronary bypass patients in the ICUs? *Medical Laboratory Observer* 1996;28:58–62.

65. Spoor PI. Traditional lab testing vs. point-of-care testing: comparing the costs. *Medical Laboratory Observer* 1996;28:4–6.

66. Steffes MW, Gillen JL, Fuhrman SA. Delivering clinical laboratory services to intensive care units. *Clin Chem* 1996;42:387–391.

67. Tortella BJ, Lavery RF, Doran JV, et al. Precision, accuracy, and managed care implications of a hand-held whole blood analyzer in the prehospital setting. *Am J Clin Pathol* 1996;106:124–127.

68. Cummings JP. *Technology report: point-of-care: portable whole-blood clinical analyzers.* Oak Brook, IL: University Health System Consortium, 1995:1–76.

69. Operational laboratory benchmarking project. Oak Brook, IL: University Hospital Consortium, 1994.

70. Fleisher M, Schwartz MK. Automated approaches to rapid response testing: a comparative evaluation of point-of-care and centralized laboratory testing. Pathology patterns. *Am J Clin Pathol* 1995;104: S18–S25.

71. Fuhrman SA, Travers EM, Handorf CR. The mobile laboratory in alternate site testing. *Arch Pathol Lab Med* 1995;119:939–942.

72. Gogola M. A joint hospital/vendor project brings CQI and point-of-care technology to home care. *Comput Nursing* 1995;13:143–150.

73. Harris NS, Chmil ME, Law T, et al. Evaluation of the APEC analyzer for whole blood glucose: testing in a pediatric setting. *Am J Clin Pathol* 1995;104:477–479.

74. Hutsko GM, Jones JB, Danielson L. Using point-of-care testing to speed patient care: one emergency department's experience. *J Emerg Nursing* 1995;21:408–412.

75. Innanen VT, Barqueira-de Campos F. Point-of-care glucose testing: cost savings and ease of use with the Ames glucometer elite. *Clin Chem* 1995;41:1537–1538.

76. Jobes DR, Aitken GL, Shaffer GW. Increased accuracy and precision of heparin and protamine dosing reduces blood loss and transfusion in patients undergoing primary cardiac operations. *J Thorac Cardiovasc Surg* 1995;110:36–45.

77. Laposata M, Lewandrowski KB. Near patient blood glucose monitoring. *Arch Pathol Lab Med* 1995;119:926–928.

78. Nosanchuck JS, Keefner R. Cost analysis of point-of-care laboratory testing in a community hospital. *Am J Clin Pathol* 1995;103: 240–243.

79. Lindsey J, Eble N. Cost analysis of point-of-care laboratory testing in a community hospital. *Am J Clin Pathol* 1995;104:107.

80. Lyon AW. The luxury of bedside testing. *Am J Clin Pathol* 1995;104: 107–108.

81. Nosanchuk JS, Keefner ER. The authors' reply. *Am J Clin Pathol* 1995;104:108.

82. Sands VM, Auerbach PS, Birnbaum J, et al. Evaluation of a portable clinical blood analyzer in the emergency department. *Acad Emerg Med* 1995;2:172–178.

83. Singal BM. Point-of-care blood testing and cost-effective emergency medicine. *Acad Emerg Med* 1995;2:163–164.

84. Cembrowski GS, Kiechle FL. Point of care testing: critical analysis and practical application. *Adv Pathol Lab Med* 1994;7:3–21.

85. Despotis GJ, Santoro SA, Spitznagel E, et al. On-site prothrombin time, activated partial thromboplastin time and platelet count: a comparison between whole blood and laboratory assays with coagulation factor analysis in patients presenting for cardiac surgery. *Anesthesiology* 1994;80:338–351.

86. Frankel HL, Rozycki GS, Ochsner MG, et al. Minimizing admission laboratory testing in trauma patients: use of a microanalyzer. *J Trauma* 1994;37:728–736.

87. Goodwin SA. Point-of-care testing in a post anesthesia care unit. *Medical Laboratory Observer* 1994;26:15–18.

88. Johnson KF. Does an on-site satellite laboratory reduce surgical delays? A study of delays in a same day surgical center. *AORN J* 1994;59:1275–1276,1279–1282,1285–1290.

89. Lee-Lewandrowski E, Laposata M, Eschenbach K, et al. Utilization and cost analysis of bedside capillary glucose testing in a large teaching hospital: implications for managing point of care testing. *Am J Med* 1994;97:222–230.

90. Haas SN. Conceptual and cost analysis errors in the evaluation of bedside capillary glucose testing. *Am J Med* 1995;99:576.

91. Lewandrowski K, Laposata M. Reply to: conceptual and cost analysis errors in the evaluation of bedside capillary glucose testing. *Am J Med* 1995;99:576–577.

92. McPeck M. A BG & E program for cardiac surgery. *Medical Laboratory Observer* 1994;26:20–25.

93. Simpson KN, Luce BR, Halpern MT, et al. *The marginal cost effectiveness of using three laboratory test production processes for the management of cardiac surgery patients in intensive care units.* Presented at: Annual Meeting of the International Society of Technological Assessment of Health Care 1994, Abst 42.

94. Travers EM, Wolke JC, Johnson R, et al. Changing the way lab medicine is practiced at the point of care. *Medical Laboratory Observer* 1994;26:33–40.

95. Tsai WW, Nash DB, Seamonds B, et al. Point of care versus central laboratory testing: an economic analysis in an academic medical center. *Clin Ther* 1994;16:898–910.

96. Winkelman JW, Wybenga DR. Quantification of medical and operational factors determining central versus satellite laboratory testing of blood gases. *Am J Clin Pathol* 1994;102:7–10.

97. Winkelman JW, Wybenga DR, Tamasijevic MJ. The fiscal consequences of central vs. distributed testing of glucose. *Clin Chem* 1994; 40:1628–1630.

98. Handorf CR. POC testing: must quality cost more? *Medical Laboratory Observer* 1993;25:28–33.

99. McCray CS. One hospital's experience with implementing POCT. *Medical Laboratory Observer* 1993;25:34–41.

100. Rink E, Hilton S, Szczepura A, et al. Impact of introducing near patient testing for standard investigations in general practice. *BMJ* 1993;307:775–778.

101. Szczepura A. *The cost-effectiveness of near-patient testing in the surgery setting.* Presented at: Annual Meeting of the International Society of Technological Assessment of Health Care 1994, Abst 57.

102. Saxena S, Wong ET. Does the emergency department need a dedicated stat laboratory? Continuous quality improvement as a management tool for the clinical laboratory. *Am J Clin Pathol* 1993;100:606–610.

103. Woo J, McCabe JB, Chauncey D, et al. The evaluation of a portable clinical analyzer in the emergency department. *Am J Clin Pathol* 1993;100:599–605.

104. Forman, DT. Controlling error in laboratory testing. *Med Lab Observ* 1993;24:8–15.

105. Greendyke RM. Cost analysis of bedside blood glucose testing. *Am J Clin Pathol* 1992;97:106–107.

106. Jacobs E, Sarkozi L, Colman N. A centralized critical care (stat) laboratory. The Mount Sinai Experience *Crit Care Rep* 1991;2:397–405.

107. Winkelman JW, Woo J, Tirabassi CP, O'Connell M. Centralization and decentralization of the hospital clinical laboratory. In Vanderschmitt DJ, ed. *Laboratory organization/automation.* New York: Walter de Gruyter, 1991: p.81–98.

108. Zaloga GP. Monitoring versus testing technologies: present and future. *Med Lab Observ* 1991;23(9S): 20–31.

109. Elliot K, Watson ID, Tsintis P, et al. The impact of near-patient testing on the organization and costs of an anticonvulsant clinic. *Ther Drug Monit* 1990;12:434–437.

110. Statland BE, Brzys K. Evaluating STAT testing alternatives by calculating annual laboratory costs. *Chest* 1990;97:198–203S.

111. Zaloga GP. Evaluation of bedside testing options for the critical care unit. *Chest* 1990;97:185S–190S.

112. Ansell JE, Hamke AK, Holden A, et al. Cost effectiveness of monitoring warfarin therapy using standard versus capillary prothrombin times. *Am J Clin Pathol* 1989;91:587–589.

113. Bernstein LH, Davis GL. The cost impact of decentralized testing: analysis of satellite laboratory expenses in support of a same-day surgery program, demonstrates dramatic savings over service by a central lab. *Medical Laboratory Observer* 1989;21:37–38,40,42.

114. Gennis P, Gallagher J, Anderson F, et al. Cost effectiveness of an accurate and rapid assay for serum human chorionic gonadotropin in suspected ectopic pregnancy. *Am J Emerg Med* 1988;6:4–6.

115. Zaloga GP, Hill TR, Strickland RA, et al. Bedside blood gas and electrolyte monitoring in critically ill patients. *Crit Care Med* 1989;17:920–925.

116. Zaloga GP. Bedside reagent testing: blood, CSF, and bacterial cultures. *J Crit Illness* 1988;3:85–94.

117. Bernstein LH. Decentralized testing: cost implications and benefits. In: Marks V, Alberti KG, eds. *Clinical biochemistry nearer the patient II.* London: Bailliere Tindall, 1986:159–165.

118. Haeckel R. Cost implications of decentralized testing—a laboratorian's view. In: Ashby JP, ed. *The patient and decentralized testing.* Lancester, England: MTP Press, 1986:109–117.

119. Trundle DS, Weizenecker RA. Capillary glucose testing: a cost-saving bedside system. *Laboratory Management* 1986:24:59–62.

120. Craig TM. The economics of point-of-care testing. In: Marks V, Alberti KG, ed. *Clinical biochemistry nearer the patient.* London: Churchill Livingstone, 1985:162–167.

121. Shapiro B, Savage PJ, Lomatch D, et al. A comparison of accuracy and estimated cost of methods for home blood glucose monitoring. *Diabetes Care* 1981;4:396–403.

122. Weil MH, Michaels S, Puri VK, et al. The stat laboratory: facilitating blood gas and biochemical measurements for the critically ill and injured. *Am J Clin Pathol* 1981;76:34–42.

SUBJECT INDEX

Page numbers followed by *f* refer to figures; page numbers followed by *t* refer to tables. Drugs are listed under their generic names. When a drug trade name is listed, the reader is referred to the generic name.

A

A-VOX, 307
A1cNow, 69*t*
AB FLU OIA, 404
ABC analysis, 579
Abciximab, efficacy of, troponin levels in monitoring, 311
Abdominal pain, emergency department evaluation of, 104*t*
ABL series, 68*t*, 69*t*, 70, 144*t*
Absorbance, optical, in point-of-care testing, 76
ABT100, 258*t*
Abuscreen Ontrak, 71*t*, 260*t*, 272, 272*t*
Abuse, drugs of. *See* Drugs of abuse
Acceava, for streptococcal antigen, 400
Acceava Mono Test, 401
Access point, 492, 493*f*, 510, 512, 512*f*
Accreditation/licensing, for point-of-care testing, 6*t*, 9, 434–443
    agencies involved in, 434–437
    agency selection and, 440
    bedside testing and, 206–207
    Centers for Medicare & Medicaid Services (CMS) and, 434–436, 435*t*, 439*t*
    College of American Pathologists (CAP) and, 436–437, 439*t*, 453–463
    cost of, 440–441
    documentation data management and, 438–439
    education/training and, 441
    inspections for, 440
        in physician office laboratory, 393, 398
    Joint Commission on Accreditation of Healthcare Organizations (JCAHO) and, 436, 439*t*, 444–452
    management/consolidation of requirements and, 438–441, 439*t*
    in operating room, 120
    in physician office laboratory, 391–392, 393, 398
    proficiency testing requirements and, 428, 439*t*
    quality assurance data management and, 438–439
    recommendations for, 419
    staff credentials and, 441
    in Veterans Affairs system, 348, 352*t*
Accu-Chek
    for cholesterol, 401
    for glucose, 403

Accu-Chek Advantage H, 70*t*, 78*t*, 198
Accu-Chek Comfort Curve, 70*t*, 77, 77*f*, 78*t*
Accu-Dx assay, 271
    for recurrent bladder cancer, 271–272
AccuLevel assay, 263
AccuMeter, 263, 401
Accuracy
    of IVD, evaluation of for premarket notification/510(k), 472–473, 473*t*
    of point-of-care testing, 6*t*, 7–8
AccuSign, 160*t*, 258*t*
Accusport portable lactate analyzer, 288, 569, 573
AccuStrip Strep A, 400
Accutest, 258*t*
Accutrend, 519
Acetaminophen, point-of-care testing for
    in emergency department, 106*t*, 109, 256*t*, 257
    spot tests, 259*t*
Acetoacetic acid, urinary, 269
Acetone
    point-of-care spot tests for, 259*t*
    urinary, 269
Acid-base disorders, intensive care unit evaluation of
    derived parameters and, 141, 142*f*, 143*f*
    future developments and, 146–148
Acidosis
    derived parameters in evaluation of, 141, 142*f*, 143*f*
    hyperlactemia and, 568, 568*f*
    in neonate/premature infant, 288–289
ACON DOA, 71*t*
ACON HBsAg, 71*t*
ACON HIV 1/2 test strips, 71*t*, 80, 80*f*
ACON Syphilis, 71*t*
Acoustic wave sensor, surface (SAW), 45*t*, 49
Acquired immunodeficiency syndrome (AIDS). *See* HIV infection/AIDS
ACS. *See* Acute coronary syndromes
ACT/ACT-Plus. *See* Activated clotting time
ACT II Plunger HepconHMS, 69*t*
Actalyke, 159*t*
Activated clotting time (ACT), 58*t*, 59*t*, 158–161, 168–169, 217, 312
    during cardiac catheterization, 171, 307–308
    celite-based, 158, 169
        versus kaolin-based assays, 158–160, 160*f*
    in Europe, 312
    during extracorporeal membrane oxygenation, 307–308, 319

during hemodialysis, 307–308, 318
    heparin responsiveness and, 158, 159*f*
    instruments for, 159, 159*t*
    in intensive care unit, 141
    kaolin-based, 158, 169
        versus celite-based assays, 158–160, 160*f*
    in operating room, 125*t*, 158–160, 159*f*, 159*t*, 160*f*, 168–169, 551
        for pediatric surgery, 307–308, 318–319
    patient factors affecting, 160
    in pediatric intensive care unit, 319
    quality control for tests of, 160–161
    venous versus arterial, 160
Activated partial thromboplastin time (aPTT), 58*t*, 59*t*, 164–165, 164*t*, 171–172
    decision making and, 588–589, 589*f*
    for heparin therapy monitoring, 171–172, 172*t*
    for hirudin therapy monitoring, 173
    in intensive care unit, 141
    in operating room, 125, 125*t*
Activity-based costing, for economic analysis, 578*t*, 579
Acute care setting. *See also* Critical care; Intensive care unit
    point-of-care testing in, nursing and interdisciplinary team and, 216–217
Acute coronary syndromes (ACS), 181. *See also* Chest pain; Myocardial infarction
    cardiac markers in risk assessment and, 186–187, 186*f*
Acute intermittent porphyria, urine tests for, 273
Acute myocardial infarction (AMI). *See* Chest pain; Myocardial infarction
Acute phase proteins, intensive care unit testing of, 148–149, 148*t*
ADH assay. *See* Alcohol dehydrogenase (ADH) assay
Adhesion molecules, single-nucleotide polymorphisms (SNPs) and, 150*t*
Admission criteria, for intensive care unit, point-of-care testing and, 137
Adult education principles, point-of-care testing training and, 225–226
Adulterants, drugs of abuse testing and, 254, 261–262, 262*f*, 272
"Advanced Care," 401
Advantage H, 70*t*, 78*t*
    characteristics of, 86*t*
aEEG. *See* Amplitude-integrated EEG

DATE DUE

#47-0108 Peel Off Pressure Sensitive